GW00381836

# COMPREHENSIVE HANDBOOK *of* Childhood Cancer and Sickle Cell Disease

EDITED BY

Ronald T. Brown

COMPREHENSIVE HANDBOOK

*of*

# Childhood Cancer and Sickle Cell Disease

## A Biopsychosocial Approach


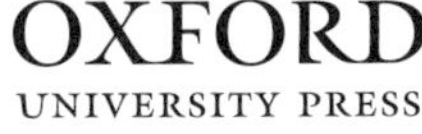

2006

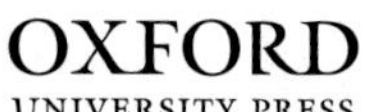

Oxford University Press, Inc., publishes works that further
Oxford University's objective of excellence
in research, scholarship, and education.

Oxford New York
Auckland Cape Town Dar es Salaam Hong Kong Karachi
Kuala Lumpur Madrid Melbourne Mexico City Nairobi
New Delhi Shanghai Taipei Toronto

With offices in
Argentina Austria Brazil Chile Czech Republic France Greece
Guatemala Hungary Italy Japan Poland Portugal Singapore
South Korea Switzerland Thailand Turkey Ukraine Vietnam



Published by Oxford University Press, Inc.
198 Madison Avenue, New York, New York 10016

www.oup.com

Oxford is a registered trademark of Oxford University Press



Library of Congress Cataloging-in-Publication Data
Comprehensive handbook of childhood cancer and sickle cell disease:
a biopsychosocial approach / edited by Ronald T. Brown.
p. cm.
ISBN-13 978-0-19-516985-0
ISBN 0-19-516985-9
1. Cancer in children—Handbooks, manuals, etc. 2. Sickle cell anemia in children—Handbooks, manuals, etc.
I. Brown, Ronald T.
[DNLM: 1. Neoplasms—psychology—Child. 2. Anemia, Sickle Cell–psychology—Child. QZ 275 C737 2006]
RC281.C4C645 2006
618.92'994–dc22 2005020559

9 8 7 6 5 4 3 2 1

Printed in the United States of America
on acid-free paper

To Raymond K. Mulhern, Ph.D., for all that he did to further knowledge about childhood cancer and sickle cell disease and for all that he contributed to psychology as a colleague and as a friend.

# Contents

# Contributors

**Melissa A. Alderfer, Ph.D.**
Department of Psychology
Children's Hospital of Philadelphia and
University of Pennsylvania
Philadelphia, Pennsylvania

**F. Daniel Armstrong, Ph.D.**
Mailman Center for Child
Development
Department of Pediatrics
University of Miami School of Medicine
Miami, Florida

**Lamia P. Barakat, Ph.D.**
Department of Psychology
Drexel University and
Department of Psychology
Children's Hospital of Philadelphia
Philadelphia, Pennsylvania

**David J. Bearison, Ph.D.**
Graduate Center
City University of New York
and Department of Pediatrics
Columbia University
College of Physicians and Surgeons
New York, New York

**Kristin Bingen, Ph.D.**
Department of Pediatrics
Medical College of Wisconsin
Milwaukee, Wisconsin

**Melanie J. Bonner, Ph.D.**
Department of Psychiatry and Behavioral
Sciences
Duke University Medical Center
Durham, North Carolina

**Rhonda C. Boyd, Ph.D.**
Department of Psychology
Children's Hospital of Philadelphia
University of Pennsylvania
Philadelphia, Pennsylvania

**Joanna Breyer, Ph.D.**
Dana Farber Cancer Institute
and Harvard Medical School
Boston, Massachusetts

**Ronald T. Brown, Ph.D.**
Departments of Public Health, Psychology,
and Pediatrics
Temple University
Philadelphia, Pennsylvania

**Robert W. Butler, Ph.D.**
Department of Pediatrics
Oregon Health Sciences Center
Portland, Oregon

**Melissa Y. Carpentier, M.S.**
Department of Psychology
Oklahoma State University
Stillwater, Oklahoma

**Cori E. Cieurzo, Ph.D.**
Dana Farber Cancer Institute
and Harvard Medical School
Boston, Massachusetts

**Daniel L. Clay, Ph.D.**
College of Education
University of Iowa
Iowa City, Iowa

**Paola M. Conte, Ph.D.**
Tomorrow's Children's Cancer
Center
Hackensack University Medical Center
Hackensack, New Jersey

**Donna R. Copeland, Ph.D.**
Department of Pediatrics
University of Texas M.D. Anderson Cancer
Center
Houston, Texas

**Michael J. Dolgin, Ph.D.**
Department of Psychology
University of Jerusalem
Jerusalem, Israel

**T. David Elkin, Ph.D.**
Department of Psychiatry and Behavioral
Sciences
University of Mississippi Medical Center
Jackson, Mississippi

**Linda J. Ewing, Ph.D.**
Western Psychiatric Institute and
Clinic and Department of
Psychology
University of Pittsburgh
Pittsburgh, Pennsylvania

**Diane L. Fairclough, Dr. Ph.**
University of Colorado Health Sciences Center
Denver, Colorado

**Celia B. Fisher, Ph.D.**
Department of Psychology
Fordham University
New York, New York

**Bernard F. Fuemmeler, Ph.D.**
National Cancer Institute
Bethesda, Maryland

**Sarah F. Griffin, Ph.D., M.P.H.**
Prevention Research Center
Department of Health Promotion, Education,
and Behavior
Norman J. Arnold School of Public Health
University of South Carolina
Columbia, South Carolina

**Kathryn E. Gustafson, Ph.D.**
Department of Psychiatry and Behavioral
Sciences
Duke University Medical Center
Durham, North Carolina

**Kristina K. Hardy, Ph.D.**
Department of Psychiatry and Behavioral
Sciences
Duke University Medical Center
Durham, North Carolina

**Momcilo Jankovic, M.D.**
The University of Milan
Bicocca, Italy

**W. Lewis Johnson, Ph.D.**
CARTE USC/Information Sciences Institute
Los Angeles, California

**Ernest R. Katz, Ph.D.**
Children's Hospital of Los Angeles
Los Angeles, California

**Anne E. Kazak, Ph.D.**
Department of Psychology
Children's Hospital of Philadelphia and
University of Pennsylvania
Philadelphia, Pennsylvania

**Mary Jo Kupst, Ph.D.**
Department of Pediatrics
Medical College of Wisconsin
Milwaukee, Wisconsin

**Laurie A. Lash, M.A.**
Department of Psychology
Drexel University
Philadelphia, Pennsylvania

**Rachel B. Levi, Ph.D.**
California Institute of Integral Studies
San Francisco, California

**Meredith J. Lutz, M.S.**
Department of Psychology
Drexel University
Philadelphia, Pennsylvania

**Avi Madan-Swain, Ph.D.**
Department of Pediatrics
University of Alabama–Birmingham
Birmingham, Alabama

**Anna L. Marsland, Ph.D., R.N.**
Western Psychiatric Institute and Clinic and Department of Psychology
University of Pittsburgh
Pittsburgh, Pennsylvania

**Giuseppe Masera, M.D.**
The University of Milan
Bicocca, Italy

**Jessica K. Masty**
Department of Psychology
Fordham University
New York, New York

**Ann M. McGrath, Ph.D.**
Department of Pediatrics
University of Kansas Medical Center
Kansas City, Kansas

**Eugene A. Meyer, Ph.D.**
Dana Farber Cancer Institute and Harvard Medical School
Boston, Massachusetts

**Monica J. Mitchell, Ph.D.**
Division of Psychology
Cincinnati Children's Hospital Medical Center
Cincinnati, Ohio

**Raymond K. Mulhern, Ph.D.**
Division of Behavioral Medicine
Saint Jude Children's Research Hospital and Department of Pediatrics
University of Tennessee School of Medicine
Memphis, Tennessee

**Larry L. Mullins, Ph.D.**
Department of Pediatrics
University of Oklahoma Medical School
Oklahoma City, Oklahoma

**Cynthia D. Myers, Ph.D.**
Department of Pediatrics
David Geffen School of Medicine at the University of California
Los Angeles, Los Angeles, California

**D. Collette Nicolaou, M.S.,**
Department of Psychology
Drexel University
Philadelphia, Pennsylvania

**Robert B. Noll, Ph.D.**
Department of Pediatrics
University of Pittsburgh School of Medicine
Pittsburgh, Pennsylvania

**Andrea Farkas Patenaude, Ph.D.**
Dana Farber Cancer Center and Harvard Medical School
Boston, Massachusetts

**Sean Phipps, Ph.D.**
Division of Behavioral Medicine
Saint Jude Children's Research Hospital
Memphis, Tennessee

**Brad H. Pollock, M.P.H., Ph.D.**
Department of Epidemiology and Biometry
University of Texas Health Sciences Center at San Antonio
San Antonio, Texas

**Scott W. Powers, Ph.D.**
Department of Psychology
Cincinnati Children's Hospital
Medical Center
Cincinnati, Ohio

**Eve S. Puffer**
Department of Psychology
University of South Carolina
Columbia, South Carolina

**Jerilynn Radcliffe, Ph.D.**
Department of Psychology
Children's Hospital of Philadelphia
and University of Pennsylvania
Philadelphia, Pennsylvania

**Michael A. Rapoff, Ph.D.**
Department of Pediatrics
University of Kansas Medical Center
Kansas City, Kansas

**Ollie Jane Z. Sahler, M.D.**
Department of Pediatrics
Strong Children's Hospital
University of Rochester
Rochester, New York

**Aurora Sanfeliz, Ph.D.**
Dana Farber Cancer Center
and Harvard Medical School
Boston, Massachusetts

**Jeffrey Schatz, Ph.D.**
Department of Psychology
University of South Carolina
Columbia, South Carolina

**Katherine A. Schneider, Ph.D.**
Dana Farber Cancer Center
and Harvard Medical School
Boston, Massachusetts

**Stephen D. Smith, M.D.**
Department of Pediatrics
University of Kansas Medical Center
Kansas City, Kansas

**John J. Spinetta, Ph.D.**
Department of Psychology
San Diego State University
San Diego, California

**Margaret L. Stuber, M.D.**
Department of Psychiatry
David Geffen School of Medicine at the
University of California, Los Angeles
Los Angeles, California

**Nicole F. Swain, Ph.D.**
Division of Psychology
Cincinnati Children's Hospital Medical Center
Cincinnati, Ohio

**Amanda Thompson, M.S.**
Western Psychiatric Institute and Clinic
and Department of Psychology
University of Pittsburgh
Pittsburgh, Pennsylvania

**Robert J. Thompson, Jr., Ph.D.**
Trinity College
Duke University
Durham, North Carolina

**Vida L. Tyc, Ph.D.**
Division of Behavioral Medicine
Saint Jude Children's Research Hospital
Memphis, Tennessee

**James W. Varni, Ph.D.**
School of Architecture
Texas A&M University
College Station, Texas

**Gary A. Walco, Ph.D.**
Palliative Care Program
Hackensack University Medical Center
Hackensack, New Jersey

**Stan F. Whitsett, Ph.D.**
Department of Psychiatry and
Behavioral Sciences
University of Washington School of Medicine
Seattle, Washington

**Dawn K. Wilson, Ph.D.**
Prevention Research Center
Department of Health Promotion, Education, and Behavior
Norman J. Arnold School of Public Health
University of South Carolina
Columbia, South Carolina

**Lonnie K. Zeltzer, M.D.**
Department of Pediatrics
David Geffen School of Medicine at the University of California, Los Angeles
Los Angeles, California

# Introduction

Ronald T. Brown

# Why a Comprehensive Handbook on Pediatric Psychosocial Oncology/Hematology

Over the past 25 to 30 years, monumental strides in national policy have been made in the management, treatment, and prevention of cancer. Rowland (2005) summarized these accomplishments, including legislation that provides for revenues and resources for research in cancer prevention and control. In addition, other pertinent policy issues have emerged from the Institute of Medicine, the National Cancer Institute, the Centers for Disease Control and Prevention, and the Lance Armstrong Foundation, all of which have served to increase the awareness of cancer, prevent the occurrence of cancer, and address cancer survivorship. Cancer policy issues have been models for increased resources and revenues for patient care, research, and quality-of-life enhancement. Nowhere is the success that we have had with policy more evident than in pediatric psychosocial oncology.

The enormous advances in the prevention, medical treatment, medical management of late effects, and quality-of-life issues in children and adolescents surviving cancer have spawned a host of research in pediatric psychosocial oncology. These investigations likely surpass most research efforts for other chronic diseases. In fact, Bearison and Mulhern (1994) observed that there are more studies related to psychosocial oncology than perhaps there have been children with the disease. In my role as editor of the *Journal of Pediatric Psychology*, I conducted an informal survey of manuscripts; it indicated we process more submissions related to cancer than any other disease or chronic illness. Bearison and Mulhern also noted that psychological studies in the area of pediatric oncology have permeated most psychology and pediatric journals. Even the most dedicated scholar in psychosocial oncology and hematology has a difficult time keeping up with the ever-burgeoning literature body.

Bearison and Mulhern published the last handbook on psychosocial issues in pediatric hematology/oncology in 1994. Since then, a proliferation of literature in the field has been concomitant with major developments in pediatric oncology, including increased use of chemotherapy, the evolution of bone marrow transplantation as a means of treating children and adolescents who have been refractory to chemotherapy and radiation therapy, and intensive investigation of survivorship and the late effects that many of these children endure. Handbooks in the late 1990s were devoted primarily to adult cancers (Holland, 1998), with some supplemental chapters devoted to pediatric cancers, but no comprehensive handbook devoted to psychosocial oncology has been published in the field since 1994. Only a special issue of the *Journal of Pediatric Psychology* published early in 2005 (Patenaude & Kupst, 2005a) has addressed this area.

Hence, the purpose of this book is to provide a comprehensive overview of and update in the field of pediatric psychosocial hematology/oncology, including neuropsychological effects of chemotherapy and radiation therapy, bone marrow transplantation, important issues about quality of life during and following treatment, collaborative research among child-focused psychologists, and standards of psychological care for children and adolescents. Indeed, accomplishments in research have already been translated to clinical practice.

We hope this book conveys the impressive growth in psychosocial research and resulting increased understanding of children and adolescents who may be at risk for adjustment difficulties, in addition to children who fare well during a cancer illness. The mere increase in chapters from 8 in the Bearison and Mulhern book published in 1994 to 30 in this handbook is a testament to this growth. It is anticipated that the length and contents of the handbook will communicate some of the lessons learned by my colleagues. These are clinicians and researchers who have devoted their professional lives to studying and understanding the psychological effects of this disease on children and adolescents. They have provided clinical services to these children to ensure optimal psychological functioning and quality of life.

## Incidence, Prevalence, and Survival Rates

Cancer is the leading cause of death by disease in children younger than 15 years. Even so, cancer in children and adolescents is fairly rare, with only 1 or 2 children per 10,000 diagnosed with cancer each year. Nearly 8,600 children were diagnosed with some type of cancer in 2001, and approximately 1,500 died from the disease (Moore, 2005). Major advances in diagnosis and treatment of many pediatric cancers have resulted in significant and impressive survival rates, particularly for some of the more common cancers (e.g., acute lymphocytic leukemia [ALL]). The 5-year survival rate for ALL is now about 90% compared to 50% survival 30 years ago.

Pediatric cancer survivorship represents less than 2% of the nearly 10 million cancer survivors in the United States. Even so, over the last 30 years cancer for children has become more of a chronic illness. The 10-year survival rate for pediatric cancers is 75%, and the 5-year survival rate is 79%. Both of these exceed the adult cancer survival rate of 64% (Rowland et al., 2004). The overall cure rate for all children and adolescents with cancer is approximately 85% (Bleyer, 1997). Thus, many young children live well into young adulthood and on to their adult years, with approximately 1 in 1,000 adults reaching the age of 20 years as a cancer survivor. Use of central nervous system (CNS) prophylaxis, multidrug regimens, delayed intensification, and maintenance intrathecal methotrexate account for the long-term survival of pediatric cancer (Gaynon et al., 2000).

## Changes in the Field

Prognosis for cancer is greatly improved, and the long-term survival rates of children and adolescents are markedly increased. These two factors have generated more psychosocial research in this field and influenced delivery of psychological services to children and adolescents who have been diagnosed with cancer. Pediatric psychosocial oncology/hematology echoes the scientist–practitioner model of inquiry and application. Science has informed practice in the field, and practice has led to important questions that subsequently were put to the test of scientific inquiry. There are several factors associated with scientific advances in the field; these are delineated next.

*Multicenter, multidisciplinary cooperative groups.* Walco (2005) observed that although there has been limited funding from the National Cancer Institute for the investigation of psychological issues in the field of pediatric cancer, productivity of investigators who have devoted research to pediatric psychosocial oncology has been high. In part, this research productivity has been because of multicenter clinical trial cooperative groups like the Children's Oncology Group (Armstrong & Reaman, 2005). Armstrong and Reaman argued that multidisciplinary, multicenter clinical trial cooperative groups provide opportunities for psychological research that would be out of reach for an individual institution. Larger cooperative groups, they noted, offer the advantage of larger numbers of participants, shared research infrastructure, and opportunities for longitudinal cohorts.

Although some have argued that barriers of cost, standardization, quality control of investigations, and competition for limited resources pose a challenge (Walco, 2005), Armstrong and Reaman (2005) insisted that the inclusion of psychological research as a component of multidisciplinary cooperative groups will contribute to a transdisciplinary science that focuses on cancer cure and optimal quality survivorship.

*Psychological adjustment and quality of life determine treatment protocols.* The advent of innovative chemotherapy and radiation therapy protocols and the use of bone marrow transplantation have led to questions about children's experience of the quality of life and the adjustment and adaptation to disease. In comparing medical therapies, similar efficacies are demonstrated. In such cases, deciding factors about which types of therapies to use include quality-of-life issues. In early studies, researchers demonstrated the deleterious effects of prophylactic radiation therapy on cognitive functioning among children being treated for ALL (Mulhern, 1994). Based on investigations conducted by Meadows and colleagues at the Children's Hospital of Philadelphia, decisions were made to use alternative chemotherapies rather than radiation therapy and to use radiation therapy only if a child relapsed (Meadows et al., 1981). These investigations underscored the importance of psychological research in making decisions about the optimal treatment for pediatric cancer patients.

There is still compelling evidence that long-term treatment using only prophylactic chemotherapy exerts significant cognitive toxicity for some children. This is particularly true for females who receive their treatment during preschool (Brown et al., 1998; Moore, 2005). More recent research has focused on intervention efforts designed to enhance cognitive functioning in children who suffer from cognitive toxicities associated with radiation therapy or chemotherapy (Butler & Copeland, 2002; Mulhern et al., 2004). In response to findings, programs of psychological and psychopharmacological research have been developed that include clinical trials designed to enhance the cognitive functioning of these children (Butler & Mulhern, 2005).

Kazak (2005) observed that the competence of children with cancer and their families is especially strong. Indeed, the number of pediatric cancer patients and their families who show overt psychopathology is small. Although there are cases of family dysfunction or problems with adjustment during the illness, this is the exception rather than the rule. Thus, Kazak noted that many investigators focused on stress processing, resilience, and predicting positive adaptation instead of using a deficit paradigm. Several models have designated living with cancer a specific stressor rather than a psychopathology (Kazak et al., 1998).

*Late effects.* Previously, the stressors associated with cancer were a paramount issue in the extant literature. In more recent years, particularly with the improved prognosis of pediatric cancers and hence the increased number of survivors, the psychosocial functioning of survivors has taken on an important role in the study of pediatric psychosocial oncology. As a result, the funding has increased for investigating late effects. An essential goal of this research has been to understand the psychosocial effects of pediatric cancer survivors. The research also has paralleled significant advances in statistical methodology that have allowed complete analysis of longitudinal designs and better means of predicting long-term outcome (Friedman & Meadows, 2002).

Patenaude and Kupst (2005b) noted the corpus of literature related to the late effects of pediatric cancers. Researchers of late effects in pediatric oncology first examined the physical sequelae of the disease and then focused on the social functioning of adolescents and young adults (Friedman & Meadows, 2002; Patenaude & Kupst, 2005b).

Major physical sequelae themes included infertility, decreased stature, and organ damage (Oberfield & Sklar, 2002). Given the toxicities associated with radiation therapy and chemotherapies, other investigations of pediatric oncology late effects included neurocognitive deficits, and radiographic studies were used to document the specific effects of radiation therapy and chemotherapy on the brain and their location in the brain (Moore, 2005). As noted, research related to the neurotoxicities associated with cancer helped with treatment protocols that mitigated the toxicities. Diminishing cognitive toxicity has been one important criterion in the development of any potential treatment protocol for children and adolescents diagnosed with cancer, particularly if there is associated CNS treatment or prophylaxis. Moore reviewed subsequent studies, including the effects of treatments on academic performance.

Physical late effects investigations were followed by research on psychosocial late effects of children and adolescents. The long-term follow-up of these survivors' psychosocial functioning into adolescence and early adulthood was a part of this emergent research (Patenaude & Kupst, 2005b). Investigators have focused on survivors' employment opportunities, relationships and marital functioning, interpersonal functioning, and the effects on the survivors' families (Boman & Bodegard, 2000; Kazak et al., 2001; Kupst et al., 1995; Mackie, Hill, Kiomdryn, & McNally, 2000; Madan-Swain et al., 2000; Zeltzer et al., 1997).

Finally, and perhaps representing a tertiary stage of investigation in the area of late effects, is the study of genetic transmission of cancer. Of primary importance to this research are the effects of genetic testing and the knowledge that one is a carrier of a cancer gene (Patenaude, 2003). In the study of such genetic transmissions is a potential for other psychosocial stressors, the knowledge of which is in infancy at this point of inquiry.

*Evidence-based interventions.* As evidence-based medicine has pervaded health care and research, a similar interest in empirical validation of psychological interventions for children with cancer and their families has occurred. However, as Kazak (2002, 2005) pointed out, much of the research in the area of pediatric psychosocial oncology has been descriptive and correlational. The result has been the expectation of good psychological care without the evidence that validates our clinical services (Kazak, 2005). Kazak reviewed intervention research in pediatric psychosocial oncology and found that cognitive behavioral approaches to manage pain and painful procedures in children with cancer have been a prototype of evidenced-based treatment research. Further, the series of investigations identifying symptoms of posttraumatic stress disorder among survivors of childhood cancer, their mothers, and siblings (Kazak, 2005; Kazak, Rourke, & Crump, 2003) has spurred a sequence of studies by Kazak and associates (Kazak, 2005) designed to evaluate an intervention integrating cognitive behavioral and family therapies.

Other studies have focused on secondary prevention efforts, including smoking prevention efforts for cancer survivors at risk for second malignancies (Tyc et al., 2003). Some research efforts have focused specifically on the late effects period in evaluating the efficacy of stimulant medication on attention and learning problems in survivors of childhood cancer. We have only begun this tertiary stage of intervention research in psychosocial oncology, and much more evidence-based research needs to be accomplished. Kazak (2005) recommended a strategic plan for future investigation, including the integration of research-based interventions into practice, interventions for families who have lost a child to cancer, inclusion of other family members in intervention studies (e.g., fathers and siblings), recruitment of ethnically diverse samples, a focus on brief treatments that are both feasible and durable within a clinical setting, and a balanced portfolio of large-scale multisite studies coupled with smaller innovative interventions for specific patients or their family members.

## A Medical Overview

An overview of pediatric psychosocial oncology follows to inform readers of essential medical issues related to cancer. We also encourage readers to consult other sources for overviews of the diagnostic, etiological, and treatment issues in this area (e.g., Granowetter, 1994).

### Etiology and Diagnosis

Little is known about the etiology of pediatric cancers. This is attributed in part to limited research because of the low incidence of the disease, making longitudinal studies difficult (Granowetter, 1994). In comparison to the adult cancers that are frequently the result of living style (e.g., lung cancer caused by smoking) and environmental causes (e.g., asbestos, radiation), there is much less evidence for any environmental or behavioral etiology for pediatric cancers. Genetic factors are likely associated with increased risk in pediatric cancers (Patenaude, 2003). In addition, specific genetic disorders like Down syndrome and neurofibromatosis are also associated with an increased risk of cancers in children, including leukemia.

Granowetter (1994) pointed out that the diagnosis of cancer is frequently made when there is a "constellation of symptoms" (p. 12) to suggest the diagnosis. A time lapse frequently occurs from the onset of symptoms to actual diagnosis of cancer. Because of the low incidence of pediatric cancers, cancer is often not immediately diagnosed by primary care physicians. Certain types of cancers, such as solid tumors, are more likely to be diagnosed earlier because they grow rapidly in comparison to leukemia.

Identification and diagnosis of cancer is almost always dependent on the type of cancer suspected. For example, cancer of the blood-forming tissues, like leukemia and lymphoma, are frequently identified by blood counts. These are followed by an examination of the bone marrow (bone marrow aspiration) and an examination of the spinal fluid (lumbar puncture) to determine whether the leukemia cells have infiltrated the CNS. Solid tumors are frequently identified by radiographic studies such as X-rays, magnetic resonance imaging, and computerized tomography. Following diagnostic tests, a biopsy is taken of the tumor to determine whether it is localized or has spread (metastasized) and to note the stage of the tumor, with stage I denoting that the tumor is localized and stage IV indicating the tumor has metastasized.

Diagnostic tests, including bone marrow aspiration and lumbar punctures, are usually conducted under sedation and repeated throughout the course of treatment and at follow-up. These tests help determine if the spread of disease has been arrested, the disease is under control (remission), and eventually if the disease continues in remission, indicating no relapse. After a definitive diagnosis is made, the family is informed of the diagnosis, the plan of treatment, and the prognosis of the disease. The diagnosis is nearly always made by pediatric oncologists and communicated by the oncologist, with a treatment team that may include a psychologist, pediatric nurse, social worker, and other support staff. After the diagnosis is communicated to caregivers, the child is usually informed in accordance with the child's developmental level. Parents or caregivers are required to provide consent for treatment. Many cancer therapies are part of research studies that are conducted nationally.

## Modalities of Treatment

Four primary modalities of therapy are available for pediatric cancer, all of which are aimed at eradication (Granwoetter, 1994). These are chemotherapy, radiation therapy, surgery, and bone marrow transplantation. For some children, treatments that include chemotherapy and radiation therapy may be best. Chemotherapeutic agents typically exert their effects by prevention of rapidly growing cancer cells. They are administered through the veins, intramuscularly, or into the spinal fluid (intrathecally). There are a number of adverse side effects associated with chemotherapy, many of which temporarily make the child feel sicker than the cancer itself. Such adverse side effects include nausea, vomiting, hair loss, diminished appetite, mouth sores, general malaise, and low blood counts that make the child susceptible to infection. Fortunately, these adverse effects are generally short term and in many cases can be alleviated by medications like antiemetic agents that help control nausea. Of greater concern are the long-term adverse side effects of the chemotherapies associated with the heart, kidneys, and liver.

Radiation therapy is often used for a tumor when surgery and chemotherapy cannot completely remove it. It is typically administered over a series of days or weeks. Similar to chemotherapy, there are a number of adverse effects. These include lethargy, loss of appetite, and irritation of the skin in areas where the radiation has been directed. Adverse effects of radiation therapy are typically dose related, with higher doses associated with greater adverse side effects. Some adverse effects are not reversible, such as those from high-dose radiation that was historically administered to pediatric patients with leukemia to prevent infiltration of the leukemia cells into the CNS. Radiation for these children was used before the development of some of the more contemporary chemotherapies. One of the adverse effects of radiation therapy administered to the CNS is a decrease in white matter in the brain, which may result in significant learning impairments and in some cases mental retardation (for review, see Mulhern and Butler, chapter 14, this volume).

Surgery is frequently used in the removal of tumors. There have been significant advances in pediatric surgery that have allowed for normal functions, particularly for children with osteosarcomas (bone tumors). Nonetheless, the use of surgery as a sole treatment is rarely sufficient because of potential metastases that must be prevented by either radiation therapy or chemotherapy.

The last treatment modality, bone marrow transplantation, has been used with increasing frequency over the past decade, particularly for children and adolescents diagnosed with leukemia and solid tumors (Granowetter, 1994). Bone marrow transplantation actually refers to the transplantation of the marrow of the bone or the cells that produce blood-forming tissue. Initially, there is administration of chemotherapy in combination with radiation therapy, which results in depletion of bone marrow functioning. Subsequently, new bone marrow is administered to the patient intravenously. The donated bone marrow may be from either the patient in remission (autologous transplant) or a transplant from a partially matched or matched donor. Typically, during the course of bone marrow transplantation the patient is at high risk for infection; protective isolation is used to prevent infection. One major complication associated with bone marrow transplantation is graft-versus-host disease, in which the recipient responds to the donor's cells as foreign. In severe forms, this can result in death.

## Common Pediatric Neoplasms

The following reviews the types of malignancies encountered in most pediatric oncology centers. For an in-depth description of these neoplasms, refer to the work of Granowetter (1994).

### *Leukemia*

The two major leukemias include acute lymphocytic leukemia (ALL) and acute nonlymphoblastic leukemia (ANLL). ALL is the most common of the pediatric neoplasms, with approximately 4 per 100,000 children in this country. ALL may occur at any age, although the peak incidence is in the preschool years (3 to 6 years of age). ALL is a cancer of the bone marrow or of the white blood cells; abnormal lymphoblasts aggregate in the bone marrow and result in the failure of bone marrow production. Symptoms of leukemia in pediatric patients include persistent fevers, infections, bruising, pain in the bones and joints, and enlargement of the lymph nodes (Granowetter, 1994). Children from ages 1 to 10 years with low white blood cell counts usually have the best prognosis and are designated as standard risk patients. Children who are younger than 12 months or older than 10 years with higher white blood cell counts are designated as high-risk ALL patients. Children and adolescents with high-risk ALL are treated more intensively than their peers with low-risk disease. Treatment for ALL typically includes a number of chemotherapies that are administered systemically (intramuscularly, intravenously, or by mouth). However, because systemic chemotherapy does not always reach the CNS, prophylactic (preventive) chemotherapy to the CNS is often necessary. Several years ago, prophylactic radiation therapy was administered to the brain, but because of significant cognitive toxicities associated with radiation therapy (Moore, 2005), chemotherapy is typically administered intrathecally (through the spinal cord to the spinal fluid). Chemotherapy in the CNS also is associated with cognitive toxicities, especially for girls (Brown et al., 1998).

ANLL, which includes acute myeloid leukemia, is cancer of the blood-forming tissues that do not include the lymphoblasts (Granowetter, 1994). The incidence of ANLL is much less overall than that of ALL but increases during adolescence. Induction therapy for this disease is very intense and lengthy, and the prognosis is much more guarded than the prognosis for ALL. For this reason, bone marrow transplantation is frequently recommended for pediatric patients with ANLL who achieve remission.

### *Brain Tumors*

The incidence of brain tumors is approximately 2.5 children per 100,000 each year. The peak age at which brain tumors occur in children is between 3 and 9 years, although such tumors may occur at any time. Symptoms usually vary in accordance with the site of the tumor and include headaches, vomiting, double vision, difficulties with balance, and cognitive or neurological deficits that cannot be explained by another disease. The prognosis of children with brain tumor is largely associated with the site of the tumor, the amount of CNS infiltration, and the specific histological subtype of the tumor.

Surgical resection of the brain tumor is the treatment of choice. In this procedure, as much of the tumor as possible is removed without impairing specific functions of the brain. Some brain tumors are removed with surgery alone, but some brain tumors are not removed because the area in which they lie affects vital functions (e.g., tumors of the spinal cord). Some tumors require radiation therapy, chemotherapy, or both, particularly those tumors that have the possibility of reoccurring. Radiation for brain tumors is typically used in high doses, and cognitive toxicities often occur. Cognitive toxicities are especially severe for children under the age of 3 years, for whom the brain is still in early stages of development. Thus, especially for younger children, attempts have been made to evaluate the effects of chemotherapy without radiation.

### *Lymphomas*

The lymphomas include non-Hodgkin's lymphomas (NHLs) and Hodgkin's lymphoma. These are cancers that have their origins in the lymph nodes. Hodgkin's lymphoma typically has a slower onset and more orderly progression than NHLs (Granowetter, 1994). This neoplasm is rare and occurs in fewer than 1 per 100,000 children per year. A subtype of NHL is Burkit's lymphoma, which is a prevalent cancer in central Africa. Common sites for NHL include the head and neck, the abdomen, and the chest. Symptoms include enlarged lymph nodes, fevers, weight loss, lethargy, and an abdominal tumor. These cancers grow rapidly and metastasize very early. Treatments for the lymphomas include chemotherapies that are administered intrathecally (directly into the spinal cord). For children with CNS involvement, cranial radiation or cranial-spinal radiation frequently is used. The cure rate for Hodgkin's lymphoma is much better than for NHL.

### *Wilms' Tumor*

Wilms' tumor, arising from embryonic tissue, virtually always occurs in children and is particularly responsive to chemotherapy (Granowetter, 1994), with cure rates of approximately 90%. The incidence of Wilms' tumor is approximately 1 in 10,000 children, with the peak age occurring between ages 2 and 3 years. The primary symptom is a lump or mass in the child's abdomen. Treatment includes chemotherapy that is followed by surgical resection of the tumor. Radiation therapy is sometimes used when there is already metastasis at diagnosis.

### *Neuroblastoma*

Neuroblastomas frequently occur in the abdomen or chest and on occasion in the neck or pelvis. For some patients, there is spontaneous regression of the tumor. Children with advanced disease often manifest a large tumor that involves the lymph nodes; frequently, the neuroblastoma has metastasized to the bone, bone marrow, distant lymph nodes, and the liver. The prognosis for advanced disease is much more guarded than for children and adolescents with more recent onset. Children who are younger than 12 months old, even with more advanced disease at diagnosis, also have a better prognosis than older children (Granowetter, 1994).

### *Retinoblastoma*

Retinoblastoma refers to a malignant cancer of the eye that is frequently congenital and recognized before the child is 3 years old (Granowetter, 1994). Again, this particular cancer is rare and has an incidence of 1 in 18,000 births. Symptoms include squinting or losing the red reflex in the eye, by which a white pupil is developed. Treatment is variable and depends on the extent of the disease. It may include photocoagulation, cryotherapy, and laser therapy to save vision. Enucleation will be performed if vision cannot be preserved. Chemotherapy and radiation therapy are most often used, particularly when retinoblastoma is advanced. Because there is a significant genetic basis for this tumor, much has been learned about the genetic basis of cancer, particularly the association between retinoblastoma and osteosarcoma tumors.

### *Bone Tumors and Soft Tissue Sarcomas*

The most frequently occurring bone tumor in children and adolescents is osteosarcoma, which typically occurs in either preadolescence or adolescence and is associated with rapid growth spurts (Granowetter, 1994). Treatment for osteosarcoma involves chemotherapy and subsequent resection of the tumor with surgery. Survival rates are approximately 75%. Significant advances in surgical techniques have allowed for limb salvaging, sparing children and adolescents the psychosocial sequelae associated with amputations.

Another bone tumor rarely found is Ewing's sarcoma, which usually occurs in preadolescence or adolescence. Treatment typically involves chemotherapy followed by surgery and radiation therapy or radiation therapy alone. The modality of treatment is contingent on the type, site, and size of the tumor.

Finally, tumors called sarcomas arise in the mesenchymal tissue and may develop anywhere in the body, although frequent sites include the head, neck, genitourinary tract, and extremities. Rhabdomyosarcoma is the most frequent soft tissue tumor and accounts for approximately 5% to 8% of children with cancer. It is more common among males, with the peak incidence at early childhood (approximately 2 to 5 years of age). Therapy for rhabdosarcoma may include surgical resection and chemotherapy with or without radiation therapy. The prognosis depends on the histological subtype, site, size, and presence of metastases and whether the tumor may be removed surgically.

## Format of the Book

The organization of this book was conceived in accordance with activities underlying the clinical course of the cancer experience. The conceptualization of psychological research in pediatric psychosocial oncology was also considered. First, introductory background material is provided for a comprehensive understanding of cancer and sickle cell disease. The biopsychosocial model that is appropriate in conceptualizing the psychosocial issues of these diseases is included. Second, factors related to being "on treatment" are provided that range from stress and coping with cancer to spirituality and complementary and alternative medicine. Third, issues pertaining to cancer late effects or "off treatment" issues are reviewed. This provides a comprehensive state of the art of the literature ranging from the transition from active treatment to survivorship and specific interventions for cancer late effects and survivorship. Although with every passing year more children and adolescents survive cancer, issues about palliative care and end of life are still realities of cancer and are appropriate for inclusion. Fourth, issues of primary and secondary prevention are routine components of the National Cancer Institute and are reviewed. Included in this section are issues that range from health promotion to genetic issues related to cancer.

Many pediatric psychologists who practice and conduct research in pediatric psychosocial oncology also provide clinical care to children and adolescents with sickle cell disease and their families. Although the diseases are very different in pathophysiology and management, they are treated in clinics that serve children and adolescents with hematological and oncology disorders. There are few comprehensive handbooks in the area of sickle cell disease. On one occasion, I proposed such a book, but no publishers were interested in publishing it because of the expected small audience. However, many issues that are important in sickle cell disease, including pain management and neuropsychological issues, also are important in cancer.

No handbook like this one would be complete without an understanding of complex training issues in the field of psychosocial hematology/oncology. Research opportunities in the field and the effect of multisite studies that have emerged are also described.

### Biopsychosocial Perspectives

In chapter 2, Armstrong extends Engel's biopsychosocial model of illness into the field of pediatric hematology/oncology and concludes that this is the standard of care for pediatric patients with any chronic illness. Armstrong concludes that the biopsychosocial model has driven the proliferation of research in this area. He notes this method has challenged investigators to use collaborative models to prevent problems that we now know will occur and provide therapy to relieve symptoms and enhance quality of life.

### The Cancer Experience "On Treatment"

Kupst and Bingen provide in chapter 3 a general overview of stress and coping as these constructs are related to cancer, the effect of pediatric cancer on children and their families, how children and their families actually cope with the stress of this disease, and how such coping is associated with overall adaptation to cancer. Theoretical and methodological issues are reviewed that are involved in the study of coping and adaptation. Kupst and Bingen suggest the next generation of investigators examine issues of coping with longitudinal methods that provide better understanding of short-term and long-term coping processes.

Extending the review of literature in chapter 4 to include the social ecology of cancer, Alderfer and Kazak provide a comprehensive and meticulous review of the family system and how it adapts and responds to the stress faced by cancer patients and their families. Included in this review are issues like treatment stabilization, illness stabilization, and end of treatment. Each of these phases affects familial adjustment and adaptation. Research in the area of family-level interventions is reviewed, and recommendations are made for some very promising research directions.

Given the recent prominence of bone marrow transplantation as a standard therapy in many children and adolescents with such high-risk cancers as leukemia, no handbook on psychosocial aspects of pediatric cancer would be complete without a chapter overview of the psychosocial issues related to stem cell transplantation. Psychological issues associated with this treatment perhaps represent a microcosm of the entire body of pediatric psychosocial oncology literature. Issues in the area of transplantation include neurocognitive and educational issues, adjustment issues, parental adjustment and adaptation to the process of transplantation, and interventions to enhance adjustment and adaptation to the transplantation process. Phipps concludes in chapter 5 that pediatric survivors of bone marrow transplants remain vulnerable in the area of psychosocial adjustment. Again, Phipps challenges investigators to embark on multisite collaborative studies designed to enhance parental and child adjustment to the transplant process.

In chapter 6, Fuemmeler, Mullins, and Carpentier provide a review of the literature related to the role that peers and friendships has on the adjustment of children and adolescents with cancer. They provide a cogent review of the association of social support to the adjustment and adaptation of survivors of childhood cancer. Challenges are made for future researchers to validate measurements across settings and informants, which will help assess children's friendships and emotional well-being. Clinical interventions that provide sufficient specificity and adequate community support will be the next direction in this area of research.

Conte and Walco in chapter 7 review literature related to cancer pain in children that is associated with procedural distress, treatment-related pain, and disease-related pain. The epidemiology of these pain problems is reviewed in addition to assessment and management issues. Conte and Walco conclude that to manage acute pain in children and adolescents adequately, a multimodal approach must be used in both assessment and management. Components of pharmacotherapeutic, physiological, and psychological treatments for the management of pain must be included. Conte and Walco conclude that structured assessments of pain in children with cancer are necessary, and that pain management, including pharmacotherapies and other analgesia, must have empirical support. Clinical trials also are necessary that demonstrate the efficacy, safety, and cost-effectiveness of pain management approaches.

Any comprehensive treatment program must necessarily consider adherence to treatment. In chapter 8, Rapoff, McGrath, and Smith review treatment for children with ALL and their families to aid in understanding the complex medical and behavioral requirements associated with medical treatments. In addition, the authors provide a comprehensive review of studies that have examined issues related to adherence, particularly for children and adolescents with ALL. Specific factors that predict good adherence to treatment are reviewed. Strategies also are provided for the assessment and improvement of adherence. The authors argue that the low incidence of cancer compared to other chronic diseases mandates that investigators collaborate on primary, secondary, and tertiary research related to adherence as part of large-scale multisite studies.

In view of the many advances in the treatment and survival rates for most childhood cancers, there has been significant interest in understanding how life is experienced for patients and their families on and off therapy. Levi reviews in chapter 9 research on the assessment of life experience and issues related to quality of life. Levi challenges future investigators in this domain to develop models that are informed by theory and that will allow for an examination of the variability of health-related quality of life during childhood, adolescence, and adulthood. It also is recommended that data be accumulated on child versus proxy ratings of child health-related quality of life. Levi recommends that issues of health-related quality of life be examined for cancers that are refractory to treatment and for children who must endure end-of-life issues.

There is rapidly increasing recognition of the role of complementary and alternative medicine in the treatment of many diseases. The National Institutes of Health has an entire institute devoted to complementary and alternative medicine that has its own funding. Myers, Stuber, and Zeltzer review medical literature on complementary and alternative medicine in chapter 10. A comprehensive definition of complementary and alternative medicine is provided as are prevalence rates of various modalities. Clinical trials assessing the efficacy and safety of complementary and alternative medicine are summarized, with discussion on spirituality and religion as it relates to complementary and alternative medicine.

This handbook includes a review of state-of-the-art extant literature on informed consent in pediatric oncology research. Nearly all pediatric patients who are treated for cancer and who have survived this disease receive their care in tertiary health science centers. In chapter 11, Fisher and Masty provide a comprehensive review of current theory and research on informed consent policies for cancer research within an ethics framework. This framework conceptualizes children's participation in such programs as a goodness of fit regarding the research context, caregivers' understanding of information provided during the informed consent process, and children's decision capabilities. Conclusions are that compassionate informed consent requires an ethic of mutual obligation, respect, and care.

Sahler and associates provide a thorough review in chapter 12 of their research that is related to problem solving among mothers of children recently diagnosed with cancer. They review their intensive problem-solving skills training and conclude that this program is effective in reducing negative affectivity in mothers during the time of cancer induction and early cancer treatment.

## Cancer Late Effects "Off Treatment"

Marsland, Ewing, and Thompson provide a review in chapter 13 of the psychological and social effects of childhood cancer survivors. They explain literature on the late psychosocial consequences of childhood cancer and provide discussion of moderating factors that may account for the variance in psychological and social adjustment of childhood cancer survivors. The authors conclude that numerous methodological issues coupled with a preponderance of cross-sectional rather than longitudinal studies make it difficult to draw any definitive conclusions on psychosocial late effects. They challenge us to embark on longitudinal investigations that will address more specifically the late effects of pediatric cancer.

In addition to psychosocial late effects that follow cancer, neuropsychological late effects frequently are associated with childhood cancer and its treatment. Chapter 14 by Mulhern and Butler provides a brief medical background on ALL and brain tumors and presents a comprehensive review of the neuropsychological literature. The authors delineate a specific analysis of the types of cognitive impairments that children sustain as well as important risk factors for these impairments. Recommendations are provided for neuropsychological assessment of survivors. Mulhern and Butler challenge us to identify specific subtypes of neurological impairments that may be associated with cancer late effects.

The most salient form of psychopathology that is associated with the late effects of cancer is posttraumatic stress disorder. In chapter 15, Stuber reviews the evidence for the presence of posttraumatic stress disorder among survivors of childhood cancer. Included are epidemiology, correlates, and predictors of posttraumatic stress disorder symptoms in cancer survivors. The scant literature on intervention research is reviewed. Suggestions for future developments are made, including endocrine and immunologic associations of posttraumatic stress disorder in children, adolescents, and young adults that may have implications for the management of symptoms related to the disorder.

The increase in survivors of childhood cancer and concomitant late effects associated with the disease and its treatment has resulted in interventions for late effects of cancer and their appropriate management. In chapter 16, Butler and Copeland review the most recent research on interventions for the late effects among long-term survivors of childhood cancer. The discussion includes physical, neurocognitive, psychosocial, and pharmacological interventions for these late effects. Recommendations are made for multimodal studies that examine the integration of cognitive remediation strategies with pharmacological approaches.

Another area needing discussion is academic and school social outcomes for cancer survivors. Reintegration to school poses a formidable task for many cancer survivors, and success at school is an important marker of functionality among survivors. Using the risk-resistance adaptation model by Wallander, authors Katz and Madan-Swain review in chapter 17 major risk factors that are posited to affect cancer survivors adversely at school. A framework is provided that delineates school reentry and interventions that might be helpful in maximizing positive school and psychosocial outcomes.

### Palliative Care and End-of-Life Issues

In chapter 18, Bearison points out that approximately 53,000 children die in this country annually, with the leading medical causes of death cancer, diseases of the heart, and lower respiratory conditions. Several topics are reviewed in this chapter, including hospice care, parents of dying children, anticipatory grief, grief counseling, end-of-life decisions, discontinuing life-sustaining treatments, and patient autonomy.

As a logical follow-up to this chapter, Breyer, Sanfeliz, Cieurzo, and Meyer provide a comprehensive overview of bereavement literature in the field of pediatric oncology in chapter 19. The authors provide a model for coping with bereavement. Anticipatory grief, acute and long-term grief, and complicated grief are reviewed and discussed, particularly as related to caregivers, siblings, and health care providers.

In chapter 20, Patenaude and Schneider discuss the concerns of survivors and their caregivers about genetics. They provide an overview of which pediatric cancers are known to have hereditary etiologies and how genetic counseling serves as an important adjunct in the care of children and adolescents who have survived cancer, particularly when these youth reach young adulthood. The work of Patenaude and Schneider is important as it underscores the importance of genetics in cancer research and more importantly for the present book highlights the importance of genetic issues in psychosocial oncology.

In chapter 21, Tyc reviews the prevalence of tobacco use, health effects associated with tobacco use, and correlates associated with tobacco use among adolescents who are treated for cancer. This is an area that has received widespread intervention efforts, and interventions that have been conducted among survivors of childhood cancer are reviewed. Information is given for health care providers on how they can assist their high-risk patients in making healthy lifestyle choices that include the reduction of or abstinence from tobacco use and avoidance of environmental tobacco exposure.

Wilson and Griffin address prevention in chapter 22 by providing a social-ecological model as a framework for promoting healthy lifestyles for children and adolescents as a means of preventing cancer. The authors review evidence suggesting an association between lifestyle risk factors and cancer. A review is provided for promoting physical activity, nutrition, sun exposure prevention, and tobacco use prevention.

### Sickle Cell Disease

In chapter 23, Gustafson, Bonner, Hardy, and Thompson provide a review of biopsychosocial and developmental issues relevant for sickle cell disease. The authors delineate the biomedical aspects of the disease itself, provide a comprehensive review of the biopsychosocial conceptual models, and outline what we know about risk and resistance factors that predict psychological adjustment in children and adolescents with sickle cell disease and their families.

Biopsychosocial issues in neurocognitive and developmental outcomes in these children also are reviewed. Consistent with much of the literature in pediatric psychology, the writers challenge us to conduct intervention studies and controlled clinical trials that will assist in the refinement of the biopsychosocial model.

Schatz and Puffer provide a review and critique in chapter 24 of knowledge of the neurological bases of sickle cell disease. The authors categorize two broad approaches that are frequently used to identify behavior correlates of brain functioning. These include psychological models and behavioral assessments. Schatz and Puffer conclude that a great deal of progress has been made in the development of technology as a means of mitigating the deleterious neurological effects of sickle cell disease. Again, recommendations are made for intervention studies to prevent or remediate the effects of these neurological insults. This remains an important endeavor destined for the next decade.

In chapter 25, Barakat, Lash, Lutz, and Nicolaou provide a thorough review of the psychological adaptation of children and adolescents with sickle cell disease. They review variables such as the influence of socioeconomic status, appraisals of stress, and family functioning, among others, on psychosocial adaptation. Again, conclusions by these authors are that intervention studies must address appraisal and coping within a familial context. The need for intervention studies seems to be a salient theme of these reviews and an area of critical importance in the years to come.

Related to the psychological adaptation of children and adolescents with sickle cell disease is the adjustment and adaptation of the families of children with this chronic illness. In chapter 26, Radcliffe, Barakat, and Boyd provide a framework for our understanding of how sickle cell disease affects family functioning. In the spirit of a biopsychosocial model, the authors present a developmental-ecological model of family functioning and use this model to characterize family system issues associated with sickle cell disease. The authors insist that an understanding of family system issues in children and adolescents with sickle cell disease is imperative in providing effective treatment for those with the disease. Family system methods facilitate psychological adjustment to stress associated with this disease and its treatment. As with the other chapters in this section, recommendations are made for intervention that are culturally sensitive in promulgating research on family-centered care for these children.

In chapter 27, Swain, Mitchell, and Powers review pain management for sickle cell disease. The authors focus on issues related to assessment and management of pain in children and adolescents with sickle cell disease; pharmacological and nonpharmacological approaches are reviewed. They suggest research in home management of sickle cell pain. This represents a novel approach for investigators who have focused on hospitalized patients and children and adolescents in outpatient clinics.

## Training, Funding, and Collaboration

Given the complexity of issues associated with pediatric psychosocial hematology/oncology, training new professionals appropriately and thoroughly is crucial. Clay and Elkin describe specific phases of training in psychosocial pediatric hematology/oncology, discuss issues that affect the training process, and delineate key content areas in which training is necessary to reach an acceptable level of competence and expertise. Chapter 28 provides a review of the process and content of specialized training in this area. Unique to the chapter is a developmental framework in Clay and Elkin's discussion of didactic issues and skills acquisition among trainees in pediatric psychosocial hematology/oncology.

As I look back on this field, the research accomplishments of behavioral scientists leave me breathless. Still, the reviews by my esteemed colleagues show how much research remains on the empirical horizon. As Whitsett, Armstrong, and Pollock remind us in chapter 29, the future of our research productivity lies in multicenter collaborative investigations. These authors review the benefits of collaborative studies and the challenges of such endeavors. It is hoped the result will be advancement in our knowledge of pediatric psychosocial oncology and direct benefits to the children and families.

## A Prospective and Retrospective View of Pediatric Hematology/Oncology

In editing this book, I became acutely aware of my diminishing youth as I looked back on the myriad accomplishments of my colleagues in this field and, more importantly, as I reflected on their career development. At the same time, some of the research that was accomplished over the past 40 years predated my graduate training. Thus, we are fortunate to have one of our senior colleagues, John Spinetta, who conducted some of the original seminal studies related to psychosocial hematology/oncology, take a look at the passage of time as this scholarship has unfolded. Spinetta, Masera, and Jankovic conclude in chapter 30 that our success as investigators may be categorized under the rubric of four preambles. Those include multidisciplinary and international efforts; an alliance among physicians and parents, research and service; and sharing of the research wealth with economically struggling countries. Spinetta and colleagues encourage us to celebrate the medical accomplishments of our physician colleagues. They also encourage behavior scientists, psychologists, and social workers to celebrate the "truly" cured child.

Many handbooks end with a challenge to readers to embark on additional research, as does this one. I also encourage us to celebrate our many accomplishments. We have furthered science and enhanced practice so that the quality of life for these children and their families also is enhanced. I do believe that we as scientists and practitioners have demonstrated through comprehensive reviews that the biopsychosocial model indeed is alive and well.

## References


Armstrong, F. D., & Reaman, G. H. (2005). Psychological research in childhood cancer: The Children's Oncology Group prospective. *Journal of Pediatric Psychology, 30,* 89–97.

Bearison, D., & Mulhern, R. K. (1994). *Pediatric psychooncology*. New York: Oxford University Press.

Bleyer, W. A. (1997). The U.S. pediatric cancer clinical trials programmes: International implications and the way forward. *European Journal of Cancer, 33,* 1439–1447.

Boman, K., & Bodegard, G. (2000). Long-term coping in childhood cancer survivors: Influence of illness, treatment and demographic background factors. *Acta Paediatrica, 89,* 105–111.

Brown, R. T., Madan-Swain, A., Walco, G. A., Cherrick, L., Ievers, C. E., Conte, P. M., et al. (1998). Cognitive and academic late effects among children previously treated for acute lymphocytic leukemia receiving chemotherapy as CNS prophylaxis. *Journal of Pediatric Psychology, 23,* 333–340.

Butler, R. W., & Copeland, D. R. (2002). Attentional processes and their remediation in children treated for cancer: A literature review and the development of a therapeutic approach. *Journal of the International Neuropsychological Society, 8,* 113–124.

Butler, R. W., & Mulhern, R. K. (2005). Neurocognitive interventions for children and adolescents surviving cancer. *Journal of Pediatric Psychology, 30,* 65–78.

Friedman, D., & Meadows, A. (2002). Late effects of childhood cancer therapy. In E. Vichinsky, M. Waters, & J. Feusner (Eds.), *Pediatric clinics of North America* (pp. 1083–1106). Philadelphia: Saunders.

Gaynon, P. S., Trigg, M. E., Heerema, N. A., Sensel, M. G., Sather, H. N., Hammond, G. D., et al. (2000). Children's Cancer Group trials in childhood acute lymphoblastic leukemia: 1983–1995. *Leukemia, 14,* 2223–2233.

Granowetter, L. (1994). Pediatric oncology: A medical overview. In D. J. Bearison & R. K. Mulhern (Eds.), *Pediatric psychooncology: Psychological perspectives on children with cancer* (pp. 9–34). New York: Oxford University Press.

Holland, J. C. (1998). *Psycho-oncology*. New York: Oxford University Press.

Kazak, A. (2002). *Surviving Cancer Competently Intervention Program–Newly Diagnosed. (SCCIP-ND) treatment manual.* Philadelphia: Children's Hospital of Philadelphia, Division of Oncology.

Kazak, A., Prusak, A., McSherry, M., Simms, S., Beele, D., & Rourke, M. (2001). The Psychosocial Assessment Tool (PAT): Pilot data on a brief screening instrument for identifying high risk families in pediatric oncology. *Family Systems and Health, 19,* 303–317.

Kazak, A., Rourke, M., & Crump, T. (2003). Families and other systems in pediatric psychology. In M. Roberts (Ed.), *Handbook of pediatric psychology* (3rd ed.) (pp. 159–175). New York: Guilford.

Kazak, A., Stuber, M., Barakat, L., Meeske, K., Guthrie, D., & Meadows, A. (1998). Predicting posttraumatic stress symptoms in mothers and fathers of childhood cancer. *Journal of the American Academy of Child and Adolescent Psychiatry, 37,* 823–831.

Kazak, A. E. (2005). Evidenced-based interventions for survivors of childhood cancer and their families. *Journal of Pediatric Psychology, 30,* 29–39.

Kupst, M. J., Natta, M. B., Richardson, C. C., Schulman, J. L., Lavigne, J. V., & Das, L. (1995). Family coping with pediatric leukemia: Ten years after treatment. *Journal of Pediatric Psychology, 20,* 601–617.

Mackie, E., Hill, J., Kiomdryn, H., & McNally, R. (2000). Adult psychosocial outcomes in long-term survivors of acute lymphoblastic leukemia and Wilm's tumor: A controlled study. *Lancet, 355,* 1310–1314.

Madan-Swain, A., Brown, R. T., Foster, M. A., Vega, R., Byars, K., & Rodenberger, W. (2000). Identity in adolescent survivors of childhood cancer. *Journal of Pediatric Psychology, 25,* 105–115.

Meadows, A. T., Massari, D. J., Fergusson, J., Gordon, J., Littman, P., & Moss, K. (1981). Declines in IQ scores and cognitive dysfunctions in children with acute lymphocytic leukemia treated with cranial irradiation. *Lancet, 2,* 1015–1018.

Moore, B. D. (2005). Neurocognitive outcomes in survivors of childhood cancer. *Journal of Pediatric Psychology, 30,* 51–63.

Mulhern, R. K. (1994). Neuropsychological late effects. In D. Bearson & R. K. Mulhern (Eds.), *Pediatric psychooncology* (pp. 99–121). New York: Oxford University Press.

Mulhern, R. K., Khan, R. B., Kaplan, S., Helton, S., Christensen, R., Bonner, M., et al. (2004). Short-term efficacy of methylphenidate: A randomized, double-blind, placebo-controlled trial among survivors of childhood cancer. *Journal of Clinical Oncology, 22,* 4743–4751.

Oberfield, S. E., & Sklar, C. A. (2002). Endocrine sequelae in survivors of childhood cancer. *Adolescent Medicine, 13,* 161–169.

Patenaude, A. F. (2003). Pediatric psychology training and genetics: What will 21st century pediatric psychologists need to know? *Journal of Pediatric Psychology, 28,* 135–145.

Patenaude, A. F., & Kupst, M. J. (2005a). Introduction to the special issue: Surviving pediatric cancer: Research gains and goals. *Journal of Pediatric Psychology, 30,* 5–8.

Patenaude, A. F., & Kupst, M. J. (2005b). Psychosocial functioning in pediatric cancer. *Journal of Pediatric Psychology, 30,* 9–27.

Rowland, J. H. (2005). Forward: Looking beyond cure: Pediatric cancer as a model. *Journal of Pediatric Psychology, 30,* 1–3.

Rowland, J. H., Mariotto, A., Aziz, N. A., Tesauro, G., Feuer, R., & Blackman, D. (2004). Cancer survivorship—United States, 1971–2001. *Morbidity and Mortality Weekly Report,* 53, 526–530.

Tyc, V., Rai, S., Lensing, S., Klosky, J., Stewart, D., & Gattuso, J. (2003). An intervention to reduce intentions to use tobacco among pediatric cancer survivors. *Journal of Clinical Oncology, 21,* 1366–1372.

Walco, G. A. (2005). Commentary: Psychologists in pediatric oncology: Kudos, criticism, and courses for the future. *Journal of Pediatric Psychology, 30,* 115–118.

Zeltzer, L. K., Chen, E., Weiss, R., Matthre, D. G., Robison, L. L., & Meadows, A. T. (1997). Comparison of psychologic outcome in adult survivors of childhood acute lymphocytic leukemia versus sibling controls: A Cooperative Children's Cancer Group and National Institutes of Health study. *Journal of Clinical Oncology, 15,* 547–556.

F. Daniel Armstrong

# Cancer and Blood Disorders in Childhood

## Biopsychosocial-Developmental Issues in Assessment and Treatment

Cancer, sickle cell disease (SCD), hemophilia, and other blood-related and immunologic disorders represent some of the most complex medical conditions of childhood. All involve a diagnosis that is directly associated with a genetic risk that is interpreted within a complex family system. All have complex biology involving multiple organ systems, and all are potentially fatal. All involve treatment that is demanding, both biologically and behaviorally. All inevitably alter the normal course of development, often during critical periods in the lives of children and families. All have potential significant economic and social consequences that include costs of treatment, indirect costs associated with disease management, and potential long-term costs associated with disability. All have potential long-term effects of treatment that may involve additional new diseases or disabilities.

Surprisingly, however, hematologic and oncologic diseases of childhood have one other commonality; despite the complexity and high potential for devastating biologic, psychosocial, family, and economic consequences, all have affected individuals and families who do not experience these devastating consequences and in fact demonstrate a biologic and psychologic resiliency that defies conventional wisdom. Understanding the complex interactions among genetic risk; biology of disease; effectiveness and outcome of treatment; child and family coping, adjustment, and resilience; developmental trajectories; and community support is the challenge for investigators and clinicians during this century, particularly as basic advances in diagnosis and treatment result in anticipation of probable survival for the vast majority of children with these conditions. It is for this reason that these diseases of childhood are frequently considered from a biopsychosocial perspective (Engel, 1980), although we argue that this term must be expanded to incorporate developmental complexity, particularly when applied to children.

### The Biopsychosocial Model

Since Engel (1980) first proposed a biopsychosocial model of illness as a conceptual model for understanding and treating functional gastrointestinal disorders, our understanding of chronic illness has increasingly incorporated this perspective. The biopsychosocial model recognizes that illness, and one's experience of illness, occurs through a dynamic interaction among biologic, psychologic, social, and environmental factors, all of which overlap as potential causes and maintenance factors of symptoms associated with the illness. Since the early 1980s, the biopsychosocial model has been applied to many different chronic illnesses of adults and children. Early applications of the model examined how a multidisciplinary perspective, one that included independent opinions of professionals from distinct disciplines, could be applied to understanding the cause of illness and how different disciplinary assessment and intervention approaches might be concurrently used to improved illness-related symptoms.

As the biopsychosocial model became more broadly recognized, a shift in approach from multidisciplinary to interdisciplinary perspectives occurred. The interdisciplinary perspective focused on bringing independent disciplinary perspectives together in an organized fashion to address complex assessment and management concerns (Guralnick, 2000). This approach relied more heavily on recognition of common considerations across discipline perspectives and integration of unique contributions by separate disciplines.

Increasingly, the interdisciplinary perspective is growing into what has been called a transdisciplinary perspective (Armstrong & Reaman, 2005). The transdisciplinary perspective has grown out of the recognition in basic science research that many research questions require a synergy of perspectives that overarch simple explanations to produce an integrated, complex understanding of multiple, concurrent, and interactive factors associated with the illness experience.

The primary outcome of the biopsychosocial model has been increased emphasis on the recognition of psychological and social factors in the individual's experience of illness and the inclusion of these factors in the development of interventions, based on psychological principles, that can alleviate illness-related symptoms and adverse health outcomes (Brown et al., 2002). Depending on the illness of interest, this focus has included assessment and treatment of psychological or social factors associated with medical regimen adherence, chronic pain, substance abuse, developmental disability, and health behaviors associated with long-term health outcomes, including smoking, alcohol use, exercise, eating, and sleeping (Brown, 2004).

Biopsychosocial conceptualizations and interdisciplinary approaches to assessment and treatment are overwhelmingly applicable to children with hematologic or oncologic disorders. Developmental change forces an additional perspective that anticipates an interaction among normal growth and development, acute events related to the disease and its treatment, and long-term changes in normal growth and development as a result of the effects and demands of the diseases and their treatment. We know that hematologic and oncologic diseases of childhood involve complex disease natural history, burdensome and prolonged treatment demands, multiple affected organ systems, acute and long-term side effects of treatment, challenges for other family members, opportunities for acquisition of behavior that is adaptive in the hospital setting but not in the natural environment, and the potential for development of long-term disabilities (Armstrong, in press).

The biopsychosocial model has been historically applied to specific disease- or treatment-related symptoms experienced by children with hematologic or oncologic diseases, such as pain or anticipatory nausea and vomiting (Powers et al., 1995; Stehbens, 1988). However, our understanding of these diseases, improvement in both direct treatment and supportive care, and increasing awareness of late consequences experienced in adolescence and adulthood now force us to expand the biopsychosocial model to include evaluation of the effectiveness of biopsychosocial interventions from a developmental perspective. The children with these diseases are rapidly becoming the adults who are survivors, the adults who live with consequences of earlier treatment decisions, or the adults who live with ongoing management requirements of diseases that cannot yet be cured (National Cancer Policy Board, 2003). The challenge today is to provide symptom relief, cure or prevent whenever possible, and make it possible for children with these diseases to both live and live well.

## The Biopsychosocial-Developmental Model in Pediatric Hematology and Oncology

The biopsychosocial model, with the added developmental perspective, can be applied to all childhood diseases in some way or another. For this chapter, two diseases, cancer and SCD, serve as the models for application of a biopsychosocial-developmental perspective. Childhood cancer is a disease that can, in most instances, be cured, but not without long-term consequences and continuing psychological and biological threat of recurrence. SCD is a disease that cannot, in most cases, be cured but can be treated or managed in a way that permits individuals with the disease to function outside the medical center setting. That these diseases are selected for illustrative purposes should not in any way discount the importance of the application of this model to other disorders involving the hematopoietic system, such as hemophilia, immune deficiency disorders, or any other disorder involving abnormalities in red or white blood cells or platelet generation, proliferation, or function. Many of the points raised in the following sections, using cancer and SCD models, are directly applicable to these other hematologic diseases and disorders.

## Childhood Cancer

Childhood cancer includes a large and diverse group of diseases. The common factor for all kinds of cancer is change in normal cells leading to (a) rapid proliferation of abnormal cells; (b) spread of these cells to other organs (termed *metastasis*); and (c) diminished, impaired, or loss of normal cell or organ function. As these abnormal cells grow or fail to function properly, the natural history of these diseases ultimately leads to death, although the speed of progression varies substantially across the different types of childhood cancer (Armstrong & Briery, 2004). Childhood cancer most often involves the hemopoietic system, with leukemias and lymphomas accounting for approximately 40% of all childhood cancer, followed by cancer of the central nervous system (CNS) (20%), neuroblastoma (8%), muscle and soft tissue sarcomas (7%), bone (5%), and tumors of other organ systems accounting for the remaining 20% (National Cancer Institute SEER Program, 1999; Ries et al., 2004). Fortunately, some of the most common cancers of adulthood (e.g., breast, lung, prostate, ovarian) are rarely seen in children, and cancer of childhood remains a relatively rare disease, affecting approximately 1 in 100,000 children or about 9,000 under the age of 15 years in the United States each year (American Cancer Society, 2003).

Treatment of childhood cancer has historically involved the use of chemotherapy, radiation therapy, or surgery to remove solid tumors. Combinations of aggressive cancer chemotherapy drugs usually result in the destruction of rapidly dividing cancer cells at the time of cell division. Radiation therapy follows the same treatment principle. This combination of treatments has led to an increase in long-term survival from approximately 60% in the early 1980s to greater than 85% in 2003 (National Cancer Policy Board, 2003; Ries et al., 2004). Unfortunately, these treatments do not discriminate between cancer and rapidly dividing normal cells, so cancer treatment often involves suppression of the immune system, hair loss, damage to the gastrointestinal system that results in nausea and vomiting, alteration of taste and appetite, and severe fatigue. In addition to these many toxic side effects, the delivery of cancer treatment is often painful and aversive. Many chemotherapy drugs require intravenous administration, and some types of cancer require multiple treatments of the CNS with chemotherapy that is delivered by intrathecal administration (using spinal taps). Finally, besides these acute problems, some of the chemotherapy drugs result in permanent injury to the heart, brain, and other organ systems (National Cancer Policy Board, 2003).

The psychosocial consequences of childhood cancer and its treatment have long been recognized (Vannatta & Gerhardt, 2003). In the 1960s and 1970s, the focus was almost exclusively on coping with the death of the child (Spinetta, 1974). In the 1980s, behavioral research expanded to include assessment of and intervention for complications associated with cancer treatment, including pain, anticipatory nausea and vomiting, and other treatment side effects, and assessment of neurocognitive outcomes following radiation and chemotherapy for cancer involving the CNS (Armstrong & Mulhern, 1999; Stehbens, 1988). Integration of the findings from these psychosocial studies had a discernable impact on the way cancer treatment was provided. For instance, the recognition of severe neurocognitive consequences of radiation therapy for very young children with brain tumors led to the development of new treatment protocols that used chemotherapy to delay radiation exposure, which led to less-severe neurocognitive consequences without a loss of survival (Duffner et al., 1993). Likewise, research on cognitive behavioral treatments of pain and distress led to greater utilization of behavioral strategies and more humane approaches to intravenous and intrathecal chemotherapy administration (Varni, Blount, Waldron, & Smith, 1995). The biopsychosocial model was clearly applicable to treatment of cancer, and psychosocial assessment and intervention became integrated into standard practice in many, but not all, clinical oncology settings, including long-term late-effects clinics (Hinkle et al., 2004).

In the 1990s, limitations of psychosocial interventions began to be understood, both in terms of short- and long-term success and cost and availability of providers. Behavioral treatments of pain began to be replaced by the use of new conscious sedation procedures and general anesthesia for invasive procedures (American Academy of Pediatrics & American Pain Society, 2001), and a new class of antiemetic medications was successful in significantly reducing acute nausea and vomiting (Tyc, Mulhern, Barclay, Smith, & Bieberich, 1997).

At the same time, new treatments for childhood cancer began to emerge that presented new challenges from a psychosocial perspective. Aggressive therapy, such as bone marrow and peripheral stem cell transplantation, became a viable and widespread alternative for children with high-risk disease, as well as those with recurrent disease, but this brought about substantial new challenges related to isolation, severe physical and emotional difficulties, and coping of family members, who experienced significant lifestyle disruption for extended periods of time (Powers et al., 1995). The need for assessment of psychosocial functioning of the child (Vannatta & Gerhardt, 2003), assessment of the coping of parents and siblings (Goldbeck, 2001), implementation of effective stress management (Sahler et al., 2002), and intervention to reduce "environment-related" toxicity in intensive care settings (Streisand, Rodrigue, Houck, Graham-Pole, & Berlant, 2000) was recognized, and the biopsychosocial perspective shifted to address these concerns. Further, we began to recognize that although not all children and families inevitably experienced long-term emotional, social, behavioral, or cognitive difficulties as a result of cancer treatment (Kazak & Barakat, 1997), there were subgroups of children and families who were clearly at risk for significant and long-term difficulties in these areas (Santacroce, 2002).

As we begin the 21st century, the way that childhood cancer is diagnosed and treated is changing, and the application of the biopsychosocial perspective will need to respond to the advancements in care. Overall survival for most types of childhood cancer is greater than 75%, and some types have survival greater than 85% (National Cancer Policy Board, 2003; Ries et al., 2004). The approach to treatment of most childhood cancers is standardized, with more than 70% of children in the United States and Canada enrolled in cooperative, multicenter clinical trials as part of the Children's Oncology Group (Liu, Krailo, Reaman, & Bernstein, 2003).

Approaches to treatment are also changing. As work on the human genome project advances, use of genetic prognostic markers makes it increasingly possible to identify subgroups for risk assessment, leading to reductions in treatment intensity without sacrificing successful outcome (M. E. Ross et al., 2003). Genetic advances are also altering the overall approach to cancer treatment. Genetic information is being used to develop individualized, targeted therapies for subgroups of children, and it is likely that these treatments will ultimately involve substantially less cost, fewer aversive procedures, less personnel demand for treatment administration, and few to no acute or long-term toxicities (Arceci & Cripte, 2002).

As these improvements in acute treatment take place, we are becoming more aware of the long-term effects of treatment provided to children of earlier times. Today, more than 270,000 adults are childhood cancer survivors, and by the year 2010, it is estimated that 1 in 900 adults will be a survivor of childhood cancer. For adults between 21 and 40 years of age, that number is 1 in 570 (National Cancer Policy Board, 2003). As this population of childhood cancer survivors grows, so does the recognition that the success has been purchased at a high price because many of these survivors will experience long-term consequences of treatment, including damage to the heart, pulmonary difficulties, endocrine abnormalities, risk of second malignancies, and neurocognitive impairment (Aziz, 2002; National Cancer Policy Board, 2003; Ries et al., 2004).

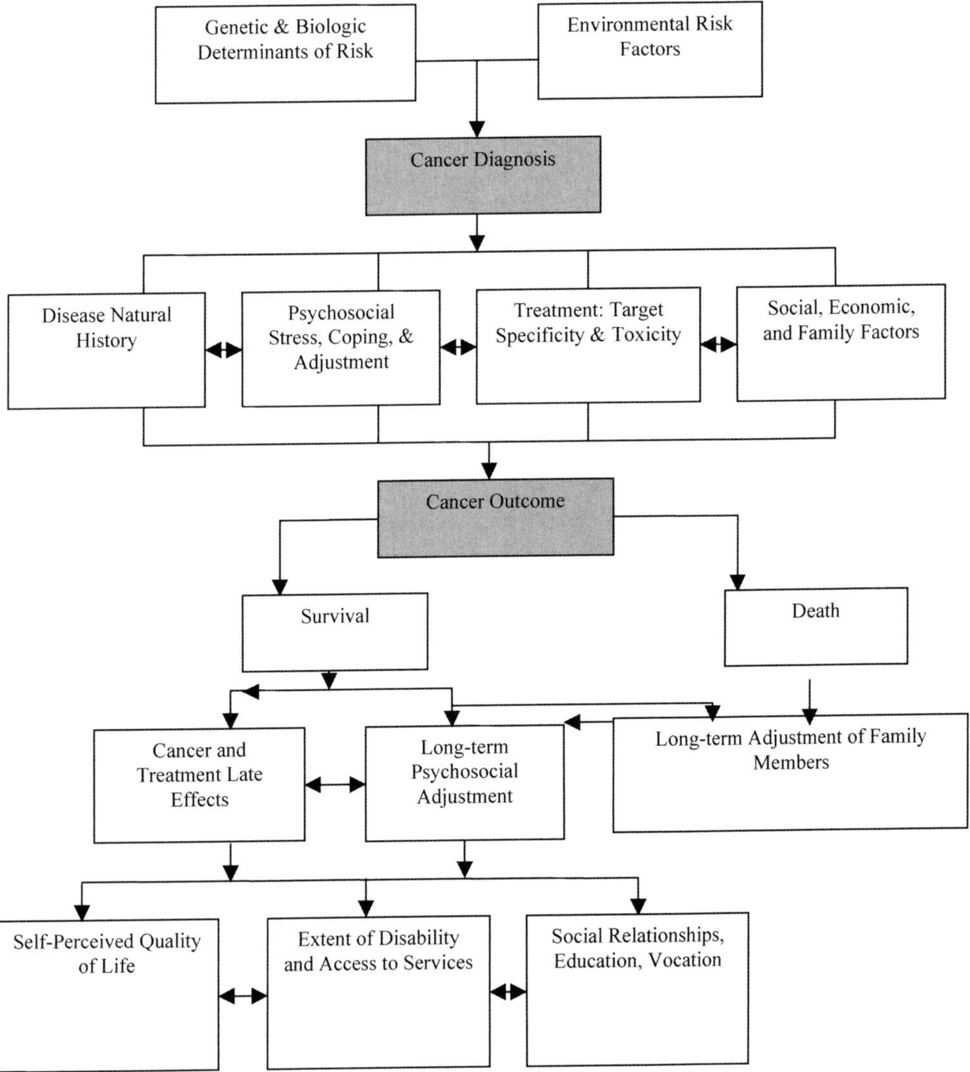


**Figure 2-1.** The biopsychosocial-developmental model of childhood cancer.

The Children's Oncology Group Late Effects Committee has developed a set of guidelines for surveillance of known late effects associated with every disease and treatment provided to children treated for cancer, along with best practice recommendations for assessment, intervention, and prevention (Landier et al., 2004). Notable in this set of guidelines is the repeated inclusion of recommendations addressing neurocognitive, behavioral, social, and emotional late effects, again reinforcing the degree to which the biopsychosocial perspective has been integrated into the care of children treated for cancer.

## Biopsychosocial-Developmental Model for the Next Decade

Better, less-aggressive treatment, combined with growing knowledge of late effects challenges us to reevaluate the way childhood cancer will be approached from a biopsychosocial-developmental perspective during the next decade. There are many opportunities for an integrated approach to continue to improve both health care delivery and the quality of long-term survival. A biopsychosocial-developmental model of childhood cancer (figure 2-1) provides one way of thinking about the synergistic interactions that currently exist and may provide a blueprint for how we will approach this disease, the children, and their families over the next generation.

## Cancer Diagnosis

The diagnosis of cancer is the starting point for a biopsychosocial-developmental perspective. Cancer diagnosis involves (a) identification of some symptoms of concern; (b) referral to a new hospital or physician; (c) medical tests that may or may not be invasive or painful, but that usually are frightening to children and parents; (d) interpretation of medical tests to arrive at a diagnosis; (e) addition of other risk information used in determining the prognosis of the illness and intensity of treatment; (f) communication of diagnostic, treatment, and prognostic information to child and family; and (g) emotional, social, and economic responses to the information and new demands brought about by the disease and its treatment. Families and children must integrate complex information based on uncertainty (Levi, Marsick, Drotar, & Kodish, 2000; Ruccione, Waskerwitz, Buckley, Perin, & Hammond, 1994). Although there are some clear genetic and biologic determinants of cancer and there are other real and believed environmental determinants, the certainty of knowing cause, and the sense of control that can come with knowing cause, can be elusive.

The diagnosis establishes the basis for a biopsychosocial-developmental approach. Complex information about genetics, blood cells, and tumor markers must be communicated to parents at a time when their ability to comprehend this information is often influenced by little background context and overwhelming emotion. Children must be provided information about the disease they have, what will be necessary to treat it, and why this must take place. How this occurs will depend on the age and developmental level of the child, with different approaches needed for children of different ages. Decisions must be made about which surgery, chemotherapy, or radiation approach will be involved, and consideration of risks of disease and consequences of therapy must be weighed against perceived and real benefits of treatment. Although information about cancer and the approach to treatment may be comprehended, parents and children may be ill prepared to cope with the aversive medical procedures and noxious side effects. For these children and families, interventions that enable them to make decisions and act on these decisions may be necessary. All of these things must occur before the first drop of chemotherapy is administered. Failure to integrate the many biologic, social, emotional, cognitive, and developmental aspects associated with cancer diagnosis may, and often does, lead to many problems with later treatment and survivorship.

## The Treatment Process

Today, most childhood cancer treatment is based on established protocols conducted within the context of a multicenter clinical trails group (see Whitsett, Armstrong, & Pollock, chapter 29, this volume). Based on laboratory, genetic, and pathology studies of the tumor, children are treated on the basis of evaluation of risk, and a "roadmap" of therapy is followed, with specific medication given at specific times in specific doses. If only treatment of cancer was that simple.

As shown in figure 2-1, there are multiple complex factors that interact to determine treatment outcome, including (a) the natural history of the type of cancer and (b) the effectiveness of targeted therapy and the toxicity, or side effects, of the treatment. In addition, there are major social, economic, family, and emotional factors that influence the outcome of cancer treatment. These may include (a) the ability of the family to access care (Himmelstein & Woolhandler, 1995); (b) the nonmedical costs of receiving treatment, such as parking, food, child care for siblings, and lost income (Cohn, Goodenough, Foreman, & Suneson, 2003); (c) the impact of the diagnosis on the coping and adjustment of the child, siblings, parents, and other family members and their need for support and information (Levi et al., 2000; Ljungman et al., 2003); and (d) external information about the decision from the Internet and others with alternative or complementary approaches to treatment (Jankovic et al., 2004). The outcome of the convergence of these factors not only may be successful completion of treatment, but also may be nonadherence, conflict with the treating medical staff, increased family conflict or adjustment problems for siblings, and possibly recurrent disease.

The easy part of treatment may be reading the treatment protocol and ordering the right medications. The difficult part is developing an integrated approach that maximizes the benefits of the treatment while concurrently reducing the aversive experience, toxicity, and disruption of life that this treatment requires. This is the point at which a biopsychosocial-developmental model may be of greatest use.

Effective use of appropriate developmental and systems education about treatment options, side effects, and supportive care strategies is a first-level intervention that can facilitate both psychosocial adjustment (of the child and family members) and lessened risk of nonadherence to treatment based on lack of information, misinterpretation of information, or fear. A number of comprehensive resources have been developed to assist with education about these concerns, including expansive Web sites such as the National Cancer Iinstitute PDQ site for pediatric cancer (National Cancer Institute, 2004). These public access educational materials are easily accessible; provide a sense of consistency in expectations about treatment, no matter which hospital or medical team provides the care; and because of the peer-review process involved in their development, strive to offer current understanding with stated levels of evidence for the information.

For some families and children, education is sufficient to allow their full participation in treatment. For others, difficulties may arise when, following education, there are problems acting on this information in a way that permits treatment to be provided in an effective manner. These families may require a second-level intervention that focuses on helping them to master obstacles to performance of what they understand, and agree, needs to be performed. Some of these obstacles may be overcome with the use of current best practice supportive care. Prescribing medications that reduce sensations of nausea (Tyc et al., 1997) and using appropriate sedation and analgesics for painful procedures (American Academy of Pediatrics & American Pain Society, 2001) are approaches that are a central part of this second-level intervention. Concurrent stress management training, crisis intervention, cognitive behavioral therapy, family therapy, pain management intervention, development of adherence habits, and training in effective parenting approaches for children with serious illness are all examples of the kind of second-level intervention that provide parents and children with the necessary skills to both understand and act on that understanding. More than 20 years of research supports the inclusion of these effective interventions for acute problems associated with cancer treatment (Vannatta & Gerhardt, 2003; Varni et al., 1995).

Cancer treatment takes place in hospitals and clinics, but the children and their families live in communities. Work, school, religion, extended family, and friends all affect and are affected by the treatment of childhood cancer. Difficulties may be encountered as health insurance is lost, income declines, and opportunities for interacting with a social network decrease, leading to real or perceived social isolation for the child with cancer and other family members. When these difficulties occur, a third level of intervention focused on impacting systems and communities, rather than individuals, may be needed. Education of teachers and classmates about childhood cancer may facilitate the flexibility needed to attend school and receive treatment (Katz, Varni, Rubenstein, Blew, & Hubert, 1992). Connecting qualified families with social service agencies that provide financial assistance or providing legal assistance related to federal or state education or employment rights may also improve a family's capacity to cope with and carry out the steps needed to effectively treat the child with cancer.

## After Treatment

At the time of diagnosis, finishing treatment successfully represents the end goal. As most children are now successfully treated for cancer, we have increasingly recognized that completing treatment is only a component of the cancer experience. As more children survive disease and treatment, the long-term biopsychosocial and developmental consequences are being identified. Cardiomyopathy, growth failure, sterility, and risk of having a second cancer represent a few of the potential long-term complications for childhood cancer survivors (Landier et al., 2004; National Cancer Policy Board, 2003). Although these are primarily physical complications, they may each have an impact on health-related quality of life, the ability to perform daily tasks, the ability to have and raise a family, and the ability to plan for a future without uncertainty (Hudson et al., 2003). Neurocognitive late effects are common in children treated for tumors of the CNS or acute leukemia, and these may include not only difficulties in school, but also problems with social relationships and long-term educational and vocational opportunities (Armstrong & Briery, 2004; Armstrong & Mulhern, 1999).

Even though studies of cancer survivors suggest that the majority experience few psychosocial or emotional adjustment problems, specific concerns related to cancer late effects have been identified (Armstrong, in press; Glover et al., 2003; L. Ross et al., 2003; Zebrack et al., 2004). The interaction among biologic, psychological, and social factors associated with cancer survivorship is magnified by developmental issues. For instance, cardiomyopathy may be seen as something that interferes with the school-aged child's ability to participate in physical education or organized sports, but this same cardiomyopathy may be seen as a barrier to meaningful employment for that same survivor when that child is an adult. The risk for a second malignancy is a distant concern for the adolescent who engages in tobacco use but may take on an immediate and compelling meaning for the young adult who is a new parent.

Family members are also cancer survivors. While it is well known that many parents and siblings experience distress during the period of active cancer treatment (Goldbeck, 2001; Levi et al., 2000), some continue to have symptoms of posttraumatic distress after treatment is finished (Alderfer, Labay, & Kazak, 2003), even when things go well. Parents of children with significant late effects of treatment may continue to experience feelings of loneliness and isolation (Van Dongen-Melman et al., 1995) for many years after treatment is completed. Adjustment difficulties may be magnified if the child with cancer dies of the disease, there is significant long-term treatment toxicity, or there are additional consequences of treatment.

## Putting the Biopsychosocial-Developmental Model to Work in Childhood Cancer

When we take a broad view of the childhood cancer experience, there are numerous opportunities for us to improve acute care, address long-term survivorship concerns, and prepare for the biopsychosocial-developmental challenges that will emerge in the future. Many improvements are occurring on the biologic and medical side of care. New medications are in development that alleviate the noxious symptoms of cancer treatment, and noninvasive techniques for assessing tumor growth and response to treatment are replacing the previous procedures that were associated with significant pain and distress.

Similar advances are needed for the psychosocial-developmental side of the biopsychosocial model for childhood cancer. Interventions for late neurocognitive effects of cancer involving the CNS are beginning to address the needs of survivors (Butler, 1998; S. J. Thompson et al., 2001), but we need to apply our biopsychosocial-developmental model of cognitive late effects to the development of strategies to prevent these difficulties in the next generation of survivors. This may involve changes in the way that these cancers are treated or providing aggressive early intervention to offset the developmental process that results from CNS treatment. Likewise, interventions that address the lingering psychological and social difficulties experienced by some survivors are needed, but we should at the same time be looking at things that can be done during the acute treatment phase to lessen or prevent some of these long-term psychosocial consequences.

We can anticipate changes in childhood cancer in the coming decade that may make many of today's biopsychosocial concerns historical relics, while new concerns never previously considered begin to emerge. Improved genetic diagnosis may lead to better decisions about how to treat a tumor optimally while minimizing toxicity in complications. Advances in fields like pharmacogenomics may lead to the development of targeted therapies that have minimal side effects and produce minimal disruption in everyday life. At the same time, the use of genetic information may produce new concerns about privacy, access to health insurance, and psychological consequences of knowing about risk before events occur (Patenaude, 2003). Many of the issues that are crucial to the care of the child with cancer today may be historical relics for the children diagnosed tomorrow. It is conceivable that things like invasive procedures, hair loss, nausea and vomiting, and CNS late learning effects will disappear from the list of major concerns for children with cancer, but new and perhaps more difficult challenges may emerge. However, it is very likely that a biopsychosocial-developmental approach to these new challenges will be as applicable tomorrow as it has been in the past.

## Sickle Cell Disease

*Sickle cell disease* is a general term used to describe a group of hemoglobinopathies involving the sickle beta globin gene, including the most frequent sickle hemoglobin variants: HbSS (sickle cell anemia), HbSC, (SC disease), and HbS$\beta$+ that or HbS$\beta^{\circ}$ that (sickle beta thalassemias). It was first described in 1910 (Herrick, 1910). Today, approximately 72,000 individuals in the United States have some form of SCD, with approximately 1 in 500 black children born in the United States diagnosed by newborn screening. This prevalence occurs largely because of a concentration of descendents of victims of slave trade from the 1700 and 1800s. In addition to the United States and Africa, SCD is found in populations in India, the Middle East, the Caribbean, and South and Central America, largely because carriers of the sickle gene are resistant to malaria (Armstrong, 2003; National Institutes of Health, 2002; Serjeant, 1985).

When sickle hemoglobin is stressed, it converts to a rigid, sickle-shaped cell that obstructs or occludes tiny blood vessels, both mechanically and through increased vascular adhesion. This occlusion may occur in any organ of the body, resulting in restricted blood flow, poor nutrition and oxygenation of healthy tissues, and eventually may lead to permanent tissue damage. This process is responsible for the many debilitating symptoms of SCD, including stroke, pain, acute chest syndrome, dactylitis, splenic sequestration, retinal injury, leg ulceration, chronic anemia, gall bladder problems, kidney damage, elevated risk of infection, growth delay, priapism, and avascular necrosis, although this is not an exhaustive list.

Some of these symptoms occur throughout the lifespan (e.g., pain), while others appear to occur more frequently during specific age periods (Armstrong, 2003; National Institutes of Health, 2002). For instance, pain is a lifetime problem for most individuals with SCD, but dactylitis is primarily seen in children younger than 4 years of age (Gill et al., 1995). Likewise, infarctive stroke occurs most frequently in children; hemorrhagic stroke is primarily seen in adults (Ohene-Frempong et al., 1998). Some of these symptoms may occur in single episodes, others may be recurrent or chronic, and still others may lead to progressive organ damage and disability (Miller et al., 2000; National Institutes of Health, 2002). For instance, a stroke is usually a single event unless untreated, but the consequences of the stroke (e.g., motor and cognitive impairment) may emerge over time and affect many areas of the child's life, well into adulthood (Armstrong et al., 1996; Boni, Brown, Davis, Hsu, & Hopkins, 2001; Bonner, Hardy, Ezell, & Ware, 2004).

Even though SCD is one of the most common genetic disorders in the United States, until the 1980s relatively little was known about its natural history and the range and severity of the symptoms experienced by individuals. At that time, a large, multicenter study of a newborn cohort of children with SCD was initiated to describe the natural history of the disease from birth through 18 years (Gaston & Rosse, 1982). The many reports from the Cooperative Study of Sickle Cell Disease stimulated a parallel interest in developing new treatments for the disease in the symptoms. Very few changes in the treatment and management of SCD had occurred before the mid-1980s. Since that time, clinical trials have demonstrated (a) the benefits of prophylactic use of penicillin for children identified by statewide newborn screening (Gaston et al., 1986); (b) the benefits of chronic transfusion therapy for prevention of second stroke (Roach, 2000); (c) the benefits of using transcranial Doppler ultrasonography to screen for children at risk for stroke and subsequently initiate chronic transfusion therapy (Adams, 2000); (d) the curative possibilities associated with bone marrow and peripheral stem cell transplantation (Hagar & Vichinsky, 2000; Walters et al., 2000); and (e) the benefits of hydroxyurea as a treatment for pain (Kinney et al., 1999) and possibly stroke prevention (Ware, Zimmerman, & Schultz, 1999).

The biopsychosocial-developmental approach was evident as these advances in medical care of children with SCD occurred. The Cooperative Study of Sickle Cell Disease emphasized the connection between biological events (e.g., stroke) and neurocognitive function, family functioning, and psychological adjustment (R. J. Thompson Jr., et al., 1999, 2003). Biopsychosocial approaches to pain assessment and management were emphasized (Gil et al., 2003; Graumlich et al., 2001), and the biopsychosocial aspects of many symptoms of SCD were examined, including pica (Lemanek et al., 2002) and enuresis (Barakat et al., 2001). Recommendations for treatment of pain often included use of comfort measures and specific relaxation skills as integral parts of a comprehensive pain treatment that included narcotic medications (Benjamin et al., 1999).

Evaluations of new treatments such as bone marrow and peripheral stem cell transplantation and hydroxyurea were planned around outcomes of previous studies of neurodevelopmental outcome as part of the natural history of SCD (Wang, Grover, Gallagher, Espeland, & Fandal, 1993; Armstrong et al., 1996), and these included an assessment of psychosocial and neurocognitive outcomes as end points (Walters et al., 2000). As new therapies have emerged, these have been compared with existing behavioral interventions to determine incremental effectiveness (Cummins & Anie, 2003) or have used psychosocial-developmental end points as primary natural history or clinical trail outcomes (Gil et al., 2003). Acknowledgment that the illness occurred within a complex cultural, ethnic, social, emotional, developmental, family, and community context led consideration of these factors as common components of nearly every study of either the natural history or the treatment of SCD (Berlew, Telfair, Colangelo, & Wright, 2000; Christian & Barbarin, 2001).

More is known about SCD, its range of symptoms, and its natural history than at any previous time. Perhaps more than with any other childhood disease, the quest for knowledge about the biological, developmental, behavioral, emotional, and social aspects of the disease has been concurrent and cohesive. Advances in medical approaches to symptoms have largely been driven by concerns about the impact that these symptoms had on a child's ability to attend school, be successful in a career, function socially, and live without pain. Changes in symptoms have been evaluated in the context of changes in the impact this has on quality of life and normal development. The biopsychosocial-developmental approach to SCD has been *the* model for research and clinical practice for two decades.

The next decades offer many more opportunities for a cohesive biopsychosocial-developmental approach to offer benefits for children with SCD. Despite the improvements in care over the past decade, children are still admitted to hospitals in pain and continue to be labeled as malingerers because of these admissions (Armstrong, Pegelow, Gonzalez, & Martinez, 1992). Despite our knowledge of the many mechanisms that can impair brain development, the transfer of this knowledge to schools where effective educational strategies can be implemented occurs infrequently. Despite the many advances in early identification of risk factors for stroke, acute chest syndrome, and life-threatening infections, children still die or become permanently disabled because of these events (Platt et al., 1994). By applying the biopsychosocial-developmental model to some of the complex problems of SCD, some of these may be corrected in the years ahead.

## Biopsychosocial-Developmental Model for the Next Decade

The complexity of SCD during childhood, adolescence, and adulthood is represented in figure 2-2. Many of the factors in this model are similar to those seen in the model presented for childhood cancer (figure 2-1), with several notable exceptions.

First, SCD is a genetic disorder, and it is possible to screen for the disease in the general population (Carreiro-Lewandowski, 2002) and to provide prenatal screening and testing for interested families (Vines, 1994). This provides an opportunity for early identification and intervention in all areas of a biopsychosocial-developmental model. Early identification allows prophylactic treatment of potential infections that have historically been associated with high mortality. Although this has resulted in a measurable decrease in mortality (Quinn, Rogers, & Buchanan, 2004), adherence with ongoing medical regimens requires comprehensive support and intervention (Teach, Lillis, & Grossi, 1998). The medical treatment will not prevent life-threatening infections if the social and behavioral system is not concurrently addressed.

Second, SCD is a chronic illness with recurrent symptoms that may cumulatively worsen. In some cases, an assessment of risk is based on developmental, biological, and functional factors, as in the case of stroke and neurocognitive impairment. We know that there are early signs of developmental delay in young children (Thompson, Gustafson, Bonner, & Ware, 2002), that most strokes occur before age 5 years (Ohene-Frempong et al., 1998), and that stroke risk can be identified by

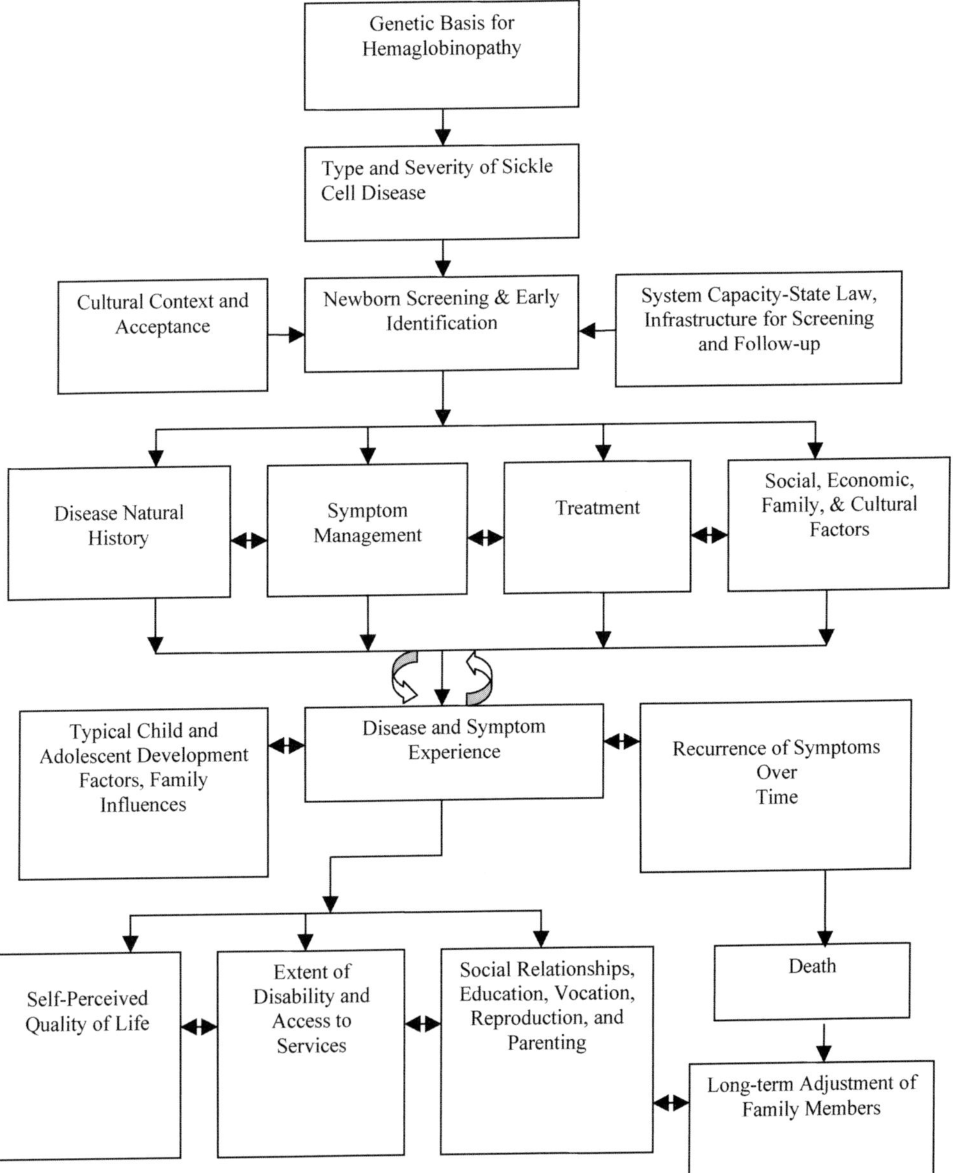


**Figure 2-2.** The biopsychosocial-developmental model of sickle cell disease.

noninvasive transcranial Doppler ultrasonography and prevented by early treatment with chronic transfusion therapy (Adams, 2000). However, we also know that children who have either a silent or a clinical stroke will have difficulties in school (Armstrong et al., 1996; Schatz, Brown, Pascual, Hsu, & DeBaun, 2001), but even those with no evidence of cerebral injury will likely have a decline in neurocognitive abilities over time (Wang et al., 2001). Known but unpredictable risk, capacity to identify at-risk children, availability of intervention, and outcome that affects school and social functioning are the biopsychosocial and developmental factors that have to be considered in an integrated and comprehensive fashion if this morbidity of SCD is to be fully addressed.

Third, many of the symptoms of SCD occur in a very public and cultural context, and the way these symptoms are viewed and treated may be affected by the cultural context. One such context is ethnic and racial. SCD occurs predominantly in individuals of African heritage in the United States, and issues ranging from access to care to acceptance and trust may determine at least a part of any child's experience with the disease (Christian & Barbarin, 2001). A second context is pain. Pain is the symptom that most often defines this disease in the community setting, and it is the symptom that is most difficult to manage and treat. It can also be a major source of social isolation and disruption of normal development for many children, particularly if failure to cope with pain in a way that others deem appropriate is viewed as a character flaw. Fortunately, education about pain is changing perspectives for many medical personnel (Armstrong et al., 1992; Benjamin et al., 1999), and children and adolescents are being aided by interventions that help them to directly affect their own pain experience (Gil et al., 2003; Powers, Mitchell, Graumlich, Byars, & Kalinyak, 2002).

The model in figure 2-2 is complex but interconnected. SCD is a biopsychosocial-developmental disease, and the solutions to its many challenges will require a transdisciplinary perspective. The synergy that can emerge from this approach will link emerging genetic research to the many psychological, social, emotional, and spiritual strengths found in the children, their families, and their communities. We will face the challenges of this disease for many years. Even if a genetic cure for the disease is identified today, we have a generation of individuals who have already experienced symptoms, injury to organs, or the social and psychological consequences of the disease. As we move toward a cure for SCD, our efforts must continue to find ways to lessen the problems and promote the abilities of those who must continue to live with the already-experienced consequences of this disease.

## Conclusions

At the time Engel (1980) proposed the biopsychosocial model of illness, the concept of integrating the biologic, psychologic, and social components of a medical illness was rather novel. Many in the fields of psychology, pediatrics, social work, nursing, and education were daunted by the many barriers that would have to be overcome to make this model work. Nearly 25 years later, the model, at least in pediatric hematology/oncology, is no longer novel but instead represents the accepted and standard approach to care of children with cancer, SCD, and other illnesses. It also drives the research in this area.

The challenge today is no longer one of needing to include a behavioral or social assessment or treatment as part of health care. Instead, we face the challenge of finding ways to use the collaborative and integrative models to (a) prevent problems we now know will occur, (b) provide treatment for existing problems that is clinically meaningful in that it relieves the symptom and has a positive effect on quality of life, and (c) anticipate and prepare for the new challenges that advancing science and clinical care will provide in the very near future. From this perspective, the biopsychosocial-developmental model shifts from one that focuses on problem solving to one that focuses on problem prevention. Collaborations in pediatric hematology and oncology provide the ideal mechanism for the future of this model.

*Acknowledgments.* This chapter was prepared with the support of the Maternal and Child Health Bureau (Leadership Education in Neurodevelopmental Disabilities Program-T73MC00013-10), the National Institute of Child and Human Development (HD-07510-04), Children's Medical Services of Florida (Contract COQ3), the Administration for Developmental Disabilities (University Center for Excellence in Developmental Disabilities Education, Research, and Service-90DD0408), and a grant from the Health Foundation of South Florida. I also acknowledge the contributions of Stuart R. Toledano, M.D., and my late colleague, Charles H. Pegelow, M.D. These two colleagues made the biopsychosocial-developmental model come to life in the care of their patients.

## References

Adams, R. J. (2000). Lessons from the Stroke Prevention Trial in Sickle Cell Anemia (STOP) study. *Journal of Child Neurology*, *15*, 344–349.

Alderfer, M. A., Labay, L. E., & Kazak, A. E. (2003). Brief report: Does posttraumatic stress apply to siblings of childhood cancer survivors? *Journal of Pediatric Psychology*, *28*, 281–286.

American Academy of Pediatrics, Committee on Psychosocial Aspects of Child and American Pain

Society, Task Force on Pain in Infants, Children, and Adolescents. (2001). The assessment and management of acute pain in infants, children, and adolescents. *Pediatrics, 108*, 793–797.

American Cancer Society. (2003). *Cancer facts and figures 2003*. Atlanta, GA: American Cancer Society.

Arceci, R. J., & Cripte, T. P. (2002). Emerging cancer-targeted therapies. *Pediatric Clinics of North America, 49*, 1339–1368.

Armstrong, F. D. (2003). Sickle cell disease. In T. H. Ollendick & C. S. Schroeder (Eds.), *Encyclopedia of clinical child and pediatric psychology* (pp. 611–614). New York: Kluwer Academic/ Plenum.

Armstrong, F. D. (in press). Emerging trends in psychological aspects of childhood cancer. *Journal of Developmental and Behavioral Pediatrics*.

Armstrong, F. D., & Briery, B. G. (2004). Childhood cancer and the school. In R. T. Brown (Ed.), *Handbook of pediatric psychology in school settings* (pp. 263–281). New York: Erlbaum.

Armstrong, F. D., & Mulhern, R. K. (1999). Acute lymphoblastic leukemia and brain tumors. In R. T. Brown (Ed.), *Cognitive aspects of chronic illness in children* (pp. 47–77). New York: Guilford Press.

Armstrong, F. D., Pegelow, C. H., Gonzalez, J. C., & Martinez, A. (1992). Impact of children's sickle cell history on nurse and physician ratings of pain and medication decisions. *Journal of Pediatric Psychology, 17*, 651–664.

Armstrong, F. D., & Reaman, G. H., (2005). Psychological research in childhood cancer: The Children's Oncology Group perspective. *Journal of Pediatric Psychology, 30*, 89–97.

Armstrong, F. D., Thompson, R. J., Jr., Wang, W., Zimmerman, R., Pegelow, C. H., Miller, S., et al. (1996). Cognitive functioning and brain magnetic resonance imaging in children with sickle cell disease. *Pediatrics, 97*, 864–870.

Aziz, N. M. (2002). Cancer survivorship research: Challenge and opportunity. *Journal of Nutrition, 132*, 3494S–3503S.

Barakat, L. P., Smith-Whitley, K., Schulman, S., Rosenberg, D., Puri, R., & Ohene-Frempong, K. (2001). Nocturnal enuresis in pediatric sickle cell disease. *Journal of Developmental and Behavioral Pediatrics, 22*, 300–305.

Benjamin, L. J., Dampier, C. D., Jacox, A. K., Odesina, V., Phoenix, D., Shapiro, B., et al. (1999). *Guideline for the management of acute and chronic pain in sickle cell disease* (APS Clinical Practice Guidelines Series, No. 1). Glenview, IL: American Pain Society.

Berlew, K., Telfair, J., Colangelo, L., & Wright, E. C. (2000). Factors that influence adolescent adaptation to sickle cell disease. *Journal of Pediatric Psychology, 25*, 287–299.

Boni, L. C., Brown, R. T., Davis, P. C., Hsu, L., & Hopkins, K. (2001). Social information processing and magnetic resonance imaging in children with sickle cell disease. *Journal of Pediatric Psychology, 26*, 309–319.

Bonner, M. J., Hardy, K. K., Ezell, E., & Ware, R. (2004). Hematologic disorders: Sickle cell disease and hemophilia. In R. T. Brown (Ed.), *Handbook of pediatric psychology in school settings* (pp. 241–261). Mahwah, NJ: Erlbaum.

Brown, R. T. (2004). Introduction: Changes in the provision of health care to children and adolescents. In R. T. Brown (Ed.), *Handbook of pediatric psychology in school settings* (pp. 1–19). Mahwah, NJ: Erlbaum.

Brown, R. T., Freeman, W. S., Brown, R. A., Belar, C., Hersh, L., Hornyak, L. M., et al. (2002). The role of psychology in health care delivery. *Professional Psychology: Research and Practice, 33*, 536–545.

Butler, R. W. (1998). Attentional processes and their remediation in childhood cancer. *Medical and Pediatric Oncology., Suppl. 1*, 75–78.

Carreiro-Lewandowski, E. (2002). Newborn screening: An overview. *Clinical Laboratory Science, 15*, 229–238.

Christian, M. D., & Barbarin, O. A. (2001). Cultural resources and psychological adjustment of African American children: Spirituality and racial attribution. *Journal of Black Psychology, 27*, 43–63.

Cohn, R. J., Goodenough, B., Foreman, T., & Suneson, J. (2003). Hidden financial costs in the treatment for childhood cancer: An Australian study of lifestyle implications for families absorbing out-of-pocket expenses. *Journal of Pediatric Hematology/Oncology, 25*, 854–863.

Cummins, O., & Anie, K. A. (2003). A comparison of the outcome of cognitive behaviour therapy and hydroxyurea. *Psychology, Health, and Medicine, 8*, 199–204.

Duffner, P. K., Horowitz, M. E., Krischer, J. P., Friedman, H. S., Burger, P. C., Cohen, M. E., et al. (1993). Postoperative chemotherapy and delayed radiation in children less than 3 years of age with malignant brain tumors. *New England Journal of Medicine, 328*, 1724–1731.

Engel, G. L. (1980). The clinical application of the biopsychosocial model. *American Journal of Psychiatry, 137*, 535–544.

Gaston M. H., & Rosse, W. F. (1982). The cooperative study of sickle cell disease: A review of study design and objectives. *American Journal of Pediatric Hematology/Oncology, 4*, 197–201.

Gaston, M. H., Verter, J. I., Woods, G., Pegelow, C. H., Kelleher, J., Presbury, G., et al. (1986). Prophylaxis with oral penicillin in children with sickle cell anemia: A randomized trial. *New England Journal of Medicine, 314*, 1593–1599.

Gil, K. M, Carson, J. W., Porter, L. S., Ready, J., Valrie, C., Lallinger, R., et al. (2003). Daily stress and mood and their association with pain, health-care use, and activity in adolescents with sickle cell disease. *Journal of Pediatric Psychology*, 28, 363–373.

Gill, F. M, Sleeper, L. A., Weiner, S. J., Brown, A. K., Bellevue, R., Grover, R., et al. (1995). Clinical events in the first decade in a cohort of infants with sickle cell disease: Cooperative Study of Sickle Cell Disease. *Blood, 86*, 776–783.

Glover, D. A., Byrne, J., Mills, J. L., Robison, L. L., Nicholson, H. S., Meadows, A. T., et al. for the Children's Cancer Group. (2003). Impact of CNS treatment on mood in adult survivors of childhood leukemia: A report form the Children's Cancer Group. *Journal of Clinical Oncology*, *21*, 4395–4401.

Goldbeck, L. (2001). Parental coping with the diagnosis of childhood cancer: Gender effects, dissimilarity within couples, and quality of life. *Psycho-oncology*, *10*, 325–335.

Graumlich, S. E., Powers, S. W., Byars, K. C., Schwarber, L. A., Mitchell, M. J., & Kalinyak, K. A. (2001). Multidimensional assessment of pain in pediatric sickle cell disease. *Journal of Pediatric Psychology*, *26*, 203–214.

Guralnick, M. J. (2000). Interdisciplinary team assessment for young children: Purposes and processes. In M. J. Guralnick (Ed.), *Interdisciplinary clinical assessment of young children with developmental disbilities* (pp. 3–15). Baltimore: Brookes.

Hagar, R. W., & Vichinsky, E. P. (2000). Major changes in sickle cell disease. *Advances in Pediatrics*, *47*, 249–272.

Herrick, J. B. (1910). Peculiar elongated and sickle-shaped red blood corpuscles in a case of severe anemia. *Archives of Internal Medicine*, 6, 517–521.

Himmelstain, D. U., & Woolhandler, S. (1995). Care denied: U.S. residents who are unable to obtain needed medical services. *American Journal of Public Health*, *85*, 341–344.

Hinkle, A. S., Proukou, C., French, C. A., Kozlowski, A. M., Constine, L. S., Lipsitz, S. R., et al. (2004). A clinic-based, comprehensive care model for studying late effects in long-term survivors of pediatric illnesses. *Pediatrics*, *113*, 1141–1145.

Hudson, M. M, Mertens, A. C., Yasui, Y., Hobbie, W., Chen, H., Gurney, J. G., et al. for the Childhood Cancer Survivor Study Investigators. (2003). Health status of adult long-term survivors of childhood cancer: A report from the Childhood Cancer Survivor Study. *Journal of the American Medical Association*, *290*, 583–592.

Jankovic, M., Spinetta, J. U. J., Martins, A. G., Pession, A., Sullivan, M., D'Angio, G., et al. for the SIOP Working Committee on Psychosocial Issues in Pediatric Oncology. (2004). Non-conventional therapies in childhood cancer: Guidelines for distinguishing non-harmful from harmful therapies: A report of the SIOP Working Committee on Psychosocial Issues in Pediatric Oncology. *Pediatric Blood and Cancer*, *42*, 106–108.

Katz, E. R., Varni, J. W., Rubenstein, C. L., Blew, A., & Hubert, N. (1992). Teacher, parent, and child evaluative ratings of a school reintegration intervention for children with newly diagnosed cancer. *Children's Health Care, 21*, 69–75.

Kazak, A. E., & Barakat, L. P. (1997). Brief report: Parenting stress and quality of life during treatment for childhood leukemia predicts child and parent adjustment after treatment ends. *Journal of Pediatric Psychology*, 22, 749–58.

Kinney, T. R., Helms, R. W., O'Branski, E. E., Ohene-Frempong, K., Wang, W., Daescher, C., et al. (1999). Safety of hydroxyurea in children with sickle cell anemia: Results of the HUG-KIDS study, a phase I/II trial. *Blood*, *94*, 1550–1554.

Landier, W., Bhatia, S., Eshelman, D., Forte, K., Sweeney, T., Hester, A., et al., for the Children's Oncology Group Late Effects Committee and Nursing Discipline. (2004). Development of risk-based guidelines for childhood cancer survivors: The Children's Oncology Group Long-Term Follow-Up Guidelines. *Journal of Clinical Oncology, 22*, 4979–90.

Lemanek, K. L, Brown, R. T., Armstrong, F. D., Hood, C., Pegelow, C. H., & Woods, G. (2002). Dysfunctional eating patterns and symptoms of pica in children and adolescents with sickle cell disease. *Clinical Pediatrics*, *41*, 493–500.

Levi, R. B., Marsick, R., Drotar, D., & Kodish, E. D. (2000). Diagnosis, disclosure, and informed consent: Learning from parents of children with cancer. *Journal of Pediatric Hematology/Oncology*, 22, 3–12.

Liu, L., Krailo, M., Reaman, G. H., & Bernstein, L. (2003). Childhood cancer patients' access to cooperative group cancer programs: a population-based study. *Cancer, 97*, 1339–1345.

Ljungman, G., McGrath, P., Cooper, E., Widger, K., Ceccolini, J., Fernancez, C. V., et al. (2003). Psychosocial needs of families with a child with cancer. *Journal of Pediatric Hematology/Oncology, 25*, 223–231.

Miller, S. T., Sleeper, L. A., Pegelow, C. H., Enos, L. E., Wang, W. C., Weiner, S. J., et al. (2000). Prediction of adverse outcomes in children with sickle cell disease. *New England Journal of Medicine, 342*, 83–89.

National Cancer Institute. (2005). PDQ cancer information summaries: Pediatric treatment. Retrieved December 7, 2005, from http://www.cancer.gov/cancertopics/pdq/pediatrictreatment.

National Cancer Institute SEER Program. (1999). *Cancer incidence and survival among children and adolescents: United States SEER Program 1975–1995* (L. A. Ries, M. A. Smith, J. G. Gurney, M. Linet, Y. Tamra, et al., Eds.) (NIH Publication No. 99-4649). Bethesda, MD: National Institutes of Health.

National Cancer Policy Board. (2003). *Childhood cancer survivorship: Improving care and quality of life* (M. Hewitt, S. L. Wiener, & J. V. Simone, Eds.). Washington, DC: National Academies Press.

National Institutes of Health. (2002). *The management of sickle cell disease* (4th ed) (NIH Publication No. 02-2117). Bethesda, MD: National Institutes of Health.

Ohene-Frempong, K., Weiner, S. J., Sleeper, L. A., Miller, S. T., Embury, S., Moohr, J. W., et al. (1998). Cerebrovascular accidents in sickle cell disease: Rates and risk factors. *Blood, 91*, 288–294.

Patenaude, A. F. (2003). Pediatric psychology training and genetics: What will 21st century pediatric psychologists need to know? *Journal of Pediatric Psychology, 28*, 135–145.

Platt, O., Branbilla, D. J., Rosse, W. F., Milner, P. F., Castro, O., Steinberg, M. H., et al. (1994). Mortality in sickle cell disease: Life expectancy and risk factors for early death. *New England Journal of Medicine, 330*, 1639–1644.

Powers, S. W., Mitchell, M. J., Graumlich, S. E., Byars, K. C., & Kalinyak, K. (2002). Longitudinal assessment of pain, coping, and daily functioning in children with sickle cell disease receiving pain management skills training. *Journal of Clinical Psychology in Medical Settings, 9*, 109–119.

Powers, S. W., Vannatta, K., Noll, R. B., Cool, V. A., & Stehbens, J. A. (1995). Leukemia and other childhood cancers. In M. C. Roberts (Ed.), *Handbook of pediatric psychology* (2nd ed., pp. 30–326). New York: Guilford Press.

Quinn, C. T., Rogers, Z. R., & Buchanan, G. R. (2004). Survival of children with sickle cell disease. *Blood, 103*, 4023–4027.

Ries, L. A. G., Eisner, M. P., Kosary, C. L., Hankey, B. F., Miller, B. A., Clegg, L., et al. (Eds.). (2004). *SEER cancer statistics review, 1975–2001*. Bethesda, MD: National Cancer Institute. Bethesda, MD. Retrieved from http://seer.cancer.gov/csr/1975_2001/.

Roach, E. S. (2000). Stroke in children. *Current Treatment Options in Neurology, 2*, 295–304.

Ross, L., Johansen, C., Dalton, S. O., Mellemkjaer, L., Thomassen, L. H., Mortensen, P. B., et al. (2003). Psychiatric hospitalizations among survivors of cancer in childhood or adolescence. *New England Journal of Medicine, 349*, 650–657.

Ross, M. E., Zhou, X., Song, G., Shurtleff, S. A., Girtman, K., Williams, W. K., et al. (2003). Classification of pediatric acute lymphoblastic leukemia by gene expression profiling. *Blood, 102*, 2951–2959.

Ruccione, K. S., Waskerwitz, M., Buckley, J., Perin, G., & Hammond, G. D. (1994). What caused my child's cancer? Parents' responses to an epidemiology study of childhood cancer. *Journal of Pediatric Oncology Nursing, 11*, 71–84.

Sahler, O. J., Varni, J. W., Fairclough, D. L., Butler, R. W., Noll, R. B., Dolgin, M. J., et al. (2002). Problem-solving skills training for mothers of children with newly diagnosed cancer: A randomized trial. *Journal of Developmental and Behavioral Pediatrics, 23*, 77–86.

Santacroce, S. (2002). Uncertainty, anxiety, and symptoms of posttraumatic stress in parents of children recently diagnosed with cancer. *Journal of Pediatric Oncology Nursing, 19*, 104–111.

Schatz, J., Brown, R. T., Pascual, J. M., Hsu, L., & DeBaun, M. R. (2001). Poor school and cognitive functioning with silent cerebral infarcts and sickle cell disease. *Neurology, 56*, 1109–1111.

Serjeant, G. R. (1985). *Sickle cell disease*. Oxford, U.K.: Oxford University Press.

Spinetta, J. J. (1974). The dying child's awareness of death: A review. *Psychological Bulletin, 81*, 256–260.

Stehbens, J. A. (1988). Childhood cancer. In D. K. Routh (Ed.), *Handbook of pediatric psychology* (pp. 135–161). New York: Guilford Press.

Streisand, R., Rodrigue, J. R., Houck, C., Graham-Pole, J., & Berlant, N. (2000). Parents of children undergoing bone marrow transplantation: Documenting stress and implementing a psychological intervention program. *Journal of Pediatric Psychology, 25*, 331–337.

Teach, S. J., Lillis, K. A., & Grossi, M. (1998). Compliance with penicillin prophylaxis in patients with sickle cell disease. *Archives of Pediatric and Adolescent Medicine, 152*, 274–278.

Thompson, R. J., Jr., Armstrong, F. D., Kronenberger, W. G., Scott, D., McCabe, M. A., Smith, B., et al.

(1999). Family functioning, neurocognitive functioning, and behavior problems in children with sickle cell disease. *Journal of Pediatric Psychology*, *24*, 491–498.

Thompson, R. J., Jr., Armstrong, F. D., Link, C. L., Pegelow, C. H., Moser, F., & Wang, W. (2003). A prospective study of the relationship over time of behavior problems, intellectual functioning, and family functioning in children with sickle cell disease: A report from the Cooperative Study of Sickle Cell Disease. *Journal of Pediatric Psychology*, *28*, 59–65.

Thompson, R. J., Jr., Gustafson, K. E., Bonner, M. J., & Ware, R. (2002). Neurocognitive development of young children with sickle cell disease through 36 months of age. *Journal of Pediatrics Psychology*, *27*, 245–244.

Thompson, S. J., Leigh, L., Christensen, R., Xiong, X., Kun, L. E., Heideman, R. L., et al. (2001). Immediate neurocognitive effects of methylphenidate on learning-impaired survivors of childhood cancer. *Journal of Clinical Oncology*, *19*, 1802–1808.

Tyc, V. L., Mulhern, R. K., Barclay, D. R., Smith, B. F., & Bieberich, A. A. (1997). Variables associated with anticipatory nausea and vomiting in pediatric cancer patients receiving ondansetron antiemetic therapy. *Journal of Pediatric Psychology*, 22, 45–58.

Van Dongen-Melman, J. E., Pruyn, J. F., De Groot, A., Koot, H. M., Hahlen, K., & Verhulst, F. C. (1995). Late psychosocial consequences for parents of children who survived cancer. *Journal of Pediatric Psychology*, *20*, 567–586.

Vannatta, K., & Gerhardt, C. A. (2003). Pediatric oncology: Psychosocial outcomes for children and families. In M. C. Roberts (Ed.), *Handbook of pediatric psychology* (3rd ed., pp. 342–357). New York: Guilford Press.

Varni, J. W., Blount, R. L., Waldron, S. A., & Smith, A. J. (1995). Management of pain and distress. In M. C. Roberts (Ed.), *Handbook of pediatric psychology* (2nd ed., pp. 105–123). New York: Guilford Press.

Vines, G. (1994). Gene tests: The parents' dilemma. *New Science*, *144*, 40–44.

Walters, M. C., Storb, R., Patience, M., Leisenring, W., Taylor, T., Sanders, J. E., et al. (2000). Impact of bone marrow transplantation for symptomatic sickle cell disease: An interim report. *Blood*, *95*, 1918–1924.

Wang, W., Enos, L., Gallagher, D., Thompson, R. J., Jr., Guarini, L., Vichinsky, E., et al. (2001). Neuropsychologic performance in school-aged children with sickle cell disease: A report from the Cooperative Study of Sickle Cell Disease. *Journal of Pediatrics*, *139*, 391–397.

Wang, W. C., Grover, R., Gallagher, D., Espeland, M., & Fandal, A. (1993). Developmental screening in young children with sickle cell disease: Results of a cooperative study. *American Journal of Pediatric Hematology Oncology*, *15*, 87–91.

Ware, R. E., Zimmerman, S. A., & Schultz, W. H. (1999). Hydroxyurea as an alternative to blood transfusions for the prevention of recurrent stroke in children with sickle cell disease. *Journal of Pediatric Hematology/Oncology*, *22*, 335–339.

Zebrack, B. J., Gurney, J. G., Oeffinger, K., Whitton, J., Packer, R. J., Mertens, A., et al. (2004). Psychological outcomes in long-term survivors of childhood brain cancer: A report from the Childhood Cancer Survivor Study. *Journal of Clinical Oncology*, *15*, 999–1006.

II

# The Cancer Experience "On Treatment"

Mary Jo Kupst and Kristin Bingen

# Stress and Coping in the Pediatric Cancer Experience

The diagnosis of pediatric cancer is one of the most stressful situations a child and family must face. It presents an overwhelming series of stressors, not the least of which is the possibility of the child's death. Although the survival rate for childhood cancer has improved significantly (from nearly always fatal in the 1950s and 1960s to nearly 75% survival at present), the treatments remain lengthy and intensive, involving fundamental changes in the child and family's lives. The chapters that follow in this book present a thorough discussion of the various psychological issues in pediatric hematology/oncology. This chapter begins with an overview of what is meant by coping and then focuses on three main questions: (a) What is the impact of pediatric cancer? That is, with what must children and families cope? (b) How do they cope? And, finally, (c) how is coping related to positive adaptation? We also discuss the theoretical and methodological issues involved in studying coping and adaptation. As there is a subsequent chapter related to families in this volume, we focus primarily on the child, adolescent, and young adult with cancer.

## The Impact of Pediatric Cancer: A Longitudinal Framework

Coping is a process that must always be considered in a situational context because it may vary across situations and over time (Compas, Worsham, & Ey, 1992; Fields & Prinz, 1997). It follows that taking a longitudinal approach toward understanding the stressors and demands placed on a child and family as they progress through the experience of cancer is essential. Despite this clinical knowledge and seemingly universal acknowledgment of the process nature of coping, most studies have assessed coping with pediatric cancer at a single point or phase (Compas et al., 1992), and it has often been necessary to extrapolate assumptions about the process by combining results from separate studies.

We present a picture of the coping tasks that children and their families face from diagnosis through and beyond treatment. In general, the descriptions of the "natural history" of adaptation (Natterson & Knudson, 1960) from early studies (Binger et al., 1969; Chodoff, Friedman, & Hamburg, 1964; Futterman & Hoffman, 1973) remain useful, although the type and duration of treatment as well as prognostic factors may have changed. It is still useful to view general coping tasks throughout the cancer experience as (a) developing a cognitive understanding of the disease and treatment demands; (b) managing emotional reactions to the disease, treatment, and their implications; and (c) seeking and using available resources to meet specific situational tasks (Koocher & O'Malley, 1981; Kupst & Schulman, 1988; Spinetta, 1977).

## Diagnosis and Early Treatment

Most of what we have learned about how children and families cope and adapt has come from research conducted in the early stages of pediatric cancer. When children are initially diagnosed with cancer, families almost universally describe feeling shocked and overwhelmed. Family members must absorb a great deal of information and make treatment decisions at a time when they are emotionally distressed (Kupst, Patenaude, Walco, & Sterling, 2003; Ruccione, Kramer, Moore, & Perin, 1991). In addition to finding out that there is a serious illness, the family must deal with thoughts of the potential death of the child. A question often raised, or at least thought about, by children and adolescents who have been informed that they have cancer is, "Am I going to die?" Often, the only familiarity that children may have with cancer is related to an older or elderly relative who previously died from cancer. Children and their caregivers often struggle with the unanswerable "wh" questions, such as "Why me (or my child)?" or "What caused me (or my child) to have cancer?" Parents or children may search for a cause, sometimes blaming themselves or others (Eiser, Havermans, & Eiser, 1995).

One of the earliest tasks for families is to achieve an intellectual understanding of the diagnosis and treatment regimen. Learning the complexities of cancer treatment protocols (the majority of children are placed on clinical trial protocols), potential adverse side effects of therapies, and medical procedures as well as interpreting results of laboratory tests ("counts") can be initially daunting. Families, particularly parents, become knowledgeable about the disease, prognosis, and what treatment will involve. They typically know less about the research involved in the clinical trials in which their children are treated (Kupst et al., 2003; Levi, Marsick, Drotar, & Kodish, 2000). However, most children and their families typically learn the necessary practical tasks related to hospital and clinic routines.

Another early task is to deal with painful or uncomfortable procedures, such as needle sticks, bone marrow aspirations (BMAs) and lumbar punctures (Peterson, Harbeck, Chaney, Farmer & Thomas, 1990). Similarly, children and families must face physical symptoms that arise as adverse side effects of treatment, such as nausea, vomiting, fatigue, and weight loss or gain. Adjustment to medical procedures and side effects of cancer treatment has significantly improved over the years with advancements in medical technology and pharmacology. Procedural distress has been reduced with surgical placement of central venous lines and portacatheters, which have decreased the frequency of needle pokes for laboratory draws or medication infusions. The introduction of the topical analgesic ointment EMLA (eutectic mixture of local anesthesia) has substantially improved the ability of children to cope with the pain of injections. Conscious sedation medications such as Versed and improvements in the use of analgesic medications for children make lumbar punctures and BMAs more tolerable for most children and adolescents. The introduction of antiemetic medications, such as Zofran, has dramatically improved coping with the adverse side effects of chemotherapy. Despite the use of these medical advancements, some children and adolescents continue to exhibit procedural distress and chronic nausea and pain. The efficacy of cognitive behavioral strategies, such as distraction techniques and relaxation, has been well documented in reducing procedural distress and managing chronic nausea and pain (Zeltzer, 1994).

Weekly and more frequent clinic visits and hospitalizations necessitate profound changes in the child and family's lives. Contrary to the developmental importance of friendships and social activities, children and adolescents frequently have to be isolated from their peers because of compromised immune systems. In addition, most pediatric cancer patients miss a substantial amount of school because of their treatment regimen or treatment-related side effects and substitute school with homebound tutoring. In addition, some children, particularly adolescents and young adults, describe altered relationships with friends while receiving cancer treatment and beyond the treatment phase.

Some friendships remain the same, some grow stronger, while others fade away. Keeping up with academics and maintaining friendships are particularly challenging tasks for children treated for cancer.

Similarly, families have to make substantial life changes and sacrifices to care for a child with cancer. Financial considerations often emerge, such as insurance, loss of a parent's income (because of the need to care for the child full time), transportation, and sometimes change of residence. There is increased strain on the caregiver who typically must accompany the child to the hospital and do home care as well and on the caregiver who must work to keep insurance and pay the bills. Because of increasing demands in terms of both the child's care and other responsibilities, an important but difficult task is to maintain communication and closeness within the family.

In addition, seeking and using available social supports is necessary, but not always easy. Many children and families receive much needed support from relatives, friends, members of their religious community, and their larger community for the first month or so after diagnosis. For some families, this burst of social response, although helpful, can be at times overwhelming. Children and their caregivers may have difficulty accepting outside help or struggle with letting others know more specifically what they do or do not need. Some caregivers are burdened by having to provide frequent updates about their sick child to a multitude of caring friends and families; others find this to be a positive diversion from stress.

## Middle-to-Later Treatment

As treatment proceeds, children and their caregivers may experience an increased sense of control over their lives when they are better able to understand the treatment regimen and generally know what to expect from therapies. However, they may also begin to process and work through a natural range of thoughts and feelings related to having cancer (Kupst, Tylke, et al., 1982). Many pediatric cancer patients grieve the loss of a "normal" life or the life that they once knew. In addition, they express sadness and anger over physical limitations or not being able to participate in activities as they had before being diagnosed with cancer. For many children and families, the overabundance of assistance and support from others begins to naturally dwindle several months after diagnosis. This may leave some children and caregivers with feelings of abandonment. The goal would be to learn to live with cancer, to try to maximize the things that one can do rather than focus on what they cannot. This involves school, peers, family, and planning for the future. Depending on their level of physical, cognitive, and psychosocial functioning, children will vary in their ability to do this. During lengthy treatment, caregivers may have less time available to spend in enjoyable activities with their adult friends, which reduces opportunities to relax or rejuvenate while still experiencing chronic stresses. Relationships with friends also may change similar to those experienced by their children with cancer.

We have learned more about sibling reactions to childhood cancer (Sahler et al., 1992, 1997). Some siblings harbor feelings of being forgotten or "passed off" on other relatives because their parents have less time or are less available to them. Some may exhibit somatic symptoms, school problems, increased social withdrawal, or acting out behaviors.

## Ending Treatment and Survival

As treatment ends, the task becomes living beyond cancer, which is often a time of ambivalence: positive feelings that treatment is over, but concern over the loss of the support of the hospital and medical team and uncertainty over the future (Kupst et al., 1982). Children and families face another transition after cancer treatment. The focus is on rebuilding versus returning to their previous lives because their perspectives have changed as a result of their cancer experiences. Children have to adjust to full-time school, whereas caregivers may have to return to part- or full-time employment. This may be a difficult transition for primary caregivers whose sole focus has been in caring for their ill child. Children do not always expect physical and emotional recovery to take as much time as it often does, which may be a source of frustration. There also is the "Damocles sword" (Koocher & O'Malley, 1981) of possible relapse or recurrence of cancer.

There has been increased awareness of the long-term stresses faced by childhood cancer survivors (Hewitt, Weiner, & Simone, 2003; Zebrack et al., 2004; Zebrack & Zeltzer, 2003), with 1 of every 900 young adults a childhood cancer survivor (Robison, 2003). Some survivors have to cope with cognitive late effects of treatment, including learning, attention, memory, and visual-motor problems (Armstrong & Mulhern, 2000; see Mulhern & Butler, chapter 14, this volume, on neuropsychological late effects), particularly brain tumor survivors and those who received chemotherapy or cranial radiation at a young age. Many pediatric cancer survivors also must cope with chronic physical complications of cancer treatment, including organ dysfunction, growth delay or deficiency, infertility, or recurrence or second malignancies. Survivors also must be more cognizant of health choices because of their medical history.

Finally, because of the increased survival rate, it is tempting to end here on an optimistic note, but children still relapse and have recurrences, and some still die. The tasks involve a shifting toward decisions about new treatment, decreasing survival rates, decreasing functioning, and moving toward acceptance and use of palliative care.

## The Impact of Pediatric Cancer: Developmental Issues

Within a temporal framework, one must consider the range of experiences and reactions that vary depending on the developmental level of the child. Coping and adaptation, including cognitive appraisal of stressful experiences, emotional-behavioral responses, and coping strategies become more differentiated and complex with cognitive-developmental maturity (Altshuler & Ruble, 1989; Compas et al., 1992; Curry & Russ, 1985; Fields & Prinz, 1997; Thies & Walsh, 1999). The transactional model (Lazarus & Folkman, 1984) posits that coping and adaptation depend on the person, the situation, and the environment in which the stressor occurs. The impact of cancer of course will be different depending on the developmental level of the person. Overlooking the importance of development in pediatric coping and adaptation may lead to faulty clinical assumptions and ineffective interventions. For example, we now know that providing a chronically ill child developmentally appropriate diagnostic and treatment information improves coping and adaptation, whereas in the past it was assumed that children should be protected from distressing medical information that likely was beyond their cognitive level of understanding (Slavin, O'Malley, Koocher, & Foster, 1982).

Unfortunately, there are few empirical studies that have examined developmental changes or perspectives in pediatric coping with chronic illness, with most focusing on responses to common medical procedures (for review, see Fields & Prinz, 1997). There are even fewer studies that exist within the context of the pediatric cancer experience despite the need for more developmental focus, particularly in pediatric cancer survivors (Eiser, Hill, & Vance, 2000; Kazak, 1992). In general, the majority of childhood cancer studies have examined stress and coping responses in a cohort of children and adolescents with a wide age range at a single time point, which fails to allow for an investigation of developmental differences in the impact of pediatric cancer over time. Much of what we know about the developmental differences in stress and coping with pediatric cancer comes from clinical experiences, observations, and extrapolation of data from normative studies of childhood coping and adaptation.

### Infancy, Toddler, and Preschool Years

Infants, toddlers, and preschoolers have to adjust to the stress of uncomfortable, painful, and frightening medical procedures during a developmental period when they may not be able to understand cognitively what is happening to them. Toddlers and preschoolers may struggle with loss of control over what happens to their bodies during a time when they are developing greater autonomy (Ritchie, Caty, & Ellerton, 1984). Fears of abandonment and separation from their primary caregivers and home environment when they have to stay in an unfamiliar hospital setting may occur during the initial adjustment period (Baum & Baum, 1989). Temporary regression or interruption in early developmental milestones (e.g., feeding, toilet training) is not uncommon. Being attached to an intravenous pole on a regular basis also may initially hamper exploration of their environment by toddlers and preschoolers. Particularly during the preschool years and beyond, some children may exhibit more behavioral reactions to the stress of cancer treatment, as evidenced by an increase in aggression or temper tantrums (Baum & Baum, 1989). Some parents feel guilty or struggle with setting limits on their ill child's misbehaviors.

Despite these stressors, at this developmental stage, hospitalizations, clinic routines, certain medical procedures, and being attached to intravenous lines and poles become "normal" over time for most children as this is their only normal experience. It has been suggested that problem-focused coping (action-oriented coping strategies) develops during the preschool years (Bull & Drotar, 1991; Compas et al., 1992). In a literature review of childhood coping with common medical procedures, Fields and Prinz (1997) described a greater dependence on behavioral distraction or avoidance during the preschool years compared to cognitive distraction or strategies used by older children.

### School-Aged Years

School-aged children may experience similar reactions as their younger cohorts as they adapt to diagnosis and treatment. Additional stressors in school-aged children include disruptions in the ability to attend school and participate in peer activities, which are essential to their cognitive and social development. Along with cognitive maturity comes the understanding of the seriousness of their medical condition. In addition, school-aged children are more aware of physical changes because of treatment-related side effects, such as hair loss, which may for some children lead to self-consciousness or feeling different from their peers (Baum & Baum, 1989).

Loss of control continues to be a significant challenge. Band and Weisz (1990) found that school-aged children who rated themselves as having greater perceived control over their diabetes were more likely to display positive adjustment. Emotion-focused coping (management of emotional reactions and cognitive appraisal of stressors) appears to emerge around late childhood and early adolescence and continues to evolve with cognitive-developmental maturity (Compas et al., 1992; Compas, Malcarne, & Fondacaro, 1988; Fields & Prinz, 1997). Similarly, results of a qualitative study of age-related differences in childhood coping with cancer found that children under age 9 years were more likely to use behavioral coping strategies, children aged 9–14 years reported using both behavioral and cognitive strategies, and adolescents 14 years and older reported using more cognitive coping strategies (Claflin & Barbarin, 1991).

### Adolescence and Young Adulthood

Adolescents also must adjust to disruptions in school and social activities during a stage of development that revolves heavily around peer interactions. The developmental importance of social support was highlighted by Nichols (1995), who found a positive association between social support and positive coping in a group of 20 adolescent cancer patients. Similarly, in a qualitative investigation of coping with cancer in 14 adolescents and young adults (aged 16–22 years), Kyngas et al. (2001) found that the majority used social support and information-seeking as their primary coping strategies. In addition, optimism about recovery and returning to a normal life were important to these adolescents and young adults (Kyngas et al., 2001).

In general, adolescents are more likely to use emotion-focused approaches that rely on cognitive strategies such as self-talk and diversion (Claflin & Barbarin, 1991; Fields & Prinz, 1997). Adolescents and young adults often express difficulties identifying with friends, who are able to be more "carefree." Furthermore, adolescent cancer patients are more vulnerable to self-image problems because of changes in physical appearance (i.e., hair loss, weight gain or loss) while they are attempting to adapt to pubertal changes (Baum & Baum, 1989).

Adolescents may display more intense emotional reactions, denial, and existential issues as they attempt to cope with cancer stressors. Thies and Walsh (1999) found that chronically ill adolescents between the ages of 14 and 16 years reported more feelings of frustration about a stressful experience related to their illness compared to two younger groups of children/preadolescents (8- to 9- and 11- to 12-year-olds).

A cancer diagnosis also promotes more dependency on caregivers, which is at odds with the developmental goal of increasing autonomy. This dependence-independence struggle sometimes leads to friction in the parent-adolescent/young adult relationship. Young adults not only may experience similar reactions to adolescents but also may have to postpone or interrupt college, work, marriage, and starting their own family to undergo treatment.

### Parents

It is important to mention the impact of pediatric cancer on parents or caregivers, which is covered more thoroughly in chapter 4 on familial issues. The impact on parents is often more intense and distressing (Coletti, 1997; for review, see Grootenhuis & Last, 1997; Kazak & Barakat, 1997) as they watch their child experience an invasive treatment process. In addition, parents are intellectually and emotionally aware of the implications of their child's cancer diagnosis and treatment and must make life-and-death treatment decisions for the child. Fears and worries about their child's acute and long-term survival are commonly experienced by caregivers. Focusing on parental stress and adaptation to their child's diagnosis and treatment is crucial because of its strong association with child adjustment (Carlson-Green, Morris, & Krawiecki, 1995; Frank, 1996; Grootenhuis & Last, 1997; Kronenberger et al., 1996; Kupst, Natta, et al., 1995; Kupst & Schulman, 1988; Noll, et al., 2000; Sawyer, Streiner, Antoniou, Toogood, & Rice, 1998; Trask et al., 2003).

## Coping and Psychological Outcome

Despite all of the stresses related to pediatric cancer and its treatment, most studies of psychological outcome have found that children with cancer and their families are not significantly different from norms, controls, or comparison groups in terms of adjustment or adaptation, and that psychopathology is relatively rare (Elkin, Phipps, Mulhern, & Fairlough, 1997; Kupst, et al., 1995; Last & Grootenhuis, 1998; Noll, Maclean, Whitt, Kaleita, Stehbens, Ruymann, et al., 1997; Sawyer, Antoniou, Toogood, Rice, & Baghurst, 2000; Sorgen & Manne, 2002; Zebrack, et al., 2002; for reviews, see Eiser et al., 2000; Kupst, 1994; Patenaude & Kupst, 2005. However, a consistent finding is that about one fourth to one third of children and adolescents and their families exhibit significant problems adjusting to the disease, treatment, and related issues. Studies of posttraumatic stress symptomatology reveal similar rates of problems (Kazak et al., 2001; Meeske, Ruccione, Globe, & Stuber, 2001), although some (Erickson & Steiner, 2001) have found higher levels of distress. The questions then become, What makes a difference? Why do some people adapt in a positive way and others have significant problems? In an attempt to address these questions, numerous studies have been conducted to determine the variables that are associated with adjustment and adaptation to the cancer experience.

### Disease-Related Factors

Adjustment has been found to be related to intensity of treatment (Zebrack & Zeltzer, 2003); severity of late effects and functional impairment in long-term survivors (Elkin et al., 1997; Fritz, Williams, & Amylon, 1988; Greenberg, Kazak, & Meadows, 1989; Koocher & O'Malley, 1981); visibility of disease or treatment effect (Koocher & O'Malley, 1981); duration of disease or time since diagnosis (Carlson-Green et al., 1995; Cella & Tross, 1986; Koocher & O'Malley, 1981; Kupst & Schulman, 1988); and degree of central nervous system involvement (Armstrong & Mulhern, 2000).

### Personal Factors

Age has been found to be related to adjustment, but in various directions. Some investigators (Barakat et al., 1997; Elkin et al., 1997; Fritz et al., 1988; Koocher & O'Malley, 1981) have found younger age at diagnosis to be positively associated with adjustment; others have found a positive relationship with older age (Cella et al., 1987; Mulhern, Wasserman, Friedman, & Fairclough, 1989). Zeltzer et al. (1997), in their review of research, noted female gender as a risk factor in adaptation to long-term survival; however, there is little research that has examined gender during treatment, with the exception of differential responses to invasive procedures. Cognitive and academic functioning in long-term survivors have been found to be related to adjustment (Boman & Bodegard, 2000; Kupst et al., 1995; Levin Newby, Brown, Pawletko, Gold, & Whitt, 2000). Psychological functioning prior to diagnosis has been a strong predictor of later functioning (Carpenter, 1992; Hubert, Jay, Saltoun, & Hays, 1988; Katz, Kellerman, & Siegel, 1980; Kupst et al., 1995; Kupst & Schulman, 1988). Although most researchers and theorists (Last & Grootenhuis, 1998; Parle, Jones, & Maguire, 1996) stress the importance of the individual's perception and appraisal of the stressors, there have been few studies that examined the effects of appraisal on adjustment.

## Family and Environmental Factors

Family variables found to be related to adjustment include adaptability (Chesler & Barbarin, 1987; Kazak & Meadows, 1989); cohesiveness (Kazak & Meadows, 1989; Levin Newby et al., 2000; Rait et al., 1992 Varni, Katz, Colegrove, & Dolgin, 1996); expressiveness (Varni et al., 1996); open communication (Fritz et al., 1988; Koocher & O'Malley, 1981; Kupst & Schulman, 1988; Spinetta & Deasy-Spinetta, 1981); family support (Fritz et al., 1988; Koocher & O'Malley, 1981; Kupst, Natta, et al., 1995; Morrow, Carpenter, & Hoagland, 1984; Trask et al., 2003); and family/environmental resources, including socioeconomic status (Canning, Harris, & Kelleher, 1996; Carlson-Green et al., 1995; Fritz et al., 1988; Koocher & O'Malley, 1981; Kupst et al., 1995). Adjustment of other family members (particularly maternal adjustment) is one of the strongest predictors of coping adequacy and adjustment in children and adolescents with cancer (Carlson-Green et al., 1995; Kupst & Schulman, 1988; Kupst et al., 1995; Sawyer et al., 1998; Trask et al., 2003). Similarly, maternal well-being has been a predictor of adjustment of siblings with cancer (Sahler et al., 1997). Social support also has been found to be a significant correlate of adjustment (Nichols, 1995; Trask et al., 2003), as has a low level of concurrent stress (Barakat et al., 1997; Kalnins, Churchill, & Terry, 1980; Kupst & Schulman, 1988).

## Coping Strategies

Although there have been numerous studies in pediatric psychology that describe the use of various coping strategies in children and their parents, the relationship of coping to psychological outcome has been less-well researched (Rudolph, Dennig, & Weisz, 1995; Thompson & Gustafson, 1996). In reviewing the studies that have been conducted, findings have typically yielded mixed results in terms of effective strategies in coping with cancer. Using the "outer-/inner-directed" overarching classifications, approach strategies (e.g., problem-focused, primary control, information-seeking) have been found to be effective in several outcomes. These include controllable situations (Altshuler & Ruble, 1989; Compas et al., 1988; Sorgen & Manne, 2002) and dealing with invasive procedures (Manne, Bakeman, Jacobson, & Redd, 1993; Peterson, 1989) and physical adverse side effects of treatment (Tyc, Mulhern, Jayawadene, & Fairclough, 1995). Avoidance coping (e.g., emotion focused, secondary control) was effective for uncontrollable stressors, such as diagnosis with a serious disease or undergoing painful procedures (Altshuler & Ruble, 1989; Compas et al., 1988), and for acute time-limited stressors (Suls & Fletcher, 1985), such as invasive procedures (Compas, 1987; Weisz, McCabe, & Dennig, 1994). Alternatively, avoidance coping has been found to increase depressive symptoms, anxiety, and distress in pediatric cancer patients and their families (Frank, Blount, & Brown, 1997; Hubert et al., 1988). Denial has been found to have both positive and negative functions, depending on the person and context (Beisser, 1979; Koocher & O'Malley, 1981; Lazarus, 1983; Zeltzer, 1980).

Of the inner-directed strategies, positive expectations and focus were related to emotional adjustment of long-term survivors of pediatric cancer (Grootenhuis & Last, 2001; Kupst & Schulman, 1988). Perceived control has also been found to be associated with adjustment (Worchel, Copeland, & Barker, 1987). Further, seeking and maintaining social support also has been found to be effective throughout treatment (Kupst et al., 1995; Kyngas et al., 2001; Morrow et al., 1984), although there is some disagreement about whether it belongs in problem-focused or emotion-focused categories. Perhaps it does not matter because Lazarus (2000) recommends that these classifications be viewed as interdependent dynamic processes rather than as independent polar opposites.

One source of the confusion in delineating effective coping strategies is the variation across studies in selection of situations, timing, consideration of personal and environmental factors, and definition and measurement of coping and outcomes. In general, the answer seems to be, "It depends." It depends upon the situation, personal characteristics (age/developmental level, gender), family variables, perception and appraisal as well as the definition and measurement of coping.

As several researchers have noted, effectiveness of a strategy or set of strategies depends on the controllability of the stressor as well as the type of stressor (Chesler & Barbarin, 1987; Compas et al., 1992). As we have seen, the progression from diagnosis through and after treatment involves many macro- and microstressors (Fields & Prinz, 1997).

For example, coping with painful procedures may be seen as one stressor; however, it can be divided into pre-, during, and postprocedure stressors. What may be effective before a procedure may not be as effective during or after the procedure. From a macro point of view, what may be effective during painful medical procedures may not be effective in dealing with later school and peer situations. For example, avoidant strategies may not be adaptive during cancer treatment but may be used by survivors as a way to focus on life after cancer (Bauld, Anderson, & Arnold, 1998). More research needs to be conducted to clarify coping both within and across these situations.

As noted, several studies (Compas et al., 1992; Spirito, Stark, & Knapp, 1992) have found that younger children tend to use more outer-directed or problem-focused strategies, with older children and adolescents employing more emotion-focused strategies. Similarly, Natta (1995) found that long-term survivors of acute lymphocytic leukemia demonstrated greater reliance on emotion-focused coping over time, which increased with age. Older adolescents and young adults have been found to verbalize more about coping than younger adolescents (Kameny & Bearison, 2002). Further, older children and adolescents tended to have more positive outcomes (i.e., less procedural distress) than younger children (Carpenter, 1992; Hubert et al., 1988; Jacobsen et al., 1990). As we have seen, there have been mixed findings in terms of adjustment and adaptation, and more research needs to be conducted to examine developmental factors across different stressful situations in pediatric cancer.

Females have been found to exhibit higher levels of pain and anxiety during procedures (Hilgard & LeBaron, 1984; Katz et al., 1980; Weisz et al., 1994). They also have been found to use more emotion management strategies overall (Bull & Drotar, 1991; Spirito, Stark, & Tyc, 1989) and a greater frequency of coping strategies than males (Spirito et al., 1989). The finding that females may in some cases be more at risk medically and for late effects (Hewitt, Weiner, & Simone, 2003) suggests that there should be more attention paid to gender in assessing coping and adaptation.

With regard to family variables, high parental anxiety/distress has been correlated with high child anxiety/distress behaviors, especially during invasive procedures (Jacobsen et al., 1990; Jay, Ozolins, Elliott, & Caldwell, 1983). In the longitudinal Coping Project (Kupst, Schulman, Honig, et al., 1982; Kupst, Schulman, Maurer, Honig, et al., 1983; Kupst, Schulman, Maurer, Morgan, et al., 1984; Kupst & Schulman, 1988; Kupst, Natta, et al., 1995), which followed the same children and families from diagnosis through long-term survival, the most consistently strong predictor of child adaptation was the adaptation of family members, particularly the mother's coping and adaptation. Similarly, Carlson-Green et al.'s (1995) study of children with brain tumors and their parents found that family variables were the best predictors of children's behavior problems and overall adaptive behavior. The work of Kazak and colleagues, particularly in the longitudinal studies (Best, Streisand, Cantania, & Kazak, 2002; Kazak & Barakat, 1997; Kazak, Penati, Brophy, & Himelstein, 1998), has done much to increase our understanding of the importance of the family in pediatric cancer studies (also see chapter 4, this volume). Finally, in clinical practice with children who have cancer, we know that little lasting progress can be made without involving and working with the family.

With regard to *perception and appraisal* of the situation (Eiser et al., 2000; Last & Grootenhuis, 1998), perception of a stressor as controllable should indicate a direction toward an outer-directed or active strategy, one that attempts to change the situation (e.g., information-seeking, efforts to fix or solve the problem), but if the stressor is in reality not controllable, it may not be effective (Sorgen & Manne, 2002). As Fields and Prinz (1997) noted in their developmental review of coping, children may be limited in the amount of control they actually have in these situations. Similarly, it is extremely important to try to understand the appraisal and meaning (Lazarus, 2000) of the situation to the individual; the effectiveness of a strategy or intervention will depend on the goals and values they place on it (Nezu, Nezu, Friedman, Faddis, & Houts, 1998). This is one reason why "one-size-fits-all" interventions often do not work well.

Studies of coping strategies frequently fail to take into account the number of different strategies that one may employ in a given situation. Several studies have found a wide variety of coping styles used by children and adolescents with cancer (Bull & Drotar, 1991; Fritz et al., 1988; Kupst & Schulman, 1988; Kupst et al., 1995; Kyngas et al., 2001; Landolt, Vollrath, & Ribi, 2002; Natta, 1995), but little information about which strategies were more effective in terms of outcome was found. Although some experts believe that having a wide repertoire of possible behaviors is optimal, others believe that it is the quality of the strategies rather than the quantity that is important (Phipps, Fairclough, Tyc, & Mulhern, 1998; Worchel et al., 1987), Thus, our early optimism about finding coping styles or strategies that would predict optimal adjustment was not well supported (Sloper, 2000).

Finally, it depends on how one approaches coping in terms of *definition and measurement*. The main difficulties in this area stem from different conceptualizations and methodological considerations.

## How Children and Families Cope: Conceptualization and Classification

At first glance, it would seem that all agree on what is meant by coping. When individuals cope, they "manage," "deal with," or "handle" some problem or situation. Definitions of coping go beyond simply managing to "endure," "persevere," and even "survive." When we try to define it operationally, however, the concept becomes more elusive. An examination of the vast body of coping research from 1996 to 2004 (over 6,500 studies with coping as a main focus) reveals considerable variation in the definitions of coping, both generally and specifically to pediatric cancer.

In many clinical studies, especially early descriptions of how families deal with cancer and other serious conditions, coping was viewed as a response or outcome synonymous with adaptation. It involves a value judgment of how well someone adjusts or adapts (e.g., Haan, 1977), sometimes defined as *coping adequacy* (Kupst & Schulman, 1988). While coping continues to be defined in this way (Boman & Bodegard, 2000; Mackie, Hill, Kondryn, & McNally, 2000), especially when the interest is in antecedents of coping, in most recent studies coping has been employed as a means (without ascribing a value) to an end (adaptation).

Coping has sometimes been viewed as an enduring trait (Loevinger, 1976; Vaillant, 1977) or adaptational style (Phipps & Srivastava, 1997), a way that a person typically reacts and responds to stressful situations. People can be classified into categories of repressor/sensitizer (Byrne, 1964; Canning, Canning, & Boyce, 1992), approacher/avoider (Frank et al., 1997; Hubert et al., 1988; Suls & Fletcher, 1985), and monitor/blunter (Compas, 1987; Miller, 1987a; Phipps, Fairclough, Tyc, & Mulhern, 1995). There has been considerable research examining how children and adolescents with cancer and other chronic conditions fall into these categories (see reviews by Fields & Prinz, 1997; Rudolph, Dennig, & Weisz, 1996), and it has been useful to examine the prevalence of these styles in cancer and other chronic conditions. For example, blunting style has been found to be prevalent in pediatric cancer patients (Phipps et al., 1995; Phipps & Srivastava, 1997).

However, type of coping style was not related to outcome (i.e., procedural distress; Phipps et al., 1998). In a rare longitudinal study of coping style, Phipps, Steele, Hall, and Leigh (2001) found a higher incidence of repressive style in children with cancer than in healthy children and children with other chronic diseases. Style remained stable over time. However, as in adult coping research (Lazarus, 1991; Parle, Jones, & Maguire, 1996), little has been done to determine how this trait view of coping relates to the way children and adolescents with cancer actually cope (i.e., state coping; Phipps et al., 1998).

The most commonly cited, and probably the most comprehensive, definition of coping was formulated by Lazarus, who defined coping as "cognitive and behavioral efforts to manage specific external or internal demands (and conflicts between them) that are appraised as taxing or exceeding the resources of the person" (1991, p. 112). Rather than an outcome, coping has been viewed by most recent theorists and researchers as an intervening variable, or mediator, between stress and adaptation, influenced by personal, situational, and environmental factors. Stress and coping theorists and researchers (Lazarus & Folkman, 1984; Thompson & Gustafson, 1996; Wallander & Varni, 1992) as well as those involved in childhood cancer (Chodoff et al., 1964; Futterman & Hoffman, 1973; Spinetta, 1977) have generally agreed with this conceptualization as well as with the process nature of coping. Spirito et al. (1992) also emphasized the dynamic nature of coping, so that a child (or adult) may cope differently in different situations and at different times.

The operative word in the definition of coping has come to be *efforts*. Fields and Prinz (1997) defined coping as a cognitive or behavioral strategy or set of strategies for the purpose of managing stressful situations. A great deal of work has been conducted to classify different types of cognitions and behaviors. Probably the classification that has been most researched in both adult and pediatric studies involves problem-focused versus emotion-focused coping (Lazarus & Folkman, 1984), in which problem-focused coping is action centered (e.g., seeking information, confrontation, planful problem solving) and is generally applicable when a situation is appraised as changeable. Emotion-focused coping attempts to change the way one attends to or interprets a stressor (e.g., denial, avoidance, minimization, distancing, positive reappraisal). Several researchers in the area of pediatric psychology have delineated typologies of coping that were associated with responses to medically oriented stressors (Blount, Davis, Powers, & Roberts, 1991; Compas et al., 1992; Spirito, Stark, & Williams, 1988).

The comprehensive review article by Rudolph et al. (1995) summarized the most frequently used classifications of coping. In general, the typologies can be grouped into two main categories: (a) outer-directed coping (behavioral, problem focused, primary control, approach coping) and (b) inner-directed coping (cognitive, emotion focused, secondary control, passive or avoidant coping). The choice of strategy is believed depend on the perception or appraisal of the stressor. If the stressor is one that is appraised as controllable, then outer-directed strategies are expected to be effective. If the stressor is not controllable, then the person must try to use inner-directed strategies to reduce distress and change focus.

A diagnosis of pediatric cancer is not a situation over which one has control. However, the experience of pediatric cancer involves myriad situations in which the person can control some aspects but not others. Some are time limited; others are more long-term. It has been postulated and examined (Sorgen & Manne, 2002) that psychological outcome (distress, adaptation) depends on whether there is a fit between the individual's perception of control and the person's preferred coping style (problem focused vs. emotion focused), as well as a fit between the type of stressor and preferred style. Despite the number of studies that have been conducted in this area, still more comprehensive work needs to be done to delineate further what, when, and how an individual copes with cancer.

## Methodology and Barriers

With the increase in research studies of pediatric psychooncology, we have learned much about how children and families adapt to the diagnosis and treatment of cancer (Patenaude & Last, 2001). Although there are some differences in findings across studies, we have learned about significant correlates of adjustment, and we have begun to study empirically the efficacy of interventions to improve adaptation. Despite the hundreds of studies that have been conducted on coping with pediatric cancer, however, the state of coping research in pediatric oncology (as well as in general child studies and in adult studies) remains fragmented and confusing.

### Timing and Determination of Stressors

A widespread problem is the lack of clarity regarding the when and what in coping research. Many early studies, and some studies today, have been cross-sectional descriptions of "children and families with cancer," utilizing convenience samples of children in different phases of treatment. Thus, we do not know to what it is they are responding (i.e., demands of diagnosis, early treatment, later treatment). An improvement over these cross-sectional studies has been the limitation to a single phase of treatment, especially early treatment, and, more recently, long-term survival. These studies, which constitute the majority of research in this field, have greatly increased our knowledge about the phases of the cancer experience.

However, a major problem is that the implications of these studies are often extrapolated to the entire cancer experience (Weisz et al., 1994). It is not sufficient to try to understand the entire trajectory of the pediatric cancer experience by piecing together results of separate studies with different samples conducted at different times. Unless we follow children and families from diagnosis through long-term survival, we cannot fully understand the entire experience of coping with cancer. We know that people can and do change over time in the way they deal with both the same and different stressors. However, there have been very few studies that actually have followed the same children or families over time (exceptions include the work of Best et al., 2002; Dahlquist, Czyzewski, & Jones, 1996;

Hoekstra-Weebers, Heuvel, Jaspers, Kamps, & Klipp, 1998; Kazak & Barakat, 1997; Kupst & Schulman, 1988; Kupst et al., 1995; Phipps et al., 2001; Sawyer et al., 2000; Varni et al., 1996). Of course, there are good reasons for this. Longitudinal studies are lengthy and time consuming, and it is difficult to maintain participation (of both participants and investigators) over many years. Collaboration of several institutions is often necessary to achieve an adequate sample size, but such studies are difficult to develop, fund, and conduct.

In studies of "coping with diagnosis" or "coping with long-term survival," researchers often fail to consider or delineate the many different stressors inherent in the experience of a particular phase. Even within a single time frame or phase of treatment, there are many different minisituations, so it is difficult to determine the precise stressor with which the person is struggling. Some studies have limited the scope to a single type of stressor, such as BMAs. Still others have asked the child or parent to specify the stressor (Spirito et al., 1992), which provides better clarification of the actual stressful event. Of course, it is difficult to compare coping across different stated stressors in the same phase or time span, but one can examine and compare types of stressors and degree of perceived stress. Some studies using problem-solving skills approaches (e.g., Nezu et al., 1998; Sahler et al., 2002) have utilized approaches that emphasize the individual perceptions of stresses and have presented promising results in terms of intervention effectiveness.

In examining stability and change in coping and adaptation, we must also consider that, although the diagnosis of cancer is a new stressor for most children and families, they are not starting at ground zero in terms of the coping they already do. As Somerfield and McCrae (2000) posited, many people already have a good coping repertoire, some near the "ceiling of their adaptive capacities." And, several studies have supported this notion in that they found that survivors of pediatric cancer and their families adapted better than originally expected (Elkin et al., 1997; Kupst et al., 1995; Verill, Schaefer, Vannatta, & Noll, 2000), and that their early functioning was a strong predictor of later functioning. Although we know that individuals vary greatly in their coping and adaptation, our studies often fail to consider how much people can actually change and the environmental constraints that make change difficult (Pearlin, 1991).

## Style, Strategy, and Behavior

Much attention has been devoted to the classification and measurement of coping styles. Similarly, there have been several classifications of coping strategies employed by children with chronic conditions. One problem is that the two often become confused. People complete a scale that really measures style or disposition, and the inference is that endorsement represents actual behavioral or emotional coping with a current stressor. Further measures of actual coping behavior are not frequently conducted. The measures of coping strategy, such as the Kidcope (Spirito et al., 1988) and Ways of Coping Questionnaire (Folkman & Lazarus, 1988), have been well researched and provide a description of strategies that people report using. Studies that have used these measures have provided a great deal of information about prevalence of different strategies in children, adolescents, and adults with chronic illness. However, as Lazarus (1996) pointed out years ago, coping disposition does not necessarily predict current coping behaviors. We have to differentiate between dispositional and situational approaches (Rudolph et al., 1995). We cannot really assume that the child who endorses using distraction during BMAs actually does so unless we can assess the behavior at that time. Another important source of confusion is between the use of coping strategies as intervening variables (between stress and adaptation) and as outcomes or responses (Rudolph et al., 1995).

## Measurement Issues

In addition to differing conceptualizations of coping, a major contributor to the muddy nature of coping research is the way coping is operationally defined. We have discussed style and strategy, which are typically measured by established coping scales. (We are not talking about standardized measures of other psychological states such as anxiety or depression because these are not measures of coping, although they are sometimes employed as such.) Such scales as the Children's Behavioral Style Scale (Miller, 1987b), which measures monitoring/blunting styles, the

Kidcope (Spirito et al., 1988), and the Ways of Coping Questionnaire (Folkman & Lazarus, 1988) are well-researched self-report scales.

The advantage of most of these scales is that they have been empirically derived, and several may be compared to normative data. They also are easy to administer and relatively easy to score, advantages in a clinical setting. Self-report measures also are the most practical way of obtaining coping data in large samples, such as in multisite studies. They are most useful when one is looking for a dispositional measure or as a self-report of what one has done previously or what one might do. A disadvantage of this procedure is that hundred of studies have been conducted that employ self-report checklists and scales, with a great deal of confusion and disparate findings regarding how people cope (Coyne & Racioppo, 2000). Reports about the child from significant others (e.g., caregivers, teachers) can be beneficial in examining similarities and differences between the child and family members (Elkin et al., 1997), although most studies have relied solely on the self-report of the child or adolescent.

Behavioral observation measures, such as the Observed Schedule of Behavioral Distress (Jay et al., 1983), the Child-Adult Medical Procedure Interaction Scale (Blount et al., 1991), and the Behavioral Approach-Avoidance Distress Scale (Hubert et al., 1988) have been well developed and have the advantage of providing descriptions of actual behavior during a stressful situation, such as a painful procedure. Much of our knowledge of how children behave before, during, and after such procedures has come from these studies, and their findings have pointed the way for effective interventions to reduce procedural distress.

Such measures are useful and go beyond the dispositional type of research cited above. However, such investigations are sometimes difficult to conduct, requiring much training of research staff, and require precise timing and coding (however, there are short forms that reduce this burden) (Blount, Bunke, Cohen, & Forbes, 2001). Although it has been relatively easy to conduct such studies in settings such as medical procedures, it is less easy to conduct systematic observation of children and families in other clinic and hospital situations. In addition, the findings of these studies are difficult to interpret in terms of coping, and few studies have made connections between observed behavior categories and coping (an exception is the work of Blount et al., 2001, who found associations between coping-promoting behaviors and child coping with procedural distress).

For pediatric cancer, for which we do not have as much information as for procedural distress, the use of qualitative questionnaires and interviews that are more open ended (e.g., Atkins & Patenaude, 1987; Kupst et al., 1995; Parle et al., 1996; Sorgen & Manne, 2002; Woodgate, 2000) is recommended. We must more fully understand the phenomena surrounding these situations before turning too quickly to standardized measures, which may not capture the important aspects of the situation. This is particularly true in situations that are emerging regarding new technology or areas of oncology research, such as genetic testing (Patenaude, Basilli, Fairclough, & Li, 1996).

The work of Haase, Heine, Ruccione, and Stutzer (1999) is a noteworthy example of proceeding from careful qualitative assessment of a phenomenon (e.g., resilience in pediatric cancer) through hypothesis generation, testing, and further conceptualization and research. The emergence of improved qualitative research methodology should not be ignored, especially when we do not fully understand the impact, appraisal, and reaction to stressful situations. It is clear that multiple methods and sources (e.g., in-depth qualitative interviews, behavioral observations, rating scales, and daily diaries) are the beginning of a comprehensive understanding of coping and adaptation, but thus far there has been little research of this type (Levin Newby, Brown, Pawletko, Gold, & Whitt, 2000).

Finally, depending on the research question, choice of outcomes is crucial and not always as easy as it might seem (Somerfield & McCrae, 2000). In many studies, researchers have typically chosen a global outcome measure such as adjustment (often defined as presence or absence of behavior problems, as in the child behavior checklist (Achenbach, 2003). However, there may be other, more relevant outcomes, such as resilience (Haase et al., 1999), that provide information on functioning outside the hospital, such as peer relationships (Noll, Bukowski, Davies, Koontz, & Kulkarni, 1997; Vannatta, Gartstein, Short, & Noll, 1998), school functioning (Katz et al., 1992), or significant other/marital relationships (Boman & Bodegard, 2000; Byrne et al., 1989). Sometimes, one outcome may even be at odds with another outcome, as when one may develop more open communication and feel more in control, but the changes produce conflicts in relationships. Although we have typically focused on reducing distress and behavioral problems, there has been less focus on positive outcomes, such as development of meaning, which can indeed coexist with negative affect (Folkman & Moskowitz, 2000).

## Challenges for Future Research

Although the barriers and difficulties mentioned here may be construed as pessimistic regarding the future of coping research, such documented barriers should really be viewed as a challenge to the next generation of researchers. Coping remains a key area in understanding adaptation to pediatric cancer, one that, if we are careful and clear, can be observed and measured, and one that is intensively linked to developing effective interventions. The bottom line is that, to truly understand coping, especially coping strategies, it is necessary to be clear about the time frame, the specific stressor, and the research question and whether coping is an antecedent, a mediator, or a consequence and how it will be assessed.

Despite the fragmentation in research studies to date, these hundreds of studies have moved the field ahead, although sometimes in a mazelike way. We need to know more about how children and families cope over time, especially in situations such as ending treatment, relapse and recurrence, during palliative care, and in long-term survival. We have to be better able to determine what are effective coping strategies both short and long term. In addition, we have to be able to determine stability and change of coping through the cancer experience. Through these findings, we will be better able to refine our interventions to help children with cancer and families in the future.

## References


Achenbach, T. M. (2003). *Manual for the Assessment Data Manager Program*. Burlington, VT: University Medical Education Associates.

Armstrong, F. D., & Mulhern, R. K. (2000). Acute lymphoblastic leukemia and brain tumors. In R. T. Brown (Ed.), *Cognitive aspects of chronic illness in children* (pp. 47–77). New York: Guilford.

Altshuler, J. L., & Ruble, D. N. (1989). Developmental changes in children's awareness of strategies for coping with uncontrollable stress. *Child Development, 60*, 1137–1149.

Atkins, D. M., & Patenaude, A. F. (1987). Psychosocial preparation and follow-up for pediatric bone marrow transplant patients. *American Journal of Orthopsychiatry, 57*, 246–252.

Band, E. B., & Weisz, J. R. (1990). Developmental differences in primary and secondary control coping and adjustment to juvenile diabetes. *Journal of Clinical Child Psychology, 19*, 150–158.

Barakat, L., Kazak, A., Meadows, A. T., Casey, R., Meeske, K., & Stuber, M. (1997). Families surviving childhood cancer: A comparison of post-traumatic stress symptoms with families of healthy children. *Journal of Pediatric Psychology, 22*, 843–859.

Bauld, C., Anderson, V., & Arnold, J. (1998). Psychosocial aspects of adolescent cancer survival. *Journal of Pediatrics and Child Health, 34*, 120–126.

Baum, B. J., & Baum, E. S. (1989). Psychosocial challenges of childhood cancer. *Journal of Psychosocial Oncology, 7*, 119–129.

Beisser, A. R. (1979). Denial and affirmation in illness and health. *American Journal of Psychiatry, 136*, 1026–1030.

Best, M., Streisand, R., Catania, L., & Kazak, A. (2002). Parental distress during pediatric leukemia and parental posttraumatic stress symptoms after treatment ends. *Journal of Pediatric Psychology, 26*, 299–307.

Binger, C. M., Ablin, A. R., Feuerstein, R. C., Kushner, J. H., Zoger, S., & Mikkelsen, C. (1969). Childhood leukemia: Emotional impact on patient and family. *New England Journal of Medicine, 280*, 414–418.

Blount, R. L., Bunke, V., Cohen, L. L., and Forbes, C. J. (2001). The Child-Adult Medical Procedure Interaction Scale-Short Form (CAMPIS-SF): Validation of a rating scale for children's and adults' behaviors during painful procedures. *Journal of Pain and Symptom Management, 22*, 591–599.

Blount, R .L., Davis, N., Powers, S. W., & Roberts, M. C. (1991). The influence of environmental factors and coping style on children's coping and distress. *Clinical Psychology Review, 11*, 93–116.

Boman, K., & Bodegard, G. (2000). Long-term coping in childhood cancer survivors: influence of illness, treatment, and demographic background factors. *Acta Paediatrica, 89*, 105–111.

Bull, B. A., & Drotar, D. (1991). Coping with cancer in remission: Stressors and strategies reported by children and adolescents. *Journal of Pediatric Psychology, 16*, 767–782.

Byrne, D. (1964). Repression-sensitization as a dimension of personality. In B. A. Maher (Ed.),

*Progress in experimental personality research* (pp. 169–220). New York: Academic Press.

Byrne, J., Fears, T. R., Steinhorn, S. C., Mulvihill, J. J., Connelly, R. R., Austin, D. F., et al. (1989). Marriage and divorce after childhood and adolescent cancer. *Journal of the American Medical Association, 262*, 2693–2699.

Canning, E. H., Canning, R. D., & Boyce, W. T. (1992). Depressive symptoms and adaptive style in children with cancer. *Journal of the American Academy of Child and Adolescent Psychiatry, 31*, 1120–1124.

Canning, R. D., Harris, E. S., & Kelleher, K. J. (1996). Factors predicting distress among caregivers to children with chronic medical conditions. *Journal of Pediatric Psychology, 21*, 735–749.

Carlson-Green, B., Morris, R. D., & Krawiecki, N. (1995). Family and illness predictors of outcome in pediatric brain tumors. *Journal of Pediatric Psychology, 20*, 769–784.

Carpenter, P. (1992). Perceived control as a predictor of distress in children undergoing invasive medical procedures. *Journal of Pediatric Psychology, 17*, 757–773.

Cella, D. F., Tan, C., Sullivan, M., Weinstock, L., Alter, R., & Jow, D. (1987). Identifying survivors of pediatric Hodgkin's disease who need psychological interventions. *Journal of Psychosocial Oncology, 5*, 83–96.

Cella, D. F., & Tross, S. (1986). Psychological adjustment to survival from Hodgkin's disease. *Journal of Consulting and Clinical Psychology, 54*, 616–622.

Chesler, M. A., & Barbarin, O. A. (1987). *Childhood cancer and the family*. New York: Brunner/Mazel.

Chodoff, R., Friedman, S. B., & Hamburg, D. A. (1964). Stress, defenses, and coping behavior: Observations in parents of children with malignant disease. *American Journal of Psychiatry, 120*, 743–749.

Claflin, C. J., & Barbarin, O. A. (1991). Does "telling" less protect more? Relationships among age, information disclosure, and what children with cancer see and feel. *Journal of Pediatric Psychology, 16*, 169–191.

Coletti, D. J. (1997). Stressful medical procedures in the context of cancer: Patterns of parent and child coping strategies and psychological adaptation. *Dissertation Abstracts International, 58*, 1523.

Compas, B. E. (1987). Coping with stress during childhood and adolescence. *Psychological Bulletin, 101*, 393–403.

Compas, B. E., Malcarne, V. L., & Fondacaro, K. M. (1988). Coping with stressful events in older children and adolescents. *Journal of Consulting and Clinical Psychology, 56*, 405–411.

Compas, B. E., Wordsham, N. L., & Ey, S. (1992). Conceptual and developmental issues in children's coping with stress. In A. LaGreca, L. J. Siegel, J. L. Wallander, & C. E. Walker (Eds.), *Stress and coping in child health* (pp. 7–24). New York: Guilford.

Coyne, J. C., & Racioppo, M. W. (2000). Never the twain shall meet? Closing the gap between coping research and clinical intervention research. *American Psychologist, 55*, 655–664.

Curry, S .L., & Russ, S. W. (1985). Identifying coping strategies in children. *Journal of Clinical Child Psychology, 14*, 61–69.

Dahlquist, L. M., Czyzewski, D. I., & Jones, C. L. (1996). Parents of children with cancer: A longitudinal study of emotional distress, coping style, and marital adjustment 2 and 20 months after diagnosis. *Journal of Pediatric Psychology, 21*, 541–554.

Eiser, C., Havermans, T., & Eiser, J. R. (1995). Parents' attributions about childhood cancer: Implications for relationships with medical staff. *Child Care Health and Development, 21*, 31–42.

Eiser, C., Hill J. J., & Vance, Y. H. (2000). Examining the psychological consequences of surviving childhood cancer: Systematic review as a research method in pediatric psychology. *Journal of Pediatric Psychology, 25*, 449–460.

Elkin, T. D., Phipps, S., Mulhern, R. K., & Fairclough, D. (1997). Psychological functioning of adolescent and young adult survivors of pediatric malignancy. *Medical and Pediatric Oncology, 29*, 582–588.

Erickson, S. J., & Steiner, H. (2001). Trauma and personality correlates in long-term pediatric cancer survivors. *Child Psychiatry and Human Development, 31*, 195–213.

Fields, L., & Prinz, R. J. (1997). Coping and adjustment during childhood and adolescence. *Clinical Psychology Review, 17*, 937–976.

Folkman, S., & Lazarus, R. S. (1988). *Manual for the Ways of Coping Questionnaire*. Palo Alto, CA: Consulting Psychologists Press.

Folkman, S., & Moskowitz, J. T. (2000). Positive affect and the other side of coping. *American Psychologist, 55*, 626–636.

Frank, N. C. (1996). Patterns of coping, attributions and adjustment in pediatric oncology patients. *Dissertation Abstracts International, 56*, 4580.

Frank, N. C., Blount, R. L., & Brown, R. T. (1997). Attributions, coping, and adjustment in children with cancer. *Journal of Pediatric Psychology, 22*, 563–576.

Fritz, G. K., Williams, J. R., & Amylon, M. (1988). After treatment ends: Psychosocial sequelae in pediatric cancer survivors. *American Journal of Orthopsychiatry, 58*, 552–561.

Futterman, E. H., & Hoffman, I. (1973). Crisis and adaptation in families of fatally ill children. In E. G. Anthony and C. Kupernik (Eds.), *The child in his family: The impact of disease and death* (Vol. 2, pp. 127–142). New York: Wiley.

Greenberg, H., Kazak, A., & Meadows, A. (1989). Psychological adjustment in 8–16 year old cancer survivors. *Journal of Pediatrics, 114*, 488–493.

Grootenhuis, M. A., & Last, B. F. (1997). Adjustment and coping by parents of children with cancer: A review of the literature. *Supportive Care Cancer*, 5, 466–484.

Grootenhuis, M. A., & Last, B. F. (2001). Children with cancer with different survival perspectives: defensiveness, control strategies, and psychological adjustment. *Psycho-Oncology*, *10*, 305–314.

Haan, N. (1977). *Coping and defending: Processes of self-environment organization*. New York: Academic Press.

Haase, J. E., Heine, S. P., Ruccione, K. S., & Stutzer, C. (1999). Research triangulation to derive meaning-based quality of life theory: Adolescent resilience model and instrument development. *International Journal of Cancer*, *22*, 125–131.

Institute of Medicine and National Research Council. (2003). *Childhood cancer survivorship: Improving care and quality of life* (M. Hewitt, S. L. Weiner, & J. V. Simone, Eds.). Washington, DC: National Academies Press.

Hilgard, J. R., & LeBaron, S. (1984). *Hypnotherapy of pain in children with cancer*. Los Altos, CA: Kaufman.

Hinds, P. S. (2000). Fostering coping by adolescents with newly diagnosed cancer. *Seminars in Oncology Nursing*, 16, 317–327.

Hoekstra-Weebers, J., Heuvel, F., Jaspers, J., Kamps, W., & Klip, E. (1998). Brief report: An intervention program for parents of pediatric cancer patients. A randomized clinical trial. *Journal of Pediatric Psychology, 23*, 207–214.

Hubert, N. C., Jay, S. M., Saltoun, M., & Hays, M. (1988). Approach-avoidance and distress in children undergoing preparation for painful medical procedures. *Journal of Clinical Child Psychology, 17*, 194–202.

Jacobsen, P. B., Manne, S. L., Gorfinke, K., Schorr, O., Rapkn, R., & Redd, W. H. (1990). Analysis of child and parent behavior during painful medical procedures. *Health Psychology, 9*, 559–576.

Jay, S. M., Ozolins, M., Elliott, C. H., & Caldwell, S. (1983). Assessment of children's distress during painful medical procedures. *Health Psychology, 2*, 139–149.

Kalnins, I. V., Churchill, M. P., & Terry, G. E. (1980). Concurrent stress in families with a leukemic child. *Journal of Pediatric Psychology*, *5*, 81–92.

Kameny, R. R., & Bearison, D. J. (2002). Cancer narratives of adolescents and young adults: A quantitative and qualitative analysis. *Children's Health Care, 31*, 143–173.

Katz, E. R., Kellerman, J., & Siegel, S. E. (1980). Behavioral distress in children with cancer undergoing medical procedures: Developmental considerations. *Journal of Consulting and Clinical Psychology, 48*, 356–365.

Katz, E. R., Varni, J. W., Rubenstein, C. L., Blew, A., et al. 1992 (1992). Teacher, parent and child evaluative ratings of a school reintegration intervention for children with newly diagnosed cancer. *Children's Health Care, 21*, 69–75.

Kazak, A., & Barakat, L. (1997). Parenting stress and quality of life during treatment for childhood leukemia predicts child and parent adjustment after treatment ends. *Journal of Pediatric Psychology,* 22, 749–758.

Kazak, A., Barakat, L., Alderfer, M., Rourke, M., Meeske, K., Gallagher, P., et al. (2001). Posttraumatic stress in survivors of childhood cancer and mothers. *Journal of Clinical Psychology in Medical Settings*, *8*, 307–323.

Kazak, A., Penati, B., Brophy, P., & Himelstein, B. (1998). Pharmacologic and psychologic interventions for procedural pain. *Pediatrics, 102*, 59–66.

Kazak, A. E. (1992). The social context of coping with childhood chronic illness: Family systems and social support. In A. LaGreca, L. Siegel, J. Wallander, & C. E. Walker (Eds.), *Stress and coping in child health* (pp. 262–278). New York: Guilford Press.

Kazak, A. E., & Meadows, A. T. (1989). Families of young adolescents who have survived cancer: Social-emotional adjustment, adaptability, and social support. *Journal of Pediatric Psychology, 14*, 175–192.

Koocher, G. P., & O'Malley, J. E. (Eds.) (1981). *The Damocles syndrome: psychological consequences of surviving childhood cancer*. New York: McGraw-Hill.

Kronenberger, W. G., Carter, B. D., Stewart, J., Morrow, C., Martin, K., Gowan, D., et al. (1996). Psychological adjustment of children in the pretransplant phase of bone marrow transplantation: Relationships with parent distress, parent stress, and child coping. *Journal of Clinical Psychology in Medical Settings, 3*, 319–335.

Kupst, M. J. (1994). Coping with pediatric cancer: Theoretical and research perspectives. In D. Bearison and R. K. Mulhern (Eds.), *Pediatric psycho-oncology* (pp. 35–59). New York: Oxford University Press.

Kupst, M. J., Natta, M. B., Richardson, C. C., Schulman, J. L., Lavigne, J. V., & Das, L. (1995). Family coping with pediatric leukemia: 10 years after treatment. *Journal of Pediatric Psychology, 20*, 601–617.

Kupst, M. J., Patenaude, A. F., Walco, G. A., & Sterling, C. (2003). Clinical trials in pediatric cancer: Parental perspectives on informed consent. *Journal of Pediatric Hematology/Oncology, 25*, 787–790.

Kupst, M. J., & Schulman, J. L. (1988). Long-term coping with pediatric leukemia: A 6 year follow-up study. *Journal of Pediatric Psychology, 13*, 7–22.

Kupst, M. J., Schulman, J. L., Honig, G., Maurer, H., Morgan, E., & Fochtman, D. (1982). Family coping with childhood leukemia: 1 year after diagnosis. *Journal of Pediatric Psychology, 7*, 157–174.

Kupst, M. J., Schulman, J. L. Maurer, H., Honig, G., Morgan, E., & Fochtman, D. (1983). Family coping with childhood leukemia: The first 6 months. *Medical and Pediatric Oncology, 11*, 269–278.

Kupst, M. J., Schulman, J. L., Maurer, H., Morgan, E., Honig, G., & Fochtman, D. (1984). Coping with pediatric leukemia: A 2 year follow-up study. *Journal of Pediatric Psychology, 9*, 149–163.

Kupst, M. J., Tylke, L., Thomas, L., Mudd, M. E., Richardson, C., & Schulman, J. L. (1982). Strategies of intervention with families of pediatric leukemia patients: A longitudinal perspective. *Social Work in Health Care, 8*, 31–47.

Kyngas, H., Mikkonen, R., Nousiainen, E. M., Rytilahti, M., Seppanen, P., Vaatvaara, R., et al. (2001). Coping with the onset of cancer: coping strategies and resources of young people with cancer. *European Journal of Cancer Care, 10*, 6–11.

Landolt, M. A., Vollrath, M., & Ribi, K., (2002). Predictors of coping strategy selection in pediatric patients. *Acta Paediatrica, 91*, 954–960.

Last, B. F., & Grootenhuis, M. A. (1998). Emotions, coping, and the need for support in families of children with cancer: a model for psychosocial care. *Patient Education and Counseling, 33*, 169–179.

Lazarus, R. S. (1966). *Psychological Stress and the Coping Process*. New York: McGraw-Hill.

Lazarus, R. S. (1983). The costs and benefits of denial. In S. Breznitz (Ed.), *The denial of stress* (pp. 1–30). New York: International Universities Press.

Lazarus, R. S. (1991). *Emotion and adaptation*. New York: Oxford.

Lazarus, R. S. (2000). Toward better research on stress and coping. *American Psychologist, 55*, 665–673.

Lazarus, R. S., & Folkman, S. (1984). *Stress, appraisal, and coping*. New York: Springer.

Levi, R. B., Marsick, R., Drotar, D., & Kodish, E. D. (2000). Diagnosis, disclosure, and informed consent: Learning from parents of children with cancer. *Journal of Pediatric Hematology/Oncology*, 22, 3–12.

Levin Newby, W., Brown, R. T., Pawletko, T. M., Gold, S. H., & Whitt, J. K. (2000). Social skills and psychological adjustment of child and adolescent cancer survivors, *Psycho-Oncology*, *9*, 113–126.

Loevinger, J. (1976). *Ego development*. San Francisco: Jossey-Bass.

Mackie, E., Hill., J., Kondryn, H., & McNally, R. (2000). Adult psychosocial outcomes in long-term survivors of acute lymphoblastic leukemia and Wilm's tumor: A controlled study. *Lancet, 355*, 1310–1314.

Manne, S. L., Bakeman, R., Jacobson, P., & Redd, W. H. (1993). Children's coping during invasive procedures. *Behavior Therapy, 24*, 143–158.

Meeske, K. A., Ruccione, K., Globe, D. R., & Stuber, M. L. (2001). Posttraumatic stress, quality of life, and psychological distress in young adult survivors of childhood cancer. *Oncology Nursing Forum, 28*, 481–489.

Miller, S. M. (1987a). Monitoring and blunting: validation of a qQuestionnaire to assess styles of information-seeking under threat. *Journal of Personality and Social Psychology*, 52, 345–353.

Miller, S. M. (1987b). *The children's behavioral style scale (CBSS)*. Unpublished manuscript, Temple University, Philadelphia, PA.

Morrow, G. P., Carpenter, P. J., & Hoagland, A. (1984). The role of social support in parental adjustment to pediatric cancer. *Journal of Pediatric Psychology*, 9, 317–325.

Morrow, G. R., Hoagland, A. C., & Morse, I. P. (1982). Sources of support perceived by parents of children with cancer: Implications for counseling. *Patient Counseling and Health Education, 4*, 36–40.

Mulhern, R. K., Wasserman, A. L., Friedman, A. G., & Fairclough, D. (1989). Social competence and behavioral adjustment of children who are long-term survivors of cancer. *Pediatrics, 83*, 18–25.

Natta, M. B. (1995). Coping strategies, psychological distress experience, and perceived adjustment of long-term survivors of pediatric leukemia. *Dissertation Abstracts International, 55*, 4127.

Natterson, J. M., & Knudson, A. G. (1960). Observations concerning fear of death in fatally-ill children and their mothers. *Psychosomatic Medicine*, 22, 456–465.

Nezu, A. M., Nezu, C. M., Friedman, S. H., Faddis, S., & Houts, P. S. (1998). *Helping cancer patients cope: A problem-solving approach*. Washington, DC: American Psychological Association.

Nichols, M. L. (1995). Social support and coping in young adolescents with cancer. *Pediatric Nursing, 21*, 235–240.

Noll, R. B., Bukowski, W. M., Davies, W. H., Koontz, K., & Kulkarni, R. (1993). Adjustment in the peer system of adolescents with cancer. *Journal of Pediatric Psychology, 18*, 351–354.

Noll, R. B., Maclean, W. E., Jr., Whitt, J. K., Kaleita, T. A., Stehbens, J. A., Ruymann, F. B., et al. (1997). Behavioral adjustment and social functioning of long-term survivors of childhood leukemia; parent and teacher reports. *Journal of Pediatric Psychology*, 22, 827–841.

Parle, M., Jones, B., & Maguire, P. (1996). Maladaptive coping and affective disorders among cancer patients. *Psychological Medicine*, *26*, 735–44.

Patenaude, A. F., Basili, L., Fairclough, D. L., & Li, F. P. (1996). Attitudes of 47 mothers of pediatric oncology patients toward genetic testing for cancer predisposition. *Journal of Clinical Oncology*, *14*, 415–421.

Patenaude, A. F., & Kupst, M. J. (2004). Psychosocial functioning of pediatric cancer survivors. *Journal of Pediatric Psychology, 30,* 9–28.

Patenaude, A. F., & Last, B. (2001). Cancer and children: Where are we coming from? Where are we going? *Psycho-Oncology*, *10*, 281–283.

Pearlin, L. I. (1991). The study of coping: An overview of problems and directions. In J. Eckenrode (Ed.), *The social context of coping* (pp. 261–276). New York: Plenum.

Peterson, L. (1989). Coping by children undergoing stressful medical procedures. Some conceptual, methodological, and therapeutic issues. *Journal of Consulting and Clinical Psychology, 57*, 380–387.

Peterson, L., Harbeck, C., Chaney, J., Farmer, J., & Thomas, A. M. (1990). Children's coping with medical procedures: A conceptual overview and integration. *Behavioral Assessment*, *12*, 197–212.

Phipps, S., Fairclough, D., Tyc, V., & Mulhern, R. K. (1995). Avoidant coping in children with cancer. *Journal of Pediatric Psychology*, *20*, 217–232.

Phipps, S., Fairclough, D., Tyc, V., & Mulhern, R. K. (1998). Assessment of coping with invasive procedures in children with cancer: State-trait and approach-avoidant dimensions. *Children's Health Care*, *27*, 147–156.

Phipps, S., & Srivastava, D. K. (1997). Repressive adaptation in children with cancer. *Health Psychology*, *16*, 521–528.

Phipps, S., Steele, R. G., Hall, K., & Leigh, L. (2001). Repressive adaptation in children with cancer: a replication and extension. *Health Psychology, 20,* 445–451.

Rait, D. S., Ostroff, J. S., Smith, K., Cella, D. F., Tan, C., & Lesko, L. M. (1992). Lives in a balance: Perceived family functioning and the psychosocial adjustment of adolescent cancer survivors. *Family Process, 31*, 383–397.

Ritchie, J. A., Caty, S., & Ellerton, M. L. (1984). Concerns of acutely ill, chronically ill, and healthy preschool children. *Research in Nursing and Health, 7*, 265–274.

Robison, L. L. (2003). *Research involving long term survivors of childhood and adolescent cancer: Methodologic considerations*. (Background paper for the Institute of Medicine.) Retrieved September 16, 2004 from http://www.iom.edu/file.asp?id=15238.

Ruccione, K., Kramer, R. F., Moore, I. K., & Perin, G. (1991). Informed consent for treatment of childhood cancer: Factors affecting parents' decision-making. *Journal of Pediatric Oncology Nursing*, *8*, 112–121.

Rudolph, K. D., Dennig, M. D., & Weisz, J. R. (1995). Determinants and consequences of children's coping in the medical setting: conceptualization, review, and critique. *Psychological Bulletin*, *118*, 328–357.

Sahler, O. J., Roghmann, O., Carpenter, P. J., Mulhern, R., Dolgin, M. J., Sargent, J. R., et al. (1992). Adaptation to childhood cancer: Sibling psychologic distress. *Pediatric Research, 31*, 137.

Sahler, O. J., Roghmann, K. J., Mulhen, R. K., Carpenter, P. J., Sargent, J. R., Copeland, D. R., et al. (1997). Sibling Adaptation to Childhood Cancer Collaborative Study: The association of sibling adaptation with maternal well-being, physical health, and resource use. *Journal of Developmental and Behavioral Pediatrics, 18*, 233–243.

Sahler, O. J., Varni, J., Fairclough, D., Butler, R., Dolgin, M., Phipps, S., et al. (2002). Problem-solving skills training for mothers of children with newly diagnosed cancer: A randomized trial. *Developmental and Behavioral Pediatrics, 23*, 77–86.

Sawyer, M., Antoniou, G., Toogood, I., Rice, M., & Baghurst, P. (2000). Childhood cancer: A 4-year prospective study of the psychological adjustment of children and parents. *Journal of Pediatric Hematology/Oncology*, 22, 214–220.

Sawyer, M. G., Streiner, D. L., Antoniou, G., Toogood, I., & Rice, M. (1998). Influence of parental and family adjustment on the later psychological adjustment of children treated for cancer. *Journal of the American Academy of Child and Adolescent Psychiatry, 37*, 815–822.

Slavin, L., O'Malley, J., Koocher, G., & Foster, D. (1982). Communication of the cancer diagnosis to pediatric patients: Impact on long-term adjustment. *American Journal of Psychiatry, 139*, 179–183.

Sloper, P. (2000). Predictors of distress in parents of children with cancer: A prospective study. *Journal of Pediatric Psychology*, *25*, 79–92.

Somerfield, M. R., & McCrae, R. R. (2000). Stress and coping research: Methodological challenges, theoretical advances, and clinical applications. *American Psychologist*, *55*, 620–625.

Sorgen, K. E., & Manne, S. L. (2002). Coping in children with cancer. Examining the goodness-of-fit hypothesis. *Children's Health Care, 31*, 191–208.

Spinetta, J. J. (1977). Adjustment in children with cancer. *Journal of Pediatric Psychology, 2*, 49–51.

Spinetta, J. J., & Deasy-Spinetta, P. (Eds.) (1981). *Living with childhood cancer*. St. Louis, MO: Mosby.

Spirito, A., Stark, L. J., & Tyc, V. (1989). Common coping strategies employed by children with chronic illness. *Newsletter of the Society of Pediatric Psychology, 13*, 3–8.

Spirito, A., Stark, L. J., & Knapp, L. G. (1992). The assessment of coping in chronically ill children: Implications for clinical practice. In A. LaGreca, L. J. Siegel, J. L. Wallander, & C. E. Walker (Eds.), *Stress and coping in child health* (pp. 327–344). New York: Guilford.

Spirito, A., Stark, L. J., & Williams, C. (1988). Development of a brief checklist to assess coping in pediatric patients. *Journal of Pediatric Psychology, 13*, 555–574.

Suls, J., & Fletcher, B. (1985). The relative efficacy of avoidant and nonavoidant coping strategies: A meta-analysis. *Health Psychology, 4*, 249–288.

Thies, K. N., & Walsh, M. E. (1999). A developmental analysis of cognitive appraisal and stress in children and adolescents with chronic illness. *Children's Health Care, 28*, 15–32.

Thompson, R. J., & Gustafson, K. E. (1996). *Adaptation to chronic illness.* Washington, DC: American Psychological Association.

Trask, P. C., Paterson, A. G., Trask, C. L., Bares, C. B., Birt, J., & Maan, C.: (2003). Parent and adolescent adjustment to pediatric cancer: Associations with coping, social support, and family function. *Journal of Pediatric Oncology Nursing, 20*, 36–47.

Tyc, V. L., Mulhern, R .K., Jayawadene, D., & Fairclough, D. (1995). Chemotherapy-induced nausea and emesis in pediatric cancer patients: An analysis of coping strategies. *Journal of Pain and Symptom Management, 10*, 338–346.

Vaillant, G. E. (1977). *Adaptation to life*. Boston: Little, Brown.

Vannatta, K., Gartstein, M. A., Short, A., & Noll, R. B. (1998). A controlled study of peer relationships of children surviving brain tumors: Teacher, peer, and self ratings. *Journal of Pediatric Psychology, 23*, 279–287.

Varni, J. W., Katz, E. R., Colegrove, R., Jr., & Dolgin, M. (1996). Family functioning predictors of adjustment in children with newly diagnosed cancer: A prospective analysis. *Journal of Child Psychology and Psychiatry and Allied Disciplines, 37*, 321–328.

Verill, J. R., Schafer, J., Vannatta, K., & Noll, R. B. (2000). Aggression, antisocial behavior, and substance abuse in survivors of pediatric cancer: possible protective effects of cancer and its treatment. *Journal of Pediatric Psychology, 25*, 493–502.

Wallander, J. L., & Varni, J. W. (1992). Adjustment in children with chronic physical disorders: Programmatic research on a disability-stress-coping model. In A. LaGreca, L. Siegal, J. L. Wallander, & C. E. Walker (Eds.), *Stress and coping with pediatric conditions* (pp. 279–298). New York: Guilford Press.

Weisz, J. R., McCabe, M., & Dennig, M. D. (1994). Primary and secondary control among children undergoing medical procedures: Adjustment as a function of coping style. *Journal of Consulting and Clinical Psychology, 62*, 324–332.

Woodgate, R. L. (2000). A review of the literature on resilience in the adolescent with cancer: Part II. *Journal of Pediatric Oncology Nursing, 16*, 78–89.

Worchel, F., Copeland, D., & Barker, D. (1987). Control-related coping strategies in pediatric oncology patients. *Journal of Pediatric Psychology, 12*, 25–38.

Zebrack, B. J. Gurney, J. G., Oeffinger, K., Whitton, J., Packer, R. J., Mertens, A., et al., & (2004). Psychological outcomes in long-term survivors of childhood brain cancer: A report form the childhood cancer survivor study. *Journal of Clinical Oncology, 22*, 999–1006.

Zebrack, B., & Zeltzer, L. (2003). Quality of life issues and cancer survivorship. *Current Problems in Cancer, 27*, 198–211.

Zebrack, B., Zeltzer, L., Whitton, J., Mertens, A., Odom, L., Berkow, R., et al. (2002). Psychological outcomes in long-term survivors of childhood leukemia, Hodgkin's disease, and non-Hodgkin's lymphoma: A report from the Childhood Cancer Survivor study. *Pediatrics, 110*, 42–52.

Zeltzer, L. (1980). The adolescent with cancer. In J. Kellerman (Ed.), *Psychological aspects of childhood cancer* (pp. 70–99). Springfield, IL: Thomas.

Zeltzer, L. (1994). Pain and symptom management. In D. Bearison and R. K. Mulhern (Eds.), *Pediatric psychooncology* (pp. 84–99). New York: Oxford University Press.

Zeltzer, L. K., Chen, E., Weiss, R., Guo, M. D., Robison, L. L., Meadows, A. T., et al. (1997). Comparison of psychologic outcome in adult survivors of childhood acute lymphoblastic leukemia versus sibling controls: A Cooperative Children's Cancer Group and National Institutes of Health Study. *Journal of Clinical Oncology, 15*, 547–556.

Melissa A. Alderfer and Anne E. Kazak

# Family Issues When a Child Is on Treatment for Cancer

When a child is diagnosed with cancer, his or her entire family is affected. Parents are shocked and devastated when they learn of the cancer diagnosis and soon after diagnosis are responsible for making difficult treatment decisions that may cause their child pain and fear. Siblings may witness the physical and emotional pain of their brother or sister and their parents and experience sudden, extended separations from them. Family roles and responsibilities shift to accommodate cancer treatment and to attend to the needs of the ill child. These new demands must be balanced with the family's previous dynamics and their implicit goals of fostering growth and development within the family. Furthermore, the reactions of individual family members have an impact on each other and can influence the way in which the child approaches cancer treatment (i.e., procedure-related distress and adherence). The purpose of this chapter is to discuss issues pertinent to the family when a child is on treatment for cancer.

Like all childhood illnesses, childhood cancers occur within a complex network of social systems, such as health care, school/peers, and the family (Kazak, Rourke, & Crump, 2003). A helpful framework for conceptualizing the important social contexts that influence and are influenced by a developing child is the social ecology model (Bronfrenbrenner, 1977). This model proposes that the child is at the center of many nested social systems, typically depicted as a series of concentric circles surrounding the child. Large *macrosystems* such as culture and societal values comprise the outermost circle, and smaller, more immediate *microsystems* such as the family, neighborhood, and school are depicted nearer to the child. Although all of these systems are important in the development of a child and useful for understanding adaptation of children with chronic illnesses (Kazak, 1989; Kazak & Christakis, 1996), the most important and immediate social system that involves the child is his or her family.

Our most basic conceptualizations of the ways in which families work stem from biologically based general systems theory (Engle, 1980; von Bertalanffy, 1968). Systems theory is inherently integrative and complex and highlights principles of organization and interrelatedness. When applied to families, systems models posit that (a) families are unified, organized systems made up of individuals, subsystems (e.g., parents), their interrelationships, and the rules that govern their behavior and patterns of interaction; (b) change in one member or aspect of the family will be associated with changes in other members and aspects of the system in a reciprocal fashion; and (c) families are self-regulating systems that develop methods for maintaining stability (homeostasis) and for accommodating change related to development (Hoffman, 1981; Kazak, 1989; Nichols & Schwartz, 2001; Wynne, 2003). These basic tenets help us to understand the ways in which families respond to childhood illnesses such as cancer.

Families, however, do not simply respond to illness; they interact with it across time. All diseases have a specific timeline with relatively distinct phases. Different challenges arise at different time points across the illness course. Various researchers and clinicians have written about the time phases of childhood cancer, and although there is considerable variability in course across the spectrum of childhood cancers, certain generalizations can be made (Gibbons, 1988; Katz & Jay, 1984; Kazak & Christakis, 1996). During treatment for childhood cancer, these phases can be identified as (a) diagnosis, (b) treatment initiation, (c) illness stabilization, and (d) end of treatment. Each of these phases poses different psychosocial challenges for the family.

The purpose of this chapter is to illustrate family issues when a child is diagnosed and treated for cancer. The first section of this chapter discusses models of individual and family-level adjustment when confronted with an extreme stressor such as childhood cancer. Next, each phase of childhood cancer is described along with qualitative and quantitative research results revealing psychosocial reactions of family members and families. Then, ways in which childhood cancer, individual adjustment, and family functioning interact to influence one another are discussed. Finally, a brief summary will be provided along with suggestions for intervention and future directions for examining family issues in the context of childhood cancer.

## Models of Family Adjustment

All families appear equally susceptible to having a child diagnosed with cancer. The cause of most childhood cancers is unknown, and it is not commonly evident which families may be at risk. Psychologically, the majority of families confronting cancer and their members are well functioning. Therefore, research into the adaptation of families to childhood cancer typically builds on models of general functioning and normal development rather than models of psychopathology or clinical dysfunction. Childhood cancer is often conceptualized as an extreme stressor to which family members and the family must adapt. Therefore, a stress and coping framework is popular in this research, and the most frequently investigated psychological outcomes for family members are anxiety and depression. A second, related model of adjustment has emerged to capture symptoms such as intrusive thoughts and hypervigilance, which are common experiences in family members of children with cancer. This traumatic stress framework (Stuber, 1995; Stuber, Kazak, Meeske, & Barakat, 1998) has been useful in understanding the long-term emotional reactions of family members of children with cancer and is now under exploration with on-treatment samples.

The family, however, is more than the reactions of individual members. A number of theorists and researchers have proposed models of the ways in which families adjust to extreme stressors such as childhood chronic illnesses. Next, a few of the more popular models of family adaptation are reviewed as an introduction to the types of constructs that have been investigated when examining family reactions to childhood cancer.

### The Circumplex Model of Marital and Family Systems

Developed by Olson and colleagues (Olson, 1993, 2000; Olson, Russel, & Sprenkle, 1983), the circumplex model of marital and family systems characterizes families on two orthogonal dimensions: cohesion and flexibility. Family *cohesion* refers to the emotional bonds between family members, and four levels of cohesion have been specified: disengaged (very low), separated (low to moderate), connected (moderate to high), and enmeshed (very high). Family *flexibility* refers to the amount of change that occurs in a family's leadership, role relationships, and relationship rules. Again, four levels of flexibility have been defined: rigid (very low), structured (low to moderate), flexible (moderate to high), and chaotic (high).

These two dimensions can be graphically depicted as perpendicular axes, and 16 family types emerge. The four family types that represent the intersection of the midlevels of cohesion and flexibility (i.e., structurally separate, flexibly separate, structurally connected, and flexibly connected) are called *balanced family types*; these family types are considered most well functioning. The four types of families described at the extremes on both dimensions (i.e., chaotically enmeshed, rigidly enmeshed, rigidly disengaged, and chaotically disengaged) are considered the least well functioning.

A third component of the model–*communication*– is considered a facilitating dimension. Communication allows the family to maintain its balance and effectively adapt its functioning to meet its changing needs (Olson et al., 1983). Open communication patterns are present in balanced families and are proposed to promote adjustment.

Family type, as defined in this model, is expected to change across the family life course. For example, families with young children are expected to be more connected and structured than families with adolescents, who are expected to be more flexible and separated. In addition, under times of family-level stress, such as the birth of a new baby or the diagnosis of a chronic illness within a family, a family may change from one family type to another. Balanced families are hypothesized to be better able to make such changes in response to stress compared to extreme families, who remain stuck and have difficulty adapting to the stressor (Olson, 1993).

Although hypotheses regarding changes in family functioning after the diagnosis of a childhood cancer are not speculated in Olson's works, he does describe expected changes in response to a physical illness in a parent. In his hypothesized example, a balanced, flexibly separated family moves to a chaotically enmeshed family when the father has a debilitating heart attack. The illness brings the family closer together emotionally and causes chaos because the family needs to dramatically shift their daily routines to accommodate the illness. After the crisis phase resolves, the family is hypothesized to remain enmeshed, but now the routine of the treatment regimen organizes the family, and they become rigid. After about 6 months, the rigidity and extreme cohesion decrease, and the family becomes balanced again, but closer and more structured. In short, in response to illness a well-functioning balanced family with good communication patterns is hypothesized to move toward the extremes and become more similar to family types that function less well while accommodating an illness. An extreme, poorly functioning family with poor communication patterns would remain entrenched in their family pattern and have difficulty adapting to the new demands of the illness.

## Family Systems Health Model

In contrast to the circumplex model, the family systems health model (Rolland, 1984, 1987, 1993) specifically provides a systemic view of healthy family adaptation to serious illness. This model highlights the complex mutual interactions among illness, the ill family member, and the family and conceptualizes adaptation to illness as a developmental process that unfolds over time. The model stresses family competence and strength, and central to this model is the idea of goodness of fit between family style and the psychosocial demands of disease over time. This model proposes that diseases have certain illness attributes and move through specific illness phases that pose different psychosocial challenges to the family.

The illness attributes that Rolland proposed are important to consider and include onset, course, outcome, and uncertainty (Rolland, 1984, 1987). Onset can be acute or gradual. Here, acuity does not necessarily reflect the actual biological development of the illness but rather the abruptness in the shift from perceived health to perceived illness (Rolland, 1984). Childhood cancers have an acute onset. Illness course can be progressive, constant, or relapsing. A progressive disease increases gradually in severity across time. A constant course illness is one in which there is an acute illness episode, followed by a period of recovery, then by a stable period, often characterized by some deficit of functioning. A relapsing illness alternates between stable periods and either actual or threatened recurrences. Childhood cancers can take any of these forms and typically include the threat of relapse, even if it does not occur.

Outcome of the illness refers to likelihood of death, shortening of life because of the illness, and incapacitation. When considering the psychosocial impact of an illness, a crucial factor is the initial expectation of whether a disease is likely to cause death (Rolland, 1984). Despite improvements in the survival rate for children with cancer, many family members appreciate the fact that without effective treatment, the diagnosed child will die. Even if the child is expected to live, childhood cancers, their treatments, and adverse side effects may result in physical, cognitive, or social limitations at various times across the disease course. Last, the predictability of the illness and the degree of uncertainty about the specific way or rate at which it will unfold is an important quality of illness when psychosocial response is considered. There is often a high degree of uncertainty in childhood cancers.

Just as illnesses are proposed to have specific characteristics and timelines, family systems are also postulated to have a developmental course with a basic sequence of events marked by family life phases and transitions. For example, during specific life cycle phases such as the birth of a first child, a family is drawn together through *centripetal forces*. Centripetal forces focus the family internally, and boundaries internal to the family are weakened to allow for more effective teamwork. At the same time, boundaries between the family and external agents are strengthened. At other times, such as when children move on to college, *centrifugal forces* come into play, pushing family members apart and allowing for shifts in family structure to accommodate goals that emphasize individual family members' lives outside the family. This centripetal–centrifugal dimension is similar to Olson's cohesion dimension.

Serious illnesses are hypothesized to exert a centripetal pull on the family system. Symptoms, loss of function, the demands of shifting or acquiring new illness-related roles, and the fear of loss through death are postulated to cause a family to refocus inward. The uncertainty of relapsing illnesses is hypothesized to keep the family in a centripetal mode, hindering the natural flow between phases of the family life cycle. This centripetal pull of the disorder causes different normative strains depending on the life cycle phase of the family. If an illness arises during a centrifugal period, it may derail family development; if it coincides with a centripetal period, it can prolong this period; if it hits during a life cycle transition, issues related to loss become particularly magnified and carried forward into the next developmental phase.

This model also proposes that family systems have characteristics that influence their ability to adapt to illness. For example, both individuals within the family and families as a whole have prior experiences with illness, loss, and crisis and health and illness beliefs. Beliefs are proposed to provide coherence to family life, facilitating continuity among past, present, and future and a way to approach new and ambiguous situations such as serious illness. At the time of medical diagnosis, a primary developmental challenge for a family is to develop an understanding of the illness (i.e., beliefs) that preserves a sense of competency and mastery in the context of partial loss, possible further physical decline, or death. This model hypothesizes that families burdened by unresolved issues and dysfunctional patterns in relation to illness are less equipped to adapt to the challenges presented by a serious medical condition.

## Family Stress Theory

Just as a stress and coping model has been proposed regarding individual adjustment to chronic illness, a number of investigators have proposed and elaborated on stress and coping models for family systems. These various models, such as Hill's ABC-X model (Hill, 1949), the double ABCX model of family stress (McCubbin & Patterson, 1983), and the family adjustment and adaptation model (Patterson, 1988; Patterson & Garwick, 1994), have been described under the umbrella term *family stress theory* (e.g., Hobfoll & Spielberger, 1992). These models have three basic elements in common: (a) the stressor, (b) family resources, and (c) family perceptions and meaning.

The stressor is defined as an environmental influence that threatens the family's well-being. For our purposes, the child's cancer is the stressor. Specific qualities of the illness as described in previous sections of this chapter partly determine its stressfulness. Family resources are defined as the strengths of individual family members and the family system. These resources may be psychological (i.e., self-esteem), social (i.e., social support), interpersonal (i.e., communication), or material (i.e., income); they are used to meet the demands imposed by the stressor (Patterson & McCubbin, 1983). Family-level resources are things such as flexibility versus rigidity, cohesion versus separateness, and mastery versus helplessness (Hobfoll & Spielberger,

1992; McCubbin & Patterson, 1983; Reiss & Oliveri, 1991). Resources can be preexisting, thus reducing a family's vulnerability to stressors, or may develop in response to the stressor. Family perceptions and meaning refers to an individual family member's or the family's conceptualization of the stressor and their conceptualization of the resources they have to cope with it (Boss, 1988; McCubbin & Patterson, 1983; Patterson & McCubbin, 1983). These perceptions may change with time.

During a crisis, new demands are placed on the family, and the family copes by fitting their resources to the demands of the stressor, seeking more resources, changing their perception of their circumstances, or removing some of the demands. Families are hypothesized to go through repeated cycles of stable adjustment, crisis, and adaptation. As proposed in the other models presented, some cycles occur naturally as part of the family life cycle. Others, like the diagnosis of illness in a family member, are not typical.

There are many similarities across these models and some agreement regarding the type of family-level constructs that are important to investigate when a family confronts a chronic illness. In the next section, the phases of childhood cancer are described along with qualitative and quantitative research results that illustrate the impact of childhood cancer on family members and families as a whole. To capture the breadth of research regarding these issues, the reactions of parents and siblings are discussed along with the impact of cancer on the marital subsystem, sibling relationships, and parenting. In addition, various aspects of general family functioning are discussed, including cohesion, flexibility, and communication.

## Family Adjustment Throughout the Phases of Childhood Cancer

### Diagnosis

Arriving at a diagnosis of childhood cancer and determining the best treatment plan is often a complicated process. Many common symptoms of childhood cancer, such as headaches, bruises, weight loss, joint pain, and fatigue, are common and easily interpreted as nonmeaningful (Janes-Hodder & Keene, 2002). Parents are usually the first to notice that something is wrong with their child but may not suspect cancer. In many cases, these vague symptoms may go on for weeks before the family seeks medical attention (Keene, 1999).

Once a medical evaluation is complete and cancer is suspected, the child may be transferred to a children's hospital or academic medical center, introduced to an unfamiliar health care team, and subjected to diagnostic tests that may be invasive, painful, and fear-inducing. These procedures may be drawn out over the course of days or weeks and may even involve early stage treatment and surgery before a definitive diagnosis is made (Janes-Hodder & Keene, 2002). Once the diagnosis is determined, a team of professionals (i.e., often several physicians, including an attending oncologist, oncology fellow, and resident; several nurses, including bedside nurses and advance practice nurses; and a social worker) may meet with the parents and possibly the patient to present the diagnosis along with treatment options. Parents may be told that without treatment their child will die, be given information about the diagnosis, and be asked to decide on treatment options (i.e., consenting to clinical trials). If a second opinion is desired, the family may need to travel to another medical center, where the child would possibly repeat diagnostic procedures.

The prediagnostic and diagnostic phase of childhood cancer has been reported by parents to be among the most stressful periods encountered (Koocher & O'Malley, 1981). As more medical professionals become involved and more medical tests endured, parents become increasingly uneasy and apprehensive (Brett & Davies, 1988). Even though many parents realize that cancer is a possibility, on confirmation most parents report feeling shocked (Brett & Davies, 1988; Chesler & Parry, 2001; McCubbin, Balling, Possin, Frierdich, & Bryne, 2002; Patistea, Makrodimitri, & Panteli, 2000). Disbelief, anxiety, sadness, denial, confusion, and fear are also common reactions of parents (Hughes & Lieberman, 1990; Patistea et al., 2000). Parents report that they feel overwhelmed by the amount of information they receive around the time of diagnosis (McCubbin et al., 2002). Despite improved survival rates for childhood cancers, many parents believe that their child will die, and this belief has been reported to linger anywhere from a week to a month after diagnosis (Brett & Davies, 1988). Such beliefs tend to be accompanied by mourning, grief, guilt, and anger (Gibbons, 1988; Patistea et al., 2000).

Quantitative research examining the reactions of parents within 1 month of diagnosis is somewhat rare but tends to show that this phase of childhood cancer is extremely stressful for parents. Magni, Carli, De Leo, Tshilolo, and Zanesco (1986) assessed parents within the first week after diagnosis using the Symptom Checklist-90 (SCL-90). Parents of children with cancer scored significantly higher than a control group for depression, anxiety, obsessive-compulsiveness, and sleep disturbance. In addition, the mean state anxiety levels that Fife, Norton, and Groom (1987) reported for parents 10 days after diagnosis were higher than norms. Within 14 days of diagnosis, Goldbeck (2001) found that parents report poorer quality of life, and Hoekstra-Weebers and colleagues found that 85.4% of parents report clinically significant psychological distress within 2 weeks of diagnosis compared to 15% of parents in a community sample (Hoekstra-Weebers, Heuvel, Klip, Bosveld, & Kamps, 1996).

Marital distress is also common around the time of diagnosis. Although couples often report feeling emotionally closer to one another (e.g., Barbarin, Hughes, & Chesler, 1985), they are often physically separated around the time of diagnosis, and this takes a toll on their relationship (McGrath, 2001). Communication patterns may be strained between spouses for a number of reasons, including physical separation, a desire to protect the spouse from feelings of fear and uncertainty, and differences in coping style (Koch, 1985; McGrath, 2001). Quantitative studies revealed that approximately 40% of couples reported marital distress around the time of diagnosis (Patistea et al., 2000; Schuler et al., 1985).

Around the time of diagnosis, siblings report knowing that something is wrong with their brother or sister but may not understand or may not be told that the diagnosis is cancer. It may be several days to a month before the siblings are informed (Brett & Davies, 1988; Havermans & Eiser, 1994). Some siblings report that, before they heard the diagnosis, they suspected something was seriously wrong because of their parents' grief and anxiety (Brett & Davies, 1988). On learning the diagnosis, siblings report feeling shock, sadness, fear, and confusion about what to expect (Brett & Davies, 1988; Breyer, Kunin, Kalish, & Petenaude, 1993; Havermans & Eiser, 1994; Koch-Hattem, 1986). Those who understand the life threat report fearing that their brother or sister would die (Havermans & Eiser, 1994; Murray, 1998). In addition, when the child with cancer is first hospitalized and the roles of parents begin to shift, some siblings report intense feelings of loneliness and marginalization (Chesler, Allswede, & Barbarin, 1991).

These feelings of marginalization seem well founded. Around the time of diagnosis, the child with cancer becomes the center of attention for the family (Koch, 1985). Schuler and colleagues (1985) found that, in the prediagnostic phase of cancer, approximately 80% of families report equal attention across their children; however, around the time of diagnosis one third of families report equal attention.

Quantitative studies of the reactions of siblings around the time of cancer diagnosis and initiation of treatment are rare. Fife and colleagues (1987) assessed state anxiety in siblings ($N=31$, age range 6 to 17 years) within a week of diagnosis and again 2–4 weeks after the cancer diagnosis and found consistently "low" scores, although numerical data were not presented or compared to norms, and their behavioral observations of siblings suggested significant levels of unreported anxiety.

Houtzager and colleagues (Houtzager, Grootenhuis, Hoekstra-Weebers, Caron, & Last, 2003) investigated the quality of life of siblings of children with cancer 1 month postdiagnosis. Overall, they found that siblings of children with cancer ($N=83$, age range 7–18 years) have more trouble concentrating and difficulties with memory and learning compared to a normative reference group. Nearly 40% of the siblings were clinically impaired on these dimensions. The siblings also reported more jealousy, anger, aggression, sadness, worry, and fear and less happiness, joy, satisfaction, relaxation, enthusiasm, and cheerfulness than the comparison group (emotional quality of life). Over half of the siblings of children with cancer (57%) scored in the clinically impaired range for emotional quality of life. In addition, 33% had clinically impaired social functioning.

Sibling relationships are another familial subsystem that may be impacted by cancer around the time of diagnosis. Sometimes, siblings feel guilt and responsibility for the diagnosis (Carr-Gregg & White, 1987; Koch-Hattem, 1986), and this may affect their behavior with the ill child. Often, siblings are separated during this phase of treatment. There are few investigations of sibling relationships during cancer treatment; however, Schuler (1985) found that approximately 94% of families indicated that their children had positive loving relationships prior to diagnosis, but around the time of cancer diagnosis, only 45% of siblings were reported to have this type of relationship. Jealousy, envy, and quarrels replaced the positive relationships between siblings, with both the child with the illness jealous of the healthy sibling for being healthy and the healthy sibling jealous of the ill child for the attention he or she receives. No quantitative studies have been identified that compare sibling relationships in families with childhood cancer to sibling relationships in healthy families.

Parenting and parent–child relationships are also influenced by cancer diagnosis. Significant levels of parenting stress have been reported in qualitative (McGrath, 2001; Young et al., 2002) and quantitative studies (Steele, Long, Reddy, Luhr, & Phipps, 2003). Overprotection is a common theme in these families (McGrath, 2001; Holm, Patterson, & Gurney, 2003). Schuler and colleagues (1985) found that, at diagnosis, there is a sharp increase in the percentage of parents reporting overprotectiveness, impatience, and trouble with self-control in a parenting context; 32% of fathers and 48% of mothers endorsed these items after diagnosis compared to 2% of fathers and 7% of mothers reporting them in the prediagnostic phase. Inconsistency in discipline and relaxed rules for the child with cancer are also common issues in these families (Chesler et al., 1991; Sargent et al., 1995). There is also confusion within families regarding appropriate communication between parent and child (McGrath, 2001). As Rolland (1984) predicted, past experiences of cancer in the family greatly impact the way in which parents choose to talk with their children about the diagnosis (Young et al., 2001).

One of the most frequent themes in qualitative research regarding family responses to childhood cancer is that families pull together, increase in cohesion, and experience the centripetal pull described in the section on the family systems health model around the time of diagnosis (Barbarin et al., 1985; Chesler & Barbarin, 1987; Koch, 1985; McGrath, 2001; Patistea et al., 2000). For example, Barbarin and colleagues (1985) found that 60% of families reported becoming closer as a result of the illness, with only 5% indicating that cancer drove the family further apart. Interestingly, siblings have indicated that the increased closeness of the family does not always apply to all members of the family and at times brings out hidden or ignored family conflicts (Chesler et al., 1991; Sargent et al., 1995). Few quantitative studies have examined cohesiveness as an individual construct at the time of diagnosis; however, Varni and colleagues (Varni, Katz, Colegrove, & Dolgin, 1996) indicated that families of children with cancer do show higher than average levels of cohesion shortly after diagnosis.

### Treatment Initiation

After the diagnosis is established, treatment is initiated, and the family's life suddenly revolves around cancer treatment. Once a course of treatment is specified, the family may be given a "roadmap" outlining the various steps in the treatment protocol, including a schedule of hospitalizations, medications, outpatient visits, and follow-up diagnostic tests. Typically, hospitalization is part of the treatment initiation phase, and parents spend a great deal of time with the child in the hospital. Early treatment may involve surgery, chemotherapy, or radiation therapy. Side effects of the treatment and possible complications (e.g., nausea, loss of appetite, severe fatigue, mouth sores, rashes, infections) may suddenly make the child feel and appear more ill than prior to treatment (Keene, 1999). During the initiation of treatment, relationships with the medical team are often under negotiation, and lines of communication are established to ensure that the child's and the family's needs are met and that treatment is progressing as planned.

The most common difficulty for parents during the treatment initiation phase of cancer treatment is dealing with their own intense emotions and psychological traumatization. In a qualitative study, nearly two thirds of parents reported this concern (Patistea et al., 2000). Feelings of helplessness, powerlessness, and a lack of control over life and the disease have been commonly reported during this phase (Enskar, Carlsson, Golsater, Hamrin, & Kreuger, 1997; Patistea et al., 2000; Young, Dixon-Woods, Finlay, & Heney, 2002). The practicalities of the treatment regimen give family members something concrete on which to focus (Katz & Jay, 1984), but the treatment is also perceived as governing everyday life (Enskar et al.,

1997; Young et al., 2001). Parents report that as treatment begins, hope regarding their child's survival rises; however, the constant uncertainty of this causes sustained anxiety (Brett & Davies, 1988; Enskar et al., 1997). During this phase, parents may begin struggling with existential questions and searching for meaning in their tragedy (Patistea et al., 2000).

During the first 3 months after diagnosis, levels of anxiety (Dahlquist et al., 1993; Santacroce, 2002; Sawyer, Antoniou, Toogood, & Rice, 1997) and depression (Barrera et al., 2004; Manne et al., 1995, 1996) are still significantly elevated above community samples for both mothers and fathers of children with cancer. Prospective studies indicated that distress does decline significantly during the first 3 months postdiagnosis (Fife, Norton, & Groom, 1987; Magni et al., 1986; Steele et al., 2003). However, between 22% and 45% of parents have clinically significant depression or anxiety within this 3-month period (Barrera et al., 2004; Fife et al., 1987; Manne et al., 1996).

Interestingly, posttraumatic stress symptoms (PTSS) seem to be even more common for parents in this phase of treatment than symptoms of general anxiety or depression. In a small sample of parents of children diagnosed with cancer 1–2 months prior to investigation, Santacroce (2002) found that 67% of parents fell into the moderate-to-severe range for PTSS. In a similarly small sample, Landolt, Vollrath, Ribi, Gnehm, and Sennhauser (2003) reported that 44.4% of mothers and 44% of fathers of children diagnosed approximately 5 to 6 weeks previously qualified for a diagnosis of posttraumatic stress disorder.

Studies examining marital variables during the treatment initiation phase have noted significant marital distress. Qualitative studies revealed that parents sometimes have difficulty because they and their partner handle the stress of cancer differently and have difficulty supporting each other given personal emotional reactions (McGrath, 2001). At 2 months postdiagnosis, 25% of mothers and 28% of fathers report clinically significant levels of marital distress (Dahlquist et al., 1993), a proportion significantly greater than that in the general population.

Brown and colleagues (1992) and Fife and colleagues (1987) reported levels of marital satisfaction for parents within 1–4 months postdiagnosis that were below norms for well-adjusted couples. In fact, Fife and colleagues found, in their longitudinal study, that there is a sharp decline in marital satisfaction between 2 and 4 months postdiagnosis. Yeh (2002) found that marital satisfaction at 2 months postdiagnosis was lower than marital satisfaction for parents in the newly diagnosed or illness stabilization phases. Increases in the number of hospitalizations during this particular phase seem to have a negative impact on marital quality (Barbarin et al., 1985).

Siblings of children with cancer report that during the treatment initiation phase the atmosphere of their family life is highly disrupted, with parents spending increasing amounts of time at the hospital with the ill child or responding to the needs of the child with cancer at home (Chesler et al., 1991). This physical or emotional unavailability of the parents contributes to siblings feeling overlooked, left out, and increasingly confused and anxious (Carr-Gregg & White, 1987; Kramer & Moore, 1983). Reactions of siblings during this phase of cancer treatment seem to be dependent on the health status of the diagnosed child. If the child with cancer returns home appearing well, siblings are quick to assume that the threat of cancer has passed; however, if the child appears ill and has many limitations on his or her behavior, the sibling is more likely to remain worried and vigilant (Brett & Davies, 1988). This reliance on observed behavior is often required as communication between the parents and healthy siblings is frequently compromised (Brett & Davies, 1988; Carr-Gregg & White, 1987). Quantitative studies examining sibling adjustment and sibling relationships specifically during this phase of treatment were not identified in the current literature.

Parenting is difficult during the treatment initiation phase, especially when families have children other than the one diagnosed with cancer. As discussed, well siblings are often pushed aside during treatment initiation, and parents report feeling that they will have time to meet the siblings' needs for attention and nurturance later in treatment or once the child with cancer is cured (Carr-Gregg & White, 1987). However, this division of attention, demanded by the cancer, is not easy for parents to accept (Birenbaum, 1995; Enskar et al., 1997; McGrath, 2001).

Difficulties also surface in the parents' relationship with their ill child. Parents report feeling helpless because they cannot protect their child from distressing medical experiences and feel implicated in inflicting the distress on the child because of their role in treatment decisions (McGrath, 2001). These feelings of guilt contribute to inconsistent discipline and differential treatment of children within the family (Chesler et al., 1992; Enskar et al., 1997).

Only one quantitative study was uncovered examining parenting during the treatment initiation period. It revealed that, although parenting consistency fluctuates over the first few months of cancer treatment, parental control, nurturance, and responsiveness are stable during this time (Steele et al., 2003).

Family organization is especially challenged during treatment initiation. Extreme changes must occur in family roles and responsibilities during this time (McCubbin et al., 2002). "Role overload" is common as families juggle their typical responsibilities with the imposed responsibilities of treatment (Chesler & Parry, 2001; Enskar et al., 1997; Koch, 1985; Young, 2001). Family separations and disruptions are seen as the biggest change that occurs during this phase from the perspective of healthy siblings (Sargent et al., 1995). Once treatment is initiated, however, the family begins to assert some control over the cancer (Katz & Jay, 1984). Quantitative studies revealed that, during the treatment initiation phase, families increase their reliance on control and rules (Fife et al., 1987).

## Illness Stabilization

Most children with cancer will experience either a remission of their disease or an otherwise favorable response to treatment, resulting in a period of illness stabilization and a fairly predictable treatment regimen. Such periods may take weeks to months to establish and may last anywhere from days to years (Katz & Jay, 1984). Even if the child does well and establishes remission quickly, treatment is rarely simple and may involve transitions (e.g., chemotherapy for a certain number of months followed by surgery) and periods of greater uncertainty (e.g., if resection will be complete). Side effects are inescapable and may include nausea, fatigue, hair loss, and a low blood count, predisposing the child to infections (Keene, 1999). Even if treatment is going as planned and the cancer is in remission, relapse remains a possibility. If relapse does occur, more intensive treatment may be needed. Sometimes, complications and serious side effects may result in additional treatments and numerous changes to the treatment roadmap. Eventually, however, the treatment typically becomes routine and the illness stabilizes.

As treatment progresses, remission is established, and certain milestones of therapy (e.g., end of chemotherapy) pass by, parents begin to settle into a new "normal" pattern that accommodates the cancer and its treatment. Of course, this new normal may be punctuated with emotionally challenging events such as relapse or the severe side effects mentioned. One qualitative study of mothers of children with cancer revealed that mothers feel an overwhelming responsibility for their children's adherence and cooperation with procedures during this phase and a need to advocate for and to continue to protect them (Young et al., 2001). During this phase, parents continue to have doubts and fears about their child's long-term survival (Brett & Davies, 1988; Gibbons, 1988; Katz & Jay, 1984), but if treatment is going well, they may come to believe survival is probable. They may also continue to search for meaning in the cancer experience (Gibbons, 1988; Young et al., 2001).

Quantitative results regarding the adjustment of parents after the initial treatment phase but within 2 years of diagnosis point toward a time when most parents return to normative levels of distress. Studies investigating parents of children with cancer at 6 months postdiagnosis continued to reveal elevated levels of anxiety and depression (Hoekstra-Weebers, Jaspars, Kamps, & Klip, 1998), with reports estimating that 43%–50% of mothers and 40%–45% of fathers remain distressed at this time point (Manne et al., 1996; Nelson, Miles, Reed, Davis, & Cooper, 1994; Sloper, 2000). Some investigations of parents 12 months postdiagnosis revealed elevated distress (e.g., Hoekstra-Weebers et al., 1998; Hoekstra-Weebers, Jaspars, Kamps, & Klip, 1999; Nelson et al., 1994), while others reported normative levels (e.g., Magni et al., 1986; Sawyer et al., 1997; Sawyer, Streiner, Antoniou, Toogood, & Rice, 1998). In addition, a few researchers found increases in anxiety and depression for parents of children with cancer about 1 year into treatment (Brown et al., 1992; Fife et al., 1987). This may reflect distress associated with complications of treatment or difficulties achieving remission (Magni et al., 1986). By 20–24 months postdiagnosis, average levels of anxiety and depressive symptoms across parents are typically reported to fall within normal limits (e.g., Dahlquist, Czyzewski, & Jones, 1996; Sawyer et al., 1997, 1998), with a small but substantial percentage of parents with continuing distress (e.g., Magni et al., 1986). Rates of PTSS have not yet been published for parents during the illness stabilization phase of treatment for childhood cancer.

The marital subsystem of the family and marital adjustment seem to be somewhat disrupted through the first year after cancer diagnosis, but then seem to improve (Lavee & Mey-Dan, 2003). Fife and colleagues (1987) found that marital adjustment in families of children with cancer at 7 and 10 months after diagnosis was poorer than norms for well-adjusted couples but better than adjustment among clinical samples. Schuler and colleagues (1985) found that once cancer remission is well established, marital distress decreases to near prediagnostic levels. Dahlquist and colleagues (1993, 1996) also found that at 20 months postdiagnosis marital adjustment was similar to norms, with 19% of mothers and 24% of fathers remaining in the clinical range.

As the initial phases of cancer diagnosis and treatment conclude, the chronicity of cancer treatment sets in, and siblings seem to feel a greater impact of the sustained attention that the ill child receives. Siblings report differential treatment by parents and others, noting that the child with cancer receives more attention, caring, and material possessions than they do. Although these discrepancies are understood cognitively, emotionally they are still upsetting and result in jealousy, envy, and anger (Chesler et al., 1991; Havermans & Eiser, 1994; Koch-Hattem, 1986). At times, perceptions of inequity and unfairness result in outbursts, avoidance, or internalization (Chesler et al., 1991; Koch-Hattem, 1986; Murray, 1998). These feelings and behaviors then serve as a source of guilt for the siblings, adding to the emotional turmoil (Chesler et al., 1991).

Some investigations reveal that siblings report the worst part of cancer is seeing their brother or sister go through treatment and endure its adverse side effects (Breyer et al., 1993; Havermans & Eiser, 1994; Sargent et al., 1995). When siblings see the pain and suffering of their brother or sister, they tend to become more vigilant of his or her well-being (Brett & Davies, 1988; Koch-Hattem, 1986), desire to help care for the child, and may wish to take on the cancer themselves to relieve their sibling (Chesler et al., 1991; Koch-Hattem, 1986). Another common theme for siblings during this phase of cancer treatment is a concern for parents and a desire to help around the house and be "extra good" so they do not add to the stress of the family (Brett & Davies, 1988; Chesler at al., 1991). In addition, some siblings, particularly adolescents, and parents report that there are benefits of the cancer experience for siblings, such as increased maturity, sympathy for others, and increased ability to cope with stressful experiences (Barbarin et al., 1995; Chesler et al., 1991; Havermans & Eiser, 1994; Murray, 1998; Sargent et al., 1995).

Descriptive studies of siblings of children with cancer on active treatment have revealed high levels of distress. For example, Heffernan and Zanelli (1997) found that over 60% of their sample of siblings (13 of 21) reported feeling afraid, a similar number reported crying "for no reason," and over 80% (17 of 21) reported thinking about running away or hiding. When parents were asked to report on the adjustment of siblings, distress was also noted. For example, Hughes and Lieberman (1990) found that 70% of parents in a small sample ($N = 10$) believed that siblings showed more distress during treatment than prior to cancer diagnosis; this was manifested in jealousy, anxiety, and poorer schoolwork.

In terms of adjustment, small studies tended to find no differences between siblings and norms or comparison groups (e.g., Evans, Stevens, Cushway, & Houghton, 1992; Horwitz & Kazak, 1990; Madan-Swain, Sexson, Brown, & Ragab, 1993). Larger studies, however, such as that of Sloper and While (1996), found that 24% of their sample had scores on the Child Behavior Checklist (CBCL) that fell into the borderline or clinical range of functioning during treatment. In another large study, Cohen and colleagues (1994) found more clinically significant internalizing and externalizing problems and less social competence among siblings of children with cancer compared to a normative sample. In the largest study to date, the Sibling Adaptation to Childhood Cancer Collaborative Study (Sahler et al., 1994; Barbarin et al., 1995; Sargent et al., 1995), parents retrospectively reported a threefold increase in behavior problems and problems of general adaptation and nearly double the incidence of emotional difficulties for siblings prior to the cancer. The reported rates of difficulties prior to cancer were consistent with norms, but the rates after the cancer diagnosis were significantly greater than rates within a nationally derived comparison group of children (Sahler et al., 1994). The only available prospective study assessing sibling self-reports of adjustment showed that at 6 months postdiagnosis there are decrements in quality of life for siblings, specifically in the areas of increased negative emotions, fewer positive emotions, and poorer social functioning than norms (Houtzager et al., 2003).

In terms of schoolwork and school behavior, Fife and colleagues (1987) investigated a group of 31 siblings within a year of diagnosis and found that 39% had a decrease of 0.5 or more in their 4-point grade point average per school records, and 55% displayed behavior problems in the classroom per teacher report. Sloper and While (1996) also documented teacher-reported behavior problems for siblings of children with cancer 5–10 months postdiagnosis.

Posttraumatic stress among siblings of children with cancer is a new area of investigation and has not been studied for siblings of children on treatment for cancer. However, we reported on PTSS in siblings of childhood cancer survivors and found that 32% had PTSS in the moderate-to-severe range, exceeding rates in a comparison sample (Alderfer, Labay, & Kazak, 2003). Investigating PTSS in siblings of children with cancer still on treatment may provide a valuable framework in which to understand distress in this population.

Although an important component of families with more than one child, very few studies have investigated sibling relationships during treatment for childhood cancer. Schuler and colleagues (1985) documented a severe decline in the quality of sibling relationships around the time of diagnosis and treatment initiation and found that sibling relationships only improve slightly during the treatment phase. Both the patient and the healthy sibling remain envious of one another. It also seems that some siblings take on caretaking roles of their ill sibling that may be qualitatively different from their previous relationships (Chesler et al., 1991). More research is needed to understand this aspect of family functioning.

Parenting also has been evaluated in this phase of childhood cancer. Schuler and colleagues (1985) found that a substantial percentage of parents (44% of mothers, 26% of fathers) continue to report overprotectiveness, impatience, and poor parental control when their child achieves remission. Similarly, Patterson and colleagues (2004) found 40% of parents reported strain in their relationships with their children, including overprotectiveness and conflicts regarding independence during treatment. Interestingly, it seems that parenting stress may increase when the child with cancer is doing better physically. Yeh (2002) found that parenting stress is higher when a child is in remission compared to when newly diagnosed.

Emotional closeness and cohesion continue throughout the treatment period (e.g., Barbarin et al., 1985; Koch, 1985; McGrath, 2001; Patistea et al., 2000). Quantitative studies conducted early in the illness stabilization phase (i.e., 6–9 months postdiagnosis) demonstrated that levels of cohesion, expressiveness, and conflict are relatively stable, more favorable than norms, and congruent with levels reported in the treatment initiation phase (Varni et al., 1996).

At some point across the treatment experience, however, families establish normative levels of functioning across most family functioning dimensions. For example, studies of families with children on treatment for cancer revealed combined levels of cohesion, expressiveness, and conflict comparable to norms (Madan-Swain et al., 1993; Noll et al., 1995). In addition, Streisand, Kazak, and Tercyak (2003), in a study of parents of children who were on average 18 months postdiagnosis (36% were off treatment), found that family functioning in the areas of communication, affective responsiveness, affective involvement, behavioral control, and general functioning were within normal limits.

During the active phase of cancer treatment, organizing the family and balancing roles and responsibilities continue to be difficult for many families. Normative family needs typically continue to be subordinated to the perceived needs and requirement of the illness throughout treatment (Ostroff, Ross, & Steinglass, 2000). According to Patterson, Holm, and Gurney (2004), 40% of families reported that they struggled with this. Plus, Horwitz and Kazak (1990) found that families of children with cancer 6 to 41 months postdiagnosis were more likely to fall into the chaotic and rigid ranges of flexibility when compared to community controls.

## End of Treatment

When all phases of treatment are complete and the child's medical tests reveal no evidence of abnormality, treatment ends. This may be months or years after the cancer was originally detected. The family is expected to return to the clinic every month or so after treatment ends for checkups, and this eventually is reduced to annual follow-up visits to scan for possible recurrence, secondary cancers, or other long-term effects of treatment.

As treatment draws to a close, parents report mixed feelings. After months or years, cancer treatment can become reassuring to families as a defense against relapse (Nitschke et al., 1982); therefore, discontinuing it can be uncomfortable (Katz & Jay, 1984). Despite this possible distress, there is still relief and joy that the treatment has been successful and is coming to an end (Gibbons, 1988). Few quantitative studies examine parental reactions to end of treatment. However, parents of children with cancer who are on active treatment have been found to have higher levels of anxiety, depression, and global distress than parents of children who have completed cancer treatment (Brown et al., 1992; Larson, Wittrock, & Sandgren, 1994; Yeh, 2002). Marital satisfaction follows a similar pattern. Parents of children who are off therapy report more marital satisfaction than parents of children who are newly diagnosed or at 1 year postdiagnosis (Brown et al., 1992; Yeh, 2002). Specific studies, however, are needed to examine parental adjustment during the months surrounding the end of treatment.

In some families, within-family emotional and behavioral coalitions that developed early in cancer treatment continue to shape family life during the transition to the off-treatment phase of cancer (Ostroff et al., 2000). This may mean that the marginalized position of the siblings is maintained within the family structure after treatment ends. Siblings' experiences of the end of treatment have not been explored. Quantitative studies have revealed that by 2 years postdiagnosis, when many families have completed cancer treatment, emotional and social problems of siblings continue, especially for younger siblings (Houtzager et al., 2003; Houtzager, Grootenhuis, Caron, & Last, 2004).

It is interesting to note that parenting stress has been found to be higher in families when the diagnosed child is off treatment compared to on treatment (Yeh, 2002). Parental fears regarding the potential return of the illness (Brett & Davies, 1988) and resulting overprotectiveness (Schuler et al., 1985) may conflict with the developmental needs of their children for autonomy and independence, resulting in greater parental stress. Our clinical experience with survivors leads us to believe that this pattern may be caused by differences in parent and child perceptions of what normal should be after cancer treatment has ended.

When comparisons are made between families on treatment and those who have completed treatment, those who are off treatment tend to be better functioning and to report more communication, affective responsiveness and involvement, behavioral control, organization, and general functioning (Brown et al., 1992; Streisand et al., 2003). However, even off treatment, there seems to be a subset of families who continue to have difficulties in functioning. For example, Cohen and colleagues (1994) found that parents of children with cancer up to 4 years postdiagnosis reported average levels of cohesion. However, when compared to normative groups, a significantly larger portion of these families scored in the enmeshed range (21% vs. 14%).

## Predictors of Family Adjustment

### Parents

Characteristics of parents have been linked to the emotional reactions that they have in response to the diagnosis and treatment of childhood cancer. For example, trait anxiety is a strong predictor of the level of cancer-related distress (Hoekstra-Weebers et al., 1999). In addition, reliance on disengaging and emotion-focused coping strategies (e.g., emotional distancing, avoidance) tends to be related to poorer adjustment (Barrera et al., 2004; Baskin, Forehand, & Sayler, 1985; Nelson et al., 1994; Wittrock, Larson, & Sandgren, 1994). Also, parents who report more concurrent stress and strain (Barrera et al., 2004; Sloper, 2000) and less social support (Speechley & Noh, 1992) have poorer adjustment.

The beliefs or cognitive appraisal of parents have also been linked to their adjustment. For example, Sloper (2000) found that less self-efficacy in managing cancer was related to poorer adjustment. We reported that parents who believe their child will suffer as a result of cancer treatment and believe their child will die and their family will be devastated have more anxiety, posttraumatic stress, and general distress. Parents who reported feeling isolated also had higher levels of hopelessness and posttraumatic stress (Kazak, McClure, et al., 2004). Qualitative studies have also revealed that optimism, faith, trust in the health care team and treatment protocol, and the ability to conceptualize the cancer experience as manageable and meaningful contribute to better adjustment (McCubbin et al., 2002; Patistea et al., 2000).

## Siblings

One major risk factor for sibling adjustment problems after cancer is the presence of major life events prior to diagnosis (Houtzager et al., 2003) and preexisting problems (Sahler et al., 1994). A lack of social support also seems detrimental to the functioning of siblings when childhood cancer has been diagnosed within their family (Barrera, Fleming, & Khan, 2004; Cohen et al., 1994; Williams et al., 2002). The perceptions of siblings also seem important. Siblings who perceived cancer as more disruptive to their family and their lives tended to adjust more poorly (Sloper & While, 1996).

There is conflicting evidence in the literature regarding how sibling age and gender relate to their adjustment to cancer. For example, Sahler and colleagues (1994) found that boys aged 4 to 11 years were most likely to develop problems, and girls aged 12 to 17 years were least likely to develop new problems per parent report. On the other hand, Houtzager and colleagues (2003), using siblings' self-reports, found that shortly after diagnosis adolescent female siblings are at greatest risk for adjustment problems, and as treatment continues, adolescent siblings have more difficulties than younger siblings. It is only near the end of treatment when the reverse seems to be true. More research is needed to explore these discrepancies as they could be caused by differences in perspective or timing of assessment.

## Family Functioning

Qualitative studies revealed that community-based social support and social support from the medical team caring for the child with cancer are helpful in family adjustment to childhood cancer (McCubbin et al., 2002; Patistea et al., 2000). Quantitative studies also have revealed that families that are functioning more poorly prior to the diagnosis of childhood cancer have more difficulty adapting to the needs of treatment and their family after the diagnosis (Fife et al., 1987). This is consistent with predictions of the family models presented in the beginning of this chapter. The factor most frequently investigated as associated with family functioning is the functioning of individual family members, discussed next.

### *Reciprocity in Family Members' Adjustment to Cancer*

When a child is diagnosed with cancer, cancer has an impact on the individuals in the family. The family systems model holds that reactions of individual family members will influence the adjustment of all other family members in a reciprocal fashion. Most of the research investigating this reciprocity has focused on the relationship between parents (typically mothers) and the child with cancer; however, linkages between the parents and healthy siblings and associations between mother and father adjustment also have been explored.

Qualitative studies revealed that parents feel they are better able to handle the challenges of cancer when the diagnosed child is handling it well (Young et al., 2001); in addition, parents indicate that it is important for them to be emotionally positive to foster their children's adjustment (Koch, 1985; Young et al., 2001). Quantitative studies seemed to demonstrate these forms of reciprocity.

For example, Brown and colleagues (Brown et al., 1993) found that children with cancer were at greater risk for anxiety when their mothers qualified for a diagnosis of depression or anxiety. Higher levels of general distress in parents also have been linked to greater hopelessness in children with cancer (Blotcky, Raczynski, Gurwitch, & Smith, 1985) and poorer adjustment (Magni, Silvestro, Tamiello, Zanesco, & Carli, 1988). Plus, Frank, Blount, and Brown (1997) found that parental anxiety was related to child depression and externalizing behaviors. Manne and colleagues (1995, 1996) found that depressive symptoms in mothers were linked to externalizing behaviors in children with cancer. Barrera and colleagues (2004) and Sawyer and coworkers (1997, 1998) extended these results, finding that the externalizing and internalizing behaviors of children with cancer covary with their mother's depression, anxiety, and global mental health.

Reciprocity between parental and sibling adjustment also has been investigated. In fact, some researchers theorized that the emotional reactions of parents and their adjustment to cancer may affect siblings more than the cancer itself (Lobato, Faust, & Spirito, 1988). Qualitative studies have revealed that parents attempt to be positive and hopeful to foster their children's adjustment (Chesler & Parry, 2001; Young et al., 2001); siblings also attempt to respond to cancer in a way that will ease the burden on their parents (Chesler et al., 1991; Koch, 1985; Sargent et al., 1995). Similar to linkages found between parents and the child with cancer, Cohen and colleagues (1994) found that depression in mothers was associated with behavioral problems in siblings. Sahler and colleagues (1997) also found that poorer sibling adaptation was linked to more maternal emotional and physical distress in response to the cancer.

Reciprocity in adjustment between mothers and fathers has been explored in various ways. First, levels of distress have been compared. During the early phases of cancer, such as at the time of diagnosis and treatment initiation, no differences are typically noted in the levels of distress reported by mothers and fathers (e.g., Fife et al., 1987; Hoekstra-Weebers et al., 1998; Nelson et al., 1994). However, when differences are uncovered, mothers report higher levels of anxiety and depression compared to fathers (Dahlquist et al., 1996; Larson et al., 1994; Yeh, 2002). These types of findings, however, do not reveal any association between distress in one parent and the other. Some researchers have revealed that distress in mothers and fathers is correlated (Hoekstra-Weebers et al.,; Landolt et al., 2003), but even these types of studies are not sensitive to subtle within-family patterns.

To try to uncover some of these subtleties, a third form of study has emerged to investigate discrepancies between the ways in which parents cope with cancer. Discrepancies between parents in certain coping styles (e.g., emotional expression, communication) have been found to relate to greater individual distress for parents (Hoekstra-Weebers et al., 1998). However, dissimilarities in other forms of coping (e.g., social support seeking) have been found to relate to better individual parent quality of life (Goldbeck, 2001). Qualitative studies also revealed that during cancer diagnosis and treatment one of the stressors that parents face is acknowledging and accepting differences in their spouse's coping style (Brett & Davies, 1988).

### *Reciprocity Between Individual Functioning and Family Functioning*

Family functioning has frequently been linked to the functioning of individual members of the family, and reciprocity is hypothesized between individual functioning and family system functioning. That is, family functioning may influence individual adjustment just as individual functioning influences family adaptation. More favorable individual family member functioning tends to co-occur with greater levels of cohesion and communication. For example, Varni and colleagues (1996) found that families with greater cohesion and expressiveness around the time of diagnosis and throughout treatment had child patients with fewer internalizing and externalizing behavioral problems and more social competence. These relationships held cross-sectionally at 1, 6, and 9 months postdiagnosis and prospectively across time.

Families higher in cohesion and expressiveness and lower in conflict also have been found to have child patients with less depression (Noojin, Causey, Gros, Bertolone, & Carter, 1999) and hopelessness (Blotcky et al., 1985). Greater cohesion or family integration also has been associated with less depression (Manne et al., 1995) and distress in parents (Sloper, 2000), both cross-sectionally and prospectively. Finally, Horwitz and Kazak (1990) found that greater cohesion and adaptability were related to fewer behavioral problems in siblings, and Dolgin, Blumensohn, and colleagues (1997) found that greater cohesion and expressiveness and less conflict was related to fewer internalizing and externalizing behavior problems in siblings.

The functioning of the marital subsystem within the family also has been linked to the functioning of individual family members, specifically to the pattern of responses across spouses. Anxiety and depression in mothers and fathers of children with cancer have been linked to greater marital distress (Dahlquist et al., 1993, 1996). Also, marital distress seems to be exacerbated in couples with greater discrepancy between their levels of state anxiety (Dahlquist et al., 1993). Discrepancies between mothers and fathers regarding the appropriateness and amount of emotional expression have been found to relate to more marital distress (Hoekstra-Weebers et al., 1998). However, complementarity (i.e., families in which only one spouse engages in the specified behavior) in problem solving (Barbarin, Hughes, & Chesler, 1985) has been found to relate to better marital adjustment. Studies specifically investigating predictors of parental functioning and sibling relational functioning were not identified in the current literature.

### *Reciprocity Between Family Members, Family Functioning, and Cancer*

Reciprocity is hypothesized between the family system and the illness system. The majority of this chapter focuses on the impact of cancer on the family; however, the reactions of individual family members, their interpersonal behavior with one another, and emergent family functioning patterns may also have an influence on the cancer experience. Next, a few examples of this interplay are be illustrated.

*Procedural Distress.* During both the diagnostic phase and the treatment phase of cancer, the child must undergo invasive painful medical procedures. Parents, typically the mother, are often present and at least somewhat involved with their child during these procedures; there seems to be a documentable interplay among individual reactions, parenting, and the cancer experience in this situation.

First, the general level of anxiety of the mother has been found to predict their child's level of procedure-related distress and cooperation with procedures such as bone marrow aspiration (Dahlquist, Power, Cox, & Fernbach, 1994; Jay, Ozolins, & Elliot, 1983) and venipuncture (Jacobson et al., 1990). The relationship between mother's distress and the child's distress is mediated at least partly by parenting strategies. More anxious parents tend to use less effective parenting strategies during procedures, including less self-reported responsiveness, consistency, nurturance, rule setting, and organization; less observed reassurance; and more observed agitation (Dahlquist et al., 1994). Ineffective parenting strategies, such as these and vague commands given during procedures, result in more procedural-related distress for the child (Dahlquist et al., 2001). Interestingly, as children become more distressed during procedures, their parents are more likely to engage in specific ineffective strategies (e.g., providing them with explanations of the procedure). When these feedback cycles of distress and ineffective parenting occur, interventions to help parents manage their anxiety and soothe their children are helpful in reducing the procedural distress and improving cooperation with procedures (e.g., Jay & Elliott, 1990; Kazak, Blackall, Himelstien, Brophy, & Daller, 1995; Powers, Blount, Bachanas, Cotter, & Swan, 1993).

*Adherence.* Nonadherence rates for adolescents with cancer have been estimated to range from 33% to 60% (Festa, Tamaroff, Chasalow, & Lanzkowski, 1992; Lansky, Smith, Cairns, & Cairns, 1983; Phipps & DeCuir-Whalley, 1990). Adherence in cancer is quite understudied but has been a consistent clinical concern given the possible fatal implications.

Kennard and colleagues (2004) examined individual adjustment, family functioning, adherence, and survival rates in a prospective study of adolescents with cancer. Adherence was measured with biological assays (serum sulfamethoxazole), adolescent self-report of behavior, and parent report. Adolescents completed measures of depression, adjustment, and self-concept. Adolescents and parents completed measures of family functioning, including subscales measuring cohesion, expressiveness, conflict, organization, and control. Adolescents who scored higher on depression and lower on self-concept had higher levels of nonadherence. In addition, adolescents who disagreed more with their parent about the functioning of the family had more nonadherence. This type of discrepancy was hypothesized to capture deficits in communication and a lack of shared environment. Finally, adolescents who were nonadherent had a poorer 6-year survival rate. Given that adherence was related to survival and that individual and family system factors influenced adherence, this study clearly suggested that familial issues may have an impact on the cancer experience.

## Family-Level Intervention Implications and Future Directions

Given the large body of literature addressing family issues during the treatment of childhood cancer, the question of how treatment teams can help patients in the context of the family is important and timely. Consistent with recommendations of pediatric and oncology groups (American Academy of Pediatrics, 2004; Noll & Kazak, 2004), most treatment centers provide some psychosocial services to families. Unfortunately, the nature and extent of interventions offered across centers is unknown, as are data regarding outcomes. Many interventions are primarily individually oriented approaches (e.g., pain management) that can be framed to include more than one member of the family (e.g., parent and child) but without a specific family therapy or intervention framework. Indeed, limiting ourselves to descriptions of family-oriented interventions that build on a specific clinical model and those for which there is empirical support unfortunately narrows the range of interventions available.

There is little question that one of the areas in which intervention is most highly developed for children with cancer is in procedural pain. Approaches that use a combination of cognitive behavioral approaches are among the most commonly studied and are well-established treatments (Powers, 1999). This literature varies in terms of the inclusion of parents in the interventions; however, research has shown that parents and staff can learn and implement these interventions effectively (Barrera, 2000; Blount et al., 1992; Kazak, Penati, Brophy, & Himelstein, 1998).

Using developmental and family systems theories, Kazak, Simms, and Rourke (2002) described an intervention approach that focuses on a systemic consultation model. This model provides an alternative to the traditional consultation framework that focuses only on the child. Building on the interrelated triad of patient–family–staff, a protocol is presented that includes four steps: referral, assessment, collaboration, and outcome. Examples are provided that illustrate how a family systems, social ecological approach can be used to reframe situations that are often otherwise viewed individually (e.g., a child's failure to eat during cancer treatment) more contextually (e.g., using the child and parents' competence to engage them in developing an approach in active collaboration with the treatment team). This clinical approach is used in the Division of Oncology at the Children's Hospital of Philadelphia but has not been tested empirically.

In general, the most promising family-oriented interventions during cancer treatment appear to be those that are carefully timed and tailored to specific outcomes rather than relying on more general outcomes (Kazak, 2005). For example, problem-solving therapy has been shown to be more effective than "treatment as usual" in reducing negative affectivity and increasing problem-solving skills for mothers of children currently in treatment (Sahler et al., 2002, 2005). This work provides a relatively easy-to-deliver treatment that helps mothers cope with stressful events related to their child's care while enhancing their emotional health. In a pilot study with mothers of children undergoing bone marrow transplantation, Streisand and colleagues (Streisand, Rodrique, Houck, Graham-Pole, & Berland, 2000) demonstrated the feasibility of providing parents with stress reduction techniques in a one-session intervention. The data comparing the intervention to standard preparation suggested that the timing of intervention may be critical, in this case prior to the admission for transplantation, when stress levels are elevated.

Interventions related to PTSS are emerging. An intervention that integrates cognitive behavioral and family therapy approaches, the Surviving Cancer Competently Intervention Program (SCCIP) was tested in a randomized clinical trial with 150 families of adolescent cancer survivors. The data suggested that PTSS can be reduced in a 1-day group intervention format (Kazak, Alderfer, et al., 2004). The SCCIP model has been adapted and is under evaluation in an ongoing randomized clinical trial for caregivers of children newly diagnosed with cancer. This three-session intervention, Surviving Cancer Competently Intervention Program–Newly Diagnosed (SCCIP-ND), is delivered within the first 2 months of treatment, with pilot data supportive of its feasibility and likely impact on PTSS (Kazak, Simms, et al., in press).

Empirically evaluated intervention programs for siblings are also rare but are important given sibling levels of adjustment difficulties during cancer treatment. Published data from two pilot studies of group interventions for siblings using small, nonrandom samples suggested that more work in this area may be valuable (Barrera, Chung, Greenberg & Fleming, 2002; Dolgin, Somer, Zaidel, & Zaizov, 1997). For example, Dolgin, Somer, and colleagues (1997) found that siblings reported fewer cancer-related relational problems, less preoccupation with cancer, better disease-related communication, more knowledge of cancer, and more positive mood after attending a 6-week intervention program. Similarly, siblings completing the 8-week program of Barrera and colleagues (2002) showed significant decreases in depression, state anxiety, and fear of disease, with desired trends seen in behavioral problems and cancer-related communication.

There are many opportunities for developing interventions across the treatment spectrum for families of children with cancer. Few intervention programs exist, but those that do tend to focus on adaptation to specific aspects of the cancer treatment (e.g., procedural pain) or adaptation of specific family members (e.g., mothers or siblings). With the exception of the SCCIP-ND study, fathers are typically not included in intervention studies yet experience levels of distress similar to mothers around the time of diagnosis (e.g., Fife at al., 1987; Hoekstra-Weebers et al., 1998; Nelson et al., 1994). It is important to investigate and intervene with fathers (Seagull, 2000) addressing their specific and unique needs (Chesler & Parry, 2001). In addition, developing interventions that target family processes (e.g., communication, accepting the discrepant coping styles of other family members) and involve multiple members of the family may be particularly effective in fostering family-level and individual adjustment.

Another reasonable approach that may promote the development of interventions that can be tailored to family needs is to attend more systematically to the assessment of families at the time of diagnosis. That is, interventions are likely to be most acceptable to families and most helpful when they match the needs of particular families. The literature clearly demonstrates the range of functioning seen in families, making general, one-size-fits-all interventions unlikely as a feasible intervention approach. A step in the direction of tailored interventions is the development of brief screening tools, such as the Psychosocial Assessment Tool (Kazak, Cant, et al., 2003). Based on brief and reliable assessment instruments, specific interventions can be provided, hence increasing the efficiency of services provided.

## References

Alderfer, M. A., Labay, L., & Kazak, A. E. (2003). Brief report: Does posttraumatic stress apply to siblings of children with cancer? *Journal of Pediatric Psychology, 28*, 281–286.

American Academy of Pediatrics. (2004). Guidelines for the pediatric cancer center. *Pediatrics, 113*, 1833–1835.

Barbarin, O. A., Hughes, D., & Chesler, M. A. (1985). Stress, coping, and marital functioning among parents of children with cancer. *Journal of Marriage and the Family, 47*, 473–480.

Barbarin, O., Sargent, J., Sahler, O. J., Roghmann, K., Mulhern, R., Carpenter, P. J., et al. (1995). Sibling adaptation to childhood cancer collaborative study: Parental views of pre- and post-diagnosis adjustment of siblings of children with cancer. *Journal of Psychosocial Oncology, 13*, 1–20.

Barrera, M. (2000). Brief clinical report: Procedural pain and anxiety management with mother and sibling as co-therapist. *Journal of Pediatric Psychology, 25*, 117–121.

Barrera, M., Chung, J. Y., Greenberg, M., & Fleming, C. (2002). Preliminary investigation of a group intervention for siblings of pediatric cancer patients. *Children's Health Care, 31*, 131–142.

Barrera, M., D'Agostino, N. M., Gibson, J., Gilbert, T., Weksberg, R., & Malkin, D. (2004). Predictors and mediators of psychological adjustment in mothers of children newly diagnosed with cancer. *Psycho-Oncology, 13*, 630–641.

Barrera, M., Fleming, C. F., & Khan, F. S. (2004). The role of emotional social support in the psychological adjustment of siblings of children with cancer. *Child: Care, Health and Development, 30*, 103–111.

Baskin, C. H., Forehand, R., & Saylor, C. (1985). Predictors of psychological adjustment in mothers of children with cancer. *Journal of Psychosocial Oncology, 3*, 43–54.

Birenbaum, L. (1995). Family research in pediatric oncology nursing. *Journal of Pediatric Oncology Nursing, 12*, 25–38.

Blotcky, A. D., Raczynski, J. M., Gurwitch, R., & Smith, K. (1985). Family influences on hopelessness among children early in the cancer experience. *Journal of Pediatric Psychology, 10*, 479–493.

Blount, R., Bachanas, P., Powers, S., Cotter, M. C., & Swan, S. C. (1992). Training children to cope and parents to coach them during routine immunizations: Effects of child, parent and staff behaviors. *Behavior Therapy, 23*, 689–705.

Boss, P. (1988). *Family stress management: Family studies text series* (Vol. 8). Thousand Oaks, CA: Sage.

Brett, K. M., & Davies, E. M. (1988). "What does it mean?": Sibling and parental appraisals of childhood leukemia. *Cancer Nursing, 11*, 329–338.

Breyer, J., Kunin, H., Kalish, L. A., & Petenaude, A. F. (1993). The adjustment of siblings of pediatric cancer patients—A sibling and parent perspective. *Psycho-Oncology, 2*, 201–208.

Bronfrenbrenner, U. (1977). Toward an experimental ecology of human development. *American Psychologist, 32*, 513–531.

Brown, R. T., Kaslow, N. J., Hazzard, A. P., Madan-Swain, A., Sexson, S. B., Lambert, R., et al. (1992). Psychiatric and family functioning in children with leukemia and their parents. *Journal of the American Academy of Child and Adolescent Psychiatry, 31*, 495–502.

Brown, R. T., Kaslow, N. J., Madan-Swain, A., Doepke, K. J., Sexson, S. B., & Hill, L. J. (1993). Parental psychopathology and children's adjustment to leukemia. *Journal of the American Academy of Child and Adolescent Psychiatry, 32*, 554–561.

Carr-Gregg, M., & White, L. (1987). Siblings of paediatric cancer patients: A population at risk. *Medical and Pediatric Oncology, 15*, 62–68.

Chesler, M. A., Allswede, J., & Barbarin, O. A. (1991). Voices from the margin of the family: Siblings of children with cancer. *Journal of Psychosocial Oncology, 9*, 19–42.

Chesler, M. A., & Barbarin, O. A. (1987). *Childhood cancer and the family: Meeting the challenge of stress and support*. Philadelphia, PA: Brunner/Mazel.

Chesler, M. A., & Parry, C. (2001). Gender roles and/or styles in crisis: An integrative analysis of the experiences of fathers of children with cancer. *Qualitative Health Research, 11*, 363–384.

Cohen, D. S., Friedrich, W. N., Jaworski, T. M., Copeland, D., et al. (1994). Pediatric cancer: Predicting sibling adjustment. *Journal of Clinical Psychology, 50*, 303–319.

Dahlquist, L. M., Czyzewski, D. I., Copeland, K. G., Jones, C. L., Taub, E., & Vaughan, J. K. (1993). Parents of children newly diagnosed with cancer: Anxiety, coping, and marital distress. *Journal of Pediatric Psychology, 18*, 365–376.

Dahlquist, L. M., Czyzewski, D. I., & Jones, C. L. (1996). Parents of children with cancer: A longitudinal study of emotional distress, coping style, and marital adjustment 2 and 20 months after diagnosis. *Journal of Pediatric Psychology, 21*, 541–554.

Dahlquist, L. M., Pendley, J. S., Power, T. G., Landthrip, D. S., Jones, C. L., & Steuber, C. P. (2001). Adult command structure and children's distress during the anticipatory phase of invasive cancer procedures. *Children's Health Care, 30*, 151–167.

Dahlquist, L. M., Power, T. G., Cox, C. N., & Fernbach, D. J. (1994). Parenting and child distress during cancer procedures: A multidimensional assessment. *Children's Health Care, 23*, 149–166.

Dolgin, M. J., Blumensohn, R., Mulhern, R. K., Orbach, J., Sahler, O. J., Roghmann, K. J., et al. (1997). Sibling Adaptation to Childhood Cancer Collaborative Study: Cross-cultural aspects. *Journal of Psychosocial Oncology, 15*, 1–14.

Dolgin, M. J., Somer, E., Zaidel, N., & Zaizov, R. (1997). A structured group intervention for siblings of children with cancer. *Journal of Child and Adolescent Group Therapy, 7*, 3–18.

Engle, G. L. (1980). The clinical application of the biopsychosocial model. *American Journal of Psychiatry, 137*, 535–544.

Enskar, K., Carlsson, M., Golsater, M., Hamrin, E., & Kreuger, A. (1997). Parental reports of changes and challenges that result from parenting a child with cancer. *Journal of Pediatric Oncology Nursing, 14*, 156–163.

Evans, C. A., Stevens, M., Cushway, D., & Houghton, J. (1992). Sibling response to childhood cancer: A new approach. *Child: Care, Health and Development, 18*, 229–244.

Festa, R. S., Tamaroff, M. H., Chasalow, F., & Lanzkowski, P. (1992). Therapeutic adherence to oral medication regimens by adolescents with cancer. *Journal of Pediatrics, 120*, 807–811.

Fife, B., Norton, J., & Groom, G. (1987). The family's adaptation to childhood cancer. *Social Science and Medicine, 24*, 159–168.

Frank, N. C., Blount, R. L., & Brown, R. T. (1997). Attributions, coping, and adjustment in children with cancer. *Journal of Pediatric Psychology, 22*, 563–576.

Gibbons, M. B. (1988). Coping with childhood cancer: A family perspective. In P. W. Power and A. E. Dell Orto (Eds.), *Family interventions throughout chronic illness and disability: Springer series on rehabilitation* (Vol. 7, pp. 74–103). New York: Springer.

Goldbeck, L. (2001). Parental coping with the diagnosis of childhood cancer: Gender effects, dissimilarity within couples, and quality of life. *Psycho-Oncology, 10*, 325–335.

Havermans, T., & Eiser, C. (1994). Siblings of a child with cancer. *Child: Health, Care and Development, 20*, 309–322.

Heffernan, S. M., & Zanelli, A. S. (1997). Behavioral changes exhibited by siblings of pediatric oncology patients: A comparison between maternal and sibling descriptions. *Journal of Pediatric Oncology Nursing, 14*, 3–14.

Hill, R. (1949). *Families under stress: Adjustment to the crisis of war, separation, and reunion.* New York: Harper and Row.

Hobfoll, S. E., & Spielberger, C. D. (1992). Family stress: Integrating theory and measurement. *Journal of Family Psychology, 6*, 99–112.

Hoekstra-Weebers, J., Heuvel, F., Klip, E. C., Bosveld, H. E. P., & Kamps, W. A. (1996). Social support and psychological distress of parents of pediatric cancer patients. In L. Baider, C. L. Cooper, and A. Kaplan De-Nour (Eds.), *Cancer and the family* (pp. 93–107). Oxford, England: Wiley.

Hoekstra-Weebers, J., Jaspars, J., Kamps, W. A., & Klip, E. C. (1998). Gender differences in psychological adaptation and coping in parents of pediatric cancer patients. *Psycho-Oncology, 7*, 26–36.

Hoekstra-Weebers, J., Jaspars, J., Kamps, W. A., & Klip, E. C. (1999). Risk factors for psychological maladjustment of parents of children with cancer. *Journal of the American Academy of Child and Adolescent Psychiatry, 38*, 1526–1535.

Hoffman, L. (1981). *Foundations of family therapy.* New York: Basic Books.

Holm, K. E., Patterson, J. M., & Gurney, J. G. (2003). Parental involvement and family-centered care in the diagnostic and treatment phases of childhood cancer: Results from a qualitative study. *Journal of Pediatric Oncology Nursing, 20*, 301–313.

Horwitz, W. A., & Kazak, A. E. (1990). Family adaptation to childhood cancer: Siblings and family systems variables. *Journal of Clinical Child Psychology, 19*, 221–228.

Houtzager, B. A., Grootenhuis, M. A., Caron, H. N., & Last, B. F. (2004). Quality of life and psychological adaptation in siblings of cancer patients, 2 years after diagnosis. *Psycho-Oncology, 13*, 499–511.

Houtzager, B. A., Grootenhuis, M. A., Hoekstra-Weebers, J. E., Caron, H. N., & Last, B. F. (2003). Psychosocial functioning in siblings of paediatric cancer patients 1 to 6 months after diagnosis. *European Journal of Cancer, 39*, 1423–1432.

Hughes, P. M., & Lieberman, S. (1990). Troubled parents: Vulnerability and stress in childhood cancer. *British Journal of Medical Psychology, 63*, 53–64.

Jacobson, P. B., Manne, S. L., Gorfinkle, K., Schorr, O., Rapkin, B., & Redd, W. H. (1990). Analysis of child and parent behavior during painful medical procedures. *Health Psychology, 9*, 559–576.

Janes-Hodder, H., & Keene, N. (2002). *Childhood cancer: A parent's guide to solid tumor cancer* (2nd ed.). Sebastopol, CA: O'Reilly.

Jay, S. M., & Elliott, C. H. (1990). A stress inoculation program for parents whose children are undergoing painful medical procedures. *Journal of Consulting and Clinical Psychology, 58*, 799–804.

Jay, S. M., Ozolins, M., & Elliot, C. H. (1983). Assessment of children's distress during painful medical procedures. *Health Psychology, 2*, 133–147.

Katz, E. R., & Jay, S. M. (1984). Psychological aspects of cancer in children, adolescents, and their families. *Clinical Psychology Review, 4*, 525–542.

Kazak, A. (2005). Evidence based interventions for survivors of childhood cancer and their families. *Journal of Pediatric Psychology, 19*, 3–5.

Kazak, A., Alderfer, M., Streisand, R., Simms, S., Rourke, M., Barakat, L., et al. (2004). Treatment of posttraumatic stress symptoms in adolescent survivors of childhood cancer and their families: A randomized clinical trial. *Journal of Family Psychology, 18*, 493–504.

Kazak, A., Cant, M. C., Jensen, M., McSherry, M., Rourke, M., Hwang, W. T., et al., & (2003). Identifying psychosocial risk indicative of subsequent resource utilization in families of newly diagnosed pediatric oncology patients. *Journal of Clinical Oncology, 21*, 3220–3225.

Kazak, A., Penati, B., Brophy, P., & Himelstein, B. (1998). Pharmacologic and psychologic interventions for procedural pain. *Pediatrics, 102*, 59–66.

Kazak, A., Simms, S., Alderfer, M., Rourke, M., Crump, T., McClure, K., et al. (in press). Feasibility and preliminary outcomes from a pilot study of a brief psychological intervention for families of children newly diagnosed with cancer. *Journal of Pediatric Psychology.*

Kazak, A., Simms, S., & Rourke, M. (2002). Family systems practice in pediatric psychology. *Journal of Pediatric Psychology, 27*, 133–143.

Kazak, A. E. (1989). Families of chronically ill children: A systems and social-ecological model of adaptation and challenge. *Journal of Consulting and Clinical Psychology, 57*, 25–30.

Kazak, A. E., Blackall, G., Himelstein, B., Brophy, P., & Daller, R. (1995). Producing systemic change in pediatric practice: An intervention protocol for reducing distress during painful procedures. *Family Systems Medicine, 13*, 173–185.

Kazak, A. E., & Christakis, D. (1996). The intense stress of childhood cancer: A systems perspective. In C. R. Pfeffer (Ed.), *Severe stress and mental disturbance in children*, (pp. 277–305). Washington, DC: American Psychiatric Press.

Kazak, A. E., McClure, K. S., Alderfer, M. A., Hwang, W. T., Crump, T. A., Le, L., et al. (2004). Cancer-related parental beliefs: The Family Illness Beliefs Inventory (FIBI). *Journal of Pediatric Psychology, 29*, 531–542.

Kazak, A. E., Rourke, M. T., & Crump, T. (2003). Families and other systems in pediatric psychology. In M. Roberts (Ed.), *Handbook of pediatric psychology* (3rd ed.). New York: Guilford.

Keene, N. (1999). *Childhood leukemia: A guide for families, friends and caregivers* (2nd ed.) Sebastopol, CA: O'Reilly.

Kennard, B. D., Stewart, S. M., Olvera, R., Bawdon, R. E., hAilin, A. O., Lewis, C. P., et al. (2004). Nonadherence in adolescent oncology patients: Preliminary data on psychological risk factors and relationships to outcome. *Journal of Clinical Psychology in Medical Settings, 11*, 31–40.

Koch, A. (1985). "If only it could be me": The families of pediatric cancer patients. *Family Relations, 34*, 63–70.

Koch-Hattem, A. (1986). Siblings' experience of pediatric cancer: Interviews with children. *Health and Social Work, 11*, 107–117.

Koocher, G., & O'Malley, J. (1981). *The Damocles syndrome: Psychological consequences of surviving childhood cancer*. New York: McGraw-Hill.

Kramer, R. F., & Moore, I. M. (1983). Living with childhood cancer: Meeting the special needs of healthy siblings. *Cancer Nursing*, 6, 213–217.

Landolt, M. A., Vollrath, M., Ribi, K., Gnehm, H. E., & Sennhauser, F. H. (2003). Incidence and associations of parental and child posttraumatic stress symptoms in pediatric patients. *Journal of Child Psychology and Psychiatry, 44*, 1199–1207.

Lansky, S. B., Smith, S. D., Cairns, N. U., & Cairns, G. F. (1983). Psychological correlates of compliance. *American Journal of Pediatric Hematology Oncology, 5*, 87–92.

Larson, L. S., Wittrock, D. A., & Sandgren, A. K. (1994). When a child is diagnosed with cancer: I. Sex differences in parental adjustment. *Journal of Psychosocial Oncology, 12*, 123–142.

Lavee, Y., & Mey-Dan, M. (2003). Patterns of change in marital relationships among parents of children with cancer. *Health and Social Work, 28*, 255–263.

Lobato, D., Faust, D., & Spirito, A. (1988). Examining the effects of chronic disease and disability on children's sibling relationships. *Journal of Pediatric Psychology, 13*, 389–407.

Madan-Swain, A., Sexson, S. B., Brown, R. T., & Ragab, A. (1993). Family adaptation and coping among siblings of cancer patients, their brothers and sisters, and nonclinical controls. *The American Journal of Family Therapy, 21*, 60–70.

Magni, G., Carli, M., De Leo, D., Tshilolo, M., & Zanesco, L. (1986). Longitudinal evaluations of psychological distress in parents of children with malignancies. *Acta Paediatrica Scandinavica, 75*, 283–288.

Magni, G., Silvestro, A., Tamiello, M., Zanesco, L., & Cerli. (1988). An integrated approach to the assessment of family adjustment to acute lymphocytic leukemia in children. *Acta Psychiatrica Scandinavica, 78*, 639–642.

Manne, S. L., Lesanics, D., Meyers, P., Wollner, N., Steinherz, P., & Redd, W. (1995). Predictors of depressive symptomatology among parents of newly diagnosed children with cancer. *Journal of Pediatric Psychology, 20*, 491–510.

Manne, S. L., Miller, D. L., Meyers, P., Wollner, N., Steinherz, P., & Redd, W. H. (1996). Depressive symptoms among parents of newly diagnosed children with cancer: A 6-month follow-up study. *Children's Health Care, 25*, 191–209.

McCubbin, H. I., & Patterson, J. M. (1983). The family stress process: The double ABCX model of adjustment and adaptation. *Marriage and Family Review, 6*, 7–37.

McCubbin, M., Balling, K., Possin, P., Frierdich, S., & Bryne, B. (2002). Family resiliency in childhood cancer. *Family Relations: Journal of Applied Family and Child Studies, 51*, 103–111.

McGrath, P. (2001). Findings on the impact of treatment for acute lymphoblastic leukaemia on family relationships. *Child and Family Social Work, 6*, 229–237.

Murray, J. S. (1998). The lived experience of childhood cancer: One sibling's perspective. *Issues in Comprehensive Pediatric Nursing, 21*, 217–227.

Nelson, A. E., Miles, M. S., Reed, S. B., Davis, C. P., & Cooper, H. (1994). Depressive symptomatology in parents of children with chronic oncologic or hematologic disease. *Journal of Psychosocial Oncology, 12*, 61–75.

Nichols, M. P., & Schwartz, R. C. (2001). *The Essentials of Family Therapy*. Boston: Pearson Education.

Nitschke, R., Humphrey, G. B., Sexauer, C. L., Catron, B., Wunder, S., & Jay, S. (1982). Therapeutic choices made by patients with end-stage cancer. *Journal of Pediatrics, 101*, 471–476.

Noll, R., & Kazak, A. (2004). Psychosocial care. In A. Altman (Ed.), *Supportive care of children with cancer: Current therapy and guidelines from the Children's Oncology Group* (pp. 337–353). Baltimore, MD: Johns Hopkins University Press.

Noll, R. B., Gartstein, M. A., Hawkins, A., Vannatta, K., Davies, W. H., & Bukowski, W. M. (1995). Comparing parental distress for families with children who have cancer and matched comparison families without children with cancer. *Family Systems Medicine, 13*, 11–27.

Noojin, A. B., Causey, D. L., Gros, B. J., Bertolone, S., & Carter, B. D. (1999). The influence of maternal stress resistance and family relationships on depression in children with cancer. *Journal of Psychosocial Oncology, 17*, 79–97.

Olson, D. H. (1993). Circumplex model of marital and family systems: Assessing family functioning. In F. Walsh (Ed.), *Normal family processes* (2nd ed., pp. 104–137). New York: Guilford Press.

Olson, D. H. (2000). Circumplex models of marital and family systems. *Journal of Family Therapy, 22*, 144–167.

Olson, D. H., Russel, C. S., & Sprenkle, D. H. (1983). Circumplex model of marital and family systems: VI. Theoretical update. *Family Process, 22*, 69–83.

Ostroff, J., Ross, S., & Steinglass, P. (2000). Psychosocial adaptation following treatment: A family systems perspective on childhood cancer survivorship. In L. Baider, C. L. Cooper, & A. K. De-Nour (Eds.), *Cancer and the Family* (2nd ed., pp. 155–173). Oxford, U.K.: Wiley.

Patistea, E., Makrodimitri, P., & Panteli, V. (2000). Greek parents' reactions, difficulties and resources in childhood leukaemia at the time of diagnosis. *European Journal of Cancer Care, 9*, 86–96.

Patterson, J. M. (1988). Families experiencing stress: I. The family adjustment and adaptation response model: II. Applying the FAAR Model to health-related issues for intervention and research. *Family Systems Medicine, 6*, 202–237.

Patterson, J. M., & Garwick, A. W. (1994). Levels of meaning in family stress theory. *Family Process, 33*, 287–304.

Patterson, J. M., Holm, K. E., & Gurney, J. G. (2004). The impact of childhood cancer on the family: A qualitative analysis of strains, resources, and coping behaviors. *Psycho-Oncology, 13*, 390–407.

Patterson, J. M., & McCubbin, H. I. (1983). The impact of family life events and changes on the health of a chronically ill child. *Family Relations: Journal of Applied Family and Child Studies, 32*, 255–264.

Phipps, S., & DeCuir-Whalley, S. (1990). Adherence issues in pediatric bone marrow transplantation. *Journal of Pediatric Psychology, 15*, 459–475.

Powers, S. (1999). Empirically supported treatments in pediatric psychology: Procedure-related pain. *Journal of Pediatric Psychology, 24*, 131–145.

Powers, S. W., Blount, R. L., Bachanas, P. J., Cotter, M. W., & Swan, S. C. (1993). Helping preschool leukemia patients and their parents cope during injections. *Journal of Pediatric Psychology, 18*, 681–695.

Reiss, D., & Oliveri, M. E. (1991). The family's conception of accountability and competence: a new approach to the conceptualization and assessment of family stress. *Family Process, 30*, 193–214.

Rolland, J. S. (1984). Toward a psychosocial typology of chronic and life-threatening illness. *Family Systems Medicine, 2*, 245–262.

Rolland, J. S. (1987). Chronic illness and the life cycle: A conceptual framework. *Family Process, 26*, 203–221.

Rolland, J. S. (1993). Mastering family challenges in serious illness and disability. In F. Walsh (Ed.), *Normal family processes* (2nd ed., pp. 444–473). New York: Guilford Press.

Sahler, O. J., Fairclough, D., Phipps, S., Mulhern, R., Dolgin, M., Noll, R., et al. (2005). Using problem-solving skills to reduce negative affectivity in mothers of children with newly diagnosed cancer: Report of a multi-site randomized trial. *Journal of Consulting and Clinical Psychology, 73*, 272–283.

Sahler, O. J., Roghmann, K. J., Carpenter, P. J., Mulhern, R. K., Dolgin, M. J., Sargent, J. R., et al. (1994). Sibling Adaptation to Childhood Cancer Collaborative Study: Prevalence of sibling distress and definition of adaptation levels. *Developmental and Behavioral Pediatrics, 15*, 353–366.

Sahler, O. J., Roghmann, K. J., Mulhern, R. K., Carpenter, P. J., Sargent, J. R., Copeland, D. R., et al. (1997). Sibling Adaptation to Childhood Cancer Collaborative Study: The association of sibling adaptation with maternal well-being, physical health, and resource use. *Journal of Developmental and Behavioral Pediatrics, 18*, 233–243.

Sahler, O. J., Varni, J., Fairclough, D., Butler, R., Dolgin, M., Phipps, S., et al. (2002). Problem-solving skills training for mothers of children with newly diagnosed cancer: A randomized trial. *Developmental and Behavioral Pediatrics, 23*, 77–86.

Santacroce, S. (2002). Uncertainty, anxiety, and symptoms of posttraumatic stress in parents of children recently diagnosed with cancer. *Journal of Pediatric Oncology Nursing, 19*, 104–111.

Sargent, J. R., Sahler, O. J., Roghmann, K. J., Mulhern, R. K., Barbarin, O. A., Carpenter, P. J., et al. (1995). Sibling Adaptation to Childhood Cancer Collaborative Study: Siblings; perceptions of the cancer experience. *Journal of Pediatric Psychology, 20*, 151–164.

Sawyer, M., Antoniou, G., Toogood, I., & Rice, M. (1997). Childhood cancer: A 2-year prospective study of the psychological adjustment of children and parents. *Journal of the American Academy of Child and Adolescent Psychiatry, 36*, 1736–1743.

Sawyer, M., Streiner, D. L., Antoniou, G., Toogood, I., & Rice, M. (1998). Influence of parental and family adjustment on the later psychological adjustment of children treated for cancer. *Journal of American Academy of Child and Adolescent Psychiatry, 37*, 815–822.

Schuler, D., Bakos, M., Zsambor, C., Polcz, A., Koos, R., Kardos, G., et al. (1985). Psychosocial problems in families of a child with cancer. *Medical and Pediatric Oncology, 13*, 173–179.

Seagull, E. (2000). Beyond mothers and children: Finding the family in pediatric psychology. *Journal of Pediatric Psychology, 25*, 161–169.

Sloper, P. (2000). Predictors of distress in parents of children with cancer: A prospective study. *Journal of Pediatric Psychology, 25*, 79–91.

Sloper, P., & While, D. (1996). Risk factors in the adjustment of siblings of children with cancer. *Journal of Child Psychology and Psychiatry and Allied Disciplines, 37*, 597–607.

Speechley, K. N., & Noh, S. (1992). Surviving childhood cancer, social support, and parents' psychological adjustment. *Journal of Pediatric Psychology, 17*, 15–31.

Steele, R. G., Long, A., Reddy, K. A., Luhr, M., & Phipps, S. (2003). Changes in maternal distress and child rearing strategies across treatment for pediatric cancer. *Journal of Pediatric Psychology, 28*, 447–452.

Streisand, R., Kazak, A. E., & Tercyak, K. P. (2003). Pediatric-specific parenting stress and family functioning in parents of children treated for cancer. *Children's Health Care, 32*, 245–256.

Streisand, R., Rodrique, J., Houck, C., Graham-Pole, J., & Berlant, N. (2000). Brief report: Parents of children undergoing bone marrow transplantation: Documenting stress and piloting a psychological intervention program. *Journal of Pediatric Psychology, 25*, 331–337.

Stuber, M. L. (1995). Stress responses to pediatric cancer: A family phenomenon. *Family Systems Medicine, 13*, 163–172.

Stuber, M., Kazak, A. E., Meeske, K., & Barakat, L. (1998). Is posttraumatic stress a viable model for understanding responses to childhood cancer? *Child and Adolescent Psychiatric Clinics of North America, 7*, 169–182.

Varni, J. W., Katz, E. R., Colegrove, R., & Dolgin, M. (1996). Family functioning predictors of adjustment in children with newly diagnosed cancer: A prospective analysis. *Journal of Child Psychology and Psychiatry, 37*, 321–328.

Von Bertalanffy, L. (1968). *General Systems Theory*. New York: Braziller.

Williams, P. D., Williams, A. R., Graff, J. C., Hanson, S., Stanton, A., Hafeman, C., et al. (2002). Interrelationships among variables affecting well siblings and mothers in families of children with a chronic illness or disability. *Journal of Behavioral Medicine, 25*, 411–424.

Wittrock, D. A., Larson, L. S., & Sandgren, A. K. (1994). When a child is diagnosed with cancer: II. Parental coping, psychological adjustment, and relationships with medical personnel. *Journal of Psychosocial Oncology, 12*, 17–32.

Wynne, L. C. (2003). Systems theory and the biopsychosocial approach. In R. M. Frankel, T. E. Quill, & S. H. McDaniel (Eds.), *The biopsychosocial approach: Past, present, and future* (pp. 219–230). Rochester, NY: University of Rochester Press.

Yeh, C. H. (2002). Gender differences of parental distress in children with cancer. *Journal of Advanced Nursing, 38*, 598–606.

Young, B., Dixon-Woods, M., Finlay, M., & Heney, D. (2002). Parenting in crisis: Conceptualizing mothers of children with cancer. *Social Science and Medicine, 55*, 1835–1847.

Sean Phipps

# Psychosocial and Behavioral Issues in Stem Cell Transplantation

Stem cell transplantation (SCT) or bone marrow transplantation (BMT) has evolved from a heroic, experimental therapy of last resort to a standard therapy for many high-risk leukemias and the preferred first option after leukemic relapse (Sanders, 1997; Santos, 2000; Treleaven & Barrett, 1998; Wingard, 1997). The indications for SCT have widened to include a number of other malignant disorders, including lymphomas, solid tumors, and even brain tumors, as well as to a growing number of nonmalignant disorders (Meller & Pinkerton, 1998; Santos, 2000; Treleaven & Barrett, 1998). The growth of bone marrow registries that allow for wider use of unrelated donor transplants and developments in stem cell selection techniques that allow for haplotype transplants using mismatched family donors, including parents, have greatly increased the availability of SCT as a viable treatment option for seriously ill children (Mehta & Powles, 2000). At the same time, advances in supportive care have led to improved survival outcomes and thus to a rapidly growing number of long-term survivors of SCT (Santos, 2000; Treleaven & Barrett, 1998). Yet, despite the extraordinary medical and technical advances that have saved the lives of many children, SCT remains a high-risk medical procedure involving a prolonged and physically demanding treatment regimen that can challenge the coping capacities of patients and their families.

Psychosocial research in pediatric SCT has progressed more slowly, but available studies indicate that SCT is a stressful experience that can have a negative impact on the social functioning, self-esteem, and general emotional well-being of survivors (Barrera, Pringle, Sumbler, & Saunders, 2000; McConville et al., 1990; Parsons, Barlow, Levy, Supran, & Kaplan, 1999; Phipps, Brenner, et al., 1995; Phipps & Barclay, 1996; Rodrigue, Graham-Pole, Kury, Kubar, & Hoffman, 1995; Stuber, Nader, Yasuda, Pynoos, & Cohen, 1991; Vannatta, Zeller, Noll, & Koontz, 1998). A number of studies have also focused on parental response to SCT (Barrera et al., 2000; Kronenberger et al., 1998; Manne et al., 2001, 2002; Phipps, Dunavant, Lensing, & Rai, 2004; Rodrigue et al., 1996; Streisand, Rodrigue, Houck, Graham-Pole, & Berlant, 2000). Much of the literature to date has focused on long-term outcomes in survivors, particularly neurocognitive and academic outcomes. The smaller number of studies that have addressed the short- and intermediate-term outcomes have focused more on the general adjustment of patients and parents and measures of transient distress.

In this chapter, we first review the literature on neurocognitive outcomes, which is the area that has been most widely addressed to date. Subsequently, we review the literature on the general adjustment and quality-of-life (QOL) outcomes in the child patient, followed by a similar review of parental responses. We conclude with a brief review of research on sibling donors and on intervention work to date, two areas in which very minimal data are available. A description of the SCT procedures and the ecology of the transplant setting will not be presented as this has been described in detail elsewhere (e.g., Phipps, 1994).

## Neurocognitive and Psychoeducational Issues

Patients undergoing SCT are at risk for a number of adverse central nervous system (CNS) events during the early post-SCT period, including cerebral hemorrhage, infectious complications such as viral encephalitis, metabolic encephalopathy, and other encephalopathies of unknown cause (Garrick, 2000; Graus et al., 1996; Marks, 1998; Meyers et al., 1994; Padovan et al., 1998; Patchell, White, Clark, Beschorner, & Santos, 1985; Wizntizer, Packer, August, & Burkey, 1984). Although the mortality associated with these complications is quite high, the surviving children are likely to recover with significant neurological impairments. Estimates of the frequency of neurological complications in SCT patients have ranged from 11% to as high as 70%, depending on survey methods (Graus et al., 1996; Meyers et al., 1994; Padovan et al., 1998; Patchell et al., 1985). However, these surveys have generally involved only adult patients or mixed adult/pediatric populations, and no surveys have been reported focusing solely on children. One of the earliest reports of late effects of SCT on the CNS in children indicated an incidence of leukoencephalopathy in 7% of patients, but this occurred only in those patients who had both previous CNS therapy and total body irradiation (TBI; Thompson, Sanders, Flournoy, Buckner, & Thomas, 1986).

More recent studies that have included new-generation diagnostic imaging have indicated the presence of abnormalities on magnetic resonance imaging (MRI) in as many as two thirds of survivors (Coley, Jager, Szydlo, & Goldman, 1999; Padovan et al., 1998). The most common findings involve white matter lesions or mild cerebral atrophy. These abnormalities have not generally been associated with the use of TBI but relate to the occurrence of graft-versus-host disease (GvHD), particularly the use of corticosteroids and cyclosporine for the treatment of GvHD (Coley, Porter, Calamante, Chong, & Connelly, 1999; Pace, Slovis, Kelly, & Abella, 1995; Padovan et al., 1998;). Again, these studies involved primarily adult patients, and it appears that the incidence of abnormal imaging may be much higher in adults than in children. Moreover, the clinical significance of these imaging abnormalities is not clear. For example, in one study involving only adults, the incidence of abnormalities in MRI exam (65%) was much higher than the incidence of cognitive deficits, and there was no significant relationship between MRI findings and cognitive function (Padovan et al., 1998).

Beyond specific neurological complications, research has focused on the risk for global cognitive and academic deficits in pediatric survivors of SCT. The concern regarding potential cognitive declines resulting from SCT has been based partly on extrapolation from studies of acute lymphocytic leukemia survivors who received CNS therapy because, until recently, empiric data from pediatric SCT survivors have been limited (Phipps & Barclay, 1996). Survivors of SCT are thought to be at risk for cognitive deficits as a result of their exposure to numerous potentially neurotoxic agents.

Among the agents used in pretransplant conditioning, TBI has been the primary focus of those assessing neurocognitive sequelae, but other cytotoxic conditioning agents, such as busulfan and other high-dose ablative chemotherapies, are potentially neurotoxic as well (Chou et al., 1996; Miale, Sirithorn, & Ahmed, 1995; Peper et al., 1993). CNS toxicities also are associated with agents (e.g., cyclosporine) commonly used for the prophylaxis or treatment of GvHD (Coley, Porter, et al., 1999; Pace et al., 1995; Padovan et al., 2001; Reece et al., 1991). More speculative is the possibility of direct effects of GvHD on the CNS (Garrick, 2000; Padovan et al., 2001; Rouah, Gruber, Shearer, Armstrong, & Hawkins, 1988).

Study of neurocognitive and academic outcomes in pediatric SCT has been hindered by a number of methodological challenges, most notably the relatively small samples of survivors at any single institution. To more comprehensively and definitively address these questions, multisite studies are in order, but to date none has been reported. Thus, while the number of published studies addressing neurocognitive outcomes in SCT is growing, most continue to be limited by small sample sizes or other methodological difficulties, such as retrospective designs.

The findings reported thus far have been somewhat contradictory, although a consensus is beginning to emerge. A few studies have indicated declines in cognitive or academic function following SCT (Cool, 1996; Kramer, Crittenden, DeSantes, & Cowan, 1997; Smedler & Bolme, 1995), but a somewhat larger number of studies have reported normal neurodevelopment, with no evidence of declines in cognitive function (Arvidson, Kihlgren, Hall, & Lonnerholm, 1999; Daniel-Llach et al., 2001; Kupst et al., 2002; Phipps, Dunavant, Srivastava, Bowman, & Mulhern, 2000; Pot-Mees, 1989; Simms, Kazak, Golumb, Goldwein, & Bunin, 2002).

Our interpretation is that many of the divergent findings in the literature may be associated with age effects within and between cohorts, and that with due consideration of age effects, a relatively coherent picture of the neurocognitive late effects of SCT can be drawn. A summary of the published literature is provided in table 5-1. Studies are presented in chronological order of publication and with a single entry per cohort; that is, multiple publications over time from ongoing longitudinal studies are included based on the most recent publication.

The earliest published reports indicated no evidence of cognitive deficits following SCT. Kalieta et al. (Kaleita, Shields, Tesler, & Feig, 1989) documented essentially normal development 2–6 years post-SCT in four children transplanted as infants: two with leukemia who were conditioned with single-dose TBI (750 cGy) and two with aplastic anemia conditioned without TBI.

Pot-Mees (1989) reported on a group of 43 children who were followed for a year post-SCT and a subset of 23 for whom pre- and post-SCT cognitive evaluations were obtained. No significant changes were found in IQ scores post-SCT.

The first study suggestive of possible post-SCT cognitive deficits was reported by Smedler, Ringden, Bergman, and Bolme (1990). They divided their initial cohort of 32 survivors into three groups based on their age at SCT: younger than 3 years, 3–11 years, and 12–17 years. They reported normal neurodevelopment post-SCT in the group 12–17 years old. The group aged 3–11 years old showed some suggestions of difficulties, particularly in the area of perceptual and fine motor skills. However, the youngest age group demonstrated clear delays in sensorimotor development.

Subsequent reports from this group on a slightly larger cohort continued to confirm this picture and to point to TBI as the crucial determinant of adverse cognitive outcomes (Smedler & Bolme, 1995; Smedler, Nilson, & Bolm, 1995). Of 10 children transplanted at younger than 3 years, all 8 who received TBI showed some evidence of developmental delay, whereas the 2 children who did not receive TBI showed normal development (Smedler & Bolme, 1995).

The age-related findings reported by Smedler and colleagues presaged the later results from larger cohorts and help to explain the apparent discrepant findings between two of the largest prospective series of neurocognitive outcome in SCT survivors to date. Kramer and colleagues (Kramer, Crittenden, Halberg, Wara, & Cowan, 1992; Kramer et al., 1997), in a well-designed, prospective longitudinal study, reported on outcomes of 67 children assessed 1 year post-SCT and a subset of 26 of these children who were reassessed at 3 years post-SCT. They reported a significant decline in IQ (a mean change of 6 points, 0.4 standard deviation units) in their cohort at 1 year post-SCT. There were no further declines in the subset followed to 3 years post-SCT, but the deficits were maintained across time. In contrast, our group (Phipps et al., 1995, 2000) found no significant declines in global IQ or academic achievement in 102 survivors assessed at 1 year post-SCT or in a subset of 54 survivors followed through 3 years post-SCT.

The discrepancies between these studies can be explained in large part by the differential age of the two cohorts. The Kramer et al. (1992, 1997) cohort had a mean age of 45 months compared with 10.5 years in our cohort. Within our cohort, the subset of children under 6 years showed declines comparable to those reported by Kramer's group (Phipps et al., 2000). In fact, our youngest patients (<3 years) showed an even greater decline than that reported by Kramer et al.; moreover, their cognitive function continued to decline through 3 years. In

**Table 5-1.** Studies of Neurocognitive Outcomes in Survivors of Pediatric Stem Cell Transplantation

| Methods | | Findings | | |
|---|---|---|---|---|
| *Study* | *Subjects* | *Design/Measures* | *Results* | *Comments* |
| Kaleita et al., 1989 | Children < 2 years old; $n = 4$ | Prospective; standardized measures of infant development administered pre- and 2–6 years post-SCT | Normal neurodevelopment in all cases; no change over time | First cases reported; 2 infants received TBI, 2 did not |
| Pot-Mees, 1989 | Children aged 5–18 years; $n = 23$ (from cohort of 75) | Prospective; standardized measures of IQ, academic achievement given pre-, 6 months, and 1 year post SCT; two comparison groups | No changes in IQ or academic achievement at 1 year post-SCT; SCT group functioned lower than control group *before* SCT | Included some patients with genetic storage disorders, which makes results more difficult to interpret |
| Smedler et al., 1990, 1995; Smedler & Bolme, 1995 | $N = 36$ in three groups; < 3 years at SCT, $n = 10$; 3–11 years, $n = 15$; 12–17 years, $n = 11$ | No pre-SCT assessment but longitudinal survey of survivors 1–6 years post-SCT; donors as controls; standardized measures of development, IQ, and neuropsychological function | No deficits found in oldest group; group aged 3–11 years showed trends toward declines in perceptual, fine-motor, and verbal skills; in group < 3 years, all treated with TBI showed moderate developmental delay | 2 children < 3 years transplanted for severe aplastic anemia without TBI showed normal development |
| McGuire, Sanders, Hill, Buckner, & Sullivan, 1991 | Children through age 18 years at SCT; $N = 178$ | Retrospective, cross-sectional survey; compared 110 patients assessed pre-SCT to 68 patients assessed 1–12 years post-SCT on standardized measures of IQ, achievement | No differences between pre- and post-SCT groups on any measures; across all patients, performance related to total amount of radiation therapy, age at first RT, and time elapsed since radiation therapy | Published only as abstract |
| Kramer et al., 1992, 1997 | Children < 18 years but with predominantly young (<6 years) population; $n = 67$ assessed at 1 year post-SCT and $n = 26$ at 3 years post-SCT (from cohort of 137 assessed pre-SCT) | Prospective, longitudinal design; standardized measures of infant development, IQ, obtained pre-SCT and at 1 and 3 years post-SCT | Significant decline in IQ at 1 year post-SCT; no relationship of post-SCT function with diagnosis, type of SCT, TBI, age, or gender. Deficits maintained at 3 years post-SCT, but no further declines | Very young sample, with mean age 45 months at SCT; restricted age range limits ability to detect age effects |
| Phipps et al., 1995, 2000 | Children through 18 years; $n = 102$ assessed at 1 year post-SCT and $n = 54$ assessed at 3 years post-SCT (from cohort of 260 assessed pre-SCT) | Prospective, longitudinal design; standardized measures of IQ, achievement, and neuropsychological function obtained pre-SCT and 1, 3, and 5 years post-SCT | In cohort as a whole, no significant declines in IQ or achievement at 1 or 3 years post-SCT; age a significant predictor of outcome, with patients < 3 years showing evidence of decline over time; TBI not related to outcome | Largest prospective study published to date; adequate power to detect small (3 IQ points) effects; concluded that SCT ± TBI entails minimal risk of neurocognitive sequelae in patients $\geq$ 6 years, but younger children may be at some risk |

| | | | | |
|---|---|---|---|---|
| Cool, 1996 | Children through 18 years; $n = ?$; maximum $n = 45$ (of cohort of 76 assessed pre-SCT) | Prospective, longitudinal study with pre-SCT assessment, and yearly follow-up through 4 years post-SCT; standardized measures of IQ, achievement, neuropsychological function; brain computed tomographic scans obtained on some survivors | At pre-SCT evaluation, children already showing some deficits in IQ and achievement related to prior CNS therapy; overall, global IQ stable at 1 year post-SCT, some trends toward decline in academic achievement | Author concluded that by 4 years post-SCT there is evidence of declines in IQ, achievement, attention, memory, and fine-motor skills; however, evidence from data is not persuasive; presented as a series of studies, which makes interpretation difficult |
| Simms et al., 1998, 2002 | $N = 47$ children assessed at pre-, 1 year, and 2 years post-SCT (from cohort of 238 assessed pre-SCT) | Prospective, longitudinal study with pre-SCT and 1, 2, and 5 years post-SCT assessments; standardized measures of IQ, achievement, and neuropsychological function | No sigificant changes in any cognitive or academic achievement measures at either 1 or 2 years post-SCT; no difference between TBI and non-TBI regimens; children < 3 years showed lower pre-SCT functioning and subseqent decline post-SCT | No evidence of any decline in function but possible risks for youngest children; despite absence of declines, evidence that parents perceive difficulties in school functioning |
| Arvidson et al., 1999 | Children < 18 years; $N = 26$ | Cross-sectional/longitudinal design; children assessed at various intervals 2–11 years post-SCT using measures of global IQ and neuropsychological function | Global IQ in normal range and generally unaffected over time; slight increase in problems in "executive function," attention, and memory; no difference between TBI and non-TBI regimens; age at diagnosis and time since SCT predictive of outcome | All patients underwent autologous transplant, but the majority conditioned with TBI in a single 7.5-Gy dose |
| Daniel Llach et al., 2001 | Children aged 4–15 years; $N = 22$ (from cohort of 54) | Prospective; children assessed pre- and 1 year post-SCT on global IQ | No significant changes in pre–post comparisons; scores in the average range | Children scoring < 100 pre-SCT showed gains, while those scoring > 100 pre-SCT showed declines; interpreted as reflective of anxiety effects |
| Kupst et al., 2002 | Children through 18 years assessed pre-SCT and at 1 year ($N = 153$) and 2 years ($N = 70$) post-SC from original cohort of 377 | Prospective, longitudinal design with standardized cognitive measures | Stable function through 2 years post-SCT; no evidence of decline in younger (< 3 years) group of children; primary predictor of cognitive outcome was pre-SCT function | Also demonstrated low prevalence of social and behavioral problems |

contrast to the report of Smedler et al. (1995), in neither the Kramer et al. nor the Phipps et al. studies was there any apparent effect of the use of TBI. In the Phipps et al. (2000) cohort, the TBI and no TBI groups were large enough to detect relatively small effects, and no such effects were apparent.

The findings from our cohort, in light of the previously published literature, led us to conclude that SCT, even with TBI, poses low-to-minimal risk for late cognitive and academic deficits in patients who are at least 6 years old at the time of transplant. For patients aged 5 years and younger, particularly for those younger than 3 years, the risk of cognitive impairment may be increased, and this appears to be the case regardless of whether TBI is used in conditioning.

The results of recently reported studies have continued to support our conclusions. Simms and colleagues (Simms et al., 2002; Sims, Kazak, Gannon, Goldwein, & Bunin, 1998) reported on a cohort of 47 patients followed prospectively through 2 years post-SCT and found normal cognitive function and academic achievement, with no evidence of decline over this time frame. However, the subset of 11 children in their cohort who were younger than 3 years at the time of SCT showed both lower pre-SCT developmental functioning and subsequent declines in developmental indices post-SCT (Simms et al., 2002).

Kupst et al. (2002) reported on a cohort of 153 children who underwent cognitive-developmental assessment pre-SCT and 1 year post-SCT and a subset of 70 who were assessed 2 years post-SCT. They reported a clear pattern of stability in IQ and developmental quotients over time (Kupst et al., 2002). In their cohort, the subgroup of children younger than 3 years did not show any greater evidence of decline, and the strongest predictor of posttransplant cognitive functioning was pre-SCT functioning (Kupst et al., 2002). Likewise, in smaller studies, Arvidson et al. (1999) and Daniel-Llach et al. (2001) have reported similar normal functioning and absence of declines over time in SCT survivors.

In summary, despite a substantial incidence of specific CNS insults and studies documenting high levels of abnormalities on diagnostic imaging, psychometric measures have generally shown survivors of SCT to be within normal limits in cognitive and academic functioning and with relatively stable performance over time. Children who are younger at the time of transplant appear to be at somewhat increased risk for cognitive impairment, while the risks for those who are above the age of 6 years at the time of SCT appear minimal. This remains a tentative conclusion that should be viewed cautiously and with a major caveat relating to the length of follow-up. No study has yet reported data beyond 3 years post-SCT. However, in our cohort, we currently have over 70 survivors who have been assessed at 5 years or more beyond transplant, and the picture of stability continues to hold (unpublished data, 2005). In the near future, additional reports from our cohort, along with those of Kramer, Simms, Kupst, and others, may allow for a more definitive confirmation of our conclusions.

## Patient Adjustment and Psychosocial Functioning

The earliest articles describing patient response to SCT focused on the acute effects of transplant hospitalization (Gardner, August, & Githens, 1977; Patenaude, Szymanski, & Rappeport, 1979; Pfefferbaum, Lindamood, & Wiley, 1977). This was understandable because the newness of the procedure and the high mortality involved at that time implied there were few long-term survivors to study. The small numbers precluded more formal, empiric study, but rather these reports organized the anecdotal data to provide a qualitative picture of the responses of patients, families, and staff to the unique challenges of SCT.

These investigations presented a fairly problematic picture of the pediatric SCT patient, suggesting high levels of affective disturbance, with increased anxiety and depression; overdependence associated with feelings of helplessness; anger toward staff and parents; reduced tolerance for medical procedures; and periodic refusal to cooperate. All stressed the need for intensive psychosocial intervention as part of the SCT program. These articles appear to have had a significant influence on clinical practice because an emphasis on psychosocial support became a standard component of pediatric transplant programs.

Perhaps owing to the benefits of the comprehensive psychosocial support programs, subsequent empiric study of patient response to transplant suggested a less-pathological picture, although not without some evidence of adjustment difficulties. In the initial report of our longitudinal study, we found significant declines in the social competence, self-esteem, and general emotional well-being of survivors from the pretransplant assessment to follow-up at 6 months after SCT (Phipps et al., 1995).

On the Child Behavior Checklist (CBCL; Achenbach & Edelbrock, 1983), children undergoing SCT demonstrated somewhat low scores on the Social Competence domain at the time of admission for transplant and showed significant decline in this domain in the period following transplant. Given the enforced isolation many patients must live with during this period, this finding might be more accurately interpreted as a decline in social opportunity rather than a true decline in social competence. However, subsequent disruption in the social functioning of survivors has also been noted in studies using peer report.

Vannatta and colleagues (Vannatta et al., 1998) found that survivors of SCT were rated by peers as more socially isolated and having fewer friends. They also found that SCT survivors were perceived by peers as less physically competent, less attractive, and less athletically skilled than their healthy peers. These outcomes were not observed by self- or teacher report but suggest potential problems with peer relations that could disrupt subsequent social and emotional development. These findings also point to significant discrepancies among peer, teacher, and self-reports. Such discrepancies are hardly unique to SCT, or even to the pediatric cancer setting, but provide an additional methodological challenge in this area. Using parent report, we found that with longer follow-up after the period of enforced isolation is lifted, there was a gradual increase in CBCL Social Competence scores back to baseline levels (Phipps, unpublished data). A similar pattern was noted in the report of Kupst and colleagues (Kupst et al., 2002).

In contrast to the Social Competence findings, children undergoing SCT showed normal levels of behavior problems on the CBCL Internalizing and Externalizing Behavior Problem domains at the time of admission, and problem behaviors decreased significantly at 6 months posttransplant (Phipps et al., 1995). At the time, we interpreted these findings to indicate that the SCT procedure leads to a diminution of *all* behavior because of both the enforced isolation and the physical debilitation of the patient. This would then lead to improvement on measures consisting entirely of negative behavior items. Other SCT investigators using the CBCL have subsequently reported similar findings (Barrera et al., 2000; Kupst et al., 2002).

However, using self-report, we found significant declines in self-concept and emotional well-being in the same period following transplant (Phipps et al., 1995; Phipps & Mulhern, 1995). Curiously, the scores on the Piers-Harris Self-Concept scale remained within normal limits despite the significant decline because pretransplant scores were indicative of exceptionally high functioning. This is consistent with studies indicating that self-reports of children with cancer tend to portray exceptionally high levels of functioning and low levels of distress (Canning, Canning, & Boyce, 1992; Phipps & Srivastiva, 1997; Phipps, Steele, Hall, & Leigh, 2001). From this perspective, it is the decline in self-esteem over time that is most concerning rather than the absolute value of the measures. These declines, coupled with findings of social disruptions and problems with peer relations, suggest the presence of some ongoing vulnerabilities in the SCT survivors that call for ongoing scrutiny and further longitudinal study.

The declines in social functioning, self-esteem, and emotional well-being that were observed at 6 months post-SCT follow-up led us to return our focus to the acute phase of transplant hospitalization and the period immediately following. Prior to our work, most of the studies addressing acute issues involved only adult patients, with the few pediatric studies involving very small samples (Gunter, Karle, Werning, & Klingbiel, 1999; Rodrigue et al., 1995). A prospective study of adult patients that involved assessment on multiple occasions during the first year following BMT reported a moderate, transient increase in symptoms of anxiety and depression during the acute isolation period, which then declined and stabilized by 4 months post-BMT (Hjermstad et al., 1999).

This pattern differs from the more commonly depicted "trajectory to recovery" following transplant, in which adult patients have been reported to show gains in functioning for up to 2 years post-SCT before leveling off (Andrykowski et al., 1995; McQuellon et al., 1998). Perhaps there are two separate trajectories, one reflecting acute processes and mood disturbances specific to the transplant procedure, which recovers more quickly, and a second trajectory related to more global QOL, which shows a longer time to recovery. The available data from children were too limited to draw any such conclusions, although a short-term prospective study by Rodrigue and colleagues (1995) showed results comparable to those of Hjermstad et al. (1999), with elevations in ratings of pain and anxiety at 2 weeks post-SCT that subsequently declined through week +5. Given the limited data on acute effects of SCT in children, we undertook a major prospective, longitudinal study designed to address some of the shortcomings of prior research, including small sample size and a limited number of observations across the transplant course.

A necessary first step for the shift in focus to acute phase issues was the development of reliable, valid, and clinically relevant measures of patient functioning during the acute setting of SCT hospitalization and thereafter. Because appropriate measures were not available, we developed a set of instruments to measure acute BMT outcomes, known as the BASES (Behavioral, Affective, and Somatic Experiences Scale; Phipps, Dunavant, Jayawardene, & Srivastava, 1999; Phipps, Hinds, Channel, & Bell, 1994). These scales were conceptualized as measures of health-related QOL for acute settings, which could serve as short-term SCT outcome measures, a prerequisite for the institution of intervention studies.

The BASES scales were developed initially as a nurse report instrument. A series of pilot studies resulted in a 38-item version, with five subscales: Somatic Distress, Mood Disturbance, Compliance, Quality of Interactions, and Activity. A parent report version (BASES-P) was created that was essentially identical to the nurse report form with a few items reworded, and an abbreviated child report version (BASES-C) was subsequently developed that provided scores on the same five subscales as the parent and nurse forms (Phipps et al., 1999). These scales were then used as the primary outcomes in a "natural history" study of children undergoing BMT (Phipps, Phipps, Dunavant, Garvie, Lensing, & Rai, 2002; Phipps, Dunavant, Lensing, & Rai, 2002).

This natural history study used a prospective, longitudinal, repeated measures design. Patients scheduled to undergo SCT were recruited prior to their admission date. At that time, we identified a "resident parent," that is, the parent who was to be physically with the patient most frequently during the transplant hospitalization. Prior to admission, patients received an abbreviated neuropsychological screening and completed a battery of self-report measures. On admission for BMT, BASES data were obtained weekly from parent and patients aged 5 years and older. A weekly assessment schedule was followed through week +6, followed by monthly assessments through month +6. This repeated measures design allows for tracking of trajectories over the course of the acute phase of transplant on BASES subscales or on any specific symptom (e.g., nausea, vomiting). Nurse report data (BASES-N) were obtained from day shift staff three times per week, beginning at admission. Nurse observations were discontinued once the patient was discharged from their initial BMT hospitalization.

Longitudinal data were obtained on a total of 153 patients/parents. Patients ranged in age from younger than 1 year to 20 years (mean 8.8 years), and 54% of patients were male. Approximately two thirds of the patients were transplanted for leukemia, 21% for solid tumors, and 17% for nonmalignant disorders. Patients underwent allogeneic transplant in 67% of cases and autologous BMT in 33%. Of those undergoing allogeneic BMT, 28% involved a matched sibling donor, 11% a mismatched family donor, and 60% an unrelated donor. TBI was used in 57% of cases.

Prior to examining outcomes, multiple methods were used to assess cross-informant consistency on the BASES scales. The identical item format of the BASES-P and BASES-N allows for calculation of a correlation coefficient between paired observations across all items of the scale. We examined paired observations on day 0 and day +14. On day 0, the median correlation $r_s$ of paired parent-nurse observations was 0.74, and on day +14 the median correlation was 0.69. To assess child report, total scores on each of the five BASES subscales were obtained, and these were correlated with the comparable subscales from the BASES-P and BASES-N. These findings are summarized in table 5-2. Although correlations were generally in the low-to-moderate range, most were statistically significant, including all parent-child correlations.

To assess patient response to SCT, we conducted a series of repeated measures analyses on the BASES subscales. Clear patterns of change over time were found on measures from all respondents. On

**Table 5-2.** Cross-Informant Correlations on BASES Subscales

| | *Parent-Nurse* | *Parent-Child* | *Nurse-Child* |
|---|---|---|---|
| Somatic Distress | $0.62^{***}$ | $0.57^{***}$ | $0.43^{**}$ |
| Mood Disturbance | $0.25^{*}$ | $0.35^{*}$ | 0.07 |
| Compliance | $0.24^{*}$ | $0.29^{*}$ | $0.36^{*}$ |
| Quality of Interaction | 0.19 | $0.49^{***}$ | 0.14 |
| Activity | $0.45^{***}$ | $0.43^{**}$ | $0.45^{**}$ |

$r_s$, $^*p<.05$; $^{**}p<.01$; $^{***}p<.001$.

the BASES-P and BASES-C, all subscales showed highly significant effects of time (all $p$ values < .0001). On nurse report, somewhat smaller effects were seen.

In addition to the BASES subscales, we also assessed change on individual items selected a priori from the BASES-N and BASES-P. All of the individual items analyzed showed significant variations over time. These data may be best appreciated graphically because the repeated measures format is particularly suited to depicting trajectories of symptomatology over time. These trajectories indicate distinct patterns of change over the course of the acute transplant period by all respondents.

In figure 5-1, it can be seen that trajectories by parent and child report are similar. Most subscales and items show an increase in distress following admission, reaching a peak in the week after SCT conditioning, followed by a pronounced decline back to or below admission levels by week +4 or +5, followed by a second decline to a presumed baseline level at months 4–6. It appears that children undergoing SCT enter the hospital with an already heightened level of distress that increases dramatically following conditioning and peaks approximately 1 week posttransplant. The trajectories indicate that, despite a standard program of supportive care, a considerable amount of distress is still experienced by patients during the acute phase of BMT, involving not only somatic discomfort, but also disturbance in mood and disruption in behavioral functions. Whether we quantify this distress in terms of peak levels experienced, change from baseline, or some function of area under the curve, there is clearly considerable room for improvement in supportive care, which suggests the need for new programs of intervention.

We also examined whether patients differing in medical or demographic characteristics (e.g., allogeneic vs. autologous SCT, age, gender, socioeconomic status [SES]) or baseline psychological measures would differ significantly in acute phase responses as measured by BASES trajectories. Many of these findings have already been reported (Phipps, Dunavant, Lensing, et al., 2002), and we present here just two examples of such analyses.

Differences in overall somatic distress according to type of SCT are illustrated on the left side of figure 5-2. Patients undergoing autologous SCT experienced significantly lower levels of Somatic Distress (by parent, child, and nurse report) than those undergoing allogeneic transplant with either a matched sibling donor or unrelated donor. The trajectories on the right side of figure 5-2 illustrate differences in somatic distress as a function of patient age. The youngest children (<6 years) experienced the lowest Somatic Distress, with adolescents experiencing the highest levels, and the group 6–12 years old had an intermediate level (figure 5-2). Similar findings were obtained by both parent and nurse report.

In summary, children undergoing SCT experience transient elevations in somatic distress and mood disturbance during the acute phase of transplant. Distress tends to peak in the early weeks following the transplant and then resolves fairly rapidly, returning to near-baseline levels within 3–4 months. As survivors reach 6 months to a year posttransplant and begin to reintegrate into their normal lifestyles, they show some mild perturbations in their self-concept and social functioning. Rarely do these disturbances reach pathological levels, but they reflect vulnerabilities in the SCT survivor population that call for continued surveillance over time. How the transient acute phase distress relates to the subsequent mild adjustment disturbances has not been clearly delineated and will be the focus of future research efforts.

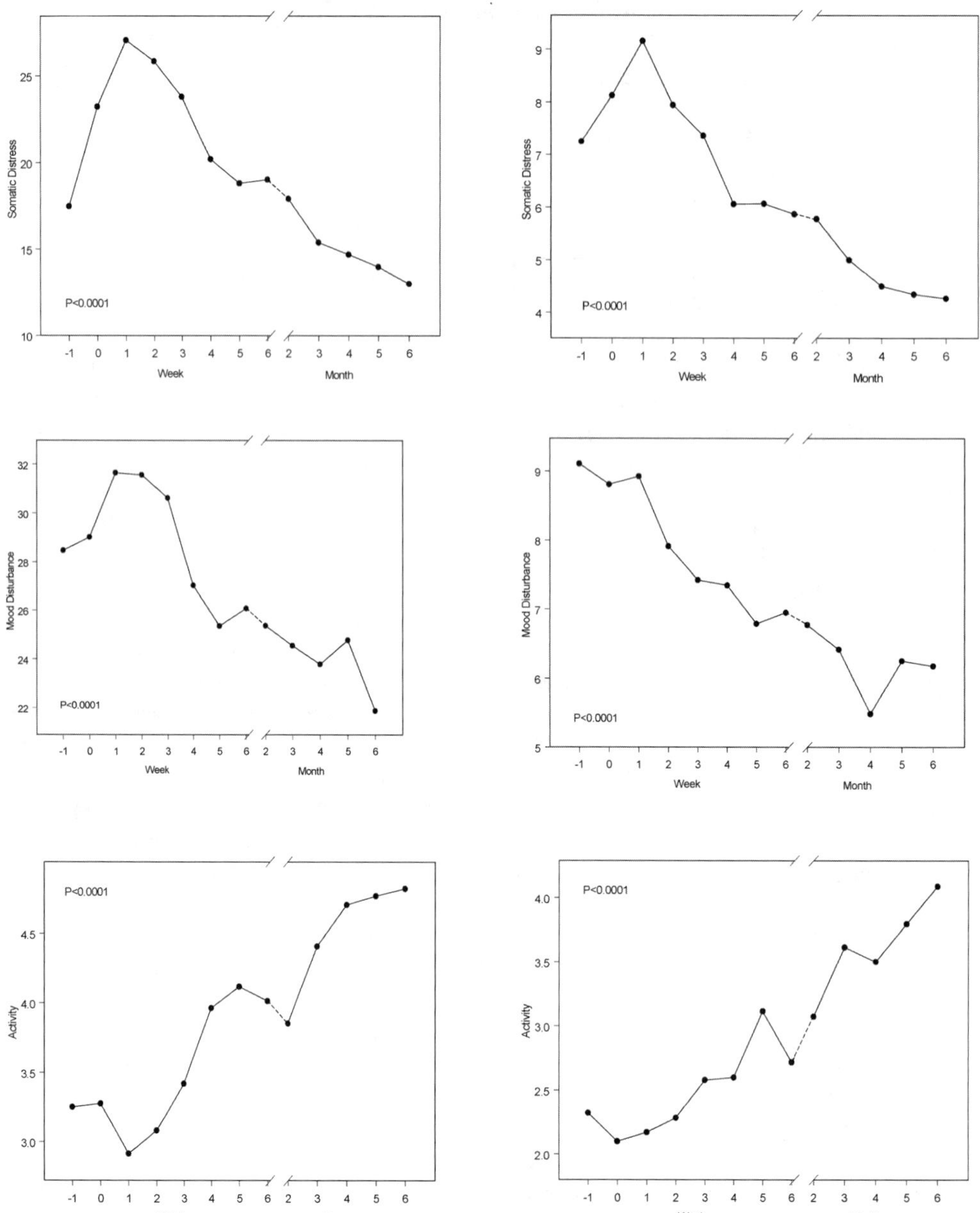


**Figure 5-1.** Trajectories of somatic distress, mood disturbance, and activity by parent and child report. Parent report is on the right; child report on the left.

## Parental Adjustment to SCT

Although the responses of the child undergoing SCT have been, appropriately, the focus of some research, there has also been considerable focus on the response of parents to the stresses of SCT. Parental response to SCT has been of interest not only because high levels of stress and psychological symptomatology have been reported in parents of children with cancer (Barakat et al., 1997; Brown et al., 1993; Dahlquist et al., 1993; Kazak et al., 1997; Sawyer, Antoniou, Toogood, Rice, & Baghurst, 1993), but also because of research demonstrating a strong relationship between parental mental health and adjustment to illness among those children (Blotcky, Raczynski,

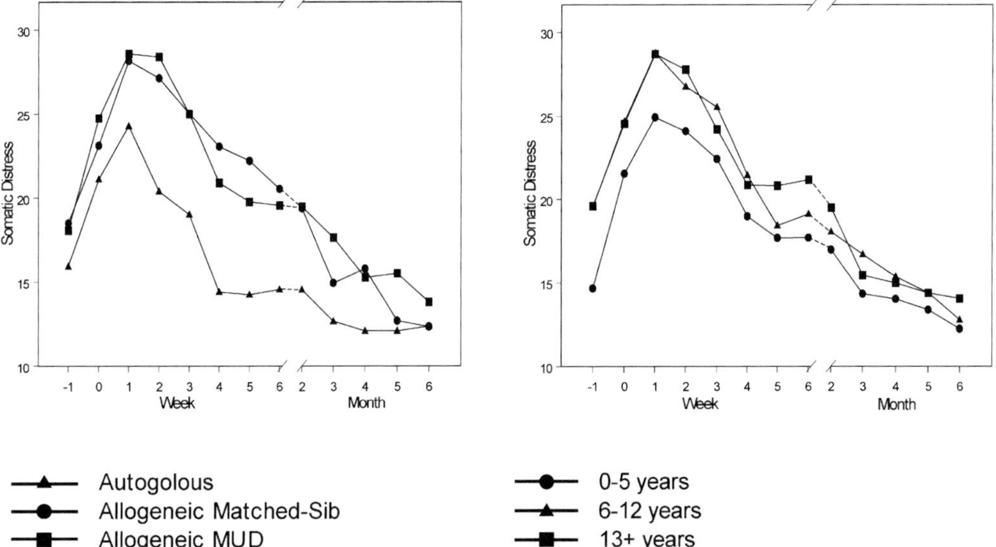


**Figure 5-2.** Left: Somatic distress trajectories by transplant type, indicating that patients undergoing autologous transplant experience significantly less distress across the acute transplant period than those undergoing allogeneic transplant with either a matched sibling or unrelated donor. Right: Somatic distress trajectories by age, illustrating that younger children experience less distress than school-aged children and adolescents.

Gurwitch, & Smith, 1985; Brown et al., 1993; Dockerty, Williams, McGee, & Skegg, 2000; Dolgin & Phipps, 1995; Sahler et al., 2002). Moreover, there is some evidence suggesting that parental and family factors may be particularly important predictors of child adjustment to the challenges of SCT (Phipps & Mulhern, 1995).

Many studies of parental response to transplant have been limited to assessment of parental functioning prior to or at the time of admission to SCT (Dermatis & Lesko, 1990; Kronenberger et al., 1998; Manne et al., 2001; Rodrigue et al., 1996); some have focused on the post-SCT functioning in parents of SCT survivors (Heiney, Newberg, Meyers, & Bergman, 1994; Sormanti, Dungan, & Reiker, 1994). A rather wide range of outcomes has been reported, from those that indicate high levels of distress and psychopathology (Dermatis & Lesko, 1990; Manne et al., 2001) to those showing very low levels of stress (Streisand et al., 2000).

In one of the first empiric studies on the topic, Dermatis and Lesko (1990) reported significantly elevated levels of psychological distress in more than 50% of parents assessed after the process of consenting for their child's transplant. Manne et al. (2001) conducted psychiatric interviews using the Structured Clinical Interview for DSD-IV (Gibbon, Spitzer, & Williams, 1996) with mothers of children at the time of their admission for transplant and found that more than 20% met the American Psychiatric Association's *Diagnostic and Statistical Manual of Mental Disorders* (*DSM-IV*) criteria for diagnosis of major depression, panic disorder, or generalized anxiety disorder. A subsequent report from that cohort also indicated elevated levels of posttraumatic stress disorder (PTSD; Manne et al., 2002).

In contrast, Barrera et al. (2000), using the Beck Depression Inventory (Beck, 1978), reported low levels of depressive symptoms in mothers at the time of their child's admission for transplant, with only 8% reaching a clinical cutoff for mild depression. This group did report mildly elevated levels of anxiety at the time of admission for SCT, but these had resolved to normative levels when reassessed at 6 months posttransplant (Barrera et al., 2000). Even more striking were the findings of Streisand et al. (2000) that mothers of children undergoing BMT reported significantly less perceived stress and parenting stress than normative samples, both at admission and at day +21 post-SCT.

Some of the discrepancies in the literature may relate to the timing of assessments because the few studies that have included assessments at more than one time point have shown significant changes over time (Barrera et al., 2000; Manne et al., 2002; Streisand et al., 2000). In the study of Manne et al., levels of both depressive symptoms and anxiety declined from admission to 6 months posttransplant. Similarly, in the Barrera et al. study, symptoms of anxiety declined significantly from pre-SCT to 6 months posttransplant, although a measure of depressive symptoms was unchanged. The declines in distress observed at 6 months posttransplant may occur much earlier than that. In the only study to include repeated assessments during this time period, Streisand et al. assessed 22 mothers of children undergoing SCT prior to admission and then obtained stress ratings weekly from admission through week +3. Stress was highest pretransplant and declined significantly from admission through week +3. Although the overall levels of stress were quite low in that study, the authors concluded that the pre-SCT period is the most difficult for parents.

Another possible explanation for some discrepancies in the literature may relate to the philosophical approach to assessment taken in the research design, that is, whether intended primarily to identify "caseness" in a psychopathology model or, alternately, to evaluate more normative responses in an adjustment or stress-and-coping model. These differing models also tend to rely on different methods of assessment, with the use of structured diagnostic interviews in a pathology approach and questionnaires assessing levels of symptomatology in general adjustment studies.

For example, the Manne et al. (2001) study was designed to ascertain the incidence of specific psychiatric disorders, and the outcome indicated a high level of problems. Other studies designed to assess issues of adjustment, and predictors of such, have reported more benign outcomes (Rodrigue et al., 1996; Streisand et al., 2000). Interestingly, in a subsequent report, when they had accrued a larger cohort for their study, Manne and colleagues (2003) reported only mildly elevated levels in depression scores at baseline that declined to normative values at 3 and 6 months posttransplant. That report was focused on maternal coping strategies and how these predicted depressive symptoms rather than diagnostic classification. Although there are advantages and disadvantages to either the pathological approach or stress-and-coping models, the apparent transience of the parents' psychological symptoms raises some question about the utility of psychopathological labels.

A few studies have identified factors that are associated with parental adjustment to the stresses of SCT. Kronenberger et al. (1998) found that avoidant and disengagement forms of coping were associated with maternal depression at the time of admission for SCT, but other personality, family environment, or social variables were not. Manne et al. (2002) found that maternal symptoms of anxiety and depression measured at the time of admission for transplant were associated with symptoms of PTSD at 6 months post-SCT. They also found that mothers who perceived more criticism from spouses or other family members at admission for BMT reported higher levels of PTSD symptoms at 6 months post-SCT. In a subsequent report, Manne et al. (2003) found that the coping behaviors of acceptance and humor were associated with declines in depression symptoms from baseline to 6 months post-SCT, while planning and substance use were associated with increases in depressive symptoms. The major impediment to this research has been sample size considerations. Aside from the Manne cohort that contained substantial numbers of participants (DuHamel et al., 2004; Manne et al., 2001, 2002, 2003), most prior studies have involved samples too small to reliably examine these associations.

As part of our natural history study described previously, we also examined changes in parental distress levels over the course of the acute phase of SCT (Phipps, Dunavant, Lensing, & Rai, 2004a, 2004b). We again used the construct of resident parent. Although we anticipated that the majority would be mothers, this group was larger than we anticipated, with better than 90% of the resident parents biological mothers.

Measures for assessing parental functioning across the acute phase of transplant were chosen based on three factors. First, we wished to depict the magnitude of symptoms of distress rather than specific diagnostic cutoffs because we assumed that the incidence of psychopathology would be relatively low, but that there would be considerable variability in levels of distress both between parents and across time. Second, because we planned to obtain measurements repeatedly, we were interested in brief measures that could be completed quickly and easily to reduce participant burden. Finally, we felt that the distress of parents in this setting would reflect a complex and dynamic composite of factors that would be difficult to capture in a single measure. Thus, we chose a triad of brief instruments assessing mood disturbance, perceived stress, and magnitude of caregiver burden, using a short-form of the Profile of Mood States scales (POMS; McNair, Lorr, & Droppleman, 1971), the Perceived Stress Scale (PSS; Cohen, Kamarck, & Mermelstein, 1983), and an adaptation of the Caregiver Burden Scale (CBS; Poulshock & Deimling, 1984). Not only does each measure of this triad provide a unique outcome, but there also is considerable overlap between them. The median intercorrelations of the measures across the study (representing over 1,100 observations) were POMS-PSS, $r = .78$; POMS-CBS, $r = .62$; PSS-CBS, $r = .66$. Given this level of common variance, we focused on the simple sum of the scores on the three instruments, which we labeled global parental distress.

Consistent with some of the previously reported findings, parents demonstrated modest but significant elevations in distress, particularly during the early period from admission through week +3 (Phipps et al., 2004a). Elevations in parental distress were transient and were largely resolved by 4–6 months post-BMT. This again may be best appreciated graphically, and a depiction of the global parental distress trajectory is illustrated in figure 5-3. Parental distress was unrelated to child age, gender, diagnosis, or type of transplant but was significantly related to parental SES. Parents from lower SES backgrounds reported greater levels of distress throughout the BMT process.

We also examined the association between parental distress (as measured by our triad of instruments) and child distress (as measured by the BASES scales). Correlations were examined concurrently (i.e., both observations were obtained on the same day) and were generally moderate. The mean correlations across the 13 observation points were parental global distress with Somatic Distress from BASES-P, $r = .36$ (median $r = .41$); with Mood Disturbance from BASES-P, $r = .49$ (median $r = .51$); and with child-reported distress from BASES-C, $r = .42$ (median $= .40$).

In addition to assessing correlations, we examined the relationship of child distress measured at admission for BMT to the trajectory of parent distress over the transplant process and, conversely, how parent distress at the time of admission for BMT is predictive of child distress trajectories over time. To facilitate interpretation of the findings and a graphical depiction of the results, the continuous predictor variables were made discrete through grouping. In both cases, the lower and upper tertiles were used as cut points, resulting in a three-level variable reflecting levels of distress at admission. Measures of child somatic distress at the time

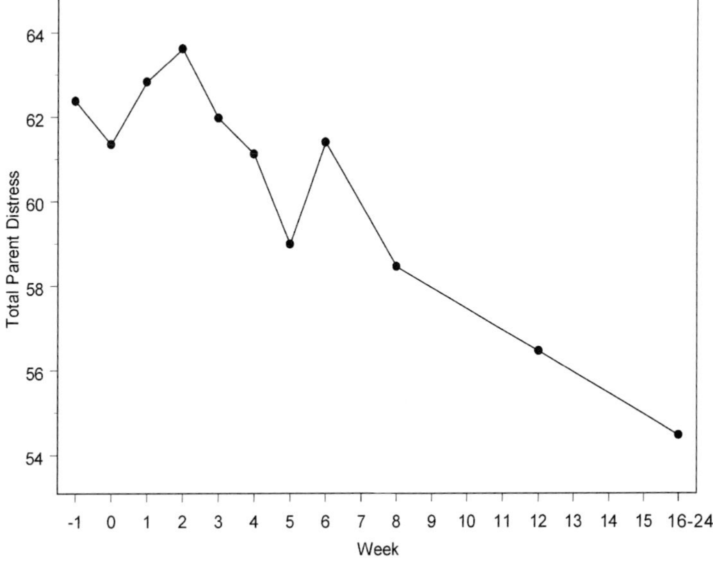


**Figure 5-3.** Global parent distress across the acute phase of SCT.

of transplant admission were not significantly predictive of parental distress trajectories. However, child mood disturbance at admission was predictive of parent global distress over time. This is illustrated in figure 5-4a, which shows that parents whose children were lower in mood disturbance at admission reported lower levels of distress throughout the transplant process. In a similar vein, parental global distress at baseline was not predictive of the child's trajectory of somatic distress but did show a relationship with child mood disturbance (figure 5-4b).

A number of psychosocial predictors of parental distress outcomes were also examined, using measures of prior illness experiences, premorbid child behavior problems, family environment, social support, and parental coping behavior obtained from the resident parents prior to the child's admission for transplant (Phipps et al., 2004b). After controlling for demographic and medical factors, several significant predictors of parental distress trajectories were identified, including prior parent and patient illness-related distress, premorbid child internalizing behavior problems, the family relationship dimensions of the family environment, and parental avoidant coping behaviors. All of the identified relationships were in the predicted direction.

One of the strongest predictors was the family relationship index (FRI) of the Family Environment Scale (FES; Moos & Moos, 1986). The FRI is obtained by summing the FES scales of cohesion and expressiveness along with the inverse of the conflict scale. Higher scores indicate a more supportive family environment. Again, for ease of interpretation and illustration, we took a tertile split on the FRI to obtain high, intermediate, and low groups. This grouping was associated with highly significant differences in parental distress trajectories, and post hoc testing indicated that all three groups differed significantly from each other. This is illustrated in figure 5-5a. Likewise, parental avoidant coping, as ascertained from the Escape-Avoidance subscale of the Ways of Coping Questionnaire (Folkman & Lazarus, 1988) was strongly predictive of parental distress. Tertile splits were used to create high, low, and intermediate avoidant coping groups; again, all three groups differed significantly from each other (figure 5-5b).

Multivariable models were developed using a hierarchical modeling approach with global distress as the dependent outcome. Adopting a strategy similar to that of a hierarchical multiple regression, variables were entered into the model according to three levels of hierarchy: (a) demographic/medical, (b) premorbid adjustment, and (c) family and parental coping. The best-fit model accounted for approximately 50% of the variance in parental global distress. The variables included in both best-fit models included time (weeks), age group, SES, the parent's prior illness-related distress, the FRI, and Ways of Coping Questionnaire Escape-Avoidance.

In summary, parents of children undergoing SCT also experience some adjustment difficulties with mild elevations in distress. These tend to be transient and largely resolve within the first few months following transplant. If assessed at the time of admission using diagnostic interviews designed to identify pathology, some increase in the incidence of depression and anxiety disorders may be noted. Many of these "cases" no longer merit a diagnosis when assessed 3–6 months post-transplant. Parent distress is associated with child distress, and the two covary when assessed across the acute phase of SCT. Factors associated with more positive parent outcomes include the use of humor and acceptance as coping strategies and a supportive family environment. Factors associated with greater parental distress include the use of avoidant coping strategies, interspousal criticism, and substance use. There have been few studies of parental functioning more than a year following SCT. Given that these parents appear to be at some risk of PTSD (Kazak et al., 1997), longer follow-up with a particular focus on symptoms of PTSD is indicated. One of the shortcomings of prior research is a focus almost exclusively on mothers. Efforts to include fathers in subsequent studies are also needed.

## Donor Issues

In the mid-1990s, in a similar chapter on BMT, the literature relating to stem cell donation was summarized in this way: "There is very little literature relating specifically to the psychological problems of BMT donors, and even less empirical information from this population" (Phipps, 1994, p. 159). Unfortunately, this still remains true. In the intervening time frame, there has been one empiric

a)

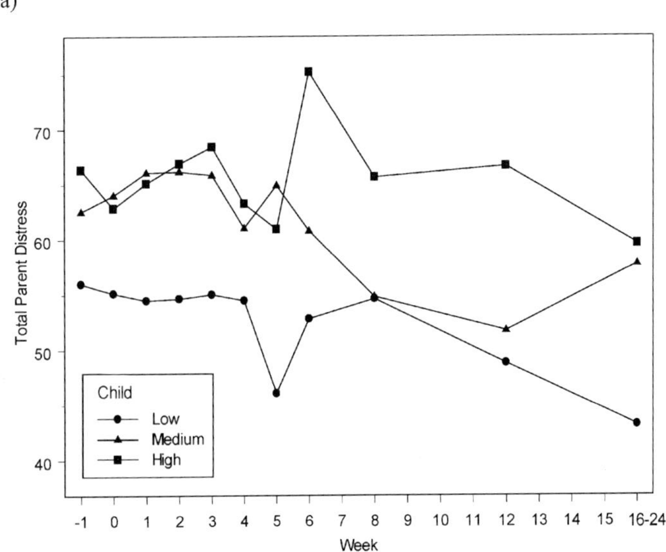


b)

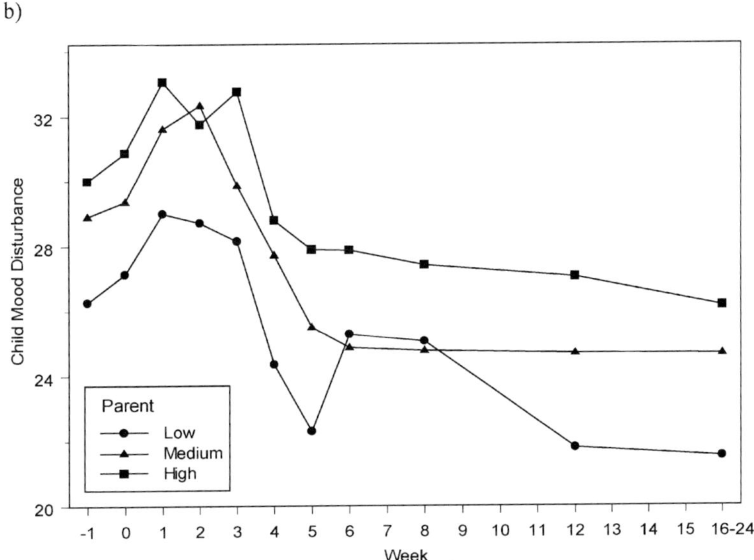


**Figure 5-4.** (a) Global parent distress across the acute phase of BMT as a function of child distress (mood disturbance) measured at admission. (b) Child mood disturbance across the acute phase of BMT as a function of parent distress measured at admission.

study comparing donor-versus-nondonor siblings of pediatric SCT survivors (Packman et al., 1997), a qualitative study comparing sibling donors of successful-versus-unsuccessful pediatric SCTs (MacLeod, Whitsett, Mash, & Pelletier, 2003), and a personal reflection of stem cell donation in childhood (Parmar, Wu, & Chan, 2003). There have been a few more studies regarding the experiences of adult sibling donors (Fortanier et al., 2002; Williams, Green, Morrison, Watson, & Buchanan, 2003), although the relevance of these to the situation of the pediatric donor is unclear.

In the only relevant empiric study to date, Packman and colleagues (1997) studied 21 donor and 23 nondonor siblings of surviving pediatric SCT patients. In their design, only one sibling was

a)

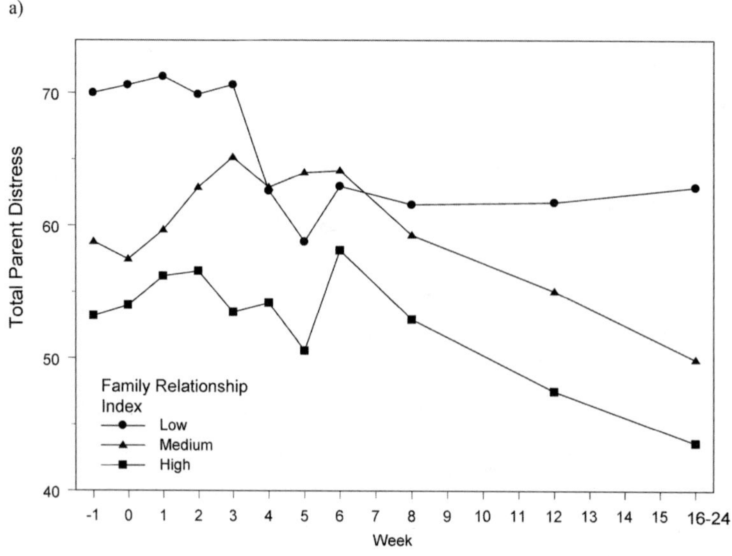


b)

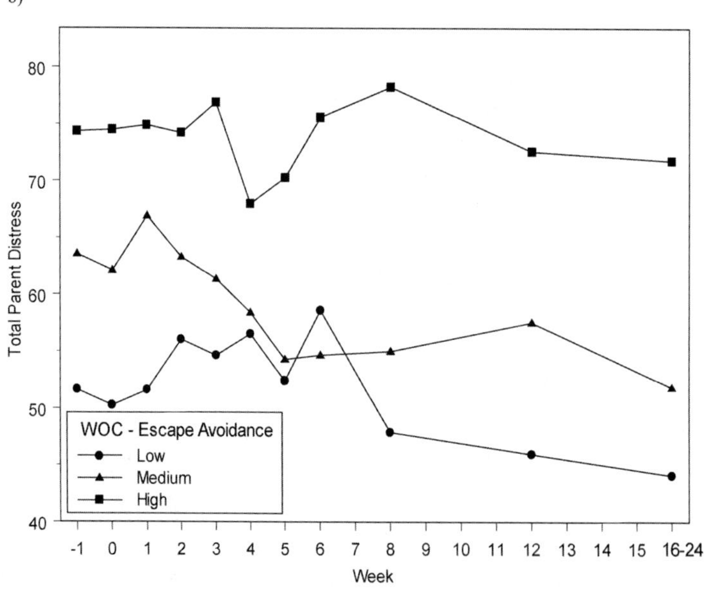


**Figure 5-5.** (a) Trajectories of global parental distress as a function of the family relationship index (FRI) of the Family Environment Scale. Higher scores reflect a more supportive family environment (higher cohesion, expressiveness, lower conflict). Parents whose families are perceived as more supportive report lower distress across the acute phase of BMT. (b) Trajectories of global parental distress as a function of Escape-Avoidant coping on the Ways of Coping Questionnaire. Parents who reported greater use of avoidant coping prior to admission experience greater distress throughout the acute phase of BMT.

studied per family, so it was not possible to compare sibling and nonsibling donors within the same family. They obtained data regarding emotional and behavioral functioning by self-, parent, and teacher report. Unfortunately, the pattern of results obtained precludes any global interpretation of the findings. By self-report, donors showed higher levels of anxiety and lower self-esteem than nondonors. There were no differences between groups on self-reported symptoms of depression or PTSD. By parent report on the Behavior Assessment System for Children (BASC; Reynolds & Kamphaus, 1992), no difference between sibling groups were found on any measure. In contrast, by teacher report on the BASC, the donor siblings were functioning significantly better than the nondonors. Donor siblings obtained significantly higher scores on the BASC adaptive behavior composite and lower scores on the school problems composite scales. Thus, in direct comparison, donors appeared to be having more difficulties than nondonors by self-report but were functioning better by teacher report. Packman et al. interpreted their findings to suggest that the donors are a very vulnerable population. However, in comparison to normative data, both groups appear to be doing relatively well, with T scores generally not much higher than 50. When significant differences were obtained, this resulted from scores indicative of exceptionally good functioning in one of the groups rather than pathology in the other.

MacLeod et al. (2003) interviewed a small group of sibling donors, approximately half of whose sibling had died following SCT. Using qualitative methods, they found, not surprisingly, that siblings in the unsuccessful transplant group reported greater negative impact of the donation experience and greater feelings of guilt and were less likely to experience any positive effects. An interesting and important finding was that both groups felt that they really had "no choice" but to consent to the procedure. In most instances, this lack of choice was self-imposed, but in others it was felt to be imposed by parents or doctors. This is similar to the perception of adult donors, who despite legally consenting to volunteer, feel that being asked by a sibling or other close family member implies there is really no option and thus no volunteer status (Williams et al., 2003).

This perceived lack of choice raises ethical issues and highlights the need for research regarding the potential psychosocial risks and benefits of stem cell donation (Weisz & Robbennolt, 1996). In the early development of SCT, when it was considered a highly experimental and heroic procedure, it was not uncommon for a guardian ad litem to be appointed by the court to help ensure that the rights of the child donor were considered appropriately. As the SCT procedure has become more commonplace and even standard, involvement of the courts has not been considered necessary. In part, this has resulted from a presumption of psychological benefit to the donor, who would benefit from a continued relationship with the sibling should the transplant be successful. However, as noted, there is very little empiric data to support or contradict this presumption of benefit. Such data have been difficult to obtain and will remain difficult to obtain because, although the number of SCTs performed continues to increase, the percentage of SCTs involving sibling donors has declined significantly as the number of unrelated donors, cord blood transplants, and parental haplotype transplants has increased (Mehta & Powles, 2000). The development of new stem cell selection procedures that allow for use of parents as donors may provide a new donor population to consider in future research (Handgretinger, Klingbiel, Lang, Gordon, & Niethammer, 2003). Any further consideration of the effects of stem cell donation on minor children will almost certainly require multisite studies.

## Behavioral Interventions

The literature on behavioral interventions in the setting of pediatric SCT also is very limited. An early report described the use of "puppet therapy" with very young children undergoing SCT, but no empiric test of the intervention was conducted (Linn, Beardslee, & Patenaude, 1986). To our knowledge, the only published study of an intervention trial in pediatric transplant is the pilot study of Streisand et al. (2000), involving an intervention with parents. In this study, mothers of children undergoing SCT were randomly assigned to a behavioral stress management intervention or standard care. Measures of stress levels were obtained weekly from admission through week +3. This pilot study was not powered to be able to definitively test between group differences, but estimates of effects were suggestive of the benefits of the intervention. No follow-up has been reported.

Given the limited literature regarding interventions in the pediatric SCT setting, we review some studies with adult transplant patients that have potential relevance for children undergoing SCT. Perhaps the best intervention work reported thus far is that of Syrjala and colleagues, who conducted two clinical trials using hypnosis, relaxation and imagery, and cognitive behavioral coping skills training to reduce pain and nausea during BMT hospitalization (Syrjala, Cummings, & Donaldson, 1992; Syrjala, Donaldson, Davis, Kippes, & Carr, 1995). In their first study, they found that patients receiving a hypnosis intervention reported less pain and distress than those receiving cognitive behavioral training or standard care controls (Syrjala et al., 1992). In their follow-up study, patients were randomly assigned to four intervention conditions: (a) relaxation and imagery training; (b) cognitive behavioral skills training, including relaxation and imagery; (c) supportive psychotherapy; or (d) treatment-as-usual control (Syrjala et al., 1995). Patients in the first two groups received two training sessions prior to admission and then participated in twice weekly booster sessions for the first 5 weeks of treatment (i.e., through BMT week +4). Results indicated that the patients in the first two groups reported less pain and used less opioid analgesics than those in the other two groups. Those studies involved only adult patients, and no comparable studies have yet been reported in pediatric populations.

A number of intervention trials in adult SCT settings have involved "complementary therapies." For example, a massage therapy intervention was tested in adults undergoing autologous SCT (Ahles et al., 1999). Patients were randomly assigned to receive either massage therapy, consisting of 20-minute sessions three times per week from admission through discharge, or standard care. Patients receiving massage showed significant immediate reductions in distress, fatigue, nausea, and anxiety relative to controls. However, when assessed at midtreatment and discharge, there were no overall group differences in distress or mood disturbance. In part, this is because both groups showed significant declines in distress measures across the study time frame. We also have piloted studies using massage with children undergoing SCT; this is discussed further in this section (Phipps, 2002, Phipps, Dunavant, Gray, & Rai, 2005).

Another complementary approach that has been tested in adult SCT settings is music therapy (Cassileth, Vickers, & Magill, 2003). Adults undergoing autologous SCT were randomly assigned to either a music therapy condition, involving multiple visits with a music therapist over a 2- to 3-week period, or standard care. Patients were assessed twice a week with a short form of the POMS through discharge or day +16. Patients who received music therapy demonstrated significantly lower total mood disturbance scores on the POMS relative to controls. Although music therapy has not been tested in children undergoing SCT, a trial was conducted in children with cancer during inpatient hospitalization (Barrera, Rykov, & Doyle, 2002). In this pilot trial, children demonstrated a significant improvement in mood after a single session of music therapy. The investigators suggested that the intervention is particularly suited to children in inpatient settings and thus would be quite appropriate for children undergoing SCT (Barrera et al., 2002).

Another intervention approach that has been tested with adults is the use of a moderate intensity aerobic exercise program introduced shortly after hospital discharge (Dimeo et al., 1996; Hayes, Davies, Parker, Bashford, & Newman, 2004). Numerous studies have been conducted examining the effects of physical exercise on QOL in cancer patients and have generally shown significant effects on overall QOL as well as on specific aspects of physical, functional, emotional, and social well-being (Courneya & Freidenriech, 1999). In the SCT setting, an aerobic exercise program resulted in a return to peak workload capacity far faster than is typically seen post-SCT (Dimeo et al., 1996). In a randomized trial, adults undergoing a 12-week exercise program showed improved peak aerobic capacity and improved QOL relative to controls (Hayes et al., 2004). Moreover, aerobic capacity was significantly associated with QOL outcomes. To our knowledge, there have been no studies examining the effects of exercise in pediatric SCT settings, but this type of intervention approach should be easily transferable to a pediatric setting.

We have conducted pilot studies of complementary interventions with children undergoing SCT and are currently conducting a multisite randomized intervention trial (Phipps, 2002, Phipps et al., 2005). Our initial pilot intervention involved exposing patients to multiple stress reduction techniques involving diverse approaches from the field of complementary medicine. The individual components were chosen based on five factors: (a) prior use in medical settings; (b) likelihood of beneficial effects on patient mood and general well-being; (c) evidence of potential to have a positive impact on physical health status (including stimulation of the immune system); (d) potential to be learned quickly; and (e) potential for application as a brief, regular practice. The components chosen included (a) relaxation training, with use of imagery (including immune-specific imagery of bone marrow engraftment); (b) massage therapy, which was taught to and administered by parents; (c) humor therapy; and (d) emotional expression therapy. In addition to these specific techniques, the intervention included a component of education, specifically the rationale and benefits of the specific intervention techniques and of the importance of taking a proactive, self-care perspective.

This initial study was designed to examine the feasibility of administering such interventions in the BMT setting and to develop and refine the intervention rather than test efficacy. As such, this was not a randomized trial; rather, a cohort of patients was enrolled, with all provided all components of the intervention. Patient, parent, and therapist perceptions of the intervention were obtained via a questionnaire designed for this study. The questionnaire included a series of questions about each of the individual components of the intervention, relating to (a) how much the patients liked that component, (b) how helpful the patient found it, and (c) how frequently they practiced it. The intervention as a whole was rated as very helpful or better by 85% of patients and parents. A clear pattern was observed regarding the individual components, indicating that massage and humor therapy were rated higher than the others.

In a subsequent study, we conducted a small-scale randomized trial comparing the benefits of massage administered by massage professionals versus massage administered by parents (Phipps et al., 2005). That study had a three-arm design, with patients randomly assigned to professional massage, parent massage, or no massage. The BASES data provided the primary outcomes, with secondary outcomes involving medical parameters such as days in hospital, time to engraftment, and use of narcotic analgesic and antiemetic medications. Initial analyses indicated no significant differences between the two massage groups. Overall, there were no differences between either intervention group and controls on the somatic distress and mood disturbance measures of the BASES scales. Curiously, however, despite the lack of significant differences by parent and child report, patients receiving either massage intervention showed a trend toward faster engraftment, earlier hospital discharge, and less use of analgesic medications (Phipps et al., 2005).

One of the biggest impediments to intervention research in the pediatric SCT setting is the difficulty in obtaining adequate samples so that studies can be powered sufficiently to definitively test intervention effects. With support from the National Cancer Institute, we are conducting a multisite controlled intervention trial. The intervention arms will provide a multicomponent, complementary health promotion intervention with one arm targeted to the child only, a second arm including the same child intervention plus a parent-targeted intervention, and a standard care control arm. Both child and parent interventions involve two primary components designed to increase positive affect states: massage and humor therapy for the child and massage and relaxation therapy for the parent. However, implicit in both interventions is a third component: education. These are framed from a positive psychology model, stressing the importance of seeking brief, positive experiences, and of taking a proactive, self-care approach to health-promoting behavior, with massage, humor, and relaxation techniques presented as examples of vehicles to achieve this. Obtaining a sufficient sample to test intervention effects necessitated a multisite study, and SCT patients will be enrolled at four large pediatric cancer centers. Even with multiple sites, it will take several years to accrue the targeted sample size.

## Conclusions

Hematopoietic SCT has evolved over the past two decades from a heroic experimental therapy of last resort to a standard therapy that is more widely available. Although the numbers of children undergoing SCT have increased substantially, the numbers undergoing transplant at any one center remain relatively small, a factor that has slowed psychosocial research considerably given the difficulties obtaining adequate samples. The most well-researched area thus far deals with the neurocognitive effects of SCT on survivors. Here, the results have been mostly good news, with the preponderance of studies suggesting minimal adverse impact. The exception involves the youngest group of children, who appear to be at somewhat higher risk for cognitive late effects. The major need in this area is for longer follow-up because results have been reported for only up to 3 years post-SCT.

There are somewhat fewer data regarding the social and emotional sequelae of SCT. The available results suggest that pathological responses are rare, but that SCT survivors remain a vulnerable population with fragile self-esteem and difficulties in social functioning. Our empiric studies of the responses of children during the acute phase of SCT indicate a typical trajectory of increased distress followed by recovery. Whether there may be additional sequelae from this transient peak in distress will require further study.

There are more data available on parents of children undergoing SCT; these show some increases in depression and anxiety disorders at the time of admission for transplant, but this also appears to be a transient phenomenon that resolves fairly quickly. This group of parents also appears to remain at higher risk for subsequent development of symptoms of PTSD.

To date, there have been very few studies of behavioral interventions in pediatric SCT, whether focused on patients or parents. Given the numbers of patients undergoing SCT at even the largest centers and the effect sizes typically expected with behavioral interventions, definitive clinical trials will necessitate multisite studies. It is hoped that such interinstitution collaborations will become easier and more commonplace in the coming decade.

*Acknowledgments.* The work described in this chapter was supported in part by grants CA 60616 and CA 82378 from the National Cancer Institute, from the Charles and Ann Morrow Lindbergh Foundation, the American Massage Therapy Foundation, and by the American Lebanese Syrian Associated Charities (ALSAC).

## References

Achenbach, T. M., & Edelbrock, C. (1983). *Manual for the Child Behavior Checklist and Revised Child Behavior Profile.* Burlington: University of Vermont Press.

Ahles, T. A., Tope, D. M., Pinkson, B., Walch, S., Hann, D., Whedon, M., et al. (1999). Massage therapy for patients undergoing autologous bone marrow transplant. *Journal of Pain and Symptom Management, 18,* 157–163.

American Psychiatric Association. (1994). Diagnostic and Statistical Manual of Mental Disorders, (2nd ed.), Washington, D.C.

Andrykowski, M. A., Brady, M. J., Greiner, C. B., Altmaier, E. M., Burish, T. G., Antin, J. H., et al. (1995). "Returning to normal: following bone marrow transplantation: outcomes, expectations, and informed consent. *Bone Marrow Transplantation, 15,* 573–581.

Arvidson, J., Kihlgren, M., Hall, C., & Lonnerholm, G. (1999). Neuropsychological functioning after treatment for hematological malignancies in childhood, including autologous bone marrow transplantation. *Pediatric Hematology Oncology, 16,* 9–21.

Barakat, L. P., Kazak, A. E., Meadows, A. T., Casey, R., Meeske, K., & Stuber, M. L. (1997). Families surviving childhood cancer: a comparison of posttraumatic stress symptoms with families of healthy children. *Journal of Pediatric Psychology 22,* 843–859.

Barrera, M., Pringle, L. A. B., Sumbler, K., & Saunders, F. (2000). Quality of life and behavioral adjustment after pediatric bone marrow transplantation. *Bone Marrow Transplantation 26,* 427–435.

Barrera, M. E., Rykov, M. H., & Doyle, S. L. (2002). The effects of interactive music therapy on hospitalized children with cancer: A pilot study. *Psycho-Oncology, 11,* 379–388.

Beck, A. T. (1978). *Depression Inventory.* Philadelphia: Center for Cognitive Therapy.

Blotcky A. D., Raczynski, J. M., Gurwitch, R., & Smitch, K. (1986). Family influences on hopelessness early in the cancer experience. *Journal of Pediatric Psychology, 10,* 479–493.

Brown, R. T., Kaslow, N. J., Madan-Swain, A., Doepke, K. J., Sexson, S. B., & Hill, L. J. (1993). Parental psychopathology and children's adjustment to leukemia. *Journal of the American Academy of Child and Adolesccent Psychiatry 32,* 554–561.

Canning, E. H., Canning, R. D., & Boyce, W. T. (1992). Depressive symptoms and adaptive style in children with cancer. *Journal of the American Academy of Child and Adolescent Psychiatry, 31,* 1120–1124.

Cassileth, B. R., Vickers, A. J., & Magill, L. A. (2003). Music therapy for mood disturbance during hospitalization for autologous stem cell transplantation. *Cancer, 98,* 2723–2729.

Chou, R. H., Wong, G. B., Kramer, J. H., Ware, D. W., Matthay, K. K., Crittenden, M. R., et al. (1996). Toxicities of total-body irradiation for pediatric bone marrow transplantation. *International Journal of Radiation Oncology, Biology and Physiology, 34,* 843–851.

Cohen, S., Kamarck, T., & Mermelstein, R. (1983). A global measure of perceived stress. *Journal of Health and Social Behavior, 24,* 385–396.

Coley, S. C., Jager, H. R., Szydlo, R. M., & Goldman, J. M. (1999). CT and MRI manifestations of central nervous system infection following allogeneic bone marrow transplantation. *Clinical Radiology, 54,* 390–397.

Coley, S. C., Porter, D. A., Calamante, F., Chong, W. K., & Connelly, A. (1999). Quantitative MR diffusion mapping and cyclosporin-induced neurotoxicity. *American Journal of Neuroradiology, 20,* 1507–1510.

Cool, V. A. (1996). Long-term neuropsychological risks in pediatric bone marrow transplant: What do we know? *Bone Marrow Transpantation, 18*(Suppl. 3), S45–S49.

Courneya, K. S., & Friedenreich, C. M. (1999). Physical exercise and quality of life following cancer diagnosis: A literature review. *Annals of Behavioral Medicine, 21,* 171–179.

Dahlquist, L. M., Czyzewski, D. I., Copeland, K. G., Jones, C. L., Taub, E., & Vaughan, J. K. (1993). Parents of children newly diagnosed with cancer: Anxiety, coping, and marital distress. *Journal of Pediatric Psychology, 18,* 365–376.

Daniel Llach, M., Perez Campdepadros, M., Baza Ceballos, N., Igual Brull, L., Badell Serra, I., Puig Reichach, T., et al. (2001). Secuelas neuropsicologicas a medio y largo plazo del trasplante de medula osea en pacientes con enfermedades heamtologicas. *Anales Pediatria, 54,* 463–467.

Dermatis, H., & Lesko, L. M. (1990). Psychological distress in parents consenting to their child's bone marrow transplantation. *Bone Marrow Transplantation, 6,* 411–417.

Dimeo, F., Bertz, H., Finke, J., Fetscher, S., Mertelsmann, R., & Keul, J. (1996). An aerobic exercise program for patients with haematological malignancies after bone marrow transplantation. *Bone Marrow Transplantation, 18,* 1157–1160.

Dockerty, J. D., Williams, S. M., McGee, R., & Skegg, D. (2000). Impact of childhood cancer on the mental health of parents. *Medical and Pediataric Oncology, 35,* 475–483.

Dolgin, M. J., & Phipps, S. (1995). Reciprocal influences in family adjustment to childhood cancer. In C. Cooper & L. Baider (Eds.), *Cancer and the family* (pp. 73–92). London: Wiley.

DuHamel, K., Manne, S., Nereo, N., Ostroff, J., Martini, R., Parsons, S., et al. (2004). Cognitive processing among mothers of children undergoing bone marrow/stem cell transplantation. *Psychosomatic Medicine, 66,* 92–103.

Folkman, S., & Lazarus, R. S. (1988). *Manual for the Ways of Coping Questionnaire.* Palo Alto, CA: Consulting Psychologists Press.

Fortanier, C., Kuentz, M., Sutton, L., Milpied, N., Michalet, M., Macquart-Moulin, G., et al. (2002). Healthy sibling donor anxiety and pain during bone marrow or peripheral blood stem cell harvesting for allogeneic transplantation: results of a randomised study. *Bone Marrow Transplantation, 29,* 145–149.

Gardner, G. G., August, C. S., & Githens, J. (1977). Psychological issues on bone marrow transplantation. *Pediatrics, 60,* 625–631.

Garrick, R. (2000). Neurologic complications. In K. Atkinson (Ed.), *Clinical bone marrow and blood stem cell transplantation* (2nd ed., pp. 958–979). New York: Cambridge University Press.

Gibbon, M., Spitzer, R. L., & Williams, J. B. W. (1996). *User's guide for the Structured Clinical Interview for* DSM-IV *Axis-I Disorders–Research Version.* New York: Biometrics Research.

Graus, F., Saiz, A., Sierra, J., Arbaiza, D., Rovira, M., Carreras, E., et al. (1996). Neurologic complications of autologous and allogeneic bone marrow transplantation in patients with leukemia: A comparative study. *Neurology, 46,* 1004–1009.

Gunter, M., Karle, M., Werning. A., & Klingbiel, T. (1999). Emotional adaptation of children undergoing bone marrow transplantation. *Canadian Journal of Psychiatry, 44,* 77–81.

Handgretinger, R., Klingbiel, T., Lang, P., Gordon, P., & Niethammer, D. (2003). Megadose transplantation of highly purified haploidentical stem cells: current results and future prospects. *Pediatric Transplantation, 7*(Suppl. 3), 51–55.

Hayes, S., Davies, P. S. W., Parker, T., Bashford, J., & Newman, B. (2004). Quality of life changes following peripheral blood stem cell transplantation and participation in a mixed-type, moderate-intensity, exercise program. *Bone Marrow Transplantation, 33,* 553–558.

Heiney, S. P., Neuberg, R. W., Myers, D., & Bergman, L. H. (1994). The aftermath of bone marrow transplantation for parents of pediatric patients: A post-traumatic stress disorder. *Oncology Nursing Forum, 21,* 843–847.

Hjermstad, M. J., Loge, J. H., Evensen, S. A., Kvaloy, S. O., Fayers, P. M., & Kaasa, S. (1999). The course of anxiety and depression during the first year after allogeneic or autologous stem cell transplantation. *Bone Marrow Transplantation, 24,* 1219–1228.

Kaleita, T. A., Shields, W. D., Tesler, A., & Feig, S. (1989). Normal neurodevelopment in four young children treated for acute leukemia or aplastic anemia. *Pediatrics, 83,* 753–757.

Kazak, A. E., Barakat, L. P., Meeske, K., Christakis, D., Meadows, A. T., Casey, R., et al. (1997). Postraumatic stress, family functioning, and social support in survivors of childhood leukemia and their mothers and fathers. *Journal of Consulting and Clinical Psychology, 65,* 120–129.

Kramer, J. H., Crittenden, M. R., DeSantes, K., & Cowan, M. J. (1997). Cognitive and adaptive behavior 1 and 3 years following bone marrow transplantation *Bone Marrow Transplantation, 19,* 607–613.

Kramer, J. H., Crittenden, M. R., Halberg, F. E., Wara, W. M., & Cowan, M. J. (1992). A prospective study of cognitive function following low-dose cranial radiation for bone marrow transplantation. *Pediatrics, 90,* 447–450.

Kronenberger, W. G., Carter, B. D., Edwards, J., Morrow C., Stewart, J., & Sender, L. (1998). Psychological adjustment of mothers of children undergoing bone marrow transplantation: the role of stress, coping, and family factors. *Children's Health Care, 27,* 77–95.

Kupst, M. J., Penatic, B., Debban, B., Camitta, B., Pietryga, D., Margolis, D., et al. (2002). Cognitive and psychosocial functioning of pediatric hematopoietic stem cell transplant patients: A prospective longitudinal study. *Bone Marrow Transplantation, 30,* 600–617.

Linn, S., Beardslee, W., & Patenaude, A. F. (1986). Puppet therapy with pediatric bone marrow transplant patient. *Journal of Pediatric Psychology, 11,* 37–46.

MacLeod, K. D., Whitsett, S. F., Mash, E. J., & Pelletier, W. (2003). Pediatric sibling donors of successful and unsuccessful hematopoietic stem cell transplants (HSCT): A qualitative study of their psychosocial experience. *Journal of Pediatric Psychology, 28,* 223–230.

Manne, S., DuHamel, K., Nereo, N., Ostroff, J., Parsons, S., Martini, R., et al. (2002). Predictors of PTSD in mothers of children undergoing bone marrow transplantation: The role of cognitive and social processes. *Journal of Pediatric Psychology, 27,* 607–617.

Manne, S., DuHamel, K., Ostroff, J., Parsons, S., Martini, R., Williams, S., et al., & (2003). Coping and the course of mother's depressive symptoms during and after pediatric bone marrow transplantation. *Journal of the American Academy of Child and Adolescent Psychiatry, 42,* 1055–1068.

Manne, S., Nereo, N., DuHamel, K., Ostroff, J., Parsons, S., Martini, R., et al. (2001). Anxiety and depression in mothers of children undergoing bone marrow transplant: Symptom prevalence and use of the Beck depression and Beck anxiety inventories as screening instruments. *Journal of Consulting and Clinical Psychology, 69,* 1037–1047.

Marks, P. V. (1998). Neurological aspects of stem-cell transplantation. In J. Barrett & J. Trealeaven (Eds.), *The clinical practice of stem-cell transplantation* (Vol. 1, pp. 787–794). Oxford, UK: ISIS.

McConville, B. J., Steichen-Asch, P., Harris, R., Neudorf, S., Sambrano, J., et al. (1990). Pediatric bone marrow transplants: Psychological aspects. *Canadian Journal of Psychiatry, 35,* 769–775.

McGuire, T., Sanders, J. E., Hill, J. D., Buckner, C. D., & Sullivan, K. (1991). Neuropsychological function in children given total body irradiation for marrow transplantation [abstract]. *Experimental Hematology, 19,* 578.

McNair, D. M., Lorr, M., & Droppleman, L. F. (1971). *Manual, Profile of Mood States.* San Diego, CA: Educational and Industrial Testing Service.

McQuellon, R. P., Russell, G. B., Rambo, T. D., Craven, B. L., Radford, J., Perry, J. J., et al. (1998). Quality of life and psychological distress of bone marrow transplant recipients: The "time trajectory" to recovery over the first year. *Bone Marrow Transplantation, 21,* 477–486.

Mehta, J., & Powles, R. (2000). The future of blood and marrow transplantation. In K. Atkinson (Ed.), *Clinical bone marrow and blood stem cell transplantation* (2nd ed., pp. 1457–1465). New York: Cambridge University Press.

Meller, S., & Pinkerton, R. (1998). Solid tumors in children. In J. Barrett & J. Trealeaven (Eds.), *The clinical practice of stem-cell transplantation* (Vol. 1, pp. 173–190). Oxford, UK: ISIS.

Meyers, C. A., Weitzer, M., Byrne, K., Valentine, A., Champlin, R. E., & Przepiorka, D. (1994). Evaluation of the neurobehavioral functioning of patients before, during and after bone marrow transplantation. *Journal of Clinical Oncology, 12,* 820–826.

Miale, T. D., Sirithorn, S., & Ahmed, S. (1995). Efficacy and toxicity of radiation in preparative regimens for pediatric stem cell transplantation. I: Clinical applications and therapeutic effects. *Medical and Pediatric Oncology, 12,* 231–249.

Pace, M. T., Slovis, T. L., Kelly, J. K., & Abella, S. D. (1995). Cyclosporin A toxicity: MRI appearance of the brain. *Pediatric Radiology, 25,* 180–183.

Packman, W. L., Crittenden, M. R., Schaaeffer, E., Bongar, B., Fischer, J. B. R., & Cowan, M. J. (1997). Psychosocial consequences of bone marrow transplantation in donor and nondonor siblings. *Developmental and Behavioral Pediatrics, 18,* 244–253.

Padovan, C. S., Gerbitz, A., Sostak, P., Holler, E., Ferrara, J. L., Bise, K., et al. (2001). Cerebral involvement in graft-versus-host disease after murine bone marrow transplantation. *Neurology, 56,* 1106–1108.

Padovan, C. S., Tarek, Y. A., Schleuning, M., Holler, E., Kolb, H. J., & Straube, A. (1998). Neurological and neuroradiological findings in long-term survivors of allogeneic bone marrow transplantation. *Annals of Neurology, 43,* 627–633.

Parmar, G., Wu, J. W. Y., & Chan, K. W. (2003). Bone marrow donation in childhood: One donor's perspective. *Psycho-oncology, 12,* 91–94.

Parsons, S. K., Barlow, S. E., Levy, S. L., Supran, S. E., & Kaplan, S. H. (1999). Health-related quality of life in pediatric bone marrow transplant survivors: According to whom? *International Journal of Cancer, 12*(Suppl.), 46–51.

Patchell, R. A., White, C. L., Clark, A. W., Beschorner, W. E., & Santos, G. W. (1985). Neurologic complications of bone marrow transplantation. *Neurology, 35,* 300–306.

Patenaude, A. F., Szymanski, L., & Rappeport, J. (1979). Psychological costs of bone marrow transplantation in children. *American Journal of Orthopsychiatry, 49,* 409–422.

Peper, M., Schraube, P., Kimming, C., Wagensommer, C., Wannenmacher, M., & Haas, R. (1993). Long-term cerebral side-effects of total body irradiation and quality of life. *Recent Results in Cancer Research, 130,* 219–230.

Pfefferebaum, B., Lindamood, B. B., & Wiley, F. (1977). Pediatric bone marrow transplantation: Psychosocial aspects. *American Journal of Psychiatry, 134,* 1299–1301.

Phipps, S. (1994). Bone marrow transplantation. In D. J. Bearison & R. K. Mulhern (Eds.), *Pediatric psychooncology: Psychological perspectives on children with cancer* (pp. 143–170). New York: Oxford University Press.

Phipps, S. (2002). Reduction of distress associated with paediatric bone marrow transplant: complementary health promotion interventions. *Pediatric Rehabilitation, 5,* 223–234.

Phipps, S., & Barclay, D. (1996). Psychosocial consequences of pediatric bone marrow transplantation. *International Journal of Pediatric Hematology/Oncology 4,* 190–201.

Phipps, S., Brenner, M., Heslop, H., Krance, R., Jayawardene, D., & Mulhern, R. K. (1995). Psychological effects of bone marrow transplantation on children: Preliminary report of a longitudinal study. *Bone Marrow Transplantation, 16,* 829–835.

Phipps, S., Dunavant, M., Garvie, P., Lensing, S., & Rai, S. N. (2002). Acute health-related quality of life in children undergoing stem cell transplant: I. Descriptive outcomes. *Bone Marrow Transplantation, 29,* 425–434.

Phipps, S., Dunavant, M., Gray, E., & Rai, S. N. (2005). Massage therapy in children undergoing hematopoietic stem cell transplant: results of a pilot trial. *Journal of Cancer Integrated Medicine, 3,* 62–70.

Phipps, S., Dunavant, M., Jayawardene, D., & Srivastava, D. K. (1999). Assessment of health related quality of life in acute inpatient settings: Use of the BASES scale in children undergoing bone marrow transplantation. *International Journal of Oncology, 12,* 18–24.

Phipps, S., Dunavant, M., Lensing, S., & Rai, S. N. (2002). Acute health-related quality of life in children undergoing stem cell transplant: II. Medical and demographic determinants. *Bone Marrow Transplantation, 29,* 435–442.

Phipps, S., Dunavant, M., Lensing, S., & Rai, S. N. (2004a). Patterns of distress in parents of children undergoing stem cell transplantation. *Pediatric Blood and Cancer* (in press).

Phipps, S., Dunavant, M., Lensing, S., & Rai, S. N. (2004b). Psychosocial predictors of distress in parents of children undergoing stem cell transplantation. *Journal of Pediatric Psychology* (in press).

Phipps, S., Dunavant, M., Srivasatava, D. K., Bowman, L., & Mulhern, R. K. (2000). Cognitive and academic functioning in survivors of pediatric bone marrow transplantation. *Journal of Clinical Oncology, 18,* 1004–1011.

Phipps, S., Hinds, P. S., Channel, S., & Bell, G. L. (1994). Measurement of behavioral, affective and somatic responses to pediatric bone marrow transplantation. Development of the BASES scale. *Journal of Pediatric Oncology Nursing, 11,* 109–117.

Phipps, S., & Mulhern, R. K. (1995). Family cohesion and expressiveness promote resilience to the stress of pediatric bone marrow transplant: A preliminary report. *Journal of Developmental and Behavioral Pediatrics, 16,* 257–263.

Phipps, S., & Srivastava, D. K. (1997). Repressive adaptation in children with cancer. *Health Psychology, 16,* 521–528.

Phipps, S., Steele, R. G., Hall, K., & Leigh, L. (2001). Repressive adaptation in children with cancer: A replication and extension. *Health Psychology 20,* 445–451.

Pot-Mees, C. C. (1989). *The psychological aspects of bone marrow transplantation in children.* The Netherlands: Eburon Delft.

Poulshock, S., & Deimling, G. (1984). Families caring for elders in residence: Issues in the measurement of burden. *Journal of Gerontology, 39,* 230–239.

Reece, D. E., Frei-Lahr, D. A., Shepherd, J. D., Dorovini-Zis, K., Gascoyne, R. D., Graeb, D. A., et al. (1991). Neurologic complications in allogeneic bone marrow transplant patients receiving cyclosporin. *Bone Marrow Transplantation, 8,* 393–401.

Reynolds, C. R., & Kamphaus, R. W. (1992). *Behavior Assessment System for Children.* Circle Pines, MN: American Guidance Service.

Rodrigue, J. R., Graham-Pole, J., Kury, S., Kubar, W., & Hoffman, G. (1995). Behavioral distress, fear, and pain among children hospitalized for bone marrow transplantation. *Clinical Transplantation, 9,* 454–456.

Rodrigue, J. R., MacNaughton, K., Hoffman, R. G., Graham-Pole, J., Andres J. M., Novak, D. A., et al. (1996). Transplantation in children: A longitudinal assessment of mothers' stress, coping, and perceptions of family functioning. *Psychosomatics, 38,* 478–486.

Rouah, E., Gruber, R., Shearer, W., Armstrong, D., & Hawkins, E. P. (1988). Graft-versus-host disease in the central nervous system. A real entity? *American Journal of Clinical Pathology, 89,* 543–546.

Sahler, O. J., Varni, J. W., Fairclough, D. L., Butler, R. W., Noll, R. B., Dolgin, M. J., et al. (2002). Problem-solving skills training for mothers of children with newly diagnosed cancer: a randomized trial. *Journal of Developmental and Behavioral Pediatrics, 23,* 77–86.

Sanders, J. E. (1997). Bone marrow transplantation in pediatric oncology. In P. A. Pizzo & D. G. Poplack (Eds.), *Principles and practices of pediatric oncology* (3rd ed., pp. 357–373). New York: Lippincott-Raven.

Santos, G. W. (2000). Historical background to hematopoietic stem cell transplantation. In K. Atkinson (Ed.), *Clinical bone marrow and blood stem cell transplantation* (2nd ed., pp. 1–12). New York: Cambridge University Press.

Sawyer, M. G., Antoniou, G., Toogood, I., Rice, M., & Baghurst, P. (1993). A prospective study of the psychological adjustment of parents and families of children with cancer. *Journal of Paediatrics and Child Health, 29,* 352–356.

Simms, S., Kazak, A. E., Gannon, T., Goldwein, J., & Bunin, N. (1998). Neuropsychological outcome of children undergoing bone marrow transplantation. *Bone Marrow Transplantation, 22,* 181–184.

Simms, S., Kazak, A. E., Golumb, V., Goldwein, J., & Bunin, N. (2002). Cognitive, behavioral, and social outcome of childhood stem cell transplantation. *Journal of Pediatric Hematology/Oncology, 24,* 115–120.

Smedler, A. C., & Bolme, P. (1995). Neuropsychological deficits in very young bone marrow transplant recipients. *Acta Pediatrica, 84,* 429–433.

Smedler, A. C., Nilsson, C., & Bolme, P. (1995). Total body irradiation: A neuropsychological risk factor in pediatric bone marrow transplant recipients. *Acta Pediatrica, 84,* 325–330.

Smedler, A. C., Ringden, K., Bergman, H., & Bolme, P. (1990). Sensory-motor and cognitive functioning in children who have undergone bone marrow transplantation. *Acta Paediatrica Scandinavica, 79,* 613–621.

Sormanti, M., Dungan, S., & Rieker, P. P. (1994). Pediatric bone marrow transplantation: Psychosocial issues for parents after a child's hospitalization. *Journal of Psychosocial Oncology, 12,* 23–42.

Streisand, R., Rodrigue, J. R., Houck, C., Graham-Pole, J., & Berlant, N. (2000). Parents of children undergoing bone marrow transplantation: documenting stress and piloting a psychological intervention program. *Journal of Pediatric Psychology, 25,* 331–338.

Stuber, M., Nader, K., Yasuda, P., Pynoos, R., & Cohen, S. (1991). Stress responses following pediatric bone marrow transplantation: Preliminary results of a prospective longitudinal study. *Journal of the American Academy of Child and Adolescent Psychiatry, 30,* 952–957.

Syrjala, K. L., Cummings, C., & Donaldson, G. W. (1992). Hypnosis or cognitive behavioral training for the reduction of pain and nausea during cancer treatment: A controlled clinical trial. *Pain, 48,* 137–146.

Syrjala, K. L., Donaldson, G. W., Davis, M. W., Kippes, M. E., & Carr, J. E. (1995). Relaxation and imagery and cognitive-behavioral training reduce pain during cancer treatment: A controlled clinical trial. *Pain, 63,* 189–198.

Thompson, C. B., Sanders, J. E., Flournoy. N., Buckner, C. D., & Thomas, E. D. (1986). The risks of central nervous system relapse and leukoencephalopathy in patients receiving marrow transplants for acute leukemia. *Blood, 67,* 195–199.

Treleaven, J., & Barrett, J. (1998). Introduction. In J. Barrett & J. Trealeaven (Eds.), *The clinical practice of stem-cell transplantation* (Vol. 1, pp. 2–16). Oxford, UK: ISIS.

Vannatta, K., Zeller, M., Noll, R. B., & Koontz, K. (1998). Social functioning of children surviving bone marrow transplantation. *Journal of Pediatric Psychology, 23,* 169–178.

Weisz, V., & Robbennolt, J. K. (1996). Risks and benefits of pediatric bone marrow donation: A critical need for research. *Behavioral Sciences and the Law, 14,* 375–391.

Williams, S., Green, R., Morrison, A., Watson, D., & Buchanan, S. (2003). The psychosocial aspects of donating blood stem cells: The sibling donor perspective. *Journal of Clinical Apheresis, 18,* 1–9.

Wingard, J. R. (1997). Bone marrow to blood stem cells: Past, present, future. In M. B. Whedon & D. Wujcik (Eds.), *Blood and marrow stem cell transplantation: Principles, practice, and nursing insights* (2nd ed., pp. 3–24). Boston: Jones and Bartlett.

Wiznitzer, M., Packer, R., August, C., & Burkey, E. D. (1984). Neurological complications of bone marrow transplantation. *Annals of Neurology, 16,* 569–576.

Bernard F. Fuemmeler, Larry L. Mullins,
and Melissa Y. Carpentier

# Peer, Friendship Issues, and Emotional Well-Being

The assertion that social relationships contribute to a child's psychological adjustment, health, and overall well-being is commonly accepted and supported by numerous investigations in the clinical child literature (Erdley, Nangle, Newman, & Carpenter, 2001). A wide variety of social phenomena have been examined, including the association between social and emotional adjustment, social network structure, how children are perceived and accepted by their peer group, and children's ability to establish friendships and close relationships. Given the importance of peer relationships to emotional well-being, it is surprising that this subject has not received greater attention in the pediatric psycho-oncology literature.

Understanding children's social relationships in the context of cancer is important for four primary reasons. First, many aspects related to having cancer and undergoing treatment for cancer, such as school absence, fatigue, interruptions in play and daily activities, changes in physical appearance, strict medical regimens and their associated adverse side effects, and neurocognitive impairments can increase children's risk for social adjustment problems. Second, positive peer relationships and social support may facilitate the adjustment of children to the experience of cancer. Third, although understudied in the pediatric literature, having positive social support from peers and friends could potentially influence the course of cancer by enhancing the functioning of the neuroendocrine and immune systems. Finally, with a broader understanding of the relevance of social relationships among children with cancer, targeted interventions can be developed and evaluated for their role on outcomes related to adjustment, quality of life, and mediating mechanisms influencing mortality and morbidity.

This chapter provides a general overview of the literature related to the role that peers and friendships have on adjustment and presents a review of the relationship of social support to adjustment and health outcomes. The impact of cancer on peer relationships and friendships also is discussed. The chapter concludes with a presentation of extant literature on interventions that have been developed to promote social adjustment and a discussion of future directions. To begin, a description is provided of the terminology and how social processes are often conceptualized. Such information is presented as a heuristic for future research in pediatric psycho-oncology.

## Definitions and Terminology

Psychologists have conceptualized and studied social relationships of children from a number of vantage points, with the notion that each perspective helps understand a child's social ecology. The constructs that are most commonly studied include social support, social networks, peer acceptance, and friendships. These perspectives are defined next.

### Social Support

Social support reflects the quality of a relationship with other individuals; it is believed that social support may enhance health and well-being in a child or individual by promoting adaptation of health behavior or enhancing the immune responses activated by stress (House, Landis, & Umberson, 1988). Often, researchers studying social support distinguish between four main functional types, including emotional support, instrumental support, informational support, and appraisal support. Emotional support reflects support provided in the form of empathy, love, trust, or caring. Instrumental support involves support in the form of tangible aid or services. Informational support is the support of advice and suggestions. Finally, appraisal support reflects what a person receives from others in the form of affirmations, constructive feedback, or social comparison (House, 1981).

### Social Networks

Social networks reflect the intricate web of social relationships and the embedded structure of these relationships. Social network analysis attempts to assess the structural characteristics of social networks, how these networks are formed, and how such social networks influence important health and psychological outcomes (Gifford-Smith & Brownell, 2003). The structural characteristics of a child's social network are an important area of inquiry in network analysis. These characteristics include size, interconnectedness, and stability. Size reflects the number of peer clusters in a child's network. Interconnectedness (sometimes referred to as density) involves the level of cohesion and the extent to which members know and interact with one another. Stability of a network reflects the level of changes in the group membership over time.

Research on the social networks of children suggests that boys generally have larger peer groups than girls, and higher social status children have larger networks than do lower status children (Gifford-Smith & Brownell, 2003). A child's position in the network also has been studied as a potential factor related to socioemotional development. For instance, perceived popularity, athletic ability (for boys), and leadership skills are characteristics associated with children who are highly central in a network (i.e., they know a great number of children and are known by many other children), and these children are predicted to function well with others and have few social and emotional adjustment difficulties (Farmer & Farmer, 1996; Farmer & Rodkin, 1996; Gest, Graham-Bermann, & Hartup, 2001). Children who are peripheral in a network (i.e., isolates) are often characterized as being shy or withdrawn and are predicted to have more social and emotional problems than their peers who are central to a network (Farmer & Rodkin, 1996).

### Peer Acceptance or Sociometric Status

Peer acceptance or sociometric status is another method of examining the social relationships of children. Common methods used to assess sociometric status involve the use of peer nominations or peer ratings (e.g., Coie & Dodge, 1983; Coie, Dodge, & Coppotelli, 1982). In this methodology, the constructs of social preference and social impact of children are assessed. Children are presented with a class roster and asked to indicate children in their class who they most like and children who they least like. Social preference reflects the number of like nominations minus the number of disliked nominations. Social impact reflects the degree to which a child is noticed by his or her peers and is the sum of the particular child's "like" and "dislike" nominations. Scores are then categorized into five sociometric categories: popular, rejected, neglected, controversial, and average (Coie & Dodge, 1983, 1988; Newcomb, Bukowski, & Pattee, 1993). These categories are described next.

#### *Popular*

Children categorized as popular receive numerous like nominations and few dislike nominations from their peers. These are children who also receive high social preference scores. Generally, popular children have many positive qualities. They are seen by their peers as being socially helpful, cooperative, considerate, and outgoing (Coie, Dodge, & Kupersmidt, 1990). They also are more likely to be children who are socially competent, demonstrating prosocial problem-solving strategies and skills (Erdley & Asher, 1999; Nelson & Crick, 1999).

### *Rejected*

Children in the rejected category receive few like nominations and numerous dislike nominations and are rated lowest on social preference. In a 5-year longitudinal study of academic achievement and psychological adjustment, Ollendick, Wiest, Borden, and Greene (1992) found that children in the rejected and controversial (discussed separately next) categories had poorer psychosocial and psychological outcomes than children in other status groups. Rejected children also demonstrate more aggressive and hostile behavior (Coie, Dodge, Terry, & Wright, 1991; Newcomb et al., 1993). Higher levels of emotional reactivity and sensation seeking also have been observed among children in the rejected category (Hinshaw & Melnick, 1995). Nonaggressive rejected children tend to be those children who are more shy and withdrawn and more prone to display socially awkward and strange behaviors than their peers who are not rejected (Bierman, Smoot, & Aumiller, 1993).

### *Neglected*

Children in the neglected category receive few dislike or like nominations. They are the children in the classroom who typically go unnoticed. Unlike children in the rejected category, children in the neglected category do not display a high frequency of externalizing or aggressive behavior; rather, they are sometimes characterized as shy and withdrawn by other children (Ollendick et al., 1992). However, some studies have found that teachers typically do not characterize these children as problematic and tend to see them as functioning independently and appropriately (Wentzel & Asher, 1995).

### *Controversial*

Children in the controversial category receive a high number of like and dislike nominations. These children share qualities of both rejected and popular children. They are viewed by their peers as leaders and sociable; however, they are also viewed as aggressive and forcefully assertive (Bagwell, Coie, Terry, & Lochman, 2000; Newcomb et al., 1993). As these children become adolescents, their leadership skills and tendency toward more aggressive behavior increase the likelihood of having a negative rather than a prosocial influence on other children around them (Bagwell et al., 2000).

### *Average*

In sociometric studies, nearly half of children do not fall into any of the aforementioned categories. These children do not appear to be at risk for poor adjustment outcomes. Rather, these children function well and display levels of externalizing and internalizing behavior that are not considered clinically significant.

Using this sociometric method provides researchers one strategy for gaining insight into the complex association between peer relationships and developmental outcomes, whether they exist in academic, psychological, behavioral, or social spheres. One consistent observation among investigators using this approach has been that there is considerable heterogeneity within these categories (Gifford-Smith & Brownell, 2003; LaGreca, 1997). That is, children in the rejected category are not always viewed as aggressive or children in the neglected category are not always seen as shy. However, these methods and the categories have been used with some success to predict development and psychological health in 5- to 10-year longitudinal studies (Bagwell, Schmidt, Newcomb, & Bukowski, 2001).

## Friendships

The study of friendships and dyadic interactions reflects another dimension that overlaps but yet is distinct from the construct of peer acceptance. Children's level of acceptance or rejection may be independent from their close reciprocal friendships (Gest et al., 2001; Ladd, Kochenderfer, & Coleman, 1997). Indeed, a friendship represents a voluntary, evolving, positive reciprocal relationship between two children (Bukowski & Hoza, 1989), whereas sociometric status represents the level of a child's acceptance within the larger peer group (Gifford-Smith & Brownell, 2003). A friendship is typically operationalized as two classmates who give mutual positive nominations (Erdley et al., 2001).

In addition, the quality of a child's friendships is important to assess as this can be relevant to the child's emotional adjustment and development (Bukowski & Hoza, 1989). High-quality friendships, such as those characterized by intimacy, loyalty, reciprocal encouragement, and validation, have been shown to be associated with overall better social adjustment (Berndt, Hawkins, & Jiao, 1999; Ladd et al., 1997). Friends also can serve as an important source of support during stressful times or transitions. Having positive friendships has been demonstrated to mitigate the stress related to family adversity and divorce (Criss, Pettit, Bates, Dodge, & Lapp, 2002; Hetherington, 1999).

Not surprisingly, children who do not have close friends appear to be at risk for poor outcomes, such as loneliness, depressive symptoms, and social anxiety (La Greca & Lopez, 1998; Parker, Rubin, Price, & De Rosier, 1995). Children who form friendships with other children who also engage in highly delinquent aggressive behaviors also appear to be at risk for poor adaptation and engaging in delinquent and aggressive behavior themselves (Newcomb, Bukowski, & Bagwell, 1999).

### Peers, Friendships, and Development

The distinct functions and behavioral differences that peer relationships have during different phases of development have been a focus of ever-increasing empirical investigation. Early theorists have suggested that age-related patterns of friendships emerge during early, middle, and late childhood (Selman, 1980; Sullivan, 1953; Youniss, 1980). Sullivan (1953) proposed that during early childhood parents remain a strong source of socialization and support for children.

However, around the age of 2 to 6 years, children begin to form companionships with other children. Small dyads are formed, and their play is characterized by sustained sessions of imaginative play (Parker & Gottman, 1989). Around the ages of 6 and 9 years, children's needs for acceptance begin to influence their social engagements. It is theorized that children at this age choose friends who are similar to them, and that they develop friendships that serve to validate their developing interpersonal awareness (Sullivan, 1953). During preadolescence (ages 9–12 years), Sullivan asserted that the need for greater intimacy begins to shape the friendships that children develop. At this age, youths begin to form relationships that are based on mutual sharing of personal information. During adolescence, sexuality and identity begin to shape their friendship relationships. Through the course of development and in the context of these friendships, Sullivan asserted that social competencies emerge.

Since that time, others have suggested that making and keeping friends requires a number of competencies and skills, such as learning to take another's perspective, regulating emotion, effective interpersonal communication, processing social information cues, and problem solving (Gifford-Smith & Brownell, 2003). Although the focus of research has largely centered on differences between individuals rather than developmental change, there is some support for Sullivan's theories. For instance, research has demonstrated that as children develop and mature their descriptions of their friendship relationships are characterized by more comments reflecting intimacy, such as sharing personal thoughts and feelings (Bigelow & La Gaipa, 1980; Furman & Bierman, 1984).

### Summary

In summary, the clinical child psychology literature offers a number of definitional frameworks for understanding and studying social relationships. Each of these frameworks and the methods of assessment differ somewhat, but together they offer a comprehensive representation of the social environment among children. Although a number of these techniques have yet to be applied to the study of social adjustment among cancer survivors, the definitions have been offered to provide a context for what follows. The following section reviews the current empirical literature on childhood cancer and peer relations.

## The Impact of Cancer on Peer Relationships and Friendships

Children with cancer experience a number of acute and long-term consequences of their illness and associated treatments that can potentially affect their social relationships. We review key areas of research related to the cancer experience and the potential impact that the experience may have on peer relationships. Specifically, our focus is on four overlapping domains: (a) social adjustment with peers, (b) the academic context and peer relations, (c) neurocognitive impairments and social adjustment, and (d) emotional well-being and impact on peer relationships. Previous work has suggested that such domains are highly relevant to children undergoing cancer treatment (Eiser, 1998; Eiser & Vance, 2002; Vannatta & Gerhardt, 2003).

## Social Adjustment With Peers

It is not uncommon for many children undergoing treatment for cancer to express concerns or worries about their relationships with peers. Such concerns may be especially salient among children with cancer (La Greca, Bearman, & Moore, 2002; Wolman, Resnick, Harris, & Blum, 1994). The question remains whether children with cancer experience significant social adjustment or peer relationship problems and, if so, of what type.

In a series of studies, Noll and colleagues used the sociometric method and asked both teachers and peers to provide information about the social relationships of children diagnosed with cancer (Noll et al., 1996, 1999; Noll, Bukowski, Davies, Koontz, & Kalkarni, 1993; Noll, Bukowski, Rogosch, LeRoy, & Kulkarni, 1990; Noll, LeRoy, Bukowski, Rogosch, & Kulkarni, 1991). In the first of these studies, Noll et al. (1990) compared teacher ratings of 24 children with cancer to a classroom comparison control group of children along three dimensions of interpersonal style: sociability-leadership, aggressive-disruptive, and sensitive-isolated. Results indicated that children with cancer were rated as less sociable and less prone to leadership, as well as more socially isolated and withdrawn than their healthy counterparts. However, it is important to note that only teacher ratings were obtained, and no child or parent data were available.

In a subsequent study, Noll and colleagues (1991) compared children with cancer to classroom controls on indices of (a) peer and self-perceptions of sociability, aggression, and social isolation; (b) overall popularity; (c) mutual friendships; (d) feelings of loneliness; and (e) self-concept. Peer report data indicated that the children with cancer were more likely to be perceived by their peers as socially isolated compared to healthy classmates. However, no significant differences between the children with cancer and the comparison control children were found in the areas of popularity, number of mutual friends, loneliness, self-worth, depression, and self-concept. Results of a longitudinal, multi-informant investigation of these variables (Noll et al., 1993) indicated that children with cancer continued to have a social reputation as more socially isolated, although no significant differences were found on measures of social acceptance or self-reported psychological functioning.

In another investigation, Noll, Ris, Davies, Bukowski, and Koontz (1992) evaluated the social reputations among children with (a) brain tumors, (b) a malignancy not primarily involving the central nervous system (CNS), and (c) sickle cell disease. Analyses comparing the child with a chronic illness to peers in each class indicated that children with cancer were nominated more often for sociability-leadership roles and less frequently for aggressive-disruptive roles by their teachers. In addition, brain tumor survivors were nominated more often for sensitive-isolated roles, while children with sickle cell disease were not significantly different from peers.

To further describe psychosocial adjustment among children with cancer, Kullgren, Morris, Morris, and Krawiecki (2003) conducted a longitudinal investigation of social and behavioral functioning among children with brain tumors at two points (1–2 years and 3–4 years post-diagnosis). The authors used the Child Behavior Checklist (CBCL) social competence (Achenbach & Edelbrock, 1983) scale as the primary measure of social functioning; items that load on the social competence scale include activity in organizations and friendships and relationships with siblings, peers, and parents. Results indicated that parents rated their children lower than average across areas of social competence at both time points. In addition, those children who experienced difficulties with social competence at Time 1 were more likely to experience these same difficulties at Time 2. Thus, the results of this study suggest that initial social competence ratings are important in predicting long-term outcomes; consequently, it may be that early intervention among children having difficulties could be important in reducing long-term social competence deficits.

Using different methodology, Spirito, Stark, Cobiella, Drigan, Androkites, and Hewett (1990) evaluated the impact of cancer treatment on peer relations of children previously treated for cancer between the ages of 2 and 5 years by examining social adjustment, peer relations, and social skills development. Specifically, 56 survivors of childhood cancer between the ages of 5 and 12 years were compared to a sample of healthy controls on measures assessing self-perception and social skills (i.e., Self-Perception Profile for Children [Harter, 1985] and specific items from the social competence scale of the CBCL [Achenbach & Edelbrock, 1983]). Teacher ratings were also obtained via the Taxonomy of Problem Situations scale (Dodge, McClaskey, & Feldman, 1985) and the Deasy-Spinetta Behavioral Questionnaire (Deasy-Spinetta, 1981) and parent ratings were obtained from the Taxonomy of Problem Situations parent form, items from the social competence scale of the CBCL, and interview questions designed specifically for the study. Results yielded few differences between cancer survivors and healthy children on measures of perceptions of competency, although there was a trend for cancer survivors to report spending more time alone than they desired compared to others of their same age. Teacher reports indicated that cancer survivors were more interested in school and less likely to argue or get teased compared to healthy children. Parent reports were similar to those of the teachers, although, interestingly, parents did not report that their children spent more time alone than their children desired. Spirito and colleagues concluded that their findings were largely consistent with other follow-up studies of cancer survivors because successful adjustment is often found in the majority of survivors. However, Spirito et al. stressed the possibility of response bias among teachers and parents, warning against over-interpreting the finding that cancer survivors were more likely to be isolated than their healthy counterparts because significant differences were found on only 2 of 23 questions.

Taken together, these studies suggest that teachers, peers, and even the children with cancer may view their social adjustment differently, thus accounting for some of the discrepancy in findings across studies. In other words, depending on who is asked, one may obtain relatively different perspectives on social adjustment. Additional investigation employing multi-informant methodology is thus needed to fully understand the nature of social adjustment of children with cancer. Certainly, research is needed to assess perceptions of social isolation and how this may have an impact on socioemotional well-being. However, the current literature would suggest that the cancer experience does not necessarily imply a course of negative social adjustment for children with cancer. Instead, it appears that considerable individual variability exists in the adjustment process, and that only a small subset of these children experience consistent difficulties.

## The Academic Context and Peer Relationships

As discussed in the previous section, peers play an important role in the social adjustment of children with cancer. Indeed, children who have undergone treatment for cancer experience a number of acute and long-term consequences related to treatment that may potentially have an impact on relationships with peers. Consequently, returning to the classroom after the diagnosis of cancer is a challenging situation for the child and the child's parents, friends, and teachers (Vance & Eiser, 2002), particularly when the child is still on treatment. We further describe social adjustment with peers among children with cancer in this section with a specific focus on reintegration into the school setting and how this relates to social relationships.

School absence becomes a salient issue among children with cancer because a majority of them attend school less regularly than do healthy children or children with other chronic conditions (Adamoli et al., 1997; Deasy-Spinetta & Spinetta, 1980; Mancini et al., 1989). Investigators have reported a significant association between the number of days missed from school and academic skills (Williams, Ochs, Williams, & Mulhern, 1991). Further, academic functioning has been associated with social skills among child and adolescent cancer survivors (Newby, Brown, Pawletko, Gold, & Whitt, 2000). Thus, it seems reasonable to conclude that successful reintegration into school is important in facilitating children's academic skills and subsequent educational progress and is crucial to the establishment of close interpersonal relationships (Vance & Eiser, 2002).

There are a number of factors that are important as children reintegrate into the school setting after diagnosis and treatment. Notably, the physical sequelae associated with cancer treatment sets some of these children apart from their peers. For example, losing their hair, puffiness or swelling, or using braces or a wheelchair may each contribute to a sense of feeling "different" or not fitting into a peer group. Such stigmas may also result in classmates pestering or teasing the child who has been ill. Fatigue and pain may also limit the child's ability to engage successfully with peers. Moreover, the child with cancer may experience limited opportunities for interaction with peers because of school absences or medical limitations.

Another important factor that may make it challenging for children, especially those with CNS involvement, to reintegrate successfully is the degree of cognitive impairment that may be associated with their illness or associated treatment. In addition, the child may be limited or even thwarted from spending much time with peers because of overprotective parents. Certainly, it appears that factors related to medical sequelae could be important in understanding how children with cancer reintegrate into their academic setting.

Although there are relatively few investigations of children's socioemotional functioning in the school context, a handful of studies have provided evidence that children with cancer are able to manage social relationships successfully as they return to school. Such studies have primarily examined differences in classroom behavior among children with cancer versus healthy comparison control children. In almost every case, no differences emerged between the two groups based on either parent or teacher report for children on or off treatment (Gartstein, Short, Vannatta, & Noll, 1999; Madan-Swain et al., 1994; Noll et al., 1999). Further, Deasy-Spinetta and Spinetta (1980) found that the children with cancer were not significantly different from their healthy peers in their willingness to attend school, teasing, or the extent to which they demonstrated age-inappropriate behaviors.

Two other studies provided largely similar results. Mancini and colleagues (1989) obtained teacher ratings of the school behavior of 91 children with cancer and healthy comparison control children chosen by the teacher to best represent class characteristics. Ratings were made using a forced-choice questionnaire that assessed teachers' perceptions of the child's interest in school, degree of learning abilities, and level of social interactions. Results revealed that children with cancer missed school more regularly and had average school behavior scores that were significantly lower than controls. Item analysis indicated that children with cancer had lower (i.e., less typical) behavior scores on only 12 of 29 items. The investigators concluded that lower attendance on the part of the children with cancer was the biggest obstacle to school performance, and they suggested that this may be caused by overprotection on the part of physicians and parents. Nonetheless, it is important to note that these conclusions were speculative, and these hypotheses deserve further empirical validation.

In another study using the same methodology with a sample of 291 children, Adamoli and colleagues (1997) found that children with cancer differed from healthy classmates in overall school functioning, including areas of learning, socialization (i.e., degree of social participation vs. social isolation), and emotionality. However, results also indicated that only a few children with cancer actually demonstrated school-related difficulties. Thus, it appears that both the Mancini et al. (1989) and Adamoli et al. (1997) studies provided further evidence to suggest that children with cancer fare well overall compared to healthy controls, and it is only a subset of this sample that may indeed exhibit school-related difficulties.

## Neurocognitive Impairments and Social Adjustment

As mentioned, children with certain forms of cancer are certainly at increased risk to experience neurocognitive impairments secondary to surgical procedures and treatment for cancer (e.g., CNS therapies for leukemia, including radiation chemotherapy). For a complete review of neuropsychological functioning in cancer survivors, see chapter 14 by Mulhern and Butler in this volume. Frequently, these neurocognitive impairments are manifested many years after cessation of treatment.

Cognition can potentially impact skills necessary for social interaction (e.g., recognition of social cues, flexibility in thinking, etc.) and affect the way in which children learn and perform in school. For instance, declines in measures of global intellectual functioning (e.g., IQ scores) have been demonstrated among children treated with radiation therapy largely because of changes in the frontal cortex of the brain (Armstrong, Blumber, & Toledano, 1999). Other common adverse effects may include slowed processing speed, difficulties with sustained attention, difficulties with visual-motor integration, memory difficulties, and some academic problems in math or reading (Armstrong & Briery, 2004). Evidence also suggests that children treated with radiation therapy to the CNS have reduced volumes of normal white matter, and that these deficits can at least partially explain deficits in children's intellectual performance (Mulhern et al., 1999).

Such cognitive impairments may create challenges for these children in their social environment. In a review of 31 studies on the social-emotional adjustment of children with brain tumors, Fuemmeler, Elkin, and Mullins (2002) concluded that cognitive impairments are a primary factor related to poor social adjustment. Such deficits may result in diminished ability to recognize subtle social cues necessary for successful interactions with peers. In addition, difficulties in attention, problem solving, decision making, and impulsivity, may lead to ineffective or inappropriate social behavior. Placement in special education classrooms (e.g., reading lab, self-contained classrooms) may inadvertently lead to social stigmatization and social isolation.

Taken together, it appears that the possibility of visible stigmas, time away from the school setting, and neurocognitive impairments result in children with cancer being at heightened risk for difficulties in social adjustment. Currently, it is difficult to determine whether the aforementioned factors directly lead to difficulties in social adjustment, as extant research has only recently begun to evaluate the effects of cancer treatment among children and adolescents reintegrating into the academic setting. Further research is needed to examine how medical sequelae can play a role in successful social reintegration among children with cancer.

### Emotional Well-Being and Peer Relationships

Research conducted with children who have survived cancer indicates that the vast majority cope well over time; however, small subsamples are at risk, primarily for internalizing types (e.g., anxiety, depression) of symptoms (Vanatta & Gerhardt, 2003). Children with cancer who are experiencing adjustment problems (e.g., internalizing symptoms) may have subsequent difficulties negotiating peer relationships and interacting with others. Specifically, the clinical child psychology literature has documented that children who are depressed perceive themselves to be less accepted by others, view their relationships with their best friends as being of lower friendship quality, or see others' neutral intentions as malevolent (Brendgen, Vitaro, Turgeon, & Poulin, 2002). In addition, research has indicated that peers rate children who are depressed as less likable and attractive as well as more likely to need therapeutic services than nondepressed peers (e.g., Peterson, Mullins, & Ridley-Johnson, 1985). Taking these findings into account, it appears that the small subset of children with cancer who experience internalizing problems may be at risk for experiencing difficulties with their peers, although this has yet to be investigated. Future research is needed to address how children with cancer who experience adjustment difficulties may also experience subtle problems with peer relations and friendships.

## Peer Support and Adjustment Outcomes

Although the cancer experience can negatively affect the child and the child's peer relationships, the potential also exists for peers and friends to provide positive social support, ultimately influencing a variety of adjustment outcomes. In this section, we focus briefly on the extent to which peer relations and friendships may buffer the impact of the cancer experience, borrowing from research conducted with other illness groups.

### Social Support and Adjustment

Social support is believed to be important in children's adjustment to their illness, functioning as a buffer for stress (Burroughs, Harris, Pontious, & Santiago, 1997; La Greca et al., 1995, 2002). Notably, few investigators have examined issues of social support in the context of childhood cancer. An early investigation by Kazak and Meadows (1989) examined the role of social support to adjustment outcomes among survivors of childhood cancer. The investigators compared young adolescent (10–15 years old) survivors of cancer to a healthy comparison control group on measures of social support, perceived self-competence, and family adaptability and cohesion at two time points (i.e., September and March of the academic year). Results revealed that scores were generally within normative limits and did not differ significantly between the survivor and comparison groups. However, survivors reported lower levels of perceived social support from family, friends, and teachers at the second assessment than earlier in the year. The investigators speculated that this perception of lower social support may be caused by subtle effects of having had cancer combined with possible parental overprotectiveness and time away from peers.

Varni, Katz, Colegrove, and Dolgin (1994) further studied the role of perceived social support on adjustment among school-aged children who were newly diagnosed with cancer (i.e., 9 months postdiagnosis). Children completed standardized measures of depression, state and trait anxiety, social anxiety, general self-esteem, and perceived social support from classmates, parents, teachers, and friends. Parental reports of internalizing and externalizing behavior problems were also assessed on the CBCL Parent Report Form (Achenbach & Edelbrock, 1983). Results revealed that perceived classmate social support significantly predicted each of the criterion variables (i.e., depressive symptoms, anxiety) with the exception of general self-esteem. Perceived social support from teachers predicted externalizing behavior problems. Perceived social support from parents and friends did not predict any criterion variables. Collectively, the results indicated that perceived classmate, parent, and teacher social support were associated with the adjustment criterion variables in the direction of greater support predicting less psychological distress and higher self-esteem. In addition, perceived classmate social support was identified as the most consistent predictor of adjustment. These data provide evidence for the potential positive effects of the school social environment and suggest that children diagnosed with cancer need continuation of their social and academic activities to normalize as much as possible an ongoing stressful experience.

In a later study, Varni and Katz (1997) prospectively examined the effects of perceived stress and social support on negative affectivity in a sample of newly diagnosed school-aged children with cancer within 1 month of diagnosis, 6 months postdiagnosis, and 9 months postdiagnosis. Negative affectivity was calculated by symptoms of depression and anxiety as measured by the Children's Depression Inventory (Kovacs, 1992) and State-Trait Anxiety Inventory for Children (Spielberger, 1973), respectively. Results revealed that higher perceived social support was predictive of lower negative affectivity at each of the assessment points. The investigators concluded that the pattern of relationships among perceived stress, perceived social support, and negative affectivity changes during the transition from an initial diagnosis of cancer through the subsequent 9 months, and that it is necessary to evaluate children's adjustment throughout this transitional period.

Consistent with other chronic illnesses (La Greca et al., 1995, 2002), it appears that perceived social support is associated with psychological adjustment among children with cancer. Unfortunately, only a small number of investigations in the pediatric psychosocial oncology literature have sought to examine the role of social support to adjustment outcomes. Further, longitudinal research is necessary to specifically examine the social support-adjustment linkage among this population.

## Social Support and Health Outcomes

There is emerging evidence bolstering the hypothesis that social support may increase survival among patients with cancer. Evidence for this relationship is found primarily in studies of adults. Several prospective studies among women with breast cancer have found that women who have greater social support (measured by frequent contact with friends) have longer survival rates than women with less social support (Funch & Marshall, 1983; Hislop, Waxler, Coldman, Elwood, & Kan, 1987; Waxler-Morrison, Hislop, Mears, & Kan, 1991). It is believed that social support buffers the association between psychological stress related to cancer and dysregulation of the immune and neuroendocrine systems, thus increasing the chances of survival from cancer (Andersen, 2002; Andersen, Kiecolt-Glaser, & Glaser, 1994; Cohen & Herbert, 1996; Helgeson, Cohen, & Fritz, 1998).

Specifically, the body's immune system functions to eradicate pathogens (such as bacteria, viruses, parasites) by generating protein molecules or antigens. The immune system also helps to rid the body of cells that have been transformed through malignancy or infection (Miller & Cohen, 2001). Stress may activate the sympathetic nervous system and neuroendocrine-immune pathways, including the hypothalamic-pituitary-adrenal axis. Aspects of antitumor immunity may be modulated or suppressed by hormones released under stress (e.g., catecholamines, cortisol, prolactin, and growth hormone) (Andersen, 2002). Accelerated tumor growth has been shown to be associated with glucocorticoids resulting from stress in animal studies, and in vitro studies have demonstrated increased tumor cell growth stimulated by cortisol (Lointier, Wildrick, & Boman, 1992).

Likewise, through their regulation of lymphocyte levels, stress-related changes in neuroepinephrine and epinephrine may also alter certain immune responses at the cellular level, such as migration, lymphocyte proliferation, antibody secretion, and cell lysis (Madden & Livant, 1991). Social support may serve to buffer this stress–immune response relationship. Turner-Cobb, Sephton, Koopman, Blake-Mortimer, and Spiegel (2000) found higher perceived social support to be associated with healthier neuroendocrine functioning (i.e., lower salivary cortisol concentrations) in women diagnosed with recurrent breast cancer.

Lutgendorf et al. (2002) found social support to be associated with important functional mechanisms involved in tumor angiogenesis among presurgical patients with ovarian carcinoma. Angiogenesis is the process related to tumor growth and metastases; one of the numerous factors related to this process is vascular endothelial growth factor. In their study, Lutgendorf et al. found that, among preoperative patients with ovarian cancer, women who reported greater social support (particularly perceived emotional support and the ability to count on others) had lower levels of serum vascular endothelial growth factor. Thus, these results suggest that perceived emotional support may be important in buffering the potential impact that stress has on cancer progression.

To date, there has been very little research examining the association between social support among children with cancer and neuroendocrine functioning or immune status. We conducted a PubMed search of the last 10 years and found only one study that directly examined the putative association between social support and immune functioning among children. Hockenberry-Eaton, Kemp, and Dilorio (1994) evaluated 44 children currently receiving treatment for cancer at two clinic visits. Participants completed a battery of questionnaires assessing psychological functioning and family and social support; epinephrine, norepinephrine, and cortisol levels were collected via urine specimens. After controlling for baseline levels, findings revealed that perceived social support from friends was associated with higher levels of norepinephrine, suggesting that perceived social support may mediate the stress–immune response among children with cancer. The investigators did not find support for the predicted relationship between social support and cortisol levels and epinephrine levels, indicating that the findings were not as robust as predicted. This study had several methodological shortcomings, including a small sample size, inclusion of children with various types of cancer (and thus a variety of treatments that could potentially influence stress differently), and infrequent physiological assessments. Clearly, a replication and extension of this study would assist in providing greater support for the hypothesis that social support mediates the impact that cancer-related stress may have on neuroendocrine and immune functioning among children with cancer.

Related studies have investigated the relationship between sense of humor and the outcomes of psychological adjustment, immune functioning, and infection among children with cancer (Dowling, Hockenberry, & Gregory, 2003). A sense of humor may be important in attracting social reinforcement, such as social support or minimizing social isolation (Cann & Calhoun, 2001; Martin, 1996). Among a sample of 43 children undergoing treatment for cancer, Dowling et al. found that children with high coping humor reported better psychological adjustment. Although no relationship was found between sense of humor and biological markers of immune function (i.e., secreted immune globulin A and absolute neutrophil counts), findings did reveal that higher coping sense of humor buffered the relationship between self-reported cancer stressors and incidence of infection. Thus, this study provides some preliminary evidence to suggest that individual characteristics associated with positive social functioning may be important in thwarting infection among children with cancer.

Although there is a compelling body of literature examining the association between social factors and immune functioning among adults, little research has been focused on children with cancer. The evidence provided by Hockenberry and colleagues gives preliminary support for the hypothesis that social support among children could be important in reducing the risk of infection. However, prior to intervention trials examining the impact of social support on health outcomes, more data are needed among children that could replicate and extend these preliminary findings.

## Interventions to Enhance Social Adjustment

Clearly, children with cancer are at risk for experiencing a number of social adjustment problems, including difficulties with social competence/social skills, isolation, restriction from certain social activities, problems with school reintegration, and peer teasing. Children with brain tumors or central nervous system involvement are perhaps at greatest risk for problems in social adjustment (e.g., Foley, Barakat, Herman-Liu, Radcliffe, & Molloy, 2000). Despite years of intervention research on social competence problems in nonchronically ill children (e.g., McFadyen-Ketchum & Dodge, 1998), unfortunately little empirical research exists that examines interventions to facilitate social functioning in children with cancer and their families. In this section, we briefly review potential levels or targets of intervention and associated studies conducted to date. These levels include individual, family, and systems-based interventions. Notably, a number of these studies involve multiple levels of intervention (e.g., both child and parents receive intervention services).

### Individual-Level Interventions

As far back as the mid-1980s, pediatric cancer researchers have recognized the potential contribution of social skills interventions to enhance psychological adjustment (Katz, Rubenstein, Hubert, & Blew, 1988). In one of the first randomized controlled trials on enhancing social competence in children newly diagnosed with cancer, Varni and colleagues compared a brief (three-session) social skills training program to a standard treatment control group who received a school reintegration program (Varni, Katz, Colegrove, & Dolgin, 1993). The social skills training intervention was individually administered and included three content areas: social cognitive problem-solving training, assertiveness training, and handling teasing and name calling. Videotaped vignettes of potentially challenging social situations coupled with the modeling of coping procedures were presented as part of these sessions. In addition, homework assignments were given to the children. Parents were involved in one of the training sessions and were encouraged to monitor and support their children's coping efforts. Child, parent, and teacher ratings were assessed at both 6 and 9 months postdiagnosis follow-up periods. Although few between-group comparisons were significant, the 9-month follow-up analyses indicated that children who received social skills training had significantly fewer behavior problems and higher levels of classmate peer social support and school competence compared to pretreatment levels. Notably, these improvements increased with time. For the children who received the school reintegration program as part of the attention control, no such effects were found at the 9-month follow-up.

As mentioned, children with CNS involvement are at particular risk for social adjustment problems. Die-Trill et al. (1996) described the development of a 16-session social skills group training program for boys aged 10–14 years who had been diagnosed with a brain tumor. The first 8 sessions were devoted to the development of specific social skills (e.g., assertiveness, making new friends, handling teasing), while the remaining 8 sessions focused on reinforcement of those skills through medical education and offering social support. A parent group also was offered at the same time that focused on support-related issues. Although no standardized measures of social skills or adjustment outcomes were administered, visual-analog ratings provided by parents and their children suggested that the sessions were helpful in skill acquisition and garnering additional social support.

Barakat and colleagues (2003) evaluated the effectiveness of a manual-based social skills training intervention using a within-group pre-posttest longitudinal design with children who had been treated for a brain tumor. Using a group format, children were trained in communication skills (e.g., starting, maintaining, and ending conversations), cooperation skills, empathy skills, and conflict resolution over six weekly sessions. Homework assignments were also employed. A parent intervention component was also included that involved a review of the targeted social skills, a discussion of barriers to practicing social skills, means of reinforcing their children's social skills and facilitating homework assignments, and discussions with the children of how the brain tumor had affected their family. Parents, children, and teachers completed measures of social skills, internalizing and externalizing behavior, and quality of life. At a 9-month follow-up, significant improvements were found for parent ratings of total competence on the CBCL (Achenbach & Edelbrock, 1983) and child ratings of social competence on the Miami Pediatric Quality of Life measure (Armstrong et al., 1999). As well, child-reported internalizing behavior problems on the Youth Self-Report Form (Achenbach & Edelbrock, 1983) were significantly decreased. Trends in the predicted direction also were found for teacher reports of social skills problems and externalizing behavior problems, as well as for children's reports of internalizing behavior.

Although preliminary, the results of these studies suggest that social skills problems in children with cancer may be effectively addressed by short-term skills-based treatment approaches. Notably, each of these studies included both children with cancer and their parents, although separate social skills interventions were provided to the children. It is difficult to discern from these preliminary results those aspects of the treatment that exerted the most influential effects given the multicomponent nature of the treatment packages. It also is unclear regarding the long-term effects of such interventions on the social relationships of these children. Future research is necessary to address such issues.

### Family-Level Interventions

Interventions that promote social functioning may also target the larger family system. Systemic interventions focus not only on the individual components of the family in isolation, but also on the interactions and relationships between family members. Family-based interventions are commonplace in the treatment of children with cancer but rarely have been subjected to empirical scrutiny. Further, although social relationships are often a focus of treatment, no data currently exist that document the effectiveness of family approaches facilitating the social adjustment of the child. However, it may be argued that parents have considerable influence in the trajectory that their child's social relationships take following the diagnosis of cancer. Although the available literature suggests that the child-rearing practices of parents of children with cancer are not significantly different from those practices for healthy children, mothers and fathers do report worries about overinvolvement and overprotectiveness (Davies, Noll, DeStefano, Bukowski, & Kulkarni, 1991). Parents of children with cancer may also experience difficulty in maintaining consistency in their parenting behavior at the time period immediately following the diagnosis of their child (Steele, Long, Reddy, Luhr, & Phipps, 2003).

Little is known about the impact of parental overprotection or overinvolvement on the social relationships of children who have survived cancer. However, other researchers have demonstrated that parental overprotection may diminish autonomy in children with a disabling condition (i.e., spina bifida) and contribute to the development of internalizing and externalizing behavior problems (Holmbeck et al., 2002). Similarly, Mullins and colleagues (2004) found that higher levels of parent-perceived child vulnerability were associated with greater depressive symptomatology in children with type 1 diabetes.

Although speculative, these studies suggested that specific parenting behaviors have the potential to contribute to problematic personal and social functioning in children with chronic health problems. To the extent that children with cancer may be vulnerable and subject to overprotection, it is likely that social interaction may occur less frequently as school attendance become sporadic. Additional research on the relationship between parent behaviors and subsequent social functioning is ripe for investigation. Such research should focus on the efficacy of general, education-based programs on enhancing parenting practices and strategies, or programs may take the form of structured, systems-based approaches such as Parent-Child Interaction Training (Hembree-Kigin & McNeil, 1995). Such structured approaches can be readily adapted to incorporate interactional strategies that maximize the development of autonomy and the furthering of social relationships.

### Multilevel Interventions: School Reintegration Programs

Perhaps the most common form of multilevel interventions is school reentry or reintegration programs (see Katz and Madan-Swain, chapter 17, this volume for a more complete review of such programs). School reintegration programs have a relatively long history in pediatric oncology (e.g., Goodell, 1984; Katz et al., 1988; McCormick, 1986) and have been posited to serve a number of important functions for the child with cancer (Madan-Swain, Fredrick, & Wallander, 1999).

First, they serve the purpose of preparing the school system (i.e., teachers, administrators, and counselors) and other children for the return and reinvolvement of the child who has survived cancer in the school context. Second, and perhaps more relevant to this particular chapter, school reentry or reintegration programs serve to facilitate social support and social relationships. Such programs vary widely in nature and may involve multiple educational/treatment components, including visits by nurses and health care workers to the school, use of videotaped vignettes for the purpose of educating peers and teachers about cancer, and provision of written information to teachers and classmates. Topics can range from discussion of the nature and impact of childhood cancer on adjustment and peer relationships to treatment effects, as well as the impact of peer teasing and safety concerns. These programs may target peer classmates, teachers and administrators, parents, the child with cancer, or some combination of these individuals. Such programs may also be relatively formal (i.e., structured and time limited) or may involve relatively informal efforts that span an indefinite amount of time.

The efficiency of such programs in enhancing the social relationships of children with cancer is unclear. The existing studies do not lend themselves well to addressing this question. Many programs were established as part of direct service provision, and outcomes either were not measured or were assessed in terms of knowledge acquisition or attitude change on the part of peers and teachers, not in terms of social adjustment of the child with cancer. Such programs do appear to diminish parental concerns and enhance teachers' awareness of safety concerns and academic performance capabilities (McCarthy, Williams, & Plummer, 1998).

Katz's research potentially bears more directly on social outcomes (Katz et al, 1988). Following institution of a school reintegration program, children diagnosed with cancer evidenced significant reductions in internalizing problems (i.e., self-esteem problems and depressive symptomatology). Although speculative, such reductions in symptoms may well reduce the likelihood of peer rejection. A follow-up report in 1992 revealed that teachers perceived such a program to benefit children, particularly females (Katz, Varni, Rubenstein, Blew, & Hubert, 1992).

Two studies targeting the behavior and attitudes of classmates of children diagnosed with cancer provided equivocal results (Vance & Eiser, 2002). Although willingness to interact with the child with cancer and cancer-related knowledge can apparently be increased following educational programs (Benner & Marlow, 1991), classmates may still continue to harbor significant health-related concerns about the child who had been diagnosed with cancer (Ellerton & Turner, 1992).

These findings are notable given analog research on attempts to manage peers' perceptions of children with various medical conditions. Gray and Rodrigue (2001) found that adolescent peers rated a hypothetical peer with cancer more favorably and were more accepting toward that individual compared to a healthy peer. Their results suggested that a cancer stereotype may not in fact exist or at least not to the extent previously believed. In contrast, Bell and Morgan (2000) found that efforts to lessen peers' negative perceptions of an obese peer by providing a medical explanation for the obesity actually resulted in either no effect or had a negative effect on intentions to interact. Based on these results, La Greca and Bearman (2000) suggested that giving classmates advanced notice of a given child's medical condition may have unexpectedly negative effects on those peers and potentially decrease the likelihood of acceptance and provision of support. In this regard, school reintegration programs may, under some circumstances, actually have the potential to create negative perceptions on the part of peers. Thus, school reintegration programs must be used with a great deal of thought.

Vance and Eiser (2002) aptly pointed out that much of the extant literature on the effectiveness of such school interventions for children, their classmates, and teachers is of questionable quality and can benefit from considerable methodological improvement. Given the improved prognosis for childhood cancer and the increasing number of children who are returning to the school setting, it is incumbent on future researchers to use these preliminary works on school reintegration as a springboard for more sophisticated designs that employ multiple outcome measures at different time points in the developmental trajectory of the disease.

## Summary and Future Directions

The experience of being diagnosed with cancer clearly has the potential to impinge on a wide variety of social aspects of childhood development, including being accepted by one's peers, maintaining old friendships, and developing new peer relationships. The nature of these social relationships, and how the cancer experience bears on their development, is clearly an understudied area in the pediatric psychology literature. Notably, the extant literature suggests that when parents or teachers are asked to assess the social functioning of these children, they often report that these children have few social adjustment difficulties during the treatment and recovery phases of cancer. Likewise, children with cancer do not appear to be wholly rejected by their peers; indeed, some research suggested they are viewed as leaders by teachers and peers. Nevertheless, it does appear that there is variability in the social adjustment process among these children, and a small subset of them experienced continued difficulties over time. For instance, even though others do not perceive children with cancer to manifest social problems, some children with cancer report feeling isolated. Further, the subset of children who do experience emotional adjustment difficulties may be at risk for developing social relationship difficulties.

Various frameworks and methods are available for conceptualizing and assessing children's social relationships, including social support, social networks, peer acceptance, and friendships. Studies of children with cancer have begun to employ a number of these methods in the last decade; however, the samples are small, and the majority of these studies are cross sectional, with the exception of those employing the sociometric methods. Indeed, the general literature regarding the development of social relationships among children could be informative in planning future studies among children with cancer.

La Greca (1997) pointed out that there is a need to use the vast amount of literature on social support and social skill acquisition in healthy children to develop interventions for children with cancer. At the same time, the unique challenges that cancer pose for children and adolescents in the social context must be acknowledged. In this regard, it may be fruitful also to borrow from the emerging literature on the social problems of children with other chronic illnesses (La Greca et al., 2002). As well, adult oncology studies that have examined the moderating influence of social support on the stress–immune response seem equally relevant to children with cancer. The importance of development and the social needs at various phases of development cannot be overlooked when studying children's adjustment. During different phases of development, the perceived stress of the cancer experience may function according to various social systems, such as family, close friends, or intimate partners.

In the assessment of children's friendships and emotional well-being, a need exists to include valid measurements, employed over long periods of time, in various settings and with multiple informants. Often, research on children's social adjustment to cancer has relied on quality-of-life measures or measures of pathology. Unfortunately, there is minimal ability for these measures to capture the intricate and more complex ways in which the cancer experience may affect social relationships and how positive social functioning can enhance physical and emotional well-being.

Likewise, the context in which children are asked about their social relationships could also be important regarding how survivors respond. Children may respond differently during clinic visits than at home or at school. Multiple assessments in various contexts are necessary to capture children's functioning in an array of social relationships.

There is a need to develop and use measures of social skills/competence that are appropriate for children with cancer. Indeed, new measures of social competence that are specific to populations of children with chronic illness are beginning to emerge (Adams, Streisand, Zawacki, & Joseph, 2002). From a measurement standpoint, assessment strategies are needed that allow more precise pinpointing of whether a given child has a skills deficit, a performance deficit, or a cognitive processing deficit that underlies a social problem. Furthermore, assessment of more precise social issues, such as intimacy during adolescence, may need to be studied in greater depth. Qualitative assessments of survivors' experiences may be useful in planning quantitative measures that can serve as screening measures to identify survivors who are having difficulty.

Finally, there is a clear need to develop cost-effective clinical interventions that facilitate the social adjustment of children with cancer. Because most studies indicated that the majority of children are not experiencing significant social problems, it is necessary to establish which subgroups of children are at highest risk. Preliminary evidence also suggests that such interventions might best target family systems and other community systems, including peers themselves. Also, because the nature and importance of peer relationships clearly change during adolescence, different interventions may need to be tailored to this group in light of developmental differences. Notably, peer group interventions for adolescents with diabetes have been successful in increasing peer and family support, decreasing diabetes-related conflict with parents, and enhancing metabolic control (Greco, Shroff-Pendley, McDonell, & Reeves, 2001). Indeed, future research among children with cancer must not only be sensitive to the unique aspects of the cancer experience, but also benefit from findings from clinical intervention research with other chronic illnesses.

## References


Achenbach, T., & Edelbrock, C. (1983). *Manual for the Child Behavior Checklist and Revised Child Behavior Profile.* Burlington: University of Vermont Press.

Adamoli, L., Deasy-Spinetta, P., Corbetta, A., Jankovic, M., Lia, R., Locati, A., et al. (1997). School functioning for the child with leukemia in continuous first remission: Screening high-risk children. *Pediatric Hematology and Oncology, 14,* 121–131.

Adams, C. D., Streisand, R. M., Zawacki, T., & Joseph, K. E. (2002). Living with a chronic illness: A measure of social functioning for children and adolescents. *Journal of Pediatric Psychology, 27,* 593–605.

Andersen, B. L. (2002). Biobehavioral outcomes following psychological interventions for cancer patients. *Journal of Consulting and Clinical Psychology, 70,* 590–610.

Andersen, B. L., Kiecolt-Glaser, J. K., & Glaser R. (1994). A biobehavioral model of cancer stress and disease course. *American Psychologist, 49,* 389–404.

Armstrong, F. D., Blumber, M. J., & Toledano, S. R. (1999). Neurobehavioral issues in childhood cancer. *School Psychology Review, 28,* 194–203.

Armstrong, F. D., & Briery, B. G. (2004). Childhood cancer and the school. In R. T. Brown (Ed.), *Handbook of pediatric psychology in school settings* (pp. 263–282). Mahwah, NJ: Erlbaum.

Bagwell, C. L., Coie, J. D., Terry, R. A., & Lochman, J. E. (2000). Peer clique participation and social status in preadolescence. *Merrill-Palmer Quarterly, 46,* 280–305.

Bagwell, C. L., Schmidt, M. E., Newcomb, A. F., & Bukowski, W. M. (2001). Friendship and peer rejection as predictors of adult adjustment. *New Directions for Child and Adolescent Development, 91,* 25–49.

Barakat, L. P., Hetzke, J. D., Foley, B., Carey, M. E., Gyato, K., & Phillips, P. C. (2003). Evaluation of a social-skills training group intervention with children treated for brain tumors: A pilot study. *Journal of Pediatric Psychology, 28,* 299–307.

Bell, S. K., & Morgan, S. B. (2000). Children's attitudes and behavioral intentions toward a peer presented as obese: Does a medical explanation for the obesity make a difference? *Journal of Pediatric Psychology, 25,* 137–145.

Benner, A. E., & Marlow, A. S. (1991). The effect of a workshop on childhood cancer on student's knowledge, concerns, and desire to interact with a classmate with cancer. *Children's Health Care, 20,* 101–107.

Berndt, T. J., Hawkins, J. A., & Jiao, Z. (1999). Influence of friends and friendships on adjustment to junior high school. *Merrill-Palmer Quarterly, 45,* 13–41.

Bierman, K. L., Smoot, D. L., & Aumiller, K. (1993). Characteristics of aggressive-rejected, aggressive (nonrejected), and rejected (nonaggressive) boys. *Child Development, 64,* 139–151.

Bigelow, B. J., & La Gaipa, J. J. (1980). The development of friendship values and choice. In H. C. Foot, A. J. Chapman, and J. R. Smith (Eds.), *Friendship and social relations in children* (pp. 15–44). New York, NY: Wiley.

Brendgen, M., Vitaro, F., Turgeon, L., & Poulin, F. (2002). Assessing aggressive and depressed children's social relations with classmates and friends: A matter of perspective. *Journal of Abnormal Child Psychology, 30,* 609–624.

Bukowski, W. M., & Hoza, B. (1989). Popularity and friendship: Issues in theory, measurement, and outcome. In T. J. Berndt and G. W. Ladd (Eds.), *Peer relationships in child development* (pp. 15–45). New York: Wiley.

Burroughs, T. E., Harris, M. A., Pontious, S. L., & Santiago, J. V. (1997). Research on social support in adolescents with IDDM: A critical review. *Diabetes Educator, 23,* 438–448.

Cann, A., & Calhoun, L. G. (2001). Perceived personality associated with differences in sense of humor: Stereotypes of hypothetical others with high and low seneses of humor. *Humor: International Journal of Humor Research, 14,* 117–130.

Cohen, S., & Herbert, T. B. (1996). Health psychology: Psychological factors and physical disease from the perspective of human psychoneuroimmunology. *Annual Review of Psychology, 47,* 113–142.

Coie, J., & Dodge, K. (1983). Continuities and changes in children's social status: A 5 year longitudinal study. *Merrill-Palmer Quarterly, 29,* 261–282.

Coie, J., & Dodge, K. (1988). Multiple sources of data on social behavior and social status in school: A cross-age comparison. *Child Development, 59,* 815–829.

Coie, J., Dodge, K., & Coppotelli, H. (1982). Dimensions and types of social status: A cross-age perspective. *Developmental Psychology, 18,* 667–570.

Coie, J., Dodge, K., & Kupersmidt, J. (1990). Peer group behavior and social status. In S. Asher, & J. Coie (Eds.), *Peer rejection in childhood* (pp.17–59). Cambridge, UK: Cambridge University Press.

Coie, J., Dodge, K., Terry, R., & Wright, V. (1991). The role of aggression in peer relations: An analysis of aggression episodes in boys' play groups. *Child Development, 62,* 812–826.

Criss, M., Pettit, G., Bates, J., Dodge, K., & Lapp, A. (2002). Family adversity, positive peer relationships and children's externalizing behavior: A longitudinal perspective on risk and resilience. *Child Development, 73,* 1220–1237.

Davies, W. H., Noll, R. B., DeStefano, L., Bukowski, W. M., & Kulkarni, R. (1991). Differences in the child-rearing practices of parents of children with cancer and controls: The perspectives of parents and professionals. *Journal of Pediatric Psychology, 16,* 295–306.

Deasy-Spinetta, P. (1981). The school and the child with cancer. In J. J. Spinetta & P. Deasy-Spinetta (Eds.), *Living with childhood cancer* (pp. 153–170). St. Louis, MO: Mosby.

Deasy-Spinetta, P. M., & Spinetta, J. J. (1980) The child with cancer in school: Teacher's appraisal. *American Journal of Pediatric Hematology and Oncology, 2,* 89–94.

Die-Trill, M., Bromberg, J., LaVally, B., Portales, L. A., SanFeliz, A., & Patenaude, A. F. (1996). Development of social skills in boys with brain tumors: A group approach. *Journal of Psychosocial Oncology, 14,* 23–41.

Dodge, K. A., McClaskey, C. L., & Feldman, E. (1985). Situational approach to the assessment of social competence in children. *Journal of Consulting and Clinical Psychology, 53,* 344–353.

Dowling, J. S., Hockenberry, M., & Gregory, R. (2003). Sense of humor, childhood cancer stressors, and outcomes of psychosocial adjustment, immune function, and infection. *Journal of Pediatric Oncology Nursing, 20,* 271–292.

Eiser, C. (1998). Practitioner review: Long-term consequences of childhood cancer. *Journal of Child Psychology and Psychiatry, and Allied Disciplines, 39,* 621–633.

Eiser, C., & Vance, Y. H. (2002). Implications of cancer for school attendance and behavior. *Medical and Pediatric Oncology, 38,* 317–319.

Ellerton, M., & Turner, C. (1992). "Back to school"—An evaluation of a re-entry program for school-aged children with cancer. *Canadian Oncology Nursing Journal, 2,* 8–11.

Erdley, C., & Asher, S., (1999). A social goals perspective on children's social competence. *Journal of Emotional and Behavioral Disorders, 7,* 156–167.

Erdley, C. A., Nangle, D. W., Newman, J. E., & Carpenter, E. M. (2001). Children's friendship experiences and psychological adjustment: Theory and research. *New Directions for Child and Adolescent Development, 91,* 5–24.

Farmer, T. W., & Farmer, E. M. Z. (1996). Social relationships of students with exceptionalities in mainstream classrooms: Social networks and homphily. *Exceptional Children, 62,* 431–450.

Farmer, T. W., & Rodkin, P. C. (1996). Antisocial and prosocial correlates of classroom social positions: The social network centrality perspective. *Social Development, 5,* 174–188.

Foley, B., Barakat, L. P., Herman-Liu, A., Radcliffe, J., & Molloy, P. (2000). The impact of childhood hypothalamic/chaiasmatic brain tumors on child adjustment and family functioning. *Children's Health Care, 29,* 209–223.

Fuemmeler, B. F., Elkin, T. D., & Mullins, L. L. (2002). Survivors of childhood brain tumors: Behavioral, emotional, and social adjustment. *Clinical Psychology Review, 22,* 547–585.

Funch, D. P., & Marshall, J. (1983). The role of stress, social support, and age in survival from breast cancer. *Journal of Psychosomatic Research, 27,* 77–83.

Furman, W., & Bierman, K. L. (1984). Children's conceptions of friendship: A multimethod study of developmental changes. *Developmental Psychology, 20,* 925–931.

Gartstein, M. A., Short, A. D., Vannatta, K., & Noll, R. B. (1999). Psychosocial adjustment of children with chronic illness: An evaluation of three models. *Journal of Developmental and Behavioral Pediatrics, 20,* 157–163.

Gest, S. D., Graham-Bermann, S. A., & Hartup, W. W. (2001). Peer experience: Common and unique features of number of friendships, social network centrality, and sociometric status. *Social Development, 10,* 23–40.

Gifford-Smith, M. E., & Brownell, C. A. (2003). Childhood peer relationships: Social acceptance, friendships, and peer networks. *Journal of School Psychology, 41,* 235–284.

Goodell, A. S. (1984). Peer education in schools for children with cancer. *Issues in Comprehensive Pediatric Nursing, 7,* 101–106.

Gray, C. C., & Rodrigue, J. R. (2001). Brief report: Perceptions of young adolescents about a hypothetical new peer with cancer: An analog study. *Journal of Pediatric Psychology, 26,* 247–252.

Greco, P., Shroff-Pendley, J., McDonell, K., & Reeves, G. (2001). A peer group intervention for adolescents with type 1 diabetes and their best friends. *Journal of Pediatric Psychology,* 26, 485–490.

Harter, S. (1985). *Manual for the self-perception profile for children.* Denver, CO: University of Denver.

Helgeson, V. S., Cohen, S., & Fritz, H. L. (1998). Social ties and cancer. In J. C. Holland (Ed.), *Psycho-Oncology* (pp. 99–109). New York: Oxford University Press.

Hembree-Kigin, T. L., & McNeil, C. B. (1995). *Parent–child interaction therapy.* New York: Plenum Press.

Hetherington, E. M. (1999). Social capital and the development of youth from nondivorced, divorced, and remarried families. In W. Collins & B. Laursen (Eds.), *Relationships as development contexts* (pp. 177–210). Mahwah, NJ: Erlbaum.

Hinshaw, S., & Melnick, S. (1995). Peer relationships in boys with attention-deficit hyperactivity disorder with and without comorbid aggression. *Development and Psychopathology, 7,* 627–647.

Hislop, T. G., Waxler, N. E., Coldman, A. J., Elwood, J. M., & Kan, L. (1987). The prognostic significance of psychosocial factors in women with breast cancer. *Journal of Chronic Disease, 40,* 729–735.

Hockenberry-Eaton, M., Kemp, V., & Dilorio, C. (1994). Cancer stressors and protective factors: Predictors of stress experienced during treatment for childhood cancer. *Research in Nursing and Health, 17,* 351–361.

Holmbeck, G. N., Johnson, S. Z., Wills, K. E., McKernon, W., Rose, B., Erklin, S., et al. (2002). Observed and perceived parental overprotection in relation to psychosocial adjustment in preadolescents with a physical disability: The mediational role of behavioral autonomy. *Journal of Consulting and Clinical Psychology, 70,* 96–110.

House, J. S. (1981). *Work stress and social support.* Reading, MA: Addison-Wesley.

House, J. S., Landis, K. R., & Umberson, D. (1988). Social relationships and health. *Science, 241,* 540–545.

Kazak, A. E., & Meadows, A. T. (1989). Families of young adolescents who have survived cancer: Social-emotional adjustment, adaptability, and social support. *Journal of Pediatric Psychology, 14,* 175–191.

Katz, E. R., Rubenstein, C., Hubert, N., & Blew, A. (1988). School and social reintegration of children with cancer. *Journal of Psychosocial Oncology, 6,* 123–40.

Katz, E. R., Varni, J. W., Rubenstein, C. L., Blew, A., & Hubert, N. (1992). Teacher, parent, and child evaluative ratings of a school reintegration intervention for children newly diagnosed with cancer. *Children's Health Care, 2,* 69–75.

Kovacs, M. (1992). *Children's depression inventory manual.* Toronto, ON: Multi-Health Systems, Inc.

Kullgren, K., Morris, R. D., Morris, M. K., & Krawiecki, N. (2003). Risk factors associated with long-term social and behavioral problems among children with brain tumors. *Journal of Psychosocial Oncology, 21,* 73–87.

Ladd, G. W., Kochenderfer, B. J., & Coleman, C. C. (1997). Classroom peer acceptance, friendship, and victimization: Distinct relational systems that contribute uniquely to children's school adjustment? *Child Development, 68,* 1181–1197.

La Greca, A. M. (1997). Children's problems with friends. *In Session: Psychotherapy in practice, 3,* 2141.

La Greca, A. M., Auslander, W. F., Greco, P., Spetter, D., Fisher, E. B., & Santiago, J. V. (1995). I get by with a little help from my family and friends: Adolescents' support for diabetes care. *Journal of Pediatric Psychology, 20,* 449–476.

La Greca, A. M., & Bearman, K. J. (2000). Commentary: Children with pediatric conditions: Can peers' impressions be managed? And what about their friends? *Journal of Pediatric Psychology, 25,* 147–149.

La Greca, A. M., Bearman, K. J., & Moore, H. (2002). Peer relations of youth with pediatric conditions and health risks: Promoting social support and healthy lifestyles. *Developmental and Behavioral Pediatrics, 23,* 271–280.

La Greca, A. M., & Lopez, N. (1998). Social anxiety among adolescents: Linkages with peer relations and friendships. *Journal of Abnormal Child Psychology, 26,* 83–94.

Lointier, P., Wildrick, D. M., & Boman, B. M. (1992). The effects of steroid hormones on a human colon cancer cell line in vitro. *Anticancer Research, 12,* 1327–1330.

Lutgendorf, S. K., Johnsen, E. L., Cooper, B., Anderson, B., Sorosky, J. I., Buller, R. E., et al. (2002). Vascular endothelial growth factor and social support in patients with ovarian carcinoma. *Cancer, 95,* 808–815.

Madan-Swain, A., Brown, R. T., Sexson, S. B., Baldwin, K., Pais, R., & Ragab, A. (1994). Adolescent cancer survivors: Psychosocial and familial adaptation. *Psychosomatics, 35,* 453–459.

Madan-Swain, A., Fredrick, L., & Wallander, J. L. (1999). Returning to school after a serious illness or injury. In R. T. Brown (Ed.), *Cognitive aspects of chronic illness in children* (pp. 312–332). New York: Guilford Press.

Madden, K. S., & Livant, S. (1991). Catecholamine action and immunologic reactivity. In R. Ader, D. L. Felten, & N. Cohen (Eds.), *Psychoneuroimmunology* (2nd ed., pp. 283–310). San Diego, CA: Academic Press.

Mancini, A. F., Rosito, P., Canino, R., Calzetti, G., Di Caro, A., Salmi, S., et al. (1989). School-related behavior in children with cancer. *Pediatric Hematology and Oncology, 6,* 145–154.

Martin, R. A. (1996). The Situational Humor Response Questionnaire (SHRQ) and Coping Humor Scale (CHS): A decade of research findings. *Humor: International Journal of Humor Research, 9,* 251–272.

McCarthy, A. M., Williams, J., & Plummer, C. (1998). Evaluation of a school re-entry nursing intervention for children with cancer. *Journal of Pediatric Oncology Nursing, 15,* 143–152.

McCormick, D. (1986). School re-entry programs for oncology patients. *Journal of the Association of Pediatric Oncology Nurses, 3,* 13–25.

McFadyen-Ketchum, S.A., & Dodge, K. A. (1998). Problems in social relationships. In E. J. Mash & R. A. Barkley (Eds.), *Treatment of childhood disorders* (2nd ed., pp. 338–365). New York: Guilford Press.

Miller, G. E., & Cohen, S., (2001). Psychological interventions and the immune system: A meta-analytic review and critique. *Health Psychology, 20,* 47–63.

Mulhern, R. K., Reddick, W. E., Palmer, S. L., Glass, J. O., Elkin, T. D., Kun, L. E., et al. (1999). Neurocognitive deficits in medulloblastoma survivors and white matter loss. *Annals of Neurology, 46,* 834–841.

Mullins, L. L., Fuemmeler, B. F., Hoff, A. L., Chaney, J. M., Van Pelt, J., & Ewing, C. (2004). The relationship of parental overprotection and perceived child vulnerability to depressive symptomatology in children with type 1 diabetes mellitus: The moderating influence of parenting stress. *Children's Health Care, 33,* 21–34.

Nelson, D., & Crick, N. (1999). Rose-colored glasses: Examining the social information processing of prosocial young adolescents. *Journal of Early Adolescence, 19,* 17–38.

Newby, W., Brown, R. T., Pawletko, T. M., Gold, S. H., & Whitt, J. K. (2000). Social skills and psychological adjustment to child and adolescent cancer survivors. *Psycho-Oncology, 9,* 113–126.

Newcomb, A. F., Bukowski, W. M., & Pattee, L. (1993). Children's peer relations: A meta-analytic review of popular, rejected, neglected, controversial, and average sociometric status. *Psychological Bulletin, 113,* 99–128.

Newcomb, A. F., Bukowski, W. M., & Bagwell, C. L. (1999). Knowing the sounds: Friendship and developmental context. In W. A. Collins and B. Laursen (Eds.), *Relationships as developmental contexts: The Minnesota symposia on child psychology* (Vol. 30, pp. 63–84). Mahwah, NJ: Erlbaum.

Noll, R. B., Bukowski, W. M., Davies, W. H., Koontz, K., & Kulkarni, R. (1993). Adjustment in the peer system of adolescents with cancer: A 2-year study. *Journal of Pediatric Psychology, 18,* 351–364.

Noll, R. B., Bukowski, W. M., Rogosch, F. A., LeRoy, S., & Kulkarni, R. (1990). Social interactions between children with cancer and their peers: Teacher ratings. *Journal of Pediatric Psychology, 15,* 43–56.

Noll, R. B., Gartstein, M. A., Vannatta, K., Correll, J., Bukowski, W. M., & Davies, W. H. (1999). Social, emotional, and behavioural functioning of children with cancer. *Pediatrics, 103,* 71–78.

Noll, R. B., LeRoy, S., Bukowski, W. M., Rogosch, F. A., & Kulkarni, R. (1991). Peer relationships and adjustment in children with cancer. *Journal of Pediatric Psychology, 16,* 307–326.

Noll, R. B., Ris, M. D., Davies, W. H., Bukowski, W. M., & Koontz, K. (1992). Social interactions between children with cancer or sickle cell disease and their peers: Teacher ratings. *Journal of*

*Developmental and Behavioral Pediatrics, 13,* 187–193.

Noll, R. B., Vannatta, K., Koontz, K., Kalinyak, K., Bukowski, W. M., & Davies, W. H. (1996). Peer relationships and emotional well-being of youngsters with sickle cell disease. *Child Development, 67,* 426–436.

Ollendick, T. H., Weist, M. D., Borden, M. C., & Greene, R. W. (1992). Sociometric status and academic, behavioral, and psychological adjustment: A 5-year longitudinal study. *Journal of Consulting and Clinical Psychology, 60,* 80–87.

Parker, J., & Gottman, J. (1989). Social and emotional development in a relational context: Friendship interaction from early childhood to adolescence. In T. Berndt & G. Ladd (Eds.), *Peer relationships in child development* (pp. 95–131). New York: Wiley.

Parker, J. G., Rubin, K. H., Price, J. M., & De Rosier, M. E. (1995). Peer relationships, child development, and adjustment: A developmental psychopathology perspective. In D. Cicchetti and D. J. Cohen (Eds.), *Developmental psychopathology, Volume 2: Risk, disorder, and adaptation* (pp. 96–161). New York: Wiley.

Peterson, L., Mullins, L. L., & Ridley-Johnson, R. (1985). Childhood depression: Peer reactions to depression and life stress. *Journal of Abnormal Child Psychology, 13,* 597–610.

Selman, R. (1980). *The growth of interpersonal understanding.* New York: Academic Press.

Spielberger, C. D. (1973). *State-trait anxiety inventory for children.* Palo Alto, CA: Consulting Psychologists Press.

Spirito, A., Stark, L. J., Cobiella, C., Drigan, R., Androkites, A., & Hewett, K. (1990). Social adjustment of children successfully treated for cancer. *Journal of Pediatric Psychology, 15,* 359–371.

Steele, R. G., Long, A., Reddy, K. A., Luhr, M., & Phipps, S. (2003). Changes in maternal distress and child-rearing strategies across treatment for pediatric cancer. *Journal of Pediatric Psychology, 28,* 447–452.

Sullivan, H. S. (1953). *The interpersonal theory of psychiatry.* New York: Norton.

Turner-Cobb, J. M., Sephton, S. E., Koopman, C., Blake-Mortimer, J., & Spiegel, D., (2000). Social support and salivary cortisol in women with metastatic breast cancer. *Psychosomatic Medicine, 62,* 337–345.

Vance, Y. H., & Eiser, C. (2002). The school experience of the child with cancer. *Child: Care, Health and Development, 28,* 5–19.

Vannatta, K., & Gerhardt, C. A. (2003). Pediatric oncology: Psychosocial outcomes for children and families. In M. C. Roberts (Ed.), *Handbook of pediatric psychology* (3rd ed., pp. 342–357). New York: Guilford.

Varni, J. W., & Katz, E. R. (1997). Stress, social support, and negative affectivity in children with newly diagnosed cancer: A prospective transactional analysis. *Psycho-oncology, 6,* 267–278.

Varni, J. W., Katz, E. R., Colegrove, R., Jr., & Dolgin, M. (1993). The impact of social skills training on the adjustment of children with newly diagnosed cancer. *Journal of Pediatric Psychology, 18,* 751–767.

Varni, J. W., Katz, E. R., Colegrove, R., & Dolgin, M. (1994). Perceived social support and adjustment of children with newly diagnosed cancer. *Journal of Developmental and Behavioral Pediatrics, 15,* 20–26.

Waxler-Morrison, N., Hislop, T. G., Mears, B., & Kan, L. (1991). Effects of social relationships on survival for women with breast cancer: A prospective study. *Social Science and Medicine, 33,* 177–183.

Wentzel, K. R., & Asher, S. R. (1995). The academic lives of neglected, rejected, popular, and controversial children. *Child Development, 66,* 754–763.

Williams, K. S., Ochs, J. Williams, J. M., & Mulhern, R. K. (1991). Parental report of everyday cognitive abilities among children treated for acute lymphoblastic leukemia. *Journal of Pediatric Psychology, 16,* 13–26.

Wolman, C., Resnick, M. D., Harris, L. J., & Blum, R. W. (1994). Emotional well-being among adolescents with and without chronic conditions. *Journal of Adolescent Health, 15,* 199–204.

Youniss, J. (1980). *Parents and peers in social development.* Chicago: University of Chicago Press.

Paola M. Conte and Gary A. Walco

# Pain and Procedure Management

## Introduction

Pediatric cancer treatment has seen an incredible increase in survival rates, so that, overall, 75% of children diagnosed with cancer will achieve long-term survival and cure (Ries et al., 2003). An estimated 9,000 new cases of childhood cancer are expected to occur each year (American Cancer Society, 2003), among which one third involve leukemia and one quarter involve a central nervous system (CNS) tumor. Other diagnoses include lymphoma, sympathetic nerve tumor, soft tissue sarcoma, bone tumor, germ cell tumor, and retinoblastoma (Gustafsson, Langmark, Pihkala, Verdier, & Lilleaas, 1998). Although less than 1% of all cancer cases are children (Stiller & Draper, 1998), pediatric cancer causes more deaths among children in industrialized nations than any other disease and after accidents is the leading cause of death among children 1–14 years of age (American Cancer Society, 2003).

Improvement in survival rates is the result of increasingly aggressive treatment protocols. With these advances, however, has come greater need for supportive care to address the array of treatment adverse side effects, including pain (Gustafsson et al., 1998). In the United States, 94% of children are treated at centers that are members of a collaborative clinical trials research consortium (American Cancer Society, 2003), implying that treatment protocols, including approaches to preventing and managing adverse side effects, are the norm. To a great degree, however, management of pain has been exempt from this standardized and rigorous approach. This is somewhat ironic and unfortunate as children with cancer reported pain to be the most feared symptom they experience (Enskar, Carlsson, Golsater, Hamrin, & Kreuger, 1997).

Undertreatment of pain in children is hardly unique to the cancer population (Schechter, Berde, & Yaster, 2003), and is generally because of limited information available to clinicians, persistence of misinformation about pain in children, and attitudes that denigrate adequate pain management. For example, there is a lack of research on pharmacological interventions for pain in children. Although it is agreed that randomized clinical trials for pain prevention and management would be helpful to address issues of safety, efficacy, pharmacodynamics, and pharmacokinetics in pediatrics, the pragmatics and ethics of such research, especially in very young children, have limited such progress (Berde, Brennan, & Raja, 2003).

Unfortunately, evidence exists that even as the field has advanced, lack of formal training in pain evaluation and treatment and poorly defined institutional standards have left children experiencing severely undertreated pain (Schechter et al., 2003). A 1996 a study by Broome, Richtsmeier, and Malkier surveyed physicians and nurses about pain assessment and management practices in U.S. teaching hospitals. It was found that 60% of respondents identified pain-specific standards of care or treatment protocols in place in their institution, but only 25% acknowledged that these protocols were used greater than 80% of the time.

Ljungman et al. (1996) surveyed all 47 pediatric hospitals in Sweden about their pain management practices with pediatric oncology patients. Of respondents, 40% indicated that moderate-to-severe pain was observed frequently in children with cancer, and 72% believed that pain could be controlled and managed more effectively. Treatment effects were reported by 41% as the greatest contributing factor to pain in these patients, and 34% identified procedural pain as more difficult to cope with than pain from the disease itself. Interview data from pediatric patients and their parents corroborated many of these views (Ljungman, Gordh, Sorensen, & Kreuger, 1999).

When disease is advanced and pain management is often at a premium, many of these same issues apply. Hilden and colleagues (2001) found that approximately 92% of pediatric oncologists sampled stated that they learned pain management strategies principally through trial and error, and that only 10% had undergone formal training in the field. Despite this, 91% viewed themselves as very competent (4 or 5 on a 5-point scale) in managing pain. These views are quite discrepant from the retrospective accounts of parents whose children succumbed to cancer; only 27% thought their child's pain was controlled adequately (Wolfe et al., 2000).

Cancer pain in children is associated with three major etiologies: (a) procedural distress, such as needle puncture, lumbar puncture (LP), bone marrow aspiration (BMA), and biopsies; (b) treatment-related pain, such as adverse side effects of chemotherapy, mucositis, infection, tumor surgery, and radiation; and (c) disease-related pain, such as tumor infiltration into organs or tissue. We first briefly examine the epidemiology of these pain problems and then discuss assessment and management issues pertaining to each in more detail.

## Epidemiology of Cancer Pain in Children

Miser, Dothage, Wesley, and Miser (1987) followed 92 children and adolescents with newly diagnosed malignancy over a 26-month period. It was reported that 62% had experienced pain as the first symptom of cancer, and 78% experienced pain that had been present for a median duration of 74 days. In a second study Miser, McCalla, Dothage, Wesley, and Miser (1987) evaluated pain experienced by 139 children and young adults with cancer. At the time of assessment, 54% of inpatients and 26% of outpatients reported some degree of pain. The predominant cause for both was treatment-related pain, and oral mucositis was most problematic, followed by postoperative pain, neuropathic pain from vincristine, and phantom limb pain from amputation. Approximately one half of inpatients and one third of outpatients were receiving opioid analgesia for pain.

In 1990, P. J. McGrath, Hsu, Cappelli, and Luke surveyed children who were outpatients at a cancer center and found that 75% experienced severe pain from BMA, 50% experienced moderate-to-severe pain from treatment, and 25% had recent pain from disease. Ljungman, Gordh, Sorensen, and Kreuger (2000) conducted interviews with 66 children and their families to investigate how the experience of pain varied over the course of cancer treatment. At diagnosis, disease-related pain was experienced by nearly one half of children. Procedural and treatment-related pains were the biggest problems initially; procedural pain gradually decreased, but treatment-related pain remained relatively constant over time.

Collins and coworkers (Collins et al., 2000, 2002) validated two versions of the Memorial Symptom Assessment Scale for children 7–12 and 10–18 years old. Both use a multidimensional approach to assess symptoms regarding prevalence, intensity, frequency and distress experienced 1 week before completing the questionnaire. In addition to low energy, children reported pain as the most prevalent symptom (49.1%). The majority of those who reported pain stated the intensity was moderate to severe. Pain was the most prevalent symptom for inpatients (84.4%) and was experienced by 35% of outpatients. In a second study, Collins and colleagues asked children to rate symptoms 48 hours prior to completing the questionnaire. Fatigue was the most frequent symptom (35.6%), followed by pain (32.4%). Of the children reporting pain, over one half reported a high degree of pain, 64% stated that pain was there all the time, and 37% reported their pain caused a high level of distress. As in the first study, pain was more prevalent in the inpatient setting as compared to outpatients.

These studies indicated that treatment-related pain is the most consistently reported type of pain experienced by children with cancer, followed by procedure-related pain, and then tumor-related pain. This is not consistent with the adult population, in which tumor-related pain is most problematic (Rawal, Hylander, & Arner, 1993; Zech, Grond, Lynch, Hertel, & Lehmann, 1995), only serving to further reinforce the need for studies specifically focused on pediatric cancer pain instead of extrapolating downward from adult clinical samples.

In the remainder of the chapter, we first describe various pain syndromes that may occur in the context of children's experiences with cancer and then provide an overview of various pharmacological, psychological, and physical strategies to address those problems. There are two additional pediatric cancer pain problems that we do not discuss in this chapter. First, there is some initial evidence to show that long-term survivors of childhood cancer endure various chronic pain problems, including chronic abdominal pain, complex regional pain syndrome Type 1 (reflex sympathetic dystrophy), diffuse musculoskeletal pain, and orthopedic difficulties such as avascular necrosis of the joints and scoliosis (Crom, Chathaway, Tolley, Mulhern, & Hudson, 1999). The epidemiology and severity of these problems are not known, but it is hoped greater insights will be gleaned as data are amassed through long-term surveillance studies. Furthermore, a discussion of interventions for these pain problems is well beyond the scope of this chapter. Second, disease-related pain at the end of life is optimally discussed in the context of palliative care and not simply the focus of pain as an isolated symptom. Chapter 18 in this text specifically addresses palliation.

## Procedure-Related Pain

For many of the cancers most common in the pediatric population (e.g., leukemia, lymphoma), invasive procedures are integral to the diagnostic and treatment process. Included are needle sticks, BMAs, and biopsies for diagnostic purposes and LPs, both for diagnostic purposes and to deliver intrathecal medication (Balis, Holcenberg, & Blaney, 2002). An LP involves the insertion of a needle between two lumbar vertebrae of the back to withdraw spinal fluid and to deliver intrathecal chemotherapy as prophylaxis against or treatment for CNS disease.

A BMA involves the insertion of a needle through the periosteum and into the bone (most often the iliac crest) to obtain a sample of marrow or aspirate. Acute pain may result from inadequate anesthetic to the skin, subcutaneous tissue, and periosteum. Intense pressure is reported as the needle pierces the bone, and severe pain is reported as withdrawal of marrow causes a vacuum within the bone. Local anesthetics do not relieve this pain. Among survivors of pediatric cancer, the trauma of undertreated procedural distress is often the most disturbing element of their entire cancer experience, sometimes severe enough to leave children and parents with posttraumatic stress symptoms (Stuber, Kazak, Meeske, & Barakat, 1998), noted even up to 12 years after cancer treatment has ended (Stuber, Christakis, Houskamp, & Kazak, 1996).

The best strategy to minimize or avoid acute distress from these procedures is to provide comfort from the first episode onward because treating high levels of distress is far more difficult than preventing them. In a placebo-controlled randomized study, children with cancer undergoing LPs or BMAs who received fentanyl citrate, a potent opioid analgesic, demonstrated significantly lower pain scores during subsequent procedures than those who received placebo for their first painful procedure, even when adequate analgesia was used subsequently (Weisman, Bernstein, & Schechter, 1998).

Pharmacological interventions combining sedating and analgesic agents along with preparatory and cognitive behavioral strategies have greatly reduced the pain and anxiety associated with invasive procedures (Berde, Billett, & Collins, 2002). Generally, the child's subjective experience is best conceptualized as *distress*, which is the cumulative effect of pain and anxiety; thus, interventions must be invoked to address both. In such circumstances, it is imperative to define outcomes; however, as recent data indicated that even when children subjectively experience or behaviorally demonstrate few or no indicators of pain or distress, there are still significant physiological indicators of distress as the procedure is conducted (Eccleston, Merlijn, Hunfeld, & Walco, 2003).

Strategies aimed at helping children cope with procedural distress involve an array of pharmacological and psychological interventions. The goal is to minimize pain and distress using as low risk and effective means as possible. Thus, by evaluating the child's coping style, providing adequate preparation, and utilizing analgesic, anxiolytic, or sedating medications, cognitive behavioral techniques, and physical interventions, optimal management techniques may be applied for each individual child. These interventions are discussed in more detail next.

## Treatment-Related Pain

From early on in the process of treatment for cancer, there are a number of potential sources of pain that should be recognized and treated. For example, in virtually all treatment centers, shortly after diagnosis children undergo a procedure to surgically implant an intravenous catheter (to avoid recurrent venipuncture for diagnostic and treatment delivery purposes), and thus postoperative pain may occur. In addition, if the diagnostic process requires a surgical biopsy or early tumor resection, one of the child's first experiences with treatment may involve postoperative pain. These acute pain syndromes are almost always time limited and may be treated aggressively with analgesic medications.

Beyond the very early phases of diagnosis, treatments for cancer include chemotherapy, radiation therapy, surgery, and stem cell transplantation, each of which potentially leads to pain problems (Collins & Weisman, 2003). Symptoms resulting from chemotherapy and radiation treatment most commonly include nausea and vomiting, fatigue, neutropenia, and the potential for infection and pain. Treatment-related pain syndromes in children with cancer are related to poor immune functioning and include mucositis or stomatitis as well as sequelae of infectious process. Pain from these ulcerations throughout the mouth and esophagus may be of very high intensity and lead to difficulty eating and swallowing. Thus, prevention of mouth sores is important, and when they do occur, treatment with anesthetic mouthwash and strong opioids may be indicated.

There are some less common but very problematic pain concerns that may also occur. For example, chemotherapeutic agents such as vincristine may elicit pain in the joints, especially the jaw, as well as peripheral neuropathy and neuropathic pain. Reasonably aggressive treatment with opioid analgesics is indicated during the acute phase, and if the neuropathy persists, treatment for chronic neuropathic pain should be considered, including the use of anticonvulsants or tricyclic antidepressants (Babul & Darke, 1993). Pain secondary to radiation is also seen in some instances and is typically managed in a fashion similar to chemotherapy-related problems. Finally, acute abdominal pain, severe enough to require administration of opioids, has been noted among patients who have undergone allogeneic bone marrow transplantation.

## Disease-Related Pain

Disease-related pain in pediatric cancer is not as common as in the adult population; thus, knowledge is limited because of the small number of children with this type of pain at single institutions. Pain may be present at the time of diagnosis because pain in the long bones is associated with leukemia, severe headache is a symptom of brain tumors, solid tumors may elicit somatic pain in the focal area of tumor growth or infiltration, and abdominal tumors may generate visceral pain. Children with cancer usually experience significant remission of pain within 2 weeks of beginning treatment (Miser, Dothage, et al., 1987; Miser, McCalla, et al., 1987). The other circumstance for which pain is problematic is in advanced illness, often in the context of end-of-life care. Neoplastic pain in these circumstances has many of the characteristics of acute pain with the exception of no expected end point. Thus, many of the same types of syndromes seen at presentation, when pain is of high intensity and unyielding, recur in advanced illness and should be treated aggressively in the service of maximizing quality of life.

## Pain Mechanisms

To further understand the assessment and treatment of pain syndromes associated with pediatric cancer, working knowledge of key elements in our current understanding of pain systems is helpful. The International Association for the Study of Pain defines pain as "an unpleasant sensory and emotional experience associated with actual or potential tissue damage" (Merskey & Bogduk, 1994). Nociceptors (pain receptors) maybe excited by mechanical, thermal, or chemical stimuli. When such stimulation occurs, biochemical mediators such as substance P and prostaglandin activate nociceptors, which initiates depolarization along the axon, leading to an action potential transmitted from the periphery and terminating in the dorsal horn of the spinal cord (Paice, 1991). Transmission of signals from the periphery to the CNS principally involves A and C class afferent nerves.

A-fibers are characterized by a moderate amount of myelin and are rapid conductors. They are involved in the transmission of pain that occurs immediately after the onset of injury. Activation of the unmyelinated C-fibers produces dull, aching, poorly localized pain sensation (Fitzgerald, 2000). Nociceptive messages are further transmitted within the CNS as substance P is released in the dorsal horn and binds to secondary receptor sites (Paice, 1991). Spinothalamic tract neurons unite in the anterolateral quadrant of the spinal cord and most ascend to the thalamus and other higher centers in the brain, such as the reticular formation, limbic system, and cerebral cortex (Fields, 1987).

Many areas in the brain appear to play a role in modifying or impacting afferent pain input (Zeltzer, Anderson, & Schechter, 1990). The gate control theory (Melzack & Wall, 1965) states that the transmission of nerve impulses from afferent fibers to the spinal cord is modulated by a spinal gating mechanism located in the dorsal horn. The relative amount of activity in large-diameter fibers that inhibit transmission (close the gate) and small fibers that facilitate transmission (open the gate) largely determine the nature of nociceptive transmission to the brain. Neurons arising in the thalamus, hypothalamus, frontal cortex, reticular formation, brain stem, limbic system, hippocampus, and amygdala have efferent pathways that can further affect the gate (Frenk, Cannon, Lewis, & Liebeskind, 1986). Hence, thoughts, emotions, memories, and attention may have a direct impact on spinal cord gating mechanisms. The descending pain system involves the release of norepinephrine and serotonin, two neurotransmitters that inhibit the transmission of nociception in the dorsal horn (Stamford, 1995). Given the role of neurotransmitters in mood regulation, intimate relationship among anxiety, depression, and pain is highlighted (Paice, 1991).

Using this conceptual model, a number of key elements of assessment and treatment may follow. First, it is clear that the context of pain must be considered. This is hardly a reflexive system that involves the simple transmission of afferent nociceptive impulses that lead to pain. Thoughts, memories, emotions, and contextual factors must be considered. Second, interventions for pain may have an impact at a number of sites in the peripheral nociceptive and central pathways. Comprehensive approaches to pain management take as many of these elements into account as possible.

## Assessment of Pain in Children

A necessary first step in pain management is the accurate assessment of the pain experience. Specific pain assessment strategies depend on the age or developmental level of the child and the nature of the pain in question (P. A. McGrath & Gillespie, 2001) and typically involve three modalities: self-report of the child, behavioral observations, and physiological indicators of stress (Walco et al., 2005). Regardless of the modality employed, it is imperative to have demonstrated reliability, validity, and clinical sensitivity for each technique that is utilized (P. A. McGrath & Gillespie, 2001).

### Self-Report

Because pain is a subjective experience, whenever possible it is optimal to use patients' verbal reports to assess their pain experience; this may be reliably done for children as young as 3 years of age (American Academy of Pediatrics and American Pain Society, 2001). During the toddler and preschool years, as children begin to use language meaningfully, increased emphasis may be placed on verbal report, but one must take care to use language and terminology that is familiar to the child.

The most common focus of assessment is pain intensity. The Poker Chip Tool (Hester, Foster, & Kristensen, 1990) is a measure that is useful with young children (4–8 years); children rate pain concretely as "pieces of hurt." Children over 4 years can reliably use a visual analogue scale, which is a line with verbal, facial, or numerical anchors at the extremes of a continuum of pain intensity. These instruments may be pencil-and-paper based or of a slide rule variety; the child is asked to indicate the level of pain on that continuum (P. A. McGrath & Gillespie, 2001). Parents or significant others may complete these scales, but only when children are too impaired or too young to reliably respond on their own.

To tap into the affective component of pain, instruments such as the Faces Scale (P. A. McGrath, 1990) provide a series of facial expressions depicting gradations of pain; children choose the one that approximates their pain experience. Although useful and reliable (P. A. McGrath & Gillespie, 2001), the limitation of this scale is that the specific affective components involved are unclear. Possibilities include general distress, mood, anxiety, unpleasantness, and perhaps even boredom in addition to pain intensity.

Body diagrams may be used to help children accurately report on the location of pain. Sensory qualities (e.g., aching, burning, tearing, gnawing, stinging, throbbing, sharp, or dull), affective elements, and tolerability of pain may be ascertained, most commonly using pain adjective checklists (Varni, Thompson, & Hanson, 1987).

### Behavioral Observation

The frequency, duration, and intensity of discretely defined pain behaviors (e.g., vocalizations, facial expressions, body movements) may be assessed systematically. The reliability and validity of behavioral observations are highest when pain is well defined, short in duration, and acute in nature, such as pain associated with procedures (Mathews, McGrath, & Pigeon, 1993). Behavioral observations should be used as a compliment to, not as a substitute for, self-report, unless the latter is not available. The relationship between pain behavior and subjective internal distress is certainly not direct, as in the case of a stoic child who demonstrates little behavioral distress while suffering intrinsically.

Developmental differences have been appreciated as well. Infants' responses to acute pain may include general body movements, specific facial expressions (furrowed brow, nasal flaring, quivering lips), and crying patterns (Grunau & Craig, 1987). Toddlers' and young children's responses to acute pain include specific body reactions that are more precisely localized and are accompanied by verbalizations. In older children, these same responses are present, but there may be some individuals who demonstrate more subtle behavioral responses, such as slight facial grimaces and brief pain reports (P. A. McGrath, 1990).

Within the area of pediatric oncology, a number of studies have assessed children's behavioral responses during painful medical procedures, and measurement strategies include two major foci, anxiety and pain. Behaviors prior to, during, and after noxious stimulation are noted to define distinct patterns that represent responses to distress. These scales operationally define specific behaviors, which are then tallied as they occur during set intervals or phases of a procedure (Mathews et al., 1993).

The Procedural Behavior Rating Scale revised (Katz, Kellerman, & Siegel, 1980) and the Observational Scale of Behavioral Distress (Jay, Ozolins, Elliott, & Caldwell, 1983) are the most utilized observational distress scales for pediatric oncology patients during LPs and BMAs. For the Procedural Behavior Rating Scale revised, the observer records the occurrence of 11 behaviors during three time periods within the medical procedure, whereas the Observational Scale of Behavioral Distress continually samples the same 11 behaviors throughout the procedure. The behaviors include crying, screaming, physical restraint, verbal resistance, requests for emotional support, muscular rigidity, verbal fear, verbal pain, flailing, nervous behavior, and information seeking.

Blount, Bunke, Cohen, and Forbes (2001) evaluated the concurrent and construct validity of the Child-Adult Medical Procedure Interaction Scale–Short Form (CAMPIS-SF), a behavior rating scale of children's acute procedural distress and coping, and the coping-promoting behaviors and distress-promoting behaviors of parents and medical personnel present during the medical procedure. Subjects were 60 preschool children undergoing immunizations at a county health department. Videotapes of the procedures were scored using three observational measures in addition to the CAMPIS-SF. Also, parent, nurse, and child report measures of child distress, fear, pain, and cooperation were obtained. The results emphasized that the CAMPIS-SF scales can be used to monitor not only children's acute procedural distress, but also their coping and the various adults' behaviors that significantly influence children's distress.

## Physiological Measurements

Finally, children's pain and distress can be evaluated through changes in specific physiological indices. Traditionally, the focus has been on sympathetic nervous system indicators of arousal, including heart rate, respiratory rate, blood pressure, and palmar sweating. It has been recognized that these factors are nonspecific for pain or stress, and increasing attention has been paid to parasympathetic responses (Walco et al., 2005), such as heart rate variability and vagal tone (Porges, 1992) and hypothalamic-pituitary-adrenocorticosteroid (HPA) responses, such as circulating cortisol levels (Gunnar, 1992).

Threats to an animal elicit a "fight-or-flight" reaction, in which the organism responds to acute stress by preparing to react with vigor. This accounts for increases in heart rate, respiration rate, blood pressure, and sweating, with concomitant decreased blood flow to the gut. Children undergoing invasive procedures demonstrate such stress responses. In addition, however, the parasympathetic nervous system works to regain a state of homeostasis. Thus, during acute threats it is relatively inactive compared to its counterpart. As the stress or pain continues, the parasympathetic nervous system may attempt to become more active in an attempt to regain homeostasis. It is through indicators of exaggerated variability, such as in heart rate and vagal tone, that one can measure the impact of stress on this system (Porges, 1992).

In addition, the body prepares itself to react to stress with hormonal and metabolic changes. Central here is the activity of the HPA system, which makes glucose more available for consumption in service of "fueling" the response. Cortisol plays a central role in this process and may be found in the blood, urine, and saliva. Thus, by measuring cortisol approximately prior to and then 20 to 30 minutes after the onset of acute stress, one has a reliable index of the HPA system response (Gunnar, 1992).

In a study at our institution, multiple modalities of measuring distress in children with cancer undergoing invasive procedures were used to measure distress: self-reported anxiety, pain, self-efficacy, and coping; behavioral observation made prior to, during, and after the procedure; and physiological parameters, including heart rate, cardiac vagal tone, and salivary cortisol. Interventions to manage pain and distress included deep sedation (propofol), conscious sedation (midazolam and opioid), and cognitive behavioral strategies with topical anesthetics. Results indicated a high degree of consistency within self-report, behavioral, and physiological parameters, but correlations between measures in different modalities were low. There were floor effects for most behavioral and self-report measures of distress. Cortisol showed marked changes pre- to postprocedure, demonstrating high levels of physiological response despite a lack of apparent or perceived discomfort. Cardiac vagal tone findings indicated that although participants received conscious or deep sedation, they still responded to stimuli associated with tissue damage. Finally, heart rate was significantly lower in the group using cognitive behavioral techniques, especially at the point of needle insertion (Walco et al., 2005).

It is recognized that physiological parameters such as vagal tone and cortisol release are not practical in most clinical settings. They are, however, potentially important factors in understanding the distress responses associated with invasive procedures. Ultimately, the goal would be to reduce pain and distress maximally while minimally introducing risk. Ongoing research is aimed at developing clinical algorithms toward that end.

# Pharmacological Management of Pain

The literature on analgesic medication trials in children with cancer is scant, especially in contrast to the parallel research base in adults. Available studies include few participants and are usually descriptive in nature rather than systematically controlled (Collins, 1998). As discussed, very few medications have been approved by the Food and Drug Administration with an indication for analgesia in children. Available data indicate that when dosing is based on body mass, the pharmacology of most analgesics is similar between adults and children beyond the neonatal period. Clearly, however, studies of safety and efficacy must be conducted for children and adolescents of all ages to use the drugs with greater confidence.

The World Health Organization (1990) proposed a three-step analgesic ladder that may serve as a useful guide in selecting various analgesic medications. Essentially, there is a match between the nature and severity of pain and the potency of analgesic regimens employed. The first step involves the recognition that mild pain exists, and it is managed with a weaker (nonopioid) analgesic with or without an adjuvant. In the second step, pain is seen as more intense, persistent, or increasing, and a weak opioid may be added to the regimen. Finally, in the third step pain is deemed to be moderate to severe, and more powerful opioid medications are utilized. It is important to note that at each step drugs may be added, not necessarily replacing others. Thus, it may be perfectly reasonable to use nonsteroidal anti-inflammatory drugs (NSAIDs) with opioids and adjuvants (Tobias, Phipps, Smith, & Mulhern, 1992).

As a general rule when prescribing these drugs, one should be familiar with the dosages, half-life, and frequency of administration, routes of administration, deleterious side effects, and interactions with other medications the child is receiving. Equianalgesic potential (the relationship among specific drugs, routes of administration, and timing) is also very important so relatively seamless changes may be made in medication regimens.

Most nonopioid drugs are prostoglandin-synthesis inhibitors and include para-amino phenol derivatives such as acetaminophen, salicylates such as aspirin and choline magnesium trisalicylate, and NSAIDs such as ibuprofen, naproxen, ketorolac, indomethacin, diclofenac, and piroxicam. At present, acetaminophen is the most commonly prescribed analgesic for mild-to-moderate pain because of the lack of serious adverse side effects on renal, gastrointestinal, and platelet functions. Acetaminophen inhibits prostaglandin synthesis mainly in the CNS. The antipyretic action of acetaminophen maybe contraindicated in children with neutropenia because of the necessity to monitor fever (Collins & Weisman, 2003).

Among the other available NSAIDs, the one with the most experience of use in children is ibuprofen. Some studies have suggested it is a more effective analgesic than acetaminophen (Maunuksela, Ryhanen, & Janhunen, 1992; Tobias, 2000). It also has been shown that continued use of NSAIDs significantly decreases the total amount of opioids needed for effective postoperative pain control (Schechter, 1989). Although NSAIDs may be considered in children with adequate platelet count and function, they are routinely contraindicated in pediatric oncology patients at risk of bleeding because of thrombocytopenia (Collins & Weisman, 2003). The newer class of NSAIDs, the cyclooxygenase-2 (Cox-2) inhibitors (celecoxib, refecoxib, valdecoxib) is not yet approved for use in children, although these new drugs do not inhibit platelet function and appear to have fewer gastrointestinal side effects (Leese et al., 2000).

Opioids are the mainstay for treatment of moderate-to-severe pain. These drugs are reliable with predictable efficacy, onset of action, half-life, and adverse side effects. One of the main barriers in the use of opioids is the misconception that they have a high incidence of causing addiction. Although it is true that sustained use of opioids will lead to tolerance and by extension physical dependency, these are expected clinical phenomena and are quite manageable. In contrast, addiction to a substance is defined as a psychological dependency that causes the use of larger amounts of that substance than originally intended and for reasons other than that for which it was intended (Craig, Lilley, & Gilbert, 1996; P. J. McGrath, 1996). Addiction to opioids is extremely rare in children when used for purposes of analgesia (P. J. McGrath & Unruh, 1987; Tobias, 2003).

The other common misconception regarding opioids is that they are associated with a high incidence of respiratory depression. When used at the appropriate dosage, respiratory depression and apnea are rarely seen, and when they do occur, they are typically manageable by withholding the drug for a period of time (Yaster, Kost-Byerly, & Maxwell, 2003). Excessive concern about either respiratory depression or addiction is not a sufficient reason to withhold opioids for a child having moderate-to-severe pain (Walco, Cassidy, & Schechter, 1994).

The weak opioid options are usually administered orally and are most often given in combination with nonopioids, such as acetaminophen.

Weaker opioids for moderate pain include codeine, which metabolizes to morphine, tramadol (a synthetic opioid), and oxycodone (a semisynthetic opioid), which may be administered in immediate or sustained relief preparations.

For moderate-to-severe pain, stronger opiates are used, the mainstay of which is morphine. It remains the most widely used opioid to treat moderate-to-severe cancer pain in children and can be administered via oral, intravenous, subcutaneous, epidural, and intrathecal routes. Two different sustained release oral preparations are available, one used every 8–12 hours and one that covers a full 24-hour period (Broomhead et al., 1997; Hunt, Joel, Dick, & Goldman, 1999). The latter preparation may be mixed with foods for children who cannot swallow pills. The advantage of using morphine is that it has the widest experience of use in the pediatric population and has a reasonably predictable onset of action and duration.

Other potent opioids may be considered when morphine adverse side effects are too severe or clinical effects are less than optimal (including effects caused by tolerance). Hydromorphone, which is available for oral, intravenous, subcutaneous, epidural, and intrathecal administration, has demonstrated efficacy for pain related to disease (Babul, Darke, & Hain, 1995; Weisman & Wishnie, 1996) and mucositis (Collins et al., 1996) in children with cancer.

Methadone is a synthetic opioid that may be a useful drug for children with cancer because of its high bioavailability by the oral route and its long half-life (Yaster, Deshpande, & Maxwell, 1989). It is especially useful for disease-related pain when there is tolerance to other opioids and clinical effect is diminishing. Caution is indicated, however, as unlike other opioids, methadone may accumulate in the system over time; thus, there is risk of delayed sedation and overdose occurring days after initiating treatment.

Fentanyl is an extremely potent analgesic (50–100 times that of morphine) and can be administered by the intravenous, intramuscular, and subcutaneous routes as well as transdermally and transmucosally (Schechter, Weisman, Rosenblum, Bernstein, & Conard, 1995). The transdermal administration is particularly effective in patients with chronic pain (Noyes & Irving, 2001) and is now approved for use in children over the age of 2 years. A study with a small sample found this administration to be feasible and tolerable in children with cancer (Collins et al., 1999).

Finally, meperidine is a short half-life synthetic opioid that has been used for procedural and postoperative pain in children. However, currently meperidine is not recommended for pediatric populations because excessive buildup of one its metabolites, normeperidine, can cause CNS irritability and seizures (American Academy of Pediatrics and American Pain Society, 2001).

For ongoing pain related to disease processes or treatment adverse side effects, opioids should be administered on an around-the-clock regimen rather than on an as-needed basis. This may be accomplished by providing the drug at regular intervals or through a continuous intravenous infusion; the latter helps to minimize peaks and valleys in the levels of the drug and to avoid significant breakthrough pain.

Patient-controlled analgesia (PCA), which enables children to have control over their analgesia and to achieve a balance between the benefits of the opioid and associated adverse side effects, has gained widespread acceptance (Mackie, Coda, & Hill, 1991). PCA is a system by which the patient can self-administer small doses of opioids at frequent intervals in response to pain. Studies have shown that children as young as 6 or 7 years can be taught this approach, and it has been used extensively for analgesia in the postoperative setting and for children with burns, sickle cell anemia, and cancer (Gureno & Reisinger, 1991). The requirements for PCA use include the medical devices necessary to administer the drug and personnel familiar with protocols for delivery of the medication. Opioids commonly used in PCA regimens include morphine, fentanyl, and hydromorphone.

In using opioids, certain predictable adverse side effects require attention, including constipation, nausea, sedation, confusion, pruritis, and urinary retention. Constipation should be anticipated, and a regimen of stool softeners and laxatives should be instituted to minimize the risk of this complication. Pruritis (itching) may be addressed with antihistamines such as diphenhydramine and hydroxyzine (Yaster et al., 2003), and sedation may be helped with the use of stimulants, such as dextroamphetamine and methylphenidate (Yee & Berde, 1994). In the rare cases of respiratory depression leading to apnea, nalaxone, which is an opioid antagonist, can be administered. However, at the same time it will also reverse the analgesia and can cause withdrawal symptoms in patients who have developed physical dependence.

Because of adverse side effects of chemotherapy, herpes zoster, or neoplastic effects on peripheral nerves, neuropathic pain may be seen in children with cancer. Medications that have greater efficacy with neuropathic pain include anticonvulsants such as gabapentin or carbamazepine and tricyclic antidepressants such as amitriptyline and nortriptyline (Backonja, 2000; Ollson, 1999; Sindrup & Jensen, 1999).

### Procedure-Related Pain

Because children with cancer frequently undergo invasive diagnostic and treatment procedures, including venipuncture, BMA and biopsy, and LP, alleviation of distress has become a priority. The American Academy of Pediatrics Subcommittee on the Management of Pain Associated with Procedures in Children With Cancer (Zeltzer et al., 1990) reported that the vast majority of pediatric oncology centers had no formal protocol for dealing with these issues. Suggestions were made to invoke various psychological strategies, as well as to use sedatives along with analgesics for the apprehensive child undergoing these procedures. Over the last decade, it has become the standard of practice in most pediatric oncology centers to offer some form of sedation to these children (Sandler et al., 1992).

The level of sedation that is employed can vary from light or "conscious" sedation, which is defined as a "medically controlled state of depressed consciousness that (1) allows protective reflexes to be maintained; (2) retains the patient's ability to maintain a patent airway independently and continuously; and (3) permits appropriate response by the patient to physical stimulation or verbal command," to deep sedation, which is defined as a "medically controlled state of depressed consciousness or unconsciousness from which the patient is not easily aroused. It may be accompanied by a partial or complete loss of protective reflexes, and includes the inability to maintain a patent airway independently and respond purposefully to physical stimulation or verbal stimuli" (p. 1110; Committee on Drugs, 1992). Ljungman, Gordh, Sorensen, and Kreuger (2001), using a prospective randomized crossover study, found that children with cancer, parents, and nurses preferred light sedation over general anesthesia for these procedures. It was also noted that light sedation saved time and medical resources.

The providers responsible for administration of these drugs should be familiar with the pharmacology of the medications. They should also be proficient in airway management and cardiopulmonary resuscitation. The child should be closely monitored with continuous pulse oximetry as well as frequent determinations of blood pressure, heart rate, and respiratory rate (Committee on Drugs, 1992). A common combination of drugs used to induce conscious sedation includes the anxiolytic drug midazalom with an opioid such as fentanyl.

An increasingly popular method of providing deep sedation in children undergoing these procedures is the use of general anesthetic agents. Until recently, these agents could only be given in the setting of an operating room or recovery room. It is now common practice in many institutions for an anesthesiologist or pediatric intensivist to administer these drugs in an outpatient area or emergency room (Valtonen, Iisalo, Kanto, & Tikkanen, 1988).

Ketamine is a general anesthetic with an extensive track record, especially in the emergency room (Hannallah et al., 1991), for procedures such as setting fractures or laceration repairs. Its main advantage is that it provides significant analgesia and can be given by the intramuscular, intravenous, or oral route. The disadvantages of ketamine are that it increases production of secretions, can cause laryngospasm (closure of the larynx), and can elevate blood pressure and intracranial pressure. Ketamine is also known to cause unpleasant dreams and hallucinations (Shapiro, Wyte, & Harris, 1972; Taylor & Towey, 1971; White, Way, & Trevor, 1982).

The preferred drug at many pediatric oncology centers across the country is propofol, an anesthetic agent that is administered intravenously. It has a rapid onset of action and a short half-life and is easy to titrate. It also has an antiemetic effect so that vomiting is unusual; it often has an amnestic effect as well (Harris et al., 1990). Because propofol has no analgesic properties, a short-acting opioid such as fentanyl is often given in conjunction. The major advantage of propofol is that it is a safe, highly effective way of achieving sedation. Because it is associated with respiratory depression and apnea, someone with experience with airway management and tracheal intubation must administer it.

Topical preparations provide effective local anesthesia prior to LP or BMA in the older cooperative child not requiring sedation or prior to venipuncture or intramuscular or subcutaneous injections. Various substances are available, including EMLA, which a eutectic mixture of lidocaine and prilocaine in a water-based cream (Halperin et al., 1989; Taddio, Shennaan, & Stevens, 1995). When applied topically under an occlusive dressing, effective local anesthesia is achieved within 60–90 minutes. An alternative treatment is Numby Stuff (Zempsky & Ashburn, 1998), which is a system for delivering topical lidocaine using iontophoresis, a technique for achieving transdermal delivery of a local anesthetic via a low-intensity electrical current. Finally, a new over-the-counter cream, ELA-Max, is a more rapidly acting topical agent that provides liposomal delivery of lidocaine. It has shown efficacy for venipuncture and dermatological procedures (Eichenfield, Funk, Fallon-Friedlander, & Cunningham, 2002) and works in approximately 30 minutes.

## Psychological Interventions

### Disease-Related Pain

Psychological interventions for pain in children with cancer have focused on two major areas: disease-related pain and procedural distress. Walco, Sterling, Conte, and Engel (1999) reviewed studies focusing on psychological interventions for disease-related pain in children. Although some controlled clinical trials were identified addressing pain and various symptoms in adults with cancer, only a small number of case studies were found for such interventions in children. Olness (1981) reported several cases in which self-hypnosis was used to reduce pain and nausea related to illness and treatment. Of the 25 cases discussed, however, only one addressed issues other than procedural pain, the case of a 13-year-old child with Ewing's sarcoma; where concerns focused on pain control and sleep problems. Using imagery techniques that focused on numbness in the areas of discomfort, the child reported less pain and utilized less analgesic medication while in the hospital.

In addition, Hilgard and LeBaron (1982) discussed the use of hypnotherapy for addressing pain and anxiety in children with cancer. In the entire report, however, only one patient was seen for other than procedure-related distress, a 20-year-old with chronic pain related to an abdominal tumor. At admission, pain intensity scores were between 6 and 9 on a 10-point scale and were reduced to 2 after teaching the patient relaxation and imagery. Morphine requirements also were reduced from 3 mg per hour to 1 mg per hour.

Finally, LaClave and Blix (1989) used hypnosis to manage cancer-related symptoms in a 6-year-old girl with astrocytoma. Over seven sessions, she was taught hypnosis to address vomiting; the treatment was successful. Two months later, when she began to develop severe headaches, the strategies were also applied for pain and appeared to be successful.

It is important to note that all of these reports were case studies. As pointed out by Walco et al. (1999), much more carefully controlled studies are needed before any meaningful conclusions may be drawn. The adult literature and case reports indicate promise, but it would be premature to conclude that psychological interventions for disease-related pain have been validated.

### Procedure-Related Distress

In contrast to the scant research on disease-related pain, a series of excellent studies over the last two decades have demonstrated the effectiveness of behavioral and cognitive behavioral strategies for children undergoing painful procedures (Powers, 1999). The aim is to provide children with a specific set of responses and behaviors that may be used to master the distressing situation, including distraction, relaxation, and imagery, ideally in a manner consistent with their basic coping strategies (Broome, Lillis, McGahee, & Bates, 1992; Liossi & Hatira, 2003; Manne et al., 1990).

Educational preparation helps children cope with anticipatory anxiety, and well-prepared children demonstrate less distress and have reduced need for analgesics. The patient is provided with information, both procedure related (what will be done) and sensory (what it will feel like) throughout the phases (pre-, during, post-) of the procedure. Procedure-related information describes the steps of the procedure in some detail; sensory descriptions focus on the child's subjective experiences. The nature and amount of information given depends on the child's developmental stage, level of anxiety, and available coping strategies (Smith, Barabasz, & Barabasz, 1996). Regarding the last, children who are principally "attenders" are focused on the pain and generally seek out information to master the challenge. Conversely, "distractors" choose to orient away from the procedure and cope more effectively when attention is diverted.

Anticipatory distress or acute fears of medical procedures can be treated with systematic desensitization (Melamed & Ridley-Johnson, 1988). With this technique, children are gradually exposed to stimuli associated with the procedure in a hierarchical fashion from least to most threatening. The key is the principal of reciprocal inhibition (Wolpe, 1981), providing an alternative response to the threatening stimuli such that what formerly resulted in acute anxiety responses is replaced with calm or relaxation.

Utilizing positive incentive techniques involves presenting children with a small token reward (e.g., stickers, prize) for their attempts at mastery during the painful procedure. Patients are encouraged to lie still, which significantly reduces the likelihood of complications in conducting the medical procedure, and to do breathing exercises that may prevent or minimize acute behavioral distress. Rewards provide incentive for engaging in positive coping behaviors and enable the child to reframe, at least partly, the meaning of the pain as a challenge. Ultimately, all children receive positive reinforcement for their efforts, thereby using tokens as an incentive rather than a reward (Jay et al., 1985; Manne et al., 1990). It is preferable to encourage the child verbally during the procedure and to present concrete rewards following the procedure, pointing out the cooperative behavior or coping efforts.

Teaching a child to implement simple relaxation strategies, such as deep breathing or progressive muscle relaxation, is especially useful for reducing anxiety. The specific approach to deep breathing techniques used depends on the child's age. For example, older children may be provided with simple verbal suggestions to take a deep breath and to let it out slowly (Jay, Elliott, Woody, & Siegel, 1991). Younger children may have trouble with these notions and may use a party blower to facilitate the same breathing patterns during painful procedures (Manne et al., 1990). Relaxation can also be achieved using imagery because children can be guided through scenes that induce relaxation, such as floating on a fluffy cloud or becoming loose like a cooked noodle (Anderson, Zeltzer, & Fanurik, 1993).

Distraction refers to activities intended to divert a patient's attention away from the painful procedure. In some cases, patients are asked to form a mental image of a strong capable character, such as a superhero. They may be given suggestions to incorporate the superhero into the painful procedure in some manner (Jay, Elliot, Ozolins, Olson, & Pruitt, 1985; Manne et al., 1990). In other cases, distraction refers to specific activities in which a child can engage, such as blowing bubbles, coloring, watching a video, or putting a puzzle together (Jay et al., 1991).

Hypnosis is a frequently used distraction technique that involves helping the child to become intensely involved in a diversional experience. Hypnosis utilizes an initial induction technique, such as eye fixation or hand levitation, followed by directions on how to progressively relax the muscles (slow rhythmic breathing, an increasing sense of well being). Finally, patients "visualize" or "experience" being in a special place, are encouraged to imagine a story around that place, and to use all the senses to feel like they are really there (Siegal, 1976). In some instances, hypnoanalgesia or hypnoanesthesia may be introduced as a means of altering the subjective sensory experience (Kellerman, Zeltzer, Ellenberg, & Dash, 1983). Once a helpful combination of strategies is found, patients are encouraged to practice on their own (self-hypnosis) in an effort to facilitate generalization to the actual distressing situation (Smith et al., 1996; Zeltzer & LeBaron, 1982). The effectiveness of hypnosis intervention on children undergoing painful procedures depends on the child's level of hypnotic susceptibility, several measures of which may be used to assess children's facility with hypnotic approaches (Olness & Kohen, 1996).

A study by Liossi and Hatira (1999) compared the efficacy of clinical hypnosis with cognitive behavioral training in the relief of BMA-induced pain and anxiety in pediatric cancer patients. Patients who received either hypnosis or cognitive behavioral training reported less pain and pain-related anxiety than did patients in the control group and less pain and anxiety than at their own baselines. Results also indicated that children in the hypnosis group reported less anxiety and exhibited less behavioral distress. In another study, Liossi and Hatira (2003) investigated the efficacy of a manual-based clinical hypnosis intervention in alleviating pain in 80 pediatric cancer patients (6–16 years of age) undergoing regular LP. Patients in the hypnosis groups reported less pain and anxiety and were rated as demonstrating less behavioral distress than those in the control group. Direct and indirect suggestions were equally effective, and the level of hypnotic susceptibility was significantly associated with treatment benefit in the hypnosis group. Therapeutic benefit was reduced when patients switched to self-hypnosis.

Modeling and rehearsal are key components for teaching and reinforcing coping prior to and during a procedure. Modeling may involve showing the patient a video of a similarly aged child who models positive coping behaviors (breathing exercises and imagery) and positive coping self statements ("I know I can do it"). Typically, a child's voice narrates the steps of the LP and BMA procedures along with thoughts and feelings at critical points (Jay et al., 1991). In medical play, children are asked to play "pretend doctor" (younger children) or to conduct a demonstration of the painful procedure using a doll (older children). While the child administers the procedure, the doll is coached to lie still and engage in deep breathing and imagery exercises (Jay et al., 1991).

Finally, data indicated that a variety of staff (physicians, nurses, social workers, child life specialists) may be taught these techniques in a systematic way and then use them successfully in clinical settings (Solomon, Walco, & Robinson, 1998). Thus, the need for individuals with advanced training in this area is reduced when children present with relatively straightforward concerns.

Cognitive behavioral interventions have a number of advantages. They facilitate a sense of mastery over a stressful situation that may be generalized to future coping. Parents may be given specific roles to assist their children with the behavioral techniques, which may be gratifying to both parents and children (Blount, Powers, Cotter, Swan, & Free, 1994). Unlike pharmacological intervention, there are no untoward side effects. These strategies are by no means a panacea, however, as some children may lack the motivation, cognitive ability, or emotional temperament to utilize them. Clearly, one does not need to choose pharmacological versus psychological strategies, but combinations tailored to the needs of individual patients are most reasonable.

There are several studies that have examined the effectiveness of cognitive behavioral therapy (CBT) and pharmacological interventions in reducing distress related to procedural pain in pediatric cancer patients. Results of a study by Jay et al. (1991) indicated that the combination of CBT and oral diazepam was no more effective in relieving procedural distress than was CBT alone. Diazepam is rarely employed at this juncture, and thus using it as a comparison modality reflects the period in which this study was conducted and is not very helpful in light of the more appropriate agents currently available (see discussion concerning the pharmacological management of pain).

Jay, Elliott, Fitzgibbons, Woody, and Siegel (1995) compared the effectiveness of a CBT protocol to the administration of halothane (a short-acting general anesthesia) in reducing procedural distress related to the treatment of cancer. Although children exhibited more behavioral distress in the CBT condition for the first minute lying down on the treatment table, parents of children in the halothane condition rated significantly more behavioral difficulties in the 24 hours following their children's painful procedure. Furthermore, no differences in children's and parents' preferences for CBT versus general anesthesia were found.

Kazak and colleagues (1996) evaluated a combined pharmacological and psychological intervention as opposed to a purely pharmacological intervention in reducing child distress during invasive procedures in pediatric leukemia. Both interventions were effective in reducing parent and child distress, highlighting the importance of integrating these approaches.

A long-standing question has focused on the benefits and limitations of parental presence during invasive procedures. Ross and Ross (1988) discovered that 99% of 994 children found parental presence to be the most helpful factor in aiding relaxation. Children have been found to respond more cooperatively during procedures if parents are present utilizing distraction, relaxation, and imagery, a finding that has been replicated many times (Manne et al., 1990; P. A. McGrath & DeVeber, 1986). It is clear, however, that when parents are present, they are most helpful if they are cued with specific behaviors to help children cope.

Power, Blount, Bachanas, Cotter, and Swan (1993) taught four preschool patients with leukemia (aged 3–5 years) to engage in specific coping behaviors before and during painful intramuscular and intravenous injections. Parents were taught to coach their children in the use of the coping behaviors. Parents and nurses rated child behavior as well. Results indicated that parents learned coping-promoting behaviors, children learned specific coping behaviors, and children displayed less behavioral distress.

## Conclusion

Although carefully controlled clinical trials have been predominant in pediatric oncology, such methodological rigor has not been applied to symptom management, including pain. To manage acute pain adequately in children, a multimodal approach to its assessment and management, which includes pharmacological, psychological, and physical components, has been recommended by the American Academy of Pediatrics and the American Pain Society (2001). Similar values are emphasized in the World Health Organization's guidelines (1990) for pain management and palliative care for pediatric cancer.

Clearly, the time has come for structured assessment of pain in children with cancer and rigorous attempts to control that pain in a systematic fashion. Pain interventions that merely reflect hospital policy or physician preference, without strong empirical support, have no place in current practice. Further research efforts are needed to demonstrate the safety and efficacy of pharmacological agents for specific use in children. Collaborative efforts among the Food and Drug Administration, the National Institutes of Health, academic clinicians, and the pharmaceutical companies are under way to begin to address this very important and mammoth problem. In addition, further validation of psychological interventions for pain are imperative. Reviews indicate that we have little more than descriptive studies; randomized controlled clinical trials are needed to show the efficacy and cost-effectiveness of these techniques.

Once we have substantiated the clinical interventions that are available, research is needed so that algorithms may emerge to guide clinicians specifically in choices of pain treatment regimens that maximize clinical efficacy and safety and minimize cost. This will require a large collaborative effort; attention to ethical issues to ensure that no child endures unnecessary pain or distress will be imperative. In the interim, careful individual assessment is important so that pain is managed with these same goals in mind.

## References


American Academy of Pediatrics Committee on Psychosocial Aspects of Child and Family Health and American Pain Society Task Force on Pain in Infants, Children, and Adolescents. (2001). The assessment and management of acute pain in infants, children, and adolescents. *Pediatrics, 108*, 793–797.

American Cancer Society. (2003). *2003 Cancer facts and figures*. Atlanta, GA: Author.

Anderson, C. T. M., Zeltzer, L. K., & Fanurik, D. (1993). Procedural pain. In N. L. Schechter, C. B. Berde, & M. Yaster (Eds.), *Pain in infants, children and adolescents* (pp. 435–458). Baltimore, MD: Williams and Wilkins.

Babul, N., & Darke, A. C. (1993). Evaluation and use of opioid analgesics in pediatric cancer pain. *Journal of Palliative Care, 9*, 19–25.

Babul, N., Darke, A. C., & Hain, R. (1995). Hydromorphone and metabolite pharmacokinetics in children. *Journal of Pain and Symptom Management, 10*, 335–337.

Backonja, M. M. (2000). Anticonvulsants (antineuropathics) for neuropathic pain syndromes. *Clinical Journal of Pain, 16*(Suppl.), 67–72.

Balis, F. M., Holcenberg, J. S., & Blaney, S. M. (2002). General principles of chemotherapy. In P. A. Pizzo & D. G. Poplack (Eds.), *Principles and practice of pediatric oncology* (4th ed., pp. 237–308). Philadelphia: Lippincott, Williams and Wilkins.

Berde, C. B., Billett, A. L., & Collins, J. J. (2002). Symptom management in supportive care. In P. A. Pizzo & D. G. Poplack (Eds.), *Principles and* practice of pediatric oncology (4th ed., pp. 1301–1332). Philadelphia: Lippincott, Williams, and Wilkins.

Berde, C. B., Brennan, T. J., & Raja, S. N. (2003). Opioids: More to learn, improvements to be made. *Anesthesiology, 98*, 1309–1312.

Blount, R. L., Bunke, V., Cohen, L. L., & Forbes, C. J. (2001). The Child-Adult Medical Procedure Interaction Scale-Short Form (CAMPIS-SF): Validation of a rating scale for children's and adults' behaviors during painful medical procedures. *Journal of Pain and Symptom Management, 22*, 591–599.

Blount, R. L., Powers, S. W., Cotter, M. W., Swan, S., & Free, K. (1994). Making the system work. Training pediatric oncology patients to cope and their parents to coach them during BMA/LP procedures. *Behavior Modification, 18*, 6–31.

Broome, M. E., Lillis, P. P., McGahee, T. W., & Bates, T. (1992). The use of distraction and imagery with children during painful procedures. *Oncology Nursing Forum, 19*, 499–502.

Broome, M. E., Richtsmeier, A., & Malkier, V. (1996). Pediatric pain practices: A national survey of health professionals. *Journal of Pain and Symptom Management, 11*, 312–320.

Broomhead, A., Kerr, R., Tester, W., O'Meara, P., Maccarrone, C., Bowles, R., et al. (1997). Comparison of a once-a-day sustained release morphine formulation with standard oral morphine treatment for cancer pain. *Journal of Pain and Symptom Management, 14*, 63–73.

Collins, J. J. (1998). Pharmacologic management of pediatric cancer pain. In R. K. Portenoy & E. Bruera (Eds.), *Topics in palliative care* (pp. 7–28). New York: Oxford University Press.

Collins, J. J., Byrnes, M. E., Dunkel, I. J., Lapin, J., Nadel, T., Thaler, H. T., et al. (2000). The measurement of symptoms in children with cancer. *Journal of Pain and Symptom Management, 19*, 363–377.

Collins, J. J., Devine, T. D., Dick, G. S., Johnson, E. A., Kilham, H. A., Pinkerton, C. R., et al. (2002). The measurement of symptoms in young children with cancer: The validation of the Memorial Symptom Assessment Scale in children aged 7–12. *Journal of Pain and Symptom Management, 23*, 10–16.

Collins, J. J., Dunkel, I. J., Gupta, S. K., Inturrisi, C. E., Lapin, J., Palmer, L. N., et al. (1999). Transdermal fentanyl in children with cancer pain: Feasibility, tolerability, and pharmacokinetic correlates. *Journal of Pediatrics, 134*, 319–323.

Collins, J. J., Geake, J., Grier, H. E., Houck, C. S., Thaler, H. T., Weinstein, H. J., et al. (1996). Patient-controlled analgesia for mucositis pain in children: A three-period crossover study comparing morphine and hydromorphone. *Journal of Pediatrics, 129*, 722–728.

Collins, J. J., & Weisman, S. J. (2003). Management of pain in childhood cancer. In N. L. Schechter, C. B. Berde, & M. Yaster (Eds.), *Pain in infants, children, and adolescents* (2nd ed., pp. 517–538). Philadelphia: Lippincott, Williams and Wilkins.

Committee on Drugs, American Academy of Pediatrics. (1992). Guidelines for monitoring and management of pediatric patients during and after sedation for diagnostic and therapeutic procedures. *Pediatrics, 89*, 1110–1115.

Craig, K. D., Lilley, C. M., & Gilbert, C. A. (1996). Social barriers to optimal pain management in children. *Journal of Palliative Care, 12*, 232–242.

Crom, D. B., Chathaway, D. K., Tolley, E. A., Mulhern, R. K., & Hudson, M. M. (1999). Health status and health-related quality of life in long-term adult survivors of pediatric solid tumors. *International Journal of Cancer, 12* (Suppl.), 25–31.

Eichenfield, L. F., Funk, A., Fallon-Friedlander, S., & Cunningham, B. B. (2002). A clinical study to evaluate the efficacy of ELA-Max (4% liposomal lidocaine) as compared with eutectic mixture of local anesthetics cream for pain reduction of venipuncture in children. *Pediatrics, 109*, 1093–1099.

Enskar, K., Carlsson, M., Golsater, M., Hamrin, E., & Kreuger, A. (1997). Life situation and problems as reported by children with cancer and their parents. *Journal of Pediatric Oncology Nursing, 14*, 18–26.

Fields, H. L. (1987). *Pain*. New York: McGraw-Hill Book Co.

Fitzgerald, M. (2000). Development of the peripheral and spinal pain system. In K. J. S. Anand, B. J. Stevens, & P. J. McGrath (Eds.), *Pain in neonates* (2nd ed., pp. 9–22). Amsterdam: Elsevier.

Frenk, H., Cannon, J. T., Lewis, J. W., & Liebeskind, J. C. (1986). Neural and neurochemical mechanisms of pain inhibition. In R. A. Sternbach (Ed.), *The psychology of pain* (2nd ed., pp. 25–47). New York: Raven Press.

Grunau, R. V. E., & Craig, K. D. (1987). Pain expression in neonates: Facial action and cry. *Pain, 28*, 395–410.

Gunnar, M. R. (1992). Reactivity of the hypothalamic-pituitary-adrenocortical system to stressors in normal infants and children. *Pediatrics, 90*, 491–497.

Gureno, M. A., & Reisinger, C. L. (1991). Patient controlled analgesia for the young pediatric patient. *Pediatric Nursing, 17*, 251–254.

Gustafsson, G., Langmark, F., Pihkala, U., Verdier, B. D., & Lilleaas, I. J. (1998). *Childhood cancer in the Nordic countries: Report on epidemiologic and therapeutic results*. Reykjavik, Iceland: Nordic Society of Pediatric Hematology and Oncology.

Halperin, D. L., Koren, G., Attias, D., Pellegrini, E., Greenberg, M. L., & Wyss, M. (1989). Topical skin anesthesia for venous, subcutaneous drug reservoir and lumbar punctures in children. *Pediatrics, 84*, 281–284.

Hannallah, R. S., Baker, S. B., Casey, W., McGill, W. A., Broadman, L. M., & Norden J. M. (1991). Propofol: Effective dose and induction characteristics in unpremedicated children. *Anesthesiology, 74*, 217–219.

Harris, C. E., Grounds, R. M., Murray, A. M., Lumley, J., Royston, D., & Morgan, M. (1990). Propofol for long-term sedation in the intensive care unit. A comparison with papaveretum and midazolam. *Anaesthesia, 45*, 366–372.

Hester, N. O., Foster, R., & Kristensen, K. (1990). Measurement of pain in children: Generalizability and validity of the pain ladder and the poker-chip tool. In D. C. Tyler & E. J. Krane (Eds.), *Pediatric pain. Advances in pain research and therapy* (Vol. 15, pp. 79–84). New York: Raven Press.

Hilden, J. M., Emanuel, E. J., Fairclough, D. L., Link, M. P., Foley, K. M., Clarridge, B. C., et al. (2001). Attitudes and practices among pediatric oncologists regarding end-of-life care: Results of the 1998 American Society of Clinical Oncology survey. *Journal of Clinical Oncology, 19*, 205–212.

Hilgard, J. R., & LeBaron, S. (1982). Relief of anxiety and pain in children and adolescents with cancer: Quantitative measures and clinical observations. *International Journal of Clinical and Experimental Hypnosis, 30*, 417–442.

Hunt, A., Joel, S., Dick, G., & Goldman, A. (1999). Population pharmacokinetics of oral morphine and its glucuronides in children receiving morphine as immediate release liquid or sustained release tablets for cancer pain. *Journal of Pediatrics, 135*, 47–55.

Jay S., Elliott, C. H., Fitzgibbons, I., Woody, P., & Siegel, S. (1995). A comparative study of cognitive behavior therapy versus general anesthesia for painful medical procedures in children. *Pain, 62*, 2–9.

Jay, S., Elliot, C. H., Ozolins, M., Olson, R., & Pruitt, S. (1985). Behavioral management of children's distress during painful medical procedures. *Behaviour Research and Therapy*, 5, 513–520.

Jay, S. M., Elliott, C. H., Woody, P. D., & Siegel, S. (1991). An investigation of cognitive-behavior therapy combined with oral Valium for children undergoing medical procedures. *Health Psychology, 10*, 317–322.

Jay, S., Ozolins, M., Elliott, C., & Caldwell, S. (1983). Assessment of children's distress during painful medical procedures. *Journal of Health Psychology, 2*, 133–147.

Katz, E. R., Kellerman, J., & Siegel, S. E. (1980). Behavioral distress in children with cancer undergoing medical procedures: Developmental considerations. *Journal of Consulting and Clinical Psychology, 48*, 356–365.

Kazak, A., Penati, B., Boyer, B., Himelstein, B., Brophy, P., Waibel, M. K., et al. (1996). A randomized controlled prospective outcome study of a psychological and pharmacological intervention protocol for procedural distress in pediatric leukemia. *Journal of Pediatric Psychology, 21*, 615–631.

Kellerman, J., Zeltzer, L., Ellenberg, L., & Dash, J. (1983). Adolescents with cancer: Hypnosis for the reduction of the acute pain and anxiety associated with medical procedures. *Journal of Adolescent Health Care, 4*, 85–90.

LaClave, L. J., & Blix, S. (1989). Hypnosis in the management of symptoms in a young girl with malignant astrocytoma: A challenge to the therapist. *International Journal of Clinical and Experimental Hypnosis, 37*, 6–14.

Leese, P. T., Hubbard, R. C., Karim, A., Isakson, P. C., Yu, S. S., & Geis, G. S. (2000). Effects of celecoxib, a novel cyclooxygenase-2 inhibitor, on platelet function in healthy adults: A randomized controlled trial. *Journal of Clinical Pharmacology, 40*,124–132.

Liossi, C., & Hatira, P. (1999). Clinical hypnosis versus cognitive behavioral training for pain management with pediatric cancer patients undergoing bone marrow aspirations. *The International Journal of Clinical and Experimental Hypnosis, 47*, 104–116.

Liossi, C., & Hatira, P. (2003). Clinical hypnosis in the alleviation of procedure-related pain in pediatric oncology patients. *The International Journal of Clinical and Experimental Hypnosis, 51*, 4–28.

Ljungman, G., Gordh, T., Sorensen, S., & Kreuger, A. (1999). Pain in paediatric oncology: Interviews with children, adolescents and their parents. *Acta Paediatrica, 88*, 623–630.

Ljungman, G., Gordh, T., Sorensen, S., & Kreuger, A. (2000). Pain variations during cancer treatment in children: A descriptive survey. *Pediatric Hematology and Oncology, 17*, 211–221.

Ljungman, G., Gordh, T., Sorensen, S., & Kreuger, A. (2001). Lumbar puncture in pediatric oncology: Conscious sedation versus general anesthesia. *Medical and Pediatric Oncology, 36*, 372–379.

Ljungman, G., Kreuger, A., Gordh, T., Berg, T., Sorensen, S., & Rawal, N. (1996). Treatment of pain in pediatric oncology: A Swedish nationwide survey. *Pain, 68*, 385–394.

Mackie, A. M., Coda, B. C., & Hill, H. F. (1991). Adolescents use patient-controlled analgesia effectively for relief from prolonged oropharyngeal mucositis pain. *Pain, 46*, 265–269.

Manne, S. L., Redd, W. H., Jacobsen, P. B., Gorfinkle, K., Schorr, O., & Rapkin, B. (1990). Behavioral intervention to reduce child and parent distress during venipuncture. *Journal of Consulting and Clinical Psychology, 58*, 565–572.

Mathews, J. R., McGrath, P. J., & Pigeon, H. (1993). Assessment and measurement of pain in children. In N. L. Schechter, C. B. Berde, & M. Yaster (Eds.), *Pain in infants, children and adolescents* (pp. 97–111). Baltimore, MD: Williams and Wilkins.

Maunuksela, E. L., Ryhanen, P., & Janhunen, L. (1992). Efficacy of rectal ibuprofen in controlling postoperative pain in children. *Canadian Journal of Anaesthesia, 39*, 226–230.

McGrath, P. A. (1990). *Pain in children: Nature, assessment and treatment*. New York: Guilford Press.

McGrath, P. A., & DeVeber, L. L. (1986). Helping children cope with painful procedures. *American Journal of Nursing, 86*, 1278–1279.

McGrath, P. A., & Gillespie, J. (2001). Pain assessment in children and adolescents. In D. C. Turk & R. Melzack (Eds.), *Handbook of pain assessment* (2nd ed., pp. 97–118). New York: Guilford Press.

McGrath, P. J. (1996). Attitudes and beliefs about medication and pain management in infants and children. *Clinical Journal of Pain, 12*, 46–50.

McGrath, P. J., Hsu, E., Cappelli, M., & Luke, B. (1990). Pain from pediatric cancer: A survey of an outpatient oncology clinic. *Journal of Psychosocial Oncology, 8*, 109–124.

McGrath, P. J. & Unruh, A. M. (1987). *Pain in children and adolescents*. Amsterdam: Elsevier.

Melamed, B. G., & Ridley-Johnson, R. (1988). Psychological preparation of families for hospitalization. *Journal of Developmental and Behavioral Pediatrics, 9*, 96–102.

Melzack, R., & Wall, P. D. (1965). Pain mechanisms: A new theory. *Science, 150*, 971–979.

Merskey, H., & Bogduk, N. (Eds.). (1994). *Classification of chronic pain: Descriptions of chronic pain syndromes and definitions of pain terms* (2nd ed.). Seattle, WA: IASP Press.

Miser, A. W., Dothage, J. A., Wesley, R. A., & Miser, J. S. (1987). The prevalence of pain in a pediatric and young adult cancer population. *Pain, 29*, 73–83.

Miser, A. W., McCalla, J., Dothage, J. A., Wesley, M., & Miser, J. S. (1987). Pain as a presenting symptom in children and young adults with newly diagnosed malignancy. *Pain, 29*, 85–90.

Noyes, M., & Irving, H. (2001). The use of transdermal fentanyl in pediatric oncology palliative care. *American Journal of Hospice and Palliative Care, 18*, 411–416.

Ollson, G. L. (1999). Neuropathic pain in children. In P. J. McGrath and G. A. Finley (Eds.), *Chronic and recurrent pain in children and adolescents: Progress in pain research and management* (Vol. 13, pp. 75–98). Seattle, WA: IASP Press.

Olness, K. (1981). Hypnosis in pediatric practice. *Current Problems in Pediatrics, 12*, 1–47.

Olness, K., & Kohen, D. P. (1996). *Hypnosis and hypnotherapy with children* (3rd ed.). New York: Guilford.

Paice, J. A. (1991). Unraveling the mystery of pain. *Oncology Nursing Forum, 18*, 843–849.

Porges, S. W. (1992). Vagal tone: A physiologic marker of stress vulnerability. *Pediatrics, 90*, 498–504.

Powers, S. W. (1999). Empirically supported treatments in pediatric psychology: Procedure-related pain. *Journal of Pediatric Psychology, 24*, 131–145.

Powers, S. W., Blount, R. L., Bachanas, P. J., Cotter, M. W., & Swan, S. C. (1993). Helping preschool leukemia patients and their parents cope during injections. *Journal of Pediatric Psychology, 18*, 681–695.

Rawal, N., Hylander, J., & Arner, S. (1993). Management of terminal cancer pain in Sweden: A nationwide survey. *Pain, 54*, 169–179.

Ries, L. A. G., Eisner, M. P., Kosary, C. L., Hankey, B. F., Miller, B. A., Clegg, L., et al. (Eds.). (2003). *SEER cancer statistics review, 1975–2000*. Bethesda, MD: National Cancer Institute.

Ross, D. M., & Ross, S. A. (1988). *Childhood pain: Current issues, research, and management*. Baltimore, MD: Urban and Schwarzenberg.

Sandler, E. S., Weyman, C., Conner, K., Reilly, K., Dickson, N., Luzins, J., et al. (1992). Midazolam versus fentanyl as premedication for painful procedures in children with cancer. *Pediatrics, 89*, 631–634.

Schechter, N. L. (1989). The undertreatment of pain in children: An overview. *Pediatric Clinics of North America, 36*, 781–794.

Schechter, N. L., Berde, C. B., & Yaster, M. (2003). Pain in infants, children, and adolescents: An overview. In N. L. Schechter, C. B. Berde, & M. Yaster (Eds.), *Pain in infants, children, and adolescents* (2nd ed., pp. 3–18). Philadelphia: Lippincott, Williams and Wilkins.

Schechter, N. L., Weisman, S. J., Rosenblum, M., Bernstein, B., & Conard, P. L. (1995). The use of oral transmucosal fentanyl citrate for painful procedures in children. *Pediatrics, 95*, 335–339.

Shapiro, H. M., Wyte, S. R., & Harris, A. B. (1972). Ketamine anesthesia in patients with intracranial pathology. *British Journal of Anaesthesia, 44*, 1200–1204.

Siegal, L. J. (1976). Preparation of children for hospitalization: A selected review of research literature. *Journal of Pediatric Psychology, 1*, 26–30.

Sindrup, S. H., & Jensen, T. S. (1999). Efficacy of pharmacological treatments of neuropathic pain: An update and effect related to mechanism of drug action. *Pain, 83*, 389–400.

Smith, J., Barabasz, A., & Barabasz, M. (1996). Comparison of hypnosis and distraction in severely ill children undergoing painful medical procedures. *Journal of Counseling Psychology, 43*, 187–195.

Solomon, R., Walco, G. A., & Robinson, M. R. (1998). Pediatric pain management: Program description and preliminary evaluation results of a professional course. *Journal of Developmental and Behavioral Pediatrics, 19*, 193–195.

Stamford, J. A. (1995). Descending control of pain. *British Journal of Anaesthesia, 75*, 217–227.

Stiller, C. A., & Draper, G. J. (1998). *The epidemiology of cancer in children*. Oxford, UK: Oxford University Books.

Stuber, M. L., Kazak, A. E., Meeske, K., & Barakat, L. (1998). Is posttraumatic stress a viable model for understanding responses to childhood cancer? *Child and Adolescent Psychiatric Clinics of North America, 7*, 169–182.

Stuber, M., Christakis, D., Houskamp, B., & Kazak, A. (1996). Post-trauma symptoms in childhood leukemia survivors and their parents. *Psychosomatics, 37*, 254–261.

Taddio, A., Shennaan, A., & Stevens, B. (1995). Safety of lidocaine-prilocaine (EMLA) in neonates > 30 weeks gestation. In T. S. Jensen, J. A. Turner, & Z. Wiesenfeld-Hallin (Eds.), *Proceedings of the Eighth World Congress on Pain* (p. 182). Seattle, WA: IASP Press.

Taylor, P. A., & Towey, R. M. (1971). Depression of laryngeal reflexes during ketamine administration. *British Medical Journal, 2*, 688–689.

Tobias, J. D. (2000). Weak analgesics and nonsteroidal anti-inflammatory agents in the management of children with acute pain. *Pediatric Clinics of North America, 47*, 527–543.

Tobias, J. D. (2003). Pain management for the critically ill child in the pediatric intensive care unit. In N. L. Schechter, C. B. Berde, & M. Yaster (Eds.), *Pain in infants, children, and adolescents* (2nd ed., pp. 807–840). Philadelphia: Lippincott, Williams and Wilkins.

Tobias, J. D., Phipps, S., Smith, B., & Mulhern, R. K. (1992). Oral ketamine premedication to alleviate the distress of invasive procedures in pediatric oncology patients. *Pediatrics, 90*, 537–541.

Valtonen, M., Iisalo, E., Kanto, J., & Tikkanen, J. (1988). Comparison between propofol and thiopentone for induction of anaesthesia in children. *Anaesthesia, 43*, 696–699.

Varni, J. W., Thompson, K. L., & Hanson V. (1987). The Varni/Thompson Pediatric Pain Questionnaire. I. Chronic musculoskeletal pain in juvenile rheumatoid arthritis. *Pain, 28*, 27–38.

Walco, G. A., Cassidy, R. C., & Schechter, N. L. (1994). Pain, hurt, and harm. The ethics of pain control in infants and children. *New England Journal of Medicine, 331*, 541–544.

Walco, G. A., Conte, P. M., Labay, L. E., Engel, R., & Zeltzer, L. K. (2005). Procedural distress in children with cancer: Self-report, behavioral observations, and physiological parameters. *Clinical Journal of Pain, 21*, 484–490.

Walco, G. A., Sterling, C. M., Conte, P. M., & Engel, R. G. (1999). Empirically supported treatments in pediatric psychology: Disease-related pain. *Journal of Pediatric Psychology, 24*, 155–167.

Weisman, S. J., Bernstein, B., & Schechter, N. L. (1998). Consequences of inadequate analgesia during painful procedures in children. *Archives of Pediatric Adolescent Medicine, 152*, 147–149.

Weisman, S. J., & Wishnie, E. (1996). Postoperative hydromorphone epidural analgesia in children. In T. S. Jensen, J. A. Turner, & Z. Wiesenfeld-Hallin (Eds.), Proceedings of the Eighth World Congress on Pain (p. 301). Seattle, WA: IASP Press.

White, P. R., Way, W. L., & Trevor, A. J. (1982). Ketamine—its pharmacology and therapeutic uses. *Anesthesiology, 56*, 119–136.

Wolfe, J., Grier, H. E., Klar, N., Levin, S. B., Ellenbogen, J. M., Salem-Schatz, S., et al. (2000). Symptoms and suffering at the end of life in children with cancer. *New England Journal of Medicine, 342*, 326–333.

Wolpe, J. (1981). Reciprocal inhibition and therapeutic change. *Journal of Behavior Therapy and Experimental Psychiatry, 12*, 185–188.

World Health Organization. (1990). *Cancer pain relief and palliative care* (Technical Report Series 804). Geneva, Switzerland: Author.

Yaster, M., Deshpande, J. K., & Maxwell, L. G. (1989). The pharmacologic management of pain in children. *Comprehensive Therapy, 15*, 14–26.

Yaster, M., Kost-Byerly, S., & Maxwell, L. G. (2003). Opioid agonists and antagonists. In N. L. Schechter, C. B. Berde, & M. Yaster (Eds.), *Pain in infants, children, and adolescents* (2nd ed., pp. 181–224). Philadelphia: Lippincott, Williams and Wilkins.

Yee, J. D., & Berde, C. B. (1994). Dextroamphetamine or methylphenidate as adjuvants to opioid analgesia for adolescents with cancer. *Journal of Pain and Symptom Management, 9*, 122–125.

Zech, D. F. J., Grond, S., Lynch, J., Hertel, D., & Lehmann, K. A. (1995). Validation of World Health Organization guidelines for cancer pain relief: A 10-year prospective study. *Pain, 63*, 65–76.

Zeltzer, L. K., Altman, A., Cohen, D., LeBaron, S., Maunuksela, E. L., & Schechter, N. L. (1990). American Academy of Pediatrics Report of the Subcommittee on the Management of Pain Associated With Procedures in Children With Cancer. *Pediatrics, 86*, 826–831.

Zeltzer, L. K., Anderson, C. T., & Schechter, N. L. (1990). Pediatric pain: Current status and new directions. *Current Problems in Pediatrics, 20*, 409–486.

Zeltzer, L. K., & LeBaron, S. (1982). Hypnosis and nonhypnotic techniques for reduction of pain and anxiety during painful procedures in children and adolescents with cancer. *Journal of Pediatrics, 101*, 1032–1035.

Zempsky, W. T., & Ashburn, M. A. (1998). Iontophoresis: Noninvasive drug delivery. *American Journal of Anesthesiology, 25*, 158–162.

Michael A. Rapoff, Ann M. McGrath,
and Stephen D. Smith

# Adherence to Treatment Demands

## Introduction

Given the life-threatening nature of cancer, one might expect that children with cancer and their parents would be especially vigilant about following prescribed medical treatments. As illustrated in this chapter, this is not always the case (Partridge, Avorn, Wang, & Winer, 2002). Nonadherence can potentially lead to outright treatment failure, relapse, compromised outcomes, bone marrow transplant failures, or resistance to drugs such as antibiotics (Rapoff, 1999).

The purpose of this chapter is to (a) review treatment demands on children with acute leukemia (the most common childhood cancer) and their families to understand better the complex behavioral requirements associated with medical treatments; (b) review studies that have investigated the extent of nonadherence to treatments for pediatric cancer, primarily leukemia; (c) examine factors predictive of adherence; (d) describe strategies for assessing adherence; (e) provide suggestions for improving adherence; and (f) suggest future directions to advance the field of adherence research in pediatric oncology. Strategies for improving adherence were gleaned from the pediatric medical adherence literature on other chronic diseases because we could not find a single adherence intervention study involving children with cancer.

## Childhood Leukemia and Treatment Demands

Acute leukemia is the most common malignancy in children (Ries et al., 1999). The specific etiology of childhood leukemia is unknown, but the causes appear to be multifactorial. Some of the factors involved in the pathogenesis of acute leukemia include exposure to ionizing radiation or certain drugs (e.g., benzene), certain chromosome abnormalities (e.g., Down syndrome), and congenital or acquired immune deficiencies (e.g., human immunodeficiency virus infection) (Golub & Arceci, 2002; Margolin, Steuber, & Poplack, 2002). The incidence of acute leukemia is 3–4 per 100,000 white children, and approximately 3,000 children will develop acute leukemia in the United States within a given year (Ries et al., 1999).

The hallmark of leukemia is bone marrow failure. The bone marrow makes red blood cells, which carry oxygen; white cells, which fight infections; and platelets, which help blood clot. Children with acute leukemia commonly present with pallor and fatigue (secondary to anemia), fever and infections (caused by reduced normal white cells), and excess bruising and bleeding (secondary to low platelets). Acute leukemia may be characterized as lymphoid (with three subtypes) or myeloid (with eight subtypes). Each subtype of leukemia has specific morphology features, monoclonal antibody profile, karyotype, or molecular markers. Acute leukemia is treated with chemotherapy, and the specific treatment is based on the specific leukemia subtype. Chemotherapy may be supplemented with radiation therapy if there is evidence of central nervous system (CNS) leukemia or testicular leukemia (Margolin et al., 2002).

## Acute Lymphoblastic Leukemia

Acute lymphoblastic leukemia (ALL) is the most common leukemia in children. When the diagnosis of ALL is suspected, the child is referred to a tertiary care center for a full evaluation. Initially, blood tests and a needle aspirate of the bone marrow are performed. When the diagnosis of ALL has been confirmed, a lumbar puncture is performed, and a central cardiac line is placed under conscious sedation or general anesthesia. The direct treatment of ALL requires systemic chemotherapy, which is started after informed consent is obtained from the parents and assent from the child. Obtaining informed consent is difficult because the treatment and monitoring of ALL is noxious (causing nausea and vomiting), painful (daily or weekly blood tests), complicated (over 10 different drugs may be used), toxic (resulting in hair loss and mouth sores), and long (over 2 years). Also, the oncologists are new to the family, some medical jargon is unavoidable, and there is high anxiety because ALL is fatal if not treated correctly. However, if full therapy can be delivered, approximately 80% of children with ALL can be cured (Margolin et al., 2002).

Although there are three subtypes of ALL (L1, L2, and L3) based on morphology, there are many different types of ALL based on the cell surface antigen profile and chromosome changes within the malignant cells. At diagnosis, children are categorized as having a good, standard, or poor prognosis based on both the child's clinical features and chromosomal abnormalities found in the lymphoblasts. The intensity of chemotherapy that a child with ALL receives is based on the prognostic group. Children with a poor prognosis receive the most aggressive chemotherapy.

The initial treatment of the different types of ALL has three general phases: induction, consolidation, and maintenance. For over 40 years, randomized clinical trials have been performed that have determined the best therapy for each stage of treatment. Randomized clinical trials sponsored by the National Cancer Institute continue to be used to improve the cure rate of ALL and to reduce the toxicity of therapy.

### *Induction Treatment Phase*

The first phase of treatment of ALL in children is called induction, and it lasts 4–5 weeks (Table 8-1). The chemotherapy agents are used to induce the leukemia cells into remission. At presentation, children with ALL have more than 25% malignant cells (called lymphoblasts) in the bone marrow. If the induction therapy is successful, then the bone marrow will have fewer than 5% lymphoblasts after the first 4–5 weeks of therapy (O'Reilly et al., 1996).

After 4–5 weeks of chemotherapy, the child with ALL is evaluated to see if the leukemia is in remission. A complete remission is defined as resolution of the signs and symptoms of leukemia, a return to normal of the blood and bone marrow values, and a leukemia cell kill resulting in fewer than 5% lymphoblasts in the bone marrow. Currently, over 95% of children with ALL achieve complete remission.

### *Consolidation Treatment Phase*

Once complete remission has been obtained, the child is started on consolidation therapy, which includes a combination of aggressive multiagent chemotherapy (Table 8-1). Consolidation chemotherapy consists of repeated cycles of drug combinations administered by mouth, in the vein (intravenous), and into the spinal canal (intrathecal).

During consolidation, children also receive treatment to prevent (or treat) overt leukemia in the CNS. At the diagnosis of ALL, a lumbar puncture is performed, some cerebral spinal fluid (CSF) is removed, and a dose of methotrexate is injected intrathecally. Methotrexate is given as an intrathecal drug after an equal volume of CSF has been removed by a lumbar puncture. The CSF is analyzed for the presence of malignant cells. If leukemia cells are

**Table 8-1.** Treatment Demands on Patients With Acute Lymphoblastic Leukemia and Their Families by Phases of Treatment

| *Induction (~4 weeks)* | *Consolidation (~6 months)* | *Maintenance (2–3 years)* |
|---|---|---|
| Intravenous chemotherapy once a week for 4 weeks (outpatient or inpatient).<br>Oral prednisone three times daily for 28 days.<br>Intramuscular injections of asparaginase, six doses over 2.5 weeks (outpatient).<br>Central catheter care: Flush line daily with saline and heparin; change dressing once or twice weekly; report any signs of inflammation at exit site.<br>Monitor food and fluid intake and signs of fever, vomiting, or diarrhea or any new symptoms of pain or discomfort.<br>Blood counts two to three times per week.<br>Avoid exposure to ill individuals or those vaccinated with a live virus.<br>Administer as-needed pain or antiemetic medications. | Oral prednisone for ~5 days; daily oral 6-MP, commonly in 2-week cycles with 6-week breaks between cycles.<br>Intravenous low-dose chemotherapy outpatient or intravenous high-dose chemotherapy inpatient (weekly or monthly).<br>Multiple doses of intrathecal methotrexate weekly with or without daily irradiation.<br>10-day courses of intravenous antibiotics (inpatient and then home) if needed.<br>Oral antibiotic for PCP prophylaxis 3 days per week.<br>Intramuscular injections of asparaginase, six doses over 2.5 weeks (outpatient).<br>Central catheter care: Flush line daily with saline and heparin; change dressing once or twice weekly; report any signs of inflammation at exit site.<br>Monitor food and fluid intake and signs of fever, vomiting, or diarrhea or any new symptoms of pain or discomfort.<br>Complete blood counts two to three times per week.<br>As-needed pain or antiemetic medications.<br>Avoid exposure to ill individuals or those vaccinated with a live virus. | Daily oral 6-MP and weekly oral or intramuscular methotrexate.<br>Additional chemotherapy is given and may include repeated cycles (every 3–4 months) of 4- to 5-day course of oral prednisone or dexamethasone; 1–3 doses of intravenous chemotherapy; 1 dose of intrathecal methotrexate.<br>Oral antibiotic for PCP prophylaxis 3 days per week.<br>Central catheter care: Flush line daily with saline and heparin; change dressing once or twice weekly; report any signs of inflammation at exit site.<br>Monitor food and fluid intake and signs of fever, vomiting, or diarrhea or any new symptoms of pain or discomfort.<br>Complete blood counts once per week.<br>Avoid exposure to ill individuals or those vaccinated with a live virus. |

*Note.* PCP, *Pneumocystis carinii* pneumonia.

present in the CNS at diagnosis, then the child will receive weekly doses of intrathecal methotrexate during induction therapy; these doses are given in addition to the induction chemotherapy. If no leukemia cells are detected, then the child will receive multiple doses of intrathecal methotrexate during the consolidation phase to prevent the overt occurrence of CNS leukemia (Lanzkowsky, 2000; O'Reilly et al., 1996).

### *Maintenance Treatment Phase*

Maintenance chemotherapy consists of daily oral mercaptopurine and weekly oral (or intramuscular) methotrexate. In addition, various other chemotherapy agents are generally given as in the consolidation phase of therapy (Table 8-1). The total duration of therapy is marked from the time when the child enters remission. Postinduction chemotherapy continues for 2–2.5 years for girls and 2.5–3 years for boys.

Some children (and their parents) misunderstand the maintenance phase of therapy and become relaxed about taking their medication and attending clinic appointments. Children may feel well and consider the chemotherapy as only a reminder of past painful experiences. Indeed, in this stage of treatment, the ALL is under excellent control (or eliminated), and the only symptoms that the child experiences may be side effects of the chemotherapy agents. Because the signs and symptoms of ALL may have been long forgotten, the child may stop taking the medications.

Children who have a subtype of ALL associated with a poor prognosis (e.g., Philadelphia chromosome-positive ALL) or children who suffer a recurrence of ALL at any site (relapse) may be treated with a bone marrow transplant. The treatment with bone marrow transplantation is covered in the next section on acute myeloblastic leukemia (AML).

### *General Treatment Recommendations*

Children with ALL usually have blood tests once or twice a week to monitor the doses of chemotherapy. Children will receive prophylaxis for *Pneumocystis carinii* pneumonia with Bactrim, administered three consecutive days a week, or monthly aerosolized pentamidine. The parents need to care for the child's Hickman central line with daily flushes of saline with heparin to keep the line patent. To avoid a line exit site infection, the Hickman dressing needs to be changed weekly or whenever the dressing gets wet. Also, sometimes bacteria will stick to the inner lumen of the line (from bacteremia or puncture cap contamination). Usually, treatment with intravenous antibiotics will clear the infection, but sometimes the central line needs to be removed and subsequently replaced (Berde, Billett, & Collins, 2002; Margolin et al., 2002).

Live virus vaccinations are contraindicated in the child with ALL because these vaccines can cause an illness. Also, children with leukemia should avoid anyone who has received a live virus vaccination. Children who have not been vaccinated with the varicella vaccine need to avoid children with chicken pox as well as adults with herpes zoster (shingles). The treatment of leukemia commonly lowers the white blood cells to a borderline low level. If the child develops a fever, the white blood cells may drop further, resulting in severe neutropenia. Treatment of fever with neutropenia commonly requires intravenous antibiotics administered in the hospital.

## Acute Myeloblastic Leukemia

AML accounts for about 20% of the acute leukemia in children. AML is a heterogeneous group of leukemia classified by cellular morphology and cytochemical stains. The etiology of AML is unclear, but there is an increased incidence of AML in children who have a bone marrow failure syndrome (e.g., Fanconi's), specific chromosome deletions (monosomy 7 or 5), or a history of previous bone marrow dysfunction (e.g., myelodysplasia). Also, children may develop AML as a partial consequence of therapy used to treat a previous malignancy. In the past, AML occurred as a second malignancy in about 5% of children treated for Hodgkin's disease (Golub & Arceci, 2002).

There are eight subtypes of AML based on the different cellular morphology, cytochemical staining patterns, cell surface antigen profile, and karyotype. All the subtypes of AML are treated with the same induction chemotherapy except for acute promyeloblastic leukemia (APL, M3) and AML in children with Down syndrome. Postinduction chemotherapy is dependent on the availability of a human lymphocyte antigen (HLA)-matched histocompatible donor.

AML is treated with intensive, sequential induction chemotherapy, which is more aggressive and toxic than ALL therapy (Table 8-2). Prolonged hospitalization is expected during the AML treatment phases. After repeated cycles of chemotherapy, most children (80%) obtain complete remission (O'Donnell, 2003).

Once complete remission is obtained, the child with AML will receive additional chemotherapy or have a bone marrow transplant. In the absence of an HLA-matched donor, intensive treatment with cytarabine and asparaginase is commonly used. Although the therapy for AML is intense, the duration of therapy is relatively short, with a total duration of therapy of about 6 months. Long-term survival is 50–60% (Golub & Arceci, 2002).

Because marrow aplasia is needed to induce AML into remission, children with AML may be hospitalized for long periods of time. They have a long period of myelosuppression, commonly need treatment for fever and neutropenia, often have mucositis, sometimes have excess neurotoxicity, and are prone to developing fungal infections.

#### *Bone Marrow Transplantation*

In contrast to ALL, children with AML are evaluated for a bone marrow transplant at diagnosis. Parents and siblings are evaluated to determine if there is a match within the family. Often, the parents, the recipient, and the potential donors all have their blood submitted at the same time to the HLA laboratory. Many oncologists recommend that if a suitable family HLA-matched donor is available, all children with AML should receive an allogeneic bone marrow transplant in first remission. There are two general exceptions to this recommendation: children with acute promyeloblastic leukemia and children with Down syndrome and AML (Golub & Arceci, 2002; Lanzkowsky, 2000).

If a donor has been identified, a child with AML is evaluated to see if the child is a potential recipient for a bone marrow transplant. To obtain the best chance of success, the child needs to be in remission, have no major organ damage, not be actively infected, not be malnourished, and have the psychological support to tolerate the transplant therapy. A countdown is started on Day –8 when chemotherapy is started and ends on Day 0 when the donor bone marrow cells are infused. Chemotherapy with or without radiation therapy is given on Days –8 to –2, Day –1 is a rest day, and Day 0 is the day when the child receives the bone marrow stem cells. A child often will need to be hospitalized for 3–5 weeks; usually has some problems with infections and requires antibiotics; can develop severe mucositis and respiratory distress, which may require intubation; and usually has anorexia, which may require parenteral feedings. After Day 0, a child will receive graft-versus-host disease prophylaxis with cyclosporine and methotrexate. Some of the special concerns after a bone marrow transplant include a diet change that avoids fresh fruits and vegetables (neutropenic diet) and the need to avoid live plants, cut flowers, and live Christmas trees. A child will need to avoid rubber balloons and cannot have contact with a cat or dog for some months (Lanzkowsky, 2000).

### Summary of Treatment Demands

As detailed in this section and in Tables 8-1 and 8-2, treatments for ALL and AML are intensive, long term, and complicated and have significant adverse side effects. These demands include oral and intravenous medications, intramuscular injections, dietary recommendations, avoidance of persons who are ill or who have received live vaccinations, and central line care. Even with a potentially life-threatening illness such as leukemia, the complexity of the regimens and the painful and bothersome adverse side effects of treatment can lead to less-than-optimal adherence, as reviewed in the next section.

## Prevalence of Nonadherence

A total of eight studies documenting nonadherence rates to regimens for pediatric cancer were located for this review (see Table 8-3). The majority of these studies involved children with ALL, and they measured adherence to prednisone or 6-mercaptopurine (6-MP). Five of these studies used a urine or serum assay to measure adherence; two primarily relied on child, parent, or provider reports; and one study used an electronic monitor.

Nonadherence rates to prednisone ranged from 18.8% to 52% (Festa, Tamaroff, Chasalow, & Lanzkowsky, 1992; Lansky, Smith, Cairns, & Cairns, 1983; S. D. Smith, Rosen, Trueworthy, & Lowman, 1979; Tebbi et al., 1986). The Tebbi et al. study monitored adherence at three occasions postdiagnosis and found that nonadherence to prednisone increased from 18.8% at 2 weeks postdiagnosis

**Table 8-2.** Treatment Demands on Patients With Acute Myeloblastic Leukemia and Their Families by Phases of Treatment

| *Induction (~3–6 weeks)* | *Consolidation (6–9 weeks)* | *Transplant and Postengraftment (~6 months)* |
|---|---|---|
| Intravenous chemotherapy for 5 days every 2 weeks (inpatient).<br>Intravenous Ara-C, VP-16, and daunorubicin; oral thioguanine; and dexamethasone (generally inpatient) for 4–6 weeks.<br>Intrathecal Ara-C, one dose with each cycle.<br>Daily subcutaneous injections of G-CSF, 2 to 3 weeks per month.<br>Central catheter care: Flush line daily with saline and heparin; change dressing once or twice weekly; report any signs of inflammation at exit site.<br>Monitor food and fluid intake and signs of fever, vomiting, or diarrhea or any new symptoms of pain or discomfort.<br>Complete blood counts two to three times per week.<br>As-needed pain or antiemetic medications.<br>Avoid exposure to ill individuals or those vaccinated with a live virus. | Intravenous chemotherapy for 5 days, every 3 weeks, with Ara-C, VP-16, and daunorubicin; oral thioguanine; and dexamethasone (generally inpatient) for 4–6 weeks.<br>Intramuscular injections of high doses of Ara-C followed by intramuscular asparaginase.<br>Intrathecal Ara-C, one dose with each cycle.<br>Daily subcutaneous injections of G-CSF, 2 to 3 weeks per month.<br>Oral antibiotic for PCP prophylaxis 3 days per week.<br>10-day courses of intravenous antibiotics (inpatient and then home) if needed.<br>As-needed pain or antiemetic medications.<br>Central catheter care: Flush line daily with saline and heparin; change dressing once or twice weekly; report any signs of inflammation at exit site.<br>Monitor food and fluid intake and signs of fever, vomiting, or diarrhea or any new symptoms of pain or discomfort.<br>Complete blood counts two to three times per week.<br>Avoid exposure to ill individuals or those vaccinated with a live virus. | Single infusion of HLA-matched bone marrow stem cells.<br>Intravenous antibiotic, antifungal, and antiviral medications for 1–6 months.<br>Intravenous immunoglobulin infusion over 6 hours, once weekly for first month and then monthly.<br>While hospitalized, neutropenic diet, no live plants, and no balloons.<br>As outpatient, no exposure to household pets and no dining out.<br>Daily oral CSA for GVHD prophylaxis for 6 months.<br>Central catheter care: Flush line daily with saline and heparin; change dressing once or twice weekly; report any signs of inflammation at exit site.<br>Monitor food and fluid intake and signs of fever, vomiting, or diarrhea or any new symptoms of pain or discomfort.<br>Complete blood counts, profile, and CSA level once per week.<br>Avoid exposure to ill individuals or those vaccinated with a live virus. |

*Note.* Ara-C, cytarabine; CSA, cyclosporine; G-CSF, granulocyte colony-stimulating factor; GVHD, graft versus host disease; 6-MP, mercaptopurine; PCP, *Pneumocystis carinii* pneumonia; VP-16, etoposide.

**Table 8-3.** Nonadherence Rates to Pediatric Cancer Regimens

| *Reference* | *Sample* | *Disease/Regimen* | *Adherence Measure* | *Results* |
|---|---|---|---|---|
| Festa et al., 1992 | $N = 50$ (two samples with $M = 15.6$ years and $M = 19.1$ years) | ALL or Hodgkin's disease/Prednisone ($N = 21$) Penicillin ($N = 29$) for postsplenectomy prophylaxis | Serum assay for prednisone<br>Urine assay for penicillin | 52% nonadherent to prednisone<br>48% nonadherent to penicillin |
| Kennard et al., 2004 | $N = 44$<br>$M = 15.3$ years | ALL and other cancers/Trimethoprim/ sulfamethoxazole | Serum assay | 27% nonadherent |
| Lancaster et al., 1997 | N=496 | ALL/6-Mercaptopurine | Assays of 6-mercaptopurine in red blood cells | Nine children (2%) had completely undetectable metabolites on one or more occasions |
| Lansky et al., 1983 | $N = 31$<br>2–14 years | ALL/Prednisone | Urine assay | 42% had subtherapeutic levels |
| Lau et al., 1998 | $N = 24$<br>($M = 7.3$ years) | ALL/6-Mercaptopurine | Electronic monitor | 17% nonadherent (<80% of doses taken) |
| Phipps & DeCuir-Whalley, 1990 | $N = 54$<br>1 month to 20 years | ALL, ANLL, tumor, SCID, aplastic anemia, or other/ Antibiotics as part of bone marrow transplant protocol | Review of patient chart and notes from psychosocial team meetings | "Significant" adherence difficulties identified in 52% of sample |
| S. D. Smith et al., 1979 | $N = 52$<br>8 months to 17 years | ALL, AML, or non-Hodgkins's lymphoma/Prednisone | Urine assay (<18.7 kg/cr defined as subtherapeutic) | 33% had subtherapeutic levels |
| Tebbi et al., 1986 | $N = 46$<br>2.5–23 years<br>($M = 6.85$ years) | ALL, Hodgkin's disease, non-Hodgkin's lymphoma, or other/Prednisone | Patient and parent report (corroborated by serum assay) | Nonadherence rates (reported missing 1–3 or more doses during preceding month) at 2 weeks postdiagnosis = 18.8%; at 20 weeks = 39.5%; and at 50 weeks = 35% |

*Note.* ALL, acute lymphoblastic leukemia; ANLL, acute nonlymphocytic leukemia; AML, acute myeloblastic leukemia; *M*, mean; SCID, severe combined immune deficiency syndrome.

to 39.5% and 35%, respectively, at 20 weeks and 50 weeks postdiagnosis. This is consistent with one study (Kovacs, Goldston, Obrosky, & Iyengar, 1992) that found increased nonadherence over time for children diagnosed with insulin-dependent diabetes. Nonadherence to 6-MP was found in 2% of the sample in one study using a blood assay (Lancaster, Lennard, & Lilleyman, 1997) but was present in 17% of the sample in the other study, which used an electronic monitor (Lau, Matsui, Greenberg, & Koren, 1998). These results illustrate a common finding in the adherence literature of cross-method variance, with generally higher rates of nonadherence as measured by electronic monitors versus assays or other methods (Rapoff, 1999).

Two studies examined adherence to antibiotic regimens for postsplenectomy or post–bone marrow transplant prophylaxis for children with cancer, with one study finding a 48% nonadherence rate by urine assay (Festa et al., 1992), and the other study finding a 52% nonadherence rate by chart review. Another study measured adherence to prophylactic oral trimethoprim/sulfamethoxazole to prevent infection with *P. carinii* by serum assay and found that 27% of a sample of adolescents with various cancers were nonadherent (Kennard et al., 2004). These studies demonstrated how difficult it is to achieve adherence to prophylactic antibiotics, particularly when they can cause nausea, diarrhea, and abdominal discomfort (Phipps & DeCuir-Whalley, 1990).

## Factors Associated With Adherence

Child and family, disease, and regimen factors often have been studied as predictors of adherence to pediatric chronic disease regimens (Rapoff, 1999). There are good reasons for examining predictors of adherence to medical regimens (Rapoff & Christophersen, 1982). First, factors that predict poor adherence can be used to develop "risk profiles" that can be used clinically (with appropriate cautions) to identify children likely to be nonadherent. Second, some correlates of adherence are potentially modifiable (such as the complexity of regimens) and therefore can suggest ways to improve adherence. Third, relatively unmodifiable correlates of adherence, such as socioeconomic status, can be used as matching or control variables in randomized, controlled adherence intervention trials. Finally, correlates of adherence can be used to support or refute existing theories about adherence or help generate new theories. A few studies have examined correlates of adherence for children with cancer.

Two studies found lower adherence to prednisone, 6-MP, and other medications for adolescents versus younger children with leukemia (S. D. Smith et. al., 1979; Tebbi et al., 1986). Lower adherence has been found among adolescents with other chronic diseases, presumably because adolescents are trying to achieve independence, and they have less parental monitoring (Rapoff, 1998). However, one study found significantly greater adherence difficulties identified by the medical team following bone marrow transplantation for preschool and school-aged children versus those under 2 years of age and adolescents (Phipps & DeCuir-Whalley, 1990).

Regarding family composition, one study found higher adherence among boys from larger families (Lansky et al., 1983); another found lower adherence among children with more siblings (Tebbi et al., 1986). One study addressed regimen factors and found a higher trend in adherence for evening versus morning doses of 6-MP (Lau et al., 1998). This may be because of more hectic schedules in the morning with school-aged children.

Those children who had better understanding of how to administer medications and what to do if they missed a dose were more likely to be adherent to oral medications in one study (Tebbi et al., 1986). A working knowledge of regimen requirements is considered a prerequisite for better adherence (Rapoff, 1999). In contrast, those children in "denial" and who had less-realistic conceptions of their illness and less perceived vulnerability to illness were less adherent (Tamaroff, Festa, Adesman, & Walco, 1992), which would be predicted by the health belief model (Rapoff, 1999). Parent, rather than child, personality variables were more predictive of adherence in one study, especially for male children (e.g., higher anxiety reported by the mother predicted better adherence; Lansky et al., 1983). This makes sense in that a cancer diagnosis is particularly stressful for parents, and they have major responsibilities for managing different aspects of the complicated treatment protocols.

Collectively, these studies suggest that demographic variables of age, gender, and family composition need to be studied further as predictors of adherence. Also, there is a need to assess parent as well as child psychological factors because parental psychological status may be as important or more important than child status in predicting adherence. More studies also are needed to determine if regimen factors, such as complexity and pain associated with treatment, are important predictors of adherence.

## Assessing Adherence

A variety of strategies exists for assessing adherence, including assays, observations, mechanical devices, pill counts, provider estimates, and child/parental reports. Each of these strategies has associated assets and liabilities, including relative costs and feasibility. Some of these strategies are only applicable to certain types of regimens, such as assays to assess medication adherence.[1]

### Drug Assays

Laboratory assays can measure drug levels, metabolic products of drugs, or markers (pharmacologically inert substances or low-dose medications) added to target drugs in bodily fluids, such as serum, urine, and saliva (Roth, 1987). Serum and urine assays have been used as the primary measure of adherence to oral medications for children with cancer and secondarily to corroborate child or parent reports (see Table 8-3).

#### *Assets*

Assays are quantifiable and clinically useful for determining subtherapeutic, therapeutic, and toxic levels of drugs, and they provide information on dose–response relationships (Rand & Wise, 1994). Also, they do not rely on potentially biased or inaccurate reports or estimates provided by children, family members, or providers. Most important, assays confirm that drugs have been ingested. Chemical markers or tracers share these same advantages and can be used with drugs for which there are no standard assays. Ideal markers should be chemically inert, nontoxic, nonradioactive, and undetectable by children (Insull, 1984).

#### *Liabilities*

Assays have some serious limitations. They measure adherence over relatively short time intervals and thus fail to provide information about consistency in medication adherence over extended periods of time. Most assays reflect medication ingestion that has occurred (at best) no further back than five half-lives (Rudd, 1993). Assays can also be expensive and invasive, which makes them less feasible for use in pediatric settings. The timing of assays relative to when the most recent dose was taken can also be a complicating factor. Samples for assays are usually drawn just before the next medication dose (at trough levels), which requires knowledge of when the last dose was taken, which in turn depends on the accuracy of children's reports of when they took their most recent dose (Backes & Schentag, 1991). Laboratory errors can also be made in transporting, analyzing, and reporting results to providers, although these are considered minimal. Low drug levels may not be diagnostic of nonadherence because they may reflect inadequacies in the prescribed regimen or pharmacokinetic variations in the way drugs are absorbed, metabolized, and excreted. Markers share some of the same disadvantages as standard assays in terms of being affected by pharmacokinetic variations. Plus, adding markers to existing drugs may require approval by the Food and Drug Administration as a "new" drug, and children may consume foods that contain markers, such as riboflavin (Rudd, 1993).

### Observation

Direct observation of child adherence is rare (Rapoff & Barnard, 1991). Observation measures, in the form of behavioral checklists, have been used to evaluate children's technique in performing skills necessary for adherence. Behavioral checklists have been developed for assessing blood or urine glucose testing (Epstein, Figueroa, Farkas, & Beck, 1981; Wing, Koeske, New, Lamparski, & Becker, 1986), insulin administration (B. O. Gilbert et al., 1982), factor replacement therapy (Sergis-Davenport & Varni, 1983), and metered dose inhaler use (Boccuti, Celano, Geller, & Phillips, 1996). Conceivably, behavioral checklists could be developed and validated for nonmedication oncology regimen requirements such as central catheter care. These checklists could be used in training and evaluating how well children and parents implement regimen components so that clinicians are assured that they have the necessary knowledge and skills to adhere.

Some studies have utilized parent or sibling observations as a primary data source, with acceptable levels of agreement with independent observers (Lowe & Lutzker, 1979; Rapoff, Lindsley, & Christophersen, 1984). Direct and unobtrusive observations in camp settings have also been used to measure dietary adherence (Lorenz, Christensen, & Pichert, 1985) and to demonstrate concurrent validity of 24-hour recall interviews (Reynolds, Johnson, & Silverstein, 1990).

### *Assets*

Unlike other strategies, observational measures are direct measures of regimen-related behaviors. They are automatically valid in the sense that they measure what they intend to measure (Johnston & Pennypacker, 1993). By directly measuring behavior, observational measures avoid subjective and potentially misleading judgments about behavior inherent in child, family, and provider ratings of adherence. Observational measures also assess important dimensions of adherence behaviors, such as frequency (e.g., how often medications are taken), duration (e.g., the amount of time intravenous medications are infused), and inter-response time (e.g., the schedule or time between medication doses taken). Finally, by focusing on public behaviors, observational measures can also reveal contemporaneous controlling variables (antecedents and consequences) related to adherence that may be amenable to intervention (Mash & Terdal, 1988). But, if observational measures have so much to offer, why are they so infrequently used in medical adherence research and less so in clinical practice?

### *Liabilities*

The major problem with observational measures is accessibility. Clinicians or researchers simply do not have sufficient access to children to measure their behavior in any consistent or representative way. At best, they have limited samples of behavior that may not reflect how children typically behave in relation to prescribed regimens. Also, observational measures can be labor intensive because they require extensive training, monitoring, and recalibration or retraining of observers (Mash & Terdal, 1988).

An oft-cited disadvantage of observational measures is their potential for reactivity (Wildman & Erickson, 1977). That is, when children are under observation, they may behave in ways that are not typical and usually in a socially desired direction (e.g., they may be more adherent). Compared to other assessment strategies, it is conceivable that directly watching someone has the potential of being more reactive than taking a blood sample, electronically monitoring their adherence, or asking them about adherence behaviors. However, reactivity is a potential problem with all measures of adherence. Another type of reactivity is relevant to those conducting observations. When observers are monitored, the quality of their observations may be higher than when they are not monitored (Wildman & Erickson, 1977).

## Microelectronic Monitors

Technological advances in microprocessors have led to the development of automated measures of adherence. Microelectronic monitors are now available to record and store information on the date and time of tablet or liquid medication removal from standard vials, removal of pills from blister packages, actuation of metered-dose inhalers, blood glucose test results, and child diary notations on adherence or other clinical events, such as pain levels (Cramer, 1991; Urquhart, 1994). These monitors can store information in real time for up to several months and can be downloaded into data files for analysis. This is one of the most important developments in adherence measurement, with some even calling electronic monitors the "new gold standard" (Cramer, 1995).

One such device for measuring removal of pills is the Medication Event Monitoring System (MEMS) available from the Aprex Corporation (Menlo Park, CA). The hardware consists of two components, the monitor and the communicator module. The monitor is a cap with self-enclosed electronic circuitry that fits on a standard pill vial. One current version is the MEMS TrackCap (with or without a child-resistant cap), which stores up to 1,800 dose events and has a battery life of approximately 18 months. Another version is the MEMS SmartCap (also available with or without a child-resistant cap), which stores up to 1,500 dose events and also has a battery life of about 18 months; it has two additional features: a visual display showing how many times the vial has been opened each day and how long (in hours) since the vial was last opened and an optional audible signal programmed for when medications are to be taken. The communicator module is attached to a serial port of a computer and allows data from the cap to be downloaded into a software program that reads, displays, and prints out dosing records. Only one study could be located that used the MEMS to monitor adherence to 6-MP in children with ALL (Lau et al., 1998).

*Assets*

Electronic monitors provide a continuous and long-term measure of medication adherence in real time that is not available with any other measure. Monitors can reveal a spectrum of adherence problems, including (a) underdosing (the most common dosing error); (b) overdosing (which can contribute to toxic effects); (c) delayed dosing (dosing that exceeds recommended dosing intervals, which can reduce therapeutic coverage); (d) drug "holidays" (omitting doses for several days in succession without provider authorization); and (e) "white coat" adherence or giving the appearance of adequate adherence by dumping medications or taking medications consistently several days before clinic visits (Urquhart, 1994).

The close monitoring conferred by electronic devices can also help distinguish probable from improbable drug reactions or side effects. For example, a drug reaction reported by a child (such as dizziness) can be correlated in real time by an electronic monitor with inappropriate medication dosing, such as shortened intervals between doses or taking extra doses. Conversely, improbable drug reactions can be revealed if the child reports a side effect when the monitor indicates low adherence (Rudd, 1993).

Monitors may also help identify "actual" drug resistance (low efficacy in spite of high adherence to an adequate dosing regimen) versus "pseudoresistance" caused by delayed or underdosing (Rudd, 1993). Combined with plasma assays, monitors can also help identify within-child variation in plasma concentrations because they provide information about the timing of drug administration (Rubio, Cox, & Weintraub, 1992).

Finally, the detailed information on adherence patterns provided by electronic monitors can be used clinically to provide feedback and counseling to children and their families during brief clinic visits or by telephone (Cramer, 1995).

*Liabilities*

When referring to the capability of electronic monitors, it is more precise to say that they measure "presumptive" dosing. The presupposition here is that children ingest what they dispense. Thus, the major drawback of electronic monitors is that they do not confirm ingestion or proper inhalation of medications and may overestimate actual adherence. Assays are needed to help confirm ingestion (Roth, 1987). Although deliberate falsification can occur if children dispense but fail to ingest medications, this seems highly unlikely because children must do this at the precise time when medications are to be taken (Urquhart, 1994). Thus, the degree of effort needed to falsify adherence would seem to present adherence problems in its own right. Monitors could also underestimate adherence if children take out several doses at once to carry with them when they are away from home or to load pill reminder boxes.

Electronic monitors, like any mechanical device, can malfunction. They may record events that did not occur, fail to record events that did occur, or simply stop working because batteries expire. However, most of these mechanical failures occurred with prototypes (Averbuch, Weintraub, & Pollock, 1990).

The clinical utility or feasibility of monitors is limited by the relatively high costs for the rental or purchasing of monitors, communicators, and proprietary software. There are also practical problems regarding the convenience and portability of the monitors. The pill monitors are somewhat oversize and heavier relative to standard vial caps, which may make them cumbersome, particularly for children on three or four times daily dosing schedules who have to transport them outside the home. Also, to download data from the monitors, they have to be retrieved; in some cases, children have lost the monitors or have not returned them.

Ethical objections can also be made to using electronic monitoring, particularly if children are not informed about the capabilities of monitoring devices. This is particularly critical for children who are not afforded the same degree of legal or ethical protection as adults.

## Pill Counts

Pill counts have a long tradition in adherence assessment and are relatively straightforward. Pills are counted at two points in time, and the initial count is subtracted from the subsequent count to determine how pills have been removed, which is then used to calculate percentage of pills removed relative to the number prescribed.

#### *Assets*

Pill counts are uncomplicated and relatively feasible for use in clinical settings. Their feasibility has been enhanced by obtaining pill counts from children or family members by phone (e.g., Pieper, Rapoff, Purviance, & Lindsley, 1989). Because pill counts have been widely used in research, they also can be used to summarize and compare adherence rates to a wide variety of medication regimens and child samples. Pill counts or measurements can also be used to validate other adherence assessment methods, such as child, parent, or provider estimates.

#### *Liabilities*

Pill counts, like electronic monitors, cannot confirm ingestion. Most often, they overestimate adherence rates, which can occur if children "dump" medications. Medications (particularly antibiotics) may also be shared with other family members. Pill counts also reveal very little about variations in drug administration, such as overdosing, underdosing, drug holidays, and the white coat effect. Sometimes, pill counts are not possible because children do not bring medication containers to clinic visits, even when reminded by telephone calls prior to the visit. Children may also dispense medications from more than one container or load them in pill reminder containers ahead of time, thus precluding an accurate count (Rudd, 1993). Because of converging evidence that pill counts overestimate adherence relative to other methods (such as assays), some have recommended that investigators cease using this as a measure of adherence (Bond & Hussar, 1991).

### Provider Estimates

Provider estimates generally involve global ratings by physicians or nurses of the degree to which children are adherent to a particular regimen. For example, clinicians may rate adherence using a 5-point Likert-type scale, with the end points 4 = almost always (95% of the time) and 0 = rarely (5% or less of the time) (Gudas, Koocher, & Wyplj, 1991). Providers are sometimes asked to make dichotomous judgments (yes or no) about whether children will be adherent.

#### *Assets*

Provider estimates are fast, simple, and inexpensive, which makes them very feasible for use in clinical practice. If providers assess adherence at all, they probably prefer this method. There is some evidence that provider estimates are better than global estimates obtained from children or family members (Rapoff & Christophersen, 1982).

#### *Liabilities*

Provider estimates are not very accurate compared to other measures, such as assays (Rudd, 1993). Furthermore, providers are inaccurate in a specific way. Although they are generally accurate in identifying adherent children, they often fail to identify nonadherent children. This is nicely illustrated in one study in which pediatric providers (nurses, resident and staff pediatricians) were asked to predict which children would be adherent to an antibiotic regimen for otitis media (Finney, Hook, Friman, Rapoff, & Christophersen, 1993). In response to the question, "Do you think this family will administer most of the prescribed medication?" providers' estimates were dichotomized as "will adhere" or "will not adhere." The objective measure of adherence was a pill count/liquid measurement conducted by the investigators in the children's homes on the Days 7–10 of the prescribed regimen, and the criterion for classifying children as nonadherent was less than 80% of medicine removed. In this study, providers' predictions were treated as a diagnostic or screening test (like a laboratory test) and nonadherence as the condition to be diagnosed (like a disease). Viewing the findings this way yielded the following results: The *sensitivity* of provider predictions (the proportion of actually nonadherent children who were predicted to be nonadherent) was quite low (28%); the *specificity* of provider predictions (the proportion of actually adherent children who were predicted to be adherent) was perfect (100%); and the overall *accuracy* of provider predictions (proportion of all predictions, both positive and negative, that were correct) was moderate (65%). These results confirmed previous studies that showed providers fail to identify children who are nonadherent and illustrated that overall accuracy does not capture the type of prediction errors made by providers. Most important, it showed that providers would not identify a fair number of children who could benefit from interventions to improve adherence.

The inaccuracy of predictions or clinical judgment has been well documented in the behavioral science literature. Clinical judgments often are biased and may actually be inferior to actuarial or statistical methods (Dawes, Faust, & Meehl, 1989). A number of clinical biases have been described (see Rock, Bransford, Maisto, & Morey, 1987, for a review). Clinicians may hold on to or become "anchored" to their initial judgments even when faced with new and disconfirmatory evidence (the "anchoring" bias). Clinicians may also base judgments on the apparent correlation of two events (e.g., adherence and child characteristics, like intelligence) when there is no direct correlation, the correlation is less than expected, or the correlation is the opposite of what is expected (the illusory correlation bias). Clinicians may also believe that judgment accuracy increases as they gain more clinical experience (the overconfidence bias). Finally, there is the correspondence bias, which is the generalized tendency for people to attribute others' behavior (but not their own behavior) to unique dispositional determinants (e.g., laziness, stupidity, or lack of motivation), while ignoring important situational determinants (see D. T. Gilbert & Malone, 1995, for an excellent review). All of these biases have the potential of reducing the accuracy of clinical judgments, and experienced clinicians may actually be more vulnerable to their effects (Rock et al., 1987).

The hall of fame catcher Yogi Berra once said, "A guy ought to be very careful in making predictions, especially about the future." As clinicians and researchers, we should acknowledge the monumental task of trying to predict adherence behaviors and try to critically analyze the basis for our predictions.

### Child/Parent Reports

Consistent with the emphasis on history taking in clinical practice, it is not surprising that child or family reports are often used to assess adherence. Reporting formats include global ratings, diaries or self-monitoring of adherence behaviors, and structured interviews.

Global ratings, like provider estimates, require that children or parents rate adherence over unspecified or varying (and sometimes lengthy) time intervals. For example, parents might be asked, "In the last 2 months, was there any time he missed taking his pills for more than 1 day?" (Gordis, Markowitz, & Lilienfeld, 1969). Parents might also be asked to rate their children's adherence on a weekly basis using a Likert-type scale, with 1 = very nonadherent to 5 = very adherent (Rapoff, Purviance, & Lindsley, 1988b).

Diaries or other monitoring formats require children or parents to record specific adherence behaviors over varying lengths of time using standardized forms. Consistent with developments in microelectronic processors, there are now software programs for portable handheld computers that children can use to record adherence events or other clinical parameters, such as pain levels (Dahlström & Eckernäs, 1991). One such software program, the *Experience Sampling Program*, was developed by Dr. Lisa Feldman Barrett at Boston College with funding from the National Science Foundation and can be downloaded at no cost (see Web site at http://www.experience-sampling.org/esp/). This program is flexible and can be individualized for particular studies or children to record answers to preprogrammed questions, store these answers, and upload data to a computer.

Significant progress has been made in the development of structured interviews for assessing adherence. An excellent example of this progress is the extension and validation of the 24-hour recall interview (a standard dietary assessment technique), which has been refined and extended to assess adherence to insulin-dependent diabetes mellitus regimens by Suzanne Bennett Johnson and colleagues (see Johnson, 1995, for a review). This method involves assessing and quantifying adherence to 13 standard components of regimens for insulin-dependent diabetes mellitus. Interviews are conducted separately with children and parents over the phone. They report the day's events in temporal sequence, from the time the child awakens in the morning until retiring to bed, but the interviewer records only diabetes-related activities. To ensure representativeness, three separate interviews are conducted over a 2-week interval, on two weekdays and one weekend day. Interviews are restricted to the previous 24 hours to minimize recall errors. Each interview takes about 20 minutes to complete (Freund, Johnson, Silverstein, & Thomas, 1991). Each of the 13 adherence measures is constructed to yield a range of scores, with higher scores indicating relative nonadherence and scores close to zero indicating relative adherence. For example, glucose testing frequency is calculated based on an ideal frequency of four times per day for a total possible frequency of 12 over the three interview days. The number of glucose testings reported is divided by the ideal and multiplied by 100 (e.g., $4 \div 12 \times 100 = 33$). This product is then subtracted from 100 (e.g., $100 - 33 = 67$), so that high scores indicate few glucose tests and low scores indicate frequent tests (e.g., a score of 67 indicates the child reported four glucose tests conducted over 3 days).

A similar structured interview format for assessing diabetes-related adherence, the Self-Care Adherence Inventory, has been reported by Cindy Hanson and colleagues (Hanson et al., 1996). In addition, a semistructured interview, the Family Asthma Management System Scale (FAMSS), has been developed for use with parents of children with asthma (Klinnert, McQuaid, & Gavin, 1997). The FAMSS assesses a variety of family-centered asthma management constructs, including adherence to medications and environmental control recommendations.

Tebbi et al. (1986) used a 49-item interview format to question children with cancer and their parents about medication adherence, knowledge of medications, understanding of the treatment regimen, treatment side effects, responsibilities for treatment adherence, and beliefs about the efficacy of treatment. They operationalized nonadherence as the number of times children or parents admitted having missed taking a medication dose during the preceding month, with nonadherers defined as those who reported missing one or more doses.

Kennard et al. (2004) found that the average score of a two-item adherence self-report measure completed by 44 adolescents with cancer positively and significantly correlated with a serum assay measure (Spearman's $\rho = .34$, $p < .03$). The two items were as follows: In the last month how many times did you forget to take a dose of medication within 1 hour of the scheduled time, but did not miss the dose? In the last month how many times did you miss a dose of medication completely? Responses were rated on a Likert scale with 0 = never, 1 = once or twice, 2 = 3 or 4 times, 3 = 5 to 10 times, and 4 = more than 10 times (pp. 33–34). Interestingly, the parent version was not significantly correlated with the assay measure.

### Assets

In general, child or proxy (such as parents) reports are relatively simple, convenient, inexpensive, and clinically feasible (Bond & Hussar, 1991). They also address the problem of accessibility to child behaviors over time and in ecologically relevant contexts (e.g., home and community).

How children or family members are questioned about adherence may be critical in the quality of data obtained by reports. Questions that are nonjudgmental, specific, and time limited are likely to yield more accurate information about adherence because they are less likely to generate evasive and defensive reactions and are less subject to recall errors or misunderstanding (Kaplan & Simon, 1990; Klinnert et al., 1997).

Diary and structured interviews offer additional advantages of providing detailed information on adherence patterns and the types of problems or obstacles encountered and can be correlated with disease symptoms or outcomes. They can also be integrated into disease management programs, which facilitate child and family involvement in health care (Rand & Wise, 1994). Computerized diary or interview methods can also facilitate the disclosing of more sensitive information, such as adherence to safe sex practices.

Structured interviews may be the best of the child or family report measures because they are less labor intensive for children and families and more comprehensive. Plus, the 24-hour recall interview, by Johnson and colleagues, has shown adequate stability, parent-child agreement, factor structure, agreement with independent observations of behavior, and predictive validity (Johnson, 1995). Similarly, adequate reliability and validity data have been reported for the Self-Care Adherence Inventory (Hanson et al., 1996) and the FAMSS (Klinnert et al., 1997).

### Liabilities

Child or family reports tend to overestimate adherence, most notably by minimizing doses that have been missed. This is likely to be truer of global estimates and diaries as compared to structured interviews. Global estimates can also tax the person's memory for adherence events. Unless they are actively rehearsed, memories fade within a short period of time. The "outer limits" of recall for events are generally 1 to 2 weeks (Rand, 2000; Rudd, 1993). Also, people tend to remember unique events (ones that are stimulating or emotionally laden) and remember events in chronological order for up to 10 days and thereafter in relation to other major events, such as holidays and birthdays. Diary methods can obviate the need for remembering events if children complete them close in time to the behavior monitored. However, about 50% of children keep complete records (Johnson, 1993). Even if diaries are complete, one cannot ascertain when and where they were completed.

Report measures are also sensitive to demand or social desirability effects. That is, children or families may tell providers what they want to hear, which could lead to overestimates or outright deception about adherence (Johnson, 1993). In this way, the child or family "protects" their relationship with the provider or at least avoids disapproval (Rand, 2000).

Proxy informants (such as parents) do not always have access to relevant behaviors, especially during adolescence. For example, only about 50% of diabetes-related activities are observed by parents (Johnson, 1995). Obviously, parents can only report on what they see.

Structured interview methods appear to be the most promising of all the child and family report measures. Parents and children are interviewed separately to obtain more representative samples of adherence behaviors, and psychometric data on reliability and validity seem to meet minimal standards. However, further work is needed to corroborate interview methods by more direct measures such as observations, assays, or electronic monitoring.

## Comparative Performance of Adherence Measures

Compared to the adult literature, there are relatively few studies that have directly compared adherence measures with children. The oldest comparative study in the pediatric literature was reported almost 30 years ago by Gordis et al. (1969). The study compared children's and mothers' reports of adherence to penicillin prophylaxis for rheumatic fever with urine assays obtained during clinic visits at least every 2 months for a 6-month period. Children were classified as compliers if they or their mother reported on at least 75% of the visits that medication had been taken on the day they were reporting. By urine assay, children were classified as compliers if at least 75% or more of urine specimens were positive for penicillin, as noncompliers if no more than 25% of specimens were positive, and as intermediate compliers if 26%–74% of specimens were positive. Using these criteria, 69%–73% of the samples were classified as compliers by child/parental report, in contrast to 33%–42% by urine assays. The major conclusion of this study was that child or parental reports of adherence are "grossly inaccurate."

Smyth and Judd (1993) compared parent reports with urine assays to assess adherence to antibiotic prophylaxis for children with urinary tract infections. Although 97% of parents reported their children took antibiotics every day, only 69% of urine assays were positive. Another study on adherence to antibiotics for otitis media found significant correlations among parent interviews, parent diaries, volume measurements, and urine assays. However, correlations between urine assays and the other adherence measures were not significant for an antihistamine-decongestant medication (Devries & Hoekelman, 1988).

Electronic monitors are becoming the gold standard for adherence measurement (Riekert & Rand, 2002). We located a total of eight studies that have compared electronic monitors to child or parental reports, pill counts, or assays. Five of these studies (Bender, Milgrom, Rand, & Ackerson, 1998; Bender et al., 2000; Gibson, Ferguson, Aitchison, & Paton, 1995; Milgrom et al., 1996; Olivieri, Matsui, Hermann, & Koren, 1991) found that child or parental reports yielded higher adherence rates compared to electronic monitors, with an average difference of 30% (range = 7%–63.4%). Two of these studies (Olivieri et al., 1991; Starr et al., 1999) found that pill counts yielded higher adherence rates compared to electronic monitors, with an average difference of 16% (range = 7%–25%). One study found that a urine assay yielded a 13% higher adherence rate compared to electronic monitoring, 79% by assay versus 66% by electronic monitoring (Starr et al., 1999).

Collectively, these studies and previous reviews of the literature suggest that assays or electronic monitors are superior measures of medication adherence compared to child, parental, or provider reports and pill counts (Bond & Hussar, 1991;

Rand & Wise, 1994; Rapoff & Barnard, 1991; Riekert & Rand, 2002; Rudd, 1993). Electronic monitors have yielded the lowest adherence rates of all measures, which may indicate they have greater sensitivity. However, there is no error-free way to assess adherence. In practice, clinicians will often have to rely on child or parent report to identify those families who can benefit from an intervention to enhance adherence.

## Treatment of Nonadherence in Pediatric Cancer

Given that children with cancer face complicated regimens and difficulties with adherence, it is surprising how little intervention research has been conducted to improve adherence rates in these children. For this chapter an extensive search of Medline and PsycINFO yielded not a single intervention study designed to improve adherence among children with cancer to any portion of their medical regimen. Therefore, this section focuses on strategies for improving adherence based on research with children who have other chronic illnesses (see Table 8-4).

### Tracking

The first step in any adherence intervention program should involve monitoring the child's adherence to each of the various components of their medical regimen. It is possible, for example, that a child may be highly adherent to pill taking but poorly adherent to activity restrictions. Tracking should take place prior to any intervention so that strategies can be directly targeted to each child's area of need.

Informing children and families that their adherence will be tracked and providing them with feedback can lead to significant improvements in adherence. For example, Eney and Goldstein (1976) informed half of their families that drug ingestion was being monitored and made a note of discussing adherence with these children; the other half of the families were treated according to typical protocol. This simple intervention improved adherence rates to therapeutic levels for 42% of families in the treatment group, while only 11% of children in the control group reached therapeutic drug levels. In a similar study, Dawson and Jamieson (1971) improved therapeutic blood levels from 25% to 80% among children over a 6-month period simply by informing children and parents that blood levels would be assessed monthly and subsequently providing them feedback on the blood levels.

### Education

Any child prescribed a medication should be informed of the reason for taking the medication and the risks associated with nonadherence. However, in the medical care of children with cancer, this message may only be provided to parents or, given the complex nature of their regimens, children and families may misunderstand it.

For these reasons, studies have been conducted to assess the effects of education on improving adherence. In a multiple-baseline, single-subject study, Lowe and Lutzker (1979) found that education alone significantly improved dietary adherence in a child with diabetes. Because parents are a key part of children's medical care, education intervention studies can be conducted solely with parents. For example, Sergis-Davenport and Varni (1983) educated parents on the medical care of their child in four to eight 2-hour visits and found skill improvement from 15% at baseline to 92% at follow-up. These data indicate that it is vital that the medical team communicate thoroughly and effectively with children and families and periodically assess their knowledge of the medical regimen and the effects of nonadherence.

### Regimen Simplification

Medical regimens for children with cancer are often extremely complicated. They typically include medications, avoidance of others with acute illness, and dietary changes at the very least. Because regimens for chronic childhood diseases can be complicated, studies have focused on simplifying medical regimens for other chronic diseases to improve adherence. For example, in one study a short-acting medication was changed to sustained-release medication, cutting the number of pills each child had to take by 50% (Tinkelman, Vanderpool, Carroll, Page, & Spangler, 1980). This simple regimen change significantly increased adherence. In a similar single-subject study, simplifying a child's regimen from four times daily to

**Table 8-4.** Adherence Intervention Studies Targeting Chronic Disease Regimens in Pediatrics

| *Reference* | *Sample/Disease* | *Regimen/Measure* | *Procedures* | *Outcome* |
|---|---|---|---|---|
| da Costa et al., 1997 | *N* = 2 (8 and 10 years old)/Asthma | Inhaled corticosteroids/ Electronic monitor | Withdrawal design. Following baseline, patients given education and token system intervention, followed by withdrawal of intervention. | Education and token system improved adherence and withdrawal, and reinstatement of token system for one patient demonstrated effectiveness of the token system. Some improvements in pulmonary function for one patient. |
| Eney & Goldstein, 1976 | *N* = 90 (3–16 years old)/Asthma | Theophylline/Serum/salivary assays | Random selection but not assignment to two groups: Group 1 had no specific intervention; Group 2 patients informed that drug ingestion was being monitored, and physicians were more "directive" in discussing adherence. | 11% of patients in Group 1 had therapeutic drug levels versus 42% in Group 2. |
| N. A. Smith et al., 1986 | *N* = 196 (5–16 years old)/Asthma | Medications/Parent and physician ratings | Pretest, posttest control group design. Intervention group received educational and behavioral strategies (written information, tailoring of regimen, and increased monitoring. | Significantly higher adherence for the intervention group (78%) versus the control group (55%). |
| N. A. Smith et al., 1994 | *N* = 53 (5–15 years)/Asthma | Medications/Investigator ratings | One group, pretest/posttest design. Baseline followed by educational and behavioral strategies (written information, tailoring of regimen, and increased monitoring. | Significant increase in adherence from pre- (73%) to postassessment (83%). Significant improvement in asthma severity and pulmonary function. |
| Tinkelman et al., 1980 | *N* = 20 (11–18 years)/Asthma | Theophylline/Serum assay and pill counts | Random assignment to short-acting (every 6 hours) or sustained-release (every 12 hours) theophylline. Dosing instructions given for both preparations. | Significantly higher adherence with sustained-release versus short-acting theophylline by pill counts. No significant difference in serum levels. |

| | | | | |
|---|---|---|---|---|
| Gordis & Markowitz, 1971 | $N = 17$/Cardiac (rheumatic fever or heart disease) | Prophylactic penicillin/ Urine assay | Random assignment to two groups: continuous care (same physician, increased accessibility, and comprehensive care) and specialty care (different physicians seen and treated only for rheumatic fever) | No significant differences between groups on adherence. |
| Stark et al., 2003 | $N = 7$ (6–12 years old)/Cystic fibrosis | Caloric intake recorded by daily diet diaries completed by parents/ Weight using a digital scale | Families randomized to behavioral (BI) or nutrition education (NE) conditions, both involving six group sessions (parents and children in separate groups for both conditions). BI condition involved nutrition information plus child behavior management strategies for parents and reward program for children. NE condition involved nutrition education only. | Children in the BI condition had greater increase in daily caloric intake (1,036 calories/ day) and weight gain (1.42 kilograms) than those in NE condition (408 calories/day, 0.78 kilograms). |
| Carney et al., 1983 | $N = 3$ (10–14 years old)/Diabetes | Blood glucose testing; patient records and used testing strips/Ghb levels | Multiple baseline across subjects; baseline followed by point system exchanged for money and special activities. | All 3 patients showed improvement in percentage of tests performed, with 2 patients improving from <5% in baseline to 87% and 93% after treatment. Gains were maintained at 4-months follow-up. Ghb levels improved from baseline (10.1%, 15.2%, and 9.1%) to follow-up (9.4%, 11.7%, and 6.0%). |
| Epstein et al., 1981 | $N = 17$ (6–16 years)/Diabetes | Urine glucose testing/Direct observation | Random assignment to practice condition (patients tested 20 prepared samples but not informed of results) or feedback condition (patients tested samples and given feedback about accuracy). | Mean number of correct urine glucose estimations were significantly higher for feedback (7.2) versus practice (3.8) conditions posttraining. |

*(continued)*

**Table 8-4.** *(continued)*

| *Reference* | *Sample/Disease* | *Regimen/Measure* | *Procedures* | *Outcome* |
|---|---|---|---|---|
| B. O. Gilbert et al., 1982 | *N* = 28 (6–9 years old)/Diabetes | Insulin injections/Direct observations (observers rating pass/fail on 27 items related to insulin injection) | Random assignment to treatment or control group; treatment group shown peer-modeling film depicting successful self-injection; control group shown nutrition film. | Older girls who viewed peer-modeling film showed greater self-injection skill compared to older girls who viewed the control film. |
| Gross, 1983 | *N* = 4 (10–12 years)/ Diabetes | Urine testing/Patient report (with parent counts of used test tablets as a reliability check) (overall agreement averaged 80%) | Multiple baseline across subjects; following baseline, patients received self-management training and developed a behavioral contract with parents. | Frequency of urine testing improved for all patients; mean percentage of days urine testing was done four times per day increased from 9% during baseline to 74% during self-management condition; at 2- and 4-week follow-ups, frequency of testing dropped for 2 of 4 patients. |
| Gross et al., 1985 | *N* = 14 (9–13 years)/ Diabetes | Diet, glucose testing, and insulin injections/Parental report | Random assignment to control or experimental group (included multiple-baseline design). Self-management training (negotiating, contracting, etc.). | Improvements noted in specific adherence behaviors for experimental group patients. No difference in metabolic control between groups. |
| Lowe & Lutzker, 1979 | *N* = 1 (9 years)/ Diabetes | Urine testing, diet, and foot care/ Direct observation by parent and sibling | Multiple baseline across behaviors. Education and token system. | Education effective in improving dietary adherence; token system increased adherence to urine testing (from baseline mean of 16% to 97%) and foot care (from baseline mean of 72% to 100%). |
| Satin et al., 1989 | *N* = 32 (mean age = 14.6 years)/Diabetes | Insulin use; urine glucose testing; diet; exercise/Parental ratings of self-care (1 = very careful to 5 = careless); Ghb levels; attitudes toward teenage with diabetes scales; Family Environment Scale | Random assignment to one of three groups: Group 1 patients and parents met for six weekly sessions to discuss diabetes and management; Group 2 identical to Group 1 plus a parent simulation of diabetes regimen; Group 3 was control group. | No significant differences between groups in self-care ratings. Significant decrease in Ghb levels at 6 weeks post-intervention for Group 2 versus Group 3. Significant difference in attitudes toward teenager with diabetes (more positive) for Groups 1 and 2. |

| | | | | |
|---|---|---|---|---|
| Schafer et al., 1982 | $N = 3$ (16–18 years)/ Diabetes | Urine glucose testing; insulin use; exercise; wearing diabetic information bracelet; blood glucose testing/Assessed by patient self-monitoring records | Multiple-baseline across-behaviors design with baseline followed by goal setting and (if needed) contingency contracting conditions. | Goal setting alone effective in improving adherence to wearing information, exercise, and urine testing for Subject 1 and for urine testing and exercise for Subject 2; goal setting plus contracting improved adherence to insulin use for Subject 2; nothing effective for Subject 3, who was experiencing severe family problems. |
| Silverman, Hains, Davies, & Parton, 2003 | $N = 6$ (11–19 years)/ Diabetes | Insulin; blood glucose testing; diet; exercise/24-hour recall interviews; glucose monitor | Multiple baseline across subjects. Baseline followed by cognitive behavioral treatment (including self-monitoring, cognitive restructuring, and problem solving) delivered individually in the home. | Of 6 subjects, 5 showed improvements in at least one self-care behavior. |
| Snyder, 1987 | $N = 1$ (14 years)/ Diabetes | Insulin use; urine glucose testing; diet/Patient self-monitoring records with independent checks by mother and school nurse | Quasi-experimental single-subject design. Following self-monitoring baseline, patient exposed to self-monitoring plus monetary incentives and then to an additional condition involving hospitalization contingent on hypo- or hyperglycemic episodes for 36 hours in a private room with no TV and the like, visitors, books, and minimal staff interaction. Behavioral contacting and communication/ conflict resolution training were also implemented for antisocial behavior and mother-child conflict. | Mean number of diabetes self-care activities performed was 5.6 during self-monitoring baseline, 6.3 during self-monitoring + reinforcement, and 8.5 during self-monitoring + reinforcement + punishment; 1-month follow-up showed maintenance of gains. Deterioration of gains at 6 months posttreatment; patient hospitalized for drug abuse. |

*(continued)*

**Table 8-4.** *(continued)*

| *Reference* | *Sample/Disease* | *Regimen/Measure* | *Procedures* | *Outcome* |
|---|---|---|---|---|
| Wysocki et al., 1989 | $N = 42$ (mean age = 14 years)/ Diabetes | Blood glucose testing; insulin use; diet; exercise/Automated recording of blood glucose (reflectance meters); 24-hour recall patient and parent interviews; Ghb levels; attitudes toward diabetes and diabetes adjustment scales | 30 patients randomly assigned to meter-alone (MA) or meter-plus-contract (MC) groups. Remaining 12 patients in conventional therapy (CT) control group. MA group patients earned money for bringing meters to clinic. MC group patients earned money contingent on glucose testing frequency. | By eighth week, MC group had significantly higher frequency of glucose testing. No differences in overall adherence, Ghb levels, or patient/parent attitudes and adjustment to diabetes. |
| Wysocki et al., 2000 | $N = 119$ (mean age = 14 years)/ Diabetes | Insulin; blood glucose testing; diet; exercise/24-hour recall interviews; Self-Care Inventory | Adolescents and parents randomized to behavioral family systems therapy (BFST) for 10 sessions that focused on problem solving, communication skills, cognitive restructuring, and the like; education and support (ES) for 10 sessions that emphasized diabetes education and social support; or current therapy (CT), which involved standard medical care only. | At 3 months posttreatment, there were no significant differences between groups on measures of adherence. There were significant improvements in parent-adolescent relations and decreased diabetes-specific conflict favoring the BFST group. |
| A. Gilbert & Varni, 1988 | $N = 1$ (10 years old)/Hemophilia | Factor replacement therapy/ Observation of patient completing factor replacement using a behavior checklist | Case study with baseline, treatment, and 4.5-month follow-up measures obtained; following baseline, nurse modeled correct performance of factor replacement skills, had patient rehearse skills, gave corrective feedback as needed, and praised for correct performance. | Mean adherence to proper technique ranged from 0% to 89% across factor replacement behavioral categories during baseline; this range improved to 83%–98% during treatment and 100% during follow-up. |

| | | | | |
|---|---|---|---|---|
| Greenan-Fowler et al., 1987 | $N = 10$ (8–15 years old)/Hemophilia | Home physical therapy program/Patient report (written records) and attendance at exercise class | One group, repeated-measures quasi-experimental design; following baseline, patients and parents were exposed to behavior management training (shaping, token system, etc.) for 12 weeks; follow-up assessments were done at 3, 6, and 9 months posttreatment. | Adherence to exercises significantly higher during treatment (mean = 96%), 3-month (mean = 91%), and 6-month (mean = 85%) follow-up compared to baseline (mean = 55%) but not at 9-month follow-up (mean = 63%); session attendance did not vary significantly between measurement periods. |
| Sergis-Davenport & Varni, 1983 | $N = 12$ parents of 10 children with hemophilia | Factor replacement therapy/Direct observation using a behavioral checklist | Nonrandom assignment to treatment or control group; parents in treatment group were given systematic training in factor replacement therapy in 2-hour weekly visits over a 4- to 8-week period; control group parents did not receive special training. | Mean percentage of correct performance in factor replacement skills increased significantly from 15% at baseline to 92% during intervention for treatment group parents; percentages significantly higher for treatment versus control group at follow-up. |
| Rapoff et al., 1984 | $N = 1$ (7 years old)/Juvenile rheumatoid arthritis | Medications, splints, and prone-lying exercise/Parent observations with interobserver reliability checks in home (mean agreement = 94% for medications and 100% for splints and prone lying) | Multiple baseline across behaviors with 10-week follow-up; token system introduced following baseline. | Baseline mean adherence was 59% for medications, 0% for splints and prone-lying exercise; improved to 95%, 77%, and 71%, respectively, during treatment and 90%, 91% and 80%, respectively, at 10-week follow-up. |
| Rapoff et al., 1988a | $N = 1$ (14 years old)/Juvenile rheumatoid arthritis | Medications/Pill counts; disease activity measures | Single-subject withdrawal design. Following baseline, regimen simplified (four times daily to three times daily); token system in the home for 10 weeks, then withdrawn for 7 weeks, reinstated for 7 weeks, and then maintenance phase for 8 weeks (with token system reintroduced if adherence was < 80% for 2 consecutive weeks). Token system then completely withdrawn. | Mean adherence levels by condition were as follows: baseline = 44%; simplified regimen = 59%; token system = 100%; withdrawal of token system = 77%; token system reinstated = 99%; maintenance phase = 92%; and 9-month follow-up = 97%. Less disease activity evident during simplified regimen and token system phases. |

(*continued*)

**Table 8-4.** *(continued)*

| *Reference* | *Sample/Disease* | *Regimen/Measure* | *Procedures* | *Outcome* |
|---|---|---|---|---|
| Rapoff et al., 1988b | $N=3$ (3, 10, and 13 years old)/Juvenile rheumatoid arthritis | Medication/Pill counts and adherence ratings on a 5-point scale (1 = very nonadherent to 5 = very adherent) from parents by phone on a weekly basis | Multiple baseline across subjects; following baseline, home visit made to provide verbal and written information on medications, importance of adherence, monitoring, and positive reinforcement; parents asked to mail completed monitoring forms on a weekly basis; 4-month follow-up. | Mean adherence by pill counts for Patients 1, 2, and 3, respectively, at baseline = 44%, 38%, and 54%; during intervention = 49%, 97%, and 92%; at follow-up = 24%, 56%, and 89%. Mean parental adherence ratings for Patients 1, 2, and 3, respectively, at baseline = 2.4, 3.4, and 3.3; during intervention = 2.2, 5, and 4.1; at follow-up = 3, 3.5, and 4.8. |
| Rapoff, Belmont, Lindsley, Olson, & Padur, 2002 | $N=34$ (mean age = 8.44 years)/ Juvenile rheumatoid arthritis (diagnosed within 1 year of study entry) | Medications/Electronic monitor | Randomized controlled trial. Subjects randomized to nurse-administered control group education intervention (received information on juvenile rheumatoid arthritis and medical treatments) or educational plus behavioral intervention (received information on juvenile rheumatoid arthritis plus strategies for enhancing adherence). Both interventions introduced during a single 30-minute clinic visit followed by phone contacts with nurse every 2 weeks for 2 months and monthly for 10 months. | Significantly higher adherence for the educational-plus-behavioral intervention group (mean = 77.7%) versus control group (mean = 56.9%) over 52-week follow-up. No significant differences between groups on disease activity or functional limitations. |
| Pieper et al., 1989 | $N=3$ (11–18 years old)/Rheumatic diseases | Medications/Pill counts | Multiple baseline across subjects. Following baseline, patients and parents given instructions in clinic about medications, adherence, and monitoring/ reinforcement strategies. | Because over- as well as underdosing occurred, patients were classified as adherent if pill counts indicated 80–120% of doses were taken. The mean percentages of pill counts in acceptable range were as follows: baseline = 38%, 7%, and 33%; intervention = 89%, 67%, and 88%; 6-month follow-up = 100% for all patients; and 12-month follow-up = 67% for 2 patients. |

| | | | | |
|---|---|---|---|---|
| Beck et al., 1980 | $N = 21$ (3–20 years old; mean = 14.6 years)/ Renal failure | Immunosuppressive drugs, posttransplant/Pill counts | One-group, pretest/posttest design. Baseline assessment followed by 6 months of physician counseling and regimen simplification when feasible. | Initially, 9 of 21 were nonadherent (43%); 4 of these 9 remained nonadherent, and 5 were adherent after 6 months of physician counseling. |
| Carton & Schweitzer, 1996 | $N = 1$ (10-year-old male)/Renal disease | Hemodialysis/Direct observation | ABAB single-subject design. Baseline followed by token system, which was withdrawn, reinstated, and faded. | Nonadherence to hemodialysis reduced with token system and worsened when the token system was withdrawn; nonadherence remained low at 3- and 6-month follow-up. |
| Magrab & Papadopoulou, 1977 | $N = 4$/Renal failure | Dietary regimen/Weight, blood, and urine tests (nitrogen and potassium levels) | Reversal design. Baseline and token system conditions. | Weight gain acceptable during treatment versus baseline. Some improvements in nitrogen and potassium levels for 2 children. |
| Dawson & Jamieson, 1971 | $N = 30$ (6 months to 12 years old)/Seizure disorder | Medications/Blood assays over a 6-month period | One group pre- and posttest quasi-experimental design; after initial blood levels were obtained, patients were monitored monthly by assays with parental and patient knowledge. | At the beginning of the study, only 25% of sample had therapeutic blood levels; this increased to 80% by the end of study. |

Adapted from M. A. Rapoff, 1999, *Adherence to pediatric medical regimens*, New York: Kluwer/Plenum, Table 6.2, pp. 133–140.

three times daily improved adherence rates from 44% to 59% (Rapoff, Purviance, & Lindsley, 1988a). Beck et al. (1980) added 6-months of physician counseling to regimen simplification. Their results indicated that 9 of 21 families were nonadherent at baseline, while only 4 remained nonadherent after the intervention. These data suggest that the medical team should review all aspects of the child's care to determine if any aspect of the regimen can be simplified or removed because decreasing the burden on children may significantly improve adherence.

## Behavioral Strategies

Of the 31 intervention studies included in this chapter (see Table 8-4), most included some behavioral component. To identify the behavioral components that were most effective, they are discussed under four categories: modeling, token systems, goal setting, and parent simulation.

### *Modeling*

Modeling involves exposing someone to another person that effectively engages in a desired behavior. Modeling is useful in a medical setting for novel or complicated behaviors, such as administering injections or testing urine or blood. In the treatment of cancer, modeling would be a valuable tool for teaching children to lie still during a bone marrow procedure or radiation therapy or how to use mouthwash for stomatitis properly.

Modeling has been used in previous pediatric adherence studies. For example, Epstein et al. (1981) used modeling to teach children with diabetes to test their urine properly. Results revealed that children who were given modeling plus feedback on their own performance significantly improved their skill and accuracy. B. O. Gilbert et al. (1982) showed children a film of peers correctly completing a successful insulin injection for diabetes. Results indicated that children who received the peer modeling demonstrated greater skill after viewing the film. Another study also has been conducted using nurses as models. The team nurse modeled correct performance of factor replacement skills for children with hemophilia, along with giving children feedback on their performance. This simple intervention led to 100% adherence to all aspects of factor replacement therapy at 4.5 months posttreatment. Thus, adherence interventions in pediatric cancer would likely benefit from the inclusion of modeling and performance feedback for the difficult and novel components of the medical regimen.

### *Token Systems*

Based on the studies reviewed for the current chapter, token systems are probably the most common behavioral component of adherence interventions. Typically, token systems involve a child receiving a token (or point) for properly completing some portion of their medical care. In cancer, this could involve a child receiving tokens for taking pills, engaging in proper central catheter care, or following dietary recommendations. These token systems can be difficult to implement because they require parent training, vigilance on the part of the family, and consistent implementation over time to be effective. In fact, they may not be recommended for families who are overwhelmed with their current medical situation, disorganized, or overextended in general.

Research indicated that when properly implemented, token systems can significantly increase adherence. Of the eight studies reviewed for this chapter that used a token system as part of their intervention, all demonstrated improvements in adherence (Carney, Schechter, & Davis, 1983; Carton & Schweitzer, 1996; da Costa, Rapoff, Lemanek, & Goldstein, 1997; Greenan-Fowler, Powell, & Varni, 1987; Lowe & Lutzker, 1979; Magrab & Papadopoulou, 1997; Rapoff et al., 1984; Snyder, 1987). Token systems can improve adherence when education alone has failed (Lowe & Lutzker, 1979). Also, token systems allow the team to target improvement across a variety of specific behaviors, such as home physical therapy, attendance at exercise class for children with hemophilia (Greenan-Fowler et al., 1987), or medications, splints, and prone-lying exercises for children with juvenile rheumatoid arthritis (Rapoff et al., 1984). It is difficult to state the duration of implementation required to receive therapeutic effect, but 8–10 weeks seems to be adequate for most children (Rapoff et al., 1988a).

Because token systems can be complicated for families, the medical team needs to teach families how to implement a token system properly and regularly consult with them (at least weekly during the first month) to answer questions and monitor their progress. The family must also sustain the token system program on a daily basis for approximately 8–10 weeks to receive maximum benefit. Given their complexity, token systems may be reserved for children who continue to have adherence problems after trying simpler interventions like modeling and for teams with a pediatric psychologist or another well-trained team member who may assist parents to implement such a program.

### *Goal Setting*

An important behavioral component of many adherence interventions involve having children and families set realistic treatment goals. Sometimes, these studies have children set goals with their parents (Gross, 1983; Gross, Magalnick, & Richardson, 1985; Snyder, 1987) and sometimes with members of the medical team (Schafer, Glasgow, & McCaul, 1982). In an interesting study using goal setting and contracting, Wysocki, Green, and Huxtable (1989) rewarded children with diabetes monetarily for testing their blood glucose levels and contracted with them ahead of time regarding the frequency of blood glucose monitoring. This led to significant improvements in child adherence.

### *Parent Simulation*

A novel component of some adherence intervention studies involves parents simulating all of the components of their child's medical regimen for a specified period of time. Satin, La Greca, Zigo, and Skyler (1989) had parents implement all components of their diabetic child's medical regimen for 6 weeks, including injections, blood glucose measurements, diet, and exercise. Results revealed that not only did parent attitudes toward their children become more positive but also children's adherence rates improved.

## Summary of Adherence Promotion Strategies

Most adherence interventions combine several of the aforementioned components (Pieper et al., 1989; Rapoff et al., 1988b; N. A. Smith, Seale, Ley, Shaw, & Braes, 1986; Smith, Seale, Ley, Mellis, & Shaw, 1994), and it is difficult to discern from previous research exactly which components are sufficient to increase adherence rates to acceptable levels. Given that some families maintain acceptable adherence rates with current standard care practices and others do not, an individualized approach seems indicated.

As part of this individualized approach to care, adherence should be tracked on an ongoing basis with all children who enter treatment for pediatric cancer. Ideally, this tracking should be completed on all aspects of the medical regimen (diet, pill taking, etc.) at regular intervals. For those individuals with low initial adherence rates or adherence rates that decrease over time, tracking should be followed by intensive education in case the lack of information is the cause of the poor adherence. As part of this consultation with the medical care team, regimen simplification options should also be considered.

Research indicated, however, that even with regular tracking, education, and regimen simplification, there will still be children who have significant difficulties with adherence. For these children, a more in-depth intervention will be necessary, including modeling, behavioral training of the parent and child, assistance with implementation of a behavioral program at home, and possible parent simulation of child treatment. A pediatric psychologist who is part of the medical care team would ideally implement these more complex interventions. However, some pediatric cancer centers may not have pediatric psychologists as part of their medical care team and will need to refer families to a pediatric psychologist in their area who is well versed in pediatric cancer treatment and can regularly assist children with adherence.

## Future Directions for Treatment Adherence in Pediatric Oncology

What is most evident from this review is that there is a dearth of studies, in general, investigating adherence to regimens for children with cancer. This is surprising given the life-threatening nature of childhood cancer. The following are suggestions for advancing the field of medical treatment adherence in pediatric oncology.

### Assessment Strategies

Reliable, valid, and clinically feasible strategies for assessing adherence are necessary to identify those in need of intervention and to document the effects of adherence promotion efforts. For research purposes, electronic monitoring plus periodic and noninvasive drug assays would be ideal (Rapoff,

1999). Electronic monitors offer the advantage of real-time assessments of adherence-related events over time, and assays are the only way to confirm short-term ingestion of medications.

Clinically, electronic monitoring and assays are not routinely available or particularly cost-effective. This may change, but in the interim clinicians must rely on child or parent report to assess adherence. As noted by Rand (2000), self-report of adherence can be enhanced by (a) directly evaluating adherence behaviors in an information-intensive way (by asking, "Which medications are you taking? What doses? How often? Have you had any adverse side-effects?"); (b) probing for nonadherence in a nonjudgmental and nonthreatening manner ("Many people have trouble remembering to take their medication. Do you ever forget to take yours?"); (c) limiting the time frame for questioning about adherence to the previous 7–10 days; and (d) asking families about personal, financial, social, and cultural barriers to adherence.

### Theoretical Models and Predictors of Adherence

The current and limited literature on predictors of adherence to medical regimens for childhood cancer lack a theoretical basis. There are a number of adherence theories that have been adapted and partially validated for pediatric chronic diseases, including the health belief model and self-efficacy theory, which might be applicable to pediatric oncology regimens (Rapoff, 1999). Longitudinal studies would be particularly useful to identify predictors of adherence across different phases of treatment (induction, consolidation, and maintenance). Examining predictors that are potentially modifiable, such as regimen complexity, would be most useful in guiding efforts to enhance adherence.

### Enhancing Adherence

We were somewhat surprised that not a single published study has reported on efforts to enhance adherence to regimens for childhood cancer. As with other chronic pediatric diseases, a three-tier approach to minimizing the potentially deleterious effects of nonadherence might be useful: primary, secondary, and tertiary prevention (Rapoff, 2000; Rapoff, McGrath, & Lindsley, 2003). Primary prevention efforts would be most relevant for those children who have not yet exhibited clinically significant nonadherence (inconsistencies in following a particular regimen that may result in compromised health and well-being), possibly those recently diagnosed or those who are able to sustain adequate adherence over phases of treatment. Interventions at this level might involve educational (e.g., stressing the importance of adherence), organizational (e.g., simplifying regimens), and relatively simple behavioral strategies (e.g., monitoring of regimen adherence by providers or parents).

Secondary prevention might be most applicable to those children for whom clinically significant nonadherence has been identified early in the treatment process or has yet to compromise their health and well-being. Interventions at this level might include more frequent monitoring of regimen adherence by parents and children, specific and consistent positive social reinforcement for adherence, and general discipline strategies (e.g., time-out for younger children). Pediatric psychologists could train primary health care providers, particularly nurses, to implement primary- and secondary-level interventions.

Tertiary prevention efforts would apply to children with an ongoing pattern of clinically significant nonadherence. Strategies at this level might include more complex interventions such as token system programs, contingency contracting, self-management training (e.g., problem solving to anticipate and manage obstacles to adherence), and possibly psychotherapy. Because of the demanding and technical nature of these strategies, pediatric psychologists would be responsible for implementing strategies at this level.

Implementing and evaluating primary, secondary, and tertiary prevention approaches to medical nonadherence depends on a number of factors. First, prevention efforts require a valid, reliable, and clinically feasible way to detect or assess nonadherence. Although no such "ideal" measure exists, 24-hour recall interviews (in clinics or by phone) may be the best option in that they have been shown to be reliable, valid, and feasible for routine and serial assessments of adherence to regimens for diabetes and cystic fibrosis and could be easily be adapted for pediatric oncology regimens (Rapoff, 1999). Second, information obtained from routine and serial assessments of adherence should also allow for the detection of clinically significant nonadherence. Previous attempts at determining levels of adherence necessary to prevent deleterious health outcomes have been arbitrary and not biologically based (e.g., adequate adherence defined as consuming 80% of prescribed medication doses). Third, because the desired outcome of adherence interventions is that children get better, feel better, and do better, there is a need for both traditional (e.g., clinical signs and symptoms) and quality-of-life measures of disease and health status that are valid, reliable, and clinically feasible (Rapoff, 1999). Finally, because childhood cancers affect relatively few children and adolescents, empirical validation of primary, secondary, and tertiary prevention interventions will require multicenter collaborative research studies.

The significant advances in the treatment of childhood cancers over the past several decades have been greatly aided by multicenter collaborative treatment studies sponsored by the National Cancer Institute. Pediatric psychologists need this type of intensive and collaborative effort on adherence promotion to make certain that children and their families benefit from these medical advances in cancer treatment.

## Note

1. This section was adapted from Rapoff (1999, chapter 3).

## References


Averbuch, M., Weintraub, M., & Pollock, D. J. (1990). Compliance assessment in clinical trials. *Journal of Clinical Research and Pharmacoepidemiology, 4*, 199–204.

Backes, J. M., & Schentag, J. J. (1991). Partial compliance as a source of variance in pharmacokinetics and therapeutic drug monitoring. In J. A. C. B. Spilker (Ed.), *Patient compliance in medical practice and clinical trials* (pp. 27–36). New York: Raven Press.

Beck, D. E., Fennell, R. S., Yost, R. L., Robinson, J. D., Geary, D., & Richards, G. A. (1980). Evaluation of an educational program on compliance with medication regimens in pediatric patients with renal transplants. *The Journal of Pediatrics, 96*, 1094–1097.

Bender, B., Milgrom, H., Rand, C., & Ackerson, L. (1998). Psychological factors associated with medication nonadherence in asthmatic children. *Journal of Asthma, 35*, 347–353.

Bender, B., Wamboldt, F. S., O'Connor, S. L., Rand, C., Szefler, S., Milgrom, H., et al. (2000). Measurement of children's asthma medication adherence by self report, mother report, canister weight, and Doser CT. *Annals of Allergy, Asthma, and Immunology, 85*, 416–421.

Berde, C. B., Billett, A. L., & Collins, J. J. (2002). Symptom management in supportive care. In P. A. Pizzo & D. G. Poplack (Eds.), *Principles and practice of pediatric oncology* (4th ed., pp. 1301–1332). Philadelphia: Lippincott, Williams and Wilkins.

Boccuti, L., Celano, M., Geller, R. J., & Phillips, K. M. (1996). Development of a scale to measure children's metered-dose inhaler and spacer technique. *Annals of Allergy, Asthma, and Immunology, 77*, 217–221.

Bond, W. S., & Hussar, D. A. (1991). Detection methods and strategies for improving medication compliance. *American Journal of Hospital Pharmacy, 48*, 1978–1988.

Carney, R. M., Schechter, K., & Davis, T. (1983). Improving adherence to blood glucose testing in insulin-dependent diabetic children. *Behavior Therapy, 14*, 247–254.

Carton, J. S., & Schweitzer, J. B. (1996). Use of a token economy to increase compliance during hemodialysis. *Journal of Applied Behavior Analysis, 28*, 111–113.

Chemlik, F., & Doughty, A. (1994). Objective measurement of compliance in asthma treatment. *Annals of Allergy, 73*, 527–532.

Cramer, J. A. (1991). Overview of methods to measure and enhance patient compliance. In J. A. Cramer & B. Spiker (Eds.), *Patient compliance in medical practice and clinical trials* (pp. 3–10). New York: Raven Press.

Cramer, J. A. (1995). Microelectronic systems for monitoring and enhancing patient compliance with medication regimens. *Drugs, 49*, 321–327.

da Costa, I. G., Rapoff, M. A., Lemanek, K., & Goldstein, G. L. (1997). Improving adherence to medication regimens for children with asthma and its effect on clinical outcome. *Journal of Applied Behavior Analysis, 30*, 687–691.

Dahlström, B., & Eckernäs, S. A. (1991). Patient computers to enhance compliance with completing questionnaires: A challenge for the 1990s. In J. A. Cramer & B. Spiker (Eds.), *Patient compliance in medical practice and clinical trials* (pp. 233–240). New York: Raven Press.

Dawes, R. M., Faust, D., & Meehl, P. E. (1989). Clinical versus actuarial judgement. *Science, 243*, 1668–1674.

Dawson, K. P., & Jamieson, A. (1971). Value of blood phenytoin estimation in management of childhood epilepsy. *Archives of Disease in Childhood, 46*, 386–388.

Devries, J. M., & Hoekelman, R. A. (1988). Comparison of four methods of assessing compliance with a medication regimen: Parent interview, medication diary, unused medication measurement, and urinary drug excretion. *American Journal of Diseases In Children, 142*, 396.

Eney, R. D., & Goldstein, E. O. (1976). Compliance of chronic asthmatics with oral administration of theophylline as measured by serum and salivary levels. *Pediatrics, 57*, 513–517.

Epstein, L. H., Figueroa, J., Farkas, G. M., & Beck, S. (1981). The short-term effects of feedback on accuracy of urine glucose determinations in insulin dependent diabetic children. *Behavior Therapy, 12*, 560–564.

Festa, R. S., Tamaroff, M. H., Chasalow, F., & Lanzkowsky, P. (1992). Therapeutic adherence to oral medication regimens by adolescents with cancer. I. Laboratory assessment. *Journal of Pediatrics, 120*, 807–811.

Finney, J. W., Hook, R. J., Friman, P. C., Rapoff, M. A., & Christophersen, E. R. (1993). The overestimation of adherence to pediatric medical regimens. *Children's Health Care, 22*, 297–304.

Freund, A., Johnson, S. B., Silverstein, J., & Thomas, J. (1991). Assessing daily management of childhood diabetes using the 24-hour recall interviews: Reliability and stability. *Health Psychology, 10*, 200–208.

Gibson, N. A., Ferguson, A. E., Aitchison, T. C., & Paton, J. Y. (1995). Compliance with inhaled asthma medication in preschool children. *Thorax, 50*, 1274–1279.

Gilbert, A., & Varni, J. W. (1988). Behavioral treatment for improving adherence to factor replacement therapy by children with hemophilia. *The Journal of Compliance in Health Care, 3*, 67–76.

Gilbert, B. O., Johnson, S. B., Spillar, R., McCallum, M., Silverstein, J. H., & Rosenbloom, A. (1982). The effects of a peer-modeling film on children learning to self-inject insulin. *Behavior Therapy, 13*, 186–193.

Gilbert, D. T., & Malone, P. S. (1995). The correspondence bias. *Psychological Bulletin, 117*, 21–38.

Golub, T. R., & Arceci, R. J. (2002). Acute myelogenous leukemia. In P. A. Pizzo & D. G. Poplack (Eds.), *Principles and practice of pediatric oncology* (4th ed., pp. 545–590). Philadelphia: Lippincott, Williams, and Wilkins.

Gordis, L., & Markowitz, M. (1971). Evaluation of the effectiveness of comprehensive and continuous pediatric care. *Pediatrics, 48*, 766–776.

Gordis, L., Markowitz, M., & Lilienfeld, A. M. (1969). The inaccuracy in using interviews to estimate patient reliability in taking medications at home. *Medical Care, 7*, 49–54.

Greenan-Fowler, E., Powell, C., & Varni, J. W. (1987). Behavioral treatment of adherence to therapeutic exercise by children with hemophilia. *Archives of Physical Medicine and Rehabilitation, 68*, 846–849.

Gross, A. M. (1983). Self-management training and medication compliance in children with diabetes. *Child and Family Behavior Therapy, 4*, 47–55.

Gross, A. M., Magalnick, L. J., & Richardson, P. (1985). Self-management training with families of insulin-dependent diabetic children: A controlled long-term investigation. *Child and Family Behavior Therapy, 7*, 35–50.

Gudas, L. J., Koocher, G. P., & Wyplj, D. (1991). Perceptions of medical compliance in children and adolescents with cystic fibrosis. *Developmental and Behavioral Pediatrics, 12*, 236–247.

Hanson, C. L., DeGuire, M. J., Schinkel, A. M., Kolterman, O. G., Goodman, J. P., & Buckingham, B. A. (1996). Self-care behaviors in insulin-dependent diabetes: Evaluative tools and their associations with glycemic control. *Journal of Pediatric Psychology, 21*, 467–482.

Insull, W. (1984). Statement of the problem and pharmacological and clinical requirements for the ideal marker. *Controlled Clinical Trials, 5*, 459–462.

Johnson, S. B. (1993). Chronic diseases of childhood: Assessing compliance with complex medical regimens. In M. A. Krasnegor, L. Epstein, S. B. Johnson, & S. J. Yaffe (Eds.), *Developmental aspects of health compliance behavior* (pp. 15–184). Hillsdale, NJ: Erlbaum.

Johnson, S. B. (1995). Managing insulin-dependent diabetes mellitus in adolescence: A developmental perspective. In J. L. Wallander & L. J. Siegel (Eds.), *Adolescent health problems: Behavioral perspectives* (pp. 265–288). New York: Guilford.

Johnston, J. M., & Pennypacker, H. S. (1993). *Strategies and tactics of behavioral research* (2nd ed.). Hillsdale, NJ: Erlbaum.

Kaplan, R. M., & Simon, H. J. (1990). Compliance in medical care: Reconsiderations of self-predictions. *Annals of Behavioral Medicine, 12*, 66–71.

Kennard, B. D., Stewart, S. M., Olvera, R., Bawdon, R. E., O hAilin, A., Lewis, C. P., et al. (2004). Nonadherence in adolescent oncology patients: Preliminary data on psychological risk factors and relationships to outcome. *Journal of Clinical Psychology in Medical Setting, 11*, 31–39.

Klinnert, M. D., McQuaid, E. L., & Gavin, L. A. (1997). Assessing the family asthma management system. *Journal of Asthma, 34*, 77–88.

Kovacs, M., Goldston, D., Obrosky, D. S., & Iyengar, S. (1992). Prevalence and predictors of pervasive noncompliance with medical treatment among youths with insulin-dependent diabetes mellitus. *Journal of the American Academy of Child and Adolescent Psychiatry, 31*, 1112–1119.

Lancaster, D., Lennard, L., & Lilleyman, J. S. (1997). Profile of non-compliance in lymphoblastic leukaemia. *Archives of Disease in Childhood, 76*, 365–366.

Lansky, S. B., Smith, S. D., Cairns, N. U., & Cairns, G. F. (1983). Psychological correlates of compliance. *The American Journal of Pediatric Hematology/Oncology, 5*, 87–92.

Lanzkowsky, P. (2000). *Manual of pediatric hematology and oncology* (3rd ed.). San Diego, CA: Academic Press.

Lau, R. C. W., Matsui, D., Greenberg, M., & Koren, G. (1998). Electronic measurement of compliance with mercaptopurine in pediatric patients with acute lymphoblastic leukemia. *Medical and Pediatric Oncology, 30*, 85–90.

Lorenz, R. A., Christensen, N. K., & Pichert, J. W. (1985). Diet-related knowledge, skill, and adherence among children with insulin-dependent diabetes mellitus. *Pediatrics, 75*, 872–876.

Lowe, K., & Lutzker, J. R. (1979). Increasing compliance to a medical regimen with a juvenile diabetic. *Behavior Therapy, 10*, 57–64.

Magrab, P. R., & Papadapoulou, Z. L. (1977). The effect of a token economy on dietary compliance for children on hemodialysis. *Journal of Applied Behavior Analysis, 10*, 573–578.

Margolin, J. F., Steuber, C. P., & Poplack, D. G. (2002). Acute lymphoblastic leukemia. In P. A. Pizzo & D. G. Poplack (Eds.), *Principles and practice of pediatric oncology* (4th ed., pp. 489–544). Philadelphia: Lippincott, Williams, and Wilkins.

Mash, E. J., & Terdal, L. G. (1988). Behavioral assessment of child and family disturbance. In E. J. Mash & L. G. Terdal (Eds.), *Behavioral assessment of childhood disorders* (2nd ed., pp. 3–65). New York: Guilford.

Milgrom, H., Bender, B., Ackerson, L., Bowry, P., Smith, B., & Rand, C. (1996). Noncompliance and treatment failure in children with asthma. *Journal of Allergy and Clinical Immunology, 98*, 1051–1057.

O'Donnell, M. R. (2003). The NCCN acute myeloid leukemia clinical practice guidelines in oncology. *Journal of the National Comprehensive Cancer Network, 1*, 52–539.

Olivieri, N. F., Matsui, D., Hermann, C., & Koren, G. (1991). Compliance assessed by the Medication Event Monitoring System. *Archives of Disease in Childhood, 66*, 1399–1402.

O'Reilly, R., Pui, C. H., Kernan, N., Sallan, S., Sanders, J., Steinherz, P., et al. (1996). NCCN pediatric acute lymphoblastic leukemia practice guidelines. The National Comprehensive Cancer Network. *Oncology, 10*, 1787–1794.

Patridge, A. H., Avorn, J., Wang, P. S., & Winer, E. P. (2002). Adherence to therapy with oral antineoplastic agents. *Journal of the National Cancer Institute, 94*, 652–661.

Phipps, S., & DeCuir-Whalley, S. (1990). Adherence issues in pediatric bone marrow transplantation. *Journal of Pediatric Psychology, 15*, 459–475.

Pieper, K. B., Rapoff, M. A., Purviance, M. R., & Lindsley, C. B. (1989). Improving compliance with prednisone therapy in pediatric patients with rheumatic disease. *Arthritis Care and Research, 2*, 132–135.

Rand, C. S. (2000). "I took the medicine like you told me, doctor": Self-report of adherence with medical regimens. In A. A. Stone, J. S. Turkkan, C. A. Bachrach, J. B. Jobe, H. S. Kurtzman, & V. S. Cain (Eds.), *The science of self-report: Implications for research and practice* (pp. 257–276). Mahwah, NJ: Erlbaum.

Rand, C. S., & Wise, R. A. (1994). Measuring adherence to asthma medication regimens. *American Journal of Critical Care Medicine, 149*, 569–576.

Rapoff, M.A. (2000). Facilitating adherence to medical regimens for pediatric rheumatic diseases: primary, secondary, and tertiary prevention. IN D. Drotar (ED.) *Promoting Adherence to Medical Treatment in Childhood Chronic Illness: Concepts, Methods, and Interventions* (pp. 329–345). Mahwah, N.J.: Lawrence Erlbaum Associates.

Rapoff, M. A. (1998). Adherence issues among adolescents with chronic diseases. In S. A. Shumaker, E. Schron, J. Ockene, & W. L. McBee (Eds.), *Handbook of health behavior change* (2nd ed., pp. 377–408). New York: Springer.

Rapoff, M. A. (1999). *Adherence to pediatric medical regimens*. New York: Kluwer/Plenum.

Rapoff, M. A., & Barnard, M. U. (1991). Compliance with pediatric medical regimens. In J. A. Cramer & B. Spilker (Eds.), *Patient compliance in medical practice and clinical trials* (pp. 73–98). New York: Raven Press.

Rapoff, M. A., Belmont, J., Lindsley, C. B., Olson, N. Y., & Padur, J. (2002). Prevention of nonadherence to non-steroidal anti-inflammatory medications for newly diagnosed patients with juvenile rheumatoid arthritis. *Health Psychology, 21*, 620–623.

Rapoff, M. A., & Christophersen, E. R. (1982). Compliance of pediatric patients with medical regimens: A review and evaluation. In R. B. Stuart

(Ed.), *Adherence, compliance, and generalization in behavioral medicine* (pp. 79–124). New York: Brunner/Mazel.

Rapoff, M. A., Lindsley, C. B., & Christophersen, E. R. (1984). Improving compliance with medical regimens: Case study with juvenile rheumatoid arthritis. *Archives of Physical Medicine and Rehabilitation, 65*, 267–269.

Rapoff, M. A., McGrath, A. M., & Lindsley, C. B. (2003). Medical and psychosocial aspects of juvenile rheumatoid arthritis. In M. C. Roberts (Ed.), *Handbook of pediatric psychology* (3rd ed., pp. 392–408). New York: Guilford.

Rapoff, M. A., Purviance, M. R., & Lindsley, C. B. (1988a). Educational and behavioral strategies for improving medication compliance in juvenile rheumatoid arthritis. *Archives of Physical Medicine and Rehabilitation. 69*, 439–441.

Rapoff, M. A., Purviance, M. R., & Lindsley, C. B. (1988b). Improving medication compliance for juvenile rheumatoid arthritis and its effect on clinical outcome: A single-subject analysis. *Arthritis Care and Research, 1*, 12–16.

Reynolds, L. A., Johnson, S. B., & Silverstein, J. (1990). Assessing daily diabetes management by 24-hour recall interview: The validity of children's reports. *Journal of Pediatric Psychology, 15*, 493–509.

Riekert, K. A., & Rand, C. S. (2002). Electronic monitoring of medication adherence: When is high-tech best? *Journal of Clinical Psychology in Medical Settings, 9*, 25–34.

Ries, L. A. G., Smith, M. A., Gurney, J. G., Linet, M., Tamara, T., Young, J. L., et al. (Eds.). (1999). *Cancer incidence and survival among children and adolescent: United States SEER Program 1975–1995*. (NIH Publication No. 99-4649). Bethesda, MD: National Cancer Institute, SEER Program.

Rock, D. L., Bransford, J. D., Maisto, S. A., & Morey, L. (1987). The study of clinical judgement: An ecological approach. *Clinical Psychology Review, 7*, 645–661.

Roth, H. P. (1987). Current perspectives: Ten year update on patient compliance research. *Patient Education and Counseling, 10*, 107–116.

Rubio, A., Cox, C., & Weintraub, M. (1992). Prediction of diltiazem plasma concentration curves from limited measurements using compliance data. *Clinical Pharmacokinetics, 22*, 238–246.

Rudd, P. (1993). The measurement of compliance: Medication taking. In M. A. Krasnegor, L. Epstein, S. B. Johnson, & S. J. Yaffe (Eds.), *Developmental aspects of health compliance behavior* (pp. 185–213). Hillsdale, NJ: Erlbaum.

Satin, W., La Greca, A. M., Zigo, M. A., & Skyler, J. S. (1989). Diabetes in adolescence: Effects of multifamily group intervention and parent simulation of diabetes. *Journal of Pediatric Psychology, 14*, 259–275.

Schafer, L. C., Glasgow, R. E., & McCaul, K. D. (1982). Increasing the adherence of diabetic adolescents. *Journal of Behavioral Medicine, 5*, 353–362.

Sergis-Davenport, E., & Varni, J. W. (1983). Behavioral assessment and management of adherence to factor replacement therapy in hemophilia. *Journal of Pediatric Psychology, 8*, 367–377.

Silverman, A., Hains, A. A., Davies, W. H., & Parton, E. (2003). A cognitive behavioral adherence intervention for adolescents with Type 1 diabetes. *Journal of Clinical Psychology in Medical Settings, 10*, 119–127.

Smith, N. A., Seale, J. P., Ley, P., Mellis, C. M., & Shaw, J. (1994). Better medication compliance is associated with improved control of childhood asthma. *Monaldi Archive of Chest Disease, 49*, 470–474.

Smith, N. A., Seale, J. P., Ley, P., Shaw, J., & Braes, P. U. (1986). Effects of intervention on medication compliance in children with asthma. *The Medical Journal of Australia, 144*, 119–122.

Smith, S. D., Rosen, D., Trueworthy, R. C., & Lowman, J. T. (1979). A reliable method for evaluating drug compliance in children with cancer. *Cancer, 43*, 169–173.

Smyth, A. R., & Judd, B. A. (1993). Compliance with antibiotic prophylaxis in urinary tract infection. *Archives of Diseases of Children, 38*, 235–236.

Snyder, J. (1987). Behavioral analysis and treatment of poor diabetic self-care and antisocial behavior: A single-subject experimental study. *Behavior Therapy, 18*, 251–263.

Stark, L. J., Opipari, L. C., Spieth, L. E., Jelalian, E., Quittner, A. L., Higgins, L., et al. (2003). Contribution of behavior therapy to diet treatment in cystic fibrosis: A randomized controlled study with 2-year follow-up. *Behavior Therapy, 34*, 237–258.

Starr, M., Sawyer, S. M., Carlin, J. B., Powell, C. V. E., Newman, R. G., & Johnson, P. D. R. (1999). A novel approach to monitoring adherence to preventive therapy for tuberculosis in adolescence. *Journal of Paediatric Child Health, 35*, 350–354.

Tamaroff, M. H., Festa, R. S., Adesman, A. R., & Walco, G. A. (1992). Therapeutic adherence to oral medication regimens by adolescents with cancer. II. Clinical and psychological correlates. *Journal of Pediatrics, 120*, 812–817.

Tebbi, C. K., Cumings, K. M., Kevon, M. A., Smith, L., Richards, M., & Mallon, J. (1986). Compliance of pediatric and adolescent cancer patients. *Cancer, 58*, 1179–1184.

Tinkelman, D. G., Vanderpool, G. E., Carroll, M. S., Page, E. G., & Spangler, D. L. (1980). Compliance differences following administration of theophylline at 6- and 12-hour intervals. *Annals of Allergy, 44*, 283–286.

Urquhart, J. (1994). Role of patient compliance in clinical pharmacokinetics: A review of recent research. *Clinical Pharmacokinetics, 27*, 202–215.

Wildman, B. G., & Erickson, M. T. (1977). Methodological problems in behavioral observation. In J. D. Cone & R. P. Hawkins (Eds.), *Behavioral assessment: New directions in clinical psychology* (pp. 255–273). New York: Brunner/ Mazel.

Wing, R. R., Koeske, R., New, A., Lamparski, D., & Becker, D. (1986). Behavioral skills in self-monitoring of blood glucose: Relationship to accuracy. *Diabetes Care, 9*, 330–333.

Wysocki, T., Green, L., & Huxtable, K. (1989). Blood glucose monitoring by diabetic adolescents: Compliance and metabolic control. *Health Psychology, 8*, 267–284.

Wysocki, T., Harris, M. A., Greco, P., Bubb, J., Danda, C. E., Harvey, L. M., et al. (2000). Randomized, controlled trial of behavior therapy for families of adolescents with insulin-dependent diabetes mellitus. *Journal of Pediatric Psychology, 25*, 23–33.

Rachel B. Levi

# Quality of Life in Childhood Cancer

## Meaning, Methods, and Missing Pieces

### Brief History of Quality-of-Life Assessment in Childhood Cancer

It is only in the last three decades that the quality of the lives of children and adolescents treated for cancer and their families has become a major focus in the field of pediatric oncology. This shift from helping families to tolerate arduous treatments and prepare for early death is a result of advances in treatment and survival rates for most pediatric disease categories. One result of this paradigm shift is that quality of life (QOL) has become a critical construct within the field of pediatric oncology.

### Development of the Quality-of-Life Construct

The construct of QOL was initially developed for use with adult populations and was based on the definition of health generated in 1948 by the World Health Organization (WHO): "a state of complete physical, mental, and social well being, and not merely the absence of disease or infirmity." Although there remains no universally adopted definition of QOL, the WHO's definition of QOL as an "individual's perceptions of their position in life in the context of the culture and value system in which they live and in relation to their goals, standards, and concerns" is frequently employed (WHO, 1993). This definition includes several domains that are considered central to the QOL construct: physical, mental/emotional, and social.

This initial construct has been expanded with adult populations to include physical symptoms and functioning, functional status (i.e., ability to participate in daily and life activities), psychological functioning, and social functioning (e.g., Ware, 1984). This more expansive definition is referred to as health-related quality of life (HRQOL). HRQOL emphasizes the impact of health on one's QOL but looks further to include other domains of life functioning that are also potentially affected by health/illness states (Jenney, 1998).

The HRQOL construct was initially developed for populations of adults living with chronic illness to assess the impacts of illness/injury/disability, medical treatment, or health care policy on an individual's life quality (for reviews, see Aaronson et al., 1991; Patrick & Erikson, 1993; Speith & Harris, 1996). Over time, there have been modifications and developments in the construct, approaches to measurement, and the measures themselves (Wilson & Cleary, 1994).

## Early Applications of the Health-Related Quality-of-Life Construct With Children and Adolescents

Multiple techniques have historically been incorporated to evaluate the functioning of children and adolescents with cancer (i.e., interviews, surveys, measures, symptom checklists). Attention to the HRQOL of children undergoing treatment for cancer first began in the 1980s (e.g., Heyn et al., 1986).[1] An investigation conducted by Bradlyn, Harris, and Speith in 1995 indicated that approximately 3% of the 70 published Phase III clinical trials from the Pediatric Oncology Group and Children's Cancer Group included data on QOL compared to 75% of the studies that included data on treatment toxicity. Although there have not been parallel studies since 1995, Bradlyn (2004) cited anecdotal reports and the Children Oncology Group's constitution, reflecting increased acknowledgment of the importance and increased inclusion of HRQOL measures into clinical trials of pediatric cancer treatments.

Many potential uses and applications of HRQOL assessment with individuals who have experienced childhood cancer have been highlighted, including evaluation of the anticipated and actual impacts of a treatment on a child's HRQOL, contribution of data to decision making and resource allocation for families of and children who are facing the end of their physical lives, and understanding the quality of the lives of children and adolescents whose lives have been impacted by childhood cancer (Eiser & Morse, 2001a; Wolfe, Friebert, & Hilden, 2002). The purpose of this chapter is to review the current state of the HRQOL construct and HRQOL assessment in pediatric oncology and to identify directions for future attention and research.

## Health-Related Quality of Life in Childhood Cancer Populations

A principle underlying the HRQOL construct is that children's perceptions of cancer and their experience with cancer are important (Eiser, 1995). The importance of such assessment is increasingly accepted in the field of pediatric oncology. There remain multiple complexities and challenges related to HRQOL assessment of individuals whose lives are impacted by childhood cancer.

## Overview of Theoretical Frameworks Guiding Health-Related Quality-of-Life Definitions

HRQOL focuses on the lived experience of childhood cancer and is consistent with a biopsychosocial model of functioning that highlights the multiple influences on a child's functioning (e.g., biological, psychological, social, familial, community, spiritual, etc.) (Bronfenbrenner, 1979; Engel, 1977). At the core of pediatric HRQOL is meaning: the meaning of cancer and its impacts on the life of a child and the child's family (Hinds et al., 2004). Acknowledgment that the meaning of the illness is separate from the disease state/experience is grounded in theory, illuminating distinctions between a disease state and the experience of living with an illness (for example, Kleinman, 1988). It has been suggested that HRQOL is an attempt to translate an individual's experience living with cancer into a format that can be used to inform care and to evaluate pediatric cancer treatments (Levi & Drotar, 1998).

It is important to note that HRQOL is a construct that aims to capture something real (life experience). It is a concept that has been developed to guide scholars working to understand how children and adolescents with cancer experience their lives. However, HRQOL has no physical or temporal basis (Wallander, 1992; Wallander, Schmitt, & Koot, 2001).

Both adult and pediatric HRQOL assessments have received criticism because of the absence of theoretical frameworks that guide the development of definitions and measures of pediatric HRQOL (Haase & Braden, 1998; Hinds et al., 2004; Levi & Drotar, 1998). Defining quality is a daunting task at best. It is difficult to measure something that is subjective, individual, and fluid (Fitzpatrick, 2000; Jenney & Levitt, 2002). Although some aspects of quality may be quantifiable, the field will benefit from acknowledging that one is inherently limited in the ability to quantify quality in the true sense (Lantos, 1998; Wallander et al., 2001). This issue is important to consider regarding definition of HRQOL in pediatric oncology populations.

## Overview of Current Definitions of Child Health-Related Quality of Life

The concept of HRQOL is organized around several principles that expand on the WHO definition of health (1948). First, child HRQOL is individual and unique and is influenced by both past and present lifestyle as well as hope, expectations, and goals. Second, child HRQOL includes multiple domains. Third, both objective and subjective aspects of each of these domains can be included in definitions and assessments of child HRQOL (Eiser & Morse, 2001). Although it remains widely accepted that HRQOL is comprised of multiple domains, there remains variability in the domains that are included in definitions and approaches to measurement of HRQOL in pediatric oncology.

### Definitions of HRQOL in Pediatric Oncology

There is no universally agreed on definition of HRQOL in pediatric oncology. Bradlyn et al. (1996) integrated a variety of QOL definitions to offer the following definition of QOL for children with cancer:

> It includes, but is not limited to, the social, physical, and emotional functioning of the child and adolescent, and when indicated, his/her family. Measurement of QOL must be from the perspective of the child, adolescent and family, and it must be sensitive to the changes that occur throughout development.
> (p. 1333–1334)

Definitions are operationalized in several ways and focus on different aspects of child/adolescent functioning.

#### *Functional Status*

Some measures use functional status as an index of HRQOL. These measures focus on the impact that an illness exerts on a child's ability to function across a variety of domains and roles. A prime example is the Play Performance Scale for Children (Lansky, List, Lansky, Ritter-Sterr, & Miller, 1987), one of the first HRQOL measures developed specifically for children with cancer. The Play Performance Scale for Children measures the functional changes experienced by children with cancer by assessing play activities.

#### *Generic Measures*

*Comprehensive Health Status.* Generic HRQOL measures aim to comprehensively assess health status typically assess a broad range of domains, such as functional status, morbidity, social functioning, psychological functioning, and, on some occasions, family functioning. They are used with broad populations of children (i.e., healthy and ill) and enable comparisons between children with cancer and healthy children or children with other illnesses. An example is the Children's Health Questionnaire (CHQ), a measure with comparable parent, child, and adolescent forms, that assesses 14 domains (Landgraf, Abetz, & Ware, 1996) and has been used internationally (e.g., Sawyer, Antoniou, G., Toogood, I., & Rice, 1999). Such measures provide a total score and scores across each domain assessed.

*Preferences/Utility-Based Measures.* These multiattribute HRQOL measures focus on a child's satisfaction with his or her health across a variety of domains. Scores are referred to as utility scores and focus on a child's satisfaction with, or preference for, various health states.

The most widely used utility-based measures in pediatric oncology are of the Health Utilities Index System Mark 2 (HUI2) (Feeny et al., 1992). The HUI2 asks respondents to rate their preferences regarding seven domains of health functioning across three to five levels of functioning. The HUI3 (Feeny, Furlong, & Barr, 1998) is another version of a generic preference/utility measure of HRQOL of children with cancer. These "preferences" allow children to identify scores for a variety of health states that reflect HRQOL on a continuum. The reports across attributes are combined to a single score.

*Disease-Specific Measures.* Disease-specific HRQOL measures are developed to obtain specific information about a child's functioning that is specific to cancer and its treatment. These measures aim to be sensitive to changes in health/functioning related to treatment and/or disease sequelae (Patrick & Erickson, 1993). Disease-specific measures are generally not comprehensive and, unlike generic HRQOL measures, do not obtain data that can be compared to children who are healthy or with other chronic conditions. An example of a disease-specific measure is the Pediatric Oncology Quality of Life Scale (Goodwin, Boggs, & Graham-Pole, 1994).

*Modular Measures.* Modular HRQOL measures incorporate elements of both generic and disease-specific scales. They include a core group of questions that are relevant to all patients and then include specific modules designed for specific groups (Nathan, Furlong, & Barr, 2004). Such measures were developed in response to recommendations to incorporate both generic and disease-specific HRQOL measures to obtain the most comprehensive assessment of the HRQOL of a child with cancer. The most widely used modular scale is the Pediatric Quality of Life Inventory, which contains modules for children with cancer (cancer, fatigue, and specific age groups) (Varni, Burwinkle, Katz, Meeske, & Dickinson, 2002).

*Qualitative Approaches.* Methods that aim to understand the nature of the individual's experience with cancer (phenomenological) via open-ended interviews, the experiences of a group of individuals with cancer (focus groups), semi-structured interviews, and profiles of instruments devised from qualitative methodologies (e.g., simultaneous concept analysis, thematic analysis) are a few examples of qualitative methods used to obtain more meaning-based data about individual experiences with childhood cancer (Haase, Heiney, Ruccione, & Stutzer, 1999; Hinds et al., 2004).

### Domains Commonly Included in Health-Related Quality-of-Life Measures for Children With Cancer

The domains of disease state, physical symptoms, functional status, and psychological and social functioning are frequently represented in measures of HRQOL in pediatric oncology (Ware, 1984; WHO, 1993). In a review of the main domains included in available measures of HRQOL of children with cancer, physical health is assessed in each of the nine measures. Social and psychological functioning are also included in the majority of the reviewed measures, and cognitive functioning and treatment-related impacts are included in fewer than half of the reviewed measures (Eiser, 2004). Other domains that some, but not all, measures of pediatric HRQOL include are adjustment to illness, perception of health, general behavior/behavior problems, pain/comfort, self-care, mobility or activity, and impact on family life/parents (Feeny et al., 1992; Landgraf et al., 1996; Starfield et al., 1993; Varni et al., 2002).

## Current Uses of Health-Related Quality-of-Life Assessment in Pediatric Oncology

Early attempts to evaluate the impact of cancer on a child's life and functioning used measures of anxiety, depression, and physical symptoms (Eiser, 2004). The current status of HRQOL measurement in pediatric oncology reflects considerable progress. HRQOL measures are currently used in clinical trials and have contributed data on two types of questions that are explored in clinical trials: (a) evaluative questions, which explore, for example, how has a child's HRQOL changed as a result of disease/treatment and (b) discriminative questions, which explore questions such as which group reports better HRQOL during or following treatment? (Bradlyn, 2004).

Another sign of progress is that a number of instruments with acceptable psychometric properties are now available for use with pediatric oncology populations are reviews of such measures (e.g., Eiser & Morse, 2001b; Levi & Drotar, 1998; Speith & Harris, 1996). Acceptable measures that reflect a variety of theoretical/conceptual orientations are now available. Investigators have declared a "moratorium" on further measure development and have recommended that research efforts focus on gathering data on the performance of available measures (Feeny, Barr, Furlong, Hudson, & Mulhern, 1999). However, a great deal remains to be determined regarding the methodological characteristics of such measures in general and as applied to groups (i.e., of children from other countries, disease types) (Bradlyn, 2004).

## Critical Considerations in Health-Related Quality-of-Life Assessment in Pediatric Oncology

### Developmental Considerations

Developmental changes are most concentrated and accentuated during childhood and adolescence

(Kamphuis, 1987). Approximately one third of children with cancer are younger than 5 years old at the time of initial diagnosis (Margolin, Steuber, & Poplack, 2002), a phase of development characterized by rapid development and change. For this and several other reasons, assessment of the HRQOL of this segment of the pediatric oncology population has been referred to as a "moving target" (Rosenbaum, Cadman, & Kirpalani, 1990). Several key developmental factors that are relevant in HRQOL assessment are described next.

### *Cognitive Ability*

HRQOL measures must take into account children's cognitive abilities across age and treatment status because of variability in children's ability to self-report. A child's comprehension of the questions asked and the accuracy of their responses are critical considerations.

Another critical factor for consideration in HRQOL measurement with children is time: Their perceptions of time and ability to understand time frames vary across development (Wallander et al., 2001). Many HRQOL measures (e.g., Children's Health Questionnaire; Landgraf et al., 1996) ask children to rate their functioning across varying time periods (e.g., 2 weeks, 1 month). Some have suggested that children under age 7 years (and older) have difficulty answering questions that ask them to comment on the last week (Juniper, Guyatt, Feeny, Ferrie, & Griffith, 1997); others have found that children 8 years and older are able to provide reliable and valid responses regarding their HRQOL (Feeny, Juniper, Ferrie, Griffith, & Guyatt, 1998).

These considerations must be balanced with the importance of accessing the individual's point of view in gauging their life experience and quality. Parents or proxies are often asked to report on the HRQOL of young cancer patients. There is a body of research documenting the differences in parental versus child report of child functioning in healthy populations as well as in populations of children and adolescents with cancer (Achenbach, McConaughy, & Howell, 1997; Eiser & Morse, 2001; Levi & Drotar, 1999). Ironically, populations for whom the child's perspective is most needed (e.g., young children, children who are severely ill) are those who are most reliant on proxy respondents (Nathan et al., 2004; Vance, Morse, Jenney, & Eiser, 2001).

### *Developmental Changes*

Despite the continuous changes characteristic of the disease process and treatment, children continue to develop throughout treatment. More so, treatment for acute lymphocytic leukemia (ALL), the most common form of cancer during childhood, lasts for at least 2–3 years and longer in cases of treatment delays or relapse (Margolin et al., 2002). Given that a large percentage of children diagnosed with ALL are under age 5 years, significant development will occur while they are on treatment. A challenge to measurement of HRQOL is thus to capture changes in HRQOL while considering and incorporating the changes in cognitive abilities and shifts in priorities and developmental milestones that occur while they are on treatment. Assessment of child HRQOL must be both dynamic and flexible (Eiser & Morse, 2001a).

## Salient Health-Related Quality-of-Life Aspects Across Development

One's subjective experience of HRQOL changes across development (Parry, 2003; Speith, 2001). The salience of HRQOL domains and the effects of the cancer treatment and illness experience also vary across development. For example, the impact of the typically short-term impacts common during cancer treatment (e.g., alopecia, school absences) can be expected to have different meaning and to have a different impact on a toddler, who may not be concerned at all about these limitations, than to a teenager, for whom school, academic performance, social relationships, and physical appearance are often of primary importance.

This differential salience of HRQOL domains throughout the childhood cancer experience also applies to late effects. As the numbers of individuals with childhood cancer live into adulthood, a large percentage of them experience some form of late effect from their treatment (Schwartz, 1999). Late effects vary based on the type and location of the cancer, associated treatments, individual physiology, and the age at which treatments were administered. The manifestation of late effects varies as a function of age and development, as may their salience (e.g., infertility) (Shover, 1999). These late effects can influence individual HRQOL and can have an impact on an individual's ability to comprehend HRQOL measures (Mostrow, Byrne, Connelly, & Muvihill, 1991).

## Multiple Informants

There are a variety of reasons why obtaining children's self-reports of their HRQOL is difficult, including inability to read, respond, or sufficiently self-reflect on their illness and health status, compromised health status, cognitive impairment because of treatment or disease, and age (Levi & Drotar, 1998; Nathan et al., 2004; Perrin & Garrity, 1981). Given these challenges, parents (especially mothers) have historically been considered to be able to provide a more reliable and valid report of their child's health status and functioning than the child. More recent history acknowledges that parents and children have unique perspectives of and experiences within a child's illness and treatment. Parents often report poorer functioning and greater disease impact than do their children/adolescents (e.g., Canning, 1994; Levi & Drotar, 1999; Parsons, Barlow, Levy, Supran, & Kaplan, 1999; Sawyer et al., 1999).

On some occasions, health care providers are also asked to provide proxy reports of children's functioning. Data indicate that health care provider proxies may be reliable reporters of visible aspects of physical health (i.e., what the child is able to do), yet are less accurate compared to children's own reports on less-visible and more internal aspects of functioning (e.g., nausea, sadness, fear) (Merkins, Perrin, Perrin, & Gerrity, 1989; Parsons et al., 1999). Questions remain regarding how to obtain the most accurate reports regarding HRQOL of all children, including those who have difficulty self-reporting (Eisner & Morse, 2001a; Nathan et al., 2004).

## Timing of Assessment

Children with cancer experience fluctuations in their illness and treatment status on a daily basis while undergoing treatment. This variability has been shown to correspond with variability in serial reports of children's HRQOL during acute intensive treatment (e.g., bone marrow transplantation [BMT]) (Phipps, Dunavant, Garvie, Lensing, & Rai, 2002).

This ongoing state of flux poses methodological challenges to the measurement of HRQOL. Some HRQOL measures that are used with childhood cancer populations inquire about functioning over long time periods (e.g., 1 month, 2 weeks, 1 week) (e.g., Goodwin, Boggs, & Graham-Pole, 1994; Landgraf et al., 1996). However, they are often cross sectional. There are measures that assess HRQOL over shorter time frames (e.g., Behavioral, Affective, and Somatic Experiences Scale; Phipps, Dunavant, Jayawardene, & Srivastiva, 1999). However, such measures require multiple administrations and may increase the burden on the respondent (Nathan et al., 2004). The relative degree of influence of a child's current state on the child or parental perception of HRQOL throughout the preceding period is difficult to determine.

## Meaning

Enduring cancer during childhood has been found to impact the meaning and values that individuals place on their lives, health, and relationships (e.g., Gray et al., 1992; Levi, 2000; Parry, 2003). The changes in one's internal values, perception of their HRQOL, and expectations that occur during treatment for cancer have been referred to as response shift (Sprangers, 2002). Response shifts have been suggested to occur in the process of accommodating to and integrating cancer and its treatment into one's life. One's perception and the barometer with which they judge the value of their life quality may change throughout the course of the illness and posttreatment yet may not correspond to changes in their functioning (Nathan et al., 2004; Schwartz, Feinberg, Jilinskaia, & Applegate, 1999).

Parents and health care providers may also experience response shifts. The process of getting "used" to the rigors associated with childhood cancer treatment may lead to changes in how one perceives life and functioning and may change the way in which they report on HRQOL.

The manifestation of response shift also varies across development, partly because of varying cognitive capacity for comparison (Sprangers, 2002). Although response shift is often considered as a source of bias in some studies, it is a critical factor to consider in attempting to understand quality of life of individuals with childhood cancer (Eiser, 2004; Nathan et al., 2004).

## Methodological Considerations

### Validity

A critical methodological factor in the utility of any measure is the validity: Is the measure actually capturing what it intends to measure? Within the field of HRQOL assessment, it is especially important that a measure is sensitive to real changes that occur in one's life, health status, and perception of personal health. Measures must be sufficiently sensitive to capture changes over short periods of time (i.e., less than 2 weeks) given that one's health and health status while on treatment changes with great frequency on a regular basis (Jenney, 1998). Sensitivity to change is a critical factor in measurement of HRQOL in these populations, and different instruments with differential sensitivities may be necessary across time/treatment periods.

### Reliability

Test-retest reliability is complicated with HRQOL assessment given that HRQOL is influenced by multiple factors and is not a stable trait. An additional complicating factor is the fact that test-retest reliability is often established on populations of individuals with stable health status. The health status of individuals enduring cancer treatment is known to be unstable and at times unpredictable both during and following the completion of treatment (Schwartz, 1999). Hence, one cannot extrapolate that such measures maintain an adequate level of test-retest reliability in these populations of individuals who have completed treatment (Nathan et al., 2004).

### Response Burden

Completing HRQOL measures may burden children and families in several ways, including the time that it takes to complete the measure and emotions that the questions may evoke related to living with cancer; cognitively, the measures may be difficult for some children and possibly parents to complete. Such response burden may have an impact on an individual's willingness to complete the measures and how they report on their HRQOL (Jenney, 1998; Nathan et al., 2004).

### Study Populations

The samples used in many studies that employ HRQOL assessments are small and heterogeneous (e.g., wide age ranges, diverse diagnoses, variability in time off treatment, etc.). Such diversity presents several difficulties in the measurement of HRQOL and in gleaning information about HRQOL in children living with cancer. First, this diversity makes it difficult to discern issues specific to disease and phase of treatment from general changes in HRQOL that occur throughout the course of life following cancer in childhood.

Second, most studies that measure HRQOL include samples of children who have completed treatment and who are disease free. Children assessed after treatment has been completed and who are older comprise a fundamentally different population from the population they represented at the time of treatment (i.e., adolescents who have survived treatment for ALL who were initially diagnosed younger than 5 years are not comparable to those younger than 5-year-olds recently diagnosed with ALL).

Finally, many of these individuals were treated with less-advanced care or were treated during an era with far lower survival rates. Children are now often treated with increasingly intense treatment protocols compared to those used a decade ago. As a result, families facing childhood cancer in the past few years do so amid a different context than families who experienced childhood cancer in the prior two decades. This different context can have an impact on their experience with and expectations about HRQOL (Engel, 1977; Kleinman, 1988). The time period in which one was treated may exert an impact on HRQOL, even within populations with the same disease.

## Cross-Cultural Utilization and Validation

The context (e.g., implicit cultural values, beliefs, ways in which medicine is practiced) within which HRQOL measures are devised and normed must be acknowledged. Perceptions of health and illness are influenced by one's context and have an impact on the ways in which HRQOL is perceived and evaluated (Felder-Puig et al., 2000; Yeh & Hung, 2003).

The context within which a child and family lives also affects the types of questions that need to be asked to assess their HRQOL. For example, administration of measures devised for health care provider reports may not be appropriate for populations of children treated for cancer in

Buenos Aires, Argentina, where nurses often do not have sufficient contact with patients to complete such questionnaires (Szecket et al., 1999). Another example is borrowed from Taiwan, a culture in which it is uncommon for Taiwanese parents to discuss cancer and its treatment with child patients. Measures that ask parents to report on their perceptions of their child's HRQOL during treatment must take this normal cultural difference into account (Yeh & Hung, 2003). Cultural variations within the United States are also important (e.g., children living in the northwest versus south) as cultural variability occurs both within and between cultures (Cheatham et al., 1997).

A second, yet related, reason to consider one's cultural context in HRQOL assessment is the issue of language. Measures developed in the United States are likely to be worded in ways that capture aspects of functioning that are relevant for children and families living in or acculturated to life in the United States. However, such wording may be irrelevant or not understood by individuals living in other cultures. For example, the ability to walk less than 1 block may have little meaning to children and families in the United Kingdom, yet makes sense to many families living in the United States (Eiser & Morse, 2001). When such questions are included in quantitative measures, participants typically respond to them, despite the fact that the nature of the question may limit the meaning and cultural appropriateness of their response.

Measures devised in English must be translated to the appropriate native language of the populations with which they will be used (e.g., Chwalow, 1995; Guillemin, Bombardier, & Beaton, 1993). While several studies report promising reliability, internal consistency, and validity data on HRQOL measures that have been translated into a variety of languages such as Dutch (Bijttebier et al., 2001); Spanish (Szecket et al., 1999); French (Le Gales et al., 1999); and German (Felder-Puig et al., 2004), the changes to the measures and associated meaning/data are rarely mentioned in reports of the methodological characteristics of translated HRQOL measures (Glaser et al., 1999). Findings that support the reliability and validity of HRQOL measures cannot overshadow or account for the cultural variability that is integral to a child's functioning.

Third, in addition to the variability in perceptions of childhood cancer between and within cultures, there is also international variability in childhood cancer treatment (Calaminus & Kiebert, 1999). Variability in resource availability for treatment centers and to individual children and families also exists. For example, Rigon, Lopes, Roasario Latorre, and Carmargo (2003) described the first pediatric oncology late-effects clinic in Brazil, which was devised in 1999. Such clinics and the need for such clinics emerged earlier in other cultures (e.g., Fochtman, 1995). The impacts of these, as well as the aforementioned culturally related characteristics, are important to acknowledge and incorporate into acquisition and interpretation of all research findings on HRQOL in pediatric oncology.

## Review of Health-Related Quality-of-Life Research in Pediatric Oncology

Research on the HRQOL of children, adolescents, young adults, and adults who have endured childhood cancer and their parents is expanding. There is wide variability in study design, populations studied, and foci.

### On Treatment

Most of the published research to date has been conducted with children, adolescents, and young adults who are off treatment. Next are reviewed some of the findings regarding HRQOL of children on treatment.

#### *Disease Type*

Most of the research conducted on children currently undergoing treatment is of children with central nervous system (CNS) tumors and leukemias (especially ALL), the two most common forms of childhood cancer (Eiser, 2004; Meeske, Katz, Palmer, Burwinkle, & Varni, 2004). Children on treatment for brain tumors have been reported to have more difficulty and poorer overall HRQOL across several domains (cognitive functioning, social functioning, and general health status) than children who are healthy or with other forms of childhood cancer (Armstrong et al., 1999; Meeske et al., 2004). These patterns of findings parallel the broad literature on the psychosocial functioning of children and adolescents with brain tumors (e.g., Fuemmeler, Elkin, & Mullins, 2002). Parent reports of children with a variety of diagnoses undergoing BMT indicated lower levels of somatic distress and higher levels of activity among children with neuroblastoma compared to those with ALL (Phipps, Dunavant, Lensing, & Rai, 2002).

In a study of parent and clinician reports of the HRQOL of Australian children on maintenance therapy for ALL, findings suggested that even during the maintenance phase of treatment, parents perceived ALL and its treatment had an impact on their child's functioning, and that clinical indicators did not fully capture this impact on children's lives as reported by parents and clinicians (Waters, Wake, Hesketh, Ashley, & Smibert, 2002).

### *Treatment Status*

Variability in HRQOL as a function of treatment status has also been reported by several researchers, for example, in samples of children in maintenance treatment for ALL (Waters et al., 2002); on treatment for any type of childhood cancer (Sawyer et al., 1999; Varni et al., 2002); and on treatment for ALL or CNS tumors (Meeske et al., 2004) and throughout the BMT process (Phipps, Dunavant, Garvie, et al., 2002; Phipps, Dunavant, Lansing, et al., 2002). Phipps, Dunavant, Lansing, et al. (2002) found similarities in parent and child report of HRQOL during BMT, with highest levels of distress after the conditioning and 1 week following the actual transplant. The group data showed HRQOL returned to HRQOL levels reported at BMT admission and to continue to improve for 4–6 months posttransplant. Phipps, Dunavant, Garvie, et al. (2002) reported that children from families of lower socioeconomic status had more difficulty (e.g., physical, emotional distress) throughout the process of BMT (conducted in the United States) than were reported for children/adolescents from backgrounds of higher socioeconomic status beginning at Week +1. Similar findings have been reported internationally in studies of adolescents and their parents from Australia (Sawyer et al., 1999) and of Taiwanese caregivers of children with brain tumors (Chien et al., 2003). Some studies have found marked differences in HRQOL of children in active treatment versus those who have been off therapy for a year or more (e.g., Meeske et al., 2004; Sawyer et al., 1999; Varni et al., 2002). However, in other research, differences in overall HRQOL were not found to vary as a function of treatment status (Vance et al., 2001).

### *Age*

Consistent with the general psychosocial research on children with cancer, studies on HRQOL have reported preschool children exhibit better HRQOL during treatment, as indicated by lower levels of distress than other age groups (Barrera et al., 2003; Phipps, Dunavant, Garvie, et al., 2002). Adolescents have been found to have poorer HRQOL throughout treatment than younger children (Barrera et al., 2003).

## After the Completion of Treatment

### *Disease Type*

Individuals who have been treated for a brain tumor during childhood have been found to report or to have proxies report poorer HRQOL as indicated by poorer scores on a variety of HRQOL domains (e.g., social functioning, physical functioning, cognitive functioning, psychological/emotional functioning) or lower achievement of expected developmental milestones than healthy samples, samples of children with other non-CNS types of cancer, those with other non-CNS involved types of chronic illness, and siblings (e.g., Eiser, Greco, Vance, Horne, & Glaser, 2004; Eiser, Vance, Horne, Glaser, & Galvin, 2003; Langeveld, Stam, Grootenhuis, & Last, 2002). Some consistent findings have emerged from studies that focused on HRQOL following childhood brain tumors, including difficulty with school/educational achievement (Hays et al., 1992; Kennedy & Leland, 1999), greater functional difficulties in individuals with supratentorial versus infratentorial tumors (Lannering, Marky, Lundberg, & Olsson, 1990; Mostrow et al., 1991), and younger age at diagnosis and treatment associated with poorer HRQOL (e.g., Barr et al., 1999).

There are wide ranges of impairment, HRQOL, and overall functioning reported in these studies and often within samples (Eiser et al., 2004; Fuemmeler et al., 2002). For example, in a review of the literature on adjustment in individuals treated for a brain tumor, ranges of maladjustment/distress ranged from 25% to 95% of the samples in included studies (Fuemmeler et al., 2002). It is key to consider premorbid functioning in differentiating the degree to which levels of functioning are influenced by cancer and its treatment versus internal and external environmental factors (e.g., Mulhern, 1999).

Several studies have found individuals off treatment for ALL reported comparable HRQOL as that reported by the general population in some domains. For example, Eiser et al. (2003) found ALL survivors reported comparable physical HRQOL to the healthy population, but lower levels of psychosocial HRQOL than physical HRQOL, and lower levels of psychosocial HRQOL than reported by the healthy norm population. The broad literature on the psychological, cognitive, and educational functioning of individuals who have been treated for ALL during childhood provides a wealth of data regarding their functioning across those domains. Few of these studies included HRQOL measures. Readers are referred to these articles for data on the functioning of individuals treated for ALL (e.g., Chen et al., 1998; Mackie, Hill, Kondryn, & McNally, 2000; Zeltzer et al., 1997).

Some studies have assessed the HRQOL of individuals following solid or bone cancer during childhood. This research has consistently reported that individuals treated for bone tumors during childhood or adolescence are generally functioning well (Felder-Puig et al., 1998; Greenberg et al., 1994; Nicholson, Mulvihill, & Byrne, 1992). Some found amputees or individuals with a bone cancer history to have more difficulty in functioning years after treatment ended than reported by controls. The domains in which such differences occur vary by study (e.g., educational achievement, employment, marriage rates, physical difficulties) (Felder-Puig et al., 1998; Nicholson, Mulvihill, & Byrne, 1992; Novakovic, Fears, Horowitz, Tucker, & Wexler, 1997).

Diagnostic heterogeneity is common in research on HRQOL of individuals following treatment for childhood cancer. In several studies of children, young adults, or adults who experienced childhood cancer, survivors reported comparable (Felder-Puig et al., 1998; Schwartz et al., 1999) or higher levels of HRQOL (De Clercq, De Fruyt, Koot, & Benoit, 2004; Zebrack, 2000) than comparison groups. Such findings parallel research findings related to response shift, growth, resilience, and changes in values that have been found in populations of individuals long term off treatment for childhood cancer (e.g., Gray et al., 1992; Zebrack, 2000), especially for those off therapy for at least several years.

These positive findings, however, must not overshadow the challenges faced by survivors of childhood cancer. The experience of childhood cancer encompasses both positive and negative aspects (Eiser & Havermans, 1994). The childhood cancer experience and the process of integrating that experience into one's life as an adult appears to leave survivors with physical and socioemotional strengths and vulnerabilities.

### *Young Adults With a Childhood Cancer History*

Although substantial data document the late medical and neoplastic complications associated with early mortality following treatment for childhood cancer, there are several gaps in knowledge regarding approaches to measuring HRQOL of childhood cancer survivors who are now adults (Eiser, 1998; Schwartz, 1999). First, the field lacks disease-specific measures that address the issues faced by such individuals. The available measures were developed for child and adolescent populations and thus do not fully capture the lived experience of young adult survivors (Zebrack & Chesler, 2001). Second, as mentioned, there is tremendous variability in approaches to treatment and in the contexts in which these individuals were treated. HRQOL measures developed more recently thus may not capture the nature of their experience with cancer during childhood.

In a review of 30 studies of the QOL of young adult survivors, Langeveld et al. (2002) reported the following trends. First, most young adults reported themselves to be in good physical and psychological health. Second, individuals who had been treated for CNS tumors or ALL reported greater risks for or problems with educational attainment and cognitive functioning. Third, despite the previously reported positive outcomes, young adults did report job discrimination, difficulties obtaining employment or health/life insurance, relationship difficulties, and lower rates of marriage and child rearing than comparison groups. Finally, concerns about fertility and the health of potential offspring were commonly reported, yet underexplored (Shover, 1999).

## Parent Versus Child Report of Child Health-Related Quality of Life

Differences in parental versus child reports of child HRQOL have been reported in many studies of

HRQOL in childhood cancer populations (Levi & Drotar, 1999; Parsons et al., 1999; Sawyer et al., 1999; Vance et al., 2001). Parents report their children to experience lower levels of HRQOL than are reported by the children themselves on multiple domains, including physical functioning (Vance et al., 2001); participation in physical activities (Sawyer et al., 1999); psychological functioning (Parsons et al., 1999; Vance et al., 2001); school functioning (Sawyer et al., 1999); functioning related to the disease and treatment (Vance et al., 2001); and overall HRQOL (Parsons et al., 1999; Vance et al., 2001).

In a study of the degree of discrepancy between the parent and child reports of child HRQOL in a group of parents and their children with cancer as compared to a group of matched parents and their children without a chronic illness history, Levi and Drotar (1999) reported statistically significant larger discrepancies in the parent versus child reports of child HRQOL in the cancer group. More specifically, on 50% of the HRQOL items assessed, parents of children/adolescents with cancer reported their child had poorer functioning/QOL than did the children themselves; in the healthy sample, such discrepancy was only present on one item.

These discrepancies and direction of discrepancy have not been replicated in all studies of parent-child report of child HRQOL (Eiser et al., 2003). For example, in the Levi and Drotar 1999 study, the reports of parents and their children with cancer on child HRQOL did not reach statistical significance on half of the items. Other studies have found good (moderate-to-high) levels of agreement between parent and child reports on a number of domains (Sawyer et al., 1999; Varni et al., 2002), including physical functioning (Eiser et al., 2003; Varni et al., 1998); social functioning (Vance et al., 2001); cognitive functioning (Vance et al., 2001); and parent and child reports of child HRQOL during BMT (Phipps, Dunavant, Lansing, et al., 2002).

Taken together, such findings suggest that although there is some overlap in parent and child reports of child HRQOL, they are not interchangeable. Different perceptions of child HRQOL are not surprising and can be expected given that parent and child reports are based on different, although mutually valuable, sources of data. Parents' reports are based on observation and communication with the child; children's reports may be based on their internal, subjective experience to which parents do not and cannot be expected to have access (Dolgin & Phipps, 1989; Parsons et al., 1999).In addition, some research suggested that there is some overlap in parent and child experience during treatment. For example, levels of child distress at the time of BMT admission have been found to be predictive of parental levels of distress across the acute phases of the BMT (Phipps, Dunavant, Lensing, & Rai, 2004). The impact of the cancer experience on parental HRQOL and the relationship between parental HRQOL and their reports of child HRQOL are relevant to the issue of parent and child report of child HRQOL.

## Parental Health-Related Quality of Life

Research on the HRQOL of people living with childhood cancer has primarily focused on the patient. It is universally accepted that having a child with cancer is traumatic and life altering for parents, and that this can continue for years after treatment is completed (Chien et al., 2003; Fuemmeler, Mullins, & Marx, 2001; Goldbeck, 2001). The daily changes, anxiety, and response shifts experienced by parents may also have an impact on the child's HRQOL and how parents report on child HRQOL. Vance et al. (2001) explored both parent and child perceptions of quality of life as well as illness-related stressors in a group of children with ALL. Parents who reported poorer quality of life in their children also reported a higher level of illness-related stressors and perceived their child as more vulnerable. In a study of Australian adolescents with a variety of cancer diagnoses, the greatest impact on quality of life within the cancer group was the impact of the cancer on the parent's quality of life (Sawyer et al., 1999).

Parents and children may also perceive the situation differently and may be focused on different aspects of the child's life. For example, parents may focus on and be influenced in their reporting more by longer term issues and risks to their child's health (e.g., death, learning problems); children may be focused on more concrete, immediate effects of the illness and treatment (e.g., missed school, pain) (Levi & Drotar, 1999; Vance et al., 2001). Parents across the world are profoundly affected by their child's diagnosis, treatment, and prognosis, and this may influence their perceptions of their child's functioning (Thomasgard & Metz, 1995).

## Summary

### Progress

The current status of HRQOL measurement reflects considerable progress in the development and employment of HRQOL assessment in pediatric oncology. HRQOL measures are currently used in clinical trials and have contributed data on evaluative and discriminative questions (Bradlyn, 2004). Another sign of formidable progress is that a number of instruments with acceptable psychometric properties are now available for use with pediatric oncology populations in a number of languages, as are reviews of such measures (e.g., Eiser & Morse, 2001b; Felder-Puig et al., 2004; Levi & Drotar, 1998; Spieth & Harris, 1996). The field of HRQOL assessment has become increasingly integrated into the field of pediatric oncology, both conceptually and methodologically, as indicated by increased participation in and attention to the science of HRQOL assessment.

### Paradigm Shift

As mentioned, assessment of HRQOL in pediatric oncology reflects a historical paradigm shift. Assessment of HRQOL is a comprehensive way to assess the lived experience of individuals who have experienced childhood cancer across multiple domains. Next are discussed a number of relevant domains that are periodically mentioned yet infrequently included in pediatric oncology HRQOL measures and research reports.

#### *Discrepancy*

Calman (1984) offered another definition of HRQOL that may be relevant to child functioning: "Quality of life measures the difference,... be-between the hopes and expectations of the individual and the individual's experience. It is concerned with the difference between perceived goals and actual goals. It is an assessment of the potential for growth." Although relevant, this definition and way to conceptualize HRQOL are infrequently used (e.g., Eiser et al., 1999, 2003).

#### *Spirituality*

Attention to the role of religious and spiritual beliefs is a relatively recent addition to the literature; however, these belief systems are salient to families and children facing cancer (e.g., Houskamp, Fisher, & Stuber, 2004). Spirituality is a force that is powerful in the lives of many children and their families, especially in the face of childhood cancer (Hart, 2003). Spirituality and the role it plays in a child's HRQOL are critical additions to HRQOL assessments in pediatric oncology.

#### *Sexuality*

Sexuality is considered an important aspect of functioning and relating for young adults and adults that is often impacted by cancer treatments (Shover, 1999). However, sexuality often is not included in assessments of well-being or HRQOL and is considered underacknowledged (Eiser & Morse, 2001; Langeveld et al., 2002).

#### *Family and Relationships*

Children are influenced substantially by the systems in which they live, such as family and friends (Bronfenbrenner, 1979). Few measures include items that directly assess the effects of cancer on the family system and how these effects have an impact on the child's HRQOL (Landgraf et al., 1996; Patterson, Holm, & Gurney, 2004). Furthermore, the HRQOL of siblings of individuals with cancer is limited (Houtzager et al., 2004).

#### *Positive Changes and Growth*

Most HRQOL measures used in populations of children with cancer provide room for respondents to communicate their experience, positive or negative. For example, on the Pediatric Oncology Quality of Life Scale measure (Goodwin et al., 1994), parents are asked to respond to questions such as "My child has been able to participate in recreational activities (sports, games, etc.)" and "My child is able to attend school," which provide room to directly report on positive aspects of a child's functioning. However, findings are often reported in comparative terms, such as parents versus children, phases of treatment, across disease or treatment groups (e.g., ALL versus CNS tumors or Wilms tumor) (Levi & Drotar, 1999; Mackie et al., 2000; Phipps et al., 1999; Phipps, Dunavant, Garvie, et al., 2002) and tend to be oriented toward where problems and difficulties in functioning remain. Positive aspects of HRQOL (i.e., increased appreciation of health, positive feelings about having increased amounts of time with family during treatment, changed priorities) and of children's functioning and resilience, while acknowledged at the core of HRQOL assessment, are underrepresented in the literature (Haase & Rostad, 1994).

### *Qualitative Themes and Meaning*

The meaning associated with difficult experiences is acknowledged as a significant factor in one's life following the experience and in understanding one's experience (Frankl, 1963; Kleinman, 1988). In the current context of HRQOL assessment in pediatric oncology, measures are primarily quantitative and oriented toward functioning (Haase et al., 1999). Several authors have suggested that such an orientation does not sufficiently address the role and influence of meaning in one's report of personal HRQOL (Haase & Braden, 1998; Lantos, 1998; Wallander et al., 2001). For example, in a qualitative study of quality of life during cancer treatment as reported by pediatric patients, six domains were identified, none of which are consistently included in current HRQOL measures. The authors highlighted that the meaning associated with being ill was the domain most frequently missing from current HRQOL measures (Hinds et al., 2004).

### *Concurrent Stressors*

Although the childhood cancer experience can be thought to impose a unique and profound set of stressors to a child and family, the variability in HRQOL that occurs as children progress through development, and in light of other non-cancer-related concurrent stressors (i.e., socioeconomic status), remains unclear. Data on concurrent, normative stressors and how these interact and influence reports of HRQOL are recommended (Parry, 2003; Phipps, Dunavant, Lansing, et al., 2002).

## Lingering Questions and Missing Pieces

The domains in which unanswered questions remain can be organized into several categories. One set of questions involves the respondent and asks: Who should we assess? Assessments of HRQOL primarily include patients themselves, mothers, and, on some occasions, health care providers. A number of people are involved in the lives of children with cancer, and their perspectives offer unique contributions. Perceptions of fathers and mothers, siblings, teachers, and possibly friends regarding the HRQOL of individuals with childhood cancer would deepen our understanding of HRQOL in the face of childhood cancer across the lifespan, while attempts to capture the child's perspective whenever possible continue.

A second set of questions involves timing: When do we assess HRQOL? To date, HRQOL assessments in pediatric oncology populations are cross sectional (Nathan et al., 2004), with few prospective studies (e.g., Phipps, Dunavant, Garvie, et al., 2002; Phipps, Dunavant, Lansing, et al., 2002; Phipps et al., 2004). Cross sectional data offer the benefit of potentially lower response burden and the ability to obtain reports from larger numbers of individuals and sacrifices the ability to capture the fluid nature of HRQOL. Few studies have assessed HRQOL across multiple time points throughout treatment (e.g., Barerra et al., 2003; Phipps, Dunavant, Garvie, et al., 2002; Phipps, Dunavant, Lansing, et al., 2002; Phipps et al., 2004). Prospective studies that incorporate repeated measures on HRQOL are strongly recommended (Bradlyn, 2004; Nathan et al., 2004). The field will benefit from clarification of ideal times to obtain these measurements across the childhood cancer trajectory (including relapse and end of life).

A third, and critical, set of questions regards what we are assessing in pediatric oncology HRQOL assessments. The field of pediatric HRQOL remains plagued by a lack of a universal definition and lack of theoretical frameworks informing the HRQOL construct (Haase & Braden, 1998; Levi & Drotar, 1998).

Although qualitative data may be more difficult to integrate into clinical trials or medical practice, the field is at a point at which further qualitative work is needed to develop the HRQOL construct and to ground it in theory. The field might consider the following questions: What does quality of life mean following a diagnosis of and throughout treatment for childhood cancer? What does quality of life mean after treatment ends? What does quality of life mean across cultures? What does quality of life mean as children are near death? (Bradlyn, 2004; Haase et al., 1999; Lantos, 1998). The issue of definition remains essential at this juncture. HRQOL measures multiple outcomes related to the functioning of individuals with childhood cancer; however, it is not clear that these multiple outcomes are equivalent to life quality (Hinds et al., 2004; Lantos, 1998).

## Future Directions and Recommendations

### Areas for Future Research

Related to the recommendations to extend qualitative work into the meaning of the HRQOL construct to patients and families, Eiser and Morse (2001) conducted an extensive review of available HRQOL measures for children and made several recommendations useful for HRQOL assessment in pediatric oncology. They recommended broader spectrum investigation into how the HRQOL measures that exist actually perform in pediatric oncology populations, across the lifespan, and in randomized national and international trials.

Further attention to issues of development in HRQOL research would strongly benefit the field of pediatric oncology in several ways. First, the field will benefit from developing models informed by theory that acknowledge and enable analysis of the variability of HRQOL across childhood, adolescence, and young adulthood (Bradlyn, 2004; Eiser & Morse, 2001; Haase et al., 1999). These data may be able to lend additional insight into the response shifts that occur throughout and following treatment (Sprangers, 2002). Second, and related to the above, is further resources invested in refining or developing new measures that can obtain self-reports of young children and children who are severely medically compromised and thus functioning at a lower cognitive level (Eiser & Morse, 2001; Nathan et al., 2004).

Third, further data regarding child versus proxy ratings of child HRQOL are needed. More specifically, data on the relationship between child and proxy ratings in general and at specific points throughout the childhood cancer process (e.g., diagnosis, relapse, informed consent, in the face of a difficult medical decision); on the influence of the family system on parental, sibling, and patient HRQOL; and reasons for discordance between parent and child reports of child HRQOL are needed (Vance et al., 2001).

A final, and imperative, domain into which research on and assessment of HRQOL needs to expand is into HRQOL in the face of refractory disease and at the end of life. Despite advances in treatment and improved rates of survival for most childhood cancers, over 2,200 children and adolescents die each year (Wolfe et al., 2002). Research on the psychological and spiritual experience of children and their families who are living with childhood cancer and facing the end of their physical lives remains limited, despite knowledge that children who are dying often experience intense pain (Bradlyn, Varni, & Hinds, 2002), and that bereavement continues for family members for an extended time period following a child's death (Chien et al., 2003).

### Clinical Applications

Many of the research recommendations also have clinical implications. Clinical applications of HRQOL assessments in pediatric oncology have only recently been reported in the literature. For example, one study examined the utility of using parent report of child HRQOL as a predictor of health care costs (Seid, Varni, Segall, & Kurtin, 2004). Another study assessed the utility of using HRQOL measures to differentiate risk of cardiac damage following anthracyclines based on patient reports of functioning (Ginsberg et al., 2004).

Other clinical applications of HRQOL data in pediatric oncology populations have been recommended, including using HRQOL data to inform the types of rehabilitation from which individuals off treatment might benefit (Eiser et al., 2004). HRQOL data have been used in populations of adults to facilitate decision making about treatment and enrollment in clinical trials. Although such interventions are rarely conducted in pediatric oncology (Jenney & Levitt, 2002), they have been recommended for future consideration (Bradlyn, 2004).

The field of pediatric HRQOL assessment has made substantial progress in working to understand the lived experience of individuals with childhood cancer. As the number of individuals whose lives have been affected by childhood cancer expands, so does the importance of refining our knowledge of the life quality that they experience.

## Note

1. The terms *children* and *child* are used to refer to individuals of all ages treated for childhood cancer (e.g., infants, toddlers, school-aged children, adolescents, young adults) unless otherwise noted.

## References


Aaronson, N. K., Meyrowitz, B. E., Bard, M., Bloom, J. R., Fawzy, F. I., Feldstein, M., et al. (1991). Quality of life research in oncology: Past achievements and future priorities. *Cancer,* Suppl. 67, 839–843.

Achenbach, T. M., McConaughy, S. H., & Howell, C. T. (1987). Child/adolescent behavioral and emotional problems: Implications of cross-informant correlations for situational specificity. *Psychological Bulletin, 101,* 213–212.

Armstrong, F. D., Toledano, S. R., Miloslavich, K., Lackman-Zeman, L., Levy, J. D., Gay, C. L., et al. (1999). The Miami Pediatric Quality of Life Questionnaire: Parent scale. *International Journal of Cancer,* Suppl. 12, 11–17.

Barr, R. D., Simpson, T., Whitton, A., Rush, B., Furlong, W., & Feeny, D. H. (1999). Health-related quality of life in survivors of tumours of the central nervous system of childhood—a preference based approach to measurement in a cross-sectional study. *European Journal of Cancer, 35,* 248–255.

Barrera, M., Wayland, L. A., D'Agostino, N. M., Gibson, J., Weksberg, R., & Malkin, D. (2003). Developmental differences in psychological adjustment and health-related quality of life in pediatric cancer patients. *Children's Health Care, 32,* 215–232.

Bijttebier, P., Vercruysse, T., Vertommen, H., Van Gool, S. W., Uyttebroeck, A., & Brock, P. (2001). New evidence on the reliability and validity of the pediatric oncology quality of life scale. *Psychology and Health, 16,* 461–469.

Bradlyn, A. S. (2004). Health-related quality of life in pediatric oncology: Current status and future challenges. *Journal of Pediatric Oncology Nursing, 21,* 137–140.

Bradlyn, A. S., Harris, C. V., & Speith, L. E. (1995). Quality of life assessment in pediatric oncology: A retrospective review of phase III reports. *Social Science and Medicine, 41,* 1463–1465.

Bradlyn, A., Ritchey, A., Harris, C., Moore, I., O'Brien, R., Parsons, S., et al. (1996). Quality of life research in pediatric oncology—research methods and barriers. *Cancer, 78,* 1333–1339.

Bradlyn, A. S., Varni, J. W., & Hinds, P. S. (2002). Assessment of health-related quality of life in pediatric end-of-life care. In M. J. Field & R. E. Behrman (Eds.), *When children die: Improving palliative and end-of-life care fore children and their families.* Washington, DC: Institute of Medicine, National Academy Press.

Bronfenbrenner, U. (1979). *The ecology of human development.* Boston: Harvard University Press.

Calaminus, G., & Kiebert, G. (1999). Studies on health related quality of life in childhood cancer in the European setting: An overview. *International Journal of Cancer,* Suppl. 12, 83–86.

Calman, K. (1984). Quality of life in cancer patients—An hypothesis. *Journal of Medical Ethics, 10,* 124–127.

Canning, E. H. (1994). Mental disorders in chronically ill children: Case identification and parent-child discrepancy. *Psychosomatic Medicine, 56,* 104–108.

Cheatham, H., Ivey, A. E., Ivey, M. B., Pederson, P., Rigazio-DiGilio, S., Simek-Morgan, L., et al. (1997). Multicultural counseling and therapy I: Metatheory—Taking theory into practice. In M. Ivey & L. Simek-Morgan (Eds.), *Counseling and psychotherapy: A multicultural perspective* (pp. 133–169). New York: Allyn and Bacon.

Chen, E., Zeltzer, L. K., Bentler, P. M., Byrne, J., Nicholson, S., Meadows, A. T., et al. (1998). Pathways linking treatment intensity and psychosocial outcomes among adult survivors of childhood leukemia. *Journal of Health Psychology, 3,* 23–38.

Chien, L. Y., Lo, L. H., Chen, C. J., Chen, Y. C., Chiang, C. C., & Chao, Y. M. Y. (2003). Quality of life among primary caregivers of Taiwanese children with brain tumor. *Cancer Nursing, 26,* 305–311.

Chwalow, A. J. (1995). Cross-cultural validation of existing quality of life scales. *Patient Education and Counseling, 26,* 313–318.

De Clercq, B., De Fruyt, F., Koot, H. M., & Benoit, Y. (2004). Quality of life in children surviving cancer: A personality and multi-informant perspective. *Journal of Pediatric Psychology, 29,* 579–590.

Dolgin, M. J., & Phipps, S. (1989). Pediatric pain: The parents' role. *Pediatrician, 16,* 103–109.

Eiser, C. (1995). Choices in measuring quality of life in children with cancer: A comment. *Psycho-oncology, 4,* 121–131.

Eiser, C. (1998). Practitioner review: Long-term consequences of childhood cancer. *Journal of Child Psychology and Psychiatry and Allied Disciplines, 39,* 621–633.

Eiser, C. (2004). Use of quality of life measures in clinical trials. *Ambulatory Pediatrics, 4,* 395–399.

Eiser, C., Cotter, I., Oades, P., Seamark, D., & Smith, R. (1999). Health-related quality of life measures for children. *International Journal of Cancer, S12,* 87–90.

Eiser, C., Greco, V., Vance, Y. H., Horne, B., & Glaser, A. (2004). Perceived discrepancies and their resolution: Quality of life in survivors of childhood cancer. *Psychology and Health, 19,* 15–28.

Eiser, C., & Havermans, T. (1994). Long term social adjustment after treatment for childhood cancer. *Archives of Disease in Childhood, 70,* 66–70.

Eiser, C., & Morse, R. (2001a). The measurement of quality of life in children: Past and future perspectives. *Journal of Developmental and Behavioral Pediatrics, 22,* 248–256.

Eiser, C., & Morse, R. (2001b). A review of measures of quality of life for children with chronic illness. *Archives of Disease in Childhood, 84,* 205–211.

Eiser, C., Vance, Y. H., Horne, B., Glaser, A., & Galvin, H. (2003). The value of the PedsQL™ in assessing quality of life in survivors of childhood cancer. *Child: Care, Health and Development, 29,* 95–102.

Engel, G. L. (1977). The need for a new medical model: A challenge for biomedicine. *Science, 196,* 129–136.

Feeny, D., Furlong, W., & Barr, R. D. (1998). Multiattribute approach to the assessment of health related quality of life: Health Utilities Index. *Medical Pediatric Oncology,* Suppl. 1, 54–59.

Feeny, D., Furlong, W., Barr, R. D., Torrance, G. W., Rosenbaum, P., & Weitzman, S. (1992). A comprehensive multi-attribute system for classifying the health status of survivors of childhood cancer. *Journal of Clinical Oncology, 10,* 923–928.

Feeny, D., Furlong, W., Mulhern, R.K., Barr, R.D., & Hudson, M. (1999). A framework for assessing health-related quality of life in children with cancer. *International Journal of Cancer,* Suppl. 12, 2–9.

Feeny, D., Juniper, E. F., Ferrie, P. J., Griffith, L. E., & Guyatt, G. H. (1998). Why not just ask the kids? Health-related quality of life in children with asthma. In D. Drotar (Ed.), *Measuring health-related quality of life in children and adolescents: Implications for research and practice* (pp. 171–186). Mahwah, NJ: Erlbaum.

Felder-Puig, R., Formann, A. K., Mildner, A., Bretschneider, W., Bucher, B., Windhager, R., et al. (1998). Quality of life and psychosocial adjustment of young patients after treatment of bone cancer. *Cancer, 83,* 69–75.

Felder-Puig, R., Frey, E., Proksch, K., Varni, J. W., Gadner, H., & Topf, R. (2004). Validation of the German version of the Pediatric Quality of Life Inventory™ (PedsQL™) in childhood cancer patients off treatment and children with epilepsy. *Quality of Life Research, 13,* 223–234.

Felder-Puig, R., Frey, E., Sonnleithner, G., Feeny, D., Gadner, H., Barr, R. D., et al. (2000). German cross cultural adaptation of the Health Utilities Index and its application to a sample of childhood cancer survivors. *European Journal of Pediatrics, 159,* 283–288.

Fitzpatrick, R. (2000). Measurement in health-related quality of life: Challenges in Parkinson's disease. *Psychology and Health, 15,* 99–108.

Fochtman, D. (1995). Follow up care for survivors of childhood cancer. *Nurse Practitioner Forum, 6,* 194–200.

Frankl, V. E. (1963). *Man's search for meaning: An introduction to logo therapy.* Oxford, UK: Washington Square Press.

Fuemmeler, B. F., Elkin, T. D., & Mullins, L. L. (2002). Survivors of childhood brain tumors: Behavioral, emotional, and social adjustment. *Clinical Psychology Review, 22,* 547–585.

Fuemmeler, B. F., Mullins, L. L., & Marx, B. P. (2001). Posttraumatic stress and general distress among parents of children surviving a brain tumor. *Children's Health Care, 38,* 169–182.

Ginsberg, J. P., Cnaan, A., Zhao, H., Clark, B. J., Paridon, S. M., Chin, A. J., et al. (2004). Using health-related quality of life measures to predict cardiac function in survivors exposed to anthracyclines. *Journal of Clinical Oncology, 22,* 3149–3155.

Glaser, A. W., Furlong, W., Walker, D. A., Fielding, K., Davies, K., Feeny, D. H., et al. (1999). Applicability of the Health Utilities Index to a population of childhood survivors of central nervous system tumours in the United Kingdom. *European Journal of Cancer, 35,* 256–261.

Goldbeck, L. (2001). Parental coping with the diagnosis of childhood cancer: Gender effects, dissimilarity within couples, and quality of life. *Psycho-oncology, 10,* 325–335.

Goodwin, D., Boggs, S., & Graham-Pole, J. (1994). Development and validation of the Pediatric Oncology Quality of Life Scale. *Psychological assessment, 6,* 321–328.

Gray, R. E., Doan, B. D., Shermer, P., FitzGerald, A. V., Berry, M. P., Jenkin, D., et al., (1992). Surviving childhood cancer: A descriptive approach to understanding the impact of life-threatening illness. *Psycho-oncology, 1,* 235–245.

Greenberg, D. B., Goorin, A., Gebhart, M. C., Gupta, L., Stier, N., Harmon, D., et al. (1994). Quality of life in osteosarcoma survivors. *Oncology, 8,* 19–25.

Guillemin, F., Bombardier, C., & Beaton. (1993). Cross-cultural adaptation of health-related quality of life measures: literature review and proposed guidelines. *Journal of Clinical Epidemiology, 46,* 1417–1432.

Haase, J., & Braden, C. J. (1998). Guidelines for achieving clarity of concepts related to quality of life. In C. King (Ed.), *Quality of life: Theory, research, and practice* (pp. 54–73). Boston: Jones and Bartlett.

Haase, J. E., Heiney, S. P., Ruccione, K., & Stutzer, C. (1999). Research triangulation to derive meaning based quality-of-life theory: Adolescent resilience model and instrument development. *International Journal of Cancer,* Suppl. 12, 125–131.

Haase, J., & Rostad, M. (1994). Experiences of completing cancer treatments: Child perspectives. *Oncology Nursing Forum, 21,* 1483–1494.

Hart, T. (2003). *The secret spiritual world of children.* Maui, HI: Inner Ocean.

Hays, D. M., Landsverk, J., Sallan, S. E., Hewett, K. D., Patenaude, A. F., Schoonover, D., et al. (1992). Educational, occupational, and insurance status of childhood cancer survivors in their fourth and fifth decades of life. *Journal of Clinical Oncology, 10,* 1397–1406.

Heyn, R., Ragab, A., Raney, R. B., Ruymann, F., Tefft, M., Lawrence, W., et al. (1986). Late effects of therapy in orbital rhabdomyosarcoma in children. *Cancer, 57,* 1738–1743.

Hinds, P. S., Gattuso, J. S., Fletcher, A., Baker, E., Coleman, B., Jackson, T., et al. (2004). Quality of life as conveyed by pediatric patients with cancer. *Quality of Life Research: An International Journal of Quality of Life Aspects of Treatment, Care, and Rehabilitation, 13,* 761–772.

Houskamp, B. M., Fisher, L. A., & Stuber, M. L. (2004). Spirituality in children and adolescents: research findings and implications for clinicians and researchers. *Child and Adolescent Psychiatric Clinics of North America, 13,* 221–230.

Houtzager, B. A., Oort, F. J., Hoekstra-Weebers, J. E. H. M., Caron, H. N., Grootenhuis, M. A., & Last, B. F. (2004). Coping and family functioning predict longitudinal psychological adaptation of siblings of childhood cancer patients. *Journal of Pediatric Psychology, 29,* 591–606.

Jenney, M. E. M. (1998). Theoretical issues pertinent to measurement of quality of life. *Medical and Pediatric Oncology,* Suppl. 1, 41–45.

Jenney, M. E. M., & Levitt, G. A. (2002). The quality of survival after childhood cancer. *European Journal of Cancer, 38,* 1241–1250.

Juniper, E. F., Guyatt, G. H., Feeny, D. H., Ferrie, P. J., & Griffith, L. E. (1997). Minimum skills required by children to complete health-related quality of life instruments for asthma: Comparison of measurement properties. *European Respiratory Journal, 10,* 2285–2294.

Kamphuis, R. P. (1987). The concept of quality of life in pediatric oncology. In N. K. Aaronson & J. Beckmann, J. (Eds.), *The quality of life in cancer patients* (pp. 141–151). New York: Raven Press.

Kennedy, C. R. & Leyland, K. (1999). Comparison of screening Instruments for disability and emotional/behavioral disorders with a generic measure of heatlh-related quality of life in survivors of childhood brain tumors. *International Journal of Cancer,* Suppl. 12, pp. 106–111.

Kleinman, A. E. (1988). *The illness narratives: Suffering, healing, and the human condition.* New York: Basic Books.

Landgraf, J. M., Abetz, L., & Ware, J. E. (1996). *The child health questionnaire (CHQ): A user's manual.* Boston: Health Institute.

Langeveld, N. E., Stam, H., Grootenhuis, M. A., & Last, B. F. (2002). Quality of life in young adult survivors of childhood cancer. *Support Care Cancer, 10,* 579–600.

Lannering, B., Marky, I., Lundberg, A., & Olsson, E. (1990). Long term sequelae after pediatric brain tumors: Their effect on disability and quality of life. *Medical Pediatric Oncology, 18,* 304–310.

Lansky, S. B., List, M. A., Lansky, L. L., Ritter-Sterr, C., & Miller, D. (1987). The measurement of performance in childhood cancer patients. *Cancer, 60,* 1651–1656.

Lantos, J. D. (1998). Some moral and political pitfalls in measuring quality of life. In D. Drotar (Ed.), *Measuring health-related quality of life in children and adolescents: Implications for research and practice* (pp. 53–60). Mahwah, NJ: Erlbaum.

Le Gales, C., Costet, N., Gentet, J. C., Kalifa, C., Frappaz, D., Edan, C., et al. (1999). Cross-cultural adaptation of a health status classification system in children with cancer. First results of the French adaptation of the Health Utilities Index Marks 2 and 3. *International Journal of Cancer,* Suppl. 12, 112–118.

Levi, R. B. (2000). Health values and behavior: Perspectives of young adults successfully treated for cancer during childhood and their peers. *Dissertation Abstracts International, 62*(09), 4224B.

Levi, R. B., & Drotar, D. (1998). Critical issues and needs in health-related quality of life assessment of children an adolescents with chronic health conditions. In D. Drotar (Ed.). *Measuring health-related quality of life in children and adolescents: Implications for research and practice* (pp. 3–24). Mahwah, NJ: Erlbaum.

Levi, R. B., & Drotar, D. (1999). Health-related quality of life in childhood cancer: Discrepancy in parent-child reports. *International Journal of Cancer,* Suppl. 12, 58–64.

Mackie, E., Hill, J., Kondryn, H., & McNally, R. (2000). Adult psychosocial outcomes in long term survivors of acute lymphoblastic leukemia and Wilms' tumor: A controlled study. *Lancet, 3555,* 1310–1314.

Margolin J., Steuber, C., & Poplack, D. (2002). Acute lymphoblastic leukemia. In P. Pizzo & D. Poplack, *Principles and practice of pediatric oncology* (4th ed., pp. 489–544). Philadelphia: Lippincott, Williams, and Wilkins.

Meeske, K., Katz, E. R., Palmer, S. N., Burwinkle, T., & Varni, J. W. (2004). Parent proxy-reported health-related quality of life and fatigue in pediatric patients diagnosed with brain tumors and acute lymphoblastic leukemia. *Cancer, 101,* 2116–2125.

Merkins, M. I., Perrin, E. C., Perrin, J. M., & Gerrity, P. S. (1989). The awareness of primary physicians of the psychological adjustment of children with a chronic illness. *Journal of Developmental and Behavioral Pediatrics, 10,* 1–6.

Mostrow, E. N., Byrne, J., Connelly, R. R., & Mulvihill, J. J. (1991). Quality of life in long term survivors of CNS tumors of childhood and adolescence. *Journal of Clinical Oncology, 9,* 592–599.

Mulhern, R. K. (1999). Correlation of the Health Utilities Index Mark 2 cognition scale and neuropsychological functioning among survivors of childhood medulloblastoma. *International Journal of Cancer,* Suppl. 12, 91–94.

Nathan, P. C., Furlong, W., & Barr, R. D. (2004). Challenges to the measurement of health-related quality of life in children receiving cancer therapy. *Pediatric Blood Cancer, 43,* 215–223.

Nicholson, H. S., Mulvihill, J. J., & Byrne, J. (1992). Late effects of therapy in adult survivors of osteosarcoma and Ewing's sarcoma. *Medical Pediatric Oncology, 20,* 6–12.

Novakovic, B., Fears, T. R., Horowitz, M. E., Tucker, M. A., & Wexler, M. A. (1997). Late effects of therapy in survivors of Ewing's sarcoma family tumors. *Journal of Pediatric Hematology/Oncology, 19,* 220–225.

Parry, C. (2003). Embracing uncertainty: An exploration of the experiences of childhood cancer survivors. *Qualitative Health Research, 13,* 227–246.

Parsons, S. K., Barlow, S. E., Levy, S. L., Supran, S. E., & Kaplan, S. H. (1999). Health related quality of life in pediatric bone marrow transplant survivors: According to whom? *International Journal of Cancer,* Suppl. 12, 46–51.

Patrick, D. L., & Erikson, P. (1993). *Health status and health policy: Quality of life in health care evaluation and resource allocation.* New York: Oxford University Press.

Patterson, J. M., Holm, K. E., & Gurney, J. G. (2004). The impact of childhood cancer on the family: A qualitative analysis of strains, resources, and coping behaviors. *Psycho-Oncology, 13,* 390–407.

Perrin, E. C., & Gerrity, P. S. (1981). There's a demon in your belly: Children's understanding of illness. *Pediatrics, 67,* 841–849.

Phipps, S., Dunavant, M., Garvie, P. A., Lensing, S., & Rai, S. N. (2002). Acute health-related quality of life in children undergoing stem cell transplant: I. Descriptive outcomes. *Bone Marrow Transplant, 29,* 425–434.

Phipps, S., Dunavant, M., Jayawardene, D., & Srivastiva, D. K. (1999). Assessment of health-related quality of life in acute inpatient settings: Use of the BASES instrument in children undergoing bone marrow transplantation. *International Journal Cancer,* Suppl. 12, 18–24.

Phipps, S., Dunavant, M., Lensing, S., & Rai, S. N. (2002). Acute health-related quality of life in children undergoing stem cell transplant: II. Medical and demographic determinants. *Bone Marrow Transplant, 29,* 435–442.

Phipps, S., Dunavant, M., Lensing, S., & Rai, S. N. (2004). Brief report: Patterns of distress in parents of children undergoing stem cell transplantation. *Pediatric Blood Cancer, 43,* 267–274.

Rigon, H., Lopes, L. F., Rosario Latorre, M. D., & Camargo, B. D. (2003). The GEPETTO program for surveillance of long-term survivors of childhood cancer: Preliminary report from a single institution in Brazil. *Medical Pediatric Oncology, 40,* 405–406.

Rosenbaum, P., Cadman, D., & Kirpalani, H. (1990). Pediatrics: Assessing quality of life. In B. Spilker (Ed.). *Quality of life assessments in clinical trials* (pp. 205–215). New York: Raven Press.

Sawyer, M., Antoniou, G., Toogood, I., & Rice, M. (1999). A comparison of parent and adolescent reports describing the health-related quality of life of adolescents treated for cancer. *International Journal of Cancer,* Suppl. 12, 39–45.

Schwartz, C. E., Feinberg, R. G., Jilinskaia, E., & Applegate, J. C. (1999). An evaluation of a psychosocial intervention for survivors of childhood cancer: Paradoxical effects of response shift over time. *Psycho-Oncology, 8,* 344–354.

Schwartz, C. L. (1999). Long term survivors of childhood cancer: the late effects of therapy. *Oncologist, 4,* 45–54.

Seid, M., Varni, J. W., Segall, D., & Kurtin, P. S. (2004). Health-related quality of life as a predictor of pediatric healthcare costs: a two-year prospective cohort analysis. *Health Quality of Life Outcomes, 2,* 48.

Shover, L. R. (1999). Psychosocial aspects of infertility and decisions about reproduction in young cancer survivors: A review. *Medical Pediatric Oncology, 33,* 53–59.

Speith, L. E. (2001). Generic health related quality of life measures for children and adolescents. In H. M. Koot and J. L. Wallander (Eds.). *Quality of life in child and adolescent illness: Concepts, methods and findings* (pp. 49–88). New York: Taylor and Francis.

Speith, L. E., & Harris, C. V. (1996). Assessment of health-related quality of life in children and adolescents: An integrative review. *Journal of Pediatric Psychology, 21,* 175–193.

Sprangers, M. A. (2002). Quality of life assessment in oncology. Achievements and challenges. *Acta Oncologica, 41,* 229–237.

Starfield, B., Bergner, M., Ensminger, M., Riley, A., Ryan, S., Green, B., et al. (1993). Adolescent health status measurement: Development of Child Health and Illness Profile. *Pediatrics, 91,* 430–435.

Szecket, N., Medin, G., Furlong, W. J., Feeny, D. H., Barr, R. D., & DePauw, S. (1999). Preliminary translation and cultural adaptation of Health Utilities Index Questionnaires for application in Argentina. *International Journal of Cancer,* Suppl. 12, 119–124.

Thomasgard, M., & Metz, W. P. (1995). The vulnerable child syndrome revisited. *Journal of Developmental and Behavioral Pediatrics, 16,* 47–53.

Vance, Y. H., Morse, R. C., Jenney, M. E., & Eiser, C. (2001). Issues in measuring quality of life in childhood cancer: Measures, proxies, and parental mental health. *Journal of Child Psychology and Psychiatry and Allied Disciplines, 42,* 661–667.

Varni, J. W., Burwinkle, T. M., Katz, E. R., Meeske, K., & Dickinson, P. (2002). The PedsQL in pediatric cancer: Reliability and validity of the Pediatric Quality of Life Inventory Generic Core Scales, Multidimensional Fatigue Scale, and Cancer Module. *Cancer, 94,* 2090–2106.

Varni, J. W., Katz, E. R., Seid, M., Quiggins, D. F. J. L., Friedman-Bender, A., & Castro, C. M. (1998). The Pediatric Cancer Quality of Life Inventory (PCQL). I. Instrument development, descriptive statistics, and cross-informant variance. *Journal of Behavioral Medicine, 21,* 179–204.

Wallander, J. L. (1992). Theory driven research in pediatric psychology: A little bit on why and how. *Journal of Pediatric Psychology, 17,* 521–535.

Wallander, J. L., Schmitt, M., & Koot, H. M. (2001). Quality of life measurement in children and adolescents: Issues, instruments, and applications. *Journal of Clinical Psychology, 57,* 571–585.

Ware, J. E., Jr. (1984). Conceptualizing disease impact and treatment outcomes. *Cancer, 15*(Suppl.), 2316–2323.

Waters, E. B., Wake, M. A., Hesketh, K. D., Ashley, D. M., & Smibert, E. (2002). Health-related quality of life of children with acute lymphoblastic leukemia: Comparisons and correlations between parent and clinician reports. *International Journal of Cancer, 103,* 514–518.

Wilson, I. B., & Cleary, P. D. (1994). Linking clinical variables with health related quality of life: A conceptual model of patient outcomes. *Journal of the American Medical Association, 273,* 59–65.

Wolfe, J., Friebert, S. E., & Hilden, J. (2002). Caring for children with advanced cancer integrating palliative care. *Pediatric Clinics of North America, 49,* 1043–1062.

World Health Organization. (1948). *Constitution of the World Health Organization.* Geneva, Switzerland: Author.

World Health Organization: Division of Mental Health. (1993). *WHO-QOL Study protocol: The development of the World Health Organization quality of life assessment instrument.* Geneva, Switzerland: Author.

Yeh, C. H., & Hung, L. C. (2003). Construct validity of newly developed quality of life assessment instrument for child and adolescent cancer patients in Taiwan. *Psycho-Oncology, 12,* 345–356.

Zebrack, B. (2000). QOL of long term survivors of leukemia and lymphoma. *Journal of Psychosocial Oncology, 18,* 39–59.

Zebrack, B. J., & Chesler, M. A. (2001). A psychometric analysis of the Quality of Life-Cancer Survivors (QOL-CS) in survivors of childhood cancer. *Quality of Life Research, 10,* 319–329.

Zeltzer, L. K., Chen, E., Weiss, R., Guo, M. D., Robison, L. L., Meadows, A. T., et al. (1997). Comparison of psychologic outcome in adult survivors of childhood acute lymphoblastic leukemia versus sibling controls: a cooperative Children's Cancer Group and National Institutes of Health study. *Journal of Clinical Oncology, 15,* 547–556.

Cynthia D. Myers, Margaret L. Stuber,

and Lonnie K. Zeltzer

# Spirituality and Complementary and Alternative Medicine

The use of complementary and alternative medicine by children with cancer appears to be common, with 31% to 84% of pediatric oncology samples reportedly using at least one complementary or alternative therapy according to surveys conducted in several regions of the world, including North America (Fernandez et al., 1998; T. Friedman et al., 1997; Kelly et al., 2000; Neuhouser et al., 2001); Australia (Sawyer et al., 1994); the Netherlands (Grootenhuis et al., 1998); Finland (Mottonen & Uhari, 1997); and Taiwan (Yeh et al., 2000). This chapter reviews the medical literature regarding complementary and alternative medicine in relation to pediatric oncology.

To begin, the issue of defining complementary and alternative medicine is addressed. Studies of complementary and alternative medicine use by the general adult population and by adults with cancer as well as by pediatric oncology samples are described to highlight issues concerning definitions of complementary and alternative medicine and to ascertain the prevalence of use of specific complementary and alternative medicine modalities. Available reports of clinical trials testing complementary and alternative medicine modalities in the context of pediatric cancer are summarized. Finally, a discussion is provided on spirituality and religion in relation to complementary and alternative medicine and the challenges faced by children with cancer and their families.

## Defining Complementary and Alternative Medicine

Complementary and alternative medicine was described by the National Center for Complementary and Alternative Medicine (NCCAM) at the National Institutes of Health as "a group of diverse medical and health care systems, practices, and products that are not presently considered to be part of conventional medicine." The NCCAM indicated that the term *complementary therapy* refers to therapies used in conjunction with conventional medicine; *alternative therapies* are those that are used in place of conventional medicine, for which *conventional medicine* is defined as medicine as practiced by holders of medical doctor (M.D.) or doctor of osteopathy (D.O.) degrees and other health professionals, including physical therapists, psychologists, and registered nurses. According to the NCCAM, additional terms for conventional medicine include allopathy, Western, mainstream, orthodox, regular medicine, and biomedicine; additional terms for complementary and alternative medicine include unconventional, nonconventional, and unproven medicine.

The NCCAM groups complementary and alternative medicine therapies into five categories or domains: biologically based therapies, manipulative and body-based therapies, energy therapies, mind-body interventions, and alternative medical systems. Biologically based therapies use substances found in nature, such as foods, herbal remedies that employ plant preparations for therapeutic effects, products derived from animals, such as shark cartilage, as well as vitamins and other dietary supplements. Manipulative and body-based methods are based on manipulation or movement of one or more parts of the body, and include chiropractic or osteopathic manipulations and massage. Energy therapies are of two types–biofield or bioelectromagnetic. Biofield therapies (e.g., Reiki, Therapeutic Touch) purport to manipulate energy fields within and around the human body. Bioelectromagnetic-based therapies involve the unconventional use of electromagnetic fields, such as pulsed, alternating current, or direct current fields. Mind-body interventions include techniques that aim to increase the mind's capacity to enhance bodily function and reduce symptoms. The NCCAM includes mental healing; expressive therapies such as music, art, or dance therapy; and spiritual practices such as meditation and prayer among the mind-body interventions and supports research on all of these as well as on medical uses of hypnosis and relaxation.

Alternative medical systems are built on complete systems of theory and practice and may make use of therapies from the biological, body-based, mind-body, and energy domains. Examples from Western cultures include homeopathic medicine, which aims to stimulate healing by administering minute doses of plant extracts and minerals, and naturopathic medicine, which aims to restore health through combined treatment that may include homeopathic remedies, herbal medicine, nutritional modification, hydrotherapy, physical therapies, and counseling. An example from Eastern cultures is traditional Chinese medicine, which incorporates the use of herbal medicine, physical therapies, acupuncture, and other therapies.

The classification scheme provided by the NCCAM provides a useful framework that may lead to more consistent use of terminology in this research area. However, in the medical literature to date, terms have been used inconsistently across studies. For example, the terms *complementary* and *alternative* have often been used interchangeably and denoted by the single abbreviated acronym CAM. An older term, *holistic*, has sometimes been used as a synonym for complementary and alternative medicine (e.g., see HolisticKids.org, discussed in Whelen & Dvorkin, 2003). Holistic medicine emphasizes the care of the whole person—body, mind, and spirit—in relation to that person's community and environment, as well as the promotion of healthy lifestyles for practitioners and patients alike (Graham-Pole, 2001b). A newer term, "*integrative medicine*," refers to the coordinated synthesis of conventional medicine and complementary therapies (e.g., see Edelblute, 2003; Faass, 2001).

Complicating matters, the boundary demarcating complementary and alternative medicine from conventional medicine is somewhat porous, with therapies once considered unconventional in Western medicine moving into acceptance as scientific evidence accumulates for their safety and effectiveness. For example, acupuncture is increasingly accepted as a legitimate therapy for chemotherapy-related nausea (see review by Weiger et al., 2002). Finally, the list of therapies considered complementary or alternative medicine has varied across studies according to the views of the investigators, contributing to the broad range of estimates of unconventional medicine use.

In two often-cited surveys by Eisenberg and colleagues (Eisenberg et al., 1993, 1998), well-established behavioral medicine interventions (e.g., relaxation training, support groups, hypnosis, biofeedback) were included as unconventional therapies, defined as "medical interventions not widely taught at U.S. medical schools or generally available at U.S. hospitals" (Eisenberg et al., 1993, p. 246). As a result, well-studied behavioral medicine interventions were effectively grouped with unproven therapies such as energy healing. Subsequent surveys conducted on the use of complementary and alternative medicine have used a similar approach. This approach obscures the fact that embedded within the frequency of use statistics for visits to professionals for unconventional medicine services are visits to professionals for conventional psychotherapy during which well-studied behavioral interventions are commonly used (R. Friedman et al., 1997).

Ernst and Cassileth (1998) reviewed literature on the use of complementary and alternative medicine by adults with cancer, and found an overall prevalence of 31.4% of adult cancer patients using complementary and alternative therapies, with a range of 7% to 64% across 26 surveys. The authors attributed the wide range across surveys to the lack of specificity and inconsistent definitions of complementary and alternative medicine and suggested that the higher prevalence in some studies may be partly caused by inclusion of mainstream interventions such as counseling and group therapy. Ernst and Cassileth's observation that these two mainstream interventions are labeled complementary and alternative medicine by some investigators highlights the lack of a universal definition of the constituent therapies comprising complementary and alternative medicine and echoes the sentiment noted by R. Friedman et al., (1997) about the inclusion of behavioral medicine in the statistics reported by Eisenberg et al. These issues highlight the importance of examining the constituent therapies when interpreting the results of survey research about complementary and alternative medicine use.

## Use of Complementary and Alternative Medicine by Pediatric Cancer Patients

A growing number of studies has been conducted to describe use of complementary and alternative medicine by children. Results indicate that the use of these therapies by pediatric oncology patients is common. Complementary and alternative medicine is used with the intention of managing symptoms or treatment side effects as well as for the intended purpose of curing disease or slowing its progression. As with use of complementary and alternative medicine by adults with cancer (e.g., Richardson et al., 2000), complementary and alternative medicine use by youths was usually not reported to physicians. Therapies were usually used to complement rather than replace conventional cancer treatment, although there have been controversial instances when parents have discontinued children's conventional treatment in favor of unproven alternative therapies (e.g., Burgio & Locatelli, 2000).

Parents of Australian pediatric oncology patients (N = 48, age 4 to 16 years) reported that nearly one half (46%) of the children had used at least one therapy these investigators termed "alternative" since receiving the cancer diagnosis (Sawyer et al., 1994). Parents viewed the alternative therapies as harmless and useful and only disclosed their use to treating physicians less than one half (44%) of the time. The most common alternative therapies employed included imagery, hypnotherapy, and relaxation. Others included diets, multivitamins, spiritualism, faith healing, meditation, megavitamins, chiropractic, and homeopathy.

In 1997, T. Friedman et al. assessed parent-reported use of "alternative therapies," which the authors defined as "any practice not prescribed by a physician or not considered a proven medical treatment" (p. 4) for their children. Parents of pediatric cancer patients ($n = 81$) and control group ($n = 80$) children attending a continuity care clinic for well-child checkups or non-cancer acute care in the southeastern United States participated. The majority of the cancer patients (65%) and 51% of the non-cancer patients used some form of alternative therapy. The most common alternative therapy parents had used for their children in both groups was prayer (64% of the cancer group, 40% of the control group). Many parents questioned the inclusion of prayer as an alternative therapy, but the investigators included it because it is not prescribed by a physician or considered to be a standard part of care. Excluding prayer, 45% of the cancer group and 42% of the non-cancer group were using alternative therapy. Parents who discussed alternative therapies with their child's physician or oncologist were most often parents of a child with cancer (53%), of higher income (59%), and white (47%).

Mottonen and Uhari (1997) collected daily diary data for 2 years to compare the use of micronutrients and alternative drugs (e.g., shark liver tablets, plant extracts) by 15 children in Finland ($n = 15$; mean age 7.3 years, range 4.3–12.6 years) with acute lymphoblastic leukemia (ALL) in the remission stage, most of whom had reached the continuation phase of therapy, and 26 randomly selected healthy children matched for age, sex, and socioeconomic status. Children who had been treated for ALL had taken preparations of multivitamins and trace elements, alternative medicines, fluoride tablets, and other minerals (except for iron) to a statistically significant greater extent than comparison controls. Of children with ALL, 40% had taken alternative medicines compared to 7.7% of the control group.

In the Netherlands, Grootenhuis et al. (1998) asked the questions "Did you ever use alternative therapies?" and "What type of alternative treatment did you use?" of parents of pediatric cancer patients 8 to18 years old. Forty-three of the children ($N=84$) were in first continuous remission, and 41 had relapsed disease or had a second malignancy. Close to one third (31%) of children used one or more alternative therapy. More children with relapsed disease used alternative therapies, compared to children whose disease was in remission (16%). One child in the remission group and seven children in the relapse group used two kinds of therapies. Homeopathy and the macrobiotic diet were the most popular of the alternative modalities ($n=15$). Next in popularity was a group that included massage, applied kinesiology, and light therapy ($n=9$). Use of imagery healing, psychic healing, or faith healers was the third most popular ($n=6$).

A retrospective population-based survey was administered by questionnaire to 366 parents of children diagnosed with cancer in British Columbia between 1989 and 1995 (Fernandez et al., 1998). An introductory letter to parents provided the investigators' definition of "alternative therapies," by which they indicated nutritional, herbal, and pharmacological or biological interventions, and their definition of "complementary therapies," in which they included psychological and behavioral approaches. Alternative therapies were further defined as lacking in empirical evaluation and lack of recognized effectiveness by conventional medicine. By contrast, complementary therapies were described as those used in addition to conventional medicine to improve the well-being of the child and relieve symptoms. Parents indicated that 42% of the children had used complementary or alternative medicine therapies, with relaxation/imagery, massage, therapeutic touch, herbal teas, plant extracts, and vitamins among the most frequently employed therapies. Predictors of increased use included prior use of complementary and alternative medicine, a positive attitude toward complementary and alternative medicine, information about complementary or alternative medicine from family, friends, or alternative caregivers, high risk of death at diagnosis, and advanced education of at least one parent. Reasons for non-utilization included lack of knowledge about complementary and alternative medicine and fear of interference with the primary medical therapy. Complementary therapies were most often used in conjunction with (as opposed to in replacement of) conventional treatment; however, parents of 8 patients with a poor prognosis reported using alternative therapies in place of recommended conventional medical treatments. Many parents reported the use of complementary and alternative medicine therapies for the intended purpose of slowing cancer progression (35%) or curing cancer (40%). Most parents (82%) indicated that they wanted to be sure to do everything possible for their child. The role of spirituality also was assessed in the questionnaire, but not as a complementary and alternative medicine therapy, because the investigators believed that many parents would view spirituality as "inseparable from one's general philosophy of life" (P. 1282).

A study of 63 pediatric oncology patients at least 2 months post-diagnosis was carried out in Taiwan to study the use of non-Western therapies including traditional Chinese medicine, spiritual practices, and folk remedies in conjunction with Western conventional oncology medicine (Yeh et al., 2000). Of children, 73% had used at least one non-Western therapy. Most common was the use by 48% of children of packaged liquid or powder remedies purported to be highly nutritious and able to limit side effects, increase immune function, and improve prognosis. Spiritual practices, including worship in Buddhist temples or consulting a shaman, were also used to complement Western treatment (41%). Folk medicine and herbal remedies (28%) were used, and their potential toxicity when used concurrently with conventional treatment was not known. Some of the children (19%) had been treated both by practitioners of Western medicine and practitioners of traditional Chinese medicine. Only 10 parents disclosed the concurrent use of non-Western therapies to the Western-trained oncologist. Parents who did not disclose were concerned that such disclosure might be interpreted as implying distrust or dissatisfaction with standard treatments or imperil their relationships with these key individuals in their child's care. Use of non-Western approaches was not predicted by education or the family's social status.

An interview study was conducted with parents of 75 cancer patients aged 3 months to 26 years, as well as with 14 of the patients themselves, who ranged in age from 10 to 26 years (Kelly et al., 2000). Patients were at least 3 months post-diagnosis and receiving conventional care for cancer or follow-up for conventional care at an urban academic hospital in the northeastern part of the United States. Of respondents, 84% reported that the patient had used one or more forms of "unconventional therapy," defined as an agent or practice initiated since diagnosis and not part of the standard care of the child with cancer. Most therapies were changes in diet or nutrition, herbal preparations, and mind-body approaches in conjunction with conventional treatment. Use of unconventional therapy was not predicted by cancer diagnosis, race, ethnicity, socioeconomic status, or education. One half of the therapies used were not reported to the treating physician. Of note, most patients using unconventional therapies (85%) were concurrently enrolled in clinical trials of experimental medical therapies for cancer. The potential impact of unconventional modalities on symptoms, quality of life, and other outcomes targeted in clinical trials is largely unknown.

In Saskatchewan, 44 parents of children age 14 or younger at the time of cancer diagnosis completed questionnaires and interviews about the child's use of "unconventional therapies," meaning therapies outside of the standard medical treatments (Bold & Leis, 2001). Sixteen families (36%) used these to complement medical treatments, with the intended goals of fighting cancer, boosting immunity, and improving quality of life. One family substituted unconventional therapy for medical treatment. Unlike most studies in this field, most treating physicians (72%) were informed of the unconventional therapies. Herbal remedies were most often used (47%), followed by 19% using foot reflexology, aromatherapy, color therapy, or massage therapy. Thirteen percent used relaxation, musical techniques, acupuncture, aboriginal healing, or other healing traditions.

Parents of 75 children in the northwestern part of the United States with a first primary neoplasm were interviewed by telephone regarding the child's use of complementary and alternative medicine (Neuhouser et al., 2001). Nearly three quarters (73%) of children in the sample had used one or more complementary and alternative therapies: 35% used herbal remedies, 28% used high-doses of vitamins, and 21% sought treatment from a complementary therapy practitioner such as an acupuncturist or naturopathic doctor. Most parents (75%) were very satisfied with their child's medical doctors. Use of complementary and alternative medicine was highest in children whose parents were not fully satisfied with the physician. Parents generally attributed substantial improvements in their child's health and well-being to complementary and alternative medicine, although two parents attributed significant adverse side effects (e.g., nausea, vomiting) to use of herbal products.

Anonymous questionnaire data were collected from 118 parents with a child at least one month post-diagnosis and currently receiving cancer treatment or having completed treatment within the past two years in the northeastern United States (Gagnon & Recklitis, 2003). Almost half (46%) of the children had used a complementary therapy during their lifetime, and a third used a complementary therapy after diagnosis. Parents' decision to use complementary therapies for children related in part to their own preferences for an active role in medical decision-making.

Molassiotis and Cubbin (2004) gathered questionnaire data in the United Kingdom from 49 parents (51% response rate) of children age 5 to 17 treated conventionally for cancer and 28 months post-diagnosis, on average. Thirty-three percent of children were using complementary therapies, most often more than one, with multivitamins (56%), aromatherapy massage (50%), and diets and dietary supplements (38%) the most common. Parents rated aromatherapy massage as the most helpful. Most parents (63%) administered complementary therapies daily for purposes of using every possible option in healthcare, improving the child's general health, helping the child relax, decreasing the child's anxiety, and reducing treatment side effects.

Results of a questionnaire study of parents in the southeastern United States indicated that nearly one half (47%) of a sample of pediatric oncology patients ($n = 195$) had used one or more complementary and alternative therapy at some time since receiving a cancer diagnosis (McCurdy et al., 2003). Among the most commonly employed therapies were faith healing (41%), megavitamins/minerals (35%), massage (25%), other dietary supplements (22%), relaxation techniques (22%), and herbal medicines/teas (20%). For those who used complementary and alternative medicine, 82% did so with the intention of treating the cancer. One fourth believed the complementary or alternative therapy would definitely help cure the condition. Complementary and alternative medicine use by 41% was not discussed with their physicians. Children in families who reported themselves to be "very" religious were more likely to use complementary and alternative medicine than those in families identifying as "somewhat" or "not at all" religious. The investigators noted that prayer has been inconsistently included in research on complementary and alternative medicine, and they chose not to identify prayer as a type of complementary and alternative medicine in their study because of the high prevalence of prayer in their geographic region. However, they did inquire about the use of prayer and found that 87% of the respondents reported regularly praying for the patient. Reanalyzing the complementary and alternative medicine data to include prayer, the prevalence of complementary and alternative medicine use in their sample increased from nearly one half to 92%.

A cross sectional survey was conducted in which questionnaires were completed by parents (80% response rate) of 92 infants and children (age range 0 to 18 years) in active treatment for cancer at a large pediatric hospital in Quebec (Martel et al., 2005). Approximately half (49%) of the children had partaken of at least one complementary therapy during the 2-month period prior to questionnaire completion. Spiritual or mental strategies were used by 35% of children, including prayer (41%), relaxation (28%), imagery (25%), and others. Physical strategies were used by 33% of patients, with massage therapy the most common (67%). Symptom reduction was most commonly the goal.

To summarize, although definitions of complementary and alternative medicine have varied across studies, making direct comparisons of prevalence of use inappropriate in some cases, it does appear clear that the use of these therapies is common among children with cancer. Motivations for their use include managing symptoms, treating underlying disease, and making sure that all avenues of potential benefit have been explored. Clinical research on these therapies is needed to judge their safety and effectiveness and to understand the predictors and mechanisms of treatment.

## Clinical Trials of Complementary and Alternative Medicine in Pediatric Oncology

To facilitate evaluation of the scientific knowledge base regarding the effects of complementary and alternative medicine modalities for children with cancer, reports of clinical trials of complementary and alternative therapies tested on this patient population were complied from two electronic databases of biomedical references: the PubMed database provided by the National Library of Medicine and the Cumulative Index of Nursing and Allied Health Literature. Reports are grouped according to the categories developed by the NCCAM and are presented in the following order: biologically based therapies, manipulative and body-based methods, energy therapies, alternative medical systems, and mind-body interventions.

### Clinical Trials of Biologically Based Therapies

No randomized clinical trials of biologically based therapies in pediatric oncology samples were located using search terms that were gleaned from prevalence studies on the use of such therapies: shark cartilage, diet, herbal, Laetrile, megavitamin, melatonin, mistletoe, phytotreatment, plant, or vitamin. One Phase II study was located on the use of homoharringtonine, a plant alkaloid derived from a Chinese evergreen tree. Children with refractory acute myelogenous leukemia (N = 37) were enrolled in the study, with 28 evaluated for response. Complete response was obtained in 4 children and a partial response in 1 (5/28 = 18% response rate). Significant toxicities included prolonged severe myelosupression in all responsive patients and neuropathic pain in 2 patients. The investigators concluded that the agent has activity with tolerable toxicity against chemotherapy-resistant acute myelogenous leukemia in children and warrants further clinical evaluation (Bell,

Chang, Weinstein, 2001). An open label study by Garami and colleagues (2004) in a sample of children under age 18 with malignant disease compared standard anticancer treatment (n = 11) to the same plus self-selected treatment with a medical nutriment made of fermented wheat germ extract (n = 11). Febrile neutropenic events were reportedly fewer and less frequent in the experimental group.

## Clinical Trials of Manipulative and Body-Based Methods

Three reports of pilot studies of massage therapy were located. Field and colleagues (2001) randomly assigned children (n = 20, mean age 6.9 years) with ALL to receive daily massages for 1 month from one of their parents in addition to medical care or to be on a waiting list and medical care. The child's complete blood count was assessed on the first and last days of the study. Parents and children rated their mood before and after the first massage and on the last day of the trial. Results suggest massage was associated with increased white blood cell count in children, short-term reduction in negative mood for children and parents, and reduced negative affect in parents over the 1-month trial.

In a pilot study involving 21 children undergoing hospitalization for stem cell transplantation, Phipps (2002) found that 15-minute massages, administered daily by parents who were provided with instruction in basic massage techniques, were a favorite component, as reported by patients and parents, of a multi-component health promotion intervention. In a follow-up study with children scheduled for stem cell transplantation, Phipps and colleagues (2005) randomized 20 children to professional massage 3 times per week (from admission to 3 weeks post-transplant), 20 children to parent-administered massage on the same schedule, and 10 to standard care. Primary outcomes were somatic distress and mood disturbance. Secondary outcomes were anti-nausea and narcotic pain medications, days spent in hospital, and days to engraftment. No significant differences were observed between professional and parent-administered massage on the primary outcomes, nor between either massage and standard care, although there were trends suggesting benefit of massage. There was a trend for the massage groups to have shorter hospital stays and to engraft faster than the standard care control.

A large-scale, National Institutes of Health-funded, multi-site randomized clinical trial is currently under way to study the effects of massage therapy provided by professional massage therapists three times per week for 30 minutes as part of multicomponent therapy for children hospitalized during bone marrow transplantation. (Phipps, accessed October 12, 2005) (see also Humor in the Clinical Trials of Mind-Body Interventions section and chapter 5, this volume, on transplantation). The National Institutes of Health is also funding a feasibility study of massage therapy for palliation of pain in children with advanced or progressive cancer (Myers, accessed October 12, 2005) and a large-scale, multi-site randomized clinical trial of massage therapy for palliation of pain, management of physical and emotional symptoms and distress, and effects on quality of life in adults with advanced cancer (Kutner, accessed October 12, 2005).

Regarding risks associated with massage, Weiger et al. (2002) found no studies reporting that massage promoted tumor metastasis. Weiger et al. recommended that massage be avoided directly over known tumors or even predictable metastasis sites without known disease, and urged caution regarding massage when patients present with bony metastases, tissues damaged by surgical or radiation therapy, thrombocytopenia or anticoagulant therapy, hypercoagulability and thrombus formation; and stents or other prosthetic devices.

## Clinical Trials of Energy Therapies

Searching the terms magnetic, healing, Reiki, Therapeutic Touch, and energy produced no records of published clinical trials of energy therapies in children with cancer. Although the clinical use of such therapies by health professionals is increasingly common (Miles & True, 2003), little research has been conducted to test these therapies. A Phase II trial of Reiki energy therapy compared pain, quality of life, and analgesic use in 24 adult patients with cancer pain who received either standard opioid management plus rest or standard opioid management plus Reiki therapy. Pain ratings, blood pressure, heart rate, and respirations were assessed both prior to and after rest or treatment periods, which took place 1 hour after the first afternoon analgesic dosage. Participants receiving Reiki reported improved pain control following treatment and improved quality of life but no overall reduction in opioid use (Olson et al., 2003).

The National Institutes of Health is currently supporting several developmental studies on the effects of energy therapies in adult patients with various medical conditions. For example, one investigation is under way examining the effects of Reiki on blood levels of prostate-specific antigen and self-report of anxiety and stress hormones in men with prostate cancer (Klein, accessed October 12, 2005). The possibility of developing a placebo intervention for use in a placebo-controlled study of Reiki has successfully been demonstrated in a sample of adults (Mansour et al., 1999). Studies are needed to test the possibility of conducting controlled research on energy therapies in pediatric samples.

### Clinical Trials of Alternative Medical Systems

Searching the terms acupuncture, Ayurvedic, homeopath, and naturopath did not lead to any records of clinical trials using these alternative medical systems in pediatric oncology samples. Studies are needed to test these modalities in pediatric samples.

### Clinical Trials of Mind-Body Interventions

#### *Hypnosis*

Clinical trials of hypnosis for symptom control in pediatric samples were located in the extant literature. This psychological intervention is used with the intended purpose of helping children to narrow and focus their attention to reduce discomfort and distress associated with medical procedures and symptoms and enhance children's feelings of control and competence. The effects of hypnosis as compared to non-hypnotic techniques (e.g., deep breathing, distraction) on pain and anxiety have been the subject of several studies. Zeltzer and LeBaron (1982) studied 33 pediatric oncology patients who ranged in age from 6 to 17 years (mean age 10.06 years, standard deviation [*SD*] ± 3.17 years) during lumbar punctures (LPs) and bone marrow aspirations (BMAs). Pain during LP was reduced only by hypnosis; anxiety was reduced by both hypnosis and non-hypnotic techniques, with greater reduction in the hypnosis group. Pain during BMA was reduced by hypnotic and non-hypnotic techniques, with greater reduction associated with hypnosis; anxiety was reduced only by hypnosis.

Results were reported for another hypnosis study of 16 adolescent oncology patients (mean age 14 years, *SD* ± 1.6 years) undergoing BMAs, LPs, and chemotherapeutic injections; the study used a multiple-baseline design with subjects as their own control, and it indicated that anxiety and discomfort were both reduced (Kellerman et al., 1983).

Katz, Kellerman, and Ellenberg (1987) studied the effects of hypnosis on pain and distress in 36 children aged 6 to 11 years with ALL, all of whom had undergone at least 3 BMAs prior to enrollment in the study and were scheduled for additional BMAs. Children were randomly assigned to a hypnosis intervention, including training in hypnosis and self-hypnosis, or to a play comparison group. Highlighting the importance of multimodal assessment, hypnosis and play were both associated with reduced self-report of pain and distress associated with BMA but were not associated with reduced observational measures.

Wall and Womack (1989) compared the effects of hypnotic and cognitive distraction strategies on pain and anxiety associated with BMA/LP in a sample of 20 pediatric oncology outpatients aged 5 to 18 years. Participants were assessed for anticipatory and procedural pain and anxiety in relation to BMA/LP procedures. Patients were taught either hypnotic or cognitive distraction procedures during two practice sessions and employed these at their next scheduled BMA/LP, with assessments again pre- and post-procedure. Both strategies were associated with pain reduction; neither was associated with anxiety reduction. The degree of hypnotizability did not predict pain reduction.

Liossi and Hatira (1999) randomly assigned 30 pediatric cancer patients (aged 5 to 15 years) to one of three groups: clinical hypnosis, cognitive behavioral coping skills training, or a no intervention control condition. Patients who received either hypnosis or cognitive behavioral coping skills training reported less pain and pain-related anxiety in association with BMAs than did patients in the control group. Hypnosis and coping skills training were similarly effective in the relief of pain.

Children reported more anxiety and exhibited more behavioral distress in the coping skills training group than in the hypnosis group.

In a second study, Liossi and Hatira (2003) assigned 80 pediatric oncology patients (6 to 16 years of age) undergoing LPs to one of four groups: direct hypnosis with standard medical treatment, indirect hypnosis with standard medical treatment, attention control with standard medical treatment, and standard medical treatment alone. Patients in the hypnosis groups reported less pain and anxiety and demonstrated less behavioral distress than those in the control groups. In contrast to the findings reported by Wall and Womak (1989), hypnotizability was associated with treatment benefit in the hypnosis groups. Therapeutic benefit declined when patients used self-hypnosis, highlighting the potentially critical importance of a therapist in such an intervention.

Hypnosis also has been studied for its usefulness in controlling nausea, vomiting, and distress when pediatric oncology patients must endure various medical procedures. Hypnosis and nonhypnotic relaxation/distraction techniques were compared to an attention-placebo control group in 54 randomly assigned pediatric cancer patients who ranged in age from 5 to 17 years. Children reported significant chemotherapy-related nausea or vomiting during baseline assessment. With anticipatory and post-chemotherapy distress, nausea, vomiting, and functional disruption assessed by observation and interview, children receiving cognitive distraction/relaxation maintained symptoms at a steady level, and those receiving hypnosis showed general reduction in symptoms over time. Children in the placebo group had generally increased symptoms over time (Zeltzer et al., 1991). In another randomized study, hypnosis and supportive counseling were equally effective in reducing chemotherapy-related nausea, vomiting, and distress, and symptomatic improvement was maintained (Zeltzer et al., 1984).

### *Expressive Therapies: Music, Art, Dance*

An uncontrolled pilot study of music therapy was conducted with 65 pediatric oncology patients ranging in age from 6 months to 17 years (mean 7 years, *SD* 4.8 years) (Barrera et al., 2002). Children were at different stages of their illness and treatment (40% newly diagnosed; 25% on chemotherapy treatment; 10% palliative care; 25% other), and diagnoses included leukemias ($n = 45$) and other malignancies ($n = 20$). When a child was experiencing difficulty with a central line, taking medication, blood work, positioning following an LP, or dressing change, one to three 15- to 45-minute therapy sessions were provided by an accredited music therapist in the inpatient hospital room. Outcomes as assessed on the faces pain scale, completed pre- and post-intervention session by children at least 3 years old or by parents of younger children, indicated an improvement following music therapy. Also, parents perceived children who actively engaged in the music sessions as more active. Comments from children and parents provided qualitative data indicating that the intervention was associated with relaxation, provided a welcome distraction from symptoms, and was well received by children and their parents. Additional small pilot studies with pediatric oncology samples (Robb, 2000; Robb & Ebberts, 2003a, 2003b), coupled with the findings from studies of psychological and physiological effects of music therapy with adult oncology patients (Burns et al., 2001; Smith et al., 2001) and healthy adults (Bittman et al., 2001), suggest that music therapy merits further study in pediatric populations.

An uncontrolled outcome study of art therapy was conducted for 32 children (aged 2–14 years) with leukemia (Favara-Scacco et al., 2001). The art therapy intervention prior to, during, and after LPs had several components, including clinical dialogue to calm children and help them cope with painful procedures; visual imagination; medical play to clarify illness, eliminate doubts, and offer control; structured and free drawing; and dramatization to help children accept body changes. Children provided with art therapy from their initial hospitalization reportedly exhibited greater collaborative behavior and fewer resistive behaviors compared to children treated before the institution of the art therapy program. They or their parents asked for art therapy when the medical intervention had to be repeated. Parents declared themselves better able to manage their child's painful procedures when art therapy was offered. The findings of this uncontrolled study are echoed in reports from existing clinical programs that incorporate the expressive arts into comprehensive care of pediatric oncology patients (Cohen & Walco, 1999; Graham-Pole, 2001a; Lane & Graham-Pole, 1994), suggesting the importance of further investigations of incorporating these therapies into caring for this patient population.

### *Humor*

Results of a pilot study testing a multi-component health promotion intervention for pediatric patients during hospitalization for bone marrow transplantation found that humor and massage were rated as more helpful than the other components typically employed for pediatric patients hospitalized with bone marrow transplants (Phipps, 2002), leading to funding by the National Institutes of Health of a large-scale, multi-site, randomized clinical trial that is currently under way to test the effects of humor and massage as adjuncts to care for children undergoing bone marrow or stem cell transplant (Phipps, accessed October 12, 2005; see also the discussion in the Clinical Trials of Manipulative and Body-Based Therapies in this chapter and see chapter 5 on transplantation).

In the ongoing three-group clinical trial, one group of children is receiving humor and the massage interventions, a second group of children is receiving the humor and massage interventions while their parents are receiving massage and relaxation training, and a third group of children is receiving standard care. The humor intervention involves education about the physical and emotional benefits of laughter and participation in humor activities (e.g., watching a comedy video). Primary outcomes measured in the study include child positive affect, somatic distress, and mood disturbance as well as parental positive affect and distress. Additional objectives of the ongoing study include the examination of the impact of interventions on short-term medical outcomes and measures at 6 months post-treatment of child adjustment and child and parent symptoms of posttraumatic stress. The role of positive affect and dispositional optimism as mediators and moderators of the intervention on child and parent well-being will be tested.

The use of humor as a medical intervention was highlighted by Norman Cousin's narrative report of his own use of comic films and television footage as an aid to cope with a painful medical condition (Cousins, 1976). Researchers have since documented what appear to be salutogenic effects on psychological and physiological parameters associated with humor or laughter in studies of healthy men (Berk et al., 2001) and women (Bennet et al., 2003), including analgesic effects reported in studies using experimental pain stimuli (Cogan et al., 1987; Hudak et al., 1991; Weisenberg et al., 1995). One investigation of 30 healthy children and teenagers found that participants watching comedy shows during laboratory pain were able to withstand the noxious stimuli longer than when they were not watching the comedy shows (Stuber, 2002). Collectively, these studies support continued investigation of humor as a potentially viable and enjoyable intervention.

### *Spiritual Practices*

One pilot study was located with the search terms prayer, spiritual healing, meditation, or distant healing. Names of 10 of 18 leukemic children from a hospital practice in the northeastern United States were randomly selected and sent to a Protestant prayer group in the northwestern United States who prayed daily for the 10 children (Collipp, 1969). After 15 months of prayer, 7 of 10 children in the group receiving prayer were alive, and 2 of 8 children in the control group were alive. Treating physicians were not informed about group membership until after data collection was completed. The result was not significant at a 95% significance level, but there was a trend favoring prayer. Systematic reviews of the existing literature on laboratory and clinical studies of distant healing in other populations (e.g., prayer, mental healing, spiritual healing) collectively suggest that distant healing is more than a placebo, although methodological weaknesses in most studies limit interpretation of the data (see Astin et al., 2000; Crawford et al., 2003; Ernst, 2003).

As an example of the type of studies that are being carried out with adult oncology patients in this relatively new area of scientific inquiry, the National Institutes of Health supported a double-blind, randomized clinical trial on the effects of *distant healing intentionality*, defined as "mental intention on behalf of one person, to benefit another at a distance," on survival time and loss of function in approximately 150 adults diagnosed with glioblastoma. Prior to beginning radiation therapy, participants were randomly assigned to either standard treatment plus distant healing or to standard treatment alone. Experienced "healers" from diverse schools and backgrounds spent

1 hour per day three times per week for 2 weeks sending a "mental intention for the health and well-being" for each participant assigned to them. Each participant in the distant healing group was assigned to another healer every 2 weeks for 20 weeks. Participants and healers did not meet in person. Hope and expectation were control variables (Freinkel, accessed October 12, 2005).

## Spiritual and Religious Practices: Complementary, Alternative, or Mainstays?

We reviewed studies on the prevalence of complementary and alternative medicine use and found that when spiritual practices such as prayer are denoted as complementary and alternative medicine, they emerge as among the most frequently used complementary and alternative medicine modalities (e.g., T. Friedman et al., 1997; McCurdy et al., 2003; Richardson et al., 2000; Yeh et al., 2000). However, we also found that survey respondents (e.g., see T. Friedman et al., 1997) and investigators alike (e.g., see Fernandez et al., 1998; McCurdy et al., 2003) have questioned the inclusion of spiritual and religious practices as complementary and alternative medicine, viewing such practices as inseparable from everyday life for most people. It has been reported that an estimated 95% of the American public professes a belief in a higher power or God (Gallup & Lindsay, 1999, cited in Miller & Thoresen, 2003).

Participation in spiritual and religious activities has been demonstrated to be protective of health (Miller & Thoresen, 2003; Seeman et al., 2003) and to contribute importantly and uniquely to the ability to cope with serious illness (Pargament, 1997; Pendleton et al., 2002). Confronting the life-changing onset of a serious illness in a loved one may increase or decrease an individual's involvement in a religious belief system and result in a profound reevaluation of one's spiritual beliefs (Penson et al., 2001). Existential questions about the meaning of life and experience arise, such as Why did this happen to me or to my child? Why do we have to go through this? How can I deal with the fact that I or my child may die, and that this has little to do with what I do?

The spiritual issues for the child are different from the issues negotiated by the parent. A young child has concrete thought processes and may view the cancer experience as punitive. They may ask, What did I do that was bad? Why are people torturing me? Why are my parents abandoning me? Why do I deserve to have these bad things to happen to me? Beliefs about ultimate reality, suffering, the divine, and the transcendent vary widely in multicultural societies, in which many conceptualizations of religion and spirituality coexist (Eisenbruch & Handelman, 1990; Fukuyama & Sevig, 1999; Kagawa-Singer & Kassim-Lakha, 2003; Yeh, 2001).

A complication in conducting quantitative research on the topic of spiritual practices relates to the challenge of defining and measuring the constructs of spirituality and religion, although progress has been made in this area (e.g., see Hill & Pargament, 2003). A collaborative effort between the Fetzer Foundation and the National Institute on Aging at the National Institutes of Health (1999/2003) resulted in the publication of a booklet devoted to the measurement of religiousness and spirituality in health research on adults. In that booklet, religiousness is described as having specific behavioral, social, doctrinal, and denominational characteristics involving a system of worship and doctrine that is shared within a group. Spirituality is described as that which is concerned with the transcendent, addressing ultimate questions about life's meaning, calling us beyond self to concern and compassion for others.

Extensive scholarship has been devoted to the issue of distinguishing between spirituality and religion. As another example, in their guidelines for assessing spirituality in religious and nonreligious families in pediatric hospice and palliative care, Davies, Brenner, Orloff, Sumner, and Worden (2002) noted that spirituality relates to meaning and transcendent connections with others and with ultimate reality and as such is relevant to persons who are religious, nonreligious, or antireligious. Religion is shared faith, beliefs, practices, and rituals that help people to express their connection to ultimate reality, which is conceptualized as God or the divine in deistic religious traditions (Davies et al., 2002).

Defining and measuring children's spirituality and religiousness are even more difficult than doing so with adults because of the cognitive and moral development that takes place during childhood. Hart and Schneider (1997) offered a definition of children's spirituality as the ability of a child, through relationships with others, to derive personal value and empowerment and, with increasing cognitive development, to build on these relationships a sense of the spiritual in their relationship to values.

Hart and Schnieder (1997) provided a framework for considering the spiritual needs of children with cancer, drawing on the cognitive developmental theories of Piaget (1971) and Erikson (1950), as well as the most widely cited theoretical formulation of children's spiritual development, which is that of Fowler (1981). To illustrate, the infant's needs center on trust versus mistrust according to Erikson, sensorimotor exploration according to Piaget, and the beginnings of faith being established through the development of basic trust in relationship with the primary caregiver according to Fowler (1981). Hart and Schneider suggested that appropriate spiritual interventions for the infant with cancer and the infant's family might include supporting the parent-child relationship by reassuring parents about the adequacy of their parenting while also attending to the physical and emotional needs of the infant.

The National Institutes of Health recently supported a study that may help to address the issue of quantitatively assessing the spirituality of children with cancer. Aimed at assessing the role of spirituality in coping used by children who have survived childhood cancer, the study had as its first goal producing a reliable and validated child measure of spiritual coping. The instrument was then used to examine the relationship between spiritual coping and psychosocial adjustment in a pediatric oncology population, testing the hypothesis that childhood cancer survivors' use of spiritual coping predicts better post-diagnosis adjustment in terms of fewer symptoms of depression and anxiety and heightened quality of life (Boeving, accessed October 12, 2005).

## In Closing

Despite scientific advances, there remains a striking disconnect between the popularity of complementary and alternative therapies and scientific evidence of their safety and efficacy. Several clinical trials of complementary therapies are under way in pediatric oncology samples. However, little is yet known, and there is a need for a great deal of additional careful study and investigation. A topic that could profitably be explored includes sociocultural aspects of complementary and alternative medicine, such as the demographics of families in which children use these therapies.

In addition, further studies are needed on the safety, cost-effectiveness, efficacy, and comparative effectiveness of complementary and alternative interventions. Research is needed pertaining to the biological and psychological mechanisms underlying the clinical effectiveness of complementary and alternative medicine practices.

Finally, the integration of complementary therapies into conventional care, termed *integrative medicine*, is an area in which little research has been undertaken to date; yet, such care is increasingly offered to young patients in conventional medical settings.

It is our hope that talented investigators will rise to the challenges of conducting research on the important topic of complementary and alternative medicine for children with cancer. We hope that investigators from several scientific disciplines will join their efforts to those of the providers of complementary and alternative therapies, resulting in collaborative endeavors to answer the many remaining questions about the potential benefits and risks of these therapies. Through such collaborations, we can continue to move toward the goal of optimizing the care of young people with cancer and enhancing their quality of life.

## References

Astin, J. A., Harkness, E., & Ernst, E. (2000). The efficacy of "distant healing": A systematic review of randomized trials. *Annals of Internal Medicine, 132*, 903–910.

Barrera, M. E., Rykov, M. H., & Doyle, S. L. (2002). The effects of interactive music therapy on hospitalized children with cancer: A pilot study. *Psycho-oncology, 11*, 379–388.

Bell, B. A., Chang, M. N., & Weinstein, H. J. (2001). A phase II study of homoharringtonine for the treatment of children with refractory or recurrent acute myelogenous leukemia: A pediatric oncology group study. *Medical and Pediatric Oncology, 37*, 103–107.

Bennett, M. P., Zeller, J. M., Rosenberg, L., & McCann, J. (2003). The effect of mirthful laughter on stress and natural killer cell activity. *Alternative Therapies in Health and Medicine, 9*, 38–45.

Berk, L. S., Felten, D. L., Tan, S. A., Bittman, B. B., & Westengard, J. (2001). Modulation of neuroimmune parameters during the eustress of humor-associated mirthful laughter. *Alternative Therapies in Health and Medicine, 7*, 62–72, 74–6.

Bittman, B. B., Berk, L. S., Felten, D. L., Westengard, J., Simonton, O. C., Pappas, J., et al. (2001). Composite effects of group drumming music therapy on modulation of neuroendocrine-immune parameters in normal subjects. *Alternative Therapies in Health and Medicine, 7*, 38–47.

Boeving, A. *Child cancer survivors—Spiritual coping and adjustment*. Grant 5R03CA090171-02. Retrieved December 20, 2003, from the National Institutes of Health CRISP database.

Bold, J. & Lies, A. (2001). Unconventional therapy use among children with cancer in Saskatchewan. *Journal of Pediatric Oncology Nursing*, 18, 16–25.

Burgio, G. R., & Locatelli, F. (2000). Alternative therapies and the Di Bella affair in pediatrics. A questionnaire submitted to Italian pediatric oncologists and hematologists. *Haematologica, 85*, 189–194.

Burns, S. J., Harbuz, M. S., Hucklebridge, F., & Bunt, L. (2001). A pilot study into the therapeutic effects of music therapy at a cancer help center. *Alternative Therapies in Health and Medicine, 7*, 48–56.

Cogan, R., Cogan, D., Waltz, W., & McCue, M. (1987). Effects of laughter and relaxation on discomfort thresholds. *Journal of Behavioral Medicine, 10*, 139–144.

Cohen, S. O., & Walco, G. A. (1999). Dance/movement therapy for children and adolescents with cancer. *Cancer Practice, 7*, 34–42.

Collipp, P. J. (1969). The efficacy of prayer: A triple-blind study. *Medical Times, 97*, 201–204.

Cousins, N. (1976). Anatomy of an illness (as perceived by the patient). *New England Journal of Medicine, 295*, 1458–1463.

Crawford, C. C., Sparber, A. G., & Jonas, W. B. (2003). A systematic review of the quality of research on hands-on and distance healing: clinical and laboratory studies. *Alternative Therapies in Health and Medicine, 9*(3 Suppl.), A96–A104.

Davies, B., Brenner, P., Orloff, S., Sumner, L., & Worden, W. (2002). Addressing spirituality in pediatric hospice and palliative care. *Journal of Palliative Care, 18*, 59–67.

Edelblute, J. (2003). Pediatric oncology patients find help and hope in New York City. *Alternative Therapies in Health and Medicine, 9*, 106–107.

Eisenberg, D. M., Davis, R. B., Ettner, S. L., Appel, S., Wilkey, S., Van Rompay, M., et al. (1998). Trends in alternative medicine use in the United States, 1990–1997. *Journal of the American Medical Association, 280*, 1569–1575.

Eisenberg, D. M., Kessler, R. C., Foster, C., Norlock, F. E., Calkins, D. R., & Delbanco, T. L. (1993). Unconventional medicine in the United States: Prevalence, costs, and patterns of use. *New England Journal of Medicine, 328*, 246–252.

Eisenbruch, M., & Handelman, L. (1990). Cultural consultation for cancer: Astrocytoma in a Cambodian adolescent. *Social Science and Medicine, 31*, 1295–1299.

Erikson, E. H. (1950). *Childhood and society*. New York: Norton.

Ernst, E. (2003). Distant healing—an "update" of a systematic review. *Wiener klinische Wochenschrift, 115*, 241–245.

Ernst, E., & Cassileth, B. R. (1998). The prevalence of complementary/alternative medicine in cancer: A systematic review. *Cancer, 83*, 777–782.

Faass, N. (Ed.). (2001). *Integrating complementary medicine into health systems*. Gaithersburg, MD: Aspen.

Favara-Scacco, C., Smirne, G., Schiliro, G., & Di Cataldo, A. (2001). Art therapy as support for children with leukemia during painful procedures. *Medical and Pediatric Oncology, 36*, 474–480.

Fernandez, C. V., Stutzer, C. A., MacWilliam, L., & Fryer, C. (1998). Alternative and complementary therapy use in pediatric oncology patients in British Columbia: Prevalence and reasons for use and nonuse. *Journal of Clinical Oncology, 16*, 1279–1286.

Fetzer Institute/National Institute on Aging Working Group Report. (2003). *Multidimensional measurement of religiousness/spirituality for use in health research: a report of the Fetzer Institute/National Institute on Aging Working Group.* Kalamazoo, MI: Fetzer Institute. (Original work published 1999).

Field, T., Cullen, C., Diego, M., Hernandez-Rief, M., Sprinz, P., Kissell, B., et al. (2001). Leukemia immune changes following massage therapy. *Journal of Bodywork and Movement Therapy, 5*, 271–274.

Fowler, J. (1981). *Stages of faith*. San Francisco: Harper and Row.

Freinkel, A. (n.d.) *Efficacy of distant healing in glioblastoma treatment*. Grant 5R01AT000644-04 Retrieved October 12, 2005 from the National Institutes of Health CRISP database http://crisp.cit.nih.gov/crisp/crisp_lib.query

Friedman, R., Sedler, M., Myers, P., & Benson, H. (1997). Behavioral medicine, complementary medicine and integrated care. Economic implications. *Primary Care, 24*, 949–962.

Friedman, T., Slayton, W. B., Allen, L. S., Pollock, B. H., Dumaont-Driscoll, M., Mehta, P., et al. (1997). Use of alternative therapies for children with cancer [Electronic version]. *Pediatrics, 100,* E1. Retrieved March 15, 2004, from http://pediatrics.aappublications.org/cgi/content/full/100/6/e1

Fukuyama, M. A., & Sevig, T. D. (1999). *Integrating spirituality into multicultural counseling.* Multicultural Aspects of Counseling Series 13. Thousand Oaks, CA: Sage.

Gagnon, E. M., & Recklitis, C. J. (2003). Parents' decision-making preferences in pediatric oncology: the relationship to health care involvement and complementary therapy use. *Psychooncology*, 12, 442–452.

Garami, M., Schuler, D., Babosa, M., Borgulya, G., Hauser, P., Muller, J., et al., (2004). Fermented wheat germ extract reduces chemotherapy-induced febrile neutropenia in pediatric cancer patients. *Journal of Pediatric Hematology Oncology*, 26, 631–635.

Graham-Pole, J. R. (2001a). The marriage of art and science in health care. *Yale Journal of Biology and Medicine, 74*, 21–27.

Graham-Pole, J. (2001b). "Physician, heal thyself": How teaching holistic medicine differs from teaching CAM. *Academic Medicine, 76,* 662–664.

Grootenhuis, M. A., Last, B. F., de Graaf-Nijkerk, J. H.,& van der Wel, M. (1998). Use of alternative treatment in pediatric oncology. *Cancer Nursing, 21,* 282–288.

Hart, D., & Schneider, D. (1997). Spiritual care for children with cancer. *Seminars in Oncology Nursing, 13,* 263–270.

Hill, P. C., & Pargament, K. I. (2003). Advances in the conceptualization and measurement of religion and spirituality: Implications for physical and mental health research. *American Psychologist, 58,* 64–74.

Hudak, D. A., Dale, J. A., Hudak, M. A., & DeGood, D. E. (1991). Effects of humorous stimuli and sense of humor on discomfort. *Psychological Reports, 69*, 779–786.

Kagawa-Singer, M., & Kassim-Lakha, S. (2003). A strategy to reduce cross-cultural miscommunication and increase the likelihood of improving health outcomes. *Academic Medicine, 78,* 577–587.

Katz, E. R., Kellerman, J., & Ellenberg, L. (1987). Hypnosis in the reduction of acute pain and distress in children with cancer. *Journal of Pediatric Psychology, 12*, 379–395.

Kellerman, J., Zeltzer, L., Ellenberg, L., & Dash, J. (1983). Adolescents with cancer. Hypnosis for the reduction of the acute pain and anxiety associated with medical procedures. *Journal of Adolescent Health Care, 4*, 85–90.

Kelly, K. M., Jacobson, J. S., Kennedy, D. D., Braudt, S. M., Mallick, M., & Weiner, M. A. (2000). Use of unconventional therapies by children with cancer at an urban medical center. *Journal of Pediatric Hematology/Oncology, 22,* 412–416.

Klein, E. (n.d.) *Effects of energy healing on prostate cancer.* Grant 1R21AT001120-01A2. Retrieved October 12, 2005 from the National Institutes of Health CRISP database http://crisp.cit.nih.gov/crisp/crisp_lib.query.

Kutner, J. (n.d.) *Efficacy of massage therapy at the end of life.* Grant 1R01AT001006-01A2. Retrieved October 12, 2005 from the National Institutes of Health CRISP database, http://crisp.cit.nih.gov/crisp/crisp_lib.query.

Lane, M. T., & Graham-Pole, J. (1994). Development of an art program on a bone marrow transplant unit. *Cancer Nursing, 17,* 185–192.

Liossi, C., & Hatira, P. (1999). Clinical hypnosis versus cognitive behavioral training for pain management with pediatric cancer patients undergoing bone marrow aspirations. *International Journal of Clinical and Experimental Hypnosis, 47*, 104–116.

Liossi, C., & Hatira, P. (2003). Clinical hypnosis in the alleviation of procedure-related pain in pediatric oncology patients. *International Journal of Clinical and Experimental Hypnosis, 51*, 4–28.

Mansour, A. A., Beuche, M., Laing, G., Leis, A., & Nurse, J. (1999). A study to test the effectiveness of placebo Reiki standardization procedures developed for a planned Reiki efficacy study. *Journal of Alternative and Complementary Medicine, 5*, 153–164.

Martel, D. Bussieres, J. F., Theoret, Y., Lebel, D., Kish, S., Moghrabi, A., et al. (2005). Use of alternative and complementary therapies in children with cancer. *Pediatric Blood Cancer,* 44, 660–668.

McCurdy, E. A., Spangler, J. G., Wofford, M. M., Chauvenet, A. R., & McClean, T. W. (2003). Religiosity is associated with the use of complementary therapies by pediatric oncology patients. *Journal of Pediatric Hematology/Oncology, 25*, 125–129.

Miles, P., & True, G. (2003). Reiki—review of a biofield therapy history, theory, practice, and research. *Alternative Therapies in Health and Medicine, 9*, 62–72.

Miller, W. R., & Thoresen, C. E. (2003). Spirituality, religion, and health: An emerging research field. *American Psychologist, 58*, 24–35.

Molassiotis, A. & Cubbin, D. (2004). "Thinking outside the box": complementary and alternative therapies use in paediatric oncology patients. *European Journal of Oncology Nursing*, 8, 50–60.

Mottonen, M., & Uhari, M. (1997). Use of micronutrients and alternative drugs by children with acute lymphoblastic leukemia. *Medical and Pediatric Oncology, 28,* 205–208.

Myers, C. (n.d.) *Massage and heat therapies for children at end of life*. Grant 1R21CA098408-01A1. Retrieved October 12, 2005, from the National Institutes of Health CRISP database http://crisp.cit.nih.gov/crisp/crisp_lib.query

National Center for Complementary and Alternative Medicine. *What is CAM?* (n.d.). Retrieved October 12, 2005, from http://nccam.nih.gov/health/whatiscam/

Neuhouser, M. L., Patterson, R. E., Schwartz, S. M., Hedderson, M. M., Bowen, D. J., & Standish, L. J. (2001). Use of alternative medicine by children with cancer in Washington State. *Preventive Medicine 33,* 347–354.

Olson, K., Hanson, J., & Michaud, M. (2003). A phase II trial of Reiki for the management of pain in advanced cancer patients. *Journal of Pain and Symptom Management, 26,* 990–997.

Pargament, K. I. (1997). *The psychology of religion and coping: Theory, research, practice.* New York: Guilford Press.

Pendelton, S. M., Cavalli, K. S., Pargament, K. I., & Nasr, S. Z. (2002). Religious/spiritual coping in childhood cystic fibrosis: A qualitative study. *Pediatrics, 109,* E8.

Penson, R. T., Yusuf, R. Z., Chabner, B. A., Lafrancesca, J. P., McElhinny, M., Axelrad, A. S., et al. (2001). Losing God. *Oncologist, 6,* 286–297.

Phipps, S. (2002). Reduction of distress associated with paediatric bone marrow transplant: Complementary health promotion interventions. *Pediatric Rehabilitation, 5,* 223–234.

Phipps, S. (n.d.) *Psychosocial impact of pediatric bone marrow transplant.* Grant 5R01CA060616-07 retrieved October 12, 2005, from the National Institutes of Health CRISP database http://crisp.cit.nih.gov/crisp/crisp_lib.query

Phipps, S., Dunavant, M., Gray, E., & Rai, S. N. (2005). Massage therapy in children undergoing hematopoietic stem cell transplantation: Results of a pilot trial. *Journal of Cancer Integrative Medicine, 3,* 62–70.

Piaget, J. (1971). *Biology and knowledge.* Chicago: University of Chicago Press.

Richardson, M. A., Sanders, T., Palmer, J. L., Greisinger, A., & Singletary, S. E. (2000). Complementary/alternative medicine use in a comprehensive cancer center and the implications for oncology. *Journal of Clinical Oncology, 18,* 2505–2514.

Robb, S. L. (2000). The effect of therapeutic music interventions on the behavior of hospitalized children in isolation: Developing a contextual support model of music therapy. *Journal of Music Therapy, 37,* 118–146.

Robb, S. L., & Ebberts, A. G. (2003a). Songwriting and digital video production interventions for pediatric patients undergoing bone marrow transplantation, part I: An analysis of depression and anxiety levels according to phase of treatment. *Journal of Pediatric Oncology Nursing, 20,* 2–15.

Robb, S. L., & Ebberts, A. G. (2003b). Songwriting and digital video production interventions for pediatric patients undergoing bone marrow transplantation, part II: An analysis of patient-generated songs and patient perceptions regarding intervention efficacy. *Journal of Pediatric Oncology Nursing, 20,* 16–25.

Sawyer, M. G., Gannoni, A. F., Toogood, I. R., Antoniou, G., & Rice, M. (1994). The use of alternative therapies by children with cancer. *Medical Journal of Australia, 160,* 320–322.

Seeman, T. E., Dubin, L. F., & Seeman, M. (2003). Religiosity/spirituality and health. *American Psychologist, 58,* 53–63.

Smith, M., Casey, L., Johnson, D., Gwede, C., Riggin, & O. Z. (2001). Music as a therapeutic intervention for anxiety in patients receiving radiation therapy. *Oncology Nursing Forum, 28,* 855–862.

Stuber, M. L. (2002, February 28). *Humor and healing: The story of Rx laughter.* The Frank and Kate Benedict Roehr Memorial Lecture, presented by The Sam and Rose Stein Institute for Research on Aging, University of California, San Diego.

Wall, V. J., & Womack, W. (1989). Hypnotic versus active cognitive strategies for alleviation of procedural distress in pediatric oncology patients. *American Journal of Clinical Hypnosis, 31,* 181–191.

Weiger, W. A., Smith, M., Boon, H., Richardson, M. A., Kaptchuk, T. J., & Eisenberg, D. M. (2002). Advising patients who seek complementary and alternative medical therapies for cancer. *Annals of Internal Medicine, 3,* 889–903.

Weisenberg, M., Tepper, I., & Schwarzwald, J. (1995). Humor as a cognitive technique for increasing pain tolerance. *Pain, 63,* 207–212.

Whelan, J. S., & Dvorkin, L. (2003). HolisticKids.org—evolution of information resources in pediatric complementary and alternative medicine projects: From monographs to Web learning. *Journal of the Medical Library Association, 91,* 411–417.

Yeh, C. H. (2001). Religious beliefs and practices of Taiwanese parents of pediatric patients with cancer. *Cancer Nursing, 24,* 476–482.

Yeh, C. H., Tsai, J. L., Li, W., Chen, H. M., Lee, S. C., Lin, C. F., et al. (2000). Use of alternative therapy among pediatric oncology patients in Taiwan. *Pediatric Hematology and Oncology, 17,* 55–65.

Zeltzer, L. K., Dolgin, M. J., LeBaron, S., & LeBaron, C. (1991). A randomized, controlled study of behavioral intervention for chemotherapy distress in children with cancer. *Pediatrics, 88,* 34–42.

Zeltzer, L., & LeBaron, S. (1982). Hypnosis and nonhypnotic techniques for reduction of pain and anxiety during painful procedures in children and adolescents with cancer. *Journal of Pediatrics, 101,* 1032–1035.

Zeltzer, L., LeBaron, S., & Zeltzer, P. M. (1984). The effectiveness of behavioral intervention for reduction of nausea and vomiting in children and adolescents receiving chemotherapy. *Journal of Clinical Oncology, 2,* 683–690.

Celia B. Fisher and Jessica K. Masty

# A Goodness-of-Fit Ethic for Informed Consent to Pediatric Cancer Research

The ethics of informed consent in pediatric cancer research are unique. First, unlike medical care for most other diseases of childhood, the majority of children with cancer receive treatment through participation in pediatric oncology research or in hospital settings in which such research is actively conducted (Ablett & Pinkerton, 2003; Aleksa & Koren, 2002; Bleyer, 2002; Ross, Severson, Pollock, & Robison, 1996). Second, for children with newly diagnosed cancers, decisions regarding entry into a clinical protocol typically occur soon after the family is informed about the initial diagnosis. Thus, in many instances consent to research participation occurs during one of the most stressful periods in a family's life. Third, because treatment decisions must be made very quickly after the initial diagnosis, there may be little opportunity for patients or parents to understand or accept the nature of the disease at the time their consent to research participation is sought.

Like other diseases of childhood for which treatments found efficacious for adults may be ineffective or toxic, the absence of pediatric research can deprive pediatric cancer patients of empirically valid therapies. Patient advocates and pediatric oncologists view the imperative of conducting pediatric cancer research with particular urgency because of the life-threatening nature of the disease and the adverse, and sometimes permanent, side effects of many current treatments. Thus, because the cancer patient's immediate treatment needs are so entwined with the research imperative, a fourth unique aspect of informed consent to pediatric oncology research is that treatment and research goals may be blurred not only by patients and parents but also by investigators, clinicians, and other care providers (Kodish et al., 1998).

Interpreting broadly worded federal regulations governing research involving children also provides challenges for developing patient- and family-appropriate consent procedures for pediatric oncology research. In most instances, federal regulations require that adequate provisions be made for soliciting the permission of parents/guardians and the child's assent (the child's affirmative agreement to participate in research) prior to conducting research involving children (Department of Health and Human Services, 2001, 45 CFR 46.408; Food and Drug Administration [FDA] 2001, 21 CFR 50.55). The regulations permit institutional review boards (IRBs) to waive the requirement for child assent when, in the IRB's judgment, the child or child population is not capable of providing assent. Assent may also be waived if the research offers the prospect of direct benefit that is important to the health or well-being of the child and is available only in the context of the research. Ongoing ethical challenges for IRBs and investigators are to develop informed consent procedures that adequately inform families about the research and decisional options and to reflect respect for both parents' right to make decisions regarding the welfare of their children and to support pediatric patients' developing autonomy and welfare

This chapter reviews current theory and research on informed consent policies for pediatric cancer research within an ethics framework that conceptualizes children's involvement in participation decisions in terms of the goodness of fit among the specific research context, parents' understanding of information provided during informed consent, and children's decisional capacities (Fisher, 2003b). Conceptualizing informed consent as a product of the relationships among the consent context, guardians, and patients shifts judgments regarding children's involvement away from an exclusive focus on their cognitive abilities to (a) an examination of those aspects of the consent setting that are creating or exacerbating child and parent consent vulnerability and (b) consideration of how the procedure can be modified to produce a consent process that best advances pediatric cancer patients' welfare, their developing autonomy, and the parent-child relationship.

## The Pediatric Research Consent Context

Ethical challenges that arise in pediatric oncology research are often tied to the specific research context. FDA approval of new therapeutic agents requires a three-phase scaled sequence of preclinical and clinical trials. Prior to testing in children, most new agents must have demonstrated potential efficacy and safety in animals and adults. However, there is growing recognition that children's physiology differs from that of adults as well as from one developmental period to another, which has led to an increase in early phase and later phase testing in children (FDA Modernization Act of 1997, followed by the Final Rule; FDA, 1998).

### Phase I Trials

At the earliest stages of testing, Phase I trials, the goal of the research is not treatment but study of the pharmacokinetic properties of an agent and demonstration of the agent's therapeutic potential by establishing the maximum dose at which biological effects are observed. Dosage levels begin low and are increased until there is evidence of toxicity. Although Phase I trials were traditionally considered to offer no prospect of direct benefit, evidence suggests that for some childhood cancers there is a small probability (5%) that a Phase I agent may delay the progression of some cancers (Blaney et al., 2003; Furman et al., 1999). A question of related ethical import is whether the shift in categorizing Phase I trials as providing potential direct benefit is a reflection of an actual change in perspective or a reaction to federal regulations that only permit IRBs to independently approve research involving more than a minor increase over minimal risk if it offers the possibility of direct benefit (DHHS, 2001, 45 CFR 46 Subpart D).

Given the very low probability of benefit and the unknown and potentially high risks associated with toxicity, many Phase I trials are conducted with children for whom other effective therapies are nonexistent or have not worked and some who may be terminally ill. With respect to informed parental permission, Phase I trials may present the greatest risk that participation decisions will be based on desperation and false hopes of cure (Aleksa & Koren, 2002). Phase I trials also raise issues regarding patient assent. Irrespective of age and maturity, pediatric patients may be too ill to make an informed decision, or parents may be concerned that fully informed assent may make the child more aware or despondent about his or her condition. On the other hand, because there is very little probability of direct benefit and a possibility of discomfort from the agent itself or from additional pharmacokinetic tests that must be conducted, a pediatric patient's dissent may be most appropriate in this instance. Phase I trials may also present the greatest potential for conflict of interest and patient exploitation because the risk–benefit ratio of participation may be more favorable for the investigator regarding the potential risks (e.g., failure to achieve professional recognition) and benefits (i.e., publication of an article, drug patents) than for the patient (Aleksa & Koren, 2002).

### Phase II Trials

The purpose of Phase II trials is to determine whether the therapeutic agent has a measurable effect on the cancer. The end point of these trials is usually the percentage of children evidencing some form of positive change, including tumor shrinkage or halt to progression of disease. Because clinical equipoise, honest professional disagreement within the expert medical community as to the preferred treatment (Freedman, 1987) is an ethical requirement for such trials, in many instances children asked to participate in Phase II trials have not responded to or have relapsed following standard therapies. Thus, as in Phase I trials, Phase II research raises challenges related to emotional, cognitive, developmental, and family factors tied to consent comprehension and decisions regarding information that would be beneficial or harmful to share with pediatric patients.

### Phase III Trials

Once an agent has been shown to be effective in a Phase II trial, a randomized clinical trial is conducted to compare the agent's effectiveness to the best-available standard treatment. Phase III trials may also consist of comparisons of different dosages of the same agent. Thus, one group of patients will be assigned to treatment with the new experimental agent and one group to treatment with the most effective standard treatment. It can be argued that Phase III trials have the most favorable risk–benefit ratio. Because clinical equipoise is required to ethically compare two forms of therapy, children will be assigned either to the best-known effective treatment or to an experimental treatment that is hypothesized to be more effective or equally effective and less toxic (Kodish et al., 1998). However, good scientific design requires that patients be randomly assigned to the different treatment arms of the trials to avoid results biased by treatment choice. Parents and patients need to understand during informed consent that neither they nor their clinician will have a choice regarding which treatment they will receive *and* the reason for the random assignment. They must also be aware of the alternative treatments.

## The Informed, Rational, and Voluntary Requirements for Informed Consent

Informed consent to pediatric oncology research represents a mutual agreement among an investigator, the patient, and the patient's family, the validity of which rests on the requirements that the consent is informed, rational, and voluntary (Faden & Beauchamp, 1986).

### Consent Must Be Informed

Informed consent for pediatric cancer research involves a series of interrelated concepts, many of which may be unfamiliar to parents and children or require perspective-taking, critical reflection, or recursive thinking skills that children have not yet adequately developed. First, parents and patients must understand that the purpose of research is to produce generalizable knowledge and not to provide direct benefit to the participant. Many parents of pediatric oncology patients and adults with cancer find this is a difficult concept to grasp (Appelbaum, Roth, Lidz, Benson, & Winslade, 1987). Moreover, in contrast to other types of clinical research, pediatric cancer research that distinguishes experimentation from treatment may not reflect an informed decision. As argued by Kodish and colleagues (1998):

> The discipline of pediatric oncology embraces the notion of therapeutic research, defining "standard treatment" as the most effective and least toxic arm of the previous study, and seeking to enroll children with cancer as subjects on the current study (in which the "experimental arm" is hypothesized to be more effective, or less toxic and equally effective). (p. 2468)

In addition, families and prospective participants must understand the specific purpose and procedures of the study for which they are being recruited, including which procedures are related to both treatment and research and which procedures are conducted exclusively for scientific purposes. For example, over the course of a 3-month clinical trial, children and their parents may not distinguish between those blood tests, spinal taps, or positron emission tomography scans that are essential for treatment monitoring and those required to obtain generalizable data to test a scientific hypothesis.

### Consent Must Be Rational

To meet the rational requirement of informed consent, parents and children need to be able not only to understand the information presented, but also to appreciate the consequences to the patient of agreeing or declining research participation (Appelbaum, Grisso, Frank, O'Donnell, & Kupfer, 1999; Grisso, Appelbaum, Mulvey, & Fletcher, 1995; Syse, 2002). This may be difficult in pediatric oncology research settings for at least two reasons. First, as noted, invitations to participate in research often occur at the same time parents learn of the child's cancer diagnosis. The emotional reaction to such news may interfere with rational comprehension of consent information irrespective of the clarity of presentation. Second, families of newly diagnosed patients do not have first-hand knowledge or familiarity with the nature of the disease, how the child will experience adverse treatment side effects, or the different paths the disease, its symptomatology, or the child's response to treatment will take over time.

### Consent Must Be Voluntary

The voluntary requirement of consent is meant to ensure that individuals are not coerced into participating and are free to withdraw from treatment or biomedical research at any time. In some contexts, patients and their guardians may be particularly vulnerable to coercion and exploitation. For example, children may fear disapproval from family caregivers, or all family members may feel they must be compliant in deference to the authority of the requesting practitioner. Some families may have little experience in exercising their rights in health care settings or may be fearful of discontinuation of other medical services if they refuse research participation.

Truly informed consent requires an understanding of human subject protections, including the right to be informed about research procedures, research risk, and potential benefits; confidentiality procedures; the voluntary nature of the participation decision; and the right to withdraw such permission once a study has begun. Children who have not had experience with independent decision making and parents from diverse cultural and economic backgrounds in which deference to authority or harmonious relations are valued and expected may not appreciate their right to refuse research participation (Fisher et al., 2002; Fisher & Ragsdale, 2006). For example, in a study by Kodish et al. (2004), between 18% and 20% of parents asked to consent to their child's participation in an oncology trial did not understand that they were free to refuse study participation, felt pressure to enroll, and did not know they could withdraw their child from the trial once it had begun.

## Parental Permission

Parents have the responsibility to make medical decisions for their children, including medical research decisions. Although the assent of the child is often sought when considering entry into a pediatric oncology clinical trial, participation in the study is ultimately the parents' choice. In the case of pediatric cancer, for which treatment often consists of participation in a clinical trial, it is assumed that parents' decision to enroll their child in a research study is based on the child's best interests. As Kopelman (1997) pointed out, by adhering to this best-interests standard, federal regulations and IRBs rely on parents' desires to "maximize the benefits and minimize the harms" to their children (p. 213). While participation in oncology clinical trials may directly benefit specific children when they are given effective treatments, research conducted with children who have cancer is also important for the advancement of clinical science and for the benefit of future pediatric cancer patients as a whole (Barrett, 2002). Despite their best intentions, some parents may not fully comprehend the distinction between treatment and clinical trials or fully comprehend the research risks and potential benefits associated with the particular investigation.

### Parental Anxiety

Because of the seriousness of pediatric cancer, parents are often asked about enrolling their child in an oncology clinical trial shortly after the child is given the cancer diagnosis. Sometimes, this issue is broached at the same time the diagnosis is first discussed with the family. Thus, it is not surprising that, when presented with the option to enroll their child in a clinical trial, some parents feel overwhelmed and report experiencing a state of shock (Kodish et al., 1998).

For example, Kupst, Patenaude, Walco, and Sterling (2003) found that all parents interviewed 1 month after giving permission for their child to participate in a clinical trial reported experiencing some level of emotional distress during the consent process. Parents commented that their distress stemmed from having just recently learned of the child's illness and from having to make a decision about research participation. Of parents in this study, 70% felt that the high level of stress was debilitating, preventing them from asking questions and seeking more information about the research and their child's illness.

Pletsch and Stevens (2001) found that the closer the timing of the initial diagnosis to the request for trial entry, the immediacy of the threat to the child's life, the belief that the clinical trial was the only option to save the child's life, and expertise in managing the health care system were critical factors influencing the informed consent experience of mothers whose children were diagnosed with cancer.

Ruccione, Kramer, Moore, and Perin (1991) formally measured parental anxiety at the time of informed consent for pediatric oncology trials. At 48 hours after giving permission for their child to enroll in a clinical trial, parents completed two questionnaires: the State-Trait Anxiety Index and the Parent Informed Consent Questionnaire. The investigators found that the measure of state anxiety for parents in the study was significantly higher than the level of anxiety previously reported for normative adult samples, and that mothers reported more anxiety than fathers. Of ethical import is the finding that higher states of anxiety were associated with parents' reports that they did not clearly understand the risks of their child's study treatment.

## The Consent Format

Another factor influencing the informed consent process is the amount of information disclosed during the consent discussion. Parents have reported both being overwhelmed by the large amount of information presented to them and wanting more information, especially pertaining to risks of the experimental treatment and alternative treatment options (Kodish et al., 1998; Kupst et al., 2003; Levi, Marsick, Drotar, & Kodish, 2000). Some parents reported feeling pressured to make a quick decision about enrolling their child in an oncology trial, often compromising their belief that participation is truly voluntary (Levi et al., 2000).

### *Timing and Terminology*

The amount of time that is available to consider the consent decision is also important. Parents report satisfaction with the amount of time to make a decision, especially when they are encouraged to take the consent form home overnight to review it more thoroughly (Kodish et al., 1998; Ruccione et al., 1991). Friebert and Kodish (2000) suggested that the difficulties parents sometimes display in reading and comprehending the consent form is a consequence of the short interval between time of diagnosis and the time when the consent form is signed. Although parents often reported that most aspects of the clinical trial they are considering for their child were adequately discussed (Kodish et al., 1998) and fairly clear (Ruccione et al., 1991), some parents complained that the medical terminology in the consent form was difficult to understand (Levi et al., 2000).

## Understanding Random Assignment

The majority of pediatric oncology patients in the United States receive treatment through randomized clinical trials (Murphey, 1995; Pui, 1999). Such trials never include placebos. As a result, random assignment to different treatment arms is often the key feature that distinguishes pediatric cancer treatment from participation in clinical trials (Kodish et al., 2004). Investigators have begun to examine the extent to which parents understand random assignment.

Kupst et al. (2003) conducted semistructured retrospective interviews with 20 parents of children enrolled in randomized clinical trials for different forms of childhood cancer. Kupst et al. found that many parents did not understand the term *randomization*. Only 5 parents of the 13 children who were receiving randomized treatment knew their child's treatment was randomized, 5 reported being unsure, and 3 stated that their children were not receiving randomized treatment. Kupst et al. also noted that although most parents were unsure of their child's diagnosis, treatment plan, and prognosis, only 55% of parents appeared to know that their child's treatment was part of research. These findings are consistent with those reported by Levi et al. (2000), who concluded that parents in their sample did not make a distinction between their child's participation in research and medical treatment.

Kodish and colleagues (2004) collected data on 137 parents' understanding of randomization in pediatric oncology trials through observation and audiotaping of the consent conference followed by parent interviews. Based on the interviews, they concluded that only 50% of parents understood randomization. Moreover, individuals from racial minority groups and lower socioeconomic status groups were significantly less likely to understand that their children's treatment was randomly allocated. Of some concern is the fact that, in 17% of the observed consent conferences, randomization was not explained to parents.

### *Randomization and Consent Decisions*

In a multisite study conducted by Wiley et al. (1999), 285 parents completed a questionnaire assessing their knowledge and perceptions about randomized clinical trials. By including parents who had not given permission for research participation, this study was able to provide insight on the relationship between parents' agreement to participate in clinical trials and their understanding of random assignment. Within 3 months of the randomization decision, parents were asked to complete the Clinical Investigation Randomization Scale, which consists of 32 items scored on a 5-point Likert scale. Wiley et al. found the following three Clinical Investigation Randomization Scale items accurately predicted whether a parent had consented to randomized treatment: "Randomization provides the best opportunity for my child to be cured of his/her cancer," "The thought of randomization was frightening for me," and "Randomization will help primarily in the treatment of my child (more than future children with cancer)" (p. 254).

Parents who refused to give permission for their child to participate in a randomized clinical trial were more likely to feel pressure to give consent, wanted control over their child's treatment, and felt that they could trust their doctor's opinion more than the randomization process to obtain the best treatment for their child. Parents who consented to randomized treatment expressed trust in the doctor who invited them to be in the randomized clinical trial and felt relief at not having to make a choice about which treatment to give their child, avoiding the possibility that they would make a poor choice. It is interesting to note that parents who chose randomization generally endorsed beliefs that randomized treatment might cure their child's cancer, and that the experimental treatment would benefit their child more than future patients (Wiley et al., 1999).

### *Involving Children in Discussion About Randomization*

Although parents' own perception of randomization may affect their decision to enroll their child in a randomized clinical trial, parents also take into consideration the opinion of the patient. Olechnowicz, Eder, Simon, Zyzanski, and Kodish (2002) conducted a multisite study to examine the involvement of parents and children in the informed consent conference with clinicians presenting leukemia treatment and research options. Children 7 years or older were typically included in the consent conference. Parents from 5 of the 14 families observed indicated that the decision to participate in a clinical trial involved a family discussion, including the patient. The patient's age was a determining factor for whether the child was asked to be present at the consent conference. Children from families who endorsed the belief that the child patient was the most important factor in making the consent decision were on average age 13 years, while the mean age of children of parents who did not believe that the child is the most important factor in making the consent decision was age 6 years.

## Parental Satisfaction With Consent Procedures

Surprisingly, despite misunderstandings, misperceptions, and the distress often associated with the informed consent process in pediatric oncology trials, parents tend to be satisfied with the informed consent process overall (Kodish et al., 1998; Kupst et al., 2003; Ruccione et al., 1991). Ruccione et al.

found that parents with higher levels of education tended to believe that research risks were adequately explained, but that insufficient time was given to consider enrolling their child in a randomized clinical trial. In contrast, Kodish et al. reported that parental level of education does not significantly affect the degree to which parents are satisfied with the consent process.

Parents' consent decisions are often influenced by their relationship with their child's physician. Wiley et al. (1999) found that regardless of parents' enrollment decision, the need to trust the physician was a frequently cited reason for agreeing to study participation. In some cases, a trusted doctor's recommendation was reported to encourage parents to enroll their child in a clinical trial. In other cases, parents decided not to enroll their children because they believed it was better to trust an expert's opinion about the best treatment for their child than to allow the child to be randomly assigned to a treatment. Similarly, 22.7% of parents in the Levi et al. (2000) study stated that trust in their physician was important in their decision to enroll their child in clinical research. Some of these parents also expressed a desire to work in a partnership with the physician and share in an open dialogue during the consent process.

## Child Assent

All children are unique individuals with unique family cultures. Although some are capable of making decisions for themselves, others may lack the capacity or experience to do so. Cancer, like other illnesses, can affect patients' cognitive, physical, and emotional abilities as well as their family environments, and these effects are not uniform across different children and families. The extent to which pediatric cancer patients should be included in research participation decisions must take into account not only the patient's ability to comprehend information presented during the consent conference, but also their emotional preparedness to process facts about their illness, short-term and long term treatment adverse side effects, and prognosis.

### Children's Competence to Consent

Voluntary informed consent is viewed by many as the best means of protecting the rights and welfare of individuals asked to participate in clinical research (Freedman, 1975). The ethical value of informed consent rests on the assumption that individuals are able to understand (a) the nature and rationale of experimentation; (b) how the risks and potential benefits of participation may directly affect them or others; and (c) their research rights, including the right to dissent to or withdraw from participation in a study (Fisher & Brokowski, 2005). In both law and ethics, minors have been presumed to lack these capacities because of immature cognitive skills, inadequate experiences in situations analogous to the research context, and the actual and perceived power differentials between adolescents, parents, and clinical researchers (Fisher, 2002a, 2003b; Fisher, Hoagwood, & Jensen, 1996; Grodin, Glantz, & Glantz, 1994).

Empirical studies of healthy children and those involved in psychiatric treatment point to mid-adolescence (14–15 years of age) as the age at which youth demonstrate the ability to understand the nature of their health condition, the nature of standard or experimental treatments, the purpose of research, and their research rights (Abramovitch, Freedman, Henry, & Van Brunschot, 1995; Abramovitch, Freedman, Thoden, & Nikolich, 1991; Bruzzese & Fisher, 2003; Grisso & Vierling, 1978; Lewis, Lewis, & Ifekwungue, 1978; Melton, 1980; Ruck, Abramovitch, & Keating, 1998; Ruck, Keating, Abramovitch, & Koegl, 1998; Weithorn & Campbell, 1982). Alderson (1993) asked children undergoing orthopedic surgery, their parents, and health professionals the age they thought children could decide for themselves if they should have surgery that was not life-saving. Children and parents mirrored the literature, suggesting that 14 years was the threshold, whereas health professionals identified 10 years. Fisher (2002a) found similar responses from parents and adolescents of diverse ethnic backgrounds concerning the age at which children had the ability to provide independent consent to participate in research on adolescent risk behaviors.

Children's health status and familiarity with their disease also influence consent capacity. For example, newly diagnosed pediatric cancer patients demonstrate more compromised comprehension of clinical trials than children of the same age diagnosed with diabetes (Broome, Richards, & Hall, 2001; Crisp, Ungerer, & Goodnow, 1996). Research also suggests that, irrespective of their more mature cognitive capacities, adolescents may not exert their research rights because of inexperience with health care decision making or fear of disapproval by parents, researchers, or health care workers (Abramovitch et al., 1991; Bruzzese & Fisher, 2003; Scherer, 1991; Susman, Dorn, & Fletcher, 1992).

## Child Welfare and Parental Rights

Is children's capacity to understand consent information a sufficient ethical justification for requiring their assent and honoring their dissent to participate in cancer research? Parents are legally responsible for the health of their minor children, and children under legal age do not have the legal right to refuse a treatment that has been approved by parents. The SIOP Working Committee on Psychosocial Issues in Pediatric Oncology (Spinetta et al., 2003) concluded that within these legal parameters children not only have a moral right to a developmentally appropriate full and thorough explanation of medical procedures, but also no medical procedure should be performed on a minor without the attempt to gain the child's assent or awareness and understanding.

Recognizing children's rights within the context of parental rights and obligations raises difficult ethical questions for pediatric oncology research. Should children's assent be sought over the parent's objections? Do investigators have the right to override parental judgment and undermine family connections? Should pediatric patients' assent be sought when their dissent will not be respected?

### Risks of Assent

Many parents are conflicted about whether children's emotional health and physical well-being may be compromised by assent information describing the nature of their disease or the pain or discomfort that may accompany experimental procedures. Some parents try to shield the adolescent from this knowledge by not including them in the research consent decision (Kunin, 1997). Little is known about the consequences of informing children or adolescents about short-term adverse side effects of cancer treatments such as hair loss, weight loss, and rashes or long-term risks such as sterility, damage to internal organs, or cognitive impairments. At the same time, there is evidence that involving children in the consent process increases their feelings of self-worth, ability to cope with anxiety over illness and treatments, and long-term emotional and social adjustment (Fletcher, van Eys, & Dorn, 1993; Grodin & Burton, 1988; Varni, Katz, Colgrove, & Dolgin, 1996). Even when parents want to involve their children in research decision making, parents often are confused and uncertain about the amount of information to share and how to do so in a way that protects their children from anxiety or depression in reaction to such information (Kunin, 1997).

### Parental Obligations and Child Autonomy

The modern doctrine of informed consent embedded in civil and criminal law and in federal regulations governing human subject research is too often grounded in a limited definition of autonomy restricted to respect for the rights of persons to self-governance and privacy. From this perspective, parents may be viewed simply as surrogate decision makers for persons with immature autonomy. However, as Childress (1990) pointed out, the ideal of autonomy must be distinguished from the conditions for autonomous choice. According to this point of view, parents have a special right and obligation to determine their children's degree of immediate research consent involvement to promote their long-term future autonomy. Conceptions of autonomy based on children's limited world experience and lack of a well-conceived life plan should not have privileged status over parental obligations to promote lifelong autonomy. As Ross (1997) argued, prioritizing children's autonomy rights over parental obligations undermines the importance of the continuity and permanence of the parent-child relationship—a significance children may not yet appreciate and investigators must be careful not to undermine.

## A Goodness-of-Fit Conception of Informed Consent

Children, like all persons, are linked to others in relationships of reciprocity and dependency (Walker, 2002). A relational ethic calls for pediatric cancer scientists to construct parent permission and child assent procedures based on moral principles of respect, care, and justice guided by responsiveness to the abilities, values, and concerns of all family stakeholders and context in which consent is sought (Fisher, 1997, 1999). Conceptualizing informed consent competence as a product of the relationship among family members, investigator, and consent context shifts assessment of decisional capacity away from an exclusive focus on pediatric patients' cognitive maturity or parents' rights and obligations to (a) an examination of those aspects of the consent setting that are creating or exacerbating parental permission and child assent vulnerability and (b) consideration of how the setting can be modified to produce a consent process that best reflects and protects the family members' hopes, values, concerns, and welfare (Fisher, 2002a, 2003b).

## Vulnerability as a Relational Construct

From a goodness-of-fit perspective, consent vulnerability is not defined solely in terms of the physical, psychological, or social characteristics of individual family members (Fisher, 1999, 2003c; Goodin, 1985). Rather, the degree to which parents and children are able to make informed, rational, and voluntary research decisions is seen to depend on the specific actions of scientists within specific experimental contexts (Fisher, 2002a, 2003b). Within this framework, both family members' susceptibility to consent misunderstandings and the specific ability of scientists to help alleviate such misunderstandings define an obligation on the part of investigators that is morally binding (Fisher, 1999, 2002a).

When pediatric cancer is the focus of scientific inquiry, investigators must consider the special life contexts that render patients and their families more or less susceptible to the harms associated with recruitment procedures and participatory requirements for each particular experimental design. For example, susceptibility to coercion and exploitation may be a particular risk for families who can only acquire high-quality cancer treatment through enrollment in a clinical trial. Failure to fully comprehend consent information may be a function of transient parental anxiety, patient illness, or insufficient time to review consent information.

A goodness-of-fit ethic obligates pediatric oncology scientists to take actions that go beyond simply protecting participants from physical or psychological risks associated with research procedures. Investigators must be willing to reconfigure experimental procedures to reduce or eliminate research vulnerability. This may include reconceptualizing traditional assumptions regarding the standards by which a child is considered competent to give informed assent and the role of guardians in consent decisions. For example, respectful and trusting relationships between children, parents, or significant others in their life may be a positive feature that investigators can draw on to enhance consent comprehension and reduce consent anxiety.

## Enhancing Consent Procedures

Within the goodness-of-fit framework, morally responsible informed consent practices require actions that go beyond simply evaluating whether pediatric patients and their parents understand the nature, risks, and benefits of procedures for which consent is sought, toward a reframing of the consent context itself. This family-context reframing may involve remedial efforts to enhance consent comprehension coupled with efforts to attain mutual understanding and support among patients, parents, and the investigator. A few studies have demonstrated that brief lessons on rights in treatment and research can improve children's and adolescents' understanding. These studies have used brief video presentations, simplified written or videotaped forms, clarification of comments by investigators, or a brief lesson on rights to increase understanding of the voluntary nature of treatment and research (Abramovitch et al., 1995; Belter & Grisso, 1984; Bruzzese & Fisher, 2003; Tymchuk, 1992).

In pediatric oncology consent contexts, investigators and clinicians can consider providing family members with age- and language-appropriate targeted preconsent educational materials and improve the readability and format of written consent and assent documents. Investigators also should be willing to repeat information and institute a respectful process of checking patient and parent comprehension or provide families with an audiotape of the consent conference and encourage them to review materials at home and to consult with trusted others before making an informed decision (American Academy of Pediatrics, 1995; Kupst et al., 2003; Ruccione et al., 1991; Spinetta et al., 2003). Presenting materials in multiple modalities, providing pictorial illustrations to increase attention to and comprehension of research procedures and participant rights, and modifying those aspects of the consent setting that may be stress provoking for that particular individual can reduce person-context consent vulnerability.

The voluntary requirement of consent is meant to ensure that patients and parents are not coerced into participating, and that they feel free to exert their right to withdraw from research at any time. In pediatric oncology settings, as in many clinical research contexts, children and families may be particularly vulnerable to coercion and exploitation. As noted, these vulnerabilities may be of special concern during recruitment for Phase I trials. For example, families may fear disapproval from the referring clinician or physicians on staff if they refuse research participation or feel they must be compliant in deference to the authority of the requesting practitioner (Fisher et al., 2002). Children and some parents may have little experience in exercising their rights in medical settings or, if they have limited health insurance, may be fearful of discontinuation of regular medical services. Modifying the consent setting to reduce the perception of power inequities, to provide opportunities to practice decision making, and to construct concrete ways of demonstrating that other services will not be compromised can strengthen the goodness of fit between family characteristics and consent setting (Fisher, 2002a).

Investigators must also be aware of aspects of the consent context that may motivate or inhibit children and parents from asking questions. For example, Olechnowicz et al. (2002) found that when children were present during pediatric oncology consent conferences, clinicians were likely to direct their discussion to the parent, parents asked fewer questions, and children's questions focused on the details of the disease and treatment rather than the research itself. In addition, investigators need to be sensitive to the possibility that they and parents may sometimes disagree on whether sharing information with a patient is in the child's best interest (Foreman, 1999; Kunin, 1997). In such situations, investigators can create contexts that encourage mutually respectful discussions with parents about the child's consent participation and strive for a consensus that reflects a concern for patient autonomy and well-being consistent with both professional standards and parental values.

## An Informed Consent Ethic of Mutual Obligation, Respect, and Care

Acutely or chronically ill pediatric cancer patients do not and should not make research participation decisions in isolation. Childrens' and adolescents' involvement in research enrollment decisions should rest on assessment of their developmental maturity, the extent to which their health is affecting their cognitive capacities, their family history of shared decision making, the extent to which the urgency of their condition precludes meaningful input, and the unique ways in which they and their parents approach stressful situations. Appropriately fitted consent procedures must also take into account the life circumstances of parents, the strategies for coping with their child's illness, the immediate demands of the research context, and the long-term consequences of parental decisions.

Investigators should not only seek to understand these patient and family characteristics, but also strive to modify the consent context to optimally fit and enhance family understandings and family-investigator dialogue. Family-context fitted consent procedures must also take into account the extent to which research offers the prospect of direct benefit to participants and the probability and degree of immediate and long-term side effects exclusive to research procedures. The rights of children and adolescents to dissent to research participation may have privileged status over concerns about children's limited assent comprehension when involvement in experimentation offers little hope of direct benefit and high probability of pain or discomfort.

All patients and families are unique. Respectful and compassionate consent procedures can be achieved through family-fitted assessment and enhancement strategies that draw on investigators' expertise and human responsiveness to pediatric patients and parents.

## References

Ablett, S., & Pinkerton, C. R. (2003). Recruiting children into cancer trials—Role of the United Kingdom Children's Cancer Study Group (UKCCSG). *British Journal of Cancer*, *88*, 1661–1665.

Abramovitch, R., Freedman, J. L., Henry, K., & Van Brunschot, M. (1995). Children's capacity to agree to psychological research: Knowledge of risks and benefits and voluntariness. *Ethics and Behavior, 5,* 25–48.

Abramovitch, R., Freedman, J. L., Thoden, K., & Nikolich, C. (1991). Children's capacity to consent to participation in psychological research: Empirical findings. *Child Development, 62,* 1100–1109.

Alderson, P. (1993). *Children's consent to surgery.* Buckingham, UK: Open University Press.

Aleksa, K., & Koren, G. (2002). Ethical issues in including pediatric cancer patients in drug development trials. *Pediatric Drugs, 4,* 267–265.

American Academy of Pediatrics. (1995). Informed consent, parental permission, and assent in pediatric practice. *Pediatrics, 95,* 314–317.

Appelbaum, P. S., Grisso, T., Frank, E., O'Donnell, S., & Kupfer, D. J. (1999). Competence of depressed patients for consent to research. *American Journal of Psychiatry, 156,* 1380–1384.

Appelbaum, P. S., Roth, L. H., Lidz, C. W., Benson, P., & Winslade, W. (1987). False hopes and best data: Consent to research and the therapeutic misconception. *Hastings Center Report, 17,* 20–24.

Barrett, J. (2002). Why aren't more pediatric trials performed? *Applied Clinical Trials,* July, 36–44. Retrieved December 3, 2003, from http://www.actmagazine.com

Belter, R. W., & Grisso, T. (1984). Children's recognition of rights violations in counseling. *Professional Psychology: Research and Practice, 15,* 899–910.

Blaney, S. M., Heideman R., Berg, S., Adamson, P., Gillespie, A., Geyer, J. R., et al. (2003). Phase I clinical trial of intrathecal topotecan in patients with neoplastic meningitis. *Journal of Clinical Oncology, 21,* 143–147.

Bleyer, A. (2002). Older adolescents with cancer in North America deficits in outcome and research. *Pediatric Clinics of North America, 49,* 1027–1042.

Broome, M. E., Richards, D. J., & Hall, J. M. (2001). Children in research: The experience of ill children and adolescents. *Journal of Family Nursing, 7,* 32–49.

Bruzzese, J. M., & Fisher, C. B. (2003). Assessing and enhancing the research consent capacity of children and youth. *Applied Developmental Science, 7,* 13–26.

Childress, J. F. (1990). The place of autonomy in bioethics. *Hastings Center Report, 20,* 12–17.

Crisp, J., Ungerer, J. A., & Goodnow, J. J. (1996). The impact of experience on children's understanding of illness. *Journal of Pediatric Psychology, 21,* 57–72.

Department of Health and Human Services. (2001, August). Title 45 Public Welfare, Part 46, *Code of Federal Regulations, Protection of Human Subjects.*

Faden, R. R., & Beauchamp, T. L. (1986). *A history and theory of informed consent.* New York: Oxford University Press.

Fisher, C. B. (1997). A relational perspective on ethics-in-science decision making for research with vulnerable populations. *IRB: Review of Human Subjects Research, 19,* 1–4.

Fisher, C. B. (1999). Relational ethics and research with vulnerable populations. In Commissioned Papers by the National Bioethics Advisory Commission, *Reports on research involving persons with mental disorders that may affect decision-making capacity* (Vol. 2, pp. 29–49). Rockville, MD: National Bioethics Advisory Commission. Retrieved October 5, 2005, from http://www.bioethics.gov/reports/past_commissions/nbac_mental2.pdf

Fisher, C. B. (2002a). A goodness-of-fit ethic of informed consent. *Urban Law Journal, 30,* 159–171.

Fisher, C. B. (2002b). Participant consultation: Ethical insights into parental permission and confidentiality procedures for policy relevant research with youth. In R. M. Lerner, F. Jacobs, & D. Wertlieb (Eds.) *Handbook of applied developmental science* (Vol. 4, pp. 371–396). Thousand Oaks, CA: Sage.

Fisher, C. B. (2003a). Adolescent and parent perspectives on ethical issues in youth drug use and suicide survey research. *Ethics and Behavior, 13,* 302–331.

Fisher, C. B. (2003b). A goodness-of-fit ethic for child assent to non-beneficial research. *American Journal of Bioethics, 3,* 27–28.

Fisher, C. B. (2003c). A goodness-of-fit ethic for informed consent to research involving persons with mental retardation and developmental disabilities. *Mental Retardation and Developmental Disabilities Research Reviews, 9,* 27–31.

Fisher, C. B., & Brokowski, C. (2005). Cancer patients, adolescent: Involvement in clinical trials decision making. In C. B. Fisher & R. M. Lerner (Eds.), *Applied developmental science: An encyclopedia of research, policies, and programs* (pp. 199–202). Thousand Oaks, CA: Sage.

Fisher, C. B., Hoagwood, K., Boyce, C., Duster, T., Frank, D. A., Grisso, T., Levine, R. J., et al. (2002). Research ethics for mental health science involving ethnic minority children and youths. *American Psychologist, 57, 1024*–1040.

Fisher, C. B., Hoagwood, K., & Jensen, P. S. (1996). Casebook on ethical issues in research with children and adolescents with mental disorders. In

K. Hoagwood, P. S. Jensen, & C. B. Fisher (Eds.), *Ethical issues in mental health research with children and adolescents* (pp. 135–266). Hillsdale, NJ: Erlbaum.

Fisher, C. B., & Ragsdale, K. (2006). A goodness-of-fit ethics for multicultural research. In J. Trimble and C. B. Fisher (Eds.), *The handbook of ethical research with ethnocultural populations and communities* (pp. 3–26). Thousand Oaks, CA: Sage Publications.

Fletcher, J., van Eys, J., & Dorn, L. (1993). Ethical considerations in pediatric oncology. In P. Pizzo & D. Poplack (Eds.), *Principles and practices of pediatric oncology* (pp. 1179–1191). Philadelphia: Lippincott.

Food and Drug Administration. (1997). The FDA Modernization Act of 1997, Public Law 105–115, 105th Congress. Federal Food, Drug, and Cosmetic Act (21 U.S.C. 301 et seq.).

Food and Drug Administration. (1998). Regulations requiring manufacturers to assess the safety and effectiveness of new drugs and biological products in pediatric patients. Final Rule, *Federal Register, 63*(231), 66,631–66,672.

Food and Drug Administration. (2001). Interim Rule: 21 CFR 50 and Section 54—Additional safeguards for children in clinical investigations of FDA-regulated products. *Federal Register, 66*(79), 20,589–20,600.

Foreman, D. M. (1999). The family rule: A framework for obtaining ethical consent for medical interventions from children. *Journal of Medical Ethics, 25*, 491–497.

Freedman, B. (1975). A moral theory of informed consent. *Hastings Center Report, 5*, 32–39.

Freedman, B. (1987). Equipoise and the ethics of clinical research. *New England Journal of Medicine, 317*, 141–145.

Friebert, S. E., & Kodish, E. D. (2000). Kids and cancer: Ethical issues in treating the pediatric oncology patient. *Cancer Treatment and Research, 102*, 99–135.

Furman, W. L., Stewart, C. F., Poquette, C. A., Pratt, C. B., Santana, V. M., Zamboni, W. C., et al. (1999). Direct translation of a protracted irinotecan schedule from a xenograft model to a phase I trial in children. *Journal of Clinical Oncology, 17*, 1815–1824.

Goodin, R. E. (1985). *Protecting the vulnerable*. Chicago: University of Chicago Press.

Grisso, T., Appelbaum, P. S., Mulvey, E. P., & Fletcher, K. (1995). The MacArthur Treatment Competence Study. II: Measures of abilities related to competence to consent to treatment. *Law and Human Behavior*, 19, 127–148.

Grisso, T., & Vierling, L. (1978). Minors consent to treatment: A developmental perspective. *Professional Psychology, 9*, 412–427.

Grodin, M., & Burton, L. A. (1988). Context and process in medical ethics: The contribution of family-systems theory. *Family Systems Medicine*, 6, 421–438.

Grodin, M. A., Glantz, L. H., & Glantz, L. E. (1994). *Children as research subjects: Science, ethics, and law*. New York: Oxford University Press.

Kodish, E., Eder, M., Noll, R. B., Ruccione, K., Lange, B., Angiolillo, A., et al. (2004). Communication of randomization in childhood leukemia trials. *Journal of the American Medical Association, 291*, 470–475.

Kodish, E. D., Pentz, R. D., Noll, R. B., Ruccione, K., Buckley, J., & Lange, B. J. (1998). Informed consent in the children's cancer group: Results of preliminary research. *Cancer, 82*, 2467–2481.

Kopelman, L. M. (1997). Children and bioethics: Uses and abuses of the best-interests standard. *The Journal of Medicine and Philosophy, 22*, 213–217.

Kunin, H. (1997). Ethical issues in pediatric life-threatening illness: Dilemmas of consent, assent, and communication. *Ethics and Behavior, 7*, 43–57.

Kupst, M. J., Patenaude, A. F., Walco, G. A., & Sterling, C. (2003). Clinical trials in pediatric cancer: Parental perspectives on informed consent. *Journal of Pediatric Hematology and Oncology*, 25, 787–790.

Levi, R. B., Marsick, R., Drotar, D., & Kodish, E. D. (2000). Diagnosis, disclosure, and informed consent: Learning from parents of children with cancer. *Journal of Pediatric Hematology and Oncology, 22*, 3–12.

Lewis, C. E., Lewis, M. A., & Ifekwunigue, M. (1978). Informed consent by children and participation in an influenza vaccine trial. *American Journal of Public Health, 68*, 1079–1082.

Melton, G. B. (1980). Children's concepts of their rights. *Journal of Clinical Child Psychology*, 9, 186–190.

Murphey, S. B. (1995). The national impact of clinical cooperative group trials for pediatric cancer. *Medical Pediatric Oncology, 24*, 279–280.

Olechnowicz, J. Q., Eder, M., Simon, C., Zyzanski, S., & Kodish, E. (2002). Assent observed: Children's involvement in leukemia treatment and research discussions. *Pediatrics, 109*, 806–814.

Pletsch, P. K., & Stevens, P. E. (2001). Children in research: Informed consent and critical factors affecting mothers. *Journal of Family Nursing, 7*, 50–70.

Pui, C. (1999). *Childhood leukemias*. Cambridge, UK: Cambridge University Press.

Ross, L. F. (1997). Health care decision making by children. Is it in their best interest? *Hastings Center Report, 27,* 41–45.

Ross, J. A., Severson R. K., Pollock, B. H. Robison, L. L. (1996). Childhood cancer in the United States: a geographical analysis of cases from the Pediatric Cooperative Clinical Trials groups. *Cancer, 77,* 201–207.

Ruccione, K., Kramer, R. F., Moore, I. K., & Perin, G. (1991). Informed consent for treatment of childhood cancer: Factors affecting parents' decision making. *Journal of Pediatric Oncology Nursing, 8,* 112–121.

Ruck, M. D., Abramovitch, R., & Keating, D. P. (1998). Children's and adolescents' understanding of rights: Balancing nurturance and self-determination. *Child Development, 69,* 404–417.

Ruck, M. D., Keating, D. P., Abramovitch, R., & Koegl, C. (1998). Adolescents' and children's knowledge about rights: Some evidence for how young people view rights in their own lives. *Journal of Adolescence, 21,* 275–89.

Scherer, D. T. (1991). The capacities of minors to exercise voluntariness in medical treatment decisions. *Law and Human Behavior, 15,* 431–449.

Spinetta, J. J., Masera, G., Jonkovic, M., Oppenheim, D., Martins, A. G., Arush, M. W., et al. (2003). Valid informed consent and participative decision-making in children with cancer and their parents: A report of the SIOP working committee on psychosocial issues in pediatric oncology. *Medical and Pediatric Oncology, 40* , 244–246.

Susman, E. J., Dorn, L. D., & Fletcher, J. C. (1992). Participation in biomedical research: The consent process as viewed by children, adolescents, young adults, and physicians. *Journal of Pediatrics, 121,* 547–52.

Syse, A. (2002). A valid (as opposed to informed) consent. *The Lancet, 356,* 1347–1348.

Tymchuck, A. (1992). Assent processes. In S. Sieber (Ed.), *Social research on children and adolescents: Ethical issues* (pp. 128–139). Thousand Oaks, CA: Sage.

Varni, J. W., Katz, E. R., Colgrove, R., & Dolgin, M. (1996). Family functioning predictors of adjustment in children with newly diagnosed cancer: A prospective analysis. *Journal of Child Psychology and Psychiatry and Allied Disciplines, 37,* 321–328.

Walker, M. U. (2002). Autonomy, beneficence, and justice in the wider context. *Ethics and Behavior, 12,* 291–293.

Weithorn, L. A., & Campbell, S. B. (1982). The competency of children and adolescents to make informed treatment decisions. *Child Development, 53,* 1589–1598.

Wiley, F. M., Ruccione, K., Moore, I. M., Mcguire-Cullen, P., Fergusson, J., Waskerwitz, M. J., et al. (1999). Parents' perceptions of randomization in pediatric clinical trials. *Cancer Practice, 7,* 248–256.

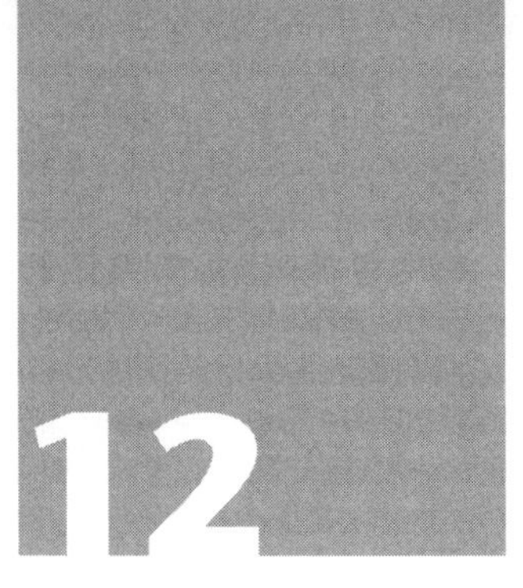

Olle Jane Z. Sahler, Diane L. Fairclough, Ernest R. Katz, James W. Varni, Sean Phipps, Raymond K. Mulhern (Deceased), Robert W. Butler, Robert B. Noll, Michael J. Dolgin, Donna R. Copeland, and W. Lewis Johnson

# Problem-Solving Skills Training for Mothers of Children With Newly Diagnosed Cancer

The diagnosis of childhood cancer is a highly stressful event for all members of the family. This chapter focuses on the responses of mothers during the first few months after the diagnosis and describes an 8-week intervention, entitled problem-solving skills training (PSST), that is efficacious in reducing features of negative affectivity in mothers during the time of induction and early treatment.

## Background

Studies examining the emotional well-being of parents of children with cancer suggested that mothers and fathers are at risk for symptoms of anxiety and depression during their child's treatment (Fife, Norton, & Groom, 1987; Hughes & Lieberman, 1990; Noll et al., 1995). In addition, some evidence suggested that mothers are at increased risk for posttraumatic stress symptoms after treatment ends (Hall & Baum, 1995; Kazak et al., 1997; Manne, DuHamel, Gallelli, Sorgen, & Redd, 1998; Manne et al., 2001, 2002; Pelcovitz et al., 1996; Stuber, Christakis, Houskamp, & Kazak, 1996). These findings are not universal. Some researchers have reported a return to normal psychological functioning among parents within months after their child was diagnosed (Dahlquist, Czyzewski, & Jones, 1996; Kupst & Schulman, 1988; Kupst et al., 1995). Regardless, consensus exists that there is a period of time immediately after a child is diagnosed with cancer when caregivers are at risk for an increase in symptoms of depression and anxiety (Kazak et al., 2001).

In addition to the specific stressors associated with a new diagnosis of cancer in her child, the wife/mother appears to be the key individual in maintaining the integrity of the entire family. For example, 74% of men reported that they talk primarily to their spouse when upset (Cutrona, 1996). Further, males will typically depend on their wives to maintain social contacts with friends, family, and the general community (Antonucci & Akiyama, 1987). Thus, mothers may be particularly vulnerable to distress because of the pivotal role they play in maintaining family social and emotional functioning.

The experience of a cancer diagnosis can be easily understood as a major negative life stressor that can cause significant psychological distress. High levels of distress in mothers at the beginning of their child's cancer treatment are problematic; it is essential that thoughtful informed decisions be made quickly regarding the administration of toxic, potentially life-threatening, and sometimes, unproven therapy. However, balancing the anxiety and fear that accompany a very serious diagnosis with the never-ceasing demands of everyday life requires energy, patience, and persistence. It is known that major stressful events can multiply and exacerbate minor stressful events (Nezu et al., 1999), and research has shown that minor, daily irritants may actually have more negative impact on psychological functioning than major events (Nezu & Ronan, 1985).

Successful coping is likely to reduce emotional distress. However, ineffective skills, especially in the face of overwhelming distress, can adversely affect an individual's enthusiasm and creativity, resulting in frustration, reduced motivation, and inhibition of otherwise adequate coping skills. These negative outcomes can lead to progressively poorer coping. Because helping mothers reduce their emotional distress as soon as possible after their child is diagnosed is critical, a major goal of intervention would be to replace the self-fulfilling prophesy of serial failure with an effective coping mechanism.

In previous work on the adaptation of siblings to cancer in the family (Sahler et al., 1997), it was found that mothers of children with cancer have a reduced sense of well-being and increased distress relative to mothers of healthy children. Furthermore, when healthy siblings were categorized according to their level of adaptation to childhood cancer in the family, less-adequate adaptation among the siblings was associated with lower levels of maternal well-being. Contrary to an expectation that more distressed mothers would be more isolated or less able to access services, it was found that mothers of the more poorly adjusted siblings accessed more resources than did mothers of siblings who were reported as adjusting well. Interestingly, however, mothers' level of satisfaction with their resources was remarkably low. Whether their dissatisfaction was caused by accessing the wrong resources, their inability to articulate their needs clearly enough to obtain appropriate help, or their inability to effectively apply whatever good and appropriate advice was offered is unknown.

These findings led to the hypothesis that a systematic method for teaching mothers of children with cancer how to identify their problems more accurately would reduce their stress levels and increase their levels of self-satisfaction and well-being. A wide variety of intervention options, including supportive counseling, brief psychotherapy, and logistical/financial assistance, are services routinely offered at children's cancer centers as part of "usual psychosocial care" (Noll & Kazak, 2004) and might potentially address this issue. However, increasing already available, but nonspecific, services appeared unlikely to address the particular problem that had been identified. That is, to enrich, rather than merely extend, existing services requires a novel approach. In particular, we were interested in directly addressing the concern our research had raised about mothers' abilities to identify their problems sufficiently well to access the best resources and use the advice they received to advantage.

Given the growing literature supporting the usefulness of problem-solving therapy (PST) for a variety of individuals in distress, we hypothesized that a PST-based intervention adapted specifically to the issues most commonly encountered in childhood cancer would increase problem-solving skills and, as a result, decrease emotional turmoil in mothers of newly diagnosed children. PST was particularly attractive because it provides an entirely different dimension of care rarely offered as part of usual psychosocial care at pediatric cancer centers.

## Problem-Solving Therapy

Problem solving is a metacognitive process by which individuals understand the nature of problems that confront them and identify or create means of coping with stressful events—either by altering the situations themselves or by altering personal reactions to them. Ineffective problem solving is the result of such obstacles as ambiguity, uncertainty, conflicting demands, lack of resources, novelty, or a combination (Nezu et al., 1999).

Classic PST has five basic components as described by D'Zurilla and Nezu (1982, 1999): (a) problem orientation (the cognitive and motivational set with which the individual approaches problems in general); (b) problem definition and formulation (delineation of a problem into concrete and specific terms and the identification of well-defined goals); (c) generation of alternatives (production of an exhaustive listing of possible solutions without regard to their consequences); (d) decision making (selection of the optimal solution); and (e) solution implementation and verification (monitoring and evaluation of the outcome after actual implementation of the selected solution). Each of the five steps makes a distinct contribution to the overall problem-solving strategy. The goal of the strategy is to clarify the specific nature of the problem; to specify a set of reasonable goals, whether they be modification of the problem situation (problem-focused goal) or modification of the individual's response to it (emotion-focused goal); and to assess the degree of success the strategy selected for the purpose of solving the problem has achieved.

PST is designed to facilitate the development of better problem-solving skills in response to specific everyday problems or stressful life events (D'Zurilla, Chang, Nottingham, & Faccini, 1998; D'Zurilla & Goldfried, 1971). It has demonstrated efficacy in the treatment of depression, anxiety, and stress-related syndromes (Arean et al., 1993; D'Zurilla & Chang, 1995; Nezu, 1986, 1987; Nezu, Nezu, & Arean, 1991; Nezu & Perri, 1989) and in facilitating adaptation to chronic health conditions (Bucher, Houts, Nezu, & Nezu, 1999; D'Zurilla & Nezu, 1999; Perri et al., 2001; van den Hout, Vlaeyen, Heuts, Zijlema, & Wijnen, 2003).

The special efficacy of PST in the treatment of depressive disorders led Nezu and colleagues to conceptualize depression as resulting from a person's ineffective attempts at coping with stressful life events, such as chronic illness (Nezu, Nezu, & Perri, 1989; Nezu, Nezu, Friedman, Houts, & Faddis, 1997). An interesting further finding is that adult patients with cancer (as an exemplar of a stressful situation) who have poor problem-solving skills have not only more depressive symptoms but also greater numbers of self-reported cancer-related problems (Nezu et al., 1999).

## Problem-Solving Skills Training

In contrast to PST, *problem-solving skills training* (PSST) is the term we have chosen to use to signify application of the PST approach to individuals who, as a group, are experiencing distress because of a challenging life event but who do not have a diagnosable psychological condition or require formal mental health intervention. PSST is grounded in the principles of PST. As a cognitive behavioral intervention, PSST is delivered as an ordered sequence of principles and exercises with review and reinforcement. Although the general paradigm is stable across interventions with many different diseases/conditions, to be most effective the context within which PSST strategies are taught to any specific learner group must be targeted to the particular psychosocial characteristics and perceived problems that are idiosyncratic to that group.

This distinction between skills training and therapy seems particularly important when providing a psychological intervention to a highly stressed but nonpsychiatric population. For example, during the course of their child's illness and treatment, mothers of children with cancer frequently make statements such as "I feel like I'm going crazy." Thus, it is important to avoid approaching these mothers in the initial stages of their experience with the notion that they require "therapy" with its attendant implication that they need mental health "treatment." Rather, the aim should be to normalize their experiences as common, reality-based reactions to the severe crisis of a cancer diagnosis in their child.

The overall model of the intervention postulates that (a) in response to a given stressor/crisis, the PSST intervention is applied; (b) the primary desired outcome of the intervention is an increase in problem-solving skills; (c) moderating factors influence how successfully problem-solving skills are mastered and implemented; and (d) higher levels of problem-solving skills decrease negative affectivity (secondary outcome) (see figure 12-1).

In the context of learning how to cope with normal reactions to stressful events, the benefit of problem-based skills training has been demonstrated in numerous populations. For example, social skills training for the newly diagnosed pediatric cancer patient has been reported by Katz and Varni (1993) and has been successfully applied by Varni, Katz, Colegrove, and Dolgin (1993) to children with cancer for such practical problems as becoming reintegrated into their school, community, and peer group. Work by a number of investigators also has led to the development of effective PSST programs for family members and friends of patients with cancer (Bucher et al., 1999; Houts, Nezu, Nezu, & Bucher, 1996; Nezu, Nezu, Felgoise, McClure, & Houts, 2003) as well as other chronic health conditions (Elliott, Shewchuk, & Richards, 1999). The success of these various interventions attests to the potential applicability of PSST across a wide population of learners, including individuals who are mildly mentally retarded (Nezu et al., 1991).

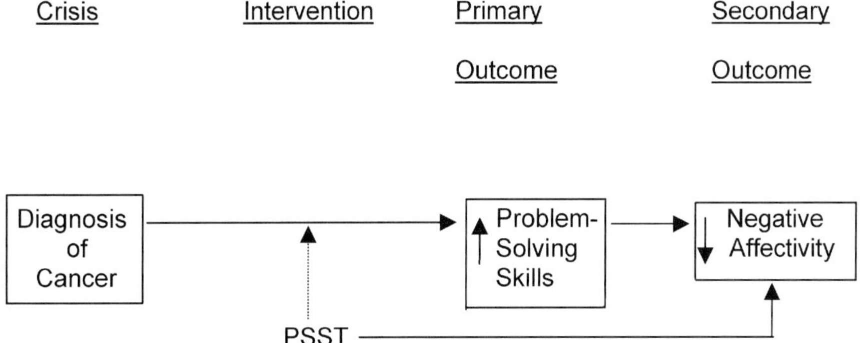


**Figure 12-1.** Conceptual model.

## Maternal Problem-Solving Skills Training: Intervention Design

### Guiding Principles

Guiding principles in designing the PSST intervention derived from the literature on adult learning are that learners should apply their own experience and knowledge to the new situation of cancer; learners should become aware of the new skills and strategies they need to acquire; adult behavior is internally motivated; different thinking and learning styles must be accommodated; deliberate feedback is essential; the instructional approach must be flexible while still meeting pedagogical goals; and learners have competing priorities (Vella, 1994).

To make the overall philosophy and steps of the PSST program more easily understood and remembered, the term *Bright IDEAS* and the logo of a lighted bulb were developed (figure 12-2). Bright signifies the sense of optimism (positive orientation) about solving problems that is essential for successful implementation. The letters *I* (identify the problem), *D* (determine the options), *E* (evaluate options and choose the best), *A* (act), and *S* (see if it worked) signify the five essential steps of problem solving as articulated by D'Zurilla and Nezu and restated by us (Varni et al., 1999). Instructional materials developed included a treatment manual, pocket-size summary brochure, worksheets for the various steps of problem solving, a refrigerator magnet with the Bright IDEAS logo, and trigger cartoons exemplifying the negative automatic thoughts to avoid (e.g., "This will never work"; "I can't do this").

### Accessibility

Few interventions are available for minority groups, yet the proportion of families seeking pediatric oncology care at border institutions who are recent immigrants, especially from Mexico and other Central and South American countries, often comprises over half of the patient population. Certainly, other areas of the country are experiencing similar influxes of other cultural groups.

Experience and research have demonstrated that Spanish-speaking mothers of pediatric cancer patients, as an example of a fast-growing immigrant group, are at increased risk for traumatic stress reactions associated with their child's illness (Hart, Katz, Stuber, Morphew, & Lopez, 2000; Saltoun-Moran, 1988). Immigrant mothers with limited English fluency have difficulty communicating and understanding complex medical systems and treatments and are more likely to perceive their child's situation as severe and life threatening (Delgado, 1981; Griffith, 1980; Heiman, Burruel, & Chavez, 1975; Saltoun-Moran, 1988; Seijo, Gomez, & Freidenberg, 1995). Even without an ill child, the difficult and often-dangerous process of immigration and acculturation experienced by immigrant mothers is associated with the loss of supportive familial, social, and cultural relationships; higher levels of poverty; interrupted maternal education; and increased emotional demands and distress (Cervantes, Salgado de Snyder, & Padilla, 1989; Cohen, 1987; Rogler, Cortes, & Malgady, 1991). These life experiences have been found to exacerbate the perceived stress of a child's illness (Saltoun-Moran, 1988; Vega, Kolody, & Valle, 1987).

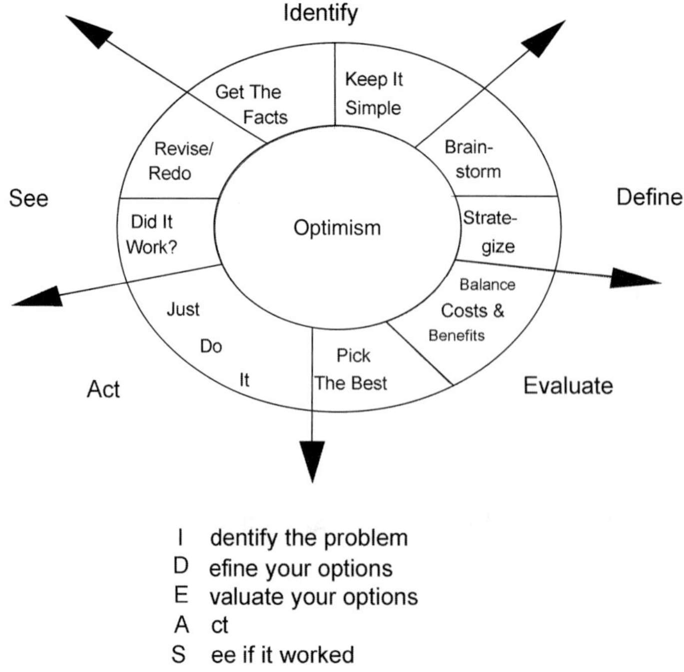


**Figure 12-2.** Bright IDEAS system for problem solving.

In the first study of traumatic stress symptoms in monolingual Spanish-speaking mothers of pediatric cancer patients using standardized assessment instruments, Hart, Katz, Stuber, Morphew, and Lopez (2000) (personal communication) found 35% of mothers reported moderate-to-high levels of distress, a rate similar to that of primarily Caucasian English-speaking mothers (Stuber et al., 1996). However, Spanish-speaking mothers experienced higher levels of severe avoidance symptoms than English-speaking parents did, and they tended to perceive lower quality of life for their ill children. Maternal education was significantly inversely associated with the development of traumatic stress symptoms.

To accommodate the large number of Mexican-Spanish mothers seeking care at several of our collaborating institutions (Childrens Hospital Los Angeles, Children's Hospital San Diego, and University of Texas/ M. D. Anderson Cancer Center), we translated all intervention and assessment materials and provided bilingual interventions. At our collaborating site in Israel, the intervention was provided in English and Hebrew.

## Resource Intensity

PSST is a human resource-intensive undertaking that requires coordination between the interventionist and the mother, who is subject to unanticipated disruptions in her daily schedule to accommodate her child's treatments and tests. Therefore, we were interested in developing an alternative method of delivery that would capitalize on new technology to provide ready access to the principles of PSST virtually any time of the day without the need for an interventionist to be present. Thus, in addition to the paper-and-pencil interventional materials, *Carmen's Bright IDEAS,* a personal computer-based interactive pedagogical drama (IPD) was developed. The goal of an IPD is to exploit the edifying power of story while promoting active learning. An IPD immerses learners in an engaging, evocative story in which they interact with realistic characters. Learners make decisions or take actions on behalf of a character in the story and view the consequences of their decisions. The story's characters are realized by autonomous agents (Marsella, Johnson, & LaBore, 2003).

The personal computer-based program consists of four related vignettes featuring the mother, Carmen, of a child with cancer and her interactions with a social worker, Gina, who instructs the mother in the steps of problem solving. *Carmen's Bright IDEAS* was used to supplement the written and in-person instruction of "classic" PSST by demonstrating and reinforcing the steps of problem solving. The ultimate goal is development of a technology-based intervention that is lifelike enough to substitute, at least in part, for an in-person intervention.

## Intervention Delivery

As noted, the Bright IDEAS PSST intervention is designed to be conducted in individual sessions with the child's mother. Although a group format is possible and has been used successfully by several investigators for other groups (e.g., caregivers of adult patients living at home), it is typically most convenient for the mother of a newly diagnosed pediatric cancer patient to schedule the instructional sessions during regular clinic appointments or during her child's extended hospitalizations. Such scheduling is too unpredictable to lend itself to a group format at this early stage of diagnosis and induction therapy, although group sessions might be possible during other phases of the illness, such as long-term survivorship. Thus, the instructional sessions are individualized, and the entire intervention program is conducted via eight 1-hour meetings over an 8- to 10-week period (see table 12-1).

## Structure of Intervention Sessions

### Session 1

The beginning of the first session is devoted to hearing the story of the child's diagnosis and the family's experiences since then. This leads naturally

**Table 12-1.** Treatment Sessions Format

Treatment Sessions 1–3

1. Introduce problem-solving steps
2. Present problem orientation philosophy (learning optimism: Bright IDEAS)
3. Define problem definition and formulation (**i**dentify the problem)
4. Describe generation of alternative solutions (**d**efine the options)
5. Delineate decision-making process (**e**valuate options)
6. Describe solution implementation (**a**ct out your choice)
7. Describe solution verification (**s**ee if it worked) and the steps in revising poor/mediocre solutions
8. Apply problem-solving steps to selected vignette in *Bright IDEAS* booklet
9. Review Current Problems Inventory to facilitate problem identification
10. Discuss parent worksheets
11. Introduce *Carmen's Bright IDEAS,* if appropriate
12. Begin problem-solving process with selected problem
13. Designate homework assignment
14. Give overview of format for subsequent sessions

Treatment Sessions 2 and 3

1. Review Session 1
2. Review homework assignment

1. Apply problem-solving steps to selected problem (either introduce or use *Carmen's Bright IDEAS,* if appropriate)
2. Steps 3–12 (without 8) for unresolved problem or new problem

Treatment Sessions 3–8

1. Review homework assignment
2. Steps 3–12 (without 8) for unresolved problem or new problem

Last Treatment Session

1. Review homework assignment
2. Discuss relapse prevention strategies

to a review of the Current Problems Inventory, developed for this intervention, which consists of 45 empirically chosen items clustered under the general headings of health (e.g., insomnia), social (e.g., attending to other children), feelings (e.g., guilt), financial (e.g., paying bills), and other problems (e.g., completing chores). Each mother is asked to identify items that are current problems for her and to rate the intensity of these problems on a 3-point scale. The Current Problems Inventory is designed to be reviewed and updated periodically. Thus, the specific problems discussed during each intervention session are identified by the individual mother as especially relevant to her and her family at that particular time. In this way, the time and effort expended in learning the problem-solving paradigm is put to good use solving an authentic personal or family problem.

During the first session, the mother is given a verbal overview of the entire intervention, in addition to the parent's manual, as well as the Bright IDEAS pamphlet summarizing the steps of problem solving with examples, the trigger cartoons, and a Bright IDEAS refrigerator magnet. *Carmen's Bright IDEAS* is also introduced if the mother is receiving the computer-enhanced intervention.

### Sessions 2–8

Worksheets are used at each session to structure problem identification, solution generation, development of a specific plan, evaluation of plan implementation, assessment of the results, and revision of unsatisfactory plans. At the end of each session, participants are given a "homework" assignment to identify and solve a problem of immediate interest to them before the next session. During the final session, mothers are coached to identify a strategy that would reinforce their usage of PSST as part of their daily coping style. Often, their solutions include the help of a support person (spouse, other family, friend) with whom they plan to share the principles of the intervention.

In the PSST-plus-*Carmen* intervention, mothers receive the same introduction to PSST that mothers in the PSST-alone intervention receive (see table 12-1). They are then introduced to the personal computer-based vignettes, which are used during at least three [of the remaining] sessions to reinforce the principles of Bright IDEAS and to provide practice with worksheets that detail the steps of problem solving.

## General Clinical Guidelines

Establishing the parent-interventionist relationship is the essential first step in conducting PSST just as it is in its more formally therapeutic counterpart, PST. Emulating warmth, empathy, trust, and genuineness sets the context for the mother's receptivity to learning the specific problem-solving strategies. Further, emphasizing the collaborative nature of the PSST approach enhances the mother's perception that the interventionist is treating her as an individual and needs her active cooperation to make PSST relevant and effective. Thus, engaging the mother in an active collaborative partnership requires a level of participation that facilitates learning the principles of PSST by immediately personalizing the application of the strategies to the mother's identified problems. This mutual collaboration fosters a sense of teamwork, in which the interventionist contributes general strategies and the overall approach to problems and the parent brings all the information and details unique to her experiences. The sense of collaboration and expectation that the mother is facing solvable problems is heightened by acknowledging that problem solving is an integral part of everyday life. The mother should also be reminded that she handled "life" quite well until faced with the relatively unique catastrophe of childhood cancer, which would strain the coping mechanisms and support networks of virtually any parent.

In this spirit of collaboration and shared expertise, the parent's manual is introduced as a method to facilitate the mother's independent and ongoing use of PSST in solving even the most mundane problems. The homework assignments are also described in this spirit of collaboration, in which the interventionist and the mother can brainstorm solutions and troubleshoot barriers together based on the mother's efforts to use PSST as recorded on the homework sheets. Thus, problem solving is presented as an eminently socially interactive interchange.

In the process of identifying problems to solve, brainstorming solutions, and troubleshooting barriers to solution implementation, it is essential that the interventionist utilize active listening techniques such as gentle probing and clarification, paraphrasing, empathic responses, and summarization. The major goal is to put the mother at ease and to have her understand that an empathic other is interested in her well-being. Throughout this process, it is essential that the interventionist emphasize a commitment to nonjudgmental, trusting, open, two-way communication. This is the essence of the collaborative empirical approach indigenous to PSST. Working closely with the parent in completing work sheets provides a concrete way of engaging in collaborative empiricism.

In implementing PSST, it is important to be aware of shortcomings that can limit the efficacy of the intervention. These include presenting PSST in a rotelike mechanistic manner and not making the process immediately relevant to the mother. As can be seen, these actions on the part of the interventionist make successful skills training dependent on excellent clinical skills even though provided from a manual.

## Maternal Problem-Solving Skills Training: Intervention Implementation

The intervention is offered to mothers between 2 and 16 weeks after the child's diagnosis with any form of cancer/brain tumor. Mothers are not approached if their child is in medical crisis (e.g., in the intensive care unit) during the period of recruitment. Mothers can choose to withdraw from the study if their child becomes critically ill or dies.

The initial plan had been to offer PSST to mothers 4–16 weeks after their child's diagnosis. The final selection of 2–16 weeks was based on the recommendation of several "experienced" mothers who participated in focus groups designed to give feedback and advice on how PSST should be implemented. These experienced mothers believed that it would be beneficial for mothers of newly diagnosed children to be aware that a program exists to help them cope and that they could access it immediately.

Mothers who agreed to participate in our studies of PSST completed the initial assessment battery consisting of a demographic inventory and three categories of measures: (a) Social Problem-Solving Inventory–Revised (SPSI-R; D'Zurilla & Nezu, 1990), a 52-item inventory of problem-solving style (rational, impulsive/careless, avoidant) and problem orientation (positive, negative); (b) Profile of Mood States (POMS; McNair, Lorr, & Droppleman, 1992), Beck Depression Inventory II (BDI-II; Beck, Steer, Ball, Ciervo, & Kabat, 1997), and the Impact of Event Scale–Revised (IES-R) (Weiss & Marmar, 1997) to assess various constructs of affectivity; and (c) the NEO-Five Factor Inventory (NEO-FFI) (Costa & McCrae, 1992), which derives its name from the first three of the five domain scales comprising the instrument, (Neuroticism, Extraversion, Openness, Agreeableness, and Conscientiousness) to investigate moderation, that is, to determine whether any personal characteristics predicted mothers who were more or less likely to benefit from the intervention. Mothers were subsequently randomly assigned to the control group (usual psychosocial care [UPC] as provided at that particular center) or one of the intervention groups (PSST + UPC; PSST + *Carmen* + UPC). The assessment battery was repeated at the end of the intervention (between Weeks 10 and 12 for the control group) and subsequently 3 months after the intervention (between Weeks 24 and 26 for the control group).

## Findings of Two Randomized Controlled Trials of Problem-Solving Skills Training

To date, 587 mothers have participated in studies of PSST: 92 mothers in the pilot feasibility study in English at five sites in the United States and in English and Hebrew at one site in Israel; and 495 English-, Hebrew-, and Spanish-speaking mothers (213 UPC, 217 PSST, and 65 PSST + *Carmen*) in the main study. The "typical" participant was Caucasian, was 35.5 years old, had at least graduated from high school, was married, and had a 7.6-year-old child with either leukemia or a solid (nonbrain) tumor. There were no significant demographic or ethnic differences between the UPC and PSST + UPC groups at baseline (*Carmen* was developed only in English). Approximately 90% of all participants completed all assessments. Lack of time was the primary reason cited for withdrawing from the study.

Table 12-2 presents the baseline frequency with which each of the five areas of potential concern listed on the Current Problems Inventory was endorsed by mothers. As may be seen, these

**Table 12-2.** Baseline Frequency of Problems

| Problem | % Endorsing as Moderate/Major/ Overwhelming | Problem | % Endorsing as Moderate/Major/ Overwhelming |
|---|---|---|---|
| Child's Needs | | Personal Physical Health | |
| Managing physical needs | 40 | Drugs/alcohol | 2 |
| Providing emotional support | 44 | Weight | 34 |
| Meeting school/social needs | 44 | Aches/pains | 30 |
| Being overprotective | 58 | Sexual functioning | 26 |
| Learning more about disease | 49 | Dizziness/faintness | 12 |
| Communicating with providers | 38 | Hot/cold spells | 15 |
| | | Heart pounding | 18 |
| Immediate Family | | Personal Mental Health | |
| Supervising other children | 43 | Anxiety | 44 |
| Emotional needs of other children | 59 | | |
| Communication among family | 44 | Personal Mental Health | |
| Conflicts with spouse | 34 | Anger | 36 |
| Financial and Occupational | | Grief | 40 |
| | | Sadness/depression | 50 |
| Medical bills | 24 | Hopelessness | 23 |
| Nonmedical bills | 41 | Guilt/self-doubt | 23 |
| Insurance | 19 | Worry | 68 |
| Job pressure | 30 | Being stressed | 60 |
| Reduced income | 47 | Helplessness | 35 |
| Social | | Poor attention | 37 |
| | | Questioning faith | 22 |
| Communication with friends | 26 | Ups-and-downs | 46 |
| Isolation from family | 35 | | |
| Social activities | 42 | Managing Daily Activities | |
| Conflict with friends | 9 | Transportation | 23 |
| Personal Physical Health | | Child care | 24 |
| | | Household management | 48 |
| Exhaustion | 57 | Time management | 48 |
| Poor sleep | 48 | Decision making | 40 |

problems ranged from concrete/logistical problem-focused issues to intense emotion-focused issues, in keeping with our notion of PSST as a generically useful approach to distressing life events.

All randomly assigned participants, regardless of whether they completed the intervention, were included in "intent-to-treat" analyses. Linear contrasts comparing the treatment groups employed *t* tests. Effect size was estimated for the change from baseline to the posttest intervention and to the 3-month follow-up using the standard deviation estimated from the baseline assessments.

## Findings for English-Speaking Mothers (Problem-Solving Skills Training Alone)

We found (Sahler et al., 2002) that there were significant differences between the control (UPC) and intervention (UPC + PSST) groups from baseline to the postintervention assessment on all measures and from baseline to 3-month follow-up on selected measures. For example, among English-speaking mothers, the POMS total score, the BDI-II score, and the IES-R total score all showed significantly greater improvement from the baseline to the follow-up assessment in the UPC + PSST group than

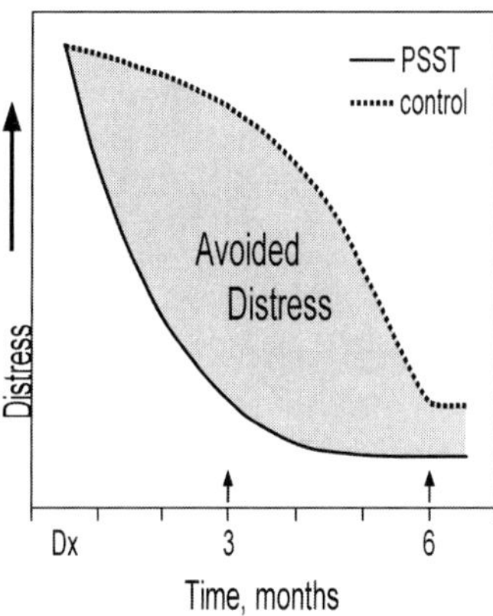


**Figure 12-3.** Distress trajectories of mothers of newly diagnosed childhood cancer patients.

in the UPC-only group. This difference was maintained at follow-up for the BDI-II and the IES-R but not for the POMS. The effect sizes obtained for the primary and secondary measures of negative affectivity (POMS, BDI-II, and IES-R) ranged from 0.31 to 0.42 (small-to-medium effect sizes). These findings were virtually indistinguishable from those of our initial pilot study, thus confirming our previous results. The findings regarding the "distress trajectory" of mothers during the first 6–8 months of their child's cancer illness with and without the PSST intervention are schematized in figure 12-3.

## Mediation

In evaluating the efficacy of PSST, we were especially interested in determining whether nonspecific effects of PSST (e.g., meeting with the interventionist in a socially supportive environment) were responsible for improvements in well-being, or whether real, objectively measured increases in problem-solving skills acquired from participation in PSST were responsible for these improvements. This question was addressed by testing the hypothesis that acquisition of problem-solving skills mediates the relationship between the PSST intervention and negative affectivity. Our analysis of the mediational model was based on our primary and secondary measures of PSST efficacy: changes from baseline to postintervention assessment in the POMS total score, the BDI-II score (square root transformation), and the IES-R total score. In the two alternative models of mediation, indirect effects of PSST are interpreted as mediation, whereas direct effects of PSST are deemed to reflect the direct impact of the intervention.

In the first model, the SPSI-R total score change from baseline to the postintervention assessment, representing an overall change in problem-solving skills, was considered the mediator. In the second model, two selected subscales of the SPSI-R, Negative Problem Orientation (NPO) and Avoidance Style (AS), were examined. All three putative mediators had been shown in the primary analysis to improve significantly more in the PSST + UPC group than in the UPC-alone group.

Evidence of partial mediation of improvement in negative affectivity as a result of PSST was provided by the following findings:

1. Improvements in problem-solving skills, as measured by the SPSI-R total score, accounted for approximately 30% of the change in the POMS total score, 20% of the change in the BDI-II score, and 21% of the change in the IES-R total score.
2. Reductions in NPO accounted for approximately 36% of the change in the POMS total score, 18% of the change in the BDI-II score, and 38% of the change in the IES-R total score.
3. Reductions in AS accounted for approximately 7% of the change in the POMS total score, 5% of the change in the BDI-II score, and 6% of the change in the IES-R total score.

The remainders, 57%, 76%, and 56%, respectively, were attributable to a direct effect of the intervention or unmeasured indirect effects. These results are consistent with our pilot study findings.

## Findings for Spanish-Speaking Mothers (Problem-Solving Skills Training Alone)

The analyses shown in table 12-3 are presented separately for English-speaking and Spanish-speaking mothers. As can be seen, although the intervention was highly successful among both groups of mothers, the results were more dramatic for Spanish-speaking mothers and some differences in negative affectivity persisted at the follow-up assessment. These findings of excellent responsivity to the intervention across cultural groups is consistent with findings reported for Israeli mothers in our pilot study (Dolgin, Peretz-Saltoun, & Eid, 2003; Peretz-Saltoun, Eid, & Dolgin, 1999).

**Table 12-3.** Change in Outcome Measures in English-Versus Spanish-Speaking Mothers (PSST Alone)

| *Outcome* | *Desired Direction* | *Language* | *T2-T1 PSST* | *T2-T1 Control* | *T3-T1 PSST* | *T3-T1 Control* | *T2-T1 p (one-tailed)* | *T3-T1 p (one-tailed)* |
|---|---|---|---|---|---|---|---|---|
| SPSI-R_T | Pos | English | 0.43 | 0.02 | 0.40 | 0.12 | .042 | |
| | | Spanish | 0.68 | 0.03 | 0.40 | 0.38 | .083 | |
| POMS_TMD | Neg | English | −22.69 | −8.16 | −20.39 | −13.32 | .001 | |
| | | Spanish | −15.69 | −11.35 | −17.67 | −18.80 | | |
| BDI-II_SQRT | Neg | English | −0.71 | −0.20 | −0.88 | −0.37 | <.001 | <.001 |
| | | Spanish | −0.88 | −0.22 | −0.79 | −0.64 | .021 | |
| IES-R_T | Neg | English | −8.77 | −5.05 | −10.56 | −6.12 | .018 | .007 |
| | | Spanish | −12.69 | −6.27 | −18.06 | −3.12 | .044 | <.001 |

SPSI-R_T, Social Problem-Solving Inventory-R—Total; POMS_TM, Profile of Mood States—Total Mood Disturbance; BDI-II_SQRT, Beck Depression Inventory II—Square Root Transformation; IES-R_T, Impact of Event Scale–Revised—Total; Neg, negative; Pos, positive. One-tailed test results are reported in keeping with our clear directional hypotheses and to uncover trend effects that might help explain the psychological mechanism of action of PSST in reducing negative affectivity.

In fact, it was the excellent results among the Israeli mothers that led us to perform only a literal translation of the PSST materials into Mexican-Spanish. We considered a culturally based modification of the intervention to accommodate the family-centered and hierarchical dynamic of Mexican families. However, based on the finding that a simple translation of PSST was accepted and used effectively at our Israeli site, which certainly represented a significantly different cultural milieu that included cosmopolitan and rural Israelis and Palestinians and nomadic Arabs, we concluded that, although the *solutions* immigrant Mexican mothers might choose to implement would likely reflect such a family system approach, the *actual steps* of problem solving did not need to be altered.

## Moderators

Clearly, congruence between the learner and the characteristics of the intervention is critical to appropriate resource utilization. For example, in the case of pain, it has been found that patients who cope best by being "vigilant monitors" prefer to observe the process, whereas patients who are "avoiders" prefer to be distracted (Schultheis, Peterson, & Selby, 1987). In the case of psychological dysfunction, the National Institute of Mental Health Treatment of Depression Collaborative Research Project reported differences in response to therapy based on level of cognitive functioning (Blatt & Felsen, 1993). Furthermore, psychotherapy researchers agree that matching an intervention to the individual's natural style requires less adjustment in usual behavior and, therefore, is more likely to be accepted and incorporated into the individual's spectrum of behavior. In contrast, a mismatch can produce no effect or even a deleterious effect (Christensen, Smith, Turner, & Cundick, 1994; Donovan & Muttson, 1994; Longabaugh, Wirtz, Beattie, Noel, & Stout, 1995; Martelli, Auerbach, Alexander, & Mercuri, 1987; Miller & Mangan, 1983; Smith & Sechrest, 1991).

Thus, we wished to identify personal characteristics and situational circumstances that moderate the feasibility and effectiveness of PSST. An exploratory analysis of patient and site characteristics associated with an enhanced impact of the intervention was conducted by adding interactions with the potential moderator into a simple regression model with change from the baseline to the postintervention assessment as the outcome. Potential moderators included age, education, marital status, language, personality style (NEO-FFI), and site (the pediatric center where the intervention was delivered).

### Problem-Solving Skills Training

Moderation was tested using a simple regression model with the change from baseline to the postintervention assessment as the outcome. Evidence of moderation consisted of a significant interaction between the moderator and an indicator of assignment to the PSST group. In the following analyses, reported $p$ values have not been adjusted for multiple comparisons.

An analysis of variables potentially moderating the impact of PSST on problem-solving skills, as measured by the SPSI-R total score, included the NEO-FFI scales and demographic factors. None of the NEO-FFI scales yielded statistically significant evidence of a moderating effect.

Among demographic factors, marital status was significant ($p < .05$). Specifically, single mothers in the PSST group (mean change = 1.02) benefited more from the intervention than mothers in the PSST group who were married or living with a partner (mean change = 0.31), whereas estimates of change in the control group were not significantly different for single (mean change = 0.27) or married mothers (mean change = 0.03). There also is a suggestion ($p = .052$) that maternal age may moderate improvements in problem-solving skills as a result of PSST. Specifically, younger mothers tended to benefit more from the PSST intervention than did older mothers. The changes in the PSST group are estimated to be 0.85, 0.47, and 0.09 in 25-, 35-, and 45-year-old mothers, respectively. Changes in the UPC group were not affected by age; estimates were 0.15, –0.02, and 0.10 in 25-, 35-, and 45-year-old mothers, respectively.

### Negative Affectivity

Demographic variables as well as the Neuroticism, Extraversion, Openness, Agreeableness, and Conscientiousness scales of the NEO-FFI were examined for moderating the effects of PSST on the measures of negative affectivity; none reached statistical significance. There is, however, a suggestion that the personality trait Extraversion, as measured by the NEO-FFI, may moderate changes in the POMS total score ($p = .08$). Specifically, participants with more *introverted* personalities obtained greater benefit from the intervention.

### Problem-Solving Skills Training Plus Carmen's Bright IDEAS

Similar changes in the acquisition of problem-solving skills were achieved by mothers in the PSST + *Carmen* arm compared to the PSST arm alone. The overall effects on negative affectivity, however, were not as strong in the combined arm as those found with the PSST condition alone.

Interestingly, in contrast to the findings with face-to-face paper-and-pencil PSST, improvements in problem-solving skills and in negative affectivity among mothers who received PSST + *Carmen* were mediated by increases in Positive Problem Orientation and Rational Problem Solving as well as significant decreases in NPO and AS.

The reasons for the difference in the mechanism of action of PSST are as yet unknown but may be based on how mothers related to the characters in the vignettes. For example, 44% of participants believed Carmen's age to be the same as their own, rather than younger or older, and 63% thought Carmen's problem was the same as theirs. Most participants (81%) believed Carmen would be able to cope with her problems to the same extent as the average person, and 75% believed that the Bright IDEAS concepts in Carmen's story were clear. At least 88% found that the story was somewhat interesting, and 69% thought the story was very believable. Most participants (56%) indicated that the particular conflict portrayed between Carmen and her daughter in the vignettes was very convincing.

The effect of *Carmen* may have been partly caused by the use of a novel learning tool. About 44% of the participants liked the animation style very much. The majority (88%) believed that the amount of interaction they had with the computer was about right. All participants thought that seeing Carmen's worksheets displayed and explained on the screen was at least somewhat useful, although only 62% thought that stopping the story to work on the worksheets was helpful. About 38% of participants agreed and an additional 38% strongly agreed that *Carmen's Bright IDEAS* helped them to remember the steps of problem solving. One half (50%) of the participants strongly agreed that using *Carmen's Bright IDEAS* helped them to understand how to apply the Bright IDEAS paradigm to their own problems.

Although these findings provoke speculation, it is important to note that *Carmen* was available only in English, and although allocation of participants to the *Carmen* group was random, assignment occurred only in the last year of the study and only in selected sites because of technical difficulties. As a result, there is greater potential for differences in demographics and initial problem-solving skills and negative affect than if the random assignment had occurred throughout the project. Interpretation of these results also is limited by the small sample size. Thus, the lack of differences should not lead to a conclusion of equivalence.

## Discussion

Our high recruitment and retention rates (~90%) confirm that mothers of newly diagnosed childhood cancer patients are eager for assistance. For our pilot project (Sahler et al., 2002), we specified the time for recruitment as 4–16 weeks after diagnosis. In focus group and other meetings with experienced mothers (mothers whose children had been diagnosed 1–2 years prior to the start of the project), we were strongly encouraged to approach mothers as early as 2 weeks after diagnosis rather than waiting until multiple problems and issues had already arisen. This modification was made for the second study. However, we found that the refusal rate prior to 4 weeks was at least twice the rate 4 weeks or longer after initial diagnosis. There appears to be a period of such great distress and disorganization that, regardless of the potential benefit of the intervention, participation by the mother in activities not directly related to caring for her child or making decisions about care seems too overwhelming. Later in the study, we continued to provide brochure and poster information about the project beginning as early as 2 weeks after diagnosis, but we did not routinely approach mothers until at least 4 weeks had passed. Our recruitment rate within the time frame of 4–16 weeks was about 85%.

The results demonstrated not only the efficacy of PSST in teaching problem-solving skills but also that administering PSST resulted in decreased negative affectivity in participants. The significant differences we found in Caucasian, African American, Spanish-speaking, Israeli, and Arab mothers attests to the universal appeal of this approach.

The overall picture is of statistically significant differences between the groups immediately following the intervention in the SPSI-R summary score and in the subscores for NPO and AS in the PSST-alone group. These same outcomes as well as desired differences for Positive Problem Orientation and Rational Problem Solving occurred in the PSST + *Carmen* group. There were also statistically significant differences on all of the measures of negative affect (POMS, BDI-II, and IES-R) for both intervention groups. Although differences were maintained at 6 months for the BDI-II and IES-R measures, other differences between the intervention and control groups diminished over time, primarily because of slow but continued improvement in mothers who were assigned to the control group (see figure 12-3). Among the group of monolingual Spanish-speaking mothers, however, the effects were both more pronounced and more sustained.

It is possible that the highly desirable effects of PSST on maternal emotional distress shortly after diagnosis may be associated with a reduction in the posttraumatic stress symptoms often reported by mothers of newly diagnosed childhood cancer patients (Hall & Baum, 1995; Pelcovitz et al., 1996). This is an area worthy of further research that includes longer-term follow-up and more precise dismantling of the most powerful components of the intervention.

A large proportion of the change in outcomes induced by the intervention is accounted for by a direct effect. There are two obvious explanations. First, there is a direct effect of the time and attention that the interventionists spend with the mothers. This possibility has been the motivation for the inclusion of a time-and-attention control for future studies that we propose to undertake. Second, the SPSI-R only partially measures the changes in functional problem-solving skills induced by the intervention. This concern has motivated our interest in an alternative measure of problem-solving skills.

Another interesting result is that, although the intervention itself seems to be affecting both NPO and AS, differential effects of PSST most likely result from the focus and content of the instructional package, especially when the results of the PSST + *Carmen* arm are considered. Based on our findings, we reviewed our written materials with respect to the individual components of the PSST intervention. Clearly, the paradigm of confronting problems by developing strategies, seeking solutions, and evaluating outcomes (avoiding "avoidance") is practiced repeatedly and strongly reinforced by our optimistic logo (glowing light bulb) and name (Bright IDEAS), all contributing to a less-negative problem orientation. Similarly, negative automatic thoughts, which can lead to a negative orientation, are addressed specifically by trigger cartoons that can be displayed as reminders to guard against certain thoughts.

In addition, AS is addressed implicitly in our training paradigm. That is, avoidance, as a way of coping with an identified problem, is not typically permitted because active solutions are considered more favorable and thus are more likely to be implemented during sessions. As a result, avoidance, even as a sometimes-useful strategy, is rarely discussed. Furthermore, given the finite time available for the intervention, the mother can actually choose not to identify issues she prefers to avoid, for whatever reason, thus bypassing direct analysis of this option.

In contrast, use of an animated story about a mother of similar age with commonly encountered problems who successfully applies the Bright IDEAS paradigm, enhances Positive Problem Orientation and Rational Problem Solving. Thus, addition of a believable role model appears to provide a complementary set of desirable effects.

A number of studies have investigated the relative contribution of the dimensions of problem-solving ability to various health outcomes. Kant, D'Zurilla, and Maydeu-Olivares (1997) found that NPO was positively and significantly associated with both depressive symptoms and anxiety. In contrast, there was a significant negative association among Positive Problem Orientation, depressive symptoms, and anxiety. Rational Problem Solving, Impulsivity/Carelessness Style, and AS also were significantly correlated, in the expected directions, with depressive symptoms and anxiety. In multiple regression analyses, the relationships among social problem solving, depression, and anxiety were primarily accounted for by NPO. In interpreting this finding, the investigators suggest that a negative problem orientation signifies that everyday problems have a threatening and pessimistic psychological significance for the individual that is likely to have a direct effect on emotional distress (symptoms of depression and anxiety). Elliott et al. (1999) found that caregiver tendencies to problem solve impulsively and carelessly were associated with lower acceptance of disability in patients with spinal cord injury and were predictive of the presence of pressure sores 1 year later.

In a dismantling investigation of the effects of PST on unipolar depression, Nezu and Perri (1989) examined the problem orientation component of the overall intervention model as distinct from the skills-oriented PST components. Findings suggested that training in problem orientation added significantly to the overall effectiveness of the PST treatment package by providing the motivational and cognitive appraisals necessary to facilitate adoption and actual performance of the PST skills-oriented components.

## Limitations

A major potential limitation of our investigation is the lack of a time-and-attention control group. Given that this investigation represents an early test of PSST in mothers of newly diagnosed pediatric cancer patients, our intent was to evaluate the efficacy of PSST in comparison to usual psychosocial care. Although our design did not control for attention effects, the mediational effects of problem-solving skills as measured by the SPSI-R do provide promising evidence of the specific effects of increasing problem-solving skills separate from merely providing attention.

A second limitation is the lack of a measure of problem-solving ability independent of the SPSI-R, which leaves the study open to the criticism that we were "teaching to the test." Although this may be true to some extent, especially regarding terminology used in the SPSI-R, the mediational effects of the PSST intervention on changes in mothers' mood state support the contention that the positive effects of the PSST intervention represent more than mere "practice effects" on the assessment measures. A more objective, real-life assessment tool is planned for future studies.

A third area necessitating greater attention is that of the effect size of our intervention. Although our findings have confirmed the efficacy of PSST, it is critical that additional research be conducted that builds on the model with innovative instructional strategies, including the use of readily accessible technology, so that we can increase the time and effort subjects put into practicing their skills. These limitations form the basis for our ongoing work.

Directions for the future study of this promising intervention include extending the conceptual framework to other family members, health care providers, and other health conditions. Addressing diagnosis-specific concerns would require only tailoring of the Current Problems Inventory; since PSST is designed to be a generic approach to teaching problem-solving skills. Thus, with little modification, this intervention is wholly applicable to managing specific as well as the myriad non-categorical, or shared-in-common, challenges characteristic of a host of chronic disorders in children (Stein & Jessop, 1982; Wallander, Varni, Babani, Banis, & Wilcox, 1988). Furthermore, although we chose to apply PSST to the crisis situation of a newly diagnosed health condition, it can be implemented at any time during the course of an illness that has the potential to overwhelm a patient's or family's capacity for successful coping.

*Acknowledgment.* This project was supported by grant R(25) CA65520 from the National Cancer Institute, National Institutes of Health.

## References

Antonucci, T. C., & Akiyama, H. (1987). An examination of sex differences in social support among older men and women. *Sex Roles, 17,* 11–12.

Arean, P. A., Perri, M. G., Nezu, A. M., Schein, R. L., Christopher, F., & Joseph, T. X. (1993). Comparative effectiveness of social problem-solving therapy and reminiscence therapy as treatments for depression in older adults. *Journal of Consulting and Clinical Psychology, 61,* 1003–1010.

Beck, A. T., Steer, R. A., Ball, R., Ciervo, C. A., & Kabat, M. (1997). Use of the Beck Anxiety and Depression Inventories for primary care with medical outpatients. *Assessment, 4,* 211–219.

Blatt, S. J., & Felsen, I. (1993). Different kinds of folks may need different kinds of strokes: The effect of patients' characteristics on therapeutic process and outcome. *Psychotherapy Research, 3,* 245–259.

Bucher, J. A., Houts, P. S., Nezu, C. M., & Nezu, A. M. (1999). Improving problem-solving skills of family caregivers through group education. *Journal of Psychosocial Oncology, 16,* 73–84.

Cervantes, R. C., Salgado de Snyder, V. N., & Padilla, A. M. (1989). Posttraumatic stress in immigrants from Central America and Mexico. *Hospital and Community Psychiatry, 40,* 615–619.

Christensen, A. J., Smith, T. W., Turner, C. W., & Cundick, K. E. (1994). Patient adherence and adjustment in renal diagnosis: A person × treatment interactive approach. *Journal of Behavioral Medicine, 17,* 549–566.

Cohen, R. E. (1987). Stressors: Migration and acculturation to American society. In M. Gaviria and J. Arana (Eds.), *Research agenda for Hispanics 1,* (pp. 59–71). Chicago: University of Illinois at Chicago, Simon Bolivar Hispanic American Psychiatric Research and Training Program.

Costa, P. T., & McCrae, R. R. (1992). Normal personality assessment in clinical practice: The NEO Personality Inventory. *Psychological Assessment, 4,* 5–13.

Cutrona, C. E. (1996). *Social support in couples: Marriage as a resource in times of stress.* Thousand Oaks, CA: Sage.

Dahlquist, L. M., Czyzewski, D. I., & Jones, C. L. (1996). Parents of children with cancer: A longitudinal study. *Journal of Pediatric Psychology, 21,* 541–554.

Delgado, M. (1981). Hispanic cultural values: Implications for groups. *Small Group Behavior, 12,* 69–80.

Dolgin, M. J., Peretz-Saltoun, N., & Eid, J. (September, 2003). *A collaborative study of maternal problem solving skills training in childhood cancer: The Israel experience.* Paper presented at the Annual Conference on Pediatric Psychooncology, Rambam Medical Center, Haifa, Israel.

Donovan, D. M., & Muttson, M. E. (1994). Alcoholism treatment matching research: Methodological and clinical approaches. *Journal of Studies on Alcohol, 12,* 5–14.

D'Zurilla, T. J., & Nezu, A. (1982). Social problem solving in adults. In P. C. KENDALL (Ed.), *Advances in Cognitive-Behavioral Research and Therapy* (Vol. 1, pp. 201–274). New York: Academic Press.

D'Zurilla, T. J., & Chang, E. C. (1995). The relations between social problem solving and coping. *Cognitive Therapy and Research, 19,* 547–562.

D'Zurilla, T. J., Chang, E. C., Nottingham, E. J., & Faccini, L. (1998). Social problem-solving deficits and hopelessness, depression, and suicidal risk in college students and psychiatric inpatients. *Journal of Clinical Psychology, 54,* 1091–1107.

D'Zurilla, T. J., & Goldfried, M. R. (1971). Problem solving and behavior modification. *Journal of Abnormal Psychology, 78,* 107–126.

D'Zurilla, T. J., & Nezu, A. M. (1990). Development and preliminary evaluation of the Social Problem-Solving Inventory. *Psychological Assessment, 2,* 156–163.

D'Zurilla, T. J., & Nezu, A. M. (1999). *Problem-solving therapy: A social competence approach to clinical intervention* (2nd ed.). New York: Springer.

Elliott, T. R., Shewchuk, R. M., & Richards, J. S. (1999). Caregiver social problem-solving abilities and family member adjustment to recent-onset physical disability. *Rehabilitation Psychology, 44,* 104–123.

Fife, B., Norton, J., & Groom, G. (1987). The family's adaptation to childhood leukemia. *Social Science and Medicine, 24,* 159–168.

Griffith, J. E. (1980). *A critique of a strategy to increase utilization of community mental health services by Mexican Americans.* Claremont, CA: Claremont University.

Hall, M., & Baum, A. (1995). Intrusive thoughts as determinants of distress in parents of children with cancer. *Journal of Applied Social Psychology, 25,* 1215–1230.

Hart, K. S., Katz, E., Stuber, M., Morphew, T. L., & Lopez, E. (November, 2000). Clinical implications for Latino mothers of children with cancer and their families. In *Latino Psychology 2000: Bridging our diversity*. San Antonio, TX: Hispanic Mental Health Society.

Heiman, E. M., Burruel, G., & Chavez, N. (1975). Factors determining effective psychiatric outpatient treatment for Mexican-Americans. *Hospital and Community Psychiatry, 26,* 515–517.

Houts, P. S., Nezu, A. M., Nezu, C. M., & Bucher, J. A. (1996). The prepared family caregiver: A problem-solving approach to family caregiver education. *Patient Education and Counseling, 27,* 63–73.

Hughes, P. M., & Lieberman, S. (1990). Troubled parents: Vulnerability and stress in childhood cancer. *British Journal of Medical Psychology, 63,* 53–64.

Kant, G., D'Zurilla, T. J., Maydeu-Olivares, A. (1997). Social problem solving as a mediator of stress-related depression and anxiety in middle-aged and elderly community residents. *Cognitive Therapy and Research, 21,* 73–96.

Katz, E. R. & Varni, J. W. (1993). Social support and social cognitive problem-solving in children with newly diagnosed cancer. *Cancer, 71,* 3314–3319.

Kazak, A. E., Barakat, L. P., Alderfer, M., Rourke, M. T., Meeske, K., Gasllagher, P. R., et al. (2001). Posttraumatic stress in survivors. *Journal of Clinical Psychology in Medical Settings, 8,* 307–323.

Kazak, A. E., Barakat, L. M., Lamia, P., Meeske, K., Cristakis, D., Meadows, A. T., et al. (1997). Posttraumatic stress, family functioning, and social support in survivors of childhood leukemia and their mothers and fathers. *Journal of Clinical Consulting and Clinical Psychology, 65,* 120–129.

Kupst, M. J., Natta, M. B., Richardson, C. C., Cathryn, C., Schulman, J. L., Lavigne, J. V., et al. (1995). Family coping with pediatric leukemia: 10 years after treatment. *Journal of Pediatric Psychology, 20,* 601–617.

Kupst, M. J., & Schulman, J. L. (1988). Long-term coping with pediatric leukemia: A 6-year follow-up study. *Journal of Pediatric Psychology, 13,* 7–22.

Longabaugh, R., Wirtz, P. W., Beattie, M. C., Noel, N., & Stout, R. (1995). Matching treatment focus to patient social investment and support: 18-month follow-up results. *Journal of Consulting and Clinical Psychology, 63,* 296–307.

Manne, S. L., DuHamel, K., Gallelli, K., Sorgen, K., & Redd, W. H. (1998). Posttraumatic stress disorder among mothers of pediatric cancer survivors: Diagnosis, comorbidity, and utility of the PTSD Checklist as a screening instrument. *Journal of Pediatric Psychology, 23,* 357–366.

Manne, S., DuHamel, K., Nereo, N., Ostroff, J., Parsons, S., Martini, R., et al. (2002). Psychological adaptation and social support of parents of pediatric cancer patients: A prospective longitudinal study. *Journal of Pediatric Psychology, 27,* 607–617.

Manne, S., Nereo, N., DuHamel, K., Ostroff, J., Parsons, S., Martini, R. et al. (2001). Posttraumatic stress symptoms and stressful life events predict the long-term adjustment of survivors of childhood cancer and their mothers. *Journal of Consulting and Clinical Psychology, 69,* 1037–1047.

Marsella, S. C., Johnson, W. L., & LaBore, C. (2003). An interactive pedagogical drama for health interventions. In U. Hoppe & F. Verdejo (Eds.), *Artificial intelligence in education: Shaping the future of learning through intelligent technologies* (pp. 341–348). Amsterdam: IOS Press.

Martelli, M. F., Auerbach, S. M., Alexander, J., & Mercuri, L. G. (1987). Stress management in the health care setting: Matching interventions with patient coping styles. *Journal of Consulting and Clinical Psychology, 55,* 201–207.

McNair, D. M., Lorr, M., & Droppleman, L. F. (1992). *Manual for the Profile of Mood States*. San Diego, CA: Educational and Industrial Testing Service.

Miller, S. M., & Mangan, C. E. (1983). Interacting effects of information and coping style in adapting to gynecologic stress: Should the doctor tell all? *Journal of Personality and Social Psychology, 45,* 223–236.

Nezu, A. M. (1986). Efficacy of a social problem-solving therapy approach for unipolar depression. *Journal of Consulting and Clinical Psychology, 54,* 196–202.

Nezu, A. M. (1987). A problem-solving formulation of depression: A literature review and proposal of a pluralistic model. *Clinical Psychology Review, 7,* 121–144.

Nezu, C. M., Nezu, A. M., & Arean, P. (1991). Assertiveness and problem solving therapy for persons with mental retardation and dual diagnoses. *Research in Developmental Disabilities, 12,* 371–386.

Nezu, A. M., Nezu, C. M., Felgoise, S. H., McClure, K. S., & Houts, P. S. (2003). Project Genesis: Assessing the efficacy of problem-solving therapy for distressed adult cancer patients. *Journal of Consulting and Clinical Psychology, 71,* 1036–1048.

Nezu, C. M., Nezu, A. M., Friedman, S. H., Houts, P. S., DelliCarpini, L., Bildner, C., et al. (1999). Cancer and psychological distress: Two investigations regarding the role of social problem-solving. *Journal of Psychosocial Oncology, 16,* 27–40.

Nezu, A. M., Nezu, C. M., Friedman, S. H., Houts, P. S., & Faddis, S. (1997). Project Genesis: Application of problem-solving therapy for distressed cancer patients. *The Behavior Therapist, 20,* 155–158.

Nezu, A. M., Nezu, C. M., & Perri, M. G. (1989). *Problem-solving therapy for depression: Theory, research, and clinical guidelines.* New York: Wiley.

Nezu, A. M., & Perri, M. G. (1989). Social problem-solving therapy for unipolar depression: An initial dismantling investigation. *Journal of Consulting and Clinical Psychology, 57,* 408–413.

Nezu, A. M., & Ronan, G. F. (1985). Life stress, current problems, problem solving, and depressive symptoms: An integrative model. *Journal of Consulting and Clinical Psychology, 53,* 693–697.

Noll, R. B., Gartstein, M. A., Hawkins, A., Vannatta, K., Davies, W. H., & Bukowski, W. M. (1995). Comparing parental distress for families with children who have cancer and matched comparison families without children with cancer. *Family Systems Medicine, 13,* 11–28.

Noll, R. B., & Kazak, A. (2004). Psychosocial care. In A. Altman (Ed.), *Supportive care of children with cancer: Current therapy and guidelines from the Children's Oncology Group*, pp. 337–353. Baltimore, MD: Johns Hopkins Press.

Pelcovitz, D., Goldenberg, B., Kaplan, S., Weinblatt, M., Mandel, F., Meyers, B., et al. (1996). Posttraumatic stress disorder in mothers of pediatric cancer survivors. *Psychosomatics, 37,* 116–126.

Peretz-Saltoun, N., Eid, J., & Dolgin, M. J. (1999). *Problem solving skills training in mothers of children with cancer.* Paper presented at the Israel Association of Medical Social Workers, Tel Aviv, Israel.

Perri, M. G., Nezu, A. M., McKelvey, W. F., Shermer, R. L., Renjilian, D. A., & Viegener, B. J. (2001). Relapse prevention training and problem-solving therapy in the long-term management of obesity. *Journal of Consulting and Clinical Psychology, 69,* 722–726.

Rogler, L. H., Cortes, D. E., & Malgady, R. G. (1991). Acculturation and mental health status among Hispanics: Convergence and new directions for research. *American Psychologist, 46,* 585–597.

Sahler, O. J., Roghmann, K. J., Mulhern, R. K., Carpenter, P. J., Sargent, J. R., Copeland, D. R., et al. (1997). Sibling Adaptation to Childhood Cancer Collaborative Study: The association of sibling adaptation with maternal well-being, physical health, and resource use. *Journal of Developmental and Behavioral Pediatrics, 18,* 233–243.

Sahler, O. J., Varni, J. W., Fairclough, D. L., Butler, R. W., Noll, R. B., Dolgin, M. W. P. S., et al. (2002). Problem-solving skills training for mothers of children with newly diagnosed cancer: A randomized trial. *Journal of Developmental and Behavioral Pediatrics, 23,* 77–86.

Saltoun-Moran, M. (1988). *Hispanic parents' adaptation to childhood cancer: Influences on language and culture.* American Cancer Society, Oakland, California Division.

Schultheis, K., Peterson, L., & Selby, V. (1987). Preparation for stressful medical procedures and person * treatment interactions. *Clinical Psychology Review, 7,* 329–352.

Seijo, R., Gomez, H., & Freidenberg, J. (1995). Language as a communicator barrier in medical care for Hispanic patients. In A. M. Padilla (Ed.), *Hispanic psychology: Critical issues in theory and research* (pp. 169–181). Thousand Oaks, CA: Sage.

Smith, B., & Sechrest, L. (1991). Treatment of aptitude * treatment interactions. *Journal of Consulting and Clinical Psychology, 59,* 233–244.

Stein, R. E., & Jessop, D. J. (1982). A noncategorical approach to chronic childhood illness. *Public Health Reports, 97,* 354–362.

Stuber, M. L., Christakis, D. A., Houskamp, B., & Kazak, A. E. (1996). Posttrauma symptoms in childhood leukemia survivors and their parents. *Psychosomatics, 37,* 254–261.

van den Hout, J. H., Vlaeyen, J. W., Heuts, P. H., Zijlema, J. H., & Wijnen, J. A. (2003). Secondary prevention of work-related disability in nonspecific low back pain: Does problem-solving therapy help? A randomized clinical trial. *Clinical Journal of Pain, 19,* 87–96.

Varni, J. W., Katz, E. R., Colegrove, R., Jr. And Dolgin, M. (1993). The impact of social skills training on the adjustment of children with newly diagnosed cancer. *Journal of Pediatric Psychology, 18,* 751–767.

Varni, J. W., Sahler, O. J., Katz, E. R., Mulhern, R. K., Copeland, D. R., Noll, R. B., et al. (1999). Maternal problem-solving therapy in pediatric cancer. *Journal of Psychosocial Oncology, 16,* 41–71.

Vega, W. A., Kolody, B., & Valle, J. R. (1987). Migration and mental health: An empirical test of depression risk factors among immigrant Mexican women. *International Migration Review, 21,* 512–530.

Vella, J. (1994). Twelve principles for effective adult learning. In J. Vella (Ed.), *Learning to listen, learning to teach: The power of dialogue in educating adults* (pp. 3–22). San Francisco: Jossey-Bass.

Wallander, J. L., Varni, J. W., Babani, L., Banis, H. T., & Wilcox, K. T. (1988). Children with chronic physical disorders: maternal reports of their psychological adjustment. *Journal of Pediatric Psychology, 13,* 197–212.

Weiss, D. S., & Marmar, C. R. (1997). The Impact of Event Scale–Revised. In J. P. Wilson & T. M. Keane (Eds.), *Assessing psychological trauma and PTSD* (pp. 399–411). New York: Guilford Press.

# Cancer Late Effects "Off Treatment"

Anna L. Marsland, Linda J. Ewing,

and Amanda Thompson

# Psychological and Social Effects of Surviving Childhood Cancer

Children diagnosed with cancer confront a series of unusually stressful life circumstances. These stressors include change from apparent health to illness, threat to the future, hospitalization, clinic visits, medical investigations and procedures, adverse side effects of treatment (e.g., hair loss, weight gain or loss, nausea, vomiting), financial strain, and the disruption of school, social supports and routines. The uncontrollable and unpredictable nature of this disease makes it the provider of a particularly potent series of stressors that may tax the coping resources of even the most resilient people. Stressors associated with childhood cancer do not stop at the end of treatment. Indeed, there is a large body of literature demonstrating that childhood cancer survivors are at substantial risk of adverse health status and physical sequelae, including neurocognitive dysfunction, cardiopulmonary toxicity, endocrinopathy, and second malignancy (Dreyer, Blatt, & Bleyer, 2002; Hudson et al., 2003).

In contrast to well-documented late physical effects, the psychosocial consequences of childhood cancer are less well understood. Although the body of literature has grown considerably, inconsistent findings and inadequate methodologies have made it difficult to draw robust conclusions. In contrast to studies showing that children with chronic physical disorders are at increased risk for psychological and social adjustment problems (Lavigne & Faier-Routman, 1993; Wallander, Varni, Babani, Banis, & Wilcox, 1988), reviews of the childhood cancer literature focusing on normative adjustment show no evidence of long-term maladjustment when compared with healthy peers or population norms and therefore conclude that the majority of survivors cope well with the stress of their disease and treatment (Eiser, Hill, & Vance, 2000; Kazak, 1994). In fact, some investigators have gone as far as to suggest that childhood cancer may play a protective role and may be associated with better-than-typical emotional health or an improvement in psychological adjustment from pre- to postdiagnosis (e.g., Gray et al., 1992; Kupst et al., 1995). Other studies have focused their attention on the significant subset of survivors (10%–20%) who do show ongoing symptoms of psychological maladjustment and social difficulties (e.g., Hobbie et al., 2000; Stuber et al., 1997). Taken together, the observed variability in psychological outcome among survivors of childhood cancers suggests individual differences in adaptation to this early stressor, with some survivors at risk for ongoing psychological and social maladjustment. Consequently, there is great need to identify risk and protective factors that may account for this variability and ultimately aid in the prediction of individual adjustment trajectories.

Given the enormous burden and disruptive nature of cancer and its treatment for both the child and the child's family, many have questioned whether methodological limitations account for the failure to find more enduring and more problematic sequelae (Eiser, 1998; Kazak, 1994). Comparisons across studies in this largely cross-sectional literature are made difficult by variability in design, type and stage of cancer, nature of treatment, demographics of the sample, age at diagnosis, length of time since diagnosis, and number of years off treatment. Other general limitations of this literature body that may explain conflicting results include small sample sizes, inconsistency in how psychosocial constructs are operationalized, and measurement of these constructs with psychometrically weak instruments that have not been validated for use with cancer populations (Eiser, 1998). Such discrepancies and variability in the characteristics of subject samples and measures may help to explain the presence of contradictory and null findings.

A couple of issues are particularly problematic regarding comparisons among studies and warrant further discussion. First, it often is erroneously assumed that cancer is a single disease entity, with common psychosocial consequences. In fact, childhood cancer shows considerable heterogeneity with respect to incidence, symptomatology, course, demographics, mortality, risk factors, treatment regimens, and etiology. Hence, the psychosocial impact of diagnosis and treatment is likely to be specific to the site and type of cancer as well as the stage of disease.

A second major limitation of this body of literature is general failure to consider the child's developmental stage at the time of both diagnosis and follow-up. Indeed, many investigators have expressed a need for research that is developmentally sensitive (Eiser et al., 2000; Hill & Stuber, 1997; Joubert et al., 2001; Kazak, Christakis, Alderfer, & Coiro, 1994; Stuber & Kazak, 1999; Woodgate, 1999). Thus far, studies examining the psychosocial late effects of treatment for childhood cancer typically employed samples that covered a wide age range; as a result, age-based differences in psychosocial adjustment have likely been obscured. Developmental constraints on outcome have not been studied systematically. Given that chronological age (a rough gauge of a child's developmental level) affects how an individual experiences and interprets his or her illness, it is likely that the long-term sequelae of childhood cancer will vary according to the developmental stage of the child during treatment and during follow-up assessment.

In this chapter, the literature body on late psychosocial consequences of childhood cancer is systematically reviewed. This review is followed by a discussion of moderating factors that may account for variance in the psychological and social adjustment of survivors. For the purposes of the review, studies published after 1985 initially were identified from a search of three databases: Medline, CancerLit, and PsycLIT. Further articles were drawn from a search of the reference sections of the identified articles. Studies were included only if they were published after 1985 and if they compared the psychological or social adjustment of cancer survivors with matched comparison controls or population norms.

This search resulted in 37 studies based on approximately 29 different samples (although the overlap was difficult to determine), which are summarized in table 13-1. Measures of psychological and social adjustment varied considerably across studies, with 28 focusing on emotional outcomes, including symptoms of depression, anxiety, posttraumatic stress, and somatic complaints; 7 studies examining self-image, body image, or self-esteem; and 8 examining social consequences, including social skills, social desirability, and loneliness. The majority of studies used self-report measures, although a few also included measures completed by parents or teachers. Age of participants at diagnosis ranged from 2 months (Greenberg, Kazak, & Meadows, 1989) to 20 years (Zebrack et al., 2002; Zeltzer et al., 1997), with the mean age at assessment ranging from 3 (Sawyer, Antoniou, Toogood, & Rice, 1997) to 26 years (Gray et al., 1992). The majority of studies included relatively small sample sizes, ranging from 19 (Noll, Bukowski, Davies, Koontz, & Kulkarni, 1993) to 5,736 (Zebrack et al., 2002). All but 7 studies included mixed cancer diagnoses. Only 1 of the studies examined participants' adjustment over a

**Table 13-1.** Summary of Studies Examining the Psychological and Social Late Effects of Childhood Cancer

| *Authors* | *Control or Population Norms (PN)* | *N (Survivors)* | *Diagnosis* | *Mean Age (years) at Diagnosis (Range)* | *Mean Assessment Age (Range)* | *Measures* | *Primary Survivor Outcomes* |
|---|---|---|---|---|---|---|---|
| Teta et al., 1986 | Control (sibling) | 450 | Multiple (50 CNS) | <19 | Not given | Interview (modified SADS-L) | No differences in frequency of lifetime major depression<br>Difficulty attaining certain major goals (i.e., college, employment, insurance) |
| Greenberg et al., 1989 | Control | 138 | Multiple | 3.6 (<1–9) | 12.5 (8–16) | PHS; CDI; FES; Norwicki-Strickland Locus of Control scale; Derogatis Stress Profile | Poorer overall self-concepts |
| Kazak & Meadows, 1989 (one study using the same sample) | Control (peer) and PN | 35 | Hematologic (83% cranial irradiation) | 3.7 | 12.2 (10–15) | FACES-II; SPP; CBCL; SSRS; LSC | Most scores on child variables within normative limits and not different from controls<br>Lower levels of school competence and less help from friends<br>Survivors rated families as "structured"; controls rated their families as "flexible" |
| Mulhern et al., 1989 | PN | 183 | Multiple (2 CNS) | 2.7 (median) (<1–8) | 12.2 (median) (7–15) | CBCL | Incidence clinically elevated scales ranged from 17% to 33%<br>Three- to fourfold increase in incidence of deficits in social competence and behavioral abnormalities<br>School problems and somatic complaints most common |
| Sanger et al., 1991 | PN | 48 | Multiple (some on treatment) | Not given | 12.5 (4–17) | PIC | High frequency of somatic concerns and academic problems<br>52% had profiles with two or more clinically significant problem areas |

*(continued)*

**Table 13-1.** *(continued)*

| *Authors* | *Control or Population Norms (PN)* | *N (Survivors)* | *Diagnosis* | *Mean Age (years) at Diagnosis (Range)* | *Mean Assessment Age (Range)* | *Measures* | *Primary Survivor Outcomes* |
|---|---|---|---|---|---|---|---|
| Gray et al., 1992, | Control (peer) | 62 | Multiple (16 CNS) | 10.7 (1–18) | 26.3 (18–37) | POMS; IES Desirability of Control Scale; Control Belief Scale; Rosenberg Self-Esteem Scale; projective drawing/ story telling | More positive affect, less negative affect, higher intimacy motivation, more perceived personal control, and greater satisfaction with control in life situations<br>More likely than peers to have repeated school grades, to be worried about fertility, to express dissatisfaction with important relationships<br>School, work, and physical symptoms caused problems for some survivors (greater representation from CNS tumor survivors)<br>Interpersonal relationships characterized by heightened sensitivity and cautiousness<br>Small minority of patients showed considerable adjustment difficulties, especially with social relations |
| Rait et al., 1992 | PN | 88 | Hematologic | 10.6 (4–17) | 15.6 (12–19) | FACES-III; CBCL-YSR; Rand Mental Health Inventory | Families less cohesive than norms<br>No differences regarding adaptability |
| Anholt et al., 1993 | Control (pediatric clinic) | 62 | Multiple | (6–18) | 13.5 | PHS; Physical Impairment Rating Scale | More positive about global self-concept and all other areas of self-concept except physical appearance and attributes |
| Noll et al., 1993 | Control (matched school peers) | 19 | Multiple (10 cranial irradiation) | Not given | 14 (11–18) | RCP; CDI; SPP; LSDQ; Sociometric Ratings | Higher on Sensitive-Isolated dimension by self- and peer report<br>No differences on friendship and social acceptance on LSDQ, CDI, or global self-worth |

| | | | | | | | |
|---|---|---|---|---|---|---|---|
| Olson et al., 1993 | Control (matched school peers) | 20 | Multiple | Not given | 9.7 (6–16) | CBCL; PHS; FES; HRI; Vineland Revised Scale of Social Maturity Health Locus of Control; Functional Status II | No differences in self-esteem, family conflicts, physical functioning, social skills, independence, or sense of control over health<br>Parents and teachers reported poorer social competence among survivors<br>Parents of survivors reported more behavior problems and teachers reported poorer school performance |
| Stern & Norman, 1993 | Control (matched healthy) | 48 | Multiple | 13.86 | 17.5 (14–23) | OSIQ; CDAI; Social Provision Scale | Less positive self-image in terms of their social and sexual self |
| Madan-Swain et al., 1994 | Control (matched healthy) | 25 | Multiple | 5.1 | 15.6 (12–18) | SPP; TRF; FACES-III; MAPI; CSI; IPAC; Marlowe-Crowne | No major difficulties in social competence, overall coping, and family communication<br>Greater body image disturbances<br>Less self-criticism than controls.<br>Endorsement of higher social desirability for cancer survivors<br>Families more rigid and less flexible |
| Kazak et al., 1994 (one study using the same sample) | PN | 59 | Hematologic (54.8% cranial irradiation) | 3.7 | 12.2 (10–15) | FACES-II; SPP; CBCL: SSRS; LSC STAIC; HSC; CSD | Levels of adjustment near normative |
| Sloper et al., 1994 | Control (school peers) | 31 | Multiple (no CNS) | Not given | 12.32 (8–18) | RCMAS; SPP; Rutter Scales A and B | No differences in self-ratings of anxiety or self esteem<br>Teachers rated survivors as lower on concentration, academic progress, popularity with peers, and behavioral adjustment |
| Kupst et al., 1995 | PN | 28 | Leukemia | 6.5 | 19.1 | FCS; CARS; BSI; WOC | All BSI T scores were within range and not significantly different from nonclinical norms |
| Sawyer et al., 1995 (two studies using the same sample) | Control (matched community) | 45 | Multiple (no CNS) | 4–16 | 8.2 | CBCL; YSR | No significant difference in prevalence of emotional and behavioral problems at 1 year after diagnosis |
| Butler et al., 1996 | PN | 72 | Multiple (10 cranial irradiation) | Not given | 8.8 (3–16) | PSS; PIC; CBCL | Incidence of PTSD no greater than general population |
| Stuber et al., 1996 | PN | 64 | Leukemia | 4.6 (1–13) | 14 (7–19) | PTSD Reaction Index | 12.5% of survivors reported symptoms of severe posttraumatic stress |

*(continued)*

**Table 13-1.** *(continued)*

| *Authors* | *Control or Population Norms (PN)* | *N (Survivors)* | *Diagnosis* | *Mean Age (years) at Diagnosis (Range)* | *Mean Assessment Age (Range)* | *Measures* | *Primary Survivor Outcomes* |
|---|---|---|---|---|---|---|---|
| Barakat et al., 1997 (three studies using the same sample) | Control (healthy peers) | 309 | Multiple | 5.83 (1–17) | (8–20) | IES; PTSD Reaction Index; STAI; FACES-IIIA; ALTTIQ; SNRDAT; RCMAS; TSC | No difference between survivors and controls in PTSD symptoms |
| Sawyer et al., 1997 (two studies using the same sample) | Control (community controls) | 38 | Multiple (no CNS) | 2–5 | 3.5 | CBCL; GHQ; FAD | More internalizing problems at diagnosis but not at 1- and 2-year time points |
| Kazak et al., 1997 (three studies using the same sample) | Control (pediatric practices) | 130 | Hematologic | 4.83 (1–16) | 13.45 (8–19) | CBCL; GHQ; FAD | No differences in family functioning, social support, or symptoms of posttraumatic stress between survivors and peers |
| Eiser et al., 1997 | PN | 41 | Primary bone tumor of the knee | Not given | 18 (8–28) | Interview; SF-36 | Below population norms on all subscales; significant on physical functioning and role performance, pain, general health, and social functioning |
| Elkin et al., 1997 | PN | 161 | Multiple (no CNS) | 10.1 median (<1–20.9) | 19 median (15–31) | SCL-90-R | Levels of distress significantly lower than population norms |
| Pendley et al., 1997 | Control (matched healthy peers) | 21 | Multiple | 12.2 | 11–21 | SIQYA; BCS; SPPA; BIAQ; SIBID; SASC-R; Self-Report Likert Ratings of Body Image; Peer Interaction Record; Loneliness Questionnaire | Less than half as many social activities as controls<br>No differences on social anxiety, loneliness, or composite body image scores |
| Zeltzer et al., 1997 (six studies using the same sample) | Control (siblings) | 580 | ALL | (Treated before age 20) | 22.6 (11.02–33.25) | Structured phone interview; POMS | Greater mood disturbance<br>Higher tension, depression, anger, and confusionNo differences in fatigue or vigor |
| Kazak, 1998 (three studies using the same sample) | Control (pediatric practices) | 130 | Hematologic | 4.83 (1–16) | 13.45 (8–19) | IES; STAI; RCMAS; PTSD Reaction Index | No difference between survivors and controls on measures of PTSD<br>Younger survivors significantly higher in worry, social anxiety, and total anxiety than same-age controls |

| | | | | | | | |
|---|---|---|---|---|---|---|---|
| Sawyer, Antoniou, Toogood, Rice, & Peter, 2000 (two studies using the same sample) | Control (community controls) | 39 | Multiple (no CNS) | 5.2 (2–12) | 9.2 (6–16) | CBCL; GHQ; FAD | Greater internalizing problems in cancer group at time of diagnosis (other time points no differences)<br>No differences in FAD scores |
| Erickson & Steiner, 2000 (four studies using the same sample) | PN | 40 | Multiple | Not given | 20.4 (12–35) | SCL-90-R somatization factor; GAF; SI-PTSD; IES-R; WAI; REMY-71 | Mean somatization score fell between nonclinical patient population and a psychiatric population<br>Majority of patients met at least partial current PTSD symptoms |
| Hobbie et al., 2000 | PN | 78 | Multiple | 11.7 | 25 (18–40) | IES; PTSD Reaction Index; STAI; SCID; BSI; ALTTIQ | 20% of sample met criteria for PTSD at some point since end of treatment<br>Clinically significant levels of intrusive and avoidant symptoms.<br>Elevated state and trait anxiety |
| Mackie et al., 2000 (five studies using the same sample) | Control (healthy controls) | 102 | ALL; Wilms | 5.9 (0.4–14.8) | 25.6 (19–30) | SADS-L; ADAPFA | No different from controls on any psychiatric disorder and overall work and performance scores<br>Poorer functioning for love/sex relationships, friendships, nonspecific social contacts, and day-to-day coping |
| Maggiolini et al., 2000 | Control (matched community) | 116 | ALL; AML | 6.6 (0.4–13) | 12–20 | OSIQ | Significantly more positive and mature self-image than controls |
| Verrill et al., 2000 | Control (matched peers) | 26 | Multiple | (12–15) | Not given | WAIS-R; CBCL; ASB; DDH | No difference in alcohol use, tobacco use, aggressive or antisocial behavior<br>Less total drug use in past year and experimented with fewer drugs than controls |
| Erickson & Steiner, 2001 (four studies using the same sample) | PN | 40 | Multiple | Not given | 20.4 (12–35) | SCL-90-R somatization factor; GAF; SI-PTSD; IES-R; WAI; REMY-71 | High levels of somatic, trauma-related symptoms when compared with nonclinic norms; 88% of sample experiencing at least one symptom of PTSD.<br>Higher than normal levels of restraint and low-to-average levels of distress |

*(continued)*

**Table 13-1.** *(continued)*

| *Authors* | *Control or Population Norms (PN)* | *N (Survivors)* | *Diagnosis* | *Mean Age (years) at Diagnosis (Range)* | *Mean Assessment Age (Range)* | *Measures* | *Primary Survivor Outcomes* |
|---|---|---|---|---|---|---|---|
| Zebrack et al., 2002 (six studies using the same sample) | Control (siblings) | 5,736 | Hematologic | 10.1 (0–20) | 26.9 (18–48) | Likert scales of psychological health | More likely to report symptomatic levels for depression and somatic distress |
| Hill et al., 2003 (five studies using the same sample) | Control (matched community) | 102 | ALL; Wilms | 4.9 | 25.9 (19–30) | ADAPFA; REFAMOS; standard interview | More likely to have impaired close relationships and poorer day-to-day coping |
| Reiter-Purtill et al., 2003 | Control (healthy peers) | 69 | Multiple (no CNS) | Not given (7–15) | 13.48 (9–17) | RCP; sociometric nominations; Like Rating Scale | Survivors described themselves as more prosocial than peers<br>Teachers described them as less aggressive<br>Peers described them as more sick, more tired, and as missing more school |

ADAPFA, Adolescent to Adult Personality Functioning Assessment; ALL, acute lymphocytic leukemia; ALTTIQ, Assessment of Life Threat and Treatment Intensity Questionnaire; AML, acute myelogenous leukemia; ASB, Antisocial Behavior Checklist; BCS, Body Cathexis Scale; BIAQ, Body Image Avoidant Questionnaire; BSI, Brief Symptom Inventory; CARS, Current Adjustment Rating Scale; CBCL (TRF, YSR), Child Behavior Checklist (Teacher Report Form, Youth Self Report); CDAI, Career Development Assessment Inventory; CDI, Children's Depression Inventory; CNS, central nervous system; CSD, Children's Social Desirability Questionnaire; CSI, Coping Strategies Inventory; DDH, Drinking and Drug History; FACES, Family Adaptability and Cohesion Evaluation Scale; FAD, Family Assessment Device; FCS, Family Coping Scale; FES, Family Environment Scale; GAF, Global Assessment of Functioning; GHQ, General Health Questionnaire; HRI, Health Resources Inventory; HSC, Hopelessness Scale for Children; IES, Impact of Event Scale; IPAC, Inventory of Parent-Adolescent Communication; LSC, Langer Symptom Checklist; LSDQ, Loneliness and Social Dissatisfaction Questionnaire; MAPI, Millon Adolescent Personality Inventory; OSIQ, Offer Self-Image Questionnaire; PHS, Pier-Harris Scale; PIC, Personality Inventory for Children; POMS, Profile of Mood States; PSS, PTSD Symptom Scale; RCMAS, Revised Children's Manifest Anxiety Scale; RCP, Revised Class Play; REFAMOS, Relationship with Family of Origin Scale; REMY-71, Response Evaluation Measure; SASC-R, Social Anxiety Scale for Children–Revised; SADS-L, Schedule of Affective Disorders; SCID, Structured Clinical Interview for *DSM-III*; SCL-90R, Symptom Checklist-90–Revised; SF-36, Short form 36 health survey questionnaire; SIBID, Situational Inventory of Body Image Distress; SI-PTSD, Structured Interview for PTSD; SIQYA, Self-Image Questionnaire for Young Adolescents; SNRDAT, Social Network Reciprocity and Dimensionality Assessment Tool; SPP, Self-Perception Profile; SSRS, Social Support Rating Scale; STAI, State-Trait Anxiety Inventory; TSC, Trauma Symptom Checklist for Children; WAI, Weinberger Adjustment Inventory; WAIS-R, Wechsler Adult Intelligence Scale–Revised; WOC, Ways of Coping.

reasonable period of time (10 years) following completion of treatment (Kupst et al., 1995); the remainder were cross sectional. In our review, findings are summarized and presented according to outcome variables.

## Emotional Consequences of Childhood Cancer

### Depression

Although it might be expected that diagnosis with a chronic physical disorder that disrupts life for long periods, results in multiple clinic visits, procedures, and hospitalizations, and that may be life threatening would be associated with an increase in rates of depression, findings have been mixed. Of the 10 studies that measured symptoms of depression or general mental health in the review, 5 compared survivors with an age-matched control group (Greenberg et al., 1989; Noll et al., 1993; Teta et al., 1986; Zebrack et al., 2002; Zeltzer et al., 1997) and the remainder with population norms (Christ, Lane, & Marcove, 1995; Eiser et al., 1997; Elkin, Phipps, Mulhern, & Fairclough, 1997; Kazak et al., 1994; Rait et al., 1992). Findings from the studies that included a control group are inconsistent, with 3 studies reporting no evidence of increased rates of depression among adolescent and young adult survivors (Greenberg et al., 1989; Noll et al., 1993; Teta et al., 1986) and 1 study reporting that older survivors are at increased risk for symptoms of depression than a comparison group of siblings (Zebrack et al., 2002). These conflicting results may be caused by the age ranges of participants in the various studies, which may differentially affect coping and emotional adjustment. Studies examining adjustment among young adolescent survivors (mean age 13–14 years) found levels of depression similar to or less than age-matched controls (Greenberg et al., 1989; Noll et al., 1993).

In contrast, a large-scale, multisite study comparing 5,736 adult survivors of childhood hematological cancer (mean age 27 years) with sibling controls found evidence of greater depressive symptoms among cancer survivors (Zebrack et al., 2002). Zebrack and colleagues (2002) found that although prevalence rates of depression fell within the normal ranges for the general population and that the majority of survivors of childhood leukemia, Hodgkin's disease, and non-Hodgkin's lymphoma do not report clinically significant levels of depression, survivors were 1.6 to 1.7 times more likely to report symptoms of depression than their siblings. Another study from the same cohort examined mood states among young adult survivors of acute lymphoblastic leukemia and found that survivors evidenced greater negative mood and more tension, depression, anger, and confusion than did sibling controls (Zeltzer et al., 1997).

It is possible that the greater power offered by the large sample size in these studies accounted for the more significant findings. Alternatively, it is feasible that young adult survivors may be at greater risk, more aware of, or more willing to acknowledge depressive symptoms than their younger counterparts. This may reflect the development of greater cognitive sophistication and emotional maturity among the adult survivors or increased insight into the life threat and potential repercussions of diagnosis and treatment for childhood cancer. These possibilities, however, have yet to be explored.

Other studies have compared levels of depression among survivors with population prevalence rates using standardized measures of depression (Christ et al., 1995; Elkin et al., 1997; Kazak et al., 1994) or general measures of mental health (Eiser et al., 1997; Rait et al., 1992). Findings from these studies were consistent and suggest that levels of depression/distress among survivors fall within population norms. Indeed, some studies have found that survivors report fewer symptoms of depression than would be suggested by normative data for clinical and nonclinical groups (Elkin et al., 1997; Greenberg et al., 1989). In sum, there is no support for levels of depressive symptoms that are greater in frequency than population norms among survivors of childhood cancer. Large-scale, multisite studies suggest that young adult survivors may be at slightly greater risk of depressive symptoms and negative affect than sibling control groups (Zebrack et al., 2002; Zeltzer et al., 1997).

### Anxiety

Findings from the seven studies that examined levels of general anxiety among survivors were consistent and suggest that survivors of childhood cancer do not report high levels of anxiety when compared to comparison controls or population norms (Barakat et al., 1997; Elkin et al., 1997; Hobbie et al., 2000; Kazak et al., 1994, 1997; Pendley, Dahlquist, & Dreyer, 1997; Sloper, Larcombe, & Charlton, 1994). Four of these studies examined young adolescent survivors and included a control group of age-matched peers (Barakat et al., 1997; Kazak et al., 1997; Pendley et al., 1997; Sloper et al., 1994). Findings were consistent and suggest no overall group differences on self-report measures of general state anxiety (Barakat et al., 1997; Kazak et al., 1997; Sloper et al., 1994) or social anxiety (Pendley et al., 1995). Similarly, two of three studies of young adult survivors suggest that levels of anxiety are well within population norms (Elkin et al., 1997; Kazak et al., 1994), with only one study to date obtaining higher than typical levels of anxiety (Hobbie et al., 2000).

As with depression, there exists some counterintuitive evidence that adolescent survivors, especially males, report lower levels of anxiety than would be expected according to normative data (Elkin et al., 1997; Kazak et al., 1994). Again, it remains unclear whether adolescent survivors are experiencing fewer symptoms of distress than the general population or whether they are underreporting those symptoms.

### Posttraumatic Stress Disorder

It has been argued that standard measures of depression and anxiety do not capture important aspects of the emotional experience of surviving childhood cancer (Erickson & Steiner, 2000; Kazak, 1998); for that reason, attention has shifted to an examination of symptoms of posttraumatic stress disorder (PTSD) among survivors (e.g., Stuber, Christakis, Houskamp, & Kazak, 1996). PTSD is a syndrome resulting from exposure to actual or perceived threat that evokes intense fear, helplessness, or horror (*Diagnostic and Statistical Manual of Mental Disorders, Fourth Edition* [*DSM-IV*]; American Psychiatric Association, 1994).

Pediatric cancer can be seen as a series of traumatic events that may evoke posttraumatic stress and its characteristic symptoms of intrusive thoughts, reexperiencing of traumatic events, avoidance of reminders or numbing of responsiveness, and increased arousal. Epidemiological data from *DSM-IV* field trials have found that 33% of 25 adolescent cancer survivors met diagnostic criteria for PTSD (Stuber et al., 1996). Observations of this sort contributed to broader PTSD inclusion criteria in the fourth edition of the *DSM* (American Psychiatric Association, 1994) and a more thorough investigation of PTSD in pediatric cancer survivors.

Six studies identified for inclusion in this review focused on symptoms of PTSD among survivors (Barakat et al., 1997; Butler, Rizzi, & Handwerger, 1996; Erickson & Steiner, 1999, 2000; Hobbie et al., 2000; Kazak et al., 1997; Stuber et al., 1996). In one of the first studies, Stuber and colleagues found that 8 of a sample of 64 survivors (12.5%) of childhood leukemia between the ages of 7 and 19 years met criteria for a clinical diagnosis of PTSD, with a further 42% endorsing subclinical symptoms of posttraumatic stress. The most common symptoms reported included reexperiencing (e.g., recurrent, distressing memories or bad dreams) and avoidance (e.g., avoiding reminders, inability to recall details of cancer and treatment). Participants identified medical procedures and the life threat of diagnosis as traumatic.

Since this initial investigation, a number of studies have confirmed that a subgroup of survivors demonstrated the full constellation of symptoms of PTSD. Among child and adolescent survivors, incidence, as measured by self- and parent report, ranged from 4.5% to 14% (Barakat et al., 1997; Butler et al., 1996; Kazak et al., 1997) and was not significantly different from same age comparison groups or population norms. However, the incidence of PTSD appears to increase among young adult survivors, suggesting the stress of childhood cancer can survive well beyond the precipitating conditions and well into the late effects period.

Hobbie and colleagues (2000) measured symptoms of posttraumatic stress among 78 adult survivors (mean age 25 years) of mixed childhood cancers who had been in remission for an average of 11 years. Overall, 20.5% met criteria for a diagnosis of PTSD, with 9% describing clinically significant symptoms of intrusion and 16.7% symptoms of avoidance. These rates are higher than estimated rates in the general population and are similar to rates reported by survivors of adult cancers (e.g., Andrykowski & Cordova, 1998). Similar findings were reported in a study of 40 long-term pediatric cancer survivors with a mean age of 20 years who had been in remission for at least 5 years (Erickson & Steiner, 2000). In this study, 88% of the sample reported at least one symptom of PTSD at a functionally significant level, and 10% met criteria for the full syndrome. Symptom severity did not change as a function of time since treatment completion.

Overall, these findings suggest that a subgroup of survivors experience clinically significant symptoms of PTSD, with rates higher among young adult survivors than child and adolescent survivors. It remains unclear whether the level of distress increases over time or whether developmentally determined cognitive maturity influences the reporting of distress during adolescence. The extent to which younger survivors can process and recall events surrounding their diagnosis and treatment also remains unclear. The majority of studies examining PTSD among child and adolescent survivors included participants who were diagnosed at a young age (5.6 years mean age at diagnosis for Barakat et al., 1997; Kazak et al., 1997; Stuber et al., 1996). In contrast, studies of young adult survivors tended to include participants who were diagnosed at older ages (12 years mean age at diagnosis for Hobbie et al., 2000). Thus, it is possible that age at diagnosis is a factor in level of distress over the course of survivorship. Alternately, changes in treatment protocols may account for differences observed across age cohorts. There is also some evidence that symptoms of PTSD decrease over the first year or two off treatment (Stuber et al., 1997), after which time they appear to persist (Erickson & Steiner, 2000). Prospective research examining the course of PTSD symptoms over time is necessary for further understanding of age-related differences in symptom patterns.

## Somatization

Somatization is characterized by multiple physical complaints that cannot be explained fully by a physical disorder and are thought to be related to underlying emotional distress. There is evidence that somatic symptoms are common after recurrent traumatic stress (Ford, 1997). As a recurrent stressor, pediatric cancer may therefore lend itself to the expression of distress through somatic complaints. Furthermore, cancer, its treatment, and exposure to the medical environment may serve to focus the child's attention on bodily symptoms and further support somatization as an acceptable coping strategy.

In support of this notion, there is evidence that a number of survivors report good global adjustment while concurrently reporting persistent illness-related concerns, including somatic preoccupation (Fritz & Williams, 1988). Five of the studies included in this review examined somatic complaints among survivors (Elkin et al., 1997; Erickson & Steiner, 2000; Mulhern, Wasserman, Friedman, & Fairclough, 1989; Sanger, Copeland, & Davidson, 1991; Zebrack et al., 2002). Four of these studies provided evidence for an increase in somatic complaints among child, adolescent, and adult survivors both when compared with population norms (Erickson & Steiner, 1999; Mulhern et al., 1989; Sanger et al., 1991) and with comparisons groups of siblings (Zebrack et al., 2002).

Indeed, the Childhood Cancer Survivor Study (Zebrack et al., 2002) examined psychological symptoms among 5,736 adult survivors of childhood cancer. Participants included those from multiple sites with leukemia, Hodgkin's disease, and non-Hodgkin's lymphoma; findings revealed that survivors were approximately 1.7 times more likely to report symptoms of somatic distress than a comparison group of 2,565 siblings. Not all findings are consistent as one study of adjustment among adolescents and young adult survivors provided no evidence of greater somatic distress when compared with normative data (Elkin et al., 1997). However, the overall majority of evidence supports greater somatization among survivors of childhood cancer compared to either comparison controls or normative data.

Findings also suggest that somatic complaints may worsen over time since the initial cancer diagnosis. In this regard, the incidence of somatic distress has been demonstrated to increase with age at follow-up evaluation (Elkin et al., 1997, Mulhern et al., 1989) and, relatedly, with time since the completion of treatment (Mulhern et al., 1989). Indeed, the largest study in the extant literature provided evidence to suggest that survivors of leukemia and lymphoma were at higher risk for symptomatic levels of somatic distress if they were more than 20 years postdiagnosis (Zebrack et al., 2002).

Thus, increasing age or time since diagnosis appears to be a risk factor for somatic distress.

Although the reasons for this finding remain unclear, it is possible that young adults, as a consequence of their past disease, perceive themselves to be at greater risk and thus are hypervigilant about physical symptoms and experience more somatic distress than adolescents, who may consider themselves less vulnerable. Alternatively, young adults may experience more general physical symptoms as a normal consequence of increasing age, which in turn reactivates memories and fears about late physical effects or recurrence of the cancer. Longitudinal studies examining the presence of somatic complaints over time may help to shed light on these possibilities.

### Comorbid Symptoms of Stress

A growing literature body suggests that cancer is a traumatic stressor for a subgroup of survivors who experience chronic trauma-related psychological distress (Baum & Posluszny, 2001). Exposure to traumatic stress is typically associated with a combination of highly correlated symptoms, including symptoms of PTSD, somatization, dissociation, and affect disregulation (Ford, 1997; van der Kolk, Pelcovitz, Roth, & Mandel, 1996). Furthermore, there is evidence that this response is more likely among adults who experienced trauma during childhood (van der Kolk et al., 1996).

The extent to which survivors of pediatric cancer are at risk for traumatic stress response remains unclear. However, there is growing evidence for comorbid symptoms of traumatic stress among pediatric cancer survivors. Erickson and Steiner (2000) interviewed 40 adult survivors of mixed cancers in remission for at least 5 years. Findings revealed that somatic symptom scores were negatively associated with general adjustment and positively correlated with symptoms of PTSD. Similarly, Hobbie et al. (2000) found that a subgroup of young adult survivors (20%) who met diagnostic criteria for PTSD also demonstrated higher levels of somatization, depression, anxiety, and general distress than survivors who did not report PTSD. These studies suggest that although the majority of adult survivors demonstrated no significant emotional problems, a subgroup struggled with ongoing emotional difficulties across a number of domains. These data are consistent with the concept of childhood cancer as a traumatic stressor. The percentage of survivors at risk of ongoing distress is similar to that observed in adult cancer survivors (Cordova et al., 1995) as well as those with other medical stressors, such as severe burn injuries (Perry, Difede, Musngi, Frances, & Jacobsberg, 1992).

Several pathways linking traumatic events to persistent distress have been proposed. In the general psychological trauma literature, one possibility is that intrusive thoughts, fears, and memories about the initiating event(s) serve to maintain the stress response (Baum, Cohen, & Hall, 1993). Alternatively, the event could have an impact on significant others, who in turn respond differently to the stressed person and serve to sustain an ongoing level of distress. A cascade of secondary stressors can result from the initial traumatic event and have an impact on the ongoing level of distress. In the case of pediatric cancer, secondary stressors could include physical and social late effects.

It also is possible that stimuli associated with the traumatic event serve as a cue and initiate a conditioned stress response or activate an emotionally charged schema from the person's memory. Anxiety-relevant stimuli can activate cognitive, behavioral, emotional, and physiological responses that can be quite strong for information that is meaningful or linked with threat (Lang, 1985). In support of this notion, the subgroup of survivors of childhood cancer who endorsed high levels of distress reported fears that their lives remained in danger (Hobbie et al., 2000). Thus, it remains possible that distress among cancer survivors is situational and associated with emotionally charged stimuli, thoughts or memories. Situational distress has not yet been examined in survivors of pediatric cancer, although it is important and may be related to survivors' willingness to seek medical care.

## Social Consequences of Childhood Cancer

### Social Competence/Interpersonal Relationships

Because of treatment-related functional impairments, changes in physical appearance, school absences, and reduced time spent with peers, survivors of childhood cancer may experience social difficulties and impaired relationships. Eight studies examining social competence were identified for inclusion in this review (Gray et el., 1992; Hill, Kondryn, Mackie, McNally, & Eden, 2003; Mackie, Hill, Kondryn, & McNally, 2000; Mulhern et al., 1989; Noll et al., 1993; Olson, Boyle, Evans, & Zug, 1993; Reiter-Purtill, Vannatta, Gerhardt, Correll, & Noll, 2003; Sloper et al., 1994).

Studies that included teacher, parent, and peer reports have provided cross-informant evidence of poorer social competence among survivors of childhood cancer (Mulhern et al., 1989; Noll et al., 1993; Olson et al., 1993; Sloper et al., 1994). Teachers, for example, have reported that survivors perform significantly worse than do controls on measures of social competence (Olson et al., 1993), earn social competence scores below the published norms (Olson et al., 1993), and are rated as less popular among peers (Sloper et al., 1994).

In a rural sample, parents identified survivors of childhood cancer as four times more likely as comparison controls to obtain social competence scores below the normative range (Olson et al., 1993). Similarly, parent report identified 54% of survivors in a school-aged sample as less functionally competent (based on population norms) on one or more Child Behavior Check List Social Competence scales; this level of impairment is significantly greater than that in the general population (Mulhern et al., 1989).

In a 2-year longitudinal study, adolescents treated for cancer did not differ from comparison controls on multiple measures of social acceptance yet were both self-identified and identified by peers as more socially isolated (Noll et al., 1993). This social isolation seems to be most salient for children who had received more intensive treatment. Despite describing themselves as more prosocial than their healthy peers, survivors were perceived by their peers as having fewer best friends 2 years after treatment (Reiter-Purtill et al., 2003). Finally, Sloper and colleagues (1994) found that survivors self-reported lower levels of close, confiding relationships, and that peers reported lower levels of social acceptance, an important finding that suggests an association between social difficulties and other domains of adjustment.

These early struggles with social competence and social isolation resulting from the cancer experience may contribute to long-term interpersonal difficulties for cancer survivors. In a descriptive study aimed at understanding the impact of surviving childhood cancer, for example, interpersonal relationships, although greatly valued by survivors, were frequently characterized by heightened sensitivity and cautiousness (Gray et al., 1992). In accordance with this descriptive evidence, a study conducted by Mackie and colleagues (2000) identified survivors as displaying *avoidant* functioning; their relationships were shorter in duration and characterized by lack of involvement or confiding.

In other studies, survivors not only were more likely than peers to express dissatisfaction with important relationships (Gray et al., 1992) such as love/sex partnerships and friendships (Mackie et al., 2000), but also were more likely to report difficulties in nonspecific social contacts (Hill et al., 2003). The tenuous nature of interpersonal relationships in survivors of childhood cancer (Gray, 1992; Mackie et al., 2000) may help explain why survivors are less likely than peers to be married (Novakovic, Fears, Horowitz, Tucker, & Wexler, 1997).

In sum, multiple reports have identified social competence as a problem for survivors of childhood cancer. Deficiencies in this area seem to have enduring effects on the development and maintenance of, and satisfaction with, future interpersonal relationships.

## Body Image

Perhaps because sexual identity and sexual relationships are critical developmental tasks during adolescence, studies assessing body image have primarily focused on adolescent populations (Anholt, Fritz, & Keener, 1993; Madan-Swain et al., 1994; Pendley et al., 1997; Sloper et al., 1994). In addition to the developmental physical changes that take place during adolescence, teenagers with cancer have to adjust to physical changes resulting from treatment (hair loss, weight gain or loss, etc.) and therefore may pay more attention to their appearance than their healthy peers. Although the actual long-term impact of cancer on physical appearance is often relatively mild, researchers have hypothesized that the adolescent's appraisal of personal appearance may be more severe (Pendley et al., 1997).

Empirical findings on body image, however, have been mixed. Some adolescent samples have reported feeling less positive about their physical appearance than healthy controls (Anholt et al.,

1994) and have indicated body comfort as a problematic and unresolved concern (Madan-Swain et al., 1994); others have not differed from peers in their self-reported perceptions of attractiveness (Pendley et al., 1997; Sloper et al., 1994). Findings have been more consistent in demonstrating that individuals who experience greater physical impairment as a result of treatment (i.e., sensory impairment, limb amputation) and those who were further from treatment termination are most vulnerable to negative body images (Anholt et al., 1993; Pendley et al., 1997). Consequently, clinicians should appreciate the challenge that cancer imposes on a patient's body image and recognize that effects of the cancer experience may not develop until several years after treatment has terminated.

## Self-Concept/Self-Image/Self-Esteem

Considered a multifaceted construct, self-concept has been defined as "a set of self-attitudes that reflect both a description and an evaluation of one's own behavior and attributes" (Piers, 1984, p. 1) and includes self-appraisal of one's intellectual abilities, academic achievement, physical appearance, popularity, and the like. A favorable self-concept, therefore, is synonymous with self-esteem and has been associated with greater capacity to adjust positively to stressors (Stern & Alvarez, 1992).

Studies examining the self-concept of individuals treated for childhood cancer similar to those studies that have assessed body image have been conducted within adolescent populations (Anholt et al., 1993; Madan-Swain et al., 1994; Maggiolini et al., 2000; Pendley et al., 1997; Sloper et al., 1994; Stern & Norman, 1993), who as a result of an emerging capacity for abstract thinking engage in increased social comparisons (Eccles et al., 1993). Adolescent cancer survivors reported having self-concepts similar to, or more positive than, healthy comparison controls in terms of both global self-concept (Anholt et al., 1993; Sloper et al., 1994) and various components of the larger construct, such as intellectual and scholastic competence, behavioral conduct, happiness/satisfaction, social acceptance, close friendships, and coping behaviors (Anholt et al., 1993; Maggiolini et al., 2000; Sloper et al., 1994). Although one study (Stern & Norman, 1993) reported less-positive social self-images in adolescent cancer survivors compared to healthy controls, the survivors were still well within normal limits and therefore considered to be relatively well adjusted.

The finding that survivors of childhood cancer report more positive self-concepts than do their healthy peers is somewhat surprising, although these data are in accord with findings of better emotional health among adolescent survivors. In interpreting these findings, some researchers have cautioned that self-report data in this population may be biased toward underreporting distress (Erickson & Steiner, 2000; Madan-Swain et al., 1994) as cancer survivors may wish to appear "supernormal." In their study of psychosocial adaptation among adolescent cancer survivors, Madan-Swain and colleagues (1994) assessed endorsement of social desirability in their sample of cancer survivors and found that, relative to healthy controls, the survivors were more eager to present themselves in a favorable light. These investigators suggested that the high degree of social desirability among the adolescents may result from the use of coping strategies, such as denial or repression (Erickson & Steiner, 2000; Madan-Swain et al., 1994).

Although the positive self-concepts reported by survivors may reflect inflation as a compensatory reaction, the endorsements may also indicate that the experience of surviving cancer results in a greater sense of appreciation for life and others, a positive and hopeful life attitude, and enhanced personal feelings of happiness and satisfaction (Anholt et al., 1994; Maggiolini et al., 2000). Research suggests that the experience of childhood cancer does not inevitably exert negative effects on adolescents' self-perceptions of their abilities. Positive self-concept in adolescent cancer survivors may result in greater confidence in facing the challenges of adolescence as a result of having overcome the challenges of a life-threatening illness. Additional research will need to be conducted to assess whether the findings within the adolescent population generalize to older age groups.

## Summary of Social and Emotional Consequences

In sum, a close examination of the existing literature reveals that although there is no evidence to suggest that the majority of survivors suffer psychosocial consequences, there is marked variability among survivors in psychological and social adjustment, with some people adapting well and others evidencing long-term psychosocial difficulties. Indeed, there is a body of evidence demonstrating that a clinically significant subgroup of survivors (estimates range from 10% to 20%) suffers long-lasting social and emotional problems (Koocher & O'Malley, 1981; Kupst et al., 1995). Furthermore, a number of survivors reported global psychological adjustment at the same time as endorsing persistent somatic complaints and preoccupation (Sanger et al., 1991), intrusive thoughts about their illness and treatment (Erickson & Steiner, 2000; Stuber et al., 1996), dissatisfaction with relationships (Gray et al., 1992), social anxiety (Pendley et al., 1997), and concerns about their body image (Anholt et al., 1993; Madan-Swain et al., 1994). A clustering of symptoms, including intrusive thoughts about the cancer experience, avoidance of illness reminders, and somatic distress have resulted in the conclusion that a significant number of survivors actually evidence posttraumatic stress responses (Erickson & Steiner, 2000; Hobbie et al., 2000).

Given the extreme level of stress surrounding a diagnosis of cancer and the disruption of routine associated with treatment, the failure to find higher levels of self-reported distress among survivors has been described as counterintuitive (Phipps & Srivastava, 1997). Indeed, there are now a number of findings suggesting that, as a group, survivors report lower levels of distress than what is suggested by published norms or comparison groups (e.g., Elkin et al., 1997; Kupst et al., 1995). A number of explanations have been posited for the better-than-normal emotional health reported by many survivors. One possibility is that some component of the cancer experience promotes resilience and children's psychological well-being. Alternately, it has been suggested that children with cancer develop psychological defenses, such as avoidance, denial, or repression, that may bias them toward minimizing affective distress (Canning, Canning, & Boyce, 1992; Elkin et al., 1997; Phipps & Srivastava, 1997). Such defensive strategies may be adaptive in the short term (i.e., during treatment), contributing to a healthy sense of mastery (Taylor, 1983); however, they may pose a burden in the long run (Canning et al., 1992; Erikson & Steiner, 2000) because the adolescent must suffer silently.

A few studies have examined defensive coping styles among pediatric cancer patients, and findings support greater use of avoidance, denial, and repression (Canning et al., 1992; Erickson & Steiner, 2000; Phipps, Fairclough, & Mulhern, 1995; Phipps & Srivastava, 1997). Phipps and colleagues (1995) found greater use of avoidant coping among children with cancer than a healthy control group, with the use of avoidance coping increasing as a function of time since diagnosis. Avoidant coping involves conscious and effortful cognitive or behavioral strategies to avoid distress. Repressive adaptation is another protective coping style, but in contrast to avoidance, repression occurs outside conscious awareness. This personality style is characterized by high levels of restraint, an investment in others' positive evaluation, an inability to express subjective distress, and a tendency to avoid disturbing affect and cognitions. When compared with healthy comparison control groups, there is evidence for higher levels of repressive adaptation among pediatric cancer patients (Canning et al., 1992; Phipps & Srivastava, 1997). Furthermore, patients high in repressive adaptation report lower levels of self-reported depression than patients with other adaptive styles (Phipps & Srivastava, 1997).

Repressive adaptation is proposed to be an enduring characteristic that persists after cancer treatment ends. In support of this notion, findings from studies of adult cancer patients support increased repression of emotions among survivors (e.g., Kneier & Temoshok, 1984; Temoshok, 1987). Furthermore, a study found high levels of repressive defensiveness and use of avoidant coping among young adult survivors of childhood cancer who had completed treatment at least 5 years previously (Erickson & Steiner, 2000). In this study, survivors who endorsed high levels of repressive adaptive coping not only were more likely to deny affective distress, but also were more likely to endorse symptoms of PTSD (specifically avoidance) and somatic complaints (Erickson & Steiner, 2000).

These findings raise the possibility that avoidance and repressive coping are learned adaptations that enable the child with cancer to cope with the threat of diagnosis and treatment and experience minimal affective distress (Erickson & Steiner, 2000). In the long term, however, this coping style may be associated with ongoing trauma symptoms, including somatization and PTSD (Erickson & Steiner, 2001). It is possible that use of psychological defenses, such as avoidance, denial, or repression, accounts at least partly for the comparatively low rates of affective distress reported among childhood cancer survivors. This possibility certainly warrants further investigation as it may have implications for treatment and long-term adaptation. Given the potential reporting bias in childhood cancer survivors, future research should incorporate multiple assessment techniques across informants (Erikson & Steiner, 2000).

## Moderators of Psychological and Social Adjustment: Disease/ Disability and Demographic Parameters

With some individuals at considerable risk for maladjustment and others adjusting well, the observed variability in psychological and social adaptation among survivors of childhood cancer raises interest in identifying those critical factors that influence adjustment and may be targeted for early intervention. Researchers have examined a variety of factors that might explain the differences in psychosocial adjustment observed among individuals. These differences include disease variables such as cancer site and treatment intensity, as well as demographic variables such as age at diagnosis or gender. However, there is little available evidence that these factors account for much of the variability in psychosocial adaptation among survivors. In contrast, there is growing support for the role of psychosocial factors such as perception of stress, coping resources, family functioning, and social support in adjustment to pediatric cancer. In the following sections, evidence for disease, demographic, and psychosocial moderators of adjustment is viewed. The model of stress and coping proposed by Lazarus and Folkman (1984) is used as a guiding framework for considering how psychosocial factors may be related to the maintenance of a traumatic stress response in a subgroup of survivors.

### Type of Cancer and Intensity of Treatment

To date, the majority of studies in this literature body have included survivors of multiple cancer types, with no real attempt to differentiate between them in terms of psychosocial outcomes. Indeed, of the 29 independent samples identified for inclusion in this review, 22 investigations included mixed cancer types, 6 limited their sample to hematologic cancers, and 1 examined osteosarcoma of the knee. Although the low incidence of pediatric cancers makes mixed samples practical, different types of cancer vary considerably regarding symptomatology, treatment regimen and intensity, course, mortality, and demographics. Hence, it is likely that the psychosocial impact of cancer may be specific to the disease type. Few studies have included sufficiently large sample sizes to have the power to compare outcomes among different cancer types. Thus, care must be taken in interpreting the available findings suggesting that adjustment is unrelated to type of cancer (Sanger et al., 1991; Sloper et al., 1994) or duration of treatment (Kazak et al., 1997; Rait et al., 1992; Zebrack et al., 2002).

Findings regarding the intensity of chemotherapy are more variable, with some studies finding no relationship between intensity and long-term adjustment (Barakat et al., 1997; Hobbie et al., 2000; Newby, Brown, Pawletko, Gold, & Whitt, 2000; Stuber et al., 1997) and other investigations suggesting that more intensive treatment regimens are associated with adjustment problems, including fewer best friends, as reported by peers (Reiter-Purtill et al., 2003) and greater somatic distress and depression (Zebrack et al., 2002). Overall, it is premature to form any conclusions on the basis of the currently available findings, and it remains possible that disease and treatment factors are related to long-term adjustment.

### Physical Late Effects

A consistent body of evidence supports poorer adjustment among survivors who experience physical late effects or ongoing functional impairments. Survivors with more severe medical late effects and greater functional impairments reported poorer self concepts (Greenberg et al., 1989), greater distress (Elkin et al., 1997; Greenberg et al., 1989), more insecure relationships (Joubert et al., 2001), and more academic and adjustment problems (Mulhern et al., 1989). Thus, there appears to be a psychosocial cost to the disability or chronic health problems that can result from some types of childhood cancer.

### Time Off Treatment

The course of psychosocial adjustment following childhood cancer remains unclear. The majority of studies in this literature were cross-sectional, making it impossible to track adjustment over time. Contrary to popular belief, studies examining groups of survivors who have been off treatment for varying periods found that adjustment does not usually improve with the passage of time. Indeed, a number of studies have found no association between longer time since diagnosis and adjustment (Barakat et al., 1997; Kazak et al., 1997; Kupst & Schulman, 1988; Zebrack et al., 2002), and others found evidence of more adjustment problems among individuals who have been off treatment longer (Elkin et al., 1997; Mulhern et al., 1989; Pendley et al., 1997; Van Dongen-Melman, 2000). Although not all study findings have been consistent (Stuber et al., 1997), the majority of studies suggested that psychosocial adjustment stays the same or worsens as survivors of childhood cancer grow into adulthood.

### Age at Assessment

There is accumulating evidence that child and adolescent survivors report better adjustment than do adult survivors. Overall, younger survivors tend to report few problems or even better adjustment than typically developing peers or than normative data would suggest (e.g., Greenberg et al., 1989; Kazak & Meadows, 1989; Noll et al., 1993). In contrast, many studies of adult survivors have found evidence of psychological and social impairment (Erickson & Steiner, 1999; Hobbie et al., 2000; Zebrack et al., 2002; Zeltzer et al., 1997; but not Gray et al., 1992).

The reasons for these age-related differences remain unclear. It is possible that the differences reflect worsening symptoms over time. Alternatively, it could be the consequence of underreporting of symptoms among adolescents or the development of greater cognitive sophistication and emotional maturity among the adult survivors. For example, adolescents and adults may appraise their cancer experience differently, with adults more concerned about recurrence, late physical effects of treatment, or threats to their life than adolescents, who are more focused in the present. Prospective research tracking adjustment over time will be necessary to further explore these possibilities.

### Age at Diagnosis

Findings from the few studies that have explored whether age at diagnosis is associated with adjustment are contradictory. Poorer adjustment has been reported both for survivors whose cancer was diagnosed at an earlier age (Eiser & Havermans, 1994) and for those who were diagnosed at an older age (Kupst et al., 1995). Others studies have found no relationship between age at diagnosis and psychosocial late effects (Barakat et al., 1997; Zebrack et al., 2002). It is likely that the psychological late effects of childhood cancer will vary according to the age of the child at diagnosis. To date, however, systematic research examining the impact of age/developmental stage at diagnosis on long-term adjustment is absent from the extant literature.

### Sex

Several investigators have examined whether one sex is more vulnerable to adjustment problems than the other. Overall, many investigations have found that male and female survivors demonstrate similar adjustment (Barakat et al., 1997; Kupst et al., 1995; Mulhern et al., 1989; Rait et al., 1992; Sloper et al., 1994; Zebrack et al., 2002). However, not all findings are consistent. More negative outcomes have been reported for survivors who are male (Teta et al., 1986) and for survivors who are female (Stuber et al., 1997; Zeltzer et al., 1997).

In sum, empirical findings from studies examining clinical and demographic correlates of psychosocial adjustment in survivor groups are inconclusive. There is some suggestion that more negative outcomes are associated with more intense treatment regimens, the presence of physical late effects or functional impairment, older age at the time of assessment, and longer time off treatment. Further research is necessary before it can be determined whether and how type of cancer or age at diagnosis have an impact on long-term psychosocial adjustment.

## A Model of Stress and Coping

The most widely accepted model of stress proposes that negative emotions arise from the belief that environmental events tax or exceed coping resources (Lazarus & Folkman, 1984). According to this model, it is not necessarily the severity of the event itself, but the appraisal of threat and of one's ability to cope with that threat that results in the perception of stress and negative mood states. Thus, in addition to biological and demographic risk factors, it has been widely proposed that psychosocial factors moderate the relationship between childhood cancer and long-term adjustment (e.g., Varni, Katz, Colegrove, & Dolgin, 1994).

Based on the Lazarus and Folkman (1984) model, it is predicted that survivors who appraise their past cancer experience as more threatening will experience more adverse emotional outcomes. Available findings support this relationship, with more traumatic stress responses reported by survivors who appraise their past treatment as more intense (Hobbie et al., 2000; Stuber et al., 1994), as "hard or scary" (Stuber et al., 1997), and of greater threat to their life (Hobbie et al., 2000; Stuber et al., 1997). Other factors that may contribute to greater appraisal of threat and have been associated with poorer psychosocial outcomes among survivors include high levels of general anxiety (Hobbie et al., 2000; Stuber et al., 1997) and the presence of other concurrent stressors (Kupst et al., 1995; Stuber et al., 1997).

The model proposed by Lazarus and Folkman also suggests that individual differences in psychological and social adjustment to stress are attributable to a number of psychosocial buffers that modulate the negative impact of life-threatening events (Lazarus & Folkman, 1984). These buffers include coping skills, perceptions of the ability to cope, personality factors, and interpersonal resources. Although few studies have examined these psychosocial moderators in pediatric cancer research, available findings do generally support the model. Prospective studies have demonstrated that more adaptive coping, lower levels of perceived stress (both disease-specific and non-disease-related, concurrent stress) and higher levels of perceived social support each predict better emotional and social adaptation among survivors (Kupst et al., 1995; Sloper et al., 1994; Varni et al., 1994; Varni, Katz, Colegrove, & Dolgin, 1996).

For example, Varni and Katz (1997) found that higher levels of non-disease-related perceived stress measured shortly after diagnosis predicted higher negative affect at 9-month follow-up in children with cancer. Similarly, higher perceived stress predicted more symptoms of anxiety and depression among long-term survivors of childhood cancer (Varni et al., 1994, 1996). Thus, perceived stress has been implicated as a risk factor, explaining some of the observed variability in adaptation to pediatric cancer (Varni & Katz, 1997). Further research is warranted examining the role that coping styles play over the course of survivorship.

Another factor associated with level of concurrent stress and the ability to cope with negative life events is socioeconomic status (SES). A growing number of studies suggest that more negative psychosocial consequences of childhood cancer are associated with lower SES (Barakat et al., 1997; Kupst et al., 1995; Kupst & Schulman, 1988; Mulhern et al., 1989). However, other studies have found no significant relationship between SES and psychosocial outcomes (Sloper et al., 1994; Varni et al., 1994; Zebrack et al., 2002).

The family is the primary unit of adaptation and functioning in which children with cancer derive the support to adjust and cope with the stress of childhood cancer. Indeed, it has been suggested that the child with a chronic illness may respond more strongly to their parents' subjective distress than to the diagnosis and severity of the condition (Sholevar & Perkel, 1990). Studies have demonstrated that high levels of parental (especially maternal) distress and family dysfunction are associated with increased behavioral, emotional, and social difficulties among childhood cancer survivors (Kazak & Barakat, 1997; Kazak et al., 1997; Newby et al., 2000; Rait et al., 1992; Sloper et al., 1994). For example, Rait and colleagues found lower levels of family cohesion among adolescent cancer survivors than healthy controls, with lower family cohesion associated with more psychological distress in the survivor group (Rait et al., 1992). Excessive control within the family also has been associated with poorer survivor adjustment (Wallander et al., 1988). Others have demonstrated that better maternal psychological adjustment and coping predicts better psychological adjustment among survivors (Kazak et al., 1997; Kupst et al., 1995; Sloper et al., 1994). In a prospective study, Sawyer, Streiner, Antoniou, Toogood, and Rice (1998) demonstrated that maternal adjustment during the period after the child's cancer diagnosis was significantly related to the child's psychological adjustment 2 years following diagnosis. In sum, parents appear to buffer the impact of stressful experiences on their children, with parental coping and better family functioning explaining at least some of the variance in the psychological adaptation among cancer survivors.

In conclusion, a number of factors have been identified that are proposed to modulate the intensity of affective responses to negative events and thus account for some of the observed variability in psychological and social adaptation to the pediatric cancer experience. In addition to disease and demographic parameters, certain psychosocial vulnerability factors characterize a child who is at increased risk of future adjustment difficulties, including high levels of perceived stress, negative appraisal of the cancer experience, lack of perceived social support, higher parental distress, and poor family cohesion and expressiveness (e.g., Hobbie et al., 2000; Kupst et al., 1995; Stuber et al., 1997; Wallander & Varni, 1998). Regarding clinical implications, taken together, non-disease-related stress and social support have been demonstrated in a prospective study to predict a substantial portion (62%) of the variance in negative affectivity 9 months postdiagnosis (Wallander & Varni, 1998). Thus, there is evidence that adequate coping with the multiple stressors that accompany cancer in children predicts future quality of life. Based on this body of literature, it may be possible to identify modifiable vulnerability factors in children with cancer and their families to target them for intervention.

## Conclusions

It is premature to form any definitive conclusions on the basis of the extant literature, which is primarily cross sectional and limited by small heterogeneous samples, lack of control for confounding factors such as developmental stage, characterized by lack of appropriate control groups, and general failure to use psychosocial measures that have been validated for this population. Possibly as a consequence, many findings are inconsistent and have not been replicated.

Yet, there are some general themes that emerge from the 30 studies reviewed in this chapter. First, it is clear that there is marked variability among individuals regarding long-term psychosocial adjustment to pediatric cancer. Although the majority of childhood cancer survivors appear to cope well and report adjustment equivalent to comparison control groups or standardized norms, a subgroup of survivors endorses maladaptive psychosocial sequelae that continues for many years after treatment is completed. Indeed, the prevalence of psychiatric morbidity among survivors of mixed childhood cancers ranges from 10% to 20%, with evidence of chronic, trauma-related psychological distress and deficiencies in social competence among this small but clinically significant subgroup. In addition, there is some evidence that yet another subgroup of survivors may exist who endorse better-than-typical adjustment, as suggested from normative data.

The presence of widespread variability in adaptation raises the need for prospective research that identifies risk and protective factors that can predict adjustment trajectories and may be targeted for intervention. Although not all findings are consistent, evidence does suggest a constellation of psychosocial factors that appear to predispose some individuals to ongoing psychosocial adjustment problems. These factors include negative appraisal of the cancer experience, perceived stress, trait anxiety, high levels of parental distress, and family dysfunction. It also has been suggested that variability in self-reported adjustment may be the consequence of defensive coping styles such as avoidance, denial, or repression that may bias some survivors toward minimizing affective distress and portraying themselves as better adjusted than peers or population norms (Canning et al., 1992; Elkin et al., 1997; Phipps & Srivastava, 1997). There is some preliminary evidence that these defensive strategies may be problematic in the long run because they are associated with increased risk of PTSD and somatic complaints (Canning et al., 1992; Erikson & Steiner, 2000).

In general, the majority of survivors of childhood cancer demonstrate resilience, which has been defined as successful adaptation in spite of challenging or threatening circumstances (Masten, Best, & Garmezy, 1990). Interestingly, developmental studies of children who overcome diversity reveal that resiliency is a common and ordinary phenomenon (Masten, 2001); in other words, resiliency is more the rule than the exception, suggesting that human psychological development is buffered (in most cases) by the action of basic human adaptational systems (Masten & Coatsworth, 1998; Masten, Morison, Pellegrini, & Tellegen, 1990). Multiple risk factors, however, may compromise these normative protective processes and lead to the emergence of maladaptive profiles.

Studies have yielded data to suggest that risk factors not only tend to co-occur, but also tend to have synergistic effects when they do. Thus, the presence of two or more risk factors has a greater deleterious effect than the sum of the factors considered in isolation (Masten, Morison, et al., 1990; Pellegrini, 1990; Sameroff & Seifer, 1990). As a result, one factor or a set of factors may attenuate or exponentially enhance the risk imposed by another factor. At this point, the late effects cancer literature has not considered the effects of multiple risk factors on the adjustment of survivors of childhood cancer. An examination of common risk factor constellations will be a vital step toward delineating individual outcome trajectories and individual differences in susceptibility to risk.

Many of the factors associated with increased risk of adjustment problems are modifiable and can be targeted for early intervention. To date, there are no published studies examining interventions aimed at reducing stress and minimizing the negative effects of stress in children with cancer or their parents. In contrast, there is a growing body of literature documenting the benefits of stress management interventions for adults with cancer (for a review, see Helgeson & Cohen, 1996). This literature body raises the need to examine whether similar types of preemptive intervention may improve the long-term adjustment of children who are at increased risk of future psychosocial adjustment difficulties.

## Recommendations for Future Research

There are multiple problems with the existing literature that make definitive conclusions difficult. These include methodological issues that may contribute to the inconsistent findings and general failure to take developmental factors into consideration.

### Methodological Considerations

Despite the growing body of research related to late psychosocial sequelae of childhood cancer, many widely noted methodological issues (e.g., Eiser et al., 2000; Kazak, 1994) remain unresolved. It is likely that the many contradictions in the literature are at least partly caused by design and methodological problems that limit the interpretation and generalization of findings. Methodological limitations include the use of small and heterogeneous samples of survivors with variations in type and stage of cancer; variability in treatment regimen and intensity and in age at diagnosis and time since diagnosis; inappropriate or no comparison control groups; and the failure to use standardized psychosocial measures normed for use with this population. It is notable that a report from the Cooperative Children's Cancer Group, a methodologically impressive, large ($N = 5{,}736$), multisite study of adult survivors of hematological cancers, found evidence for symptomatic levels of depression and somatic distress among survivors when compared with sibling controls (Zebrack et al., 2002). This study has sufficient power to detect effects that may not have been present in many other studies with much smaller samples and mixed cancer types.

Another concerning limitation of the extant literature is the predominance of cross-sectional rather than longitudinal studies. To date, only one study of 28 survivors of childhood leukemia has followed the adjustment of survivors over a reasonable period of time (Kupst et al., 1995). The cross-sectional nature of the majority of studies in this literature and the variability across studies in the ages of participants and time since diagnosis make it impossible to document changes in adjustment over time. Further longitudinal research is necessary to track individual pathways of adjustment and to examine factors that moderate different outcomes.

Aside from the methodological limitations, it is difficult to interpret positive associations between past cancer diagnosis and current psychosocial morbidity. Although it is frequently assumed that psychosocial problems result from the cancer experience, causation cannot be attributed on the basis of correlational data. Psychosocial problems could antecede the diagnosis of cancer. Alternately, both psychosocial factors and risk of cancer may be related to a third factor, such as genetic predisposition or environmental situations. To specify causation, large-scale prospective studies are necessary, tracking changes within individuals over time.

## Developmental Considerations

Future research in the field also needs to focus on whether psychosocial outcomes are related to developmental factors both at the time of diagnosis and at the current assessment period. It is likely that developmental level will affect how an individual experiences and interprets his or her illness and thus have an impact on long-term psychosocial sequelae. The value of incorporating theoretical underpinnings from child development literature cannot be underestimated (Woodgate, 1999) because the challenges presented by childhood cancer may interfere with a child's ability to accomplish major developmental tasks. Illness and hospitalization in the first few years of life, for example, may disrupt normal parent-infant bonding, interfere with a toddler's struggle for mastery, or interrupt a preschooler's developing sense of initiative. As school-aged children are striving to become more independent and adjust to classroom demands, they may be especially affected by isolation from peers and school problems like absenteeism and school reentry. The diagnosis and treatment of cancer during adolescence may add to the usual challenges of puberty. Specifically, typical adolescent concerns of autonomy seeking, identity consolidation, peer relations, self-esteem, sexuality, and future orientation may be complicated by the dependency of the patient role, the isolating effects of the illness, treatment-related physical changes and bodily discomfort, and the potential uncertainty of chronic or relapsing conditions (Apter, Farbstein, & Yaniv, 2003; Kazak, 1994; Stuber & Kazak, 1999).

A child's developmental stage at the time of diagnosis is also likely to affect interpretation of the cancer experience. With increasing cognitive sophistication comes a new understanding of the illness and a wider (or at least different) array of coping strategies from which to draw. As Gibbons (1993) described, the limited cognitive skills of a preschooler prevent this child from understanding the meaning of the disease, making the child particularly vulnerable to fears associated with cancer and to an interpretation of the disease as punishment. Although the awareness of what the illness is has increased by school age, the understanding of why the illness has occurred remains limited (Gibbons, 1993). Adolescents, however, are generally mature enough to understand the implications of a diagnosis and prognosis but may not be equipped with the range of coping mechanisms possessed by an older adult. It is possible that they are at greater risk of using denial and avoidance as a means of remaining in control.

Just as the long-term effects of treatment for childhood cancer may differ as a function of developmental stage, so too might the various risk and protective factors that moderate the relationship between childhood cancer and later adjustment. In other words, the variables that may exacerbate maladjustment in a toddler may not be particularly detrimental to adolescents, and those variables that buffer adolescents from experiencing long-term psychological distress may not protect a toddler. Recognizing this possibility, Woodgate (1999) observes that the study of social support in childhood cancer in relation to the developing child has been almost completely ignored. Research focusing on how social support is received by children at different stages of development may provide valuable opportunities and efficient avenues for intervention.

At this time, it is not clear whether there is a critical period when the traumatic aspect of childhood cancer has more significant long-term consequences (Stuber & Kazak, 1999). Small samples involving individuals from a wide age range have prevented the detection of potential developmental differences (Woodgate, 1999). In other words, we have not yet been able to assess the extent that the developmental phase of the survivors may have affected study findings. Statistically controlling for age, however, does not mitigate the problems created when salient developmental issues are neglected (Kazak et al., 1997). Instead, future research should either include a wide age range while ensuring a large enough sample size to assess developmental differences or, consistent with the program of research conducted by Kazak and colleagues (Kazak et al., 1994), narrow the age range to capture a specific developmental stage (Woodgate, 1999), such as adolescence. In conjunction, these sampling practices may facilitate our understanding of the developmental impact of treatment for childhood cancer.

In sum, because the challenges children face vary according to their developmental period, it seems likely that both the long-term effects of treatment for childhood cancer and moderators of those effects also will demonstrate distinct developmental differences. Stuber and Kazak (1999) recognized that it no longer seems sufficient to ask the somewhat simplistic question whether there are adverse psychiatric sequelae of childhood cancer. Instead, because individuals across the age range may differ in their susceptibility to maladjustment, time-related and developmental issues should become a research priority. Sampling procedures that permit analyses at different developmental stages will provide an important first step toward delineating individual outcome trajectories and identifying age-dependent mechanisms that contribute to risk susceptibility.

## References

American Psychiatric Association. (1994). *Diagnostic and statistical manual of mental disorders*. Washington, DC: Author.

Andrykowski, M. A., & Cordova, M. (1998). Factors associated with PTSD symptoms following treatment for breast cancer: Test of the Anderson model. *Journal of Traumatic Stress, 11*, 189–201.

Anholt, U. V., Fritz, G. K., & Keener, M. (1993). Self-concept in survivors of childhood and adolescent cancer. *Journal of Psychosocial Oncology, 11*, 1–16.

Apter, A., Farbstein, I., & Yaniv, I. (2003). Psychiatric aspects of pediatric cancer. *Child and Adolescent Psychiatric Clinics of North America*, 12, 473–492.

Barakat, L. P., Kazak, A. E., Meadows, A. T., Casey, R., Meeske, K., & Stuber, M. L. (1997). Families surviving childhood cancer: A comparison of posttraumatic stress symptoms with families of healthy children. *Journal of Pediatric Psychology, 22*, 843–859.

Baum, A., Cohen, L., & Hall, M. (1993). Control and intrusive memories as possible determinants of chronic stress. *Psychosomatic Medicine, 55*, 274–286.

Baum, A., & Posluszny, D. M. (2001). Traumatic stress as a target for intervention with cancer patients. In A. Baum & B. L. Andersen (Ed.), *Psychosocial interventions for cancer* (pp. 143–173). Washington, DC: American Psychological Association.

Butler, R. W., Rizzi, L. P., & Handwerger, B. A. (1996). Brief report: The assessment of posttraumatic stress disorder in pediatric cancer patients and survivors. *Journal of Pediatric Psychology, 21*, 499–504.

Canning, E. H., Canning, R. D., & Boyce, W. T. (1992). Depressive symptoms and adaptive style in children with cancer. *Journal of American Academy of Child and Adolescent Psychiatry, 31*, 1120–1124.

Christ, G. H., Lane, J. M., & Marcove, R. (1995). Psychosocial adaptation of long-term survivors of bone sarcoma. *Journal of Psychosocial Oncology, 13*, 1–22.

Cordova, M., Andrykowski, M., Kenady, D., McGrath, P., Sloan, D., & Redd, W. (1995). Frequency and correlates of posttraumatic-stress-disorder-like symptoms after treatment for breast cancer. *Journal of Consulting and Clinical Psychology, 63*, 981–986.

Dreyer, Z. E., Blatt, J., & Bleyer, A. (2002). Late effects of childhood cancer and its treatment. In P. A. Pizzo (Ed.), *Principles and practice of pediatric oncology* (4th ed., pp. 1421–1461). Philadelphia: Lippincott, Williams, and Wilkins.

Eccles, J. S., Midgley, C., Wigfield, A., Buchanan, C. M., Reuman, D., Flanagan, C., et al. (1993). Development during adolescence: The impact of stage-environment fit on young adolescents' experiences in schools and in families. *American Psychologist, 48*, 90–101.

Eiser, C. (1998). Practitioner review: Long term consequences of childhood cancer. *Journal of Child Psychology and Psychiatry, 39*, 621–633.

Eiser, C., Cool, P., Grimer, R. J., Carter, S. R., Cotter, I. M., Ellis, A. J., et al. (1997). Quality of life in children following treatment for a malignant primary bone tumor around the knee. *Sarcoma, 1*, 39–45.

Eiser, C., & Havermans, T. (1994). Long-term social adjustment after treatment for childhood cancer. *Archives of Disease in Childhood, 70*, 66–70.

Eiser, C., Hill, J., & Vance, Y. H. (2000). Examining the psychological consequences of surviving childhood cancer: Systematic review as a research method in pediatric psychology. *Journal of Pediatric Psychology, 25*, 449–460.

Elkin, T. D., Phipps, S., Mulhern, R. K., & Fairclough, D. (1997). Psychological functioning of adolescent and young adult survivors of pediatric malignancy. *Medical and Pediatric Oncology, 29*, 582–588.

Erickson, S. J., & Steiner, H. (1999). Somatization as an indicator of trauma adaptation in long-term pediatric cancer survivors. *Clinical Child Psychology and Psychiatry, 4*, 415–426.

Erickson, S. J., & Steiner, H. (2000). Somatic symptoms in long-term pediatric cancer survivors. *Psychosomatics, 41*, 339–346.

Erickson, S. J., & Steiner, H. (2001). Trauma and personality correlates in long-term pediatric cancer survivors. *Child Psychiatry and Human Development, 31*, 195–213.

Ford, C. V. (1997). Somatic symptoms, somatization, and traumatic stress: An overview. *Nordic Journal of Psychiatry, 51*, 5–14.

Fritz, G. K., & Williams, J. R. (1988). Issues of adolescent development for survivors of childhood cancer. *Journal of the American Academy of Child and Adolescent Psychiatry, 27*, 712–715.

Gibbons, M. B. (1993). Psychosocial aspects of serious illness in childhood and adolescence. In A. Armstrong-Dailey & S. Goltzer (Eds.), *Hospice care for children* (pp. 60–74). London: Oxford University Press.

Gray, R. E., Doan, B. D., Shermer, P., Vatter Fitzgerald, A., Berry, M. P., Jenkin, D., et al. (1992). Psychosocial adaptation of survivors of childhood cancer. *Cancer, 70*, 2713–2721.

Greenberg, H. S., Kazak, A. E., & Meadows, A. T. (1989). Psychological functioning in 8- to 16-year-old cancer survivors and their parents. *Journal of Pediatrics, 114*, 488–493.

Helgeson, V., & Cohen, S. (1996). Social support and adjustment to cancer: Reconciling descriptive, correlational, and intervention research. *Health Psychology, 15*, 135–148.

Hill, J., Kondryn, H., Mackie, E., McNally, R., & Eden, T. (2003). Adult psychosocial functioning following childhood cancer: The different roles of sons' and daughters' relationships with their fathers and mothers. *Journal of Child Psychology and Psychiatry, 44*, 752–762.

Hill, J. M., & Stuber, M. L. (1997). Long-term adaptation, psychiatric sequelae and PTSD. In J. C. Holland (Ed.), *Psycho-Oncology* (pp. 923–929). New York: Oxford University Press.

Hobbie, W., Stuber, M. L., Meeske, K., Wissler, K., Rourke, M. T., Ruccione, K., et al. (2000). Symptoms of posttraumatic stress in young adult survivors of childhood cancer. *Journal of Clinical Oncology, 18*, 4060–4066.

Hudson, M. M., Mertens, A. C., Yasui, Y., Hobbie, W., Chen, H., Gurney, J., G., et al. (2003). Health status of adult long-term survivors of childhood cancer. *Journal of the American Medical Association, 290*, 1583–1592.

Joubert, D., Reza Sadeghi, M., Elliot, M., Devins, G. M., Laperriere, N., & Rodin, G. (2001). Physical sequelae and self-perceived attachment in adult survivors of childhood cancer. *Psycho-oncology, 10*, 284–292.

Kazak, A. E. (1994). Implications of survival: Pediatric oncology patients and their families. In A. Bearison & R. Mulhern (Eds.), *Pediatric psychooncology*. New York: Oxford University Press.

Kazak, A. E. (1998). Posttraumatic distress in childhood cancer survivors and their parents. *Medical and Pediatric Oncology Supplement, 1*, 60–68.

Kazak, A. E., & Barakat, L. P. (1997). Brief report: Parenting stress and quality of life during treatment for childhood leukemia predicts child and parent adjustment after treatment ends. *Journal of Pediatric Psychology, 22*, 749–758.

Kazak, A. E., Barakat, L. P., Meeske, K., Christakis, D. A., Meadows, A. T., Casey, R., et al. (1997). Posttraumatic stress, family functioning, and social support in survivors of childhood leukemia and their mothers and fathers. *Journal of Consulting and Clinical Psychology, 65*, 120–129.

Kazak, A. E., Christakis, D. A., Alderfer, M., & Coiro, M. (1994). Young adolescent cancer survivors and their parents: adjustment, learning problems, and gender. *Journal of Family Psychology, 8*, 74–84.

Kazak, A. E., & Meadows, A. T. (1989). Families of young adolescents who have survived cancer: Social-emotional adjustment, adaptability, and social support. *Journal of Pediatric Psychology, 14*, 175–191.

Kneier, A. W., & Temoshok, L. (1984). Repressive coping reactions in patients with malignant melanoma as compared to cardiovascular disease patients. *Journal of Psychosomatic Research, 28*, 145–155.

Koocher, G. P., & O'Malley, J. E. (1981). *The Damocles syndrome: Psychological consequences of surviving childhood cancer*. New York: McGraw-Hill.

Kupst, M. J., Natta, M. B., Richardson, C. C., Schulman, J. L., Lavigne, J. V., & Das, L. (1995). Family coping with pediatric leukemia: 10 years after treatment. *Journal of Pediatric Psychology, 20*, 601–617.

Kupst, M. J., & Schulman, J. L. (1988). Long-term coping with pediatric leukemia: A 6-year follow-up study. *Journal of Pediatric Psychology, 13*, 7–22.

Lang, P. (1985). The cognitive psychophysiology of emotion: Fear and anxiety. In A. Tuma & J. Maser (Eds.), *Anxiety and the anxiety disorders* (pp. 131–170). Hillsdale, NJ: Erlbaum.

Lavigne, J. V., & Faier-Routman, J. (1993). Correlates of psychological adjustment to pediatric physical disorders: A meta-analytic review and comparison with existing models. *Journal of Developmental and Behavioral Pediatrics, 14*, 117–123.

Lazarus, R. S., & Folkman, S. (1984). *Stress, appraisal, and coping*. New York: Springer.

Mackie, E., Hill, J., Kondryn, H., & McNally, R. (2000). Adult psychosocial outcomes in long-term survivors of acute lymphoblastic leukemia and Wilms' tumor: A controlled study. *The Lancet, 355*.

Madan-Swain, A., Brown, R., Sexson, S. B., Baldwin, K., Pais, R., & Ragab, A. (1994). Adolescent cancer survivors: psychosocial and familial adaptation. *Psychosomatics, 35*, 453–459.

Maggiolini, A., Grassi, R., Adamoli, L., Corbetta, A., Charmet, G. P., Provantini, K., et al. (2000).

Self-image in adolescent survivors of long-term childhood leukemia. *Journal of Pediatric Hematology Oncology, 22*, 417–421.

Masten, A. S. (2001). Ordinary magic: Resilience processes in development. *American Psychologist, 56*, 227–238.

Masten, A. S., Best, K. M., & Garmezy, N. (1990). Resilience and development: Contributions from the study of children who overcome adversity. *Development and Psychopathology, 2*, 425–444.

Masten, A. S., & Coatsworth, J. D. (1998). The development of competence in favorable and unfavorable environments: Lessons from research on successful children. *American Psychologist, 53*, 205–220.

Masten, A. S., Morison, P., Pellegrini, D., & Tellegen, A. (1990). Competence under stress: Risk and protective factors. In J. Rolf, A. S. Masten, D. Cicchetti, K. H. Neuchterlein, & S. Weintraub (Eds.), *Risk and protective factors in the development of psychopathology* (pp. 236–256). New York: Cambridge University Press.

Mulhern, R. K., Wasserman, A. L., Friedman, A. G., & Fairclough, D. (1989). Social competence and behavioral adjustment of children who are long-term survivors of cancer. *Pediatrics, 83*, 18–25.

Newby, W. L., Brown, R. T., Pawletko, T. M., Gold, S. H., & Whitt, J. K. (2000). Social skills and psychological adjustment of child and adolescent cancer survivors. *Psycho-Oncology, 9*, 113–126.

Noll, R. B., Bukowski, W. M., Davies, W. H., Koontz, K., & Kulkarni, R. (1993). Adjustment in the peer system of adolescents with cancer: A 2-year study. *Journal of Pediatric Psychology, 18*, 351–364.

Novakovic, B., Fears, T. R., Horowitz, M. E., Tucker, M. A., & Wexler, L. H. (1997). Late effects of therapy in survivors of Ewing's sarcoma family tumors. *Journal of Pediatric Hematology Oncology, 19*, 220–225.

Olson, A. L., Boyle, W. E., Evans, M. W., & Zug, L. A. (1993). Overall function in rural childhood cancer survivors: The role of social competence and emotional health. *Clinical Pediatrics, 32*, 334–342.

Pellegrini, D. S. (1990). Psychosocial risk and protective factors in childhood. *Developmental and Behavioral Pediatrics, 11*, 201–209.

Pendley, J. S., Dahlquist, L. M., & Dreyer, Z. (1997). Body Image and psychosocial adjustment in adolescent cancer survivors. *Journal of Pediatric Psychology, 22*, 29–42.

Perry, S., Difede, J., Musngi, G., Frances, A., & Jacobsberg, L. (1992). Predictors of posttraumatic stress disorder after burn injury. *American Journal of Psychiatry, 149*, 931–935.

Phipps, S., Fairclough, D., & Mulhern, R. K. (1995). Avoidant coping in children with cancer. *Journal of Pediatric Psychology, 20*, 217–232.

Phipps, S., & Srivastava, D. K. (1997). Repressive adaptation in children with cancer. *Health Psychology, 16*, 521–528.

Piers, E. V. (1984). *Piers-Harris Children's Self-concept Scale: Revised manual*. Los Angeles: Western Psychological Services.

Rait, D. S., Ostroff, J. S., Smith, K., Cella, D. F., Tan, C., & Lesko, L. M. (1992). Lives in balance: Perceived family functioning and the psychosocial adjustment of adolescent cancer survivors. *Family Process, 31*, 383–397.

Reiter-Purtill, J., Vannatta, K., Gerhardt, C. A., Correll, J., & Noll, R. B. (2003). A controlled longitudinal study of the social functioning of children who completed treatment of cancer. *Journal of Pediatric Hematology Oncology, 25*, 467–473.

Sameroff, A. J., & Seifer, R. (1990). Early contributors to developmental risk. In J. Rolf, A. S. Masten, D. Cicchetti, K. H. Neuchterlein, & S. Weintraub (Eds.), *Risk and protective factors in the development of psychopathology* (pp. 52–66). New York: Cambridge University Press.

Sanger, M., Copeland, D., & Davidson, E. (1991). Psychosocial adjustment among pediatric cancer patients: A multidimensional assessment. *Journal of Pediatric Psychology, 16*, 463–474.

Sawyer, M., Antoniou, G., Toogood, I., & Rice, M. (1997). Childhood cancer: A 2-year prospective study of the psychological adjustment of children and parents. *Journal of the American Academy of Child and Adolescent Psychiatry, 36*, 1736–1743.

Sawyer, M., Antoniou, G., Toogood, I., Rice, M., & Peter, B. (2000). Childhood cancer: A 4-year prospective study of the psychological adjustment of children and parents. *Journal of Pediatric Hematology Oncology, 22*, 214–220.

Sawyer, M. G., Antoniou, G., Nguyen, A., Toogood, I., Rice, M., & Baghurst, P. (1995). A prospective study of the psychological adjustment of children with cancer. *American Journal of Pediatric Hematology/Oncology, 17*, 39–45.

Sawyer, M. G., Streiner, D.L., Antoniou, G., Toogood, I., & Rice, M. (1998). Influence of parental and family adjustment on later psychological adjustment of children treated for cancer. *Journal of the American Academy of Child and Adolescent Psychiatry, 37*, 815–822.

Sholevar, G. P., & Perkel, R. (1990). Family systems intervention and physical illness. *General Hospital Psychiatry, 12*, 363–372.

Sloper, T., Larcombe, I. J., & Charlton, A. (1994). Psychosocial adjustment of 5-year survivors of childhood cancer. *Journal of Cancer Education, 9*, 163–169.

Stern, M., & Alvarez, A. (1992). Pregnant and parenting adolescents: A comparative analysis on style of coping, self-image, and family environment. *Journal of Adolescent Research, 7*, 469–493.

Stern, M., & Norman, S. L. (1993). Adolescents with cancer: Self-image and perceived social support as indexes of adaptation. *Journal of Adolescent Research, 8*, 124–142.

Stuber, M. L., Christakis, D. A., Houskamp, B., & Kazak, A. E. (1996). Posttrauma symptoms in childhood leukemia survivors and their parents. *Psychosomatics, 37*, 254–261.

Stuber, M. L., Gonzalez, S., Meeske, K., Guthrie, D., Houskamp, B. M., Pynoos, R., et al. (1994). Post-traumatic stress after childhood cancer II: A family model. *Psycho-oncology, 3*, 313–319.

Stuber, M. L., & Kazak, A. E. (1999). The developmental impact of cancer diagnosis and treatment for adolescents. In M. Sugar (Ed.), *Trauma and adolescence: Monograph series of the International Society for Adolescent Psychiatry* (Vol. 1, pp. 143–162). New York: International Universities Press, Inc.

Stuber, M. L., Kazak, A. E., Meeske, K., Barakat, L. P., Guthrie, D., Garnier, H., et al. (1997). Predictors of posttraumatic stress symptoms in childhood cancer survivors. *Pediatrics, 100*, 958–964.

Taylor, S. E. (1983). Adjustment to threatening events: a theory of cognitive adaptation. *American Psychologist, 38*, 1161–1173.

Temoshok, L. (1987). Personality, coping style, emotion and cancer: Towards an integrative model. *Cancer Surveys, 6*, 545–567.

Teta, M. J., Del Po, M. C., Kasl, S. V., Meigs, J. W., Myers, M. H., & Mulvihill, J. J. (1986). Psychosocial consequences of childhood and adolescent cancer survival. *Journal of Chronic Disease, 39*, 751–759.

van der Kolk, B. A., Pelcovitz, D., Roth, S., & Mandel, F. S. (1996). Dissociation, somatization, and affect dysregulation: The complexity of adaptation to trauma. *American Journal of Psychiatry, 153 (Suppl.)*, 83–93.

van Dongen-Melman, J. E. W. M. (2000). Developing psychosocial aftercare for children surviving cancer and their families. *Acta Oncologica, 39*, 23–31.

Varni, J. W., & Katz, E. R. (1997). Stress, social support, and negative affectivity in children with newly diagnosed cancer: A prospective transactional analysis. *Psycho-Oncology, 6*, 267–278.

Varni, J. W., Katz, E. R., Colegrove, R., & Dolgin, M. (1994). Perceived stress and adjustment of long-term survivors of childhood cancer. *Journal of Psychosocial Oncology, 12*, 1–16.

Varni, J. W., Katz, E. R., Colegrove, R., & Dolgin, M. (1996). Family functioning predictors of adjustment in children with newly diagnosed cancer: A prospective analysis. *Journal of Child Psychology and Psychiatry, 37*, 321–328.

Wallander, J. L., & Varni, J. W. (1998). Effects of pediatric chronic physical disorders on child and family adjustment. *Journal of Child Psychology and Psychiatry, 39*, 29–46.

Wallander, J. L., Varni, J.W., Babani, L., Banis, H.T. & Wilcox, K.T. (1988). Children with chronic physical disorders: Maternal reports of their psychological adjustment. *Journal of Pediatric Psychology, 13*, 197–212.

Woodgate, R. L. (1999). Social support in children with cancer: A review of the literature. *Journal of Pediatric Oncology Nursing, 16*, 201–213.

Zebrack, B. J., Zeltzer, L. K., Whitton, J., Mertens, A. C., Odom, L., Berkow, R., et al. (2002). Psychological outcome in long-term survivors of childhood leukemia, Hodgkin's disease, and non-Hodgkin's lymphoma: A report from the childhood cancer survivor study. *Pediatrics, 110*, 42–52.

Zeltzer, L. K., Chen, E., Weiss, R., Guo, M. D., Robison, L. L., Meadows, A. T., et al. (1997). Comparison of psychologic outcome in adult survivors of childhood acute lymphoblastic leukemia versus sibling controls: A Cooperative Children's Cancer Group and National Institutes of Health Study. *Journal of Clinical Oncology, 15*, 547–556.

# 14

Raymond K. Mulhern and Robert W. Butler

# Neuropsychological Late Effects

This chapter reviews neuropsychological late effects associated with childhood cancer and its treatment. The study of late effects presupposes that patients are long-term survivors, if not permanently cured, of their disease. Late effects are temporally defined as occurring after the successful completion of medical therapy, usually 2 or more years from the time of diagnosis, and it is generally assumed that late effects are chronic, if not progressive, in their course. This definition serves to separate late effects from those effects of disease and treatment that are acute or subacute and time limited, such as chemotherapy-induced nausea and vomiting or temporary cognitive changes induced by cancer therapy.

Research interest in neuropsychological outcomes, as well as neurological and other functional late effects, has shown an increase commensurate with improvements in effective therapy. For example, 30 years ago when few children were cured of acute lymphoblastic leukemia (ALL), questions related to the ultimate academic or vocational performance of long-term survivors were trivial compared to the need for improved therapy. In contrast, today more than 80% of children diagnosed with ALL can be cured, and issues related to their quality of life as long-term survivors have now received increased emphasis. There is at least comparable attention to neuropsychological status in primary brain tumors.

We first provide a brief medical background on the two most frequent forms of childhood cancer, ALL and malignant brain tumors, followed by a review of the current neuropsychological literature. The literature review provides an in-depth analysis of the types of cognitive impairments observed and known or suspected risk factors for impairments. When neurobiological substrates are known, particularly from neuroimaging studies, they are discussed. Finally, we conclude the review with sections that discuss current recommendations for a core battery of neuropsychological assessment of survivors and recommendations for future research.

## Acute Lymphoblastic Leukemia

### Medical Background

Approximately 20,000 children and adolescents under the age of 20 years were diagnosed with cancer in 1999 (Steen & Mirro, 2000). The most commonly diagnosed cancer in this age group is

ALL, a malignant disorder of lymphoid cells found in the bone marrow that migrates to virtually every organ system, including the central nervous system (CNS), via the circulatory system. ALL accounts for one fourth of all childhood cancers and 75% of all cases of childhood leukemia (Margolin, Steuber, & Poplack, 2002). In the United States, approximately 3,000 children are diagnosed with ALL each year, with an incidence of 3–4 cases per 100,000 white children. ALL is more common among white than black children and is more common among boys than girls, with a peak incidence at 4 years of age. Although genetic, environmental, viral, and immunodeficiency factors have been implicated in the pathogenesis of ALL, the precise causes of most cases of ALL remain largely unknown.

Presenting symptoms include fever, fatigue, pallor, anorexia, bone pain, and bruising. Because the symptoms of ALL can mimic a number of nonmalignant conditions, definitive diagnosis, usually made by bone marrow aspiration, is sometimes delayed. The duration of treatment varies from 30 to 36 months, and in the modern era is usually restricted to intervention with combination chemotherapy, reserving cranial irradiation for patients who experience a CNS relapse. A better prognosis is associated with female gender, age at diagnosis between 2 and 10 years, a lower white blood cell count, and an earlier positive response to treatment.

Treatment can be divided into four phases: remission induction, CNS preventive therapy, consolidation, and maintenance. The purpose of the remission induction phase is to eradicate leukemia cells rapidly from the bone marrow and circulatory system. CNS preventive therapy is necessary because the CNS is a sanctuary for occult leukemia. Traditionally, CNS therapy has included cranial radiation therapy (RT) and intrathecal chemotherapy, usually with methotrexate or methotrexate combined with other drugs. However, because of the risks for CNS toxicity (discussed in the following section of this review), treatment is now usually restricted to intrathecal and systemic chemotherapy with equivalent success in the prevention of CNS relapses.

Consolidation may be used to intensify therapy following remission induction. Maintenance therapy is required for a prolonged period, usually 30–36 months, because of the presence of undetectable levels of leukemia that nevertheless have the capacity to be fatal. After the completion of treatment, approximately 20% of those children who will eventually relapse will do so in the first year off therapy, with a subsequent risk of relapse in the remaining patients of 2%–3% per year for the next 3–4 years.

## Neuropsychological Late Effects and Risk Factors

The effects of CNS prophylactic treatments in ALL have been extremely well studied. From a historical perspective, Soni, Marten, Pitner, Duenas, and Powazek (1975) reported the first study on the effects of 2,400-cGy cranial irradiation as a prophylactic treatment on measured intelligence in survivors of ALL. Their study did not note any significant impact of this treatment. Meadows and colleagues (1981) published a study that came to the opposite conclusion: Radiation to the brain did result in declines in intellectual functioning, particularly in younger children. These discrepant findings stimulated numerous studies on the effects of whole brain irradiation and intrathecal chemotherapy on intelligence and subsequently neuropsychological functions.

Initial studies on the neuropsychological effects of CNS prophylactic treatment were summarized by Butler and Copeland (1993). Building on previous work (Fletcher & Copeland, 1988), over 50 studies were reviewed, most of which were case and descriptive. There were, however, exceptions. The St. Jude group (Mulhern et al. 1987; Ochs et al., 1991; Ochs, Parvey, & Mulhern, 1986) studied a group of cancer survivors who had been randomly assigned to intrathecal versus cranial irradiation prophylactic treatments. Initial results indicated no significant differences between the two groups; however, as the survivors were studied longitudinally, it was revealed that both groups showed evidence of equivalent deterioration in intellectual functioning.

One of the first studies to investigate neurocognitive processes subsequent to CNS prophylactic treatments was reported by Rowland et al. (1984). This study suggested a negative impact from CNS treatments and was original in that the comparative effects of intrathecal chemotherapy and whole brain irradiation, which was administered at a dose of 2400 cGy at that time, were evaluated. The investigators reported global intellectual and neurocognitive deficits secondary to 2400-cGy whole brain irradiation, but evidence began to implicate maximal deficit in nondominant hemisphere functions. In terms of neurocognitive involvement, there was evidence of shortened attention span, poor concentration, distractibility, and impaired school performance, particularly within the area of arithmetic computation. The detrimental effects on fine motor dexterity likely secondary to peripheral neuropathy associated with vincristine were discussed. The report is significant as it assessed discreet neuropsychological deficits apart from intellectual functioning.

A series of studies conducted at the University of Texas/M. D. Anderson Cancer Center in Houston documented clear evidence of primary deterioration in nondominant hemisphere functions following irradiation to the whole brain (Copeland, Dowell, Fletcher, Bordeau, et al., 1988; Copeland, Dowell, Fletcher, Sullivan, et al., 1988, Copeland et al., 1985). This series of studies laid the foundation for our current knowledge on the effects of whole brain irradiation. Evidence clearly suggested that this treatment modality had a maximal impact on nondominant hemisphere functions, including performance intelligence, nonverbal reasoning, arithmetic academic achievement, and visual-motor integration, in addition to reduced speed of information processing. These studies were the first to involve comprehensive assessments of many higher cortical and subcortical neuropsychological functions.

The findings of the M. D. Anderson group were subsequently replicated in a large sample of pediatric cancer survivors (Butler, Hill, Steinherz, Meyers, & Finlay, 1994). This study reproduced and further delineated the specific nature of nondominant hemisphere dysfunction following irradiation to the brain. Intrathecal chemotherapy, however, was not associated with significant neuropsychological deficits. All treatments, however, did tend to result in decreased information-processing speed, which is likely associated with the demyelination effects of CNS treatments. Irradiation to the brain was reported to have a maximal effect on visual-perceptual abilities, visual-motor integration, and spatial awareness. The results documented significant support for the detrimental effects of whole brain irradiation in pediatric cancer patients, even after chronological age, socioeconomic status, age at diagnosis, time since first and last CNS treatment, missed schooling, and type of CNS cancer were statistically controlled. The study is also significant for its inclusion of a comparison group of pediatric patients treated for malignancies without CNS involvement.

It remains somewhat unclear why whole brain irradiation would differentially affect the nondominant hemisphere. Nevertheless, this appears to be a clear and consistent finding across studies. Whole brain irradiation most commonly results in declines in performance intelligence, nonverbal memory, visual-motor integration abilities, perceptual abilities, and attentional functions, particularly under conditions of vigilance, premature disengagement, and working memory (Brouwers, Riccardi, Poplack, & Fedio, 1984; Butler, Kerr, & Marchand, 1999; Lockwood, Bell, & Colegrove, 1999; Rodgers, Horrocks, Britton, & Kernahan, 1999).

One attractive hypothesis advanced by Rourke (1989) suggests that irradiation to the brain has its primary effect on white matter; thus, there may be more tissue to damage in the nondominant hemisphere. It has been documented that the nondominant hemisphere does have a higher ratio of white to gray matter when compared to the dominant hemisphere (Goldberg & Costa, 1981). Alternatively, or perhaps as an additive function, it is possible that the dominant hemisphere has greater brain reserve capacity because of its language-based functions (Satz, 1993). Current work on irradiation-influenced white matter damage in patients with a brain tumor (reviewed in this chapter) will likely have relevance for the ALL population.

Largely because of the above findings, irradiation as a CNS prophylactic treatment in ALL is typically avoided whenever possible. Although it remains an appropriate treatment for patients with poor prognosis and under conditions of a CNS relapse, most children receive intrathecal chemotherapy as a CNS prophylaxis. As documented by the St. Jude study, at very high doses intrathecal therapy has been shown to be detrimental to intellectual functioning. Initial studies on lower dose intrathecal chemotherapy suggested minimal neurocognitive impact (Butler et al., 1994; Copeland, Moore, Francis, Jafe, & Culbert, 1996). Nevertheless, there were suggestions that some children might be susceptible to neuropsychological dysfunction following this CNS treatment modality.

There is increasing evidence that intrathecal chemotherapy does result in cognitive dysfunction in a significant proportion of patients. Reviews of studies suggest that at least 30% of the survivors exhibit some degree of evidence of impairment. The severity of the dysfunction, however, may be less than that found following irradiation (Brown et al., 1998; Copeland, et al., 1996).

Moleski (2000) reviewed the neuropsychological, neurological, and neurophysiological consequences of intrathecal chemotherapy as an ALL CNS prophylactic treatment. The overall conclusions were in agreement with the above observations. Thus, it appears that pediatric oncologists have decreased the neurocognitive impact of CNS prophylactic treatments.

Nevertheless, a significant proportion of children continue to experience dysfunction, albeit often less severe than that reported with cranial irradiation. The pattern of neuropsychological involvement is similar to that following irradiation in that nondominant hemisphere functions appear to suffer the brunt of observed deterioration. A number of risk factors increase the likelihood of neuropsychological declines, and these are likely relevant for both CNS prophylactic modalities.

Younger age at diagnosis has long been known to be a risk factor for increased neuropsychological involvement following CNS prophylactic treatments (Butler et al., 1994; Meadows et al., 1981). In fact, in our clinical experience, receiving these treatments in infancy often results in global neuropsychological dysfunction rather than the above-described differential impairment in nondominant hemisphere functions. As a prophylaxis, the standard dose of cranial irradiation is 1,800 cGy, and the effects of this have been well studied. However, there has been more variation in the dosages of intrathecal chemotherapy used, and high doses are likely associated with greater impairment (Mulhern, Wasserman, Fairclough, & Ochs, 1988; Mulhern, Fairclough, & Ochs, 1991).

Interestingly, gender also appears to be a risk factor, with females showing evidence of greater impairment compared to males, given equivalent dosages of prophylaxis. This finding was originally reported by Waber and coworkers (1990) and subsequently replicated (Butler, Rizzi, & Bandilla, 1999; Ris, Packer, Goldwein, Jones-Wallace, & Boyett, 2001). The underlying processes behind this effect are not understood. There are, however, known differences in normal neurocognitive development across genders, and this may provide clues regarding sex as a risk factor for CNS prophylactic treatment.

Finally, there is emerging evidence that the use of steroids may interact with CNS prophylactic treatments to further impair cognitive abilities (Waber et al., 2000). The need for further research on risk factors for neuropsychological deficits in ALL is imperative. Not uncommonly, pediatric oncologists and parents are faced with difficult decisions regarding a choice between irradiation and intrathecal chemotherapy. Current Children's Oncology Group protocols for standard-risk ALL have emphasized the increased use of systemic methotrexate; the manner in which this might interact with CNS functioning remains unclear. This is particularly important given isolated evidence that systemic methotrexate may have an indirect, but significant, effect on brain integrity via its metabolic cascade (Quinn et al., 1997).

## Malignant Brain Tumors

### Medical Background

Pediatric brain tumors are considerably more heterogeneous than ALL in that they vary by histology as well as location. Next to ALL, brain tumors are the second most frequently diagnosed malignancy of childhood and the most common pediatric solid tumor, with an annual incidence of 2.2 to 2.5 per 100,000 (Strother et al., 2002). The etiology of most pediatric brain tumors is unknown, although brain tumors can appear as a second malignancy following the treatment of ALL with cranial irradiation. Tumors are often characterized as above (supratentorial) or below (infratentorial) the tentorium, a membrane that separates the cerebellum and brain stem from the rest of the brain. In approximate decreasing order of incidence, the most common tumors are supratentorial low-grade tumors, medulloblastoma, brain stem glioma, cerebellar astrocytomas, supratentorial high-grade tumors, and craniopharyngioma.

Among the more common symptoms of a brain tumor are morning headaches, nausea, and lethargy resulting from tumor obstruction of the ventricles and increased intracranial pressure. Problems with balance and cranial nerve findings are more common among patients with infratentorial tumors, whereas seizures are more common among patients with supratentorial tumors. Computed tomography and magnetic resonance imaging (MRI) are critical to the diagnosis of pediatric brain tumors, although surgical resection or biopsy of tissue is usually necessary for definitive histological diagnosis. In addition to maximal safe surgical resection of the tumor, chemotherapy with or without cranial or craniospinal irradiation (CSI) is indicated for malignant tumors. Cranial irradiation is delivered once daily, 5 days each week for up to 6 weeks. The total dose delivered to the brain can be more than twice that traditionally given in the treatment of ALL.

Prognosis varies with the tumor type. For example, medulloblastoma, the most common malignant brain tumor in childhood, has a prognosis of approximately 65% long-term survival, whereas children with intrinsic brain stem glioma have a prognosis of less than 10% survival. Although this review focuses on the neuropsychological toxicity of cranial irradiation, other potentially serious complications from irradiation (e.g., hormone deficiencies, growth retardation, second malignancies) are recognized in the literature, as well as sensory deficits such as hearing loss from treatment with cisplatin chemotherapy and optic atrophy from RT or increased intracranial pressure.

## Neuropsychological Late Effects and Risk Factors

The quality of life of survivors of pediatric brain tumors has been previously reported by Mostow, Byrne, Connelly, and Mulvihill (1991), who studied 342 adults who had been treated for brain tumors before the age of 20 years and who had survived 5 years or longer. When compared to their siblings, survivors were at significantly greater risk for unemployment, chronic health problems, and inability to operate a motor vehicle. Specific risk factors included male gender, supratentorial tumors, and treatment that included RT. Treatment at a younger age was associated with greater risk of poor school achievement, never being employed, and never being married.

What, specifically, can account for the unacceptably high incidence of social and vocational problems among these survivors of pediatric brain tumors? The analysis of risk factors for neuropsychological impairments is more complex among patients treated for brain tumors than among those treated for ALL because of the increased number and variety of putative sources of brain damage. Unlike patients treated for ALL, those treated for brain tumors are exposed to the mechanical trauma of an invasive, space-occupying lesion of the CNS as well as the trauma associated with surgical resection and secondary effects (e.g., visual field cuts, seizures, hemiplegia, etc.) of both of these processes. It has been demonstrated that secondary, perioperative deficits adversely affect neuropsychological performance after controlling for the effects of treatment (Ris & Noll, 1994). In general, a young age at diagnosis, more aggressive CNS therapy, and tumor-associated factors such as location, seizures, and hydrocephalus are the most frequently cited risk factors.

One early review of intellectual outcomes among children treated for brain tumors included 22 studies of the neuropsychological status in 544 children surviving treatment for brain tumors (Mulhern, Hancock, Fairclough, & Kun, 1992). A quantitative reanalysis of intelligence (IQ) data from 403 children investigated the impact of age, tumor location, and RT. Although the mean IQ was 91.0, particular subgroups were clearly at greater risk. In particular, children who received RT when younger than 4 years were very vulnerable to loss of intellectual functioning when compared to older children (means 73.4 vs. 87.0).

A comprehensive assessment of risk factors in children was conducted in a longitudinal design by Ellenberg, McComb, Siegel, and Stowe (1987). A total of 43 children with various brain tumors were followed with serial IQ testing. Univariate analyses found significantly lower IQs among those children who were younger at treatment, received greater RT volume, and had cerebral (vs. posterior fossa) tumors. IQ deficits were greater with more time elapsed posttreatment. Multivariate analysis revealed that IQ at 1 month following diagnosis, age at treatment, and RT volume accounted for 80% of the variance in IQ scores 1–4 years later.

Jannoun and Bloom (1990) provided neuropsychological follow-up 3–20 years following irradiation in 62 children with a variety of brain tumors. Tumor location, RT volume (limited vs. full RT), and patient gender had no discernible effect on IQ outcomes. The age of the patient at the time of treatment was the most powerful determinant of ultimate IQ, with those younger than 5 years at greatest risk (mean IQ = 72), those 6–11 years at intermediate risk (mean IQ = 93), and those older than 11 years functioning solidly in the normal range of intellectual functioning (mean IQ = 107). Although not statistically significant, children presenting with hydrocephalus had a 10-point decrement in IQ compared to those with normal pressure.

Investigators from France reported on a cohort of 42 consecutively diagnosed children with low-grade cerebral hemispheric gliomas (Hirsch, Rose, Pierre-Kahn, Pfister, & Hoppe-Hirsch, 1989). Children were treated with surgery alone, comprising an important "standard" for evaluating the late effects of other forms of treatment, such as RT. Long-term follow-up revealed that 29% of children had IQ levels below 80, often with major problems in school. Although the authors did not associate a 20% incidence of poorly controlled postoperative seizures with low IQ or school problems, this additional influence cannot be ruled out.

## Posterior Fossa Tumors

Tumors of the posterior fossa region (cerebellum and brain stem), such as medulloblastoma (primitive neuroectodermal tumor of the posterior fossa) and ependymoma, are among the most common brain tumors in childhood (Figure 14-1). Because of their frequency and noncerebral location, studies of surviving children provide some of the clearest information about radiation-induced late effects and other variables, such as age, that may moderate these effects.

In the first randomized study comparing standard (36 Gy) and reduced (23.4 Gy) RT in medulloblastoma (Pediatric Oncology Group; Mulhern et al., 1998), the authors reported on the neuropsychological performance of 22 of 35 surviving eligible patients divided into four groups based on RT dose and age at RT (younger or older than 9 years). Although the number of patients in each of the four groups was small, there was a clear suggestion of both age and dose effects at the most

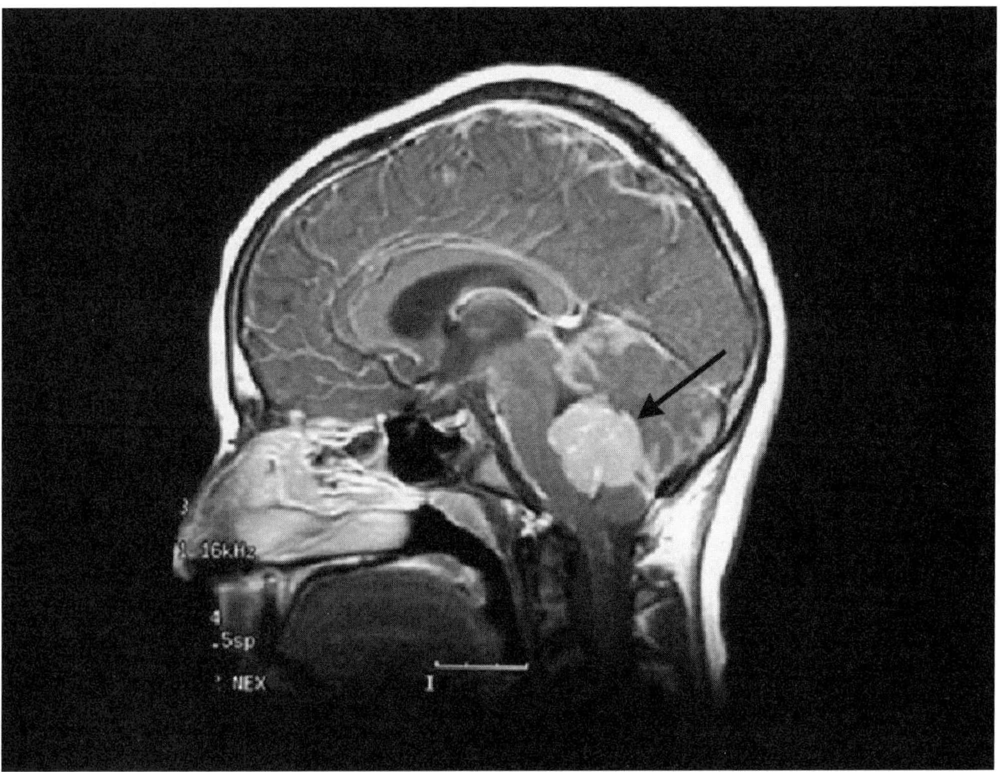


**Figure 14-1.** Saggital view of MRI of a patient with medulloblastoma. Tumor, located above the brain stem, is indicated by the arrow.

recent testing: Younger children with standard-dose RT had a median IQ of 70, younger children with reduced-dose RT had a median IQ of 85, older children with standard-dose RT had a median IQ of 83, and older children with reduced-dose RT had a median IQ of 92. Similar, although not necessarily statistically significant, differences between groups were found regarding measures of attention and academic achievement. Overall, the authors concluded that the 35% dose reduction resulted in a measurable sparing of IQ for children diagnosed between the ages of 4 and 9 years of age.

A more recent longitudinal study was published by the Children's Cancer Group; it involved 43 children who were survivors of average-risk medulloblastoma treated with 23.4-Gy RT and adjuvant chemotherapy at age 3 years or older (Ris et al., 2001). Overall, Full-Scale IQ declined a mean of 17.4 points or 4.3 points per year, Verbal IQ declined a mean of 16.8 points or 4.2 points per year, and Nonverbal IQ declined a mean of 16 points or 4.0 points per year. Although no significant age effects were found for Full-Scale IQ changes, children younger than 7 years at the time of receiving RT lost a mean of 20.8 points over the interval of observation, placing in question the notion that younger children benefit from lower doses of RT. However, without an internal comparison group, no definitive answer could be drawn.

Another longitudinal study of children surviving treatment for medulloblastoma elucidated the changes in learning that underlie often-noted declines in IQ in this group of children (Palmer et al., 2001). Forty-four children treated with RT with or without chemotherapy received serial assessments of their IQ up to 12 years posttreatment. The mean IQ score of the sample was 83.6 at the most recent testing, with a rate of decline from diagnosis estimated at 2.2 points per year. Children younger than 8 years at RT had a more rapid decline than older children (means, –3.2 vs. –1.2 points/year), and patients who received RT doses of 36 Gy or higher had a more rapid decline than those receiving lower RT doses (–3.6 vs. –1.6 points/year). Importantly, the analysis of patient's performance using raw score values (uncorrected for age) demonstrated a positive learning slope that was only 50%–60% of that necessary to maintain their original IQ scores. The above finding gives hope to the notion that the rate of learning could be accelerated in affected patients.

The results from these and other studies are summarized in Table 14-1. Despite considerable variability in methodology, several conclusions can be drawn from the existing literature:

1. Longitudinal studies consistently show significant declines in IQ over time among patients treated for medulloblastoma with CSI.
2. Cross-sectional studies that compared patients treated for medulloblastoma to those treated for ependymoma with posterior fossa RT alone or to patients treated for low-grade astrocytoma with surgery alone showed greater IQ deficits among those treated with CSI for medulloblastoma.
3. A young chronological age at the time of treatment increases the risk for IQ loss. Among studies that focused on very young patients, typically those younger than 3 or 4 years of age at diagnosis, the IQ changes can be devastating, with one series showing a median IQ of 62 at 5 years posttreatment (Walter et al., 1999). One study reported minimal neuropsychological toxicity with 1,800 cGy CSI, although the long-term outcomes in terms of survival and IQ have not yet been reported (Goldwein et al., 1996).

Although IQ loss has been primarily attributed to RT, other factors such as hydrocephalus and posterior fossa syndrome are also known to have an impact on development (Chapman et al., 1995). Furthermore, it has been observed that very young children have pre-RT scores that are depressed compared to their older counterparts, implying greater vulnerability to the impact of tumor, surgery, and perioperative factors (Walter et al., 1999). Also, one must appreciate that, because of the assumptions of the normal distribution of IQ in the general population, 50% of patients would be predicted to have an IQ less than 100.

IQ loss has frequently been associated with a commensurate decline in areas of basic academic achievement (Copeland, deMoor, Moore, & Ater, 1999; Mulhern et al., 1998, 1999; Ris et al., 2001), but these neuropsychological outcomes are not sufficiently functionally specific to be of use in determining the neural network(s) involved or for rehabilitation purposes. Increasingly, knowledge-based measures of IQ and academic achievement are viewed as the distal products of a pathological

**Table 14-1.** Summary of Studies of Intellectual Development Among Survivors of Medulloblastoma and Ependymoma

| *Reference* | *Sample* | *N* | *Treatment* | *Design* | *Results* |
|---|---|---|---|---|---|
| Palmer et al. (2003) | MED | 50 | 50/50 RT | Longitudinal | Mean loss of 2.2 IQ points/year post-RT |
| | | | CSI: 35–40 Gy | | Greater IQ deficits with younger age at RT |
| | | | PF: 51–59 Gy | | Greater IQ deficits among female patients |
| Palmer et al. (2001) | MED | 44 | 44/44 RT | Longitudinal | Mean loss of 2.6 IQ points/year post-RT |
| | | | CSI: 23.4–48 Gy | | Rate of learning 50%–60% of normal |
| | | | PF: 49–55 Gy | | Greater IQ deficits with younger age at RT |
| | | | 23/44 chemo | | |
| Mulhern et al. (2001) | MED | 42 | 42/42 RT | Cross sectional | Greater IQ deficits with younger age at RT |
| | | | CSI: 49–54 Gy | | Greater IQ deficits with increasing time from RT |
| | | | PF: 23.4–36 Gy | | |
| | | | 29/42 chemo | | |
| Ris et al. (2001) | MED | 43 | 43/43 RT | Longitudinal | Mean IQ loss of 4.3 points/year post-RT |
| | | | CSI: 23.4 Gy | | Greater IQ deficits with younger age at RT |
| | | | PF: 32.4 Gy | | |
| Mulhern et al. (1999) | MED | 18 | 9/18 chemo | Cross sectional | Mean IQ of MED < LGA (age matched) |
| | | | 18/18 RT | | |
| | | | CSI: 23.4–36 Gy | | |
| | | | PF: 49–54 Gy | | |
| | LGA | 18 | Surgery only | | |
| Mulhern et al. (1998) | MED | 22 | 22/22 RT | Cross sectional | Greater IQ deficits with younger age at RT |
| | | | 22/22 PF: 54 Gy | | Greater IQ deficits in those receiving 36-Gy CSI |
| | | | 13/22 CSI: 36.0 Gy | | |
| | | | 9/22 CSI: 23.4 Gy | | |
| Dennis, Spiegler, Hetherington, & Greenberg (1996) | MED | 25 | 25/25 RT<br>RT not specified<br>7/25 chemo | Cross sectional | Greater IQ deficits with younger age at RT<br>Greater IQ deficits with increasing time from RT |
| Grill et al. (1999) | MED | 19 | 19/19 RT | Cross sectional | Medulloblastoma IQ < ependymoma IQ |
| | | | 19/19 CSI: 25–35 Gy | | MED with 25-Gy CSI performed better than those with 35 Gy CSI |
| | | | 19/19 PF: 55 Gy | | |
| | | | 17/19 chemo | | |

*(continued)*

**Table 14-1.** *(continued)*

| *Reference* | *Sample* | *N* | *Treatment* | *Design* | *Results* |
|---|---|---|---|---|---|
| | EPEN | 12 | 12/12 RT<br>11/12 PF: 25 Gy<br>4/12 chemo | | |
| Hoppe-Hirsch et al. (1995) | MED<br>EPEN | 59<br>37 | 59/59 CSI, PF RT<br>28/37 PF RT | Cross sectional | 10% IQ > 90 in MED<br>60% IQ > 90 in EPEN |
| Copeland et al. (1999) | Very young PF | 27 | 7/27 RT<br>CSI: 30–40 Gy<br>PF: 40–50 Gy<br>20/27 Chemo | Longitudinal | Greater decline in IQ with RT |
| Walter et al. (1999) | Very young MED | 19 | 19/19 Chemo<br>19/19 RT<br>CSI: 35.2 Gy<br>PF: 53.4 Gy | Longitudinal | Mean IQ loss of 3.9 points/year post-RT |
| Kiltie, Lashford, & Gattamaneni (1997) | Very young MED | 37 | 37/37 RT<br>CSI, PF doses varied<br>15/37 chemo | Cross sectional | 8/16 long-term survivors in special schools |
| Goldwein et al. (1996) | Very young MED | 10 | 10/10 RT<br>CSI: 18 Gy<br>PF: 54 Gy<br>10/10 chemo | Longitudinal | No change in baseline IQ at 3 years post-RT |

MED, medulloblastoma; EPEN, ependymoma; PF, posterior fossa; chemo, chemotherapy; RT, radiation therapy; CSI, craniospinal irradiation; IQ, intelligence quotient; LGA, low-grade astrocytoma.

process that affects "core" cognitive functions such as attention, processing speed, and working memory that provide the foundations for the ability to efficiently learn and retain information (Copeland et al., 1999; Mulhern et al., 1998, 2001). This conceptualization is reinforced by evidence that normal, age-related improvement in processing speed and working memory account for nearly half of the age-related improvements in fluid intelligence (Fry & Hale, 1996).

Studies that have emphasized assessment of these core deficits among patients surviving medulloblastoma are summarized in Table 14-2. In general, these studies confirmed that deficits in the core areas of attention and memory are prevalent, and similar to IQ, that the more severe core deficits are associated with a younger age at RT, increasing time from RT, and increasing RT dose. However, whether these deficits truly result in IQ and academic achievement declines has not yet been demonstrated among children surviving brain tumors.

## Insights from Neuroimaging

The shared neurobiological substrate for neuropsychological deficits attributed to RT is thought to be loss of normal white matter or the failure to develop normal white matter at an age-appropriate rate (Mulhern et al., 1999). The adverse effects of ionizing RT on the cerebral microvasculature is thought to be the primary pathway leading to white matter loss as opposed to the direct effects of irradiation on glial cells or their precursors (Hopewell & van der Kogel, 1999). However, the pathophysiology of late, RT-induced CNS damage is incompletely understood, especially regarding the predilection of white matter to injury. Hypotheses attributing primary mechanisms to neu-

**Table 14-2.** Studies of Core Cognitive Deficits among Survivors of Medulloblastoma.

| *Reference* | *Sample* | *N* | *Treatment* | *Core Deficits* | *Findings* |
|---|---|---|---|---|---|
| Mulhern et al. (2001) | MED | 42 | 42/42 RT | Memory (verbal) | Greater deficits with increased time from RT |
| | | | CSI: 49–54 Gy | Attention (visual) | Greater deficits with younger age at RT |
| | | | PF: 23.4–36 Gy | | |
| | | | 29/42 chemo | | |
| Mulhern et al. (1998) | MED | 22 | 22/22 RT | Attention | Greater deficits in younger patients |
| | | | 22/22 PF: 54 Gy | | Greater deficits in those receiving 36 Gy CSI |
| | | | 13/22 CSI: 36.0 Gy | | |
| | | | 9/22 CSI: 23.4 Gy | | |
| Copeland et al. (1999) | Very young PF | 27 | 7/27 RT | Attention | Overall decline (RT > no RT) |
| | | | CSI: 30–40 Gy | Memory (verbal) | Overall decline |
| | | | PF: 40–50 Gy | Memory (spatial) | Overall decline (RT > no RT) |
| | | | 20/27 chemo | | |

MED, medulloblastoma; PF, posterior fossa; chemo, chemotherapy; RT, radiation therapy; CSI, craniospinal irradiation.

ronal, oligodendrocyte, or endothelial cell death are insufficient. Secondary processes, such as damage to the myelin membrane from oxidative stress following RT, have been proposed as alternative mechanisms (Trofilon & Fike, 2000).

Current imaging research has progressed beyond just diagnosis and surveillance to begin assessing neuropathological and neurodevelopmental correlates. One mechanism thought to account at least partially for the rate of IQ decline in survivors is the loss of cerebral white matter or failure to develop white matter at a developmentally appropriate rate. Studies that have quantified toxic effects on white matter and investigated the association between neurotoxicity and cognitive deficits in children have focused primarily on survivors of medulloblastoma of the posterior fossa.

One such study compared patients treated for medulloblastoma with age-similar controls who had received surgery alone for low-grade tumors of the posterior fossa; the survivors of medulloblastoma had a significantly smaller volume of cerebral white matter, a substantially greater volume of cerebrospinal fluid, and an equal volume of gray matter (Reddick, Mulhern, Elkin, Glass, & Langston, 1998). As was expected, the survivors of medulloblastoma had significantly lower IQs, which had a positive and statistically significant association with the cerebral white matter volumes (Mulhern et al., 1999). However, because of their cross-sectional design, these studies could not discern whether the smaller cerebral white matter volume reflected loss of tissue, failure to develop white matter at an appropriate rate, or both.

A subsequent longitudinal study revealed a significant loss of cerebral white matter volume in patients undergoing treatment for medulloblastoma; this loss was more rapid among those patients who received a CSI dose of 36 Gy versus CSI of 23.4 Gy (Reddick et al., 2000). These findings relating cerebral white matter with radiation dose were confirmed in another longitudinal study of corpus callosum volumes that found that the greatest deviation from normal development occurred in the most posterior subregions, which also received the highest total dose of irradiation (Palmer et al., 2002).

The previous studies established relationships between cerebral white matter volume and both irradiation dose and IQ. The next study established that cerebral white matter volume can explain approximately 70% of the association between IQ and age at the time of irradiation (Mulhern et al., 2001). Even more recently, a cross-sectional study of patients treated for medulloblastoma demonstrated significantly impaired performance on all neuropsychological measures of intellect, attention, memory, and academic achievement (Reddick et al., 2003). The study produced a developmental model in which academic achievement was predicted by cerebral white matter volume, attentional ability, and IQ; these factors explained approximately 60% of the variance observed in reading and spelling and almost 80% of the variance observed in mathematics. The primary consequence of reduced cerebral white matter volume was decreased attentional ability, which reduced patients' IQ and academic achievement. More detailed investigation of this relationship between attention and cerebral white matter in this same patient sample using a self-administered computer test of visual attention revealed that, after statistically controlling for the effects of age at diagnosis and time elapsed since treatment, there was a significant association between attentional functioning and cerebral white matter volumes or specific regional white matter volumes of the prefrontal/frontal lobe and cingulate gyrus (Mulhern et al., in press).

In addition to neurostructural volumes, other measures of white matter integrity, such as diffusion tensor imaging of fractional anisotropy and apparent diffusion coefficients, should be incorporated. A pilot study of medulloblastoma survivors found significant reductions in white matter fractional anisotropy that were significantly correlated with younger age at treatment, longer time since treatment, and deterioration of school performance (Khong et al., 2003).

Although methods to quantify leukoencephalopathy in children treated for ALL have been developed (Reddick, Glass, Langston, & Helton, 2002), no clinical correlations with neuropsychological function have yet been published. Functional MRI, a method of mapping human brain activation that has been used extensively to investigate and characterize the basic neural networks that support normal cognitive function and disease-associated alterations in the networks, may also provide important insights into the relationship between disease- and treatment-induced morphological abnormalities and the behavioral deficits that negatively affect the quality of life of medulloblastoma survivors (Ogg et al., 2002).

## Recommended Core Battery

The two major cooperative groups that coordinate childhood cancer therapy in the United States (Children's Cancer Group, Pediatric Oncology Group) have consolidated into the Children's Oncology Group (COG). This action has enabled the national standardization of pediatric cancer therapy and studies of late effects of treatment. One of the additional benefits has been the development of a consensus among participating COG psychologists regarding a set of core neuropsychological domains and the specific tests to assess these domains (B. D. Moore, personal communication, 2004).

The advantages of this initiative are twofold: First, it will facilitate comparisons among patients treated for the same disease (e.g., ALL) on different generations of protocols, providing historical controls for currently treated patients; second, it will allow for the comparison of patients with different malignancies (e.g., ALL vs. medulloblastoma) to identify subsets of patients who are experiencing more severe neuropsychological deficits. In both of these situations, the standardization of the core battery should lead to better identification of demographic and clinical variables that place children at risk for neuropsychological deficits.

A summary of the relevant neuropsychological domains and tests for the core battery is presented in Table 14-3. The tests were chosen because of psychometric properties in terms of reliability and validity as well as to increase the likelihood of reimbursement by third-party payers to psychologists who perform the testing. This battery is not intended to replace clinically driven decisions regarding patient assessment. Therefore, the examining psychologist is encouraged to build on this framework according to individual patient needs and clinical questions.

Although it is extremely important to have a standardized series of neuropsychological tests that are age appropriate and that will allow for important comparisons across different treatment regimens within pediatric cancer diagnostic categories, there is also a need for flexibility in terms of diagnostic and treatment variables from a neuroanatomical perspective. Thus, the COG basic battery is designed not only to assess many higher cortical and subcortical functions in an efficient and logistically reasonable manner, but also to provide freedom for the inclusion of specific neuropsychological measures that can test for specific hypotheses when necessary. It is also recognized that some patients may exhibit neurological deficits (e.g., hemiplegia, blindness, somnolence) that

**Table 14-3.** Children's Oncology Group Core Neuropsychological Test Battery

| *Functional Domain* | *Tests* | *Reference* |
|---|---|---|
| Intelligence | Bayley Infant Neurodevelopmental Screener | Aylward (1995) |
| | Child Development Inventory[a] | Ireton & Thwing (1992) |
| | Wechsler Preschool and Primary Scales of Intelligence | Wechsler (2002) |
| | Wechsler Abbreviated Scales of Intelligence | Psychological Corporation (1999) |
| Language | Expressive One Word Picture Vocabulary Test | Gardner (2000a) |
| | Receptive One Word Picture Vocabulary Test | Gardner (2000b) |
| Memory | Children's Memory Scale (selected subtests) | Cohen (1997) |
| | California Verbal Learning Test | Delis, Kramer, Kaplan, & Ober (1994) |
| | Wechsler Memory Scale | Wechsler (1997) |
| Attention | Conners' Continuous Performance Test | Conners (2000) |
| Executive function | NEPSY | Korkman, Kirk, & Kemp (1998) |
| | Delis-Kaplan Executive Function System | Delis, Kaplan, & Kramer (2001) |
| | Tower of London—DX | Culbertson & Zimmer (2000) |
| | Behavior Rating Inventory of Executive Function[a] | Gioia, Isquith, Guy, & Kenworthy (2000) |
| Academic achievement | Wide Range Achievement Test | Wilkinson (1993) |
| Adjustment and quality of life | Behavioral Assessment System for Children[a]<br>Adaptive Behavior Assessment System[a]<br>Pediatric Quality of Life Inventory[a] | Reynolds & Kamphaus (1997)<br>Harrison & Oakland (2003)<br>Varni, Burwinkle, Seid, & Skarr (2003) |

*Notes.* [a]Parent report measure. Tests are listed in ascending order according to patient age within their primary domain, although some assess aspects of multiple domains. The most recently published version is recommended. Adapted with permission from Moore, 2004.

would prevent valid assessment with some of the tests listed. Nevertheless, this represents an important first effort to standardize neuropsychological assessment of patients participating in COG treatment protocols.

## Future Directions

With the rise in survival rates among children diagnosed with cancer, we believe that research priorities will involve at least two major changes. First, even within medical treatment protocols, the design and end points will necessarily be driven by quality of life rather than survival considerations. Second, neuropsychological testing, and the integration of neuropsychological testing with modalities at other levels of analysis such as neurotransmitter assays or MRI, will allow for a more thorough examination of the neurobiological mechanisms and sequence of changes that are associated with neuropsychological late effects. These issues are discussed in more detail next.

The "gold standard" of research designs in pediatric oncology has been the randomized clinical trial (RCT). The widespread use of RCTs is arguably one factor responsible for the vast improvement in prognosis. However, disease-specific RCTs may soon become a victim of their own success. Because of the limited number of children diagnosed with cancer each year and the current high levels of cure for the most common forms of cancer, it is becoming extremely difficult to design RCTs to demonstrate incremental improvements in survival as a primary outcome. From our perspective, this barrier will hasten the already-growing focus on quality of life as a primary outcome in therapeutic trials of new cancer therapies.

This shift from an emphasis on increasing survival rates to reducing the adverse consequences of treatment is already palpable in COG protocols. As behavioral scientists, we must be prepared to meet this challenge in terms of our knowledge of RCT design and reporting requirements (Stinson, McGrath, & Yamada, 2003) as well as supporting our colleagues in conducting and reporting the results of RCTs (Brown, 2003; McGrath, Stinson, & Davidson, 2003). Consensus statements, such as the COG core testing guidelines presented in this chapter (Moore, personal communication, 2004), will need to be developed in the future to address questions that relate primarily to psychosocial rather than neuropsychological aspects of quality of life.

Developmental models of neuropsychological toxicity secondary to childhood cancer treatments have only recently begun to evolve. Some (e.g., Schatz, Kramer, Ablin, & Matthay, 2000) test mediational hypotheses using sophisticated measures of cognitive processes derived from experimental laboratory techniques. Other models incorporate neuroimaging and neuropsychological data in an attempt to discover the association between brain damage and specific functional outcomes (e.g., Reddick et al., 2003). Both of these research reports illustrate what we think will be a growing trend toward increasing our knowledge regarding biological changes in the brain and their associated consequences in terms of basic cognitive processes. Because most clinical measures have not been developed from cognitive theory, we expected increased reliance on tasks derived from experimental psychology that can measure more focused aspects of cognitive processing. Because such measures are not normed, studies using these measures will need to incorporate healthy age peers in the design.

Even within subgroups of children known to be at greater risk for neuropsychological damage following their cancer therapy, there exists considerable variability in their outcomes. Demographic factors such as age, gender, and parental education have been shown to moderate the effects of cancer therapy, but how? Is it likely that variables such as these are merely proxies for processes that we do not appreciate? For example, age at the time of treatment is clearly understood as a proxy for stages of brain development that make children more vulnerable biologically and neuropsychologically to certain forms of treatment toxicity (e.g., Mulhern et al., 2001). It is also possible that particular genotypes yet unknown may provide a protective effect to certain neurotoxins. Understanding the underlying mechanisms responsible for neuropsychological toxicity will be essential to the development of targeted biological and cognitive behavioral interventions for those patients for whom brain damage cannot be avoided. Some of these interventions may be restorative, compensatory, or environmental involving multiple targeted systems. Issues relating to intervention are discussed more fully by Butler and Copeland in chapter 16, this volume.

Continued efforts toward the detailed definition and description of discrete neuropsychological impairment in the pediatric cancer population remain imperative. As treatment protocols change, it is necessary to document alterations in neurocognitive dysfunction. On a very positive note, oncology protocol advances have resulted in lessened neuropsychological involvement, but many children continue to suffer cognitive and learning deficits associated with their oncology treatment, as documented in this chapter. As oncologists continue to reduce CNS toxicity, it is incumbent on the pediatric psychologists and neuropsychologists to develop interventions designed to further lessen and alleviate difficulties associated with treatment. The synergistic combination of oncology treatment advancement, knowledge of the neuropathological and correlated neuropsychological changes that occur following disease and treatments to the CNS, and our ability to effectively remediate neurocognitive deficits associated with the above-noted disease variables are defining the next "era" of pediatric oncology.

*Acknowledgments.* Preparation of this chapter was supported in part by the American Lebanese Syrian Associated Charities and grants CA 21765, CA 20180, CA78957, and CA83936 from the National Cancer Institute.

## References

Aylward, G. P. (1995). *Bayley Infant Neurodevelopmental Screener*. New York: Psychological Corporation.

Brouwers, P., Riccardi, R., Poplack, D., & Fedio, P. (1984). Attentional deficits in long-term survivors of childhood acute lymphoblastic leukemia (ALL). *Journal of Clinical Neuropsychology*, 6, 325–336.

Brown, R. T. (2003). Editorial: The *Journal of Pediatric Psychology* will support the publication of clinical trials. *Journal of Pediatric Psychology*, 28, 173.

Brown, R. T., Madan-Swain, A., Walco, G. A., Cherrick, I., Levers, C. E., Conte, P. M., et al. (1998). Cognitive and academic late effects among children previously treated for acute lymphocytic leukemia receiving chemotherapy as CNS prophylaxis. *Journal of Pediatric Psychology*, *23*, 333–340.

Butler, R. B., & Copeland, D. R. (1993). Neuropsychological effects of central nervous system prophylactic treatment in childhood leukemia: Methodological considerations. *Journal of Pediatric Psychology*, *18*, 319–338.

Butler, R. W., Hill, J. M., Steinherz, P. G., Meyers, P. A., & Finlay, J. L. (1994). The neuropsychologic effects of cranial irradiation, intrathecal methotrexate, and systemic methotrexate in childhood cancer. *Journal of Clinical Oncology*, *12*, 2621–2629.

Butler, R., Kerr, M., & Marchand, A. (1999). Attention and executive functions following cranial irradiation in children. *Journal of the International Neuropsychological Society*, *5*, 108.

Butler, R. W., Rizzi, L. P., & Bandilla, E. B. (1999). The effects of childhood cancer treatment on two objective measures of psychological functioning. *Children's Health Care*, *28*, 311–327.

Chapman, C. A., Waber, D. P., Bernstein, J. H., Pomeroy, S. L., LaVally, B., Sallan, S. E., et al. (1995). Neurobehavioral and neurologic outcome in long-term survivors of posterior fossa brain tumors: Role of age and perioperative factors. *Journal of Child Neurology*, *10*, 209–212.

Cohen, M. (1997). *Children's Memory Scale*. New York: Psychological Corporation.

Conners, K. (2000). *Conners' continuous performance test* (2nd ed.). North Tonawanda, NY: MHS.

Copeland, D. R., DeMoor, C., Moore, B. D., & Ater, J. L. (1999). Neurocognitive development of children after a cerebellar tumor in infancy: A longitudinal study. *Journal of Clinical Oncology*, *17*, 3476–3486.

Copeland, D. R., Dowell, R. E., Jr., Fletcher, J. M., Bordeau, J. D., Sullivan, M. P., Jaffe, N., et al. (1988). Neuropsychological effects of childhood cancer treatment. *Journal of Child Neurology*, *3*, 53–62.

Copeland, D. R., Dowell, R. E., Jr., Fletcher, J. M., Sullivan, M. P., Jaffe, N., Cangir, A., et al. (1988). Neuropsychological test performance of pediatric cancer patients at diagnosis and one year later. *Journal of Pediatric Psychology*, *13*, 183–196.

Copeland, D. R., Fletcher, J. M., Pfefferbaum-Levine, B., Jaffe, N., Reid, H., & Maor, M. (1985). Neuropsychological sequelae of childhood cancer in long-term survivors. *Pediatrics*, *75*, 745–753.

Copeland, D. R., Moore, B. D., Francis, D. J., Jafe, N., & Culbert, S. J. (1996). Neuropsychologic effects of chemotherapy on children with cancer: A longitudinal study. *Journal of Clinical Oncology*, *14*, 2826–2835.

Culbertson, W. C., & Zillmer, E. A. (2000). *Tower of London—DX*. North Tonawanda, NY: MHS.

Delis, D., Kaplan, E., & Kramer, J. (2001). *Delis-Kaplan executive function system*. New York: Psychological Corporation.

Delis, D., Kramer, J., Kaplan, E., & Ober, B. (1994). *California verbal learning test*. New York: Psychological Corporation.

Dennis, M., Spiegler, B. J., Hetherington, C. R., & Greenberg, M. L. (1996). Neuropsychological sequelae of the treatment of children with medulloblastoma. *Journal of Neuro-oncology*, *29*, 91–101.

Ellenberg, L., McComb, J. G., Siegel, S. E., & Stowe, S. (1987). Factors affecting intellectual outcome in pediatric brain tumor patients. *Neurosurgery*, *21*, 638–644.

Fletcher, J. M., & Copeland, D. R. (1988). Neurobehavioral effects of central nervous system prophylactic treatment of cancer in children. *Journal of Clinical and Experimental Neuropsychology*, *10*, 495–538.

Fry, A. S., & Hale, S. (1996). Processing speed, working memory, and fluid intelligence: Evidence for a developmental cascade. *Psychological Science*, *4*, 237–241.

Gardner, M. F. (2000a). *Expressive one word vocabulary test—2000 edition*. Wood Dale, IL: Stoelting.

Gardner, M. F. (2000b). *Receptive one word vocabulary test—2000 edition*. Wood Dale, IL: Stoelting.

Gioia, G., Isquith, P., Guy, S., & Kenworthy, L. (2000). *Behavior Rating Inventory of Executive Function*. Lutz, FL: Psychological Assessment Resources.

Goldberg, E., & Costa, L. D. (1981). Hemisphere difference in the acquisition and use of descriptive systems in the brain. *Brain and Language*, *14*, 144–173.

Goldwein, J. W., Radcliffe, J., Johnson, J., Moshang, T., Packer, R. J., Sutton, L. N., et al. (1996). Updated results of a pilot study of low dose craniospinal irradiation plus chemotherapy for children under five with cerebellar primitive neuroectodermal tumors (medulloblastoma). *International Journal of Radiation Oncology and Biological Physics*, *34*, 899–904.

Grill, J., Renaux, V. K., Bulteau, C., Viguier, D., Levy-Piebois, C., Sainte-Rose, C., et al. (1999). Long-term intellectual outcome in children with posterior fossa tumors according to radiation doses and volumes. *International Journal of Radiation Oncology and Biological Physics, 45*, 137–145.

Harrison, P., & Oakland, T. (2003). *Adaptive behavior assessment system* (2nd ed.). New York: Psychological Corporation.

Hirsch, J. F., Rose, C. R., Pierre-Kahn, A., Pfister, A., & Hoppe-Hirsch, E. (1989). Benign astrocytic and oligodendrocytic tumors of the cerebral hemispheres in children. *Journal of Neurosurgery, 70*, 568–572.

Hopewell, J. W., & van der Kogel, A. J. (1999). Pathophysiological mechanisms leading to the development of late radiation-induced damage to the central nervous system. In T. Wiegel, W. Hinkelbein, M. Brock, & T. Hoell (Eds.), *Controversies in neuro-oncology: Frontiers of radiation therapy and oncology* (pp. 265–275). Basel, Switzerland: Karger.

Hoppe-Hirsch, E., Brunet, L., Laroussinie, F., Cinalli, G, Pierre-Khan, A., Renier, D., et al. (1995). Intellectual outcome in children with malignant tumors of the posterior fossa: Influence of the field of irradiation and quality of surgery. *Child's Nervous System, 11*, 340–346.

Ireton, H. R., & Thwing, E. J. (1992). *Child Development Inventory*. Circle Pines, MN: AGS.

Jannoun, L., & Bloom, H. J. G. (1990). Long-term psychological effects in children treated for intracranial tumors. *International Journal of Radiation Oncology and Biological Physics, 18*, 747–753.

Khong, P.-L., Kwong, D. L. W., Chan, G. C. F., Sham, J. S., Chan, F. L., & Ooi, G. C. (2003). Diffusion-tensor imaging for the detection and quantification of treatment-induced white matter injury in children with medulloblastoma: A pilot study. *American Journal of Neuroradiology, 24*, 734–740.

Kiltie, A. E., Lashford, L. S., & Gattamaneni, H. R. (1997). Survival and late effects in medulloblastoma patients treated with craniospinal irradiation under 3 years old. *Medical and Pediatric Oncology, 28*, 348–354.

Korkman, M., Kirk, V., & Kemp, S. (1998). *NEPSY: A developmental neuropsychological assessment*. New York: Psychological Corporation.

Lockwood, K. A., Bell, T. S., & Colegrove, R. W. (1999). Long-term effects of cranial radiation therapy on attention functioning in survivors of childhood leukemia. *Journal of Pediatric Psychology, 24*, 55–66.

Margolin, J. F., Steuber, C. P., & Poplack, D. G. (2002). Acute lymphoblastic leukemia. In P. A. Pizzo & D. G. Poplack (Eds.), *Principles and practice of pediatric oncology* (3rd ed., pp. 489–544). Philadelphia: Lippincott-Raven.

McGrath, P. J., Stinson, J., & Davidson, K. (2003). Commentary: The *Journal of Pediatric Psychology* should adopt the CONSORT statement as a way of improving the evidence base in pediatric psychology. *Journal of Pediatric Psychology, 28*, 169–172.

Meadows, A. T., Massari, D. J., Ferguson, J., Gordon, J., Littman, P., & Moss, K. (1981). Declines in IQ scores and cognitive dysfunctions in children with acute lymphocytic leukemia treated with cranial irradiation. *Lancet, 2*, 1015–1018.

Moleski, M. (2000). Neuropsychological, neuroanatomical, and neurophysiological consequences of CNS chemotherapy for acute lymphoblastic leukemia. *Archives of Clinical Neuropsychology, 5*, 603–630.

Mostow, E. N., Byrne, J., Connelly, R. R., & Mulvihill, J. J. (1991). Quality of life in long-term survivors of CNS tumors of childhood and adolescence. *Journal of Clinical Oncology, 9*, 592–599.

Mulhern, R. K., Fairclough, D., & Ochs, J. (1991). A prospective comparison of neuropsychologic performance of children surviving leukemia who received 18-Gy, 24-Gy, or no cranial irradiation. *Journal of Clinical Oncology, 9*, 1348–1356.

Mulhern, R. K., Hancock, J., Fairclough, D., & Kun, L. E. (1992). Neuropsychological status of children treated for brain tumors: A critical review and integrative analysis. *Medical and Pediatric Oncology, 20*, 181.

Mulhern, R. K., Kepner, J. L., Thomas, P. R., Armstrong, F. D., Friedman, H. S., & Kun, L. E. (1998). Neuropsychologic functioning of survivors of childhood medulloblastoma randomized to receive conventional or reduced-dose craniospinal irradiation: A Pediatric Oncology Group study. *Journal of Clinical Oncology, 16*, 1723–1728.

Mulhern, R. K., Ochs, J., Fairclough, D., Wasserman, A. L., Davis, K. S., & Williams, J. M. (1987). Intellectual and academic achievement status after CNS relapse: A retrospective analysis of 40 children treated for acute lymphoblastic leukemia. *Journal of Clinical Oncology, 5*, 933–940.

Mulhern, R. K., Palmer, S. L., Reddick, W. E., Glass, J. O., Kun, L. E., Taylor, J., et al. (2001). Risks of young age for selected neurocognitive deficits in medulloblastoma are associated with white matter loss. *Journal of Clinical Oncology, 19*, 472–479.

Mulhern, R. K., Reddick, W. E., Palmer, S. L., Glass, J., Elkin, D., Kun, L. E., et al. (1999). Neurocognitive deficits in medulloblastoma survivors and white matter loss. *Annals of Neurology*, *46*, 834–841.

Mulhern, R. K., Wasserman, A. L., Fairclough, D., & Ochs, J. (1988). Memory function in disease-free survivors of childhood acute lymphocytic leukemia given CNS prophylaxis with or without 1,800 cGy cranial irradiation. *Journal of Clinical Oncology*, *6*, 315–320.

Mulhern, R. K., White, H. A., Glass, J. O., Kun, L. E., Leigh, L., Thompson, S. J., et al. (2004). Attentional functioning and white matter integrity among survivors of malignant brain tumors of childhood. *Journal of the International Neuropsychological Society*, *10*, 180–189.

Ochs, J., Mulhern, R., Fairclough, D., Parvey, L., Whitaker, J., Ch'ien, L., et al. (1991). Comparison of neuropsychologic functioning and clinical neurotoxicity in long-term survivors of childhood leukemia given cranial radiation or parenteral methotrexate: A prospective study. *Journal of Clinical Oncology*, *9*, 145–151.

Ochs, J., Parvey, L. S., & Mulhern, R. (1986). Prospective study of central nervous system changes in children with acute lymphoblastic leukemia receiving two different methods of central nervous system prophylaxis. *Neurotoxicity*, *7*, 217–226.

Ogg, R., Zou, P., White, H., Cooper, T., O'Grady, J., Butler, R., et al. (2002). Attention deficits in survivors of childhood cancer: An MRI study. *Journal of the International Neuropsychological Society*, *8*, 494.

Palmer, S. L., Gajjar, A., Reddick, W. E., Glass, J. O., Kun, L. E., Wu, S., et al. (2003). Predicting intellectual outcome among children treated with 35–40 Gy craniospinal irradiation for medulloblastoma. *Neuropsychology*, *17*, 548–555.

Palmer, S. L., Goloubeva, O., Reddick, W. E., Glass, J. O., Gajjar, A., Kun, L., et al. (2001). Patterns of intellectual development among survivors of pediatric medulloblastoma: A longitudinal analysis. *Journal of Clinical Oncology*, *19*, 2302–2308.

Palmer, S. L., Reddick, W. E., Glass, J. O., Goloubeva, O., Gajjar, A., & Mulhern, R. K. (2002). Decline in corpus callosum volume among pediatric patients with medulloblastoma: Longitudinal MR imaging study. *American Journal of Neuroradiology*, *23*, 1088–1094.

Psychological Corporation. (1999). *Wechsler Abbreviated Scale of Intelligence*. New York: Author.

Quinn, C. T., Griener, J. C., Bottiglieri, T., Hyland, K., Farrow, A., & Kamen, B. A. (1997). Elevation of homocysteine and excitatory amino acid neurotransmitters in the CSF of children who receive methotrexate for the treatment of cancer. *Journal of Clinical Oncology*, *15*, 2800–2806.

Reddick, W. E., Glass, J. O., Langston, J. W., & Helton, K. J. (2002). Quantitative MRI assessment of leukoencephalopathy. *Magnetic Resonance in Medicine*, *47*, 912–920.

Reddick, W. E., Mulhern, R. K., Elkin, T. D., Glass, J. O., & Langston, J. W. (1998) A hybrid neural network analysis of subtle brain volume differences in children surviving brain tumors. *Magnetic Resonance Imaging*, *16*, 413–421.

Reddick, W. E., Russell, J. M., Glass, J. O., Xiong, X, Mulhern, R. K., Langston, J. W., et al. (2000). Subtle white matter volume differences in children treated for medulloblastoma with conventional or reduced-dose cranial-spinal irradiation. *Magnet Resonance Imaging*, *18*, 787–793.

Reddick, W. E., White, H., Glass, J. O., Wheeler, G. C., Thompson, S. J., Gajjar, A., et al. (2003). Developmental model relating white matter volume with neurocognitive deficits in pediatric brain tumor survivors. *Cancer*, *97*, 2512–2519.

Reynolds, C. R., & Kamphaus, R. W. (1997). *Behavioral Assessment Scale for Children*. Circle Pines, MN: AGS.

Ris, M. D., & Noll, R. B. (1994). Long-term neurobehavioral outcome in pediatric brain-tumor patients: Review and methodological critique. *Journal of Clinical and Experimental Neuropsychology*, *16*, 21–42.

Ris, M. D., Packer, R., Goldwein, J., Jones-Wallace, D., & Boyett, J. M. (2001). Intellectual outcome after reduced-dose radiation therapy plus adjuvant chemotherapy for medulloblastoma: A Children's Cancer Group study. *Journal of Clinical Oncology*, *19*, 3470–3476.

Rodgers, J., Horrocks, J., Britton, P. G., & Kernahan, J. (1999). Attentional ability among survivors of leukaemia. *Archives of Diseases of Childhood*, *80*, 318–323.

Rourke, B. P. (1989). *Nonverbal learning disabilities: The syndrome and the model*. New York: Guilford.

Rowland, J. H., Glidewell, O. J., Sibley, R. F., Holland, J. C., Tull, R., Berman, A., et al. (1984). Effects of different forms of central nervous system prophylaxis on neuropsychologic function in childhood leukemia. *Journal of Clinical Oncology*, *12*, 1327–1355.

Satz, P. (1993). Brain reserve capacity on symptom onset after brain injury: A formulation and review of evidence for threshold theory. *Neuropsychology*, *7*, 273–295.

Schatz, J., Kramer, J., Ablin, A., & Matthay, K. K. (2000). Processing speed, working memory, and IQ: A developmental model of cognitive deficits following cranial radiation therapy. *Neuropsychology*, *14*, 189–200.

Soni, S. S., Marten, G. W., Pitner, S. E., Duenas, D. A., & Powazek, M. (1975). Effects of central-nervous system irradiation on neuropsychologic functioning of children with acute lymphocytic leukemia. *New England Journal of Medicine*, *293*, 113–118.

Steen, G., & Mirro, J. (2000). *Childhood cancer: A handbook from St. Jude Children's Research Hospital.* Cambridge, MA: Perseus.

Stinson, J. N., McGrath, P. J., & Yamada, J. T. (2003). Clinical trials in the *Journal of Pediatric Psychology*: Applying the CONSORT statement. *Journal of Pediatric Psychology*, *28*, 159–168.

Strother, D. R., Pollack, I. F., Fisher, P. G., Hunter, J. V., Woo, S. Y., Pomeroy, S. L., et al. (2002). Tumors of the central nervous system. In P. A. Pizzo and D. G. Poplack (Eds.), *Principles and practice of pediatric oncology* (4th ed., pp. 751–784). Philadelphia: Lippincott.

Tofilon, P. J., & Fike, J. (2000). The radioresponse of the central nervous system: A dynamic process. *Radiation Research*, *153*, 357–370.

Varni, J. W., Burwinkle, T. M., Seid, M., & Skarr, D. (2003). The PedsQL™ 4.0 as a pediatric population health measure: Feasibility, reliability, and validity. *Ambulatory Pediatrics*, *3*, 329–341.

Waber, D. P., Carpentieri, S. C., Klar, N., Silverman, L. B., Schwenn, M., Hurwitz, C. A., et al. (2000). Cognitive sequelae in children treated for acute lymphoblastic leukemia with dexamethasone or prednisone. *Journal of Pediatric Hematology/Oncology*, *22*, 206–213.

Waber, D. P., Gioia, G., Paccia, J., Sherman, B., Dinklage, D., Sollee, N., et al. (1990). Sex differences in cognitive processing in children treated with CNS prophylaxis for acute lymphoblastic leukemia. *Journal of Pediatric Psychology*, *15*, 105–122.

Walter, A. W., Mulhern, R. K., Gajjar, A., Heideman, R., Reardon, D., Sanford, R. A., et al. (1999). Survival and neurodevelopmental outcome of young children with medulloblastoma at St. Jude Children's Research Hospital. *Journal of Clinical Oncology*, *17*, 3720–3728.

Wechsler, D. (1997). *Wechsler Memory Scale* (3rd ed.). New York: Psychological Corporation.

Wechsler, D. (2002). *Wechsler Preschool and Primary Scale of Intelligence.* (rd ed.). New York: Psychological Corporation.

Wilkinson, G. (1993). *Wide Range Achievement Test 3.* Wilmington, DE: Jastak.

Margaret L. Stuber

# Posttraumatic Stress and Posttraumatic Growth in Childhood Cancer Survivors and Their Parents

Few would disagree that a diagnosis of childhood cancer is shocking and frightening to the child and to the child's family. In addition to the sudden and dreadful diagnosis, the intensive and often lengthy treatment is extremely stressful. The combination of diagnosis and subsequent treatment frequently leaves children and parents feeling helpless. However, life-threatening illness has historically been categorized as stressful but not "traumatic" in the way that interpersonal violence or natural disasters are traumatic. In fact, the third edition of the *Diagnostic and Statistical Manual of Mental Disorders* (*DSM-III*) (American Psychiatric Association [APA], 1987) stated that "chronic medical illness" was specifically excluded as a potential precipitant of a formal psychiatric diagnosis of posttraumatic stress disorder (PTSD). This was important because PTSD is the only diagnosis in the *DSM* that includes a cause or precipitating event within the diagnostic criteria rather than simply offering a description of typical symptoms.

Clinical observations challenging the perception that cancer was not sufficiently "traumatic" to precipitate the symptoms of PTSD began to be described in the psychiatric literature in the 1980s and prompted a series of field trials in preparation for the fourth edition of the *DSM*. A group of 24 adolescent cancer survivors and their mothers were interviewed, and findings revealed that a substantial minority of both groups met criteria for a diagnosis of PTSD (Alter et al., 1996). Life-threatening medical illness was subsequently included as a potential precipitating event for PTSD in the text of the fourth edition of the *Diagnostic and Statistical Manual of Mental Disorders* (*DSM-IV*) in 1994. The accompanying text specified not only that the person experiencing the medical life threat might respond with posttraumatic stress but also that this might also be a precipitant for family members. This allowed a common framework for researchers to investigate posttraumatic stress responses to medical life threat in adult patients, spouses of patients, and childhood patients, their siblings, and their parents.

In this chapter, we review the growing body of literature that has emerged regarding the epidemiology, correlates, and predictors of posttraumatic stress symptoms in those exposed to medical life threat. We examine the provocative biological studies and the more limited intervention research. A relatively new area of investigation, posttraumatic growth after a life-changing event, also is reviewed as it may apply to childhood cancer. Future research directions are highlighted, and implications for clinical practice are discussed. For those interested in posttraumatic stress research, excellent summaries are available (Ballenger et al., 2004; Yehuda, 1999).

## Posttraumatic Stress Disorder

One of the largest changes in the diagnostic criteria for PTSD in *DSM-IV* was the change in the conceptualization of what constituted a traumatic event. It had previously been believed that the traumatic magnitude of the event and the degree of exposure were the primary determinants of the response. As such, the previous version of the *DSM*, the *DSM-III*, stated that the individual was required to have been exposed to an event that was "outside of the range of ordinary human experiences." However, the intervening research demonstrated that it was the individual's perception of life threat that was significantly associated with the symptoms. Thus, in the *DSM-IV*, the precipitating event could be a threat to life *or* physical integrity, and it could be experienced, witnessed, or even just heard about if it happened to someone who was important to the affected person. This signified that parents or spouses of cancer patients might also be at risk. More important, however, exposure was necessary but not sufficient to precipitate PTSD. A response that included helplessness, horror, or extreme fear was also required. This indicated that a simple diagnosis of cancer would not be sufficient to trigger PTSD, but that a specific type of emotional response was necessary to set off the presumed neurological consequences that culminated in the brain changes of PTSD.

The other criteria for PTSD require a certain number of symptoms from among three clusters of symptoms: reexperiencing, avoidance, and arousal. Reexperiencing symptoms, commonly known as flashbacks or nightmares, are familiar to most laypeople from movies about PTSD and are well known by those caring for cancer patients. Conditioned responses have long been seen in response to the chemotherapeutic treatment of cancer, in which the mere smell of the hospital setting is sufficient to elicit a conditioned wave of nausea for many patients. Nightmares in response to treatment also are well known. Less apparent to many clinicians in oncology is the idea of reenactment of the traumatic event in play, a relatively common manifestation of reexperiencing in children.

Similarly, the idea of avoidance makes intuitive sense to most clinicians. Oncologists are well aware of how reluctant many families are to come in to clinic even when there are no procedures scheduled or how anxious they become the night before a follow-up visit. Some parents will report taking relatively extensive detours so they do not drive past the hospital where their child was diagnosed or treated. However, in addition to the physical avoidance of reminders of the traumatic event, this symptom cluster includes emotional numbing, an internal avoidance of strong feelings. This is consistent with the observations made in the literature on coping with cancer that has found that avoidance strategies are more commonly employed by childhood cancer survivors than healthy controls (Frank, Blount, & Brown, 1997; Phipps & Srivastava, 1997; Phipps & Srivastava, 1999). Avoidance has been seen as one of the methods children and parents employ to protect themselves from unpleasant reminders of past or potential events.

Symptoms of increased arousal are familiar to anyone who works with children or parents in the hospital or outpatient settings. Both the increased reactivity to stimuli and the increased baseline anxiety would be easy for most clinicians to recognize and understand. Increased watchfulness for medical symptoms or errors of omission or commission by medical personnel are generally seen as irritating but common behaviors of children and parents who are fearful about the meaning of any small bruise. Again, this is largely viewed as an understandable response to reminders and of perceived danger.

However, no set of psychiatric symptoms is considered a "disorder" unless it leads to functional impairment or clinical distress. Maybe cancer survivors have been traumatized by the cancer experience, but does it really cause significant distress or impairment? Repeated studies over the years have found that children do not report significant levels of depression or anxiety. Indeed, in some cases they appear to report fewer symptoms of emotional distress than do comparison controls (Zebrack et al., 2002). It could be argued that many of the symptoms described above are "normal" or adaptive response to an extremely stressful situation. This chapter reviews the evidence that these types of symptoms have an impact on function or persistent distress.

Notice that some of the studies reviewed refer to PTSD the disorder; others refer to posttraumatic stress symptoms. This reflects the lack of resolution to date regarding whether posttraumatic stress is best considered as a dichotomous condition, present or absent, or as a continuous variable, a measure of severity. At this early stage in the development of the field, both types of analyses yield useful information. The potential significance of the distinction is discussed.

## Posttraumatic Growth

Meanwhile, a separate set of investigations was ongoing. These were also based on the assumption that the experience of childhood cancer diagnosis and treatment was traumatic for children and their parents. However, these investigators argued that not only stress but also growth could result from traumatic disruption of life. The challenge of cancer to the basic assumptions and values of an individual or family could result in new and possibly healthier priorities following the cancer experience. Cancer was conceptualized as a psychosocial transition with the potential for both positive and negative outcomes (Cordova & Andrykowski, 2003).

For example, a study of quality of life in 176 childhood cancer survivors (aged 16–28 years) found that the survivors rated themselves high on happiness, feeling useful, life satisfaction, and their ability to cope and viewed these positive attributes as a result of having had cancer. The results of this study suggest that survivors who reported feeling a sense of purpose in life and perceiving positive changes as a result of cancer were more likely to report a positive quality of life (Zebrack & Chesler, 2002). A similar finding was revealed in a study comparing 70 adult breast cancer survivors to 70 age- and education-matched healthy comparison women on self-reports of depression, well-being, and posttraumatic growth. The two groups did not differ in depression or well-being, but the group of survivors demonstrated a pattern of greater posttraumatic growth, particularly in relating to others, appreciation of life, and spiritual change. Posttraumatic growth was unrelated to distress or well-being but was positively associated with perceived life threat, prior talking about breast cancer, income, and time since diagnosis (Cordova, Cunningham, Carlson, & Andrykowski, 2001).

Both posttraumatic growth and posttraumatic stress require that the person be exposed to a traumatic event of sufficient magnitude to change the way in which the person approaches life. However, little is known about the relationship between these two types of responses. They do not appear to be mutually incompatible. A study that examined both posttraumatic stress and posttraumatic growth found that avoidance (one component of the posttraumatic stress response) was significantly associated with posttraumatic growth (Best, Streisand, Catania, & Kazak, 2002).

## Posttraumatic Stress Symptoms in Adult Cancer Survivors

There is already considerable evidence of posttraumatic stress symptoms in response to adult cancer, particularly breast cancer (Green et al., 1998; Hampton & Frombach, 2000; Malt & Tjemsland, 1999; Neel, 2000; Smith, Redd, Peyser, & Vogl, 1999). These studies have found a broad range of prevalence of PTSD, which does not appear to be strongly associated with objective measures of life threat or treatment intensity. For example, as one might expect, only 3% of node-negative and 6% of Stage 0–IIIA breast cancer survivors reported current levels of symptoms meeting criteria for PTSD (Andrykowski, Cordova, Studts, & Miller, 1998; Hampton & Frombach, 2000). However, there was little difference between the 12%–14% with PTSD in women treated for breast cancer with surgery alone (Tjemsland, Soreide, & Malt, 1998) and the 12%–19% with PTSD in women treated with aggressive chemotherapy, resection, and a bone marrow transplant (Jacobsen et al., 1998). Another study of PTSD in breast cancer patients, using a somewhat different measure, reported PTSD in approximately 35% of the sample, again with no significant difference between those who underwent bone marrow transplant and those who had more conventional treatment (Mundy et al., 2000).

The studies support a model in which the individual's appraisal of the cancer and the treatment is more predictive of posttraumatic stress symptoms than the stage of the cancer or the type and duration of treatment. A study of 23 men and 79 women who were 3–26 months post–bone marrow transplant found only 5% of the patients met full diagnostic criteria for PTSD using a structured interview. Similar to the other studies examining predictors, the variables that accounted for significant variability in symptoms of posttraumatic stress above the relevant demographic and medical variables were negative appraisals of the bone marrow transplant experience, avoidance-based coping strategies, lower levels of social support, and greater social constraint (Jacobsen et al., 2002; Widows, Jacobsen, & Fields, 2000).

## Posttraumatic Stress Symptoms in Childhood Cancer Patients and Survivors

Initial studies in the area of posttraumatic stress in pediatric oncology employed small samples and descriptive, rather than diagnostic, measures. The first such research study of posttraumatic stress responses of children during and after the acute phase of treatment was a small, longitudinal descriptive study published in 1991 (Stuber, Nader, Yasuda, Pynoos, & Cohen, 1991). Nine children aged 7 to 18 years who were undergoing bone marrow transplantation for hematological and malignant disorders were administered semistructured clinical interviews in the hospital, days prior to the transplant. Some posttraumatic stress symptoms were reported or observed in each of the nine patients. However, only three of the children met the full *DSM* (at that time, *DSM-III*) diagnostic criteria for PTSD.

A second semistructured interview was conducted in the child's home 3 months after returning home posttransplant (Stuber, Nader, Yasuda, Pynoos, & Cohen, 1991). On average, the nine children reported or demonstrated more symptoms and more severity of symptoms at the 3-month visit than in the first interview prior to the transplant. This was not surprising. All of the children at the time of initial interview were familiar with their diagnosis, had received some treatment, and had been informed that they faced a significant threat of mortality and morbidity from the bone marrow transplant itself, so some symptoms were expected. However, during the hospitalization they had been separated from their friends in protective isolation for an average of 8 weeks and had endured intense radiation therapy and chemotherapy with significant morbidity and pain. The actual transplant procedure, rather than the diagnosis, appeared to be the traumatic event. What was more counterintuitive for the research team was that the number and severity of symptoms had not dropped back to pretransplant levels when these patients were interviewed for a third time 1 year after the transplant. Given that most of the 50% risk of death after a bone marrow transplant is in the first year, one might conclude that these 1-year survivors had "beaten the odds." However, the children continued to report nightmares and to participate in traumatic play (e.g., pretending to poison the interviewer with an injection or having monsters invade a play hospital room and kill all the occupants). By both their report and that of their parents, they actively avoided discussion of the transplant with their parents or friends. On observation, the children were hypervigilant and easily startled. Interestingly, the parents also had not initiated conversations about the transplant experience with their children. Some of the parents interpreted the advice they had received from the oncologists to "go out and live a normal life and put this behind you" as meaning they should try to forget about all that had occurred previously (Stuber et al., 1991).

Most of the subsequent studies of posttraumatic stress symptoms have focused on survivors who have been off active treatment for at least 1 year and have included children undergoing less-intensive cancer treatments as well as bone marrow transplantation. Alter et al. (1996) employed self-report measures in a cross-sectional comparison of three groups: 23 adolescent cancer survivors, 27 adolescents who had been physically abused, and 23 healthy, nonabused adolescents. Of the cancer survivors, 35% met lifetime PTSD criteria; only 7% of the abused adolescents met lifetime PTSD criteria. These findings were instrumental in getting the *DSM* criteria changed in the fourth version so they included serious medical illness.

Some questions have been subsequently raised, however, about the relative importance of considering the prevalence of full PSD versus the severity of symptoms of posttraumatic stress in childhood cancer survivors. A pilot study, using parents as the proxy reporters of symptoms, examined 30 pediatric cancer patients and 42 off-treatment survivors of pediatric cancer. Although findings revealed that some parents of children on active treatment did report symptoms in their children that were consistent with a diagnosis of PTSD, the prevalence of full PTSD among the off-treatment survivors was not higher than epidemiological estimates from the general population (Butler, Rizzi, & Handwerger, 1996).

Similar findings came from a cross-sectional, self-report study that examined 309 childhood cancer survivors, 8–20 years old, contacted an average of almost 6 years after the end of successful cancer treatment. Diagnoses included 38% with acute lymphoblastic leukemia, 10% Wilm's tumor, 9% sarcomas, 8% acute nonlymphoblastic leukemia, 8% lymphomas, and 6% Hodgkin's disease. A comparison group of 219 healthy children 8–20 years old was recruited from the pediatric clinics of the same hospitals. Both groups completed the PTSD Reaction Index, a self-report measure of the presence and severity of symptoms of posttraumatic stress. Of the 309 cancer survivor children, only 2.6% reported severe PTSD symptoms; 12.1% reported symptoms in the moderate range. This was not statistically significantly different from the comparison group, in which 3.4% reported severe PTSD symptoms, and 12.3% reported symptoms in the moderate range (Kazak et al., 1997).

Finally, a study that included a smaller sample employing similar methods compared 52 adolescent cancer survivors and their mothers to 42 healthy adolescents and their mothers. Although 36% of the survivors reported some symptoms of posttraumatic stress, none of them met full *DSM-IV* diagnostic criteria for PTSD (Brown, Madan-Swain, & Lambert, 2003).

Despite the low reporting prevalence of full PTSD, researchers are interested in understanding the prediction of symptoms in those children who did report symptoms. In a path analysis of 186 childhood cancer survivors (aged 8–10 years, off treatment at least 1 year) and their parents, the significant, independent predictors of posttraumatic stress symptoms were (a) the survivor's retrospective subjective appraisal of life threat at the time of treatment and the degree to which the survivor experienced the treatment as "hard" or "scary"; (b) the child's general level of anxiety; (c) history of other stressful experiences; (d) time since the termination of treatment (negative association); (e) female gender; and (f) family and social support. The mother's perception of treatment intensity and life threat contributed to anxiety and subjective appraisal of life threat and treatment intensity for the cancer survivor but did not independently contribute to the child's posttraumatic stress symptoms. It appears that the mothers' impact on the survivors was mediated through modeling the appraisal of life threat and treatment intensity rather than directly through modeling symptoms of posttraumatic stress. Contrary to what had been predicted, the "objective" life threat and treatment intensity (as estimated by the medical staff) was not significantly associated with the survivor's appraisal of life threat and treatment intensity or with the survivor's reported symptoms of posttraumatic stress (Stuber et al., 1997).

Other investigations have raised questions about the low prevalence of self-reported posttraumatic stress symptoms in childhood cancer survivors. A study of 78 young adult (aged 18–37 years) survivors of childhood cancer found that approximately 20% of the survivors reported symptoms meeting diagnostic criteria for PTSD. The diagnosis of PTSD was associated with higher self-reported distress and with an increased appraisal of life threat. However, the physician's rating of the severity of the child's illness did not correlate significantly with a diagnosis of PTSD (Hobbie et al., 2000).

This was further explored in a substudy of 51 of the young adult survivors of childhood cancer. Physician ratings of moderate and severe adverse toxicity or late effects of treatment were more common in the group with PTSD. Such problems often do not occur for 5 years following termination of treatment. Thus, ongoing medical problems might act to activate or sustain symptoms of PTSD either by increasing traumatic reminders or by serving as markers of severity of exposure (Meeske et al., 2001).

Another way of understanding these findings of PTSD in young adults but not in younger survivors is that posttraumatic stress symptoms emerge in young adult pediatric cancer survivors as part of the developmental process. A history of cancer and the resulting long-term toxic effects of treatment have considerable impact on negotiating normal developmental tasks such as completing education, finding a job or career, finding a mate, or establishing a family.

A study compared 9,535 adults who were long-term survivors of pediatric cancer to a randomly selected group of 2,916 siblings and found moderate-to-severe impairment in mental health functioning in the survivors. Those who had been diagnosed with Hodgkin's disease, sarcomas, or bone tumors reported the highest levels of cancer-related fears and anxiety, adversely affecting their health status. These are diagnoses that tend to occur in older children and adolescents. It may be that many children are able to avoid acknowledging the life threat or at least avoid the symptoms of posttraumatic stress until they encounter the specific challenges of young adulthood (Hudson et al., 2003). Further exploration is needed as to how symptoms of posttraumatic stress manifest over time.

### Posttraumatic Stress Symptoms in Parents of Cancer Survivors

Parents have been long known to report significant distress both during and after their children's cancer treatment (Best et al., 2002). The initial *DSM-IV* field trial results (Pelcovitz et al., 1996, 1998) found that mothers of pediatric cancer survivors exhibited significantly more PTSD symptoms than mothers of healthy children. These findings were replicated in a study that compared 309 mothers and 213 fathers of childhood cancer survivors to 211 mothers and 114 fathers of a healthy comparison control group. Of the survivors' mothers, 10% reported severe levels of current symptoms of PTSD, and 27% reported moderate levels of symptoms. This was significantly more than the mothers in the comparison group, of whom 3% reported severe symptoms, and 18.2% reported moderate symptoms. Of the fathers of survivors, 7% reported severe and 28.3% reported moderate symptoms of PTSD, compared to 0% severe and 17.3% moderate for the fathers in the comparison group. Trait anxiety was the strongest predictor of posttraumatic stress symptoms for both mothers and fathers. Objective medical data did not contribute significantly to the variance, but perceived life threat, perceived treatment intensity, and social support were significant independent contributors (Barakat et al., 1997; Kazak et al., 1998).

In another study of 72 mothers of childhood cancer survivors, symptoms of posttraumatic stress reported were comparable to those of adult cancer survivors (Manne, DuHamel, Gallelli, Sorgen, & Redd, 1998). Posttraumatic stress symptoms were associated with reports of more perceived social constraints and less perceived belonging support. Surprisingly, lifetime traumatic events were not predictive of posttraumatic stress symptoms in mothers of survivors (Manne, DuHamel, & Redd, 2000).

One of the few studies to compare the impact of pediatric cancer to other types of medically traumatic events was a study of the parents of 209 children (aged 6.5–14.5 years) in Switzerland who had recently been diagnosed with pediatric cancer or diabetes mellitus or had been recently hospitalized for an accidental injury. This study also examined the relationships between posttraumatic stress symptoms in these children and their mothers ($n = 180$) and fathers ($n = 175$). Parents and children were administered self-report questionnaires on posttraumatic stress symptoms 5–6 weeks after the potentially traumatic event. Full *DSM-IV* diagnostic criteria for current PTSD were met by 16% of the mothers and 23.9% of the fathers, which is very similar to that observed in the other studies of parents of childhood cancer survivors. The parents of children recently diagnosed with cancer reported more posttraumatic stress symptoms than parents of children with diabetes mellitus or accidental injuries. The posttraumatic stress scores for mothers were significantly associated with those of the fathers. However, the symptoms of the children were not associated with those of their mothers or fathers. The children reported posttraumatic stress symptoms in the mild range overall, with accident-related injury associated with the highest scores. These data suggest again that childhood cancer has a more immediate impact on parents than on children, and that children are responding to different aspects of the event than are parents (Landolt, Vollrath, Ribi, Gnehm, & Sennhauser, 2003).

One published report has documented symptoms of posttraumatic stress in siblings of childhood cancer survivors. Nearly one half of 78 adolescent siblings reported mild symptoms of posttraumatic stress, and 32% reported moderate-to-severe symptoms. These rates of posttraumatic stress symptoms were significantly higher than those reported by a comparison group of non-affected teens, although the two groups did not differ in reported levels of anxiety. Over one half of the siblings found the cancer experience frightening and difficult, and 25% reported that they believed their sibling would die during treatment. As has been found with survivors and with parents, these appraisals of life threat and treatment intensity were significantly associated with reported symptoms (Alderfer, Labay, & Kazak, 2003).

## Consequences of Posttraumatic Stress

With so many differing reports regarding the prevalence of posttraumatic stress in childhood cancer survivors, it is reasonable to inquire about the significance of such symptoms. First, posttraumatic stress appears to be a significant correlate of negative functional and emotional status. In a study of 51 young adult survivors of childhood cancer (18–37 years old), a categorical diagnosis of PTSD was predictive of adverse consequences in several areas of functioning. The young adult survivors who met criteria for PTSD were less likely to be married (none, compared to 23% of the non-PTSD group) and reported more psychological distress and poorer quality of life across all domains. The greatest differences reported were in social functioning, emotional well-being, and role limitations because of emotional health and pain. Survivors without PTSD did not differ from population norms, and all subscales on the psychological distress measure were higher for those with PTSD. In fact, the summative score for psychological distress was in the upper 97th percentile compared to a normative population. Some of these differences may be related to the fact that moderate and severe late effects of treatment were more common in the group with PTSD. Thus, ongoing medical problems may sustain chronic symptoms of PTSD or may be indictors of more traumatic exposure (Meeske et al., 2001).

Similar findings were reported from a study of 40 adolescents and young adults who were survivors of pediatric cancer. Survivors who reported symptoms meeting the diagnostic threshold for PTSD also reported more somatic symptoms and greater psychological distress and received a lower Global Assessment of Functioning (GAF score than the survivors not meeting criteria for PTSD (Erikson & Steiner, 2000, 2001).

Additional suggestions of adverse outcomes related to posttraumatic stress come from the studies of physiological correlates of chronic PTSD. It has been established that stress activates the sympathetic nervous system and the hypothalamic-pituitary-adrenal axis. How the body responds to a given stressor depends on the genetic vulnerability of the individual, the exposure to environmental factors, and the timing of the stressful events. Animal studies of mice exposed to a cat suggested that this fearful stimulus initiated neural changes that mediated lasting increases in anxiety following severe stress, providing support for predator stress as a model of aspects of posttraumatic stress disorder (Adamec, Burton, Shallow, & Budgell, 1999). Another animal model suggested that corticosterone is instrumental in the pathogenesis of chronic anxiety following acute psychological stress (H. Cohen, Benjamin, Kaplan, & Kotler, 2000).

In human studies, there is evidence of change in the structure and function of the brain that is not only a response to exposure to a traumatic event, but also appears to be related to the specific symptoms of posttraumatic stress. In a study of 33 women, measures of hippocampal structure and function were compared for 10 women with early childhood sexual abuse and PTSD, 12 with abuse histories but no PTSD, and 11 without abuse or PTSD. Hippocampal volume was measured with magnetic resonance imaging for all participants and was 16% less in the women with abuse and PTSD compared to women with abuse without PTSD and 19% less than for the women without abuse or PTSD. Hippocampal function during the performance of hippocampal-based verbal declarative memory tasks was measured by positron emission tomography in abused women with and without PTSD. Activation of the hippocampus was less in the women with abuse and PTSD compared to women with abuse without PTSD (Bremner, Vythilingam, Vermetten, et al., 2003).

Changes in activation of the autonomic nervous system and adrenal glands also have been documented in adults with PTSD. The results of a study of 16 adults with non-combat-related stress compared to 16 age-matched comparison controls suggested that patients with non-combat-related PTSD have peripheral noradrenergic dysregulation (Yatham, Sacamano, & Kusumakar, 1996).

This type of investigation is now under way with mothers of childhood cancer survivors. One study compared 21 mothers of pediatric cancer survivors with ($n$ =14) and without ($n=7$) PTSD symptoms to comparison control mothers of healthy children ($n=8$). Cortisol and norepinephrine levels assessed from a 12-hour overnight urine collection differed significantly by group (Glover et al., 2003). The 14 mothers of pediatric cancer survivors who reported symptoms of PTSD had higher urinary dopamine levels ($p=.01$) than

7 mothers of cancer survivors who did not report symptoms of PTSD and 8 comparison control mothers of healthy children (Glover & Poland, 2002). These types of changes are consistent with a model of posttraumatic stress as causing a form of accelerated aging of the brain (Pitman et al., 2001).

Studies in children and young animals suggested that exposure of the developing brain to severe or prolonged stress may result in increases in the basal rate of response of the stress system or increased reactivity to stressors. This may be manifest as amygdala hyperfunction (fear reaction); decreased activity of the hippocampus (defective glucocorticoid-negative feedback); decreased activity of the mesocorticolimbic dopaminergic system (dysthymia, novelty seeking, addictive behaviors); hyperactivation of the hypothalamic-pituitary-adrenal axis (hypercortisolism); suppression of reproductive, growth, thyroid, and immune functions; and changes in pain perception (Charmandari, Kino, Souvatzoglou, & Chrousos, 2003). However, some of the brain changes observed in adults are not seen in children. For example, a longitudinal study of hippocampal volume in children with PTSD associated with physical abuse used magnetic resonance imaging to measure temporal lobes, amygdala, and hippocampal volumes in nine prepubertal children and nine sociodemographically matched healthy nonmaltreated yoked control participants at baseline and after at least 2 years of follow-up (during the later stages of pubertal development) using identical equipment and measurement methodology. No differences were found in temporal lobe, amygdala, and hippocampal volumes at baseline, follow-up, or across time (De Bellis, Hall, Boring, Frustaci, & Moritz, 2001).

The long-term biological impact of adverse childhood experience is illustrated by an interesting study of adults aged 40–80 years in the United Kingdom. Peripheral leukocyte counts were conducted on 11,367 participants and, after a mean interval of 44 months, on 11,857 at a second health check. Participants completed self-report questionnaires assessing adverse experiences in childhood during the interval between health checks. Significant associations were found between self-report of adverse experiences and lymphocyte counts at both health checks. Lifestyle factors accounted for about half of this association (Surtees et al., 2003).

Immunological and endocrine changes may account for some of the long-term impact of medical trauma. In a study of 52 women with and without a history of early childhood sexual abuse and PTSD, the abused women with PTSD had lower levels of cortisol during the afternoon hours (12:00–8:00 p.m.) of a 24-hour period than the non-PTSD women. The corticotropin response to a cortisol-releasing factor challenge of the abused women with PTSD was blunted compared with nonabused, non-PTSD (but not abused, non-PTSD) women. No differences in cortisol response to cortisol-releasing factor and corticotropin challenges were found between the three groups. Increased PTSD symptom levels were associated with low afternoon cortisol levels, suggesting that PTSD changes the baseline circadian rhythm of serum cortisol (Bremner, Vythilingam, Anderson, et al., 2003).

This same research group in the Netherlands used trauma-specific stimuli to determine if there were cortisol changes in response to reminders. Twelve abused women with PTSD and 12 abused women without PTSD were assessed for salivary cortisol levels before, during, and after exposure to personalized trauma scripts. Compared to controls, patients with PTSD had 122% higher cortisol levels during script exposure, 69% higher cortisol levels during recovery, and 60% higher levels in the period leading up to the script exposure. PTSD symptoms were highly predictive of cortisol levels during trauma script exposure but not during periods of rest. This study also assessed memory for neutral and emotional material immediately after trauma script exposure and 3 days later. In both PTSD patients and comparison controls, memory consolidation after the trauma scripts was impaired relative to baseline with no differences between the two groups on memory performance. There was no association between memory performance and cortisol levels (Elzinga, Schmahl, Vermetten, van Dyck, & Bremner, 2003).

Alterations in cortisol may be one way of understanding the results of a longitudinal, prospective study of 101 adult survivors of heart transplantation, which found that self-reported symptoms of PTSD were the strongest predictor of cardiac morbidity in this group (Dew et al., 1999). This would be an important finding because earlier studies documented PTSD in response to myocardial infarction (Doerfler, Pbert, & DeCosimo, 1994; Kutz, Garb, & David, 1988; Kutz, Shabtai,

Solomon, Neumann, & David, 1994). A cumulative adversity model has been postulated to explain an association between PTSD and myocardial infarction (Alonzo, 1999). However, the association between cardiac morbidity and PTSD may be linked to nonadherence as well as to biological changes secondary to PTSD. This was suggested in a study in which PTSD was associated with nonadherence to prescribed aspirin and with second cardiac events among survivors of myocardial infarction (Shemesh et al., 2001).

This link between nonadherence and PTSD also has been reported in children. In a study of 19 pediatric liver transplant recipients, 6 met criteria for PTSD on the Posttraumatic Stress Reaction Index. Three of these 6, and none of the others, were considered by the transplant team to be significantly nonadherent to treatment recommendations. A high avoidance score on the Posttraumatic Stress Reaction Index was highly correlated with nonadherence. Perception of disease threat and demographic variables did not differ significantly between patients with PTSD and the others (Shemesh et al., 2000).

However, the physiological changes in adults have not been replicated in studies of children and adolescents. In a study of 48 adolescents (20 with current PTSD, 9 trauma controls without PTSD, and 19 healthy nontraumatized controls), adolescents reporting current PTSD symptoms demonstrated no difference in the suppression of salivary cortisol in response to low-dose (0.5 mg) dexamethasone compared to trauma controls without PTSD and nontraumatized controls. More severely affected PTSD participants with co-occurring major depression demonstrated higher pre- and postdexamethasone salivary cortisol levels in relation to comparison controls. This indicates that the response of the hypothalamic-pituitary axis to trauma differs in children and adolescents compared to adults (Lipschitz et al., 2003)

## Interventions for Posttraumatic Stress

With the accumulating data to suggest that posttraumatic stress responses are relatively common in parents of children with cancer and that posttraumatic stress can lead to medical as well as psychological morbidity, appropriate interventions for the prevention and treatment of traumatic stress responses to medical life threat are emerging (Donnelley & Amaya-Jackson, 2002). Specific problem-solving therapy has been effective in assisting mothers manage the stressor of treatment (Sahler et al., 2002; 2003) as have brief stress reduction techniques (Streisand et al., 2001). Preventive interventions target decreasing helplessness through psychoeducational interventions and the provision of training in appropriate coping techniques. Many of the potentially traumatic aspects of medical treatment of life-threatening conditions can be anticipated, allowing interventions to decrease the fear, helplessness, and horror associated with the treatment events. There is an extensive body of literature on the preparation of children for medical procedures (see Conte, Walco, Sterling, Engel, & Kuppenheimer, 1999, and Powers, 1999, for review). However, the impact of preparation on posttraumatic stress symptoms in childhood cancer patients has not been investigated systematically. Specific suggestions have been made for empirical examination based on clinical experience, primarily having to do with family assessment and intervention (Kazak et al., 2003; Kazak, Simms, & Rourke, 2002).

Trauma-focused cognitive behavioral therapy has been documented to reduce posttraumatic stress symptoms in several studies of children exposed to sexual abuse when treatment is provided 1–6 months after the traumatic event. However, it is not yet clear what the optimal dosage or critical components are for effective trauma-focused cognitive behavioral therapy (J. A. Cohen, 2003). An adaptation of a trauma-focused cognitive behavioral intervention used for other types of traumatic events in adults has been successfully employed in pediatric liver transplant recipients (Shemesh et al., 2000). Of note in this case is the suggestion that intervention for posttraumatic stress symptoms can improve adherence to medical instruction. This might be a result of decreased avoidance of the medications as a traumatic reminder of the transplant or a decrease in the autonomic arousal caused by decreased helplessness. Further investigation of this intriguing finding is ongoing.

Pharmacotherapy for posttraumatic stress symptoms has been tested in adults with some success. A variety of medications has been tried with the goal of decreased hyperarousal and sleep disturbance in veterans with combat-related PTSD. These trials were prompted by the poor clinical outcome of the use of benzodiazepines, often in large doses, to manage these symptoms. Pharmacological agents investigated were chosen for their effect on target symptoms and included medications usually used for hypertension, insomnia, seizure control, depression, or anxiety (Viola et al., 1997). The majority of the published reports are case studies or small, open-label trials. Guanfacine has been used for nightmares with some anecdotal success (Horrigan & Barnhill, 1996). Naltrexone was found to have some minimal but statistically insignificant effect on chronic posttraumatic stress symptoms in a small, open-label study with eight adults over a 2 week period. However, the adverse effects of the medication were not well tolerated, and the investigators concluded that therapeutic use of naltrexone was not to be encouraged (Lubin, Weizman, Shmushkevitz, & Valevski, 2002). A case study of the use of gabapentin in an adult woman suggested that it was helpful for intrusive memories or flashbacks (Malek-Ahmadi, 2003). Propranolol was effective in treating reemergent symptoms in a 44-year-old woman after multiple car accidents (Taylor & Cahill, 2002). Citalopram reduced symptoms of posttraumatic stress in two Persian Gulf War veterans (Khouzam, el-Gabalawi, & Donnelly, 2001). Sertraline is one of the few medications relatively rigorously tested and found to be effective, safe, and well tolerated in the treatment of posttraumatic stress symptoms in adults (Schwartz & Rothbaum, 2002; vander Kolk et al., 1994).

Most of the studies with children have been uncontrolled trials or case studies (Putnam & Hulsmann, 2002). Many different medications have been attempted, including prazosin (Brkanac, Pastor, & Storck, 2003), carbamazine (Looff, Grimley, Kuller, Martin, & Schonfield, 1995), and mirtazapine (Good & Petersen, 2001). The earliest medications more formally tested in children were propranolol and clonidine because it was hypothesized that a $\beta$-adrenergic antagonist or an adrenergic receptor blocker might reduce many of the symptoms associated with posttraumatic stress. Eleven children with hyperarousal symptoms after physical or sexual abuse were treated with propranolol, with a significant decrease in symptoms (Famularo, Kinscherff, & Fenton, 1988).

In an open-label trial of use of clonidine and imipramine with 68 severely traumatized Cambodian refugees, chronic symptoms of depression and PTSD improved. A subsequent prospective pilot study of 9 children used the same combination of pharmacotherapies, with decreases in nightmares, sleep disorders, depressed mood, and startle response. The medications were well tolerated (Kinzie & Leung, 1989). A case report described the successful use of clonidine alone for posttraumatic stress symptoms (Porter & Bell, 1999).

The most meticulously studied medications for symptomatic treatment of children with PTSD have been the specific serotonin reuptake inhibitors (SSRIs) and clonidine (Harmon & Riggs, 1996). There is one randomized, double-blind study of imipramine with 25 children (Robert, Blakeney, Villarreal, Rosenberg, & Meyer, 1999) and a randomized trail of clonidine (Lustig et al., 2002) demonstrating some efficacy for symptoms of PTSD.

In a review of all of the literature on pharmacological treatment of PTSD in children, the recommendation based on current evidence was to treat symptomatically. In general, this would mean starting with an SSRI, targeting anxiety, mood, and reexperiencing symptoms. Sertraline has been found to improve social and occupational functioning and the individual's perceived quality of life. Clonidine could be used alone or with an SSRI to address symptoms of impulsivity or hyperarousal. Mood stabilizers would be used when affective dyscontrol is severe and neuroleptic medications used in cases involving aggression, psychosis, dissociation, or self-injurious behaviors (Donnelley, 2003).

The theoretical basis for most of the medications used to treat PTSD in children is the reduction of autonomic arousal, resulting in reduced intrusive symptoms. An intriguing longitudinal study of 24 children who had been hospitalized with burns examined the relationship between dose of morphine administered for the acute burn and the course of posttraumatic stress symptoms over 6 months after discharge. A significant association was found, indicating that the higher the mean dose of morphine, the greater the reduction of posttraumatic stress symptoms over a 6-month period. The finding is interpreted to suggest the utility of morphine to reduce fear conditioning and consolidation of traumatic memory (Saxe et al., 2001). Although no one would suggest that morphine be used to treat PTSD in general, it does suggest that adequate pain control could be an important element in prevention of medical traumatic stress.

## Posttraumatic Growth in Adults

The study of growth and perceived benefit after traumatic events has evolved over the past decade into a major research area. Studies have now examined responses to many types of traumatic events, including natural disasters like tornadoes, interpersonal violence such as mass killings, and large accidental events such as plane crashes. A review cited 39 empirical studies documenting positive change following trauma and adversity. Consistent factors associated with such "adversarial growth" included cognitive appraisal variables (threat, harm, and controllability), problem-focused coping, acceptance and positive reinterpretation coping, optimism, religion, cognitive processing, and positive affect (Tedeschi & Calhoun, 1996). Somewhat counterintuitively, sociodemographic variables (gender, age, education, and income) and psychological distress variables (e.g., depression, anxiety, posttraumatic stress disorder) were not significantly associated with adversarial growth. It did appear that people who reported and maintained adversarial growth over time became less distressed over time (Linley & Joseph, 2004).

An example of a study of posttraumatic growth is a survey of 174 bereaved human immunodeficiency virus/acquired immunodeficiency syndrome (HIV/AIDS) caregivers. Spirituality, social support, and stressors were all found to have independent positive relationships with growth (Cadell, Regehr, & Hemsworth, 2003). Another study surveyed 54 young adults who had experienced a variety of traumatic events. Two variables were related to posttraumatic growth: the degree of rumination about the events soon after the event and the degree of openness to religious change (Calhoun, Cann, Tedeschi, & McMillan, 2000). Dimensions that may be seen as genetic predisposing factors, or "dimensions of wisdom" in the words of one author (Linley, 2003), that have been seen as playing crucial roles in such growth include the recognition and management of uncertainty, the integration of affect and cognition, and the recognition and acceptance of human limitations.

The association between posttraumatic stress and posttraumatic growth has been the focus of some studies, and this relationship appears to be complex. In one study that compared reactions to several different types of traumatic events, perception of benefit appeared to moderate the impact of event severity on emotional recovery over time. Perceived benefit as measured 4–6 weeks after traumatic exposure predicted posttraumatic stress disorder 3 years later. If benefit was perceived, as the severity of the traumatic exposure increased, the amount of recovery increased. If no benefit was perceived, severity of traumatic exposure was negatively associated with recovery (McMillen, Smith, & Fisher, 1997). In another study, 85 survivors of bone marrow transplants were evaluated, examining the association between perception of "global meaning" (the belief that life has purpose and coherence) and psychological adjustments. Although posttraumatic growth was not directly assessed, global meaning appeared to have a protective effect for the survivors. After controlling for physical functioning, stressor severity, and gender, global meaning was inversely related to global psychological distress and symptoms of posttraumatic stress (Johnson et al., 2001).

One study of parents of childhood cancer survivors examined both posttraumatic stress and posttraumatic growth. A longitudinal study of pain control during active treatment as a predictor of posttraumatic stress followed 113 parents of children who had been treated for leukemia. Anxiety during treatment was a significant predicator of posttraumatic stress symptoms in mothers but not fathers who were followed after the end of treatment. In particular, symptoms of avoidance were associated with anxiety, self-efficacy, posttraumatic growth, and length of time since treatment ended (Best et al., 2002).

In adult oncology, a study of 72 husbands of breast cancer survivors found that posttraumatic growth was associated with general social support, greater marital support and depth of commitment, greater posttraumatic growth in the wife, and shorter time since diagnosis (Weiss, 2004). A longitudinal study of women with early-stage breast cancer followed for 3 ($n = 92$) and 12 ($n = 60$) months posttreatment found that 83% of the women reported at least one benefit of the breast cancer experience. Positive reappraisal coping at study entry predicted positive mood and perceived health at 3 and 12 months and posttraumatic growth at 12 months. Finding a benefit of the cancer experience, however, was not predictive of positive mood, perceived health, or posttraumatic growth at either 3 or 12 months (Sears, Stanton, & Danoff-Burg, 2003).

A recent study of 150 adolescent survivors of cancer, ages 11 to 19 years, and their mothers ($n = 146$) and fathers ($n = 107$) found that a majority of the adolescents and their mothers and fathers reported posttraumatic growth. Perceptions of greater treatment severity and life threat were related to more reported posttraumatic growth, but objective disease severity was not. Adolescents who were more than 5 years old at diagnosis were more likely to recieve benefit, and reported more posttraumatic stress symptoms, than were those diagnosed earlier (Barakat, Alderfer, & Kazak, 2005).

## Consequences of Posttraumatic Growth

The impact of a positive perspective on health may be large. In a study of 407 men with HIV infections, positive affect was examined as a separate marker from other aspects of depression. When risk estimates were adjusted for significant medical variables, positive affect remained a significant predictor of AIDS mortality. This remained significant even when adjusted for potential that better health was simply reflected by a more positive mood (Moskowitz, 2003).

Other HIV studies have found similar findings in the relationships between mortality and positive expectancies. Men with HIV infections who reported finding meaning in the AIDS-related loss of a close friend demonstrated less rapid declines in CD4 T-cell levels and lower rates of AIDS-related mortality over a 2- to 3-year follow-up period, independent of heath status at baseline, health behaviors, and other potential confounds (Bower, Kemeny, Taylor, & Fahey, 1998). Men who were positive for HIV but asymptomatic over 3 years ($n = 72$) were followed for an additional period of years. There was a significant interaction between bereavement and negative HIV-specific expectancies on symptoms onset. Negative HIV-specific expectancies predicted the subsequent development of symptoms among bereaved men, even after controlling for immunological status, use of zidovudine, high-risk sexual behavior, substance use, and depression (Reed, Kemeny, Taylor, & Visscher, 1999).

Obviously, at this point any application to children with cancer requires systematic investigation. However, given what has been noted with the adverse biological impact of posttraumatic stress and the positive health effects of posttraumatic growth, this is an area in need of careful research given the medical vulnerability of these children after their exposure to chemotherapy and radiation.

## Interventions to Enhance Posttraumatic Growth

Little research has been conducted with intervention studies for the purpose of increasing posttraumatic growth compared to efforts to decrease symptoms of posttraumatic stress. One group of investigators employed individual narratives to explore themes that were associated with positive change processes and found that an inner drive toward growth, psychological changes, and vehicles of change were common themes in those who experience posttraumatic growth. The challenge then for clinicians is to find or to serve as a "vehicle of change" (Woodward & Joseph, 2003).

One intriguing study examined 32 women with breast cancer who were participating in an Internet-based support group. The women met in groups of 8, with a trained facilitator, for 90 minutes once a week for 16 weeks. Participants reported significant reductions in symptoms of depression and reactions to pain on self-report inventories after treatment compared to baseline. There also was a trend toward increases in two subscales on the posttraumatic growth measure: New Possibilities and Spirituality (Lieberman et al., 2003).

Another study pointed to the possible benefits to be gained if the right intervention can be found. Emotional disclosure writing was used in an effort to increase the finding of positive meaning in loss. Forty-three women who had lost a close relative to breast cancer wrote about the death or about nonemotional topics for 4 weeks. The written disclosure group did not demonstrate an increase in either positive meaning-related goals or in natural killer cell cytotoxicity relative to the other group. However, the women in both groups who reported positive changes in meaning-related goals also demonstrated increases in natural killer cell cytotoxicity (Bower, Kemeny, Taylor, & Fahey, 2003). Although the original hypothesis was not supported, it does provide evidence of the impact of positive perceptions on immune parameters.

## Summary and Implications for Clinical Practice

A key finding in all of the studies of posttraumatic stress and posttraumatic growth is that clinicians cannot depend on their own impressions of risk to assess the impact of cancer diagnosis and treatment on childhood cancer patients and their parents. It is the appraisal of the life threat or treatment intensity of the child or parent that is important to the development of symptoms of posttraumatic stress and the individual's appraisal of benefit that leads to posttraumatic growth. Preexisting trait anxiety and long-term medical sequelae of treatment are more salient for the cancer survivors than the statistical risk of relapse. It is important for a clinician trying to assist a child and family to assess their anxiety and to understand how they perceive life threat and treatment intensity as well as the meaning and potential benefit of the cancer experience. Although it may seem obvious, one must also keep in mind that these particular variables are not the same for all members of a given family. Each individual must be evaluated and considered on an individual basis.

The relationship of the appraisal and of symptoms between the child and parents is complex. What is clear, however, is that parents are in general more traumatized and more symptomatic than the childhood cancer patients and survivors themselves. This suggests that a major clinical goal needs to be to assist the parents so they can be sufficiently stable to provide the parenting that the children need (Wolmer et al., 2000). This is an area of potential increasing intervention research. It appears likely that some type of psychoeducational intervention would be useful as a preventive measure for most or all families, with more intense cognitive behavioral interventions for those families at high risk or for those who are symptomatic.

One provocative study (Saxe et al., 2001) suggested use of analgesics that decrease pain without causing confusion or perceived loss of control may be helpful in decreasing trauma symptoms as well as treatment avoidance and nonadherence in both survivors and parents. Pain and anxiety appear to amplify the imprinting of traumatic reminders and the conditioning of specific reactions. The full implications of these findings are the subject of current study, but clinical attention to unnecessary suffering is clearly indicated.

The endocrine and immunological implications of posttraumatic stress symptoms in childhood cancer survivors and their parents are still far from clear. However, there is now sufficient evidence to mark posttraumatic stress and posttraumatic growth as important areas to consider in caring for pediatric cancer patients and their families.

*Acknowledgment.* This work was supported by the Substance Abuse and Mental Health Services Administration funding to the National Child Traumatic Stress Network.

## References

Adamec, R. E., Burton, P., Shallow T., & Budgell, J. (1999). Unilateral block of NMDA receptors in the amygdala prevents predator stress-induced lasting increases in anxiety-like behavior and unconditioned startle—Effective hemisphere depends on the behavior. *Physiology of Behavior, 65*, 739–51.

Alderfer, M. A., Labay, L. E., Kazak, & A. E. (2003). Brief report: Does posttraumatic stress apply to siblings of childhood cancer survivors? *Journal of Pediatric Psychology, 28*, 28–186.

Alonzo, A. A. (1999). Acute myocardial infarction and posttraumatic stress disorder: The consequences of cumulative adversity. *Journal of Cardiovascular Nursing, 13*, 33–45.

Alter, C. L., Pelcovitz, D., Axelrod, A., Goldenberg, B., Harris, H., Meyers, B., et al. (1996). Identification of PTSD in cancer survivors. *Psychosomatics, 37*, 137–143.

American Psychiatric Association. (1987). *Diagnostic and statistical manual of mental disorders* (3rd ed.). Washington, DC: Author.

American Psychiatric Association. (1994). *Diagnostic and statistical manual of mental disorders* (4th ed.). Washington, DC: Author.

Andrykowski, M. A., Cordova, M. J., Studts, J. L., & Miller, T. W. (1998). Posttraumatic stress disorder after treatment for breast cancer: Prevalence of diagnosis and use of the PTSD Checklist–Civilian Version (PCL-C) as a screening instrument. *Journal of Consulting and Clinical Psychology, 66*, 586–590.

Ballenger, J. C., Davidson, J. R., Lecrubier, Y., Nutt, D. J., Marshall, R. D., Nemeroff, C. B., et al. (2004). Consensus statement update on posttraumatic stress disorder from the international consensus group on depression and anxiety. *Journal of Clinical Psychiatry*, *65*(Suppl. 1), 55–62.

Barakat, L. P., Kazak, A. E., Meadows, A. T., Casey, R., Meeske, K., & Stuber, M. L. (1997). Families surviving childhood cancer: a comparison of posttraumatic stress symptoms with families of healthy children. *Journal of Pediatric Psychology*, *22*, 843–859.

Barakat, L. P., Alderfer, M. A., & Kazak, A. E. (2005). Posttraumatic Growth in Adolescent Survivors of Cancer and Their Mothers and Fathers. *Journal of Pediatric Psychology*. Published ahead of print, August 10. doi: 10.1093/jpepsy/jsj058. Retrieved from http://jpepsy.oxfordjournals.org

Best, M., Streisand, R., Catania, L., & Kazak, A. (2002). Parental distress during pediatric leukemia and parental posttraumatic stress symptoms after treatment ends. *Journal of Pediatric Psychology*, *26*, 299–307.

Bower, J. E., Kemeny, M. E., Taylor, S. E., & Fahey, J. L. (1998). Cognitive processing, discovery of meaning, CD4 decline, and AIDS-related mortality among bereaved HIV-seropositive men. *Journal of Consulting and Clinical Psychology*, *66*, 979–986.

Bower, J. E., Kemeny, M. E., Taylor, S. E., & Fahey J. L. (2003). Finding positive meaning and its association with natural killer cell cytotoxicity among participants in a bereavement-related disclosure intervention. *Annals of Behavioral Medicine*, *25*, 146–155.

Bremner, J. D., Vythilingam, M., Anderson, G., Vermetten, E., McGlashan, T., Heninger, G., et al. (2003). Assessment of the hypothalamic-pituitary-adrenal axis over a 24-hour diurnal period and in response to neuroendocrine challenges in women with and without childhood sexual abuse and posttraumatic stress disorder. *Biological Psychiatry*, *54*, 710–718.

Bremner, J. D., Vythilingam, M., Vermetten, E., Southwick, S. M., McGlashan, T., Nazeer, A., et al. (2003). MRI and PET study of deficits in hippocampal structure and function in women with childhood sexual abuse and posttraumatic stress disorder. *American Journal of Psychiatry*, *160*, 924–932.

Brkanac, Z., Pastor, J. F., & Storck, M. (2003). Prazosin in PTSD. *Journal of the American Academy of Child Adolescent Psychiatry*, *42*, 384–385.

Brown, R. T., Madan-Swain, A., & Lambert, R. (2003). Posttraumatic stress symptoms in adolescent survivors of childhood cancer and their mothers. *Journal of Traumatic Stress*, *16*, 309–318.

Butler, R. W., Rizzi, L. P., & Handwerger, B. A. (1996). Brief report: The assessment of posttraumatic stress disorder in pediatric cancer patients and survivors. *Journal of Pediatric Psychology*, *21*, 499–504.

Cadell, S., Regehr, C., Hemsworth, D. (2003). Factors contributing to posttraumatic growth: A proposed structural equation model. *American Journal of Orthopsychiatry*, *73*, 279–287.

Calhoun, L. G., Cann, A., Tedeschi, R. G., & McMillan, J. (2000). A correlational test of the relationship between posttraumatic growth, religion, and cognitive processing. *Journal Traumatic Stress*, *13*, 521–527.

Charmandari, E., Kino, T., Souvatzoglou, E., & Chrousos, G. P. (2003). Pediatric stress: Hormonal mediators and human development. *Hormonal Research*, *59*, 161–179.

Cohen, H., Benjamin, J., Kaplan, Z., & Kotler, M. (2000). Administration of high-dose ketoconazole, an inhibitor of steroid synthesis, prevents posttraumatic anxiety in an animal model. *European Neuropsychopharmacology*, *10*, 429–435.

Cohen, J. A. (2003). Treating acute posttraumatic reactions in children and adolescents. *Biological Psychiatry*, *53*, 827–833.

Conte, P. M., Walco, G. A., Sterling, C. M., Engel, R. G., & Kuppenheimer, W. G. (1999). Procedural pain management in pediatric oncology: A review of the literature. *Cancer Investigations*, *17*, 448–459.

Cordova, M. J., & Andrykowski, M. A. (2003). Responses to cancer diagnosis and treatment: Posttraumatic stress and posttraumatic growth. *Seminars in Clinical Neuropsychiatry*, *8*, 286–296.

Cordova, M. J., Cunningham, L. L., Carlson, C. R., & Andrykowski, M. A. (2001). Posttraumatic growth following breast cancer: a controlled comparison study. *Health Psychology*, *20*, 176–185.

De Bellis, M. D., Hall, J., Boring, A. M., Frustaci, K., & Moritz, G. (2001). A pilot longitudinal study of hippocampal volumes in pediatric maltreatment-related posttraumatic stress disorder. *Biological Psychiatry*, *50*, 305–309.

Dew, M. A., Kormos, R. L., Roth, L. H., Murali, S., DiMartini, A., & Griffith, B. P. (1999). Early post-transplant medical compliance and mental health predict physical morbidity and mortality one to three years after heart transplantation. *Journal of Heart and Lung Transplantation*, *18*, 549–562.

Doerfler, L. A., Pbert, L., & DeCosimo, D. (1994). Symptoms of posttraumatic stress disorder following myocardial infarction and coronary artery bypass surgery. *General Hospital Psychiatry*, *16*, 193–199.

Donnelly, C. L. (2003). Pharmacologic treatment approaches for children and adolescents with posttraumatic stress disorder. *Child and Adolescent Psychiatric Clinics of North America, 12*, 251–269.

Donnelly, C. L., & Amaya-Jackson, L. (2002). Posttraumatic stress disorder in children and adolescents: epidemiology, diagnosis and treatment options. *Paediatric Drugs, 4*, 159–170.

Elzinga, B. M., Schmahl, C. G., Vermetten, E., van Dyck, R., & Bremner, J. D. (2003). Higher cortisol levels following exposure to traumatic reminders in abuse-related PTSD. *Neuropsychopharmacology, 28*, 1656–1665.

Erickson, S. J., & Steiner, H. (2000). Trauma spectrum adaptation: Somatic symptoms in long-term pediatric cancer survivors. *Psychosomatics, 41*, 339–346.

Erickson, S. J., & Steiner, H. (2001). Trauma and personality correlates in long-term pediatric cancer survivors. *Child Psychiatry and Human Development, 31*, 195–213.

Famularo, R., Kinscherff, R., & Fenton, T. (1988). Propranolol treatment for childhood posttraumatic stress disorder, acute type. A pilot study. *American Journal of Diseases in Children, 142*, 1244–1247.

Frank, N. C., Blount, R. L., & Brown, R. T. (1997). Attributions, coping, and adjustment in children with cancer. *Journal of Pediatric Psychology, 22*, 563–576.

Glover, D. A., & Poland, R. E. (2002). Urinary cortisol and catecholamines in mothers of child cancer survivors with and without PTSD. *Psychoneuroendocrinology, 27*, 805–819.

Glover, D. A., Powers, M. B., Bergman, L., Smits, J. A., Telch, M. J., & Stuber M. (2003). Urinary dopamine and turn bias in traumatized women with and without PTSD symptoms. *Behavioral Brain Research, 144*, 137–141.

Good, C., & Petersen, C. (2001). SSRI and mirtazapine in PTSD. *Journal of the American Academy Child and Adolescent Psychiatry, 40*, 263–264.

Green, B. L., Rowland, J. H., Krupnick, J. L., Epstein, S. A., Stockton, P., Stern, N. M., et al. (1998). Prevalence of posttraumatic stress disorder in women with breast cancer. *Psychosomatics, 39*, 102–111.

Hampton, M. R., & Frombach, I. (2000).Women's experience of traumatic stress in cancer treatment. *Health Care Women International, 21*, 67–76.

Harmon, R. J., & Riggs, P. D. (1996). Clonidine for posttraumatic stress disorder in preschool children. *Journal of the American Academy Child and Adolescent Psychiatry, 35*, 1247–1249.

Hobbie, W., Stuber, M., Meeske, K., Wissler, K., Rourke, M., Ruccione, K., et al. (2000). Symptoms of posttraumatic stress in young adult survivors of childhood cancer. *Journal of Clinical Oncology, 18*, 4060–4066.

Horrigan, J. P., & Barnhill, L. J. (1996). The suppression of nightmares with guanfacine. *Journal of Clinical Psychiatry, 57*, 371.

Hudson, M. M., Mertons, A. C., Yasui, Y., Hobbie, W., Chen, H., Gurney, J. G., et al. (2003). Health status of adult long-term survivors of childhood cancer. *Journal of the American Medical Association, 290*, 1583–1592.

Jacobsen, P. B., Sadler, I. J., Booth-Jones, M., Soety, E., Weitzner, M. A., & Fields, K. K. (2002). Predictors of posttraumatic stress disorder symptomatology following bone marrow transplantation for cancer. *Journal of Consulting and Clinical Psychology,* 2002 *70*, 235–40.

Jacobsen, P. B., Widows, M. R., Hann, D. M., Andrykowski, M. A., Kronish, L. E., & Fields, K.K. (1998). Posttraumatic stress disorder symptoms after bone marrow transplantation for breast cancer. *Psychosomatic Medicine, 60*, 366–371.

Johnson, Vickberg, S. M., DuHamel, K. N., Smith, M. Y., Manne, S. L., Winkel, G., et al. (2001). Global meaning and psychological adjustment among survivors of bone marrow transplant. *Psycho-oncology, 10*, 29–39.

Kazak, A. E., Barakat, L. P., Meeske, K., Christakis, D., Meadows, A. T., Casey, R., et al. (1997). Posttraumatic stress symptoms, family functioning, and social support in survivors of childhood leukemia and their mothers and fathers. *Journal of Consulting and Clinical Psychology, 65*, *120–129.*

Kazak, A. E., Cant, M. C., Jensen, M. M., McSherry, M., Rourke, M. T., Hwang, W. T., et al. (2003). Identifying psychosocial risk indicative of subsequent resource use in families of newly diagnosed pediatric oncology patients. *Journal of Clinical Oncology, 21*, 3220–3225.

Kazak, A. E, Simms, S., & Rourke, M. T. (2002). Family systems practice in pediatric psychology. *Journal of Pediatric Psychology, 27*, 133–143.

Kazak, A. E., Stuber, M. L., Barakat, L. P., Meeske, K., Guthrie, D., & Meadows, A. T. (1998). Predicting posttraumatic stress symptoms in mothers and fathers of survivors of childhood cancers. *Journal of the American Academy of Child and Adolescent Psychiatry, 3*, 823–831.

Khouzam, H. R., el-Gabalawi, F., & Donnelly, N. J. (2001). The clinical experience of citalopram in the treatment of post-traumatic stress disorder: A report of two Persian Gulf War veterans. *Military Medicine, 166*, 921–923.

Kinzie, J. D., & Leung, P. (1989). Clonidine in Cambodian patients with posttraumatic stress disorder. *Journal of Nervous and Mental Disorders, 177*, 546–550.

Kutz, I., Garb, R., & David, D. (1988). Post-traumatic stress disorder following myocardial infarction. *General Hospital Psychiatry*, *10*, 169–176.

Kutz, I., Shabtai, H., Solomon, Z., Neumann, M., & David, D. (1994). Post-traumatic stress disorder in myocardial infarction patients: prevalence study. *Israel Journal of Psychiatry and Related Sciences, 31*, 48–56.

Landolt, M. A., Vollrath, M., Ribi, K., Gnehm, H. E., & Sennhauser, F. H. (2003). Incidence and associations of parental and child posttraumatic stress symptoms in pediatric patients. *Journal of Child Psychology and Psychiatry, 44*, 1199–1207.

Lieberman, M. A., Golant, M., Giese-Davis, J., Winzlenberg, A., Benjamin, H., Humphreys, K., et al. (2003). Electronic support groups for breast carcinoma: A clinical trial of effectiveness. *Cancer*, *97*, 920–925.

Linley, P. A. (2003). Positive adaptation to trauma: wisdom as both process and outcome. *Journal of Traumatic Stress, 16*, 601–610.

Linley, P. A., & Joseph, S. (2004). Positive change following trauma and adversity: A review. *Journal of Traumatic Stress, 17*, 11–21.

Lipschitz, D. S., Rasmusson, A. M., Yehuda, R., Wang, S., Anyan, W., Gueoguieva, R., et al. (2003). Salivary cortisol responses to dexamethasone in adolescents with posttraumatic stress disorder. *Journal of the American Academy of Child and Adolescent Psychiatry, 42*, 1310–1317.

Looff, D., Grimley, P., Kuller, F., Martin, A., & Shonfield, L. (1995). Carbamazepine for PTSD. *Journal of the American Academy of Child and Adolescent Psychiatry*, *34*, 703–704.

Lubin, G., Weizman, A., Shmushkevitz, M., & Valevski, A. (2002). Short-term treatment of post-traumatic stress disorder with naltrexone: an open-label preliminary study. *Human Psychopharmacology*, *17*, 181–185.

Lustig, S. L., Botelho, C., Lynch, L., Nelson, S. V., Eichelberger, W. J., & Vaughan, B. L. (2002). Implementing a randomized clinical trial on a pediatric psychiatric inpatient unit at a children's hospital: the case of clonidine for post-traumatic stress. *General Hospital Psychiatry*, *24*, 422–429.

Malek-Ahmadi, P. (2003). Gabapentin and posttraumatic stress disorder. *Annals of Pharmacotherapy, 37*, 664–666.

Malt, U. F., & Tjemsland, L. (1999). PTSD in women with breast cancer. *Psychosomatics*, *40*, 89.

Manne, S. L., DuHamel, K., Gallelli, K., Sorgen, K., & Redd, W. H. (1998). Posttraumatic stress disorder among mothers of pediatric cancer survivors: Diagnosis, comorbidity, and utility of the PTSD checklist as a screening instrument. *Journal of Pediatric Psychology*, *23*, 357–366.

Manne, S. L., DuHamel, K., & Redd, W. H. (2000). Association of psychological vulnerability factors to posttraumatic stress symptomatology in mothers of pediatric cancer survivors. *Psycho-oncology*, *9*, 372–384.

McMillen, J. C., Smith, E. M., & Fisher, R. H. (1997). Perceived benefit and mental health after three types of disaster. *Journal of Consulting and Clinical Psychology*, *65*, 733–739.

Meeske, K., Ruccione, K., Globe, D. R., & Stuber, M. L. (2001). PTSD, Quality of life and psychological outcome in young adult survivors of pediatric cancer. *Oncology Nursing Forum, 28*, 481–489.

Moskowitz, J. T. (2003). Positive affect predicts lower risk of AIDS mortality. *Psychosomatic Medicine, 65*, 620–626.

Mundy, E. A., Blanchard, E. B., Cirenza, E., Gargiulo, J., Maloy, B., & Blanchard, C. G. (2000). Posttraumatic stress disorder in breast cancer patients following autologous bone marrow transplantation or conventional cancer treatments. *Behavioral Research and Therapeutics*, *38*, 1015–1027.

Neel, M. L. (2000). Posttraumatic stress symptomatology and cancer. *International Journal of Emergency Mental Health*, *2*, 85–94.

Pelcovitz, D., Goldenberg, B., Kaplan, S., Weinblatt, M., Mandel, F., Meyers, B., et al. (1996). Posttraumatic stress disorder in mothers of pediatric cancer survivors. *Psychosomatics, 37*, 116–126.

Pelcovitz, D., Libov, B. G., Mandel, F., Kaplan, S., Weinblatt, M., & Septimus, A. (1998). Posttraumatic stress disorder and family functioning in adolescent cancer. *Journal of Traumatic Stress*, *11*, 205–221.

Phipps, S., & Srivastava, D. K. (1997). Repressive adaptation in children with cancer. *Health Psychology*, *16*, 521–528.

Phipps, S., & Srivastava, D. K. (1999). Approaches to the measurement of depressive symptomatology in children with cancer: Attempting to circumvent the effects of defensiveness. *Development and Behavioral Pediatrics, 20*, 150–156.

Pitman, R. K., Lanes, D. M., Williston, S. K., Guillaume, J. L., Metzger, L. J., Gehr, G. M., et al. (2001). Psychophysiologic assessment of posttraumatic stress disorder in breast cancer patients. *Psychosomatics, 42*, 133–140.

Porter, D. M., & Bell, C. C. (1999). The use of clonidine in post-traumatic stress disorder. *Journal of the National Medical Association, 91*, 475–477.

Powers, S. W. (1999). Empirically supported treatments in pediatric psychology: Procedure-related pain. *Journal of Pediatric Psychology*, *24*, 131–145.

Putnam, F. W., & Hulsmann, J. E. (2002). Pharmacotherapy for survivors of childhood trauma. *Seminars in Clinical Neuropsychiatry*, *7*, 129–136.

Reed, G. M., Kemeny, M. E., Taylor, S. E., & Visscher, B. R. (1999). Negative HIV-specific expectancies and AIDS-related bereavement as predictors of symptom onset in asymptomatic HIV-positive gay men. *Health Psychology, 18*, 354–363.

Robert, R., Blakeney, P. E., Villarreal, C., Rosenberg, L., & Meyer, W. J., 3rd. (1999). Imipramine treatment in pediatric burn patients with symptoms of acute stress disorder: A pilot study. *Journal of the American Academy of Child and Adolescent Psychiatry*, *38*, 873–882.

Sahler, O. J., Varni, J. W., Fairclough, D. L., Butler, R. W., Noll, R. B., Dolgin, M. J., et al. (2002). Problem-solving skills training for mothers of children with newly diagnosed cancer: A randomized trial. *Journal of Developmental and Behavioral Pediatrics*, *23*, 77–86.

Saxe, G., Stoddard, F., Courtney, D., Cunningham, K., Chawla, N., Sheridan, R., et al. (2001). Relationship between acute morphine and the course of PTSD in children with burns. *Journal of the American Academy of Child and Adolescent Psychiatry, 40*, 915–921.

Schwartz, A. C., & Rothbaum, B. O. (2002). Review of sertraline in post-traumatic stress disorder. *Expert Opinion in Pharmacotherapy*, *3*, 1489–1499.

Sears, S. R., Stanton, A. L., & Danoff-Burg, S. (2003). The yellow brick road and the emerald city: benefit finding, positive reappraisal coping and posttraumatic growth in women with early-stage breast cancer. *Health Psychology*, *22*, 487–497.

Shemesh, E., Lurie, S., Stuber, M. L., Emre, S., Patel, Y., Vohra, P., et al. (2000). A pilot study of posttraumatic stress and nonadherence in pediatric liver transplant recipients. *Pediatrics, 105*, E29.

Shemesh, E., Rudnick, A., Kaluski, E., Milovanov, O., Salah, A., & Alon, D. (2001). A prospective study of posttraumatic stress symptoms and nonadherence in survivors of a myocardial infarction (MI). *General Hospital Psychiatry, 23*, 215–222.

Smith, M. Y., Redd, W. H., Peyser, C., & Vogl, D. (1999). Post-traumatic stress disorder in cancer: A review. *Psycho-Oncology, 8*, 521–537.

Streisand, R., Braniecki, S., Tercyak, K. P., & Kazak, A. E. (2001). Childhood illness-related parenting stress: The pediatric inventory for parents. *Journal of Pediatric Psychology, 26*, 155–162.

Stuber, M. L., Kazak, A. E., Meeske, K., Barakat, L., Guthrie, D., Garnier, H., et al. (1997). Predictors of posttraumatic stress symptoms in childhood cancer survivors, *Pediatrics, 100*, 958–964.

Stuber, M. L., Nader, K., Yasuda, P., Pynoos, R. S., & Cohen, S. (1991). Stress responses after pediatric bone marrow transplantation: preliminary results of a prospective longitudinal study. *Journal of the American Academy of Child and Adolescent Psychiatry, 30*, 952–957.

Surtees, P., Wainwright, N., Day, N., Brayne, C., Luben, R., & Khaw, K. T. (2003). Adverse experience in childhood as a developmental risk factor for altered immune status in adulthood. *International Journal of Behavioral Medicine, 10*, 251–268.

Taylor, F., & Cahill, L. (2002). Propranolol for reemergent posttraumatic stress disorder following an event of retraumatization: A case study. *Journal of Traumatic Stress, 15*, 433–437.

Tedeschi, R. G., & Calhoun, L. G. (1996). The Posttraumatic Growth Inventory: Measuring the positive legacy of trauma. *Journal of Traumatic Stress, 9*, 455–471.

Tjemsland, L., Soreide, J. A., & Malt, U. F. (1998). Posttraumatic distress symptoms in operable breast cancer III: Status 1 year after surgery. *Breast Cancer Research and Treatment, 47*, 141–151.

van der Kolk, B. A., Dreyfuss, D., Michaels, M., Shera, D., Berkowitz, R., Fisler, R., et al. (1994). Fluoxetine in posttraumatic stress disorder. *Journal of Clinical Psychiatry*, *55*, 517–522.

Viola, J., Ditzler, T., Batzer, W., Harazin, J., Adams, D., Lettich, L., et al. (1997). Pharmacological management of post-traumatic stress disorder: clinical summary of a 5-year retrospective study, 1990–1995. *Military Medicine, 162*, 616–619.

Weiss, T. (2004). Correlates of posttraumatic growth in husbands of breast cancer survivors. *Psycho-oncology, 13*, 260–268.

Widows, M. R., Jacobsen, P. B., & Fields, K. K.(2000). Relation of psychological vulnerability factors to posttraumatic stress disorder symptomatology in bone marrow transplant recipients. *Psychosomatic Medicine*, *62*, 873–882.

Wolmer, L., Laor, N., Gershon, A., Mayes, L. C., & Cohen, D. J. (2000). The mother-child dyad facing trauma: a developmental outlook. *Journal of Nervous and Mental Diseases, 188*, 409–415.

Woodward, C., & Joseph, S. (2003). Positive change processes and post-traumatic growth in people who have experienced childhood abuse: Understanding vehicles of change. *Psychology and Psychotherapy*, *76*(Part 3), 267–283.

Yatham, L. N., Sacamano, J., & Kusumakar, V. (1996). Assessment of noradrenergic functioning in patients with non-combat-related posttraumatic stress disorder: A study with desmethylimipramine and orthostatic challenges. *Psychiatry Research, 63*, 1–6.

Yehuda, R. (Ed.). (1999). *Risk factors for posttraumatic stress disorder.* Washington, DC: American Psychiatric Press.

Zebrack, B., Zeltzer, L., Whitton, J., Mertons, A., Odom, L., Berkow, R., et al. (2002). Psychological outcomes in long-term survivors of childhood leukemia, Hodgkin's disease, and non-Hodgkins's lymphoma: A report from the Childhood Cancer Survivors Study. *Pediatrics, 110*, 42–52.

Zebrack, B. J., & Chesler, M. A. (2002). Quality of life in childhood cancer survivors. *Psycho-Oncology, 11*, 132–141.

Robert W. Butler and Donna R. Copeland

# Interventions for Cancer Late Effects and Survivorship

## Overview

It is now generally accepted that the diagnosis of many pediatric cancers and their treatments result in significant and long-lasting neurocognitive, psychological, and psychosocial impairments and difficulties. The current status of research in this field has been addressed by other chapters in this text. We would, however, like to emphasize at the onset of our chapter that we firmly believe pediatric cancer is truly a family affair. The effects of the diagnosis of a life-threatening illness and its often-chronic treatment not only result in significant impact on the child's or adolescent's neuropsychological and psychological state, but also cause psychological ramifications for the parents, siblings, and extended family members.

In healthy, well-functioning families, this major life obstacle can serve as an impetus to rally family members in support of the child. When this happens, interventions for late effects are beginning to be identified as effective and of potential benefit. This field, however, is clearly in its infancy. If the family is chaotic and struggling with relationship issues, the prognosis is less positive. Our clinical observations of these relationships are supported both by preliminary data from studies conducted by our research group and others, and by published manuscripts in the field of pediatric traumatic brain injury (Yeates et al., 1997, 2001).

In one of the only studies investigating the impact of familial variables on psychosocial and neuropsychological outcome in pediatric brain tumor patients, the results are extremely consistent with the traumatic brain injury population (Carlson-Green, Morris, & Krawjecki, 1995). Reduced maternal dependence on external coping resources, higher parental socioeconomic status, dual-parent families, and familial cohesion were all identified as improving long-term outcome in this population, as documented by intellectual and behavioral integrity.

The late effects of pediatric cancer and its treatment are physical, cognitive, psychological, and social. When multiple effects are present, they can be expected to result in a synergistic impact not only on the child, but also on other family members. The important point is that late effects should not be viewed in isolation or summated but should be appreciated for their interrelatedness. For example, in cognitive remediation, a psychological treatment program designed to improve neurocognitive deficits following childhood cancer treatment, physical deficits associated with disease and its treatments, such as motoric disabilities and visual dysfunction, have an impact on our ability to work with the patient in a therapeutically effective manner. Correspondingly, family dysfunction often results in failure to complete cognitive remediation homework sessions and an increased incidence of missed treatment sessions. All areas of the patient's life need to be considered. In the pediatric population, this includes the school environment: teachers and peers.

The theory behind rehabilitation after brain injury can be traced to the writings of Luria (1963), who posited that the brain is not a static organ. Luria recognized that, following an insult to the central nervous system (CNS), a period of spontaneous recovery occurs that typically extends 1–2 years. During this period of spontaneous recovery, it was believed that functional reorganization occurs within the brain, and that new neuronal pathways develop to compensate for terminally damaged neurons. Growing evidence within the field of brain injury clearly supports the likelihood of structural and functional changes in the brain secondary to damage (Levin & Grafman, 2000). Cognitive rehabilitation and remediation on an outpatient basis historically involved efforts to stimulate the process of spontaneous recovery. Thus, the initial approaches to brain injury rehabilitation were very similar to a cognitive form of physical therapy: exercising the brain's abilities. As elucidated in this chapter, the initial approach, while still relevant, has been significantly broadened to include the use of memory strategies, metacognitive strategies, psychological treatments, and particularly for children and adolescents, interventions directed toward the family.

Research and clinical efforts to improve neurocognitive and psychological functioning in childhood cancer survivors are only now becoming a reality because successful medical treatment for many malignancies by pediatric oncologists is a recent accomplishment (Pizzo & Poplack, 1997). Although our initial attempts at neurocognitive and psychological treatment have borrowed heavily from the field of brain injury rehabilitation, there are significant differences between the pediatric cancer population and the patients more commonly seen in outpatient brain injury rehabilitation. More specifically, most brain injury rehabilitation treatments have been developed for adults. Very little work has been directed toward child/adolescent brain injury survivors. In addition, the most common adult and noncancer-related brain injuries involve an acute insult to the brain, for example, closed/open head injury and stroke. In the case of adult degenerative disorders, treatments tend to rely on pharmacology and support rather than rehabilitation-based interventions. As described in this volume's chapter 14 on neuropsychological late effects, the effects of irradiation and chemotherapy on the developing brain tend to be chronic, degenerative, and deteriorating rather than acute. We are only now beginning to modify and individualize our intervention efforts to make them more specific to this unique population.

This chapter reviews research on interventions for the late effects of many childhood cancers and their treatment. The focus is on long-term survivorship. Within the context of this chapter, long-term survivorship refers to posttreatment late effects or effects that are only addressed following successful treatment for the malignancy. Although the National Cancer Institute and American Cancer Society are now conceptualizing cancer survivorship at diagnosis, endorsement of that position within the context of the current text would result in considerable redundancy with other chapters. Thus, although we heartedly support this new conceptualization of survivorship at diagnosis, for practical purposes we address posttreatment interventions. In keeping with the interdisciplinary approach, we discuss physical, neurocognitive, psychosocial, and pharmacological interventions. It is frankly a pleasure to write this chapter because it represents the future, not just of pediatric oncology, but also of life.

## Interventions

### Physical

In a large study of adult survivors of childhood cancer ($N = 9{,}535$) in which participants completed questionnaires, 44% reported at least one adversely affected health status domain (general health, mental health, activity limitations, and functional impairment) (Hudson et al., 2003). Physical findings might involve abnormalities in the hormonal, reproductive, or nervous systems; bone; soft tissue; heart; kidneys; liver; and blood (Blatt, Copeland, & Bleyer, 1993). In addition, there may be long-term effects on speech, language, motor functions, and hearing that often overlap with psychological functions.

Survivors of brain tumors are at greatest risk because of tumor location and multimodal treatment. Further, all those who received the chemotherapy cisplatin as part of their treatment are at risk for hearing loss and visual-motor deficits because it may damage the inner ear as well as specific parts of the brain (Blatt et al., 1993; Children's Oncology Group Web site; Schell et al., 1989). If the survivor was treated in infancy, the hearing loss might have affected the development of speech. In this case, immediate intervention with a certified speech-language therapist is essential to minimize more extensive effects.

Survivors of brain tumors, who tend to have more adverse long-term effects caused by disease factors and the intensity and types of treatment, may have slurred speech, dysarthria, and word-finding difficulties. Tumors in specific locations of the brain specialized for speech or hearing will likely create dysfunction, if not from the tumor itself, then from the surgery. If vocal cords have been damaged, resulting in voice changes or swallowing problems, a speech-language pathologist or speech therapist will be very helpful in providing therapeutic interventions.

Occupational therapists are especially skilled in alleviating detrimental effects on visual-spatial awareness and skills. A complete neuropsychological assessment is often extremely helpful in measuring speech/language, hearing, and fine-motor and visual-motor deficits as well as more purely cognitive (e.g., intellectual, academic) functions. If problems are identified, the survivor can be referred to other specialists.

It is important for the health care providers who are treating survivors of childhood cancer to be aware of the potential late effects so that when a problem is identified, a timely referral to the appropriate provider can be instigated. As a clinical example of this process, speech and language difficulties may be subtle or not recognized for some reason (Beal, Mabbot, & Bouffet, 2003). This was true for Giraldo (not really the patient's name).

Giraldo was a 7-year-old survivor of acute lymphocytic leukemia who had been treated with chemotherapy. He was very active when he came to the clinic and required individual treatment from the child life specialists and psychologists. At that time, it was apparent that he had an attention deficit, which did not present a major problem until he was enrolled in school. When his mother expressed her frustration about his behavior at home, at school, and at church, he was evaluated and enrolled in the cognitive remediation program (CRP) at his treatment center. This is an intensive psychologically based treatment program that is described in detail in this chapter. The degree of distractibility and impulsivity that he exhibited, however, interfered with attempts to modify his behavior in cognitive remediation.

Initially, Giraldo's mother was not in favor of his taking additional medication after his cancer treatment, but when the doctors and therapists she trusted recommended giving it a try, she relented. It was at this point that the therapists learned that despite Giraldo's age, he was not eating solid foods; his mother would grind everything up for him, including medications in tablet form. She had never mentioned this to anyone on the treatment team. It became apparent when he was prescribed a stimulant medication that was in a timed-release capsule form. At the recommendation of the psychologist and his attending physician, Giraldo was evaluated by the speech-language pathologist to be sure he did not have a swallowing abnormality. When it was found he did not, the psychologist began working with Giraldo and his mother, using cognitive-behavioral techniques, on reducing his fear of choking. She helped him with a slight articulation problem as well. During this time, Giraldo continued in the CRP, and his mother was seen by the psychologist and speech therapist to coach her in reinforcing the teaching at home. The benefits of these multidisciplinary interventions were that Giraldo began eating regular foods, and he eventually achieved honor roll status at school.

This case illustrates the following points regarding rehabilitation interventions for pediatric cancer survivors:

1. Long-term survivors may have subtle difficulties that are not immediately apparent.
2. Multidisciplinary collaboration and communication are essential when survivors have multiple problems.
3. Parent involvement is crucial in the remediation therapy of children.
4. The sources of survivors' difficulties may or may not be directly attributable to cancer and its treatment.

## Cognitive Remediation

Very few studies have been published on efforts to improve cognitive functioning following disease- and treatment-related deficits in pediatric cancer. To our knowledge, one of the first studies was conducted by Butler (1998) and described a treatment approach that involved combined massed practice, instruction in metacognitive strategies, and cognitive behavioral psychotherapy with a single participant. Massed practice refers to drill exercises that are designed to strengthen cognitive abilities such as attention and information-processing speed. Metacognitive strategies involve teaching individuals to be conscious of their own styles of thinking and to incorporate the use of new styles and strategies that will result in superior performance. Cognitive behavioral psychotherapy (Meichenbaum, 1977) refers to an intervention approach that recognizes the importance of self-thought and self-talk and uses behavioral principles to strengthen appropriate, positive internal dialogues. Thus, an individual is taught to avoid unproductive and irrational self-thinking and to become one's "best coach" rather than "worst enemy." These three techniques were respectively selected from the fields of brain injury rehabilitation, educational psychology, and clinical psychology. Butler's case study used this innovative tripartite model for brain injury rehabilitation, and he reported significant improvement in cognitive functions following the remediation process.

An additional case study appeared in the literature at about this same time. Kerns and Thomson (1998) investigated the potential effectiveness of a compensatory memory device. These researchers, working with an adolescent who was suffering significant memory impairment secondary to a brain tumor and its treatment, reported that the participant, while continuing to demonstrate significantly impaired memory, did show some acceleration in academic achievement. It also was reported that the research participant used the compensatory device over 1 year following the initial training. Improved classroom adjustment appeared to be an outcome of the intervention. Instruction in the use of the compensatory device was reasonably intensive as the memory notebook had been assembled into different parts. There was a memory log in which the participant could make notes to assist episodic memory. A calendar section allowed for the recording of future activities and events and provided for a time record of past events. There also was a "things to do" section. An orientation portion of the device included names of teachers, classroom location, the participant's counselor's name, and other important personal information. Finally, there was a transportation section that included maps of the school and bus schedules. Training was divided into three stages: acquisition, application, and adaptation.

An effort has been made to supplement traditional educational procedures with a more intensive tutorial approach directed toward arithmetic concept instruction in pediatric cancer survivors (Moore et al., 2000). A pilot study was conducted that consisted of eight survivors who received a special education intervention, and there were seven comparison participants. The intervention involved 40–50 hours of instruction in math concepts and, possibly, calculation abilities. The article does not describe the intervention process in detail but does report the results of both pre- and posttesting of academic achievement using standardized psychological tests. The results indicated that the intervention group was able to maintain stable achievement over time, but the comparison group declined in arithmetic over the course of the study.

To date, the most comprehensive report of an intervention designed to improve neurocognitive functioning in pediatric cancer survivors has been published by Butler and Copeland (2002). This study described in greater detail the approach used in the aforementioned case study by Butler (1998). Continuing to use the tripartite model, brain injury rehabilitation training exercises were applied. Techniques developed by Sohlberg and Mateer (1996), entitled attention process training (APT), were administered to pediatric cancer survivors. These exercises are multidimensional and directed to strengthen attentional abilities in the areas of sustained, selective, divided, and executive attentional control.

The APT treatment exercises were combined with activities designed to be more intrinsically interesting to children. APT exercises were developed for adults, and they tend to be demanding. It was believed that using these activities exclusively would result in decreased motivation in our population, particularly the younger children. Thus, various toys and games were selected that not only had a significant attentional component, but also stimulated active participation. These included games such as "Simon" and computer-administered exercises. An alternating rule was adopted in which an APT activity was maintained for no more than 15 minutes, at which time one of the more intrinsically interesting activities was then selected with the participant's input. We would then progress alternately in this manner. Also, to maximize the participant's internal perception of progress and success, a 50%–80% rule was adopted. To maintain engagement in a single activity, the individual had to achieve at least 50% successful responding. When 80% successful responding was achieved, the exercises were advanced to the next level of difficulty.

Intensive instruction in metacognitive strategies was provided. Strategies were divided into three arenas (task preparedness, on-task performance, and posttask behavior). Depending on the level of functioning of the participant, it was expected that at least 10 strategies be incorporated, preferably 15. The above-described brain rehabilitation exercises were used to document the effectiveness of an individual strategy. An exercise was administered, a strategy was taught, and if improvement on the exercise was noted, the strategy was incorporated into the participant's dictionary of metacognitive resources. Strategies were individualized for the participant, and the individual's own terminology and language were used whenever possible. While a dictionary of metacognitive strategies exists (Butler & Copeland, 2002), therapists were encouraged to observe the participant very closely to identify new potential strategies that would be effective for the individual child's cognitive difficulties.

Cognitive behavioral psychotherapeutic techniques and principles were also employed. Participants were instructed initially to talk out loud to themselves following the therapist's modeling. When appropriate successful internal dialogue patterns and structures were obtained, the individual was subsequently allowed to silently use his or her self-statements. We also used this technique to assist the children/adolescents in their ability to resist distraction. During this part of therapy, following modeling, the therapist served as a very active distractant to the participant, thus allowing for the verification of skill acquisition.

The CRP was administered as a team approach intervention. The team consisted of the therapist and participant as well as the parents and teachers. Therapy was administered in an individualized manner, and treatment occurred over a 4- to 6-month period. The CRP initially consisted of 2-hour weekly sessions of therapy for 25 weeks. The length of the intervention was based on traditional outpatient brain injury rehabilitation practice. Each week, parents were provided with the metacognitive strategies that had been taught in the session and prompted to promote their use during homework and household chores at home. Parents were requested to provide the strategies to teachers, and teachers were contacted on a regular basis by the child/adolescent's therapist.

Based on a case control study, individuals who received the CRP exhibited significant improvement on a continuous performance test and other measures of attention/concentration (Butler & Copeland, 2002). There was not, however, evidence to suggest that these benefits in neurocognitive functioning resulted in significantly improved arithmetic academic achievement. It was reported that potential problems regarding treatment generalizability would need to be addressed to promote success in this area. Nevertheless, there was evidence that benefits had been realized by most children/adolescents who received the CRP, and a more intensive, scientifically sophisticated design to assess effectiveness was recommended.

A randomized, multi-institutional clinical trial of cognitive remediation for survivors of pediatric brain cancer and its treatments has been concluded. At the time of preparing this chapter, the study has just been completed; unfortunately, results were not available for publication at this time. Interim data analysis, however, does indicate an overall improvement in academic achievement and self-image in children/adolescents who did receive the CRP as compared to a waiting list control group.

Although our initial results are encouraging and positive regarding the beneficial effects of the CRP, the treatment approach needs to become more potent. Data analyses will provide evidence to suggest hypotheses of why certain individuals benefit maximally from our intervention, as opposed to those who do not recognize significant measurable treatment gains. As noted, we suspect that familial factors have not been appropriately addressed, and plans are being finalized to alter our treatment approach to include a direct intervention with the parents and caregivers of the pediatric cancer survivors.

Psychotherapeutic interventions as part of the cognitive remediation process for patients, and their family members, have long been recognized as essential and beneficial (Lezak, 1978). This work, however, has almost exclusively been conducted with adults, most commonly those suffering a traumatic brain injury. Although likely pertinent to the pediatric population, including cancer survivors, research within this population has been surprisingly deficient. Prigatano (1999) wrote extensively on the importance and relevance of psychotherapeutic interventions for adults who have suffered a brain injury. Questions regarding why the injury occurred to the person, whether they regain normality, and how they can continue their functioning following the brain damage lend themselves well to supportive and explorative psychotherapy. Although many childhood cancer survivors who experience neurocognitive deficits remain in their developmental stages, increased survival rates are resulting in young adult and adulthood survivors of the more common malignancies of childhood: leukemias and brain tumors. This further amplifies the need for increased investigations on how psychotherapy can be of benefit to these individuals.

One of the essential goals of psychotherapy with all patients involves exploration and instruction in the most effective means of adjusting self-interest (Prigatano, 1999). There are many different theories of how psychotherapeutic change occurs, with their respective techniques and approaches. Nevertheless, the overall goal is to reduce intrapsychic suffering and promote intra- and interpersonal adjustment, with presumed positive reverberations into the familial, vocational, and especially children's and adolescents' academic arenas.

While most work is being conducted with brain injured adults, Butler and Satz (1999) have addressed the need for therapeutic interventions with children and adolescents who have suffered a brain injury. Concerns for this population were directly addressed by these authors. In particular, it is important to assess the possible presence of dysphoria and depression. Language functions are especially relevant with younger populations. Reduced facility with expressive speech and comprehension coupled with the possibility of neuropsychological deficits suggest that these individuals often lack the ability for self-reflection or verbal expression of mood. Although cognitive behavioral therapy is frequently a very appropriate treatment for psychological disturbance, language deficits may make this treatment modality difficult to accomplish.

Nevertheless, it is our position that there is a strong psychotherapeutic component to cognitive remediation. At the very least, this relationship begins to emerge when a patient and the patient's family realizes that the therapist has concerns regarding the patient's successful adjustment to life's challenges whether they are educational, vocational, or inter-/intrapersonal. Our approach to cognitive remediation with brain-injured cancer survivors is not only reasonably structured, but also individualized. In short, while we have an agenda, any problem is "grist for the mill." If a patient arrives for therapy upset or perturbed or if a parent points out a new problem area, this becomes a focus of intervention in addition to our overall treatment plan.

## Vocational Counseling

The prospect of leaving school and entering into adult employment is somewhat intimidating for most students, but especially for those who have gone through the cancer experience and have developed neurosensory or learning deficits as a result. For these young people, anticipation of that challenge can be daunting. Planning for this eventuality should begin early, perhaps in middle school. For instance, younger survivors planning to enroll in higher education (junior college, college/university) need to be informed about the high school courses required for entry. Vocational planning is especially important for students in special education. Their neurocognitive abilities and interests should be assessed and monitored—preferably for several years—by a qualified professional with experience in pediatric oncology.

If a student is not planning to attend college or if this is not a viable option, the school district may have a work-study program with mentors in specific fields of work and job placements with local employers. The high school student's enrollment in occupationally oriented vocational courses has important long-term implications according to a study conducted by the National Longitudinal

Transition Study of Special Education Students, completed in 1994 (Blackorby & Wagner, 1997). This study demonstrated that those concentrating on vocational courses were less likely to drop out of high school and had a better chance of employment at a higher wage than students with disabilities whose coursework was restricted to academically oriented pursuits.

All survivors should receive aptitude testing, and when appropriate, vocational counselors should discuss with them their interests and abilities, work values, personality, and skills. Finally, these individuals should be provided information about study and work possibilities and how to apply and interview for these opportunities. Survivors will likely benefit from working with a vocational counselor or coach who will ensure that the appropriate assessments are conducted, guide the student in finding appropriate placements for which to apply, and coach the student in how to interview for financial aid, college entrance, and employment.

Parents have a role in this domain as well. Key factors in students' success in general are the parent's encouragement in their learning, appropriate expectations for their performance, and involvement in school and community life (Henderson, 1994).

Next, we address the social issues that confront the families of pediatric cancer survivors and available interventions. Interventions directed to parents, mothers in particular, of newly diagnosed patients have shown promise in reducing stress and promoting healthy psychological adjustment in critical caregivers.

## Problem-Solving Skills Training for Parents

Parents have an essential role in the psychosocial outcome for children who survive cancer. The mother is commonly the parent who brings the child with cancer to treatment. For this reason, we focus primarily on mothers in this chapter; however, as fathers assume more child care roles in our society, some of the issues and interventions may need to be modified to take fathers into account. Mothers express great interest in how they can help their children and express frustration about not being able to provide more support. They appreciate being coached and guided in developing strategies that will increase their children's efforts to participate in their psychosocial milieu. Mothers play a key role in another respect. A number of studies have demonstrated an association between parental, particularly mothers', sense of well-being and that of their children (Hetherington & Martin, 1986; Perrin, Ayoub, & Willett, 1993; Sahler et al., 1997; Silver, Bauman, & Ireys, 1995; Wallander & Varni, 1998).

A key role mothers typically assume is getting the child to medical and therapy appointments. In the event that logistic or other situations arise that make it difficult for the mother to access assistance, we have found that her problem-solving skills often influence the difference between the child continuing or canceling treatment sessions. When parents are able to conceptualize the difficulties associated with psychosocial and school-related problems, they appreciate the importance of their children's consistent participation in treatment (i.e., compliance is improved). Second, they are more likely to explore various approaches for addressing cognitive and academic problems, are more likely to provide helpful responses to the child at home (e.g., reinforcement strategies, provision of helpful activities and games), and are more likely to advocate for their child at school. Finally, they seem better prepared to identify and access helpful resources in their schools and communities (e.g., special treatments and academic programs).

We have used the problem-solving skills training (PSST) approach, originally developed by D'Zurilla and Nezu (1999) and reinterpreted for specific application to pediatric oncology (Varni et al., 1999), as an effective approach in helping parents reduce treatment-related stress. PSST is a generic program for teaching adults how to cope with a range of problem- and emotion-based stressful situations commonly encountered during treatment by patients and families affected by cancer. It is a five-step process in which the person approaches a difficult situation by identifying the problem, considering various options, evaluating those options and choosing the one most likely to succeed, implementing the selected option, and then reassessing to see if the solution was effective. If it is unsuccessful, the five-step process is reiterated until success is achieved. Throughout the process, a spirit of optimism is encouraged. In parental PSST, the parent is provided instructional materials that detail the steps of problem solving and give examples. In general, six to eight training sessions with homework between each session are sufficient for the parent to learn the techniques.

Because school has such importance in childhood, parents will receive not only direct instruction in the five steps of problem-solving skills, but also instruction on how to improve their ability to navigate the educational system as an advocate for their child/adolescent. Thus, the intervention has been modified to include education in federal laws that are relevant to requirements that schools meet the special needs of children who have neurocognitive impairments (i.e., 504, individual education plan [IEP]). In addition, the PSST paradigm addresses familial stability and the parents' ability to manage family-based issues such as economic distress, marital discord, and sibling distress.

In a multisite, randomized controlled trial (Sahler et al., 2004), this model has been successful in alleviating maternal distress during the initial stages of cancer treatment. After receiving eight sessions of PSST, mothers reported significantly enhanced problem-solving skills and reduced negative affectivity compared with the control group of mothers.

## Psychosocial

According to the Children's Oncology Group (Childhood Cancer Survivor Long-Term Follow-Up Guidelines, 2003), potential psychosocial late effects of the cancer experience include mild forms of depression, anxiety symptoms, posttraumatic stress, and social withdrawal. This information was gleaned from a thorough search of the literature, including two of the following studies. Research teams from the Children's Cancer Group assessed the impact of CNS treatments on psychological functioning in adult survivors of childhood leukemia and found that a subset reported mood disturbances (Glover et al., 2003; Zebrack et al., 2002).

One large group of researchers with a sizable sample investigated the incidence and predictors of symptoms of posttraumatic stress among pediatric cancer survivors and their families and reported that these symptoms persist in a subset of survivors (Alderfer, Labay, & Kazak, 2003; Barakat, Kazak, Gallagher, Meeske, & Stuber, 2000; Best, Streisand, Catania, & Kazak, 2001; Hobbie et al., 2000; Kazak et al., 1997, 2001; Stuber et al., 1997). Interestingly, results also indicate that parents and siblings are at greater risk than the survivors for developing symptoms, but the investigators concluded that the incidence in all groups was sufficient to warrant routine psychological screening in the childhood cancer survivor clinic. At least one cancer center found this practice to be feasible (Recklitis, O'Leary, & Diller, 2003); however, in view of the aforementioned findings, the family as a whole, or at least the parents, should be included in screening.

Noll and colleagues (Gartstein, Short, Vannatta, & Noll, 1999; Noll, Bukowski, Rogosch, LeRoy, & Kulkarni, 1990; Noll, Leroy, Bukowski, Rogosch, & Kulkarni, 1991; Noll et al., 1999) take issue, to some extent, with the findings of the increased incidence of psychosocial sequelae among pediatric cancer survivors, except in the case of brain tumor survivors. Results, obtained from studies of peers and teachers at school, indicate that most survivors are generally accepted by peers, have a good self-concept, and are not lonely, although they may be somewhat more socially isolated. Researchers generally agree, however, that survivors of brain tumors are at greater risk for long-term psychosocial difficulties (Anderson et al., 2001; Nicholson & Butler, 2001; Vannatta, Gartstein, Short, & Noll, 1998).

The types of negative psychosocial effects that some pediatric cancer survivors experience are understandable because these children frequently have encountered multiple shortcomings and failures that can potentially erode their self-confidence and sense of competency, which may reinforce their social withdrawal. The extent to which these problems exist is becoming increasingly clear. The psychosocial issues that arise during and following childhood cancer will need to be further elucidated, particularly regarding efforts at the formation of successful psychotherapeutic interventions.

## Social Skills

The existence of social skills deficits in some survivors of childhood cancer has only recently been fully recognized. This appears to be a particular issue in pediatric patients who have completed treatment for brain tumors (Vannatta et al., 1998). Considerable effort has been directed toward the assessment of social functioning in children with cancer and chronic illness under the rubric of quality of life (Gartstein et al., 1999; Spieth & Harris, 1996; Varni, Burwinkle, Katz, Meeske, & Dickinson, 2002; Varni, Seid, & Kurtin, 2001). Clinical trials on interventions directed toward improving social skills in childhood cancer survivors, however, are virtually nonexistent. This is partly because difficulties in the area of socialization with brain tumor patients have only recently been identified and recognized. Past research in the childhood leukemia population has generally indicated that survivors of this disease do not suffer difficulties in socialization with peers (Butler, Rizzi, & Handwerger, 1996; Noll, Bukowski, Davies, Koontz, & Kulkarni, 1993; Noll et al., 1997).

Research with children who suffer chronic illness other than childhood cancer supports the efficacy of efforts to improve socialization both at home and with peers. Encouraging flexibility and teaching family members how to establish clear boundaries, balancing competing needs, and providing positive meanings to life events are predictive of psychological health and social adjustment (Patterson & Blum, 1996). Enlarging social support networks also appears to benefit children with chronic illness (Ellerton, Stewart, Ritchi, & Hirth, 1996).

Specific interventions designed to improve social skills and socialization in children and adolescents include pet therapy (Hall & Malpus, 2000), cognitive behavioral interventions (Kendall, 1991), group interventions (Roberts, Turney, & Knowles, 1998), and specific techniques directed toward teaching social competency, self-evaluation skills, and appropriate affect expression (Reed, 1994). All of these approaches likely have relevance to childhood cancer survivors. As more information emerges about the specific nature of social difficulties in individuals who have completed treatment for a pediatric malignancy, brain tumors in particular, we will be better positioned to tailor individual therapies and conduct experimental outcome studies. We now discuss the importance of more traditional psychotherapeutic interventions with pediatric cancer survivors.

## Psychotherapy/Counseling

Cognitive behavioral, psychodynamic, and family therapy techniques have the potential for effectively supporting long-term survivors of childhood cancer. Behavioral approaches such as reinforcement and positive reframing are routinely used to help children and families in this population. In addition, improvements in self-concept can be accomplished in a psychotherapeutic relationship and in the interactions that occur within that framework (Altman, Briggs, Frankel, Gensler, & Pantone, 2002). For instance, the child/adolescent has the therapist's full attention during a session, which implies that he or she is important. The therapist also redefines the student's identity by pointing out observed aspects or characteristics such as "You did a fine job!" "I see you are very careful in your work." "I see you enjoy playing with other children." "You are very articulate in expressing yourself." The child and therapist form a bond during psychotherapeutic sessions, out of which may emerge a survivor's new sense of oneself and others. Ideally, the child adds new behaviors or ways of interacting with others that reflect improvement: increased confidence, self-direction, expressiveness, and organization.

Following are our clinical observations based on our considerable experience at both M. D. Anderson Cancer Center in the Department of Pediatrics and in the Division of Pediatric Hematology/Oncology at Oregon Health and Science University. These reflect approaches and methods employed in the supervision of students and engaging children and adolescents in psychotherapy. These are based on principles of psychotherapy as explicated by the authors of *Relational Child Psychotherapy* (Altman et al., 2002).

Survivors whose treatment included cranial radiation therapy tend to become more withdrawn and self-focused than others, partly because of slowed brain processing speed and deficits in working memory (Schatz, Kramer, Ablin, & Matthay, 2000). Often, their speech is laborious, so others talk faster, answer for their peers, or ignore the child during group conversations. Over the course of a therapy session, the therapist can encourage the child/adolescent to converse by creating an atmosphere in the treatment room that seems special in its clear sense of safety and promotes the freedom to express oneself freely. The therapist does this by listening attentively, asking leading questions, and waiting patiently for the response. Having someone listen to him or her without interrupting is frequently a new experience for these students.

An essential element in good psychotherapy is for the therapist to take an empathic, sympathetic stance. Letting patients know you understand and sympathize with their difficulties gives them a sense of belonging and importance. Staying in this mode for some time before offering direct suggestions will also be a new experience for the individual. In their interactions with others, the survivor may frequently encounter advice given with the best of intentions but with little or no sympathy expressed. The students subsequently become accustomed to "tuning out" others' suggestions. Engaging them in problem solving might then be a novel experience because the children may be asked to engage in an active process of expressing their opinions.

In our clinical experience, many survivors respond better in environments that are structured and consistent. This is the case for both home and school environments. Ideally, appointments and many activities and chores will be set for the same time each week for a specified amount of time. As much as possible, unusual events—such as prolonged teacher/parent absences, consequences of behavior, and major life changes—should be discussed beforehand and the child/adolescent given the opportunity to plan and make decisions. As with all children/adolescents, expectations of behaviors should be stated clearly, and consequences for complying/not complying should be clearly defined. Follow-up and adherence to whatever plan is devised is essential.

Metaphors provide an excellent means of helping children remember their coping strategies and add a kind of playfulness that is interesting and appealing. According to Lakoff and Johnson (1980), metaphor is one way the human mind structures experience. It gives our experience shape and substance by defining it in physical and sensory terms. Some examples they give are when we say that what someone has said was "right on target," or when we say to someone who has an idea, "Shoot," or we might say that by using the wrong strategy "You might get wiped out." The authors have noted that we use metaphors every day; they underlie assumptions by which we live. And, that is the purpose of devising metaphors in psychotherapy and cognitive remediation that can be used in coping—to create automatic "pictures" that come to mind when the child/adolescent is presented with a challenge.

Andy (not his real name) had trouble sitting still and frequently fidgeted in his chair and hopped around. He and his trainer devised a magic bubble for him to go inside (another example) and feel a sense of quiet. He knew he had to be careful not to fidget because if he hit the sides of the bubble it could burst. Another child found that reminding herself to "send oxygen to her brain" when she was struggling with a problem helped her focus and think more logically. This child was more scientifically minded than most, and as with Andy, this was a metaphor she conceived on her own. Metaphors are best when chosen by the student, although sometimes they are suggested by the therapist. Most important is that the metaphor is meaningful to the child and facilitates coping. One child used the image of a cheetah in the jungle as a way of reminding himself to pay attention and stay on track toward a goal, or the cheetah might get lost (i.e., the student might not hear what the teacher has said.)

Following cancer treatment, many parents have trouble backing off from caring for their child. This affects the child's sense of competency and responsibility, as demonstrated in the following case.

Joe (not his real name) was a 14 year-old survivor of a brain tumor who was socially withdrawn and sometimes taunted by bullies at school, and he frequently called his mother to retrieve him from school because of headaches or some type of physical complaint. He had a documented attention deficit and was enrolled in a CRP, but it was also apparent that Joe's parents perceived him as needing more help than others his age, despite the fact that he was primarily at age level in his physical and cognitive development.

Joe's mother was seen in separate individual sessions during his attention training to encourage his mother to regard him in a more realistic light. Joe's mother was first introduced to the concept that as long as she and her husband treated him as if he were much younger, Joe would continue to be overly dependent (i.e., change would be beneficial to *him*.) Next, she was encouraged to observe her and her husband's actions at home that reinforced dependent behaviors (e.g., helping Joe when he did not need the help, accompanying him on school and church field trips, picking him up from school for emotional rather than physical reasons). A significant step was taken when Joe's parents were persuaded to allow him to accompany the cancer center group on a 3-day field trip to another city. He enjoyed his time and functioned appropriately. As the parents gained insight and began "letting go" of Joe, encouraging more independence, and the cognitive remediation therapist prompted him to take more responsibility for himself, Joe became more socially outgoing, self-responsible, and less angry than he had been.

Frequent conversations with parents of survivors and assessment of family functioning are essential in achieving positive results from psychotherapy. It would be most unusual in the general population to find a parent who would jump up to get a child or adolescent a glass of water, race up the stairs to find and bring down the child's missing shoe, or assist the child into his or her shirt. But, this type of overparenting is not uncommon among caregivers of childhood cancer survivors, and because children and adolescents do not recognize it as outside the norm, they are not likely to talk about it; hence, an individual child therapist would not be aware of parental practices. In addition, parents need to be given permission from the therapist to expect more from the survivor and to develop insight into the insidious effects of overindulgence. Generally, it takes several weeks or months for parents to develop insight into the matter and achieve a stance that is more age appropriate for their preteen and teenage children. Moreover, as noted, family and marital conflicts may need to be addressed to minimize the effects of these issues on the child.

The relationship between parent and child is complex, as documented by researchers attempting to improve child compliance and mother-child satisfaction by teaching mothers positive parenting practices, such as mirroring and praise (Wahler & Meginnis, 1997). Results demonstrated that there was significantly improved child compliance and dyadic satisfaction in the learner group compared with a control group; however, the only significant predictor of the improved compliance and dyadic satisfaction was the mother's responsiveness to her child, a basic process in effective parenting practices, as opposed to the specific behaviors taught. Rather than indulging a child who has been ill, parents may be effectively responsive to their children by listening to them, setting appropriate limits, being consistent in their expectations and following through on contingencied or desired behaviors, and generally showing respect to their children.

## Pharmacological

Given that attentional deficits, delayed information-processing speed, and processing efficacy are some of the most common neurocognitive impairments following the treatments of cranial irradiation and intrathecal chemotherapy, researchers have begun to explore the potential effectiveness of stimulant medications in the pediatric cancer survivor population. Methylphenidate hydrochloride (MPH) has been the classic medication used for children with attention deficit disorder with and without hyperactivity (Brown, 1998; Brown, Dingle, & Dreelin, 1997). Although newer forms of stimulant medications are being introduced into the market, MPH and its close molecular cousins remain a mainstay for the treatment of attentional difficulties for children and adults. MPH is a mixed dopaminergic-noradrenergic agonist that enhances function of the frontostriatal attentional network (Weber & Lutschg, 2002). Beneficial effects of MPH have been documented on measures of vigilance and sustained attention (Rapport, Denny, DuPaul, & Gardner, 1994) and in hastening reaction time and improved learning (Brown, 1998). Thus, given that these are also some of the more common deficits observed in survivors of many childhood cancers, it is intuitively attractive to expect that this medication would be effective in improving neurocognitive functioning in school performance in this population.

Although childhood cancer survivors as a group do not exhibit the behavioral difficulties of impulsivity and there is no evidence that these individuals have neurotransmitter system deficiencies, the behavioral phenotype does suggest that the stimulant medications may be beneficial in ameliorating attentional deficits in these children. Three studies have now been conducted using MPH as an intervention for childhood cancer survivors. A pilot study (DeLong, Friedman, Friedman, Gustafson, & Oakes, 1992) reported that 8 of 12 participants demonstrated a "good" response to MPH, two manifested a "fair" response, and two participants had a "poor" response. The researchers did not provide dose information, and the behavioral objective definition of response was not well defined. A second pilot study (Torres et al., 1996) reported on six participants who had received cranial irradiation for brain tumors. No significant immediate or delayed benefits to the patients were reported.

From a methodological perspective, the most sophisticated study was published by Thompson and coworkers (2001). This study investigated the effects of MPH using a randomized, double-blind trial with survivors of childhood cancer. Participants were over the age of 6 years and had completed all treatment at least 2 years prior to entry into the study. Potential participants with a diagnosis of attention deficit hyperactivity disorder prior to the occurrence of the malignancy were excluded from the trial. In addition, individuals under treatment with other psychotropic medications were excluded, as were those children with uncorrected endocrine difficulties or abnormal brain electrical activity. Thompson et al. reported significantly greater improvement following the administration of MPH when compared to a placebo condition on a continuous performance test of sustained attention. This was particularly salient in errors of omission. Reaction time remained unchanged, as did tendencies toward impulsivity. The two groups were not significantly different on measures of verbal and auditory learning.

Preliminary results suggest that pharmacological interventions may be appropriate and beneficial for some, if not many, survivors of childhood cancer. These survivors will have suffered neurocognitive involvement in attention and processing speed secondary to disease, CNS treatment, or a combination of both processes. The availability of newer medications that have fewer adverse side effects is especially attractive for this population. This is particularly important because, in our clinical experience, many parents do not wish to avail themselves of the option of stimulant medication. We have observed that these parents become averse to the continued use of various medications, likely, and not surprisingly, because of their experiences with extended chemotherapy treatments of their children. In relation to more demanding treatment regimens, such as cognitive remediation, pharmacological interventions may be a logistically attractive alternative, particularly if patients and their families live great distances from treatment centers. Alternatively, the combination of stimulant medication with cognitive remediation and psychotherapeutic efforts may result in synergistic benefits to some, if not many, patients.

In sum, preliminary results from both psychological and pharmacological interventions for childhood cancer survivors provide us with a beginning armamentarium of interventions that may be offered to families who have a child expressing neurocognitive deficits associated with their cancer diagnosis or treatment. These interventions were not available to families until the years immediately preceding publication of this book. Continued efforts at refinement and amplification of treatment benefits are likely to occur in the near future, and ongoing research is directed toward these endeavors.

## Integration and Future Directions

Given the significant advances realized by pediatric oncologists, many children are appreciating long-term survival and even cure from the two most common malignancies of childhood: acute lymphoblastic leukemia and brain tumors. Although oncologists are working toward increased survival rates and reduced treatment toxicities, pediatric psychologists now enjoy the luxury of developing interventions and treatment programs specifically tailored for this population. As documented in this text, a vast body of literature has accumulated on the nature of the neurocognitive and psychosocial impairment that may result following cancer and CNS child-related treatment. While a young field, brain injury rehabilitation directed toward pediatric patients after these CNS insults and resultant cognitive toxicities is rapidly expanding.

The traditional model of brain injury rehabilitation in adults and children has emphasized a team approach that includes physical therapy, occupational therapy, speech and language therapy, brain injury rehabilitation, psychotherapeutic interventions, and particularly for children and adolescents, familial interventions. Given the aforementioned evidence that family factors are extremely relevant for brain-injured pediatric patients, this traditional model will likely serve the pediatric oncology survivor well. We are, however, only now directing specific interventions for the family to reduce chaos and interpersonal dysfunction. In addition, the beneficial effects of pharmacological treatments along with cognitive remediation have not been systematically examined for empirical efficacy.

There is much work to be done, and randomized clinical trials are needed. A multidisciplinary approach is essential, in our view, for maximal treatment and intervention gains to be realized. We are on the frontier of an exciting field that will combine medical advances designed to manage treatment toxicity and psychological/pharmacological interventions that will enable maximal academic achievement and advancement in children and adolescents treated for a malignancy that involves brain function. Obviously, the goal of childhood cancer treatment is the eradication of the disease and cure without significant physical, fiscal, cognitive, and psychosocial dysfunction. While progress is being rallied, it is the aim of pediatric neuropsychologists and psychologists to maximize child and family functioning, adjustment, and quality of life if impairment is present.

*Acknowledgment.* Preparation of this manuscript was supported by grant NIH/NCI RO1 CA83936.

## References


Alderfer, M. A., Labay, L. E., & Kazak, A. E. (2003). Brief report: Does posttraumatic stress apply to siblings of childhood cancer survivors? *Journal of Pediatric Psychology, 28*, 281–286.

Altman, N., Briggs, R., Frankel, J., Gensler, D., & Pantone, P. (2002). *Relational child psychotherapy*. New York: Other Press.

Anderson, D. M., Rennie, K. M., Ziegler, R. S., Neglia, J. P., Robison, L. R., & Gurney, J. G. (2001). Medical and neurocognitive late effects among survivors of childhood central nervous system tumors. *Cancer, 92*, 2709–2719.

Barakat, L. P., Kazak, A. E., Gallagher, P. R., Meeske, K., & Stuber, M. (2000). Posttraumatic stress symptoms and stressful life events predict the long-term adjustment of survivors of childhood cancer and their mothers. *Journal of Clinical Psychology in Medical Settings, 7*, 189–196.

Beal, D., Mabbott, D., & Bouffet, E. (2003). Speech, language, and hearing difficulties. In N. Keene (Ed.), *Educating the child with cancer: A guide for parents and teachers* (pp. 69–76). Kensington, MD: Candlelighters Childhood Cancer Foundation.

Best, M., Streisand, R., Catania, L., & Kazak, A. E. (2001). Parental distress during pediatric leukemia and posttraumatic stress symptoms (PTSS) after treatment ends. *Journal of Pediatric Psychology, 26*, 299–307.

Blackorby, J., & Wagner, W. M. (1997). The employment outcomes of youth with learning disabilities: A review of findings from the National Longitudinal Transition Study of Special Education Students. In P. J. Gerber & D. S. Brown (Eds.), *Learning disabilities and employment* (pp. 57–74). Austin, TX: Pro-Ed.

Blatt, J., Copeland, D. R., & Bleyer, W. A. (1993). Late effects of childhood cancer and its treatment. In P. A. Pizzo & D. G. Poplack (Eds.), *Principles and practice of pediatric oncology* (2nd ed., pp. 1091–1114). Philadelphia: Lippincott.

Brown, R. T. (1998). Short-term cognitive and behavioral effects of psychotropic medications. In R. T. Brow & M. Sawyer (Eds.), *Medication for school children: Cognitive, academic, and behavioral effects*. New York: Guildford.

Brown, R. T., Dingle, A., & Dreelin, B. (1997). Neuropsychological effects of stimulant medication on children's learning and behavior. In C. R. Reynolds & E. Fletcher-Janzen (Eds.), *Handbook of clinical child pharmacology*. New York: Wiley.

Butler, R. W. (1998). Attentional processes and their remediation in childhood cancer. *Medical and Pediatric Oncology*, Suppl. 1, 75–78.

Butler, R. W., & Copeland, D. R. (2002). Attentional processes and their remediation in children treated for cancer: A literature review and the development of a therapeutic approach. *Journal of the International Neuropsychological Society, 8*, 113–124.

Butler, R. W., Rizzi, L. P., & Bandilla, E. B. (1999). The effects of childhood cancer treatment on two objective measures of psychological functioning. *Children's Health Care, 28*, 311–327.

Butler, R. W., & Satz, P. (1999). Depression and its diagnosis and treatment. In K. Langer, L. Laatsch, & L. Lewis (Eds.), *Psychotherapeutic interactions for adults with brain injury or stroke: A clinician's treatment resource* (pp 97–112). Madison, CT: Psychological Press.

Carlson-Green, B., Morris, R. D., & Krawiecki, N. (1995) Family and illness predictors of outcome in pediatric brain tumors. *Journal of Pediatric Psychology, 20*, 769–784.

*Childhood cancer survivor long-term follow-up guidelines*. (2003). Retrieved from www.childrens oncologygroup.org/disc/LE/pdf/SurvivorGuidelines9-03.pdf

DeLong, R., Friedman, H., Friedman, N., Gustafson, K., & Oakes, J. (1992). Methylphenidate in neuropsychological sequelae of radiotherapy and chemotherapy of childhood brain tumors and leukemia [letter]. *Journal of Child Neurology, 7*, 462–463.

D'Zurilla, T. J., & Nezu, A. M. (1999). *Problem-solving therapy: A social competence approach to clinical intervention*. New York: Springer.

Ellerton, M. L., Stewart, M. J., Ritchie, J. A., & Hirth, A. M. (1996). Social support in children with a chronic condition. *Canadian Journal of Nursing Research, 28*, 15–36.

Gartstein, M. A., Short, A. D., Vannatta, K., & Noll, R. B. (1999). Psychosocial adjustment of children with chronic illness: an evaluation of three models. *Journal of Developmental and Behavioral Pediatrics, 20*, 157–163.

Glover, D. A., Byrne, J., Mills, J. L., Robison, L. L., Nicholson, H. S., Meadows, A., et al. (2003). Impact of CNS treatment on mood in adult survivors of childhood leukemia: A report from the Children's Cancer Group. *Journal of Clinical Oncology, 21*, 4395–4401.

Hall, P. L., & Malpus, Z. (2000). Pets as therapy: Effects on social interaction in long-stay psychiatry. *British Journal of Nursing, 9*, 2220–2225.

Henderson, A. (1994). *A new generation of evidence: The family is critical to student achievement*. Washington, DC: National Committee for Citizens in Education.

Hetherington, E. M., & Martin, B. (1986). Family factors and psychopathology in children. In H. D. Quay and J. S. Werry (Eds.), *Psychopathological disorders of childhood* (pp. 332–389). New York: Wiley.

Hobbie, W. L., Stuber, M., Meeske, K., Wissler, K., Rourke, M. T., Ruccione, K., et al. (2000). Symptoms of posttraumatic stress in young adult survivors of childhood cancer. *Journal of Clinical Oncology, 18*, 4060–4066.

Hudson, M. M., Mertens, A. C., Yasui, Y., Hobbie, W., Chen, H., Gurney, J. G., et al. (2003). Health status of adult long-term survivors of childhood cancer. *Journal of the American Medical Association, 290*, 1583–1592.

Kazak, A. E., Barakat, L. P., Alderfer, M., Rourke, M. T., Meeske, K., Gallagher, P. R., et al. (2001). Posttraumatic stress in survivors of childhood cancer and mothers: Development and validation of the Impact of Traumatic Stressors Interview Schedule (ITSIS). *Journal of Clinical Psychology in Medical Settings, 8*, 307–323.

Kazak, A. E., Barakat, L. P., Meeske, K., Christakis, D., Meadows, A. T., Casey, R., et al. (1997). Posttraumatic stress, family functioning, and social support in survivors of childhood leukemia and their mothers and fathers. *Journal of Consulting and Clinical Psychology, 65*, 120–129.

Kendall, P. C. (Ed.). (1991). *Child and adolescent therapy: Cognitive-behavioral procedures*. New York: Guilford Press.

Kerns, K. A., & Thomson, J. (1998). Case study: Implementation of a compensatory memory system in a school age child with severe memory impairment. *Pediatric Rehabilitation, 2*, 77–87.

Lakoff, G., & Johnson, M. (1980). *Metaphors we live by*. Chicago: University of Chicago Press.

Levin, H. S., & Grafman, J. (Eds.). (2000). *Cerebral reorganization of function after brain damage*. New York: Oxford Press.

Lezak, M. D. (1978). Living with the characterological altered brain injured patient. *Journal of Clinical Psychiatry, 39*, 592–598.

Luria, A. R. (1963). *Restoration of function after brain injury*. New York: Pergamon.

Meichenbaum, D. (1977). *Cognitive-behavior modification: An integrative approach*. New York: Plenum Press.

Moore, I. M., Espy, K. A., Kaufmann, P., Kramer, J., Kaemingk, K., Miketova, P., et al. (2000). Cognitive consequences and central nervous system injury following treatment for childhood leukemia. *Seminars in Oncology Nursing, 16*, 279–290.

Nicholson, H. S., & Butler, R. (2001). Late effects of therapy in long-term survivors. In R. F. Keating, J. T. Goodrich, and R. Packer (Eds.), *Tumors of the pediatric central nervous system* (pp. 535–540). New York: Thieme.

Noll, R. B., Bukowski, W. M., Davies, W. H., Koontz, K., & Kulkarni, R. (1993). Adjustment in the peer system of children with cancer: A 2 year follow up study. *Journal of Pediatric Psychology, 18*, 351–364.

Noll, R. B., Bukowski, W. M., Rogosch, F. A., LeRoy, S., & Kulkarni, R. (1990). Social interactions between children with cancer and their peers: Teacher ratings. *Journal of Pediatric Psychology, 15*, 43–56.

Noll, R. B., Gartstein, M. A., Vannatta, K., Correll, J., Bukowski, W. M., & Davies, W. H. (1999). Social, emotional, and behavioral functioning of children with cancer. *Pediatrics, 103*, 71–78.

Noll, R. B., LeRoy, S., Bukowski, W. M., Rogosch, F. A., & Kulkarni, R. (1991). Peer relationships and adjustment in children with cancer. *Journal of Pediatric Psychology, 16*, 307–326.

Noll, R. B., MacLean, W. E., Jr., Whitt, J. K., Kaleita, T. A., Stehbens, J. A., Waskerwitz, M.J., et al. (1997). Behavioral adjustment and social functioning of long-term survivors of childhood leukemia: Parent and teacher reports. *Journal of Pediatric Psychology, 22*, 827–841.

Patterson, J., & Blum, R. W. (1996). Risk and resilience among children and youth with disabilities.

*Archives of Pediatrics and Adolescent Medicine, 150*, 692–698.

Perrin, E. C., Ayoub, C. C., & Willett, J. B. (1993). In the eyes of the beholder: Family and maternal influences on perceptions of adjustment of children with a chronic illness. *Journal of Developmental and Behavioral Pediatrics 14*, 94–105.

Pizzo, P. A., & Poplack, D. G. (Eds.), (1997). *Principles and practice of pediatric oncology*. Philadelphia: Lippincott.

Prigatano, G. P. (1999). *Principles of neuropsychological rehabilitation*. New York: Oxford University Press.

Rapport, M. D., Denny, C., DuPaul, G. J., & Gardner, M. J. (1994). Attention deficit disorder and methylphenidate: Normalization rates, clinical effectiveness, and response prediction in 76 children. *Journal of the American Academy of Child and Adolescent Psychiatry, 33*, 882–893.

Recklitis, C., O'Leary, T., & Diller, L. (2003). Utility of routine psychological screening in the childhood cancer survivor clinic. *Journal of Clinical Oncology, 21*, 787–792.

Reed, M. K. (1994). Social skills training to reduce depression in adolescents. *Adolescence, 29*, 293–302.

Roberts, C. S., Turney, M. E., & Knowles, A. M. (1998). Psychosocial issues of adolescents with cancer. *Social Work in Health Care, 27*, 3–18.

Sahler, O. J., Roghmann, K. J., Mulhern, R. K., Carpenter, P. J., Sargent, J. R., Copeland, D. R., et al. (1997). Sibling Adaptation of Childhood Cancer Collaborative Study: The association of sibling adaptation with maternal well being, physical health, and resource use. *Journal of Developmental and Behavioral Pediatrics, 18*, 233–243.

Sahler, O. J., Fairclough, D. L., Phipps, S., Mulhem, R. K., Dolgin, M. J., Noll, R. B., et al. (2005). Using problem-solving skills training to reduce negative affectivity in mothers of children with newly diagnosed cancer: report of a multisite randomized trial. *J Consult Clin Psychol, 73(2)*, 272–283.

Schatz, J., Kramer, J., Ablin, A., & Matthay, K. K. (2000). Processing speed, working memory, and IQ: A developmental model of cognitive deficits following cranial radiation therapy. *Neuropsychology, 14*, 189–200.

Schell, M. J., McHaney, V. A., Green, A. A., Kun, L. E., Hayes, F. A., Horowitz, M., et al. (1989). Hearing loss in children and young adults receiving cisplatinum with or without prior cranial irradiation. *Journal of Clinical Oncology, 7*, 754–760.

Silver, E. J., Bauman, L. J., & Ireys, H. T. (1995). Relationships of self-esteem and efficacy to psychological distress in mothers of children with chronic physical illnesses. *Health Psychology, 14*, 333–340.

Sohlberg, M. M., & Mateer, C. A. (1996). *Attention Process Training II (APT-II)*. Puyallup, WA: Association for Neuropsychological Research and Development.

Spieth, L. E., & Harris, C. V. (1996). Assessment of health-related quality of life in children and adolescents: An integrative review. *Journal of Pediatric Psychology, 21*, 175–193.

Stuber, M. L., Kazak, A. E., Meeske, K., Barakat, L., Guthrie, D., Garnier, H., et al. (1997). Predictors of posttraumatic stress symptoms in childhood cancer survivors. *Pediatrics, 100*, 958–964.

Thompson, S. J., Leigh, L., Christensen, R., Xioing, X., Kun, L. E., Heideman, R., et al. (2001). Immediate neurocognitive effects of methylphenidate on learning-impaired survivors of cancer. *Journal of Clinical Oncology, 19*, 1802–1808.

Torres, C., Korones, D., Palumbo, D., Wissler, K., Vadasz, E., & Cox, C. (1996). Effect of methylphenidate in the postradiation attention and memory deficits in children [abstract]. *Annals of Neurology, 40*, 331–332.

Vannatta, K, Gartstein, M. A., Short, A., & Noll, R. B. (1998). A controlled study of peer relationships of children surviving brain tumors: Teacher, peer and self ratings. *Journal of Pediatric Psychology, 23*, 279–287.

Varni, J. W., Burwinkle, T. M., Katz, E. R., Meeske, K., & Dickinson, P. (2002). The PedsQL™ in pediatric cancer: Reliability and validity of the Pediatric Quality of Life Inventory™ Generic Core scales, Multidimensional Fatigue scale, and Cancer module. *Cancer, 94*, 2090–2106.

Varni, J. W., Sahler, O. J., Katz, E. R., Mulhern, R. K., Copeland, D. R., Noll, R. B., et al. (1999). Maternal problem-solving therapy in pediatric cancer. *Journal of Psychosocial Oncology, 16*, 41–71.

Varni, J. W., Seid, M., & Kurtin, P. S. (2001). The PedsQL™ 4.0: Reliability and validity of the Pediatric Quality of Life Inventory™ Version 4.0 Generic Core scales in healthy and patient populations. *Medical Care, 39*, 800–812.

Wahler, R. G., & Meginnis, K. L. (1997). Strengthening child compliance through positive parenting practices: What works? *Journal of Clinical Child Psychology, 26*, 433–440.

Wallander, J. L., & Varni, J. W. (1998). Effects of pediatric chronic physical disorders on child and family adjustment. *Journal of Child Psychology and Psychiatry and Allied Disciplines, 39*, 29–46.

Weber, P., & Lutschg, J. (2002). Methylphenidate treatment. *Pediatric Neurology, 26*, 261–266.

Yeates, K. O., Taylor, H. G., Barry, C. T., Drotar, D., Wade, S. L., & Stancin, T. (2001). Neurobehavioral symptoms in childhood closed-head injuries: Changes in prevalence and correlates during the first year postinjury. *Journal of Pediatric Psychology*, *26*, 79–91.

Yeates, K. O., Taylor, H. G., Drotar, D., Wade, S. L., Stancin, T., Klein, S., et al. (1997). Pre-injury family environment as a determinant of recovery from traumatic brain injuries in school-age children. *Journal of the International Neuropsychological Society*, *3*, 617–630.

Zebrack, B. J., Zeltzer, L. K., Whitton, J., Mertens, A. C., Odom, L., Berkow, R., et al. (2002). Psychological outcomes in long-term survivors of childhood leukemia, Hodgkin's disease, and non-Hodgkin's lymphoma: A report from the Childhood Cancer Survivor Study. *Pediatrics, 110*, 42–52.

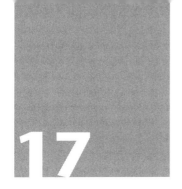

Ernest R. Katz and Avi Madan-Swain

# Maximizing School, Academic, and Social Outcomes in Children and Adolescents With Cancer

Medical advances incorporating intensive and difficult multimodal therapies have resulted in improved rates of survival in childhood cancer (Institute of Medicine, 2003). With improvements in disease management and survival, maintaining and enhancing maximal quality of life in young people living with cancer is the accepted psychosocial goal of comprehensive care (Armstrong & Briery, 2004; Institute of Medicine, 2003; Madan-Swain, Katz, & LaGory, 2004). As the primary venue for academic, cognitive, social, and emotional development during childhood and adolescence, ongoing participation and success in school are essential for positive health outcomes in young people (Brown, 2004; Madan-Swain et al., 2004). Actively engaging in school activities is an opportunity for the young person living with cancer and its often-difficult treatment to normalize an otherwise-disrupted life experience. School participation enhances quality of life and provides youths with hope for the future (Katz, 1980; Katz, Dolgin, & Varni, 1990; Katz, Kellerman, Rigler, Williams, & Siegel, 1977; Madan-Swain, Fredrick, & Wallender, 1999).

Cancer and its treatment have been associated with multiple school-related difficulties, including attendance problems, fatigue, pain, teasing and social isolation from peers, neurocognitive impairments, and academic deficiencies (Armstrong, 2003; R. Butler & Copeland, 2002; Katz, 1980; Katz et al., 1977; Katz, Rubinstein, Hubert, & Blew, 1988; Keene, 2003; Madan-Swain et al., 1999; Mitby et al., 2003; Spinetta & Deasy-Spinetta, 1986). Psychosocial factors such as single-parent families, high levels of maternal distress, and non-English-speaking immigrant families each may further negatively impact a family's ability to manage school and social difficulties experienced by their children (Madan-Swain et al., 2004; Madan-Swain, Katz, LaGory, 2004; Kazak et al., 1998; Mulhern, Wasserman, Friedman, & Fairclough, 1989; Sahler et al., 2005; Varni, Burwinkle, Katz, Meeske, & Dickinson, 2002).

School and social difficulties in children and adolescents with cancer can best be understood within the disability, stress, and coping theoretical model of pediatric chronic physical disorders proposed by Varni and Wallender (Varni & Wallender, 1988; Wallender & Varni, 1989). Cancer produces chronic strains for both children and parents. *Strains* are defined as persistent objective conditions that require continual readjustment, repeatedly interfering with the adequate

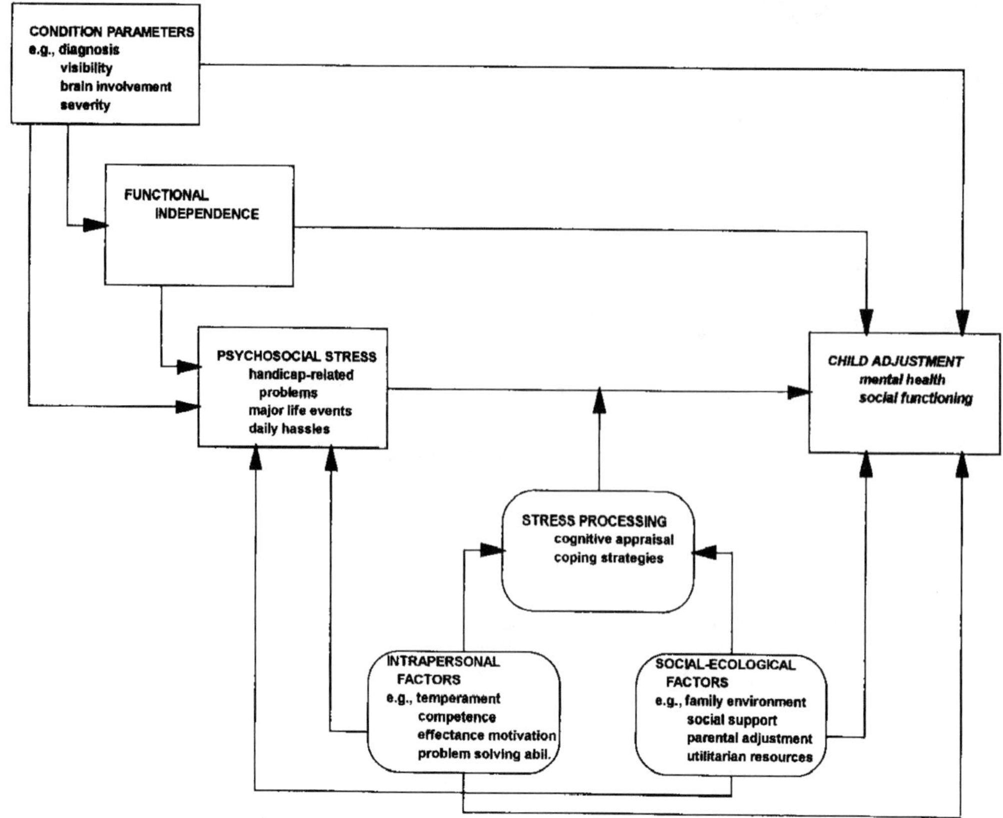


**Figure 17-1.** Varni-Wallender (1988) disability-stress-coping model of child adjustment to chronic illness.

performance of ordinary role-related activities such as school and social relationships. The chronic strains associated with childhood cancer include severe treatment-related pain and distress (e.g., recurrent bone marrow aspirations, lumbar punctures, chemotherapy); recurrent nausea/vomiting and fatigue; visible treatment-related adverse side effects (e.g., hair loss, weight gain, surgical disfigurement); multiple hospitalizations and clinic visits, leading to repeated and extended absences from school and peers; and neurocognitive/learning difficulties associated with illness or treatment of the central nervous system (CNS). These synergistically combine to have a negative impact on school and social adjustment (Varni & Katz, 1997; Varni, Katz, Colegrove, & Dolgin, 1994a, 1994b).

A major tenet of the Varni-Wallender model is that modifiable risk and resistance factors can be empirically identified. These factors provide heuristic guidance for the development of new treatment interventions for children with chronic physical disorders or chronic illness to promote and enhance resilience and positive health outcomes (see figure 17-1; Varni & Katz, 1997; Varni & Wallender, 1988). Risk factors include disease/disability parameters, functional independence, and psychosocial stress. Resistance factors are delineated into three categories: *intrapersonal factors* such as competence, temperament, and problem-solving ability; *sociologic factors* such as family and community social support; and *stress-processing factors* such as cognitive appraisal and coping strategies. Controlling and minimizing risk factors while increasing resistance and resilience factors through effective school and social intervention strategies can help improve school and social adjustment outcomes (Katz et al., 1988; Varni & Katz, 1997; Varni et al., 1994a, 1994b).

The Varni-Wallender model suggests that improving school and associated psychosocial functioning through effective support and intervention can have a positive impact on overall perceived quality of life and general health outcomes (Varni et al., 2002). A current measurement strategy in health-related quality of life (HRQOL) in children with cancer, the Pediatric Cancer Quality of Life Inventory (PedsQL), has incorporated school and social functioning as primary components in a multifactorial self-report and parent proxy report with children and adolescents at all stages of the illness experience (i.e., on treatment, off treatment, and long-term survivors). With data on healthy as well as multiple chronic illness populations, these measures indicate that children on active cancer treatment protocols have significantly more school, cognitive, and social difficulties than most comparison groups, with youths diagnosed with brain tumor experiencing the most problems (Eiser, Vance, Horne, Glaser, & Galvin, 2003; Meeske, Katz, Palmer, Burwinkle, & Varni, 2005; Varni et al., 2002; Varni, Burwinkle, Seid, & Skarr, in press).

HRQOL assessment that incorporates school and social experiences as integral components of overall adjustment and health outcomes in young people with cancer emphasizes the importance of these domains. Using brief HRQOL measures for screening and identification of youths experiencing school and social problems as well as for evaluating outcomes associated with school intervention strategies makes these measures an excellent choice as surveillance tools (www.pedsql.org; Varni et al., 2003).

This chapter review the major risk factors that may have an adverse impact on the child or adolescent with cancer in school participation, academic performance, and social interactions, as well as resistance factors associated with school and social adjustment. This heuristic framework is used to delineate a school reentry and intervention approach across various temporal phases constructed to maximize positive school and social outcomes. Finally, suggestions for future research and clinical directions in school and social reintegration are presented.

## Potential Risk Factors of Cancer on Learning and School Performance

### Disease or Treatment Involving the Central Nervous System

Findings from clinical investigations clearly indicated that some children and adolescents with cancer are at increased risk for school-related learning problems (Madan-Swain, & Brown, 1991; Madan-Swain et al., 2004; Mitby et al., 2003). This risk is greatest in youths who experience cognitive toxicities as a direct consequence of cancer affecting the brain (i.e., a brain tumor) or secondary to treatment, such as surgery, cranial irradiation, whole body radiation, or intrathecal chemotherapy used to prevent infiltration of the leukemia cells into the CNS (Armstrong, 2003; Brown et al., 1992, 1998; Mulhern & Palmer, 2003). The locus and extent of direct brain damage through disease or treatment will generally correlate with the level of school and functional impairment experienced by the child (Aicardi, 1998; Mulhern & Palmer, 2003; Raymond-Speden, Tripp, Lawrence, & Holdaway 2000). Females and children who are younger at time of treatment (generally under age 6 years) tend to have greater neruocognitive deficits (Armstrong & Briery, 2004; Brown et al., 1998; Mulhern & Palmer, 2003).

The well-documented body of literature examining the effects of radiation therapy and chemotherapy on cognitive functioning in children treated for brain tumors and leukemia indicates that the effects may be global for some children, although typically nonverbal abilities are affected more intensely than verbal abilities (Armstrong & Briery, 2004; Eiser & Tillman, 2001). The full impact of neurocognitive deficits usually takes several years to completely emerge and requires ongoing evaluation and advocacy to ensure that proper educational assistance is provided (Mulhern & Palmer, 2003; Ris, Packer, Goldwein, Jones-Wallace, & Boyett, 2001; Taylor, Buckner, Cascino, O'Fallon, Schaefer, Dinapoli, et al., 1998).

In the classroom setting, these neurocognitive deficits often result in the child or adolescent experiencing specific academic difficulties associated with underlying neural pathways, including the following:

1. *Variabilities in attention.* With impairments in one or more aspects of attention (i.e., sustained, selective, alternating, or divided), students may miss the beginning of statements or directions, may fail to orient themselves toward a new important signal (such as an assignment about to be given by the teacher), or may be easily distracted by noises or peer

behaviors. Inconsistency in the ability to focus and concentrate may cause them to miss out on important information throughout the school day. Patterns of school and learning performance may reveal idiosyncratic errors caused by fluctuating attention.

2. *Difficulties in memory.* The various dimensions of memory can be impaired by illness and treatment and may be further compromised by stress and anxiety. Short-term memory problems can make it difficult to remember multiple components of an instruction. Working memory difficulties can disrupt the sequential processing of a word or math problem. Long-term memory difficulties in storage and retrieval make it difficult to perform well on tests of cumulative knowledge.
3. *Difficulties completing tasks quickly secondary to decreased processing speed.* This can result in difficulty keeping pace with new material, taking notes during lectures, and requiring more time to complete assignments and examinations.
4. *Poor planning and organizational skills having an impact on the ability to self-monitor and complete projects independently.* This contributes to not bringing books and materials needed to class or home and consequently results in falling further behind classmates academically. Students also may have difficulty successfully completing long-term assignments such as projects and are inefficient in studying for tests.
5. *Difficulty writing quickly and accurately.* This will have an impact on written language skills and the ability to complete written assignments within a prescribed period of time.
6. *Difficulty copying or writing visual information, such as assignments written on a blackboard.* Difficulty with visual-motor integration will likely contribute to errors copying information or completing worksheets with a great deal of information.
7. *Difficulty learning visual information that is not verbally meaningful.* This may have an impact on mathematics involving symbols and sequencing.
8. *Problems with mathematics calculation skills.* Although affected children may understand math concepts, these children may experience difficulty with the smooth application of arithmetical algorithms (e.g., multiplication, division).
9. *Increased difficulty with reading comprehension.* Despite average-to-above-average word recognition and decoding skills, survivors may have difficulty with reading comprehension, particularly inferential comprehension. This is most apparent when material is increasingly long and complex (Armstrong & Briery, 2004; R. Butler & Copeland, 2002; Copeland & Butler, 2003; Cousens, Ungerer, Crawford, & Stevens, 1991; Deasy-Spinetta, 1981; Mulhern & Palmer, 2003; White, 2003).

Neurocognitive deficits may also impair social interactions. Problems maintaining social discourse that relies on detecting and responding to subtle social cues have been associated with difficulties in peer and social relationships, particularly for youths diagnosed with brain tumors (Vanatta, Gartstein, & Noll, 1998). Such nonverbal learning disabilities may impair the child's abilities to comprehend subtle social and emotional cues from peers, leading to inappropriate responses. This behavior may result in either teasing or social isolation by peers (LaGreca, Bearman, & Moore, 2004; Nassau & Drotar, 1997). Uninformed teachers may interpret the child's difficulties with social and academic tasks as a lack of motivation or interest in complying with classroom requirements rather than associating them with the diagnosis or treatment (Mulhern & Palmer, 2003). Such unsupportive responses from teachers and school personnel may further impair the child's self-esteem and adaptability (Madan-Swain et al., 2004).

## General Effects of Illness and Treatment

Children and adolescents receiving medical treatment for cancer may experience a number of acute and long-term consequences of the disease and treatment that have an impact on emotional, social, and academic functioning. Chemotherapy and radiation therapy may have acute adverse side effects that are transient as well as other adverse side effects that may be lifelong, with the magnitude of adverse effects increasing over time (Keene, Hobbie, & Ruccione, 2000).

The most common adverse side effects are those that alter the appearance of children and adolescents. Loss of hair, bloating and puffiness secondary to treatment with steroids, weight loss or gain, chemotherapy-related nausea and vomiting, decreased stature, or use of prosthetic limbs because of amputation are obvious physical signs to the child's classmates and teachers that they are undergoing cancer treatment. These may lead to social interactional difficulties (Katz & Varni, 1993). In a prospective study of children with cancer undergoing treatment, Varni, Katz, Colegrove, and Dolgin (1995) determined that perceived physical appearance has direct and indirect effects on depressive symptoms and social anxiety, mediated by general self-esteem.

Hearing deficits are associated with specific chemotherapy agents and may adversely impact the understanding of spoken language necessary for learning and social discourse (Keene et al., 2000). Visual impairments may occur as a direct result of disease involving the eye or optic nerves (e.g., retinoblastoma or brain tumor) or cataracts associated with total body irradiation for stem cell transplantation (Keene et al., 2000). Less-obvious adverse side effects associated with treatment also may occur, such as fatigue, emotional difficulties, hormonal deficiencies, sterility, and increased susceptibility to life-threatening infections. Although some of these adverse side effects may be short term, they also represent sources of disability that may persist throughout the child's life (Armstrong & Horn, 1995; Armstrong & Briery, 2004; Deasy-Spinetta, 1997; Keene et al., 2000; Varni et al., 2002).

## Immigrant Parents With Limited Educational Background

Healthy children from immigrant families have been found to experience many challenges to their educational success (Hernandez & Charney, 1998). Coming from homes where English is not the main spoken language, children and their parents may not have the ability to communicate easily or directly with school personnel. Parents from many foreign countries do not understand the culture of schools, and that it is acceptable for parents to request services for their child even when they may not be offered by school authorities. Immigrant families tend to settle in large urban areas that may have troubled school districts that cannot easily meet the needs of healthy immigrant children. When a serious childhood illness is added into the mix of adjustment issues facing an immigrant family, difficulties in communication with school personnel and obtaining specialized support or services for their child can easily be overwhelming (Katz et al., 1988; Madan-Swain et al., 2004).

For some immigrant parents who themselves have had very limited schooling, maintaining the ill child or adolescent at home rather than returning to a regular school campus may appear to be a simpler option. Cultural norms may dictate that these parents be more inclined to shelter the ill child within a supportive family. They also may perceive continued school experience as too taxing for the ill child rather than a positive component of the child's overall adjustment and quality of life (Madan-Swain et al., 2004).

Having a child diagnosed with cancer may be viewed as a benefit by some families in that the family may receive access to services and resources that they otherwise might not have had prior to their child's illness (Madan-Swain et al., 2004). Hospital personnel may assist in helping the family to access community resources for all family members, including school (e.g., securing necessary special education services for a sibling of a child with cancer). Care must be taken to help such families maintain the benefits gained secondary to the cancer diagnosis so that they do not sabotage the child's recovery (Katz, 1980).

## Preexisting Academic or Social Problems

Children and adolescents with preexisting learning problems such as a learning disability, attention-deficit/hyperactivity disorder, or a developmental delay are at greater risk for school reentry and continuing problems because cancer and its treatments may exacerbate these premorbid difficulties (Katz, 1980; Katz et al., 1977; Madan-Swain et al., 2004). In addition, children whose parents were only minimally involved with their child's school prior to the illness may also experience educational disadvantages after a cancer diagnosis. These parents may lack the knowledge, communication skills, or experience regarding school procedures to know how to access help when problems are encountered (Madan-Swain et al., 2004). This difficulty may be compounded when parents do not speak English (Hernandez & Charney, 1998).

Academic deficits after the onset of disease and treatment are most likely to be manifested in skill areas that build on previous knowledge, which may have initially been weak (Chekryn, Deegan, & Reid, 1987). Academic difficulties will be compounded by gaps in knowledge and classroom experiences sustained during absences, periods of not feeling well, and neurocognitive effects of illness and treatment (Madan-Swain et al., 2004). Similarly, gaps in social and peer relationships make it difficult for many students with cancer to make a smooth transition back to school without assistance (Bessel, 2001; Katz et al., 1988). Youths who are cognizant of changes in their school performance become increasingly anxious, and this serves to exacerbate learning difficulties and social relationships (White, 2003). For children who were only marginally academically or socially successful prior to the onset of the illness, the effects of prolonged or even brief absences may be especially disruptive to learning and social relationships (Katz, 1980; Madan-Swain et al., 2004).

### Absenteeism

Children and adolescents with cancer often miss extended periods of school because of illness, adverse side effects associated with treatment and immunosuppression, hospitalizations, and outpatient clinic appointments. Rates of absenteeism that are four times higher than that of the general school-age population have been found for children with cancer (Stehbens, Kisker, & Wilson, 1983). This is characterized by one prolonged period of absence at the time of diagnosis and treatment initiation, followed by periodic or short-term absences for chemotherapy, medical procedures, treatment side effects (e.g., fever and neutropenia), or clinic visits to monitor progress (Charlton et al., 1991).

Numerous factors have been associated with absenteeism in children with cancer. Demographic factors also have been associated with lower rates of school attendance, including parental education (Charlton et al., 1991; Cook, Schaller, & Krischer, 1985); gender (i.e., female) (Cairns, Klopovich, Hearne, & Lansky, 1982; Charlton et al., 1991; Fowler, Johnson, & Atkinson, 1985); and birth position (Cairns et al., 1982). Psychosocial factors associated with increased absenteeism include parental reluctance to allow their ill child to return to school, even when medically approved, secondary to their lack of confidence in the school's capacity to be responsive to their child's needs, fears that school attendance may worsen the medical condition, or a sense of hopelessness about their child's future and doubts regarding the benefits of regular school attendance (Katz, 1980). Difficulties coordinating communication among hospital, home, and school, resulting in a perceived lack of support and understanding from school personnel, also contribute to increased absenteeism (Bessel, 2001; Katz et al., 1977, 1980; Katz et al., 1988; Lansky, Lowman, Vata, & Gyulay, 1975).

### Intraindividual Psychological Adjustment

Psychosocial and emotional factors have a significant impact on attendance and influence the child's ability to engage effectively in the academic process or social milieu while at school. Prolonged absences with little peer contact create social discomfort for the child or adolescent with cancer (Bessel, 2001). Illness-related stress, generalized psychological distress, concerns about peer reactions to physical changes, and the lack of confidence in both physical and academic abilities may detract from the child's willingness to attend school and to perform when present (Davis, 1989). Frequently, these issues are developmentally related, with adolescents more sensitive to treatment-related adverse side effects that make them seem different from their peers (Zeltzer, 1993).

Anxiety over returning to school is typical for a child or adolescent confronted with major physical changes, such as hair loss secondary to chemotherapy, disfigurement, or amputation (Armstrong & Briery, 2004; Katz, 1977, 1980). Physical limitations hindering full participation in regular school and extracurricular activities may contribute to difficulties in self-concept and a willingness to interact with peers that ultimately hamper school return and participation (Henning &

Fritz, 1983; Varni et al., 1994a, 1995). While the fear of peer rejection associated with physical changes and being "different" may peak prior to the child's initial return to school, difficult peer reactions such as shunning or avoidance because of inaccurate information and attitudes may add to the child's emotional distress after returning to the school setting (Chekryn et al., 1987; Davis, 1989; Katz, Varni, Rubinstein, Blew, & Hubert, 1992).

A fairly complicated emotional obstacle to school reentry is parent and child separation anxiety following a lengthy period of restriction from regular school attendance because of immunosuppression or disease instability (Katz, 1980; Madan-Swain et al., 1999). It may be very difficult for parents to shift their mind-set from hypervigilance and protection of the medically fragile child to encourage school attendance and independence when the child is deemed medically able after months or even years of vulnerability (Katz, 1980: Madan-Swain et al., 2004; Nessim & Katz, 2003). Parents who experience greater feelings of vulnerability regarding their child tend to have children with higher levels of separation anxiety and school avoidance (Katz, 1980; Madan-Swain et al., 1999). The symptom onset of separation anxiety may begin with somatic complaints, initially leading to parent-sanctioned school absences and ultimately to school refusal.

## Socioecological Resistance Factors

### Maternal Adjustment

Studies of social and emotional adjustment among parents of children with cancer suggested that mothers are at risk for anxiety and depression as well as posttraumatic stress symptoms (Hall & Baum, 1995; Overholser & Fritz, 1990; Noll et al., 1995; Pelcovitz et al., 1996; Stuber, Christakis, Houskamp, & Kazak, 1996). Maternal symptoms of distress appear to be most prevalent during the period immediately following their child's diagnosis (Sahler et al., 2002; Wallender & Varni, 1992) but may persist even years after completion of treatment.

The emotional adjustment of children has been associated with parental, especially maternal, reports of their own mental and physical health (Hetherington & Martin, 1986; Zeltzer et al., 1996); health beliefs (Perrin, Ayoub, & Willet, 1993); coping strategies (Sanger, Copeland, & Davidson, 1991); and perceptions of family and community social support (Morrow, Hoagland, & Carnrike, 1981). Research to date suggested that increased social support of parents (especially mothers) serves as a buffer to protect parents from the adverse impact of stress. In turn, better adjusted parents serve as a buffer for their children, helping to protect them from the deleterious stressful effects of the cancer diagnosis and its associated treatment. In fact, family functioning and extrafamilial social support are significant predictors of adjustment in children newly diagnosed with cancer (Varni, Katz, Colegrove, & Dolgin, 1996; Varni & Katz, 1997) and their siblings (Sahler et al., 1997).

### Peer Social Support

Peers play a critical protective and supportive role in facilitating the school reentry and adjustment of chronically ill children and adolescents (La Greca et al., 2004). The impact of cancer on school experience is decreased if peer support is encouraged and not disrupted (Varni, Katz, Colgrove, & Dolgin, 1993; Varni et al., 1994a). However, this protective factor may become a risk factor if the child or adolescent with cancer becomes socially isolated because of frequent absenteeism (Varni et al., 1994b).

Any major physical change threatens the child's body image, self-concept, and ultimately self-esteem, potentially causing discomfort in peer relations (LaGreca et al., 2004). Adolescents particularly express specific concerns about the changes in their appearance, fears of peer ridicule or teasing, and discomfort in discussing the illness with classmates and teachers (Zeltzer, 1993).

Varni et al. (1994a) studied the association between various types of social support and psychological adjustment in 32 newly diagnosed school-aged children with cancer, excluding brain tumors. Perceived classmate social support was the most consistent predictor of adaptation, providing evidence for the essential function of the school's social environment. The child's perceived stress and social support accounted for 62% of the variance in negative affectivity (anxiety and depression) at 9 months following diagnosis.

These investigators also conducted a randomized trial of a social skills intervention program for newly diagnosed children with cancer (Varni, Katz, Colgrove, & Dolgin, 1993). Findings revealed that social skills training was associated with higher perceived classmate and teacher social support and better overall psychological adjustment. Therefore, decreasing a child's perceived stress and increasing the child's perceived social support through effective school intervention can help increase adjustment and improve health-related quality of life.

A growing body of literature indicates that children with brain tumors experience significantly greater difficulties in peer relationships. This is related to problems with cognitive processing, more obvious academic impairments, and difficulties in understanding and reacting to subtle social cues (Mitby et al., 2003; Vanatta et al., 1998). Therefore, the need for effective cognitive remediation and social skills intervention in school is significantly more acute for this group of children and adolescents than for the cancer population at large (Butler & Copeland, 2002).

### Familial and Cultural Resources

Among children previously treated for leukemia, several studies have demonstrated that higher familial socioeconomic status is positively associated with intellectual functioning and other neurocognitive outcomes (Butler, Hill, & Steinherz, 1994; Mulhern & Palmer, 2003; Rubinstein, Varni, & Katz, 1990). These findings are similar to studies of healthy children, which demonstrated that up to 28% of the variance in intelligence can be predicted by parental education. School performance and adjustment is generally facilitated in families and cultures that place high emphasis on education and educational pursuits (Hernandez & Charney, 1998). Established families and communities are generally better able than are immigrant families to serve the educational needs of youths in providing a consistent and supportive environment for learning (Gortmaker, Walker, Weitzman, & Sobel, 1990). However, immigrant families who have succeeded in their acculturation process and acclimation to life in their new country, including the mastery of systems and processes associated with their child's education, have children who achieve better educational outcomes (Fuligni, 1997). Together, these data suggest that a child's family environment may modify secondary neurocognitive deficits in children with cancer, even among children with similar core deficits (Mulhern & Palmer, 2003).

### School and Academic Environment

Teachers and school administrators are the individuals most directly responsible for the school experience of a child with a special health care need. Educating school personnel regarding the child's reentry and ongoing school and socioemotional needs enables the teacher to better assist the child and family in school adjustment by helping peers be more accepting and to facilitate accessing necessary special services (Katz et al., 1992). Teachers need to be aware of personal reactions to an emotionally charged "cancer" diagnosis in a student because this will have an impact on their ability to set fair and realistic educational goals (Varni et al., 1993). Some teachers may require assistance to ensure that personal feelings do not adversely impact their relationship with the child (Katz et al., 1990; Madan-Swain et al., 2004).

### Stress Processing

Preeminent among the potentially modifiable resistance factors identified in the Varni-Wallender model is the concept of perceived stress (Varni et al., 1994b). Perceived stress derives from the theoretical model of Lazarus and Folkman (1984), in which the individual's subjective cognitive appraisal determines which events are perceived as stressful and which may be perceived as manageable. It is the *meaning* of an event or experience, rather than its mere occurrence, that may result in a child's perception of it being stressful or not. In a study of 39 survivors of childhood cancer, Varni et al. (1994b) demonstrated that higher perceived stress was associated with increased psychological distress and lower general self-esteem, even after controlling for relevant demographic and medical variables. These findings support the notion that children with cancer who perceive less stress associated with their illness and treatment will adjust better in their school and social relationships (Wallender & Varni, 1992).

## Intervention to Maximize School and Social Outcomes

### Federal Laws Protecting the Educational Rights of Children With Disabilities

Ensuring reentry and adjustment to school requires careful understanding and examination of a child's academic needs and available resources through general and special education programs. The goal of school intervention is to meet the child's learning and social needs in the least-restrictive educational environment (i.e., most like a regular classroom with nondisabled peers; Monaco & Smith, 2003). Four federal laws protect the educational rights of children between birth and 21 years of age who have disabilities that impede their ability to benefit from their educational environment. These laws are the Individuals With Disability Education Act (IDEA; 1990), the Rehabilitation Act (Section 504), the Americans With Disabilities Act (ADA), and the No Child Left Behind Act. These laws apply to every level of education, from early intervention to college and vocational training, and the laws guarantee every child a right to education regardless of physical, mental, or health impairment (Deasy-Spinetta, 1997; Wright & Wright, 2002; Wright, Wright, & Heath, 2003).

#### *IDEA: Overview*

IDEA is a revision of an earlier law, P.L. 94-142 (Education of the Handicapped Act) and establishes an array of educational services available for children who have disabilities who require special education so that they may maximize their potential and attain the educational goals set for all students. To receive special education under the provision of IDEA, children with cancer must qualify for 1 of 13 special education classifications that delineate criteria for eligibility (Deasy-Spinetta, 1997). "Other health impaired" is the classification commonly applied to youths diagnosed with cancer when their disease or treatment have an adverse impact on their ability to perform in school.

*Determining Eligibility.* Children suspected of needing services are referred to the multidisciplinary evaluation team at the child's regular school. If the child with cancer has received neuropsychological, physical, or occupational therapy evaluations while in the hospital, the parent or school liaison, with parental permission, can provide these reports to the appropriate school personnel. A letter from the treating oncologist regarding diagnosis, treatment course, and any illness or treatment-related impairments also is helpful. Some school systems require the oncologist to complete a standard form verifying the eligibility to receive services through the classification of other health impaired.

*Individualized Education Plan Development and Monitoring.* The multidisciplinary evaluation team reviews the data, and if the child is deemed eligible for special education services, a meeting is scheduled to design their individualized education plan (IEP). At minimum, this meeting should include the parents, the child's regular and special education teachers, and a school administrator. It is helpful to have someone from the hospital, possibly the school liaison, at the meeting to ensure that the pertinent aspects of the child's medical care, illness, and any transient and chronic impairment are well understood by the IEP team. The IEP constructed at the meeting must consist of certain elements: present level of cognitive and academic functioning and statement of need as identified by the assessments; annual goals and objectives, including procedures for evaluating whether the objectives are met; and educational placement and the amount of time allocated for participation in the regular classroom. The plan also should address the child's ability to participate in the state- or districtwide achievement tests and a statement regarding necessary accommodations (e.g., increased time). Also necessary is the delineation of transition services for youths aged 14 years and older.

After the IEP is signed by all participants at the meeting, it becomes a legal document that by law the state is required to carry out. The plan is evaluated on a yearly basis with a reevaluation of appropriateness of eligibility for special education services performed no less than every 3 years. The parents can call for an IEP meeting at any time to review their child's educational program.

IDEA also mandates early intervention services for infants and toddlers who are either disabled or at risk of developmental delays. These services are provided either by the school systems or by the state health department. The law requires that services be provided to affected children and their families. Hence, rather than an IEP, an individual family service plan is written.

### *Section 504*

*Overview.* Although Section 504 of the Rehabilitation Act of 1973 (reauthorized in 1998) is not an education law or a federal grant program, it does contain a provision that allows schools to develop intervention plans specific to meeting student needs without necessarily identifying these students as eligible for special education services. Students requiring only minor environmental and instructional accommodation services are best served through this law. Section 504 protects all qualified students with disabilities, defined as those having any "physical or mental impairment that substantially limits one or more major life activities (including learning)." Students who meet this definition are covered, even if they do not fall within the IDEA-designated categories and even if they do not participate in specific special education programs. For example, a newly diagnosed student with leukemia may not be covered under IDEA if he does not require specially designed instruction (special education services). However, for the purposes of Section 504, this student may be considered disabled because he is limited in the performance of a life activity (e.g., learning, because of frequent treatment-related absences). This law applies to private schools, colleges, and universities that receive federal funds.

*Determining Eligibility and Obtaining Services.* A referral should be made to the Section 504 coordinator for the school system by either the parent or a member of the medical treatment team. To expedite a quick review, the school should be provided with all pertinent medical information as well as neuropsychological or psychological testing completed at the hospital. Following data collection, the Section 504 coordinator convenes a meeting to analyze the evaluation data and determine the child or adolescent's eligibility to receive services. If eligibility criteria are met, then necessary accommodations are designated in a personalized education plan and implemented in the classroom. Each student's accommodations and or services are reviewed periodically.

Because the legal obligations of 504 plans are outside the perview of IDEA 1997, the law governing provision of services in special education programs, the opportunities to develop, prescribe, and obtain such plans are usually not as difficult as when special education services are needed. However, by the same token, the level and frequency of developing 504 plans is variable across school districts and somewhat dependent on the degree of child advocacy. Because school districts do not view 504 plans as having the full force of legal protections for either the child or the school, many districts do not readily agree to the development and implementation of 504 plans and prefer instead to have students identified under the legal mandate of IDEA.

### *Americans With Disabilities Act*

The ADA of 1990 provides a wide range of protection for all individuals with disabilities. All students with cancer, even long-term survivors, are eligible for protection under the provisions of ADA. It prohibits discrimination against individuals with disabilities and applies to all state and local agencies (not just those receiving federal funds), including private businesses. Although it is not an education law, its provisions do apply to education, including nonsectarian private schools. It provides a second layer of protection, in addition to Section 504, to ensure that public schools provide reasonable accommodations for students with disabilities.

### *No Child Left Behind*

The federal No Child Left Behind Act requires schools to teach all children to proficiency in reading, mathematics, and science by 2014. Key requirements of the law include proficiency testing in Grades 3–8; highly qualified teachers in every classroom; research-based instruction; increased parental rights; public school choice; and state, district, and school report cards (Wright et al., 2003). This law includes children with special health care needs and provides parents, school personnel, and advocates more leverage to help ensure that a child with cancer is meeting educational objectives.

## School Support Services Available Through General and Special Education

Based on their needs and as mandated by the laws outlined here, youths diagnosed with cancer may need minor-to-major modifications in their educational programs. The level and intensity of school accommodations will vary based on the child's pre-illness academic and social functioning, the impact of illness and treatment on learning, and the ability of adults assisting the child to access available resources and ensure their successful application, as discussed next.

### *Assessment Process*

To ensure that every child continues to receive an appropriate education, a careful assessment of learning needs and social functioning should be completed (Armstrong & Briery, 2004). This is particularly important for youth receiving CNS treatment for cancer or brain tumors. Conventional approaches to evaluation and determination of educational needs are often based on static concepts of learning disabilities that rely heavily on discrepancies between intellectual functioning and academic achievement. Learning deficits also are considered stable. For children treated for CNS cancer, these assumptions may be inaccurate and may lead to psychological assessments that do not provide information helpful to the child or school system. It is inappropriate to rely on a one-time assessment to determine the academic functioning and educational needs of these children. Rather, evaluation of the child with CNS cancer should be considered a process, with planned reevaluations every 18–24 months, or as clinically indicated, to appropriately track the developmental emergence of new areas of difficulty.

To appropriately plan for the educational needs of the child receiving CNS treatment for cancer or brain tumors, thorough baseline and serial evaluations need to be conducted. In addition, assessment should be carefully planned and completed by a pediatric psychologist, a neuropsychologist, or a school psychologist knowledgeable about the neurocognitive difficulties. Formal assessment should be complemented with criterion-referenced assessment completed by the classroom teacher (Madan-Swain et al., 2004). Reliance on age-appropriate measures of intellectual functioning and academic achievement, although necessary to meet local, state, and federal eligibility guidelines, often provide insufficient data for education planning. For these children, the evaluation should also include tests of specific functional abilities likely to be affected by craniospinal radiation or intrathecal chemotherapy over time, as well as tests of specific functional abilities that are unlikely to be affected, representing strengths of the child in the educational setting. In addition, the assessment battery should include evaluation of potential areas of functioning that may not be detected as impaired at the time of the evaluation but will likely be expected to demonstrate impairment at some point in time.

The assessment tools selected for the psychoeducational evaluation are critical. Typically, global measures of intellectual and cognitive functioning are not likely to be adequate indicators of the needs of children who receive CNS treatment or have brain tumors. Instead, the assessment battery should include neurocognitive measures of processing speed, cognitive flexibility, attention and concentration, language, memory, and visual-spatial and visual-motor abilities. This will allow the development of an educational plan that not only targets weaknesses but also builds on areas of strength. Teachers need to be aware that the child may have difficulty with the development of skills, and for this reason the educational program should strengthen those skills present at the time of treatment and foster the development of strategies to aid in the acquisition of later skills.

### *Categories of Learning and Social Needs*

Based on the nature of the child's pre-illness school and social functioning, along with potential illness- and treatment-related learning and social deficits, appropriate educational planning is necessary. The following categories outline degree of impairment and potential educational intervention for both learning and social deficits.

1. *No preexisting learning or social difficulties.* Students with cancer who have no premorbid learning or social difficulties will likely experience *transient* school problems. Planning for school reentry should focus on returning to their general education classrooms and school, with potential minor modifications that can be implemented by the teachers and staff.

   For the majority of youths, these modifications may be made through Section 504. Some typical accommodations because of frequent absences caused by hospitalizations may include dual homebound/school-based schooling during treatment, a modified class schedule of only half days or a 2- to 3-day week, and decreased or modified classroom and homework assignments. Resource teachers and tutors on a school campus can assist children and adolescents in bridging the repeated gaps associated with absences. However, this requires considerable coordination to ensure continuity of instruction and opportunities for social interactions. Occasionally, environmental adaptations for children requiring walking devices or adjustments in school rules (e.g., allowing hats for those students who have lost their hair secondary to medical treatment and the provision of a quiet rest when children become fatigued during periods of low counts or pain crises) are necessary (Armstrong & Horn, 1995).

In addition to instructional program consideration, children should be allowed to use technology as an aid or to adapt procedures as needed (e.g., tape recorders for lectures, word processors to complete written assignments; and calculators for mathematics). Equally important is the removal of time constraints and writing requirements in test taking.

2. *Preexisting learning or social problems.* Children and adolescents with premorbid learning problems, such as attention-deficit disorder, specific learning disabilities, developmental disabilities, or visual or hearing impairments, will likely experience more difficulty returning to their regular school programs secondary to treatment-related absences and exacerbation of premorbid difficulties. Typically, youths in this category will have had some level of formal classroom accommodations or special education services prior to their illness that may need to be adjusted to account for new illness- and treatment-related challenges. Educational services for youths in this group will likely include a combination of special education services through IDEA or services through Section 504.
3. *Previously undetected preexisting learning and social difficulties.* Some children may have had previously undetected learning problems that have now been identified during their intensive medical treatment and individualized contact with homebound teachers and hospital specialists (e.g., pediatric psychologists, child life specialists, social workers). Children from immigrant, non-English-speaking households or families who have moved frequently before the illness with the child having no continuous school connections tend to be overrepresented in this category. Depending on the severity of the difficulties, these children and adolescents will require school accommodations and services through Section 504 or special education services through IDEA.
4. *Acquired disease- or treatment-related learning or social problems.* Children who have acquired functional disabilities because of illness or treatment, progressive medical complications, or the end stage of their illness will require more individualized educational assistance to maintain their involvement in school and maximize their potential (Katz & Ingle-Nelson, 1989; Madan-Swain et al., 1999). For example, neurocognitive impairments associated with brain tumors or CNS therapy for leukemia, which have an impact on learning new information or mobility, are at greatest risk for acquired disabilities (cf. Disease or Treatment Involving the Central Nervous System. Visible changes may go beyond hair loss and include the use of a wheelchair, prosthesis, or assistive technology.

Although a child may have been in a regular education program prior to his or her illness, the child may now require specialized instructional services through special education as well as related therapies (i.e., occupational and physical therapy, speech and language therapy, etc.). Service delivery is organized on a continuum of inclusion, ranging from providing all services within the general education classroom through full residential treatment services. Typically, in schools the nature of services includes some combination of services in the regular classroom as well as resource (through either inclusion or pull-out) and support services.

School reentry is likely to be more complex for this group, requiring intensive cooperative efforts among health care providers, school personnel, the child or adolescent, and the family (Madan-Swain et al., 1999; Shields, Heron, Rubenstein, & Katz, 1995).

## Systematic Phases of School Intervention

The process of school reentry during active treatment, and ongoing academic success as a student throughout the illness experience and beyond, requires ongoing cooperation, coordination, and vigilance among the child and family, health care team, teachers and school personnel, and peers (Katz et al., 1988; Sexson, & Madan-Swain, 1993; Shields et al., 1995). Each participant is an integral component to effective school and social adjustment in children and adolescents with cancer. Successful school reentry requires an appreciation for the unique needs of each individual child or adolescent, ensuring maximal academic and social skills development through appropriate modifications of the school environment and assisting parents to be effective advocates for their children.

School reentry programs typically share the common goal of preparing the child diagnosed with cancer, the family, and school personnel for transition back into the routine of attending school (Davis, 1989; Henning & Fritz, 1983; Katz et al., 1988; McCarthy, Willimas, & Plumer, 1998; Ross, 1984). These programs serve to establish a formal liaison function between various systems. Programs vary in terms of the formality and structure of services provided, but all approaches emphasize intersystem coordination (Katz et al., 1988, 1992; McCarthy et al., 1998).

The eco-triadic model of educational consultation (Shields et al., 1995) provides a framework for a designated school liaison person who is a member of the health care team in conducting multisystemic collaboration for young people with cancer. Because educational and medical systems are so complex and confusing to parents and professionals alike, a designated liaison can help facilitate intersystem cooperation. By closely collaborating and exchanging information among the child and the child's family, medical team, and school, the liaison helps anticipate potential difficulties in the school reentry and maintenance process and assists in increasing the likelihood of successful school and social outcomes.

Katz and colleagues developed a comprehensive approach to school and social reintegration of children with cancer that includes the following components (Katz et al., 1977, 1988; Nessim & Katz, 2003):

1. Early preventive education of children, parents, and school personnel about the realities of cancer and its treatment, the importance of ongoing school participation, and planning for continued school involvement.
2. Short-term counseling for children and parents to help them cope with the emotional demands of returning to school and to prepare for likely educational and social challenges. This helps to empower children and parents to succeed by creating a positive expectation for success at school.
3. Establishing a working liaison among the health care team, the child and family, and the teachers to ensure that accurate information is readily available and the child's medical and academic needs are considered conjointly.
4. Informing and supporting classmates to understand what their peer is going through and dispelling myths and misconceptions about cancer and its treatment. Open communication and dialogue are facilitated to support cancer as a treatable, noncontagious disease.
5. Assisting in the accurate assessment of children with special learning needs and ensuring their access to remedial educational interventions at school.
6. Providing ongoing follow-up with the child, parents, and school to ensure that continuing school success is achieved and to deal proactively with any school or learning issues that may arise later as a result of the illness and treatment.

In the only controlled investigation to date of a school reentry program for children with cancer, Katz and colleagues (1988) found that children and adolescents who received a structured intervention program exhibited fewer parent-reported internalizing problems than nonparticipants and, according to their classroom teachers, were socially better adjusted relative to the comparison group. More important, children, parents, and teachers reported a high degree of satisfaction with the intervention in promoting school adjustment (Katz et al., 1992).

The process of school intervention in pediatric cancer follows a temporal trajectory based on the child's needs during phase-specific periods. Five major phases of the school reentry and follow-up process are currently delineated based on the clinical experience of the authors and the extant literature (Katz, 1980; Katz et al., 1988; Katz & Ingle-Nelson, 1989; Madan-Swain et al., 1999; Madan-Swain, Austin, & Taylor-Cook, 2003). Each phase is constructed around the unique challenges facing the child, family, school, and health care team at different points in the illness trajectory. These phases are not necessarily orthogonal and may overlap or transpire almost simultaneously. They are discussed next.

### *Phase 1: Initial Diagnosis, Hospitalization, and Homebound Instruction*

During the initial diagnostic period, usually coinciding with hospitalization, the oncologist and health care team play a primary role in establishing the foundation for the continuation of normal life and school experience for both the child and the family. By stressing the importance of school participation, the health care team conveys the message that cancer and its treatment are a life disruption that may require modifications and delays in school involvement but not the cessation of basic requirements of childhood such as school. The critical importance of school to quality of life must be clearly communicated to parents, especially when working with diverse ethnic minority populations.

Information should be elicited from the child and family regarding their preillness experience with the child's school and education. With the parents' permission, a member of the treatment team should contact the child's school to notify school personnel of the child's health status, obtain premorbid information regarding the child's academic and social functioning, and elicit any concerns from the school's perspective. As soon as the child or adolescent is medically stable, school instruction should be incorporated into the child's daily inpatient treatment program. Hospital-based school programs vary greatly in terms of how educational instruction is provided. In some hospital settings, children receive individual instruction if they are physically or emotionally unable to attend school in a classroom setting. If hospitals do not have school programs, then school work can be forwarded from the school, and a parent or staff member can function as a teacher.

*Homebound Instruction.* Very often after the onset of an illness, the child will not be medically ready to return to school for a period of time. This will be true if a child is recovering from surgery, is receiving intensive chemotherapy and is severely immunosuppressed, or if a child requires a period of convalescence and rehabilitation. Homebound school programs are mandated by federal and state laws to continue a child's school program at home until the child is medically able to return to school. Ensuring that this initial postillness school experience is a positive one, in which the teacher is able to help motivate the student and be perceived as helpful, can serve as a "gateway" to successful reintegration and encourage a child to maintain the structure of normal life (Katz, 2004).

Generally, most hospital teachers working with the newly diagnosed child or adolescent will help arrange homebound teaching prior to discharge from the initial hospitalization. However, at other centers a designated member of the medical team such as the social worker or nurse practitioner will assist with establishing services. If the center does not have personnel resources focused on school issues, then it is critical that families be provided with the necessary information to contact schools and initiate teaching as well as a letter from their treating oncologist establishing the medical basis for the request.

Larger school districts will usually have specially trained homebound teachers ready to be dispatched to a child's home, whereas smaller districts might not have teachers immediately available. The quality and sophistication of teachers providing homebound instruction can vary tremendously, and care needs to be given to the "fit" between the teacher and child the teacher is assigned to teach. Non-English-speaking families will need assistance negotiating the teaching sessions and scheduling with a homebound teacher who may not speak their language. Variability also exists between school districts regarding the number of hours of homebound instruction they will provide, from a minimum of 1 hour per week to a few hours per day.

A study by Bessell (2001) indicated that many families have been dissatisfied with the quality and quantity of homebound teaching their ill child received prior to returning to school. To be effective, the homebound teacher should work to maintain the child's academic performance with that of classmates in the regular classroom to facilitate a smooth reentry. The homebound teacher should ideally have ongoing contact with the regular teacher to coordinate the individualized program and participate in the reentry preparation when the child is ready to return to school.

It is essential that a homebound teaching program be monitored by parents and members of the health care team to ensure that a teacher is coming on a regular basis, the child is participating actively, the teaching experience is productive, and the child is continuing to grow as a student. When the teacher does not speak the same language as the parents, additional oversight by the medical team is necessary to monitor progress and accountability (Katz, 2003).

Using technology to help homebound students maintain contact with their classroom peers or to communicate with other young people experiencing similar life circumstances holds great promise. The Starbright World, available on the Internet through wired hospital connections or through home versions (www.starbright.org), represents the largest sustained effort to create content and connectivity that could augment home teaching and social interactions for children with health problems. Homebound teachers and parents also can use multiple instructional sites on the Internet that are geared to various content areas as well as general homework assistance. Using technology to assist homebound students maintain contact with their classroom peers or to communicate with other young people experiencing similar life experiences holds great promise.

The following Internet sites are illustrative of the types of Web-based resources available to augment educational instruction and socialization for children with cancer:

A to Z's Cool Homeschooling: www.gomilpitas.com/homeschooling
Bandaids and Blackboard: www.faculty.fairfield.edu/fleitas/contents.html
Cancer Source Kids: www.cancersourcekids.com
Captain Chemo: www.royalmarsden.org/captchemo/adventures.asp
General educational topics for preschool to Grade 6: www.funschool.com
General educational topics for kindergarten to Grade 12: www.funbrain.com and www.brainpop.com
Kids Cancer Network: www.kidscancernetwork.org
NOVA Interactive Archives/PBS: www.pbs.org/wgbh/nova/hotscience

### *Phase 2: Preparing for Return to School*

*Preparing Parents.* When a child's medical condition stabilizes and the child's physician provides approval for returning to school, parents may be reluctant to allow the child with a chronic illness or injury back to school for a variety of reasons. Parents may not agree with the medical team when they determine the child or adolescent is physically ready to return to school. They also may want to protect their child from potential hurt, ridicule, or rejection by other children. Parents are susceptible to their own emotions and feelings of guilt and may become too protective and overly responsive to their child's physical complaints or expressions of anxiety related to rejection and ridicule. Understanding the importance of the child's reintegration, parents may provide support by also contacting the child's school, keeping the teacher and classmates informed of medical progress, and encouraging mutual communication between the ill or injured child and his or her peers (Davis, 1989; Katz, 1980). In addition, the parents of youths receiving homebound instruction should work with the teacher providing that instruction to ensure a smooth transition back to school.

*Preparing Children.* The child or adolescent who has been out of school because of illness and treatment may benefit from individual counseling and preparation for the emotional experience of returning to school (Katz, 1980; Katz et al., 1988). Preparing the child for academic and social challenges and developing a joint plan for informing and supporting peers and teachers about the child's experience needs to happen during this phase. In facilitating the child's cooperation and support for the reentry process, videos such as the *Back to School Video* in the Videos with Attitude Series of the Starbright Foundation (1999), The Cancervive *Back to School Videos* (1997:www.cancervive.org), or *Why Charlie Brown? Why?* (1986; distributed by the Leukemia/Lymphoma Society: www.leukemia-lymphoma.org/all_page.adp?item_id=360118 - 43k) can be very helpful. These videos and others similar to them can be used in schools and classrooms to help the other children understand their peer's experience with greater precision.

*Preparing School Staff.* Teachers and school administrators need to be closely apprised and prepared regarding the child's medical condition and to begin their preparation for the child's return (Madan-Swain et al., 2004). With the family's consent, the child's teacher and staff should be prepared with basic medical and treatment information that might have an impact on the child's learning and social performance. This should include information about potential immunosuppression related to chemotherapy and the need for parents of other children to be informed and vigilant regarding communicable diseases (Katz et al., 1988).

*Preparing Peers.* The teacher or school counselor should inform the class about their classmate's illness in general terms. Communication with the hospitalized child may be encouraged through cards, electronic mail, phone calls, weekly newsletters, class meetings conducted with a speakerphone to include the classmate, audiotaped class discussions of a high-interest topic with comments from the teacher to include the classmate, and when possible, visits from classmates to the hospital. If peers stay in close contact with the ill child during protracted absences, then the child may feel more connected and supported by the class and find it easier to return to school with less negative affect (Sexson & Madan-Swain, 1995; Varni & Katz, 1997).

### *Phase 3: Returning to School*

The extent to which school personnel can successfully facilitate the reentry process will be partially determined by their attitudes (Sexson & Madan-Swain, 1995). It is likely that many teachers lack the necessary information or experience with chronic illnesses and are susceptible to all the fears, anxieties, and failings of the general public. A child with a serious chronic illness or injury returning to the classroom is a new experience for most teachers. Preconceived notions about certain cancer diagnoses, limited knowledge about cancer, and the vulnerability communicated by the change in a child's appearance or energy level may cause teachers to arrive at the premature or erroneous conclusion that the child is likely to die (Ross, 1984). Teachers may be overwhelmed, unsure of how to approach the child, and uncomfortable in seeking information from parents who are already stressed from the illness experience and unable to deal with their own anxieties about the situation. Lacking this information, teachers may be overly sympathetic and reluctant to challenge the student to his or her potential (Ross, 1984). Conversely, teachers may be unable to recognize true limitations, thus exerting unrealistic expectations that may lead to frustration and discouragement on the part of the child and the family. Teachers also may worry that they will be unable to manage the medical issues that could arise (Katz, 1980; Madan-Swain, Katz, & LaGory, 2004; Nessim & Katz, 2003). These fears may cause the teacher to be increasingly more protective, overreact to even minor complaints, isolate the child, decrease the child's self-confidence, limit peer acceptance, and as a result further hamper the child's normalization process (Ross, 1984).

To provide a reinforcing classroom in which students are successful, teachers need specific information regarding the illness or injury and its possible impact on school performance and general development (Nessim & Katz, 1999). This allows the teacher to adapt instruction to ensure that the child is successful. Initially, teacher verbal reinforcement should be provided to the chronically ill child reentering the classroom simply for returning to school and for participating in classroom activities. This reinforcement should be delivered at a rapid pace at the beginning of each instructional session (Zanily, Dagged, & Pestine, 1995). In addition, teachers need to analyze the function of behaviors in which the child is likely to engage on returning to the classroom. Many of these behaviors may actually reinforce school avoidance, such as requiring the ill child to sit in a designated place or making a fuss over the ill child's special needs, which will likely elicit negative peer reactions (e.g., Iwata, Dorsey, Slifer, Bauman, & Richman, 1994). Avoidance may also be reinforced if the child is required to perform tasks that are academically too difficult because of either missed instruction or the cognitive difficulties associated with the illness or because of adverse side effects of treatments, such as fatigue.

*Classroom Presentations.* To ease the transition back into the classroom, members from the medical team may visit the school and present information regarding the chronic illness. The child is generally given the opportunity to provide "expert" information during the presentation to encourage peers to communicate directly with the child or adolescent if they have questions, but the ill child may elect not to do so if this poses a discomfort (Katz et al., 1988; Nessim & Katz, 1999). Components of the classroom presentation, presented in developmentally appropriate terms, include providing a basic understanding of cancer and the specific type involved; basic approaches to cancer treatment; demystification (i.e., cancer is not contagious, it is not caused by bad or inappropriate behavior); adverse side effects of treatment that students might notice in the chronically ill child at school (i.e., hair loss, weight gain, absences); and the critical role of peer support and how peers can help in the process (Katz, 1980; Katz et al., 1988; Nessim & Katz, 1999). Classroom presentations will help demystify the illness or accident, facilitating open communication and peer social support that will likely result in a more reinforcing environment for the child (Katz et al., 1988).

*Parental Support.* If the school provides a reinforcing environment for the child's return and if the parents' behavior of encouraging the child to return to school is reinforced by school personnel, the transition will proceed more smoothly. One way to reinforce the parents' efforts is to provide frequent positive communication about the school reentry process. For the first few days, it may be necessary for the classroom teacher or school counselor to phone the parents several times during the day to assure them that the reentry is progressing well and to reassure them that the child is experiencing no adjustment difficulties. Over time, the frequency of the contacts may decrease as the parents view the success of their child's return to the classroom. For children and teenagers who are returning to school with significant learning difficulties requiring special education services, parents will need to learn how to become educational advocates for their children throughout their school experience. Parents need to be provided with information regarding their child's rights to educational programs and services (cf. Phase 4, Parent Educational Advocacy Training).

### Phase 4: Early and Long-Term Follow-Up

Central to this phase is continued communication among the family, school personnel, and medical team. Even after the child returns to school, it is important that school personnel remain in close contact with an identified medical team member so that school-related concerns can be easily discussed. Such communication allows the school to inform the medical team of increasing absences and to seek information on how to address the issue. The medical team can assist with the development of decision rules that are acceptable to the school and family. These rules can be used to determine when a child may stay home from school and when attendance is mandatory. Because the decision rules may change depending on the course of the illness, continued contact must be maintained, particularly for children with unstable disease.

In the largest educational follow-up study to date of over 12,000 childhood cancer survivors (Mitby et al., 2003), almost one quarter of all survivors surveyed used special education services at some point during their educational careers. This contrasts to only 8% of matched sibling controls using special education services. The greatest risk factors associated with school performance for survivors included diagnosis before age 6 years and diagnosis of a brain tumor, leukemia (with radiation therapy to the CNS or intrathecal chemotherapy), or Hodgkin's disease. With increasing survival rates and a greater number of survivors receiving special education services, the annual IEP meeting conducted by the school to review the child's or adolescent's progress and educational needs is a critical step to ensure that their educational needs are met and not ignored. One should consider writing into the IEP the requirement that the health care team be consulted on an annual basis to determine if the child's or adolescent's medical needs have changed and to get their input into the ongoing educational program. The annual IEP meeting and review of educational progress should become an automatic time for parents to consult with the medical team and review how the child or adolescent is progressing at school to determine if the child's educational needs are adequately met.

*Social Skills Training for Children and Teens.* Once back in school, children and teens with cancer who are experiencing difficulties in their social interactions with peers should have access to empirically supported intervention strategies such as social skills training. In the only randomized, controlled trial to date with elementary students with cancer, Varni et al. (1993) used a manualized treatment program that focused on training children in the following core skills:

1. *Social cognitive problem solving*: Children were taught to problem solve cancer-related interpersonal difficulties regarding peers, teachers, parents, and siblings as they occurred. Steps in the problem-solving model included promoting optimism in one's ability to improve things, identifying specific problems, considering antecedents and associated factors, brainstorming alternative solutions, planning, implementation, and outcomes evaluation to guide future behavior.
2. *Assertiveness training*: Children were taught how to identify their thoughts, wishes, and concerns and how to express these issues effectively to others in a forthright, respectful manner.
3. *Handling teasing and name calling*: Children were taught how to cope with verbal and physical teasing associated with changes in their physical appearance related to illness or treatment (e.g., hair loss, weight gain or loss, surgical disfigurement). Strategies included extinguishing inappropriate peer behaviors through withdrawal of attention, giving age-appropriate explanations for physical changes, and using authoritative adults for support and assistance.

Training was delivered individually to each child during three 1-hour training sessions. In addition to didactic discussions and role playing, the children used specially developed video vignettes. During the viewing session, the vignettes were periodically stopped, and the child was encouraged to process and practice the skill learned. Results indicated that the participants, relative to the control group, mastered the strategies taught and experienced higher degrees of perceived social support from classmates and teachers at 9 months posttraining. Parents of youths in the intervention group reported significant decreases in behavior problems along with an increase in school competence. This study demonstrated the efficacy of providing explicit social skills training to elementary school children and should be replicated with adolescents to explore the usefulness of this approach to older patients (Katz & Varni, 1993).

*Parent Educational Advocacy Training.* Parents play a particularly critical role in promoting the educational needs of their child, especially when their child has special education needs (Dane, 1990; Flood, 1999; Wright & Wright, 2002). Parental participation regarding special education services has been mandated by federal legislation, resulting in the expectation that parents will actively participate in assessment, planning, and program evaluation (Brantlinger, 1987). However, Brantlinger noted that parents frequently demonstrate passive involvement when participating in educational conferences. Reasons for this minimal engagement include lack of knowledge, confusion about the parental role in the school setting, uncertainty regarding the child's academic ability, and perceived unfavorable attitudes toward parental participation by the educational staff (Brantlinger, 1987).

Lack of effective parental participation in educational planning for their child will hinder the establishment of a collaborative relationship among the child, parents, teachers, administrators, and health care team, leading to less-successful educational and social outcomes for their child. Frequent and effective communication with the child's teacher is essential in ensuring that appropriate services are rendered (Stephenson, 1992). As discussed by Allen and Hudd (1987), to be effective in this advocacy role, parents require specialized knowledge and skills. This is especially true in families that have difficulty communicating with their child's school because of linguistic or sociocultural barriers (Madan-Swain et al., 2004).

School intervention approaches for children with cancer have long included preparing the child for the return to school and preparing the school for the special needs of the child (Katz et al., 1992). Parents have been identified as needing support and information to assist their child in transitioning back to school after an extended absence for cancer treatment. Parental interventions to date have tended to focus on the emotional issues they and their child will experience when returning to school. Because parents are the primary adults monitoring the long-term school progress of their child, it is essential that parents learn how to help their children succeed in school throughout the child's educational experience by developing successful school advocacy skills (Smith, 2003; Wright & Wright, 2002).

Flood (1999) developed and pilot tested a program to train parents of children with cancer in educational advocacy skills to help them meet the needs of their children. Using a manualized approach delivered to 21 English-speaking mothers who participated in the pilot, training was delivered over the following five core content areas:

1. Identification of potential school and social problems encountered by children with cancer and introduction to parental educational advocacy training to help improve their child's educational outcomes
2. Identification of regular and special education school professionals who are mandated to help children with special learning needs
3. An overview of basic special education and disability laws (including the IEP and Section 504 modifications) that require school districts to assist children with unique educational needs
4. Information on how classroom modifications or special educational services are accessed
5. A review of all previously presented content areas

Results of this initial pilot study indicated that parents trained in educational advocacy skills demonstrated statistically significant improvements over pretraining levels in knowledge of their rights under special education law, their perception of their own ability to apply this knowledge, and finally the ability to apply this knowledge to vignettes developed for this purpose.

*Compensatory educational interventions.* Children and adolescents who have specific educational deficits may benefit from focused educational therapy at home and at school to strengthen their abilities and compensate for weaknesses (Levine, 1994). Young people with cognitive deficits associated with cancer or cancer-related treatment may need specialized educational interventions that have been termed *cognitive remediation* (Butler & Copeland, 2002; Butler & Rizzi, 1995). These interventions identify the specific underlying cognitive deficit rather than merely the academic weakness a particular child may be experiencing, and they attempt to help the child develop the underlying skills that can facilitate academic success. In addition to focusing on strengthening attention and concentration skills, which are often weak in children with acquired cognitive impairments, interventions that include learning strategies for the child (e.g., getting ready to learn), teaching the child social-cognitive problem-solving skills, and teaching parents and teachers how to support these skills in the school and home settings show great promise for improving school and social performance (Butler & Copeland, 2002; Varni et al., 1992).

*Transition Services.* The transition from pediatric to adult medical care and ongoing health surveillance throughout adulthood is an increasingly important topic in pediatric oncology (Keene et al., 2000). In a similar vein, the adolescent's educational transition from high school to college or vocational training also requires intensive consideration (Betz, 2003; Deasy-Spinetta, 1997; Schulzinger, 1999). Federal law, under the IDEA legislation, requires that schools provide services for the student receiving special education who will be exiting high school that promote the adolescent's transition to postsecondary education, work, and community integration (Deasy-Spinetta, 1997; deFur, 2002). These transition services are part of the student's IEP and are mandated to begin between the ages of 14 and 16 years. The goal of transition is meaningful employment and a quality of adult life for all students with disabilities (Deasy-Spinetta, 1997).

This critical planning for the adolescent's future usually takes place at the annual school review of each student's IEP, and school districts have identified transition coordinators to ensure that this type of planning occurs. Each special education student should have an individual transition plan developed for him or her that carefully outlines the plans of the team to prepare the adolescent for college, vocational training, or community support programs and ensure that any needed support services will be there when the child arrives. Transition services should focus on educational and social needs, including preparing the student for independent living (i.e., grooming, mobility, managing finances, recreation, etc.) (Deasy-Spinetta, 1997; deFur, 2002).

Many long-term survivors with learning disabilities who are college bound may need learning assistance to succeed in that setting. Other survivors who have more intensive problems may need alternative learning and vocational options that must be planned well in advance of graduation. Parents may need assistance from their child's health care and school professional teams to advocate for effective transition services to prepare their child for life after high school (Deasy-Spinetta, 1997; deFur, 2002; Hayes, Landsverk, Sallan, Hewett, Patenaude, Schoonover, et al., 1992).

### *Phase 5: Disease Progression and Death*

Although the majority of children diagnosed with cancer will be long-term survivors, cancer still remains the leading cause of death by illness in childhood. In the year 2000, the American Cancer Society estimated that approximately 2,300 children and adolescents would die of cancer (American Cancer Society, 2000). Although many children who relapse or have a secondary malignancy later in life may still be cured, many of these children will experience progressive decline in health, leading to death, which may occur rapidly but more often transpires over months or even years (Pizzo & Poplack, 2002).

If the child has been disease free for many years, the return of active disease may be similar to the initial diagnosis, especially if the child was very young when first diagnosed and does not have a strong recollection of that period (Sourkes, 1982). Older children and parents will often experience a relapse as even more emotionally traumatic than the initial diagnosis because of their increased knowledge of what lies ahead and fears regarding survival (Spinetta, 1980). Continuing school during this phase provides the same hope and structured normal experience as at diagnosis, with many of the same interventions described here useful.

For the child whose illness is no longer controllable and is expected to die within a period of weeks or months, school participation continues to be of critical importance to the child's sense of well-being (American Academy of Pediatrics, 2000; Katz & Ingle-Nelson, 1989). During this end stage of the child's life, involvement in academic pursuits and school activities is often one of the few parts of the child's life that may continue to have structure and be hopeful.

For the child in declining health and facing death, maximal communication among the family, teachers and school, and the health care team will help ensure the flexibility in scheduling and reasonable expectations for the child and all those around the child (Katz & Ingle-Nelson, 1989; Madan-Swain et al., 2003). Whenever possible, the child should be given opportunities to participate in classroom and school activities, especially special events such as holiday parties and graduation. Many adolescents and their families find that the opportunity to complete high school is a major life goal that helps them cope with impending death with increased hopefulness and dignity. Special education services may be needed to ensure that the child can transition between home and regular education settings, depending on their medical condition at that point in time.

School personnel and peers will need assistance processing the child's declining health and maintaining their focus on the child's ongoing inclusion in class experiences to the maximum degree possible. Although completion of academic tasks may diminish in importance at this time, the importance to quality of life for ongoing school involvement may actually be increasing during this period (Katz & Ingle-Nelson, 1989). Teachers and school peers need information and support to process their emotional experiences as they see their classmate in a continually weakening physical state. This is a period when rumors and inaccurate and frightening information may be rife within the school community, and a proactive approach by teachers and administrators may be necessary to maintain emotional balance on the campus. Some ill children with very strong connections to school and with maximal family support will continue a periodic presence at school until literally their last days of life. Other children with weaker attachments to school and less encouragement from parents, school, and health care team may not be in school for months preceding their death. Each situation must be handled uniquely and with the utmost sensitivity to accommodate the individual needs of the child, family, and school. Special consideration should also be directed toward the ill child's siblings and close relatives who may attend the same school or other schools in the same community because their school performance and emotional well-being may also suffer (Deasy-Spinetta, 1997). Although outside the scope of this particular chapter, the school needs of siblings of seriously ill and dying children are a topic of critical significance and import to their long-term adjustment (Chesler, Allswede, & Barbarin, 1993).

When a child dies, either at home or in the hospital, it is important to provide the school of the ill child with information and support to assist in the natural process of bereavement and expression of grief (Madan-Swain et al., 2003; Reynolds, Miller, Jelalian, & Spirito, 1995). The intensity of grief that will likely be encountered by the schoolmates and staff will usually be proportional to the intensity of their ongoing relationship during the last few months of the child's life. Teachers and adults in the school setting may need separate opportunities and support to process their emotions because the death of a student will likely lead to the renewal of strong feelings associated with other grief and loss experiences they have encountered (Katz & Ingle-Nelson, 1989). Teachers need to be able to support their students at a time of loss rather than reacting strongly in a manner that students may find confusing and frightening.

If the ill child who has died did not have direct contact with the class or school for months and years prior to death, this experience may be relatively weak for most classmates. Some individual children from the child's immediate neighborhood may have very strong reactions that may not be predicted by school personnel unaware of such connections. If the ill child was a regular part of the class through direct participation or through visitation at home, cards and letters, and the like, the school's grief reaction should be expected to be significant, and active steps to facilitate bereavement should be provided. School-based mental health staff should work together with members of the health care team knowledgeable about grief and bereavement in children and adolescents to assist the school community to process their loss. Planned memorial activities such as tree plantings, assemblies to remember their friend, and acts of communal charity in the deceased child's memory have proven very useful (Madan-Swain et al., 2003; Reynolds, Miller, Jelalian, & Spirito, 1995).

## Conclusions and Future Directions

To maximize school and social outcomes in young people with cancer as well as long-term survivors of cancer, it is useful to apply the risk-and-resistance model of Varni and Wallender (1988) to each individual child and adolescent. School participation and success are part of a dynamic process that must be monitored and supported in children and adolescents affected by cancer. Although this chapter reviewed general approaches to helping ensure that young people with cancer are supported in their school and social experiences after the onset of illness, our challenge is to consider how best to individualize these approaches to a particular situation. Individual circumstances require specific considerations of a particular child's risk and resistance factors, the child's ability to process and adapt to stress, and an overall determination of which resources and services could be most beneficial to the long-term adjustment of that child.

Theoretically based empirical research is needed to continue evaluating assumptions of the risk-and-resistance model as applied to school and social outcomes. The following recommendations for a research agenda are advanced to help support the development of evidence-based interventions that may be tailored to the needs of individual children and families to maximize overall adjustment and adaptation.

1. Develop an empirically based predictive model of successful reentry based on Wallander and Varni's risk/resistance framework and test its ability to successfully predict children at risk for school and social difficulties who may be targeted for early intervention.
2. Develop and evaluate specific educational curriculum materials and methods that can remediate identified cognitive deficits associated with disease and treatment at school, at home, and in the oncology clinic. Explore interactive Web-based methods for delivering these materials.
3. Evaluate the efficacy of home teaching for homebound students to help prepare students for reentry into regular school environments. Explore methods for training home teachers, incorporating Web-based pedagogic and social interactiveness technology, and monitoring progress.
4. Evaluate the impact on quality of life of effective identification and remediation of school and learning difficulties in children living with cancer and long-term survivors.
5. Evaluate the long-term impact on quality of life (including educational, vocational, and

psychological functioning) of school and social intervention during illness and treatment. Develop a predictive model that matches risk and resilience factors with specific intervention strategies.

## References


Aicardi, J. (1998). *Diseases of the nervous system in childhood (2nd ed.)*. London: MacKeith Press.

American Academy of Pediatrics. (2000). Palliative care for children. *Pediatrics, 106,* 351–357.

Allen, D.A., & Hudd, S.S. (1987). Are we professionalizing parents? Weighing the benefits and pitfalls. *Mental Retardation, 25,* 133–139.

American Cancer Society. (2000). *Cancer facts and figures*. American Cancer Society, Atlanta, GA.

Armstrong, F. D. (2003). Childhood cancer and education. In N. Keene (Ed.), *Educating the child with cancer: A guide for parents and teachers* (pp. 15–24). Bethesda, MD: Candlelighters Childhood Cancer Foundation.

Armstrong, F. D., & Briery, B.G. (2004). Childhood cancer and the School. In R. T. Brown (Ed.), *Handbook of* Psychology in School Settings (pp. 263–282). Mahwah, NJ: Erlbaum.

Armstrong, F. D., & Horn, M. (1995). Educational issues in childhood cancer. *School Psychology Quarterly, 10,* 292–304.

Bessel, A. G. (2001). Children surviving cancer: Psychosocial adjustment, quality of life, and school experiences. *Exceptional Children, 67,* 345–359.

Betz, C. (2003). High school and beyond. In N. Keene (ed.), *Educating the child with cancer: A guide for parents and teachers* (pp. 241–251). Bethesda, MD: Candlelighters Childhood Cancer Foundation.

Brantlinger, E. A. (1987). Making decisions about special education placement: Do low-income parents have the information they need? *Journal of Learning Disabilities, 20,* 94–101.

Brown, R. T. (2004). Introduction: Changes in the provision of health care to children and adolescents. In R. T. Brown (Ed.), *Handbook of pediatric psychology in school settings* (pp. 1–19). Mahwah, NJ: Erlbaum.

Brown, R. T., Madan-Swain, A., Pais, R., Lambert, R. G., Sexson, S. B., & Ragab, A. (1992). Chemotherapy for acute lymphocytic leukemia: Cognitive and academic sequelae. *Journal of Pediatrics, 121,* 885–889.

Brown, R. T., Madan-Swain, A., Walco, G. A., Cherrick, I., Ievers, C. E., Conte, P. M., et al. (1998). Cognitive and academic late effects among children previously treated for acute lymphocytic leukemia receiving chemotherapy as CNS prophylaxis. *Journal of Pediatric Psychology, 23,* 333–340.

Butler, R., & Copeland, D. (2002) Attentional processes and their remediation in children treated for cancer: A literature review and development of a therapeutic approach. *Journal of the International Neuropsychological Society, 8,* 115–124.

Butler, R., Hill, J. M., & Steinherz, P. G. (1994) Neuropsychologic effects of cranial irritation, intrathecal methotrexate, and systemic methotrexate in childhood cancer. *Journal of Clinical Oncology, 12,* 2621–2629.

Butler, R. W., & Namerow, N. S. (1988). Cognitive retraining in brain injury rehabilitation: A critical review. *Journal of Neurological Rehabilitation, 2,* 97–101.

Butler, R. W., & Rizzi, L. P. (1995). The remediation of attentional deficits secondary to treatment for childhood cancer: Progress notes. *Society of Pediatric Psychology, 19,* 5–13.

Cairns, N. U., Klopovich, P., Hearne, E., & Lansky, S. B. (1982). School attendance of children with cancer. *Journal of School Health, 52,* 152–155.

Charlton, A., Larcombe, I. J., Meller, S. T., Morris-Jones, P. H., Mott, M. G., Potton, M. W., et al. (1991). Absence from school related to cancer and other chronic conditions. *Archives of Diseases in Childhood, 66,* 1217–1222.

Chekryn, J., Deegan, M., & Reid, J. (1987). Impact on teachers when a child with cancer returns to school. *Children's Health Care, 15,* 161–165.

Chesler, M., Allswede, J., & Barbarin, O. (1993). Voices from the margin: Siblings of children with cancer. In P. Deasy-Spinetta and E. Irvin (Eds.), *Educating the child with cancer* (pp. 97–116). Bethesda, MD: Candlelighters Childhood Cancer Foundation.

Cook, B. A., Schaller, K., & Krischer, J. P. (1985). School absence among children with chronic illness. *Journal of School Health, 55,* 265–267.

Copeland, D., & Butler, R. W. (2003). Cognitive remediation. In N. Keene (Ed.), *Educating the child with cancer: A guide for parents and teachers* (pp. 165–173). Bethesda, MD: Candlelighters Childhood Cancer Foundation.

Cousens, P., Ungerer, J. A., Crawford, J. A., & Stevens, M. (1991). Cognitive effect of childhood leukemia therapy: A case for four specific deficits. *Journal of Pediatric Psychology, 16,* 475–488.

Dane, E. (1990). *Painful passages: Working with children with learning disabilities*. Silver Springs, MD: NASW Press.

Davis, K. G. (1989). Educational needs of the terminally ill student. *Issues in Comprehensive Pediatric Nursing, 12,* 235–245.

Deasy-Spinetta, P. (1981). The school and the child with cancer. In J. J. Spinetta & P. Deasy-Spinetta (Eds.), *Living with childhood cancer* (pp. 153–166). Toronto: Mosby.

Deasy-Spinetta, P. (1997). Educational issues for children with cancer. In P. A. Pizzo & D. G. Poplack (Eds.), *Principles and practice of pediatric oncology* (3rd ed., pp. 1331–1342). Philadelphia: Lippincott-Raven.

DeFur, S. H. (2002). Transition planning: A team effort. National Information Center for Children and Youth with Disabilities, TS10. Retrieved from www.nichcy.org, 2/14/2004.

Eiser, C., & Tillmann, V. (2001). Learning difficulties in children treated for acute lymphoblastic leukemia. *Pediatric Rehabilitation, 4,* 105–118.

Eiser, C., Vance, Y. H., Horne, B., Glaser, A., & Galvin, H. (2003). The value of the PedsQL™ in assessing quality of life in survivors of childhood cancer. *Child Heath and Development, 29, 2,* 95–102.

Flood, G. (1999). *Advocacy training: A look towards the future of pediatric cancer patients and their families.* Unpublished doctoral dissertation, Pepperdine University, Culver City, California.

Fowler, M. G., Johnson, M. P., & Atkinson, S. S. (1985). School achievement and absence in children with chronic health conditions. *Journal of Pediatrics, 106,* 683–687.

Fuligni, A. J. (1997). The academic achievement of adolescents from immigrant families: The roles of family background, attitude, and behavior. *Child Development, 68,* 351–363.

Gortmaker, S. L., Walker, D. K., Weitzman, M., & Sobel, A. M. (1990). Chronic conditions, socioeconomic risks and behavioral problems in children and adolescents. *Pediatrics, 85,* 267–276.

Hall, M., & Baum, A. (1995). Intrusive thoughts as determinants of distress in parents of children with cancer. *Journal of Applied Social Psychology 25,* 251–272.

Hayes, D. M., Landsverk, J., Sallan, S. E., Hewett, K. D., Patenaude, A. F., Schoonover, D., et al. (1992). Educational, occupational, and insurance status of childhood cancer survivors in their fourth and fifth decades of life. *Journal of Clinical Oncology, 10,* 1397–1406.

Henning, J., & Fritz, G. K. (1983). School reentry in childhood cancer. *Psychosomatics, 24,* 261–269.

Hernandez, D. J., & Charney, E. (1998). *From generation to generation: The health and well-being of children in immigrant families.* Washington, DC: National Academy Press.

Hetherington, E. M., & Martin, B. (1986). Family factors and psychopathology in children. In H. C. Quay & J. S. Werry (Eds.), *Psychopathological disorders of childhood* (pp. 332–389). New York: Wiley.

Individuals With Disabilities Education Act of 1990, Pub. L. No. 101-456. (1990). *Reauthorization of Public Law 94-142.* Washington, DC: U.S. Government Printing Office.

Institute of Medicine, National Research Council. (2003). *Childhood cancer survivorship: Improving care and quality of life.* Washington, DC: National Academies Press.

Iwata, B. A., Dorsey, M. F., Slifer, K. J., Bauman, K. E., & Richman, G. S. (1994). Towards a functional analysis of self-injury. *Journal of Applied Behavior Analysis, 27,* 197–209.

Katz, E. R. (1980). Illness impact and social reintegration. In J. Kellerman (Ed.), *Psychological aspects of cancer in children* (pp. 14–46). Springfield, IL: Thomas.

Katz, E. R. (2004). Education in the hospital and at home. In N. Keene (Ed.), *Educating the child with cancer: A guide for parents and teachers* (pp. 27–34). Bethesda, MD: Candlelighters Childhood Cancer Foundation.

Katz, E. R., Dolgin, M. J., & Varni, J. W. (1990). Cancer in children and adolescents. In A. M. Gross & R. S. Drabman (Eds.), *Handbook of clinical behavioral pediatrics* (pp. 129–146). New York. Plenum Press.

Katz, E. R., & Ingle-Nelson, M. J. (1989). School and the seriously ill child. In B. B. Martin (Ed.), *Pediatric hospice care: What helps* (pp. 145–167). Los Angeles: Childrens Hospital Los Angeles[no apostrophe in Childrens].

Katz, E. R., Kellerman, J., Rigler, D., Williams, K. O., & Siegel, S. E. (1977). School intervention with pediatric cancer patients. *Journal of Pediatric Psychology, 2,* 72–76.

Katz, E. R., Rubenstein, C. L., Hubert, N. C., & Blew, A. (1988). School and social reintegration of children with cancer. *Journal of Psychosocial Oncology, 6,* 123–140.

Katz, E. R., & Varni, J. W. (1993). Social support and social cognitive problem solving in children with newly diagnosed cancer. *Cancer, 71,* 3314–3319.

Katz, E. R., Varni, J. W., Rubenstein, C. L., Blew, A., & Hubert, N. (1992). Teacher, parent, and child evaluative ratings of school reintegration intervention for children with newly diagnosed cancer. *Children's Health Care, 21,* 69–75.

Kazak, A. E., Steuber, M., Barakat, L. P., Meeske, K., Gutherie, D., & Meadows, A. T. (1998). Predicting posttraumatic stress symptoms in mothers and fathers of survivors of childhood cancers. *Journal of American Academy of Child and& Adolescent Psychiatry, 37,* 823–831.

Keene, N. (Ed.). (2003). *Educating the child with cancer: A guide for parents and teachers.* Bethesda, MD: Candlelighters Childhood Cancer Foundation.

Keene, N., Hobbie, W., & Ruccione, K. (2000) *Childhood cancer survivors: A practical guide to your future.* Sebastopol, CA: O'Reilly.

Kun, L. E., Mulhern, R. K., & Crisco, J. J. (1983). Quality of life in children treated for brain tumors: Intellectual, emotional, and academic function. *Journal of Neurosurgery, 58,* 1–6.

La Greca, A. M., Bearman, K. J., & Moore, H. (2004). Peer Relations. In R. T. Brown (Ed.), *Handbook of psychology in school settings* (pp. 657–678). Mahwah, NJ: Erlbaum.

Lansky, S. B., Lowman, J. T., Vata, T., & Gyulay, J. (1975). School phobia in children with malignant neoplasms. *American Journal of Diseases of Children, 129,* 42–46.

Lazarus, R. S., & Folkman, S. (1984). *Stress, appraisal, and coping.* New York: Springer.

Levine, M. (1994). *Educational care: A system for understanding and helping children with learning problems at home and in school.* Cambridge, MA: Educators Publishing Service.

Madan-Swain, A., Austin, H., & Taylor-Cook, P. (2003). Grief in the classroom. In N. Keene (Ed.), *Educating the child with cancer: A guide for parents and teachers* (pp. 287–298). Bethesda, MD: Candlelighters Childhood Cancer Foundation.

Madan-Swain, A., & Brown, R. T. (1991). Cognitive and psychosocial sequelae for children with acute lymphocytic leukemia and their families. *Clinical Psychology Review, 11,* 267–294.

Madan-Swain, A., Fredrick, L. D., & Wallander, J. L. (1999). Returning to school after a serious illness or injury. In R. T. Brown (Ed.), *Cognitive aspects of chronic illness in children* (pp. 312–332). New York, NY: Guilford Press.

Madan-Swain, A., Katz, E. R., & LaGory, J. (2004). School and social reintegration after serious illness or injury. In R. T. Brown (Ed.), *Handbook of psychology in school settings* (pp. 637–655). Mahwah, NJ: Erlbaum.

McCarthy, A. M., Williams, J., & Plumer, C. (1998). Evaluation of a school re-entry nursing intervention for children with cancer. *Journal of Pediatric Oncology Nursing, 15,* 143–152.

Meeske, K., Katz, E. R., Palmer, S. N., Burwinkle, T., & Varni, J. W. (2005) Parent and proxy-reported health related quality of life and fatigue in pediatric cancer patients diagnosed with brain tumors and acute lymphoblastic leukemia. *Cancer, 101,* 2116–2125.

Mitby, P. A., Robison, L. L., Whitton, J. A., Zevon, M. A., Gibbs, I. C., Tersak, J. M., et al. (2003). Utilization of special education services and educational attainment among long-term survivors of childhood cancer: A report from the Childhood Cancer Survivor Study. *Cancer, 97,* 1115–1126.

Monaco, G. P., & Smith, G. P. (2003). Special education: The law. In N. Keene (Ed.), *Educating the child with cancer: A guide for parents and teachers* (pp. 193–205). Bethesda, MD: Candlelighters Childhood Cancer Foundation.

Morrow, G. R., Hoagland, A., & Carnrike, C. L. J. (1981). Social support and parental adjustment to pediatric cancer. *Journal of Consulting and Clinical Psychology, 49,* 763–765.

Mulhern, R. K., & Palmer, S. L. (2003, July/August) Neurocognitive late effects in pediatric cancer. *Current Problems in Cancer,* 177–197.

Mulhern, R. K., Wasserman, A. L., Friedman, A. G., & Fairclough, D. (1989). Social competence and behavioral adjustment of children who are long term survivors of cancer. *Pediatrics, 83,* 1, 18–25.

Nassau, J. H., & Drotar, D. (1997). Social competence among children with central nervous system-related chronic health conditions: a review. *Journal of Pediatric Psychology, 22,* 771–793.

Neesim, S., & Katz, E. R. (2003). *Can[cervive] teacher guide for kids with cancer,[ 2nd edition. Distributed by the Leukemia-Lymphoma Society,* New York, NY. www.leukemia-lymphoma.org/all_page.adp?item_id=360118 - 43k]

Noll, R. B., Gartstein, M. A., Hawkins, A., Vannatta, K., Taylor, J., & Passo, M. (1995). Comparing parental distress for families with children who have cancer and matched comparison families without children with cancer. *Family Systems Medicine, 13,* 11–27.

Noll, R. B., Gartstein, M. A., Vannatta, K., Correll, J., Bukowski, W. M., & Davies, W. H. (1999). Social, emotional, and behavioral functioning of children with cancer. *Pediatrics, 103,* 71–78.

Overholser, J. C., & Fritz, G. K. (1990). The impact of childhood cancer on the family. *Journal of Psychosocial Oncology, 8,* 71–85.

Pelcovitz D, Goldenberg B, Kaplan S, Weinblatt, M., Mandel, F., Meyers, B., et al. (1996). Posttraumatic stress disorder in mothers of pediatric cancer survivors. *Psychosomatics, 37,* 116–126.

Perrin, E. C., Ayoub, C. C., & Willett, J. B. (1993). In the eyes of the beholder: family and maternal influences on perceptions of adjustment of children with a chronic illness. *Journal of Developmental and Behavioral Pediatrics, 14,* 94–105.

Pizzo, P. A., & Poplack, D. G. (Eds.). (2002). *Principles and practice of pediatric oncology* (4th ed.). Philadelphia: Lippincott, Williams and Wilkins.

Raymond-Speden, E., Tripp, G., Lawrence, B., & Holdaway, D. (2000). Intellectual, neuropsychological, and academic functioning in long-term survivors of leukemia. *Journal of Pediatric Psychology, 25,* 59–68.

Reynolds, L. A., Miller, D. L., Jelalian, E., & Spirito, A. (1995). Anticipatory grief and bereavement. In M. C. Roberts (Ed.), *Handbook of pediatric psychology* (2nd ed., pp. 142–166). New York: Guilford Press.

Ris, M. D., Packer, R., Goldwein, J., Jones-Wallace, D., & Boyett, J. M. (2001). Intellectual outcome after reduced-dose radiation therapy plus adjuvant chemotherapy for medulloblastoma: A children's cancer study group study. *Journal of clinical Oncology, 19,* 3470–3476.

Ross, J. W. (1984). Resolving nonmedical obstacles to successful school reentry for children with cancer. *Journal of School Health, 54,* 84–86.

Rubinstein, C. L., Varni J. W., & Katz, E. R. (1990). Cognitive functioning in long-term survivors of childhood leukemia: A prospective analysis. *Journal of Developmental and Behavioral Pediatrics,* 11, 301–305.

Sahler, O. J., Roghmann, K. J., Mulhern, R. K., Carpenter, D., Sargent, L., Copeland, D., et al. (1997) Sibling Adaptation to Childhood Cancer Collaborative Study: The association of sibling adaptation with maternal well-being, physical health, and resource use. *Journal of Developmental and Behavioral Pediatrics, 18,* 233–243.

Sahler, O. J., Varni, J. W., Fairclough, D. L., Butler, R. W., Noll, R. B., Dolgin, M. J., et al. (2002). Problem-solving skills training for mothers of children with newly diagnosed cancer: A randomized, clinical trial. *Journal of Developmental and Behavioral Pediatrics, 23,* 77–65.

Sahler O. J., Fairclough, D. L., Phipps, S., Mulhern, R. K., Katz E. R., Varni J. W., et al. (2005). Maternal problem solving skills training in childhood cancer: Results of a randomized clinical trial. *Journal of Consulting and Clinical Psychology 73,* 272–283.

Sanger, M. S., Copeland, D. R., & Davidson, E. R. (1991). Psychosocial adjustment among pediatric cancer patients: A multidimensional assessment. *Journal of Pediatric Psychology, 16,* 463–474.

Schulzinger, R. (1999). *Key transition issues for youth with disabilities and chronic health conditions: Report on the Healthy and Ready to Work Project.* Institute for Child Health Policy, Gainsville, FL. Retrieved from www.mchbhrtw.org, 2/15/2004.

Sexson, S. B., & Madan-Swain, A. (1993). School reentry for the child with chronic illness. *Journal of Learning Disabilities, 26,* 115–125.

Sexson, S. B., & Madan-Swain, A. (1995). The chronically ill child in the school. *School Psychology Quarterly, 10,* 359–368.

Shields, J. D., Heron, T. E., Rubinstein, C. L., & Katz, E. R. (1995). The eco-triadic model of educational consultation for students with cancer. *Education and Treatment of Children, 18,* 184–200.

Smith, K. (2003). Special education: Navigating the system. In N. Keene (Ed.), *Educating the child with cancer: A guide for parents and teachers* (pp. 215–223). Bethesda, MD: Candlelighters Childhood Cancer Foundation.

Sourkes, B. (1982). *The deepening shade: Psychological aspects of life-threatening illness.* Pittsburgh, PA: University of Pittsburgh Press.

Spinetta, J. (1980) Disease related communication: How to tell. In J. Kellerman (Ed.), *Psychological aspects of childhood cancer* (pp. 257–269). Springfield, IL: Thomas.

Spinetta, J. J., & Deasy-Spinetta, P. (1986). The patient's socialization in the community and school during therapy. *Cancer, 58,* 512–515.

Stehbens, J. A., Kisker, C. T., & Wilson, B. K. (1983). School behavior and attendance during the first year of treatment for childhood cancer. *Psychology in the Schools, 20,* 223–228.

Stephenson, J. (1992). The perspectives of mothers whose children are in special day classes for learning disabilities. *Journal of Learning Disabilities, 25,* 539–543.

Stuber, M. L., Christakis, D. A., Houskamp, B., & Kazak, E. (1996). Posttrauma symptoms in childhood leukemia survivors and their parents. *Psychosomatics, 37,* 254–261.

Taylor, B. V., Buckner, J. C., Cascino, T. L., O'Fallon, J. R., Schaefer, P. L., Dinapoli, R. P., et al. (1998). Effects of radiation and chemotherapy on cognitive function in patients with high-grade glioma. *Journal of Clinical Oncology, 16,* 2195–2201.

Vannatta, K., Gartstein, M. A., & Noll, R. B. (1998). Peer relationships of children surviving brain tumors. *Journal of Pediatric Psychology, 23,* 279–288.

Varni, J. W., Burwinkle, T. M., Katz, E. R., Meeske, K., & Dickinson, P. (2002). The PedsQL in pediatric cancer: Reliability and validity of the Pediatric Quality of Life Inventory Generic Core Scales, Multidimensional Fatigue Scale, and Cancer Module. *Cancer, 94,* 2090–2106.

Varni, J. W., Burwinkle, T. M., Seid, M., & Skarr, D. (2003). The PedsQL TM 4.0 as a pediatric population health measure: Feasibility, reliability, and validity. Ambulatory Pediatrics, 3, 329–341.

Varni, J. W., & Katz, E. R. (1997). Stress, social support and negative affectivity in children with newly diagnosed cancer: A prospective transactional analysis. *Psycho-Oncology, 6,* 267–278.

Varni, J. W., Katz, E. R., Colgrove, R., & Dolgin, M. J. (1993). The impact of social skills training on the adjustment of children with newly diagnosed cancer. *Journal of Pediatric Psychology, 18,* 751–767.

Varni, J. W., Katz, E. R., Colgrove, R., & Dolgin, M. J. (1994a). Perceived social support and adjustment of children with newly diagnosed cancer. *Journal of Developmental and Behavioral Pediatrics, 15,* 20–26.

Varni, J. W., Katz, E. R., Colegrove, R., & Dolgin, M. (1994b). Perceived stress and adjustment of long-term survivors of childhood cancer. *Journal of Psychosocial Oncology, 12,* 1–16.

Varni J. W., Katz, E. R., Colegrove, R. J., & Dolgin, M. J. (1995). Perceived physical appearance and adjustment of children with newly diagnosed cancer: A path analytic model. *Journal of Behavioral Medicine, 18,* 261–278.

Varni, J. W., Katz, E. R., Colegrove, R. J., & Dolgin, M. J. (1996). Family functioning predictors of adjustment in children with newly diagnosed cancer: A prospective analysis. *Journal of Child Psychology and Psychiatry and Allied Disciplines, 37,* 321–328.

Varni, J. W., & Wallender, J. L. (1988) Pediatric chronic disabilities. In D. K. Routh (Ed.), *Handbook of pediatric psychology* (pp. 190–221). New York: Guilford.

Wallander, J. L., & Varni, J. W. (1989). Social support and adjustment in chronically ill and handicapped children. *American Journal of Community Psychology, 17,* 185–201.

Wallander, J. L., & Varni, J. W. (1992). Adjustment in children with chronic physical disorders: Programmatic research on a disability-stress-coping model. In A. M. LaGreca, L. J. Siegel, J. L. Wallender, & C. E. Walker (Eds.), *Stress and coping in child health* (pp. 279–298). New York: Guilford.

White, N. C. (2003). Educational related problems for children with cancer. *Journal of Pediatric Oncology Nursing, 20,* 50–55.

Wright, P. W. D., & Wright, P. D. (2002). *From emotions to advocacy: The special education survival guide.* Hartfield, VA: Harbor House Law Press.

Wright, P. W. D., Wright, P. D., & Heath, S. W. (2003). *No child left behind.* Hartfield, VA: Harbor House Law Press.

Zanily, L., Dagged, J., & Pestine, H. (1995). The influence of the pace of teacher attention on preschool children's engagement. *Behavior Modification, 19,* 339–356.

Zeltzer, L. K. (1993). Cancer in adolescents and young adults: Psychosocial aspects of long term survivors. *Cancer, 71*(10 Suppl.), 3463–3468.

Zeltzer, L. K., Dolgin, M. J., Sahler, O. J., Mulhern, R. D., Carpenter, D., Sargeant, L., et al. (1996) Sibling adaptation to childhood cancer collaborative study: Health outcomes of siblings of children with cancer. *Medical and Pediatric Oncology, 27,* 98–107.

# Palliative Care and End-of-Life Issues

18

David J. Bearison

# Palliative Care at the End of Life

## Introduction

Consider the following advice given to parents whose children are dying in hospitals: "If your child has to die, he can die peacefully. You can make sure he is free of pain. You can make sure that everyone has a chance to say good-bye" (Hilden & Tobin, 2003, p. 3). To offer parents this kind of unconditional assurance (i.e., "You can make sure . . . ") dismisses the confusing and disturbing realities of actually having to care for a child when it becomes increasingly apparent that curative intent is failing and staff begin to question how best to proceed. The complexity of symptom control in various clinical conditions sometimes precludes children from having peaceful deaths. However, when you read findings from the few palliative care studies that exist (and there are few that consider children as participants), issues of pain management and psychosocial support at the end of life do not seem to be so difficult to resolve. These findings promote ideas that, when satisfactory end-of-life care is not achieved, it is because mistakes were made, staff were inadequately trained, and children thereby were made to suffer unnecessarily. Such ways of thinking in turn lead bereft parents to feel guilty at not having empowered themselves to have taken greater control in the care of their child and to have done the right thing for their child.

Although mistakes occur, staff can be better trained, and children might unnecessarily suffer, there are very few guarantees of a comfortable way of dying from medical causes. Most textbooks and studies about end-of-life care simply ignore the messy realities and uncertainties, particularly as they pertain to children and their families. The Report to the Board of Directors of the American Psychological Association from its Working Group on Assisted Suicide and End-of-Life Decisions (2003) raised a clarion call to document publicly what it is like, in practical day-by-day terms, for people who die in hospitals and how it affects end-of-life decisions for the staff, patients, and families. We all prefer to die quickly, without protracted suffering and pain and without humiliation. Deaths during sleep are particularly preferred. However, such kinds of death are not so common.

When considering end-of-life issues, there is a need to capture the sense of immediacy and involvement of those who, day by day, make the critical decisions regarding end-of-life care of children. Such people have to account for how issues evolve in the press of hospital-based pediatric practice where dying often is messy, muddled, unduly complicated, sometimes painful, possibly degrading, wildly uncertain, meandering, mystifying, circuitous, dirty, and debilitating. For example, it is far from uncommon for children at the end of their lives to have the following, sometimes uncontrollable, symptoms: pain, anorexia, fatigue, dyspnea (i.e., gasping for air), constipation, vomiting food and blood (hematemesis), bleeding, seizures, fear, anxiety, and terminal agitation (Gawande, 2002; Nuland, 1994; Portenoy & Bruera, 2003; see Bearison, 2005, regarding particular cases of children dying in hospitals).

In the United States, each year 53,000 children die (Institute of Medicine [IOM], 2003). About half of all children's deaths occur in the neonatal and perinatal periods, most soon after birth because of congenital abnormalities. Among children and adolescents, unintentional (and sometimes intentional [i.e., suicidal]) accidents are the leading cause of death. Among medical conditions, the leading causes of death are cancers, diseases of the heart, and lower respiratory conditions (IOM, 2003). About 85% of children who die from medical causes do so in hospitals, and their median length of stay at the end is 7–9 days. This trend toward children dying in hospitals took hold after World War II, with increasing emphasis on acute care and the medicalization of death.

## Hospice

Despite the rise in hospice care in the United States, less than 1% of dying children receive hospice services (American Academy of Pediatrics, 2000; Frager, 1996). In the Netherlands, by contrast, approximately 80% of children dying of medical causes do so at home or out-of-hospital hospice care (Huijier, 2003). Current regulations in this country require that a child, to be eligible for hospice care, has 6 months or less to live—a difficult prediction for physicians to make given the prognostic uncertainties in pediatric care because of children's greater recuperative abilities (Levetown, 1996). A further barrier to adequate palliative care in this country has been a system that focuses on either active therapy with curative intent or hospice care, and this does not allow an appropriate interface between these two approaches. For example, to enter hospice care, patients must agree to forego any care with curative intent and accept strictly palliative care. This model of hospice benefits was developed by Medicare in 1982 for adult patients with no regard for children and adolescents.

Further barriers to out-of-hospital care for children at the end-of-their lives are fears and culturally grounded reluctance of parents in this country to wrestle with the idea of allowing their child to die at home. This is a particularly critical issue in a country such as ours with such a diverse amalgam of cultural beliefs and values about death and dying. It makes it difficult to establish uniform standards about what is important during the dying process and in end-of-life decision making. Despite arguments in favor of allowing children to die at home (Stajduhar & Davies, 1998) and at times the stated preferences of parents for home versus hospital palliative care (Lauer & Camitta, 1980; Martinson, 1993), little research has been conducted to explore systematically why this has not been practical or easy to accomplish in this country. There are no comprehensive current studies of whether families who had their child die at home versus in a hospital had an easier or more comfortable experience with their child's death or adjusted better to their loss (see Martinson & Papadatou, 1994).

## Informing Dying Children

Twenty years ago, those of us in the field of pediatric psychology spoke of a conspiracy of silence that existed between children who had cancer and adults caring for them. This situation portends the story of how we presently need to be with children who are dying. Then, children generally were reluctant to talk to adults (especially their parents), who in turn were reluctant to talk to them about common fears and uncertainties about having a life-threatening diagnosis such as cancer. Each, in their own way, thought that they were protecting the other, which of course led children to too readily seem to accept adults' false reassurances that everything is all right and there is nothing to worry about. Adults continued to offer such reassurances because children so readily seemed to accept them.

Since then, we have learned from children that what they know about having cancer and being treated profoundly affects their adjustment. It leads them on a powerful journey to find out as much as they can about cancer despite adults' reluctance to be open and honest with them. It is a journey in search of personal meanings and making sense of what is happening to them. Regardless of what, how, and when they are told, we find that even very young children with cancer are able to gather enough incidental cues from parents, peers, siblings, and medical staff to realize that their condition is serious enough to be life threatening. Often, they display a seemingly precocious discernment of the medical procedures, the biomedical implications of sequentially more toxic forms of chemotherapy, and the prognostic consequences of relapses following progressively briefer periods of remission (D. Bearison & Pacifici, 1989; D. J. Bearison, 1991; Bluebond-Langner, 1978; Nitschke et al., 1982). Although such a conspiracy of silence is still the norm in some countries, thankfully it no longer is in ours, where it is generally acknowledged that children have a fundamental right to know why they are hospitalized and under treatment (American Academy of Pediatrics, 1996).

Beyond the endemic problems of communicating with children about frightening topics, in the case of children who might be dying there are even greater barriers and more peculiar and distorted ways of communicating. Most children quickly come to perceive that adults simply are not able to talk to them about death, dying, and end-of-life decisions, so they begin to feel isolated and alienated. Despite their own fears, children's hesitancies to talk spontaneously about issues about their dying in such situations are more a reflection of the fears and anxieties they experience among others around them than their own. Parents and caregivers, largely because of their own fears about facing complicated and difficult issues and uncertainties about death and dying in both their own lives and the lives of others who are close to them, are quick to rationalize that children's hesitancy to pursue questions is a sign of their disinterest in learning about the limits of their care. What stronger evidence could there be of our collective fears about death and dying than the range of euphemisms we use to avoid facing this forbidden topic directly and honestly in discourse.

There is sufficient evidence today to concede that all children in hospitals know when they are dying, and that they are able to discern the extraordinary distress among family and caregivers around them when death becomes imminent (Bluebond-Langner, 1985; Faulkner, 2001; Lansdown & Benjamin, 1985; Sourkes, 1996; Spinetta & Maloney, 1975; Waechter, 1987). They therefore have the right to supportive and developmentally appropriate means to express their concerns about end-of-life issues (J. M. Hilden, Waterson, & Chrastek, 2003; Masera et al., 1999). This can be done by talking alone or in combination with various kinds of play activities, music, art, video, and so on. In ways appropriate to their level of social, cognitive, and emotional development, children should be included in discussions about withholding or withdrawing life-sustaining medical treatment (American Academy of Pediatrics, 1994). The American Academy of Pediatrics goes even further than not only endorsing the need for physicians to provide to children information needed to make decisions about health care, but also advises those physicians who choose to withhold information to assume the burden of justifying the decision not to disclose and document it in the medical record.

## Parents of Dying Children

The death of a child remains for any parent a constant presence in everything they do for the rest of their lives; it can never be fully resolved because there is no tolerable answer to why their child has died. It is unquestionably the most abominable anomaly in our sense of life and human development. Parents are an integral part of their child's health care team and are so acknowledged by the term *family-centered medicine*, the hallmark of pediatric practice in major medical centers.

However, in the course of a chronic and prolonged illness, when parents come to recognize that hope for a cure for their child is receding, they approach a new phase that portends profound changes in how they relate to the medical staff. We find that they begin to question, if not abandon, the premise that they, their child, and the medical staff are all inseparable in a common struggle to fight the illness and find a cure. While trying to protect their child from what they perceive as increasingly more frightening realities of death and dying, they press the medical staff to assume ever-more-heroic, invasive, and uncertain kinds of treatment protocols.

This press for increasingly more aggressive care means that attention often is diverted for parents (and medical staff) from addressing the child's feelings about death and dying. Even when physicians, however reluctant, go beyond established procedures to uncharted and highly experimental treatment protocols, it is only natural that, when their child dies, parents question whether they did all they possibly could to have saved their child. Although pediatric subspecialists often are seen as unwilling to accept death as a likely outcome and to pursue curative intent, if nothing else than as an experiment from which to learn and apply to other cases, parents typically are much less able than physicians to accept the idea that treatment ought to be withheld or withdrawn because there is no realistic chance of cure (Wolfe, Grier, et al., 2000).

Even when prior relations between parents and staff had been optimal, the ending of hope for cure imposes conflicting and frustrating issues on the relationship. Parents, who are feeling guilty for the looming death of their child, inevitably question if things could have been better if they had made other treatment decisions or had pursued care for their child at other medical centers. Other emotions at this time include intense anxiety, anger, and depression. Parents' relationships during this time can be either mutually supportive or alienating (Klass, 1988; Martinson & Papadatou, 1994; Miles & Demi, 1986; Rosof, 1994; Rubin, 1993).

## Anticipatory Grief

The idea of anticipatory grief as a coping mechanism for diminishing hope for cure has received special attention. It is a reaction by which parents begin to detach or distance themselves from their dying child. Others, however, have not reported widespread incidences of anticipatory grieving in parents. There is a long-running debate about whether it is related to bereavement outcomes in parents and families and how to deal with it if and when it does occur (Benfield, Leib, & Reuter, 1976; Binger et al., 1969; Friedman, Chodoff, Mason, & Hamburg, 1963; Spinetta, Swarner, & Sheposh,1981). Rando (1983), for example, found that the time parents spent in anticipatory grief affected bereavement outcome. Parents who had anticipatory grief beyond 18 months often left their child feeling abandoned, while those with less than 6 months had more intense grief reactions at the time of death and later.

## Grief Counseling

A related field of study is the effectiveness of bereavement interventions for parents and siblings who have lost a child. Although most bereavement counselors assume that their interventions are helpful, the research findings suggest otherwise. The efficacy of grief counseling is distressingly low compared to other kinds of psychotherapeutic interventions and in some cases is more debilitating than therapeutic (such as association with heightened symptoms of posttraumatic stress disorder; Murphy et al., 1998).

Allumbaugh and Hoyt (1999), in a meta-analysis of 35 bereavement intervention studies, found an overall effect size of only .43. Kato and Mann (1999), in a meta-analysis of 13 studies, reported effects sizes of .05, .27, and .09 for the reduction of depression, somatic symptoms, and other psychological symptoms, respectively. (We expect effect sizes of about .85 for most kinds of psychotherapeutic interventions.) They concluded that these effect sizes "suggest that psychological interventions for bereavement are not effective interventions" (p. 293).

Jordan and Neimeyer (2003), in an extensive review of several meta-analyses regarding the efficacy of bereavement interventions concluded that "it should no longer be taken for granted that grief counseling is necessary and necessarily helpful for all or most mourners.... grief counseling does not appear to be very effective.... (and) many of the people who receive it would do just as well (and perhaps, in some cases, better) without it" (p. 781). Bonanno (2004) also found that resilience to loss is much more common than it had previously been acknowledged.

It is not unusual for family, friends, and neighbors of parents whose children have died to be at a loss for words to express their feelings or to be able to appropriately comfort them. This leads to parents feeling anomic in their grief and mourning (Finkbeiner, 1996; Galli, 2000). Institutions involved in the welfare of children and families have not been very effective in providing ways to help parents cope with their reactions about their children dying and the grief and mourning that follows death. Only religious mysticism and rituals seem oriented to explicitly and systematically recognize the restorative roles of grief and mourning. That is why parents and children, regardless of their levels of prior religiosity, seek spiritual succor when coping with issues of death and dying (Bohannon, 1991; Miller & Thoresen, 2003).

## Medical Practice

Physicians generally are reluctant to consider anything but clearly tested methods of care because, when they are wrong, the consequences are too great. However, end-of-life care presents physicians with inescapable opportunities to move beyond established methods of medical practice. When it involves children, such opportunities rise exponentially, and caring for children who are dying is one of the most difficult struggles for hospital-based clinicians. For many complex reasons, it is something not easily addressed in medicine beyond what might be framed as the so-called good deaths and bad deaths. Good deaths are quick, uncomplicated, expected, progressive, and without pain and suffering, and all caregivers among all subspecialties are on the same page regarding end-of-life questions; bad deaths are the opposite of all that. Any death is seen among physicians and nurses as a failure of treatment because treatment, according to how they are trained, always is viewed as a cure from illness. The death of a patient, particularly when it is a child, can be a powerful impetus to seek new and more effective treatment protocols. Khaneja and Milrod (1998) found that a majority of attending physicians considered a patient's death as a personal failure. According to Epstein (2003), "This is a tough lesson for me and for doctors like me who were trained in a medical model that posited a cure as the only acceptable goal and death as a failure" (p. 41).

## Uncertain Consequences

Until the early part of the 20th century, most serious diseases, including cancer, took a fairly rapid course to death. Over time, however, medicine has become increasingly more complex. Despite substantially improved prognoses, greater complexity has led to more uncertain consequences for dying patients and their families. It is ironic that while the introduction of increasingly more effective kinds of treatments, medications, medical imaging technologies, and surgical procedures have produced remarkable improvements in prognoses and longer survival times, new uncertainties and risks have appeared because the chances of cure and survival in individual cases have become more unpredictable. It is these kinds of uncertainties that constitute the psychological impact of having to cope with increasingly protracted and complicated ways of dying. The growing sophistication of advanced medical practices (knowledge about which is increasingly accessible to patients and families on the Internet) has meant that people are living longer with knowledge that they may be dying while struggling to deny it at the same time.

A retrospective study of end-of-life care for children dying of cancer from 1990 to 1997 found that, in their last month of life, parents reported that 89% of children suffered a lot or a great deal; they suffered from pain or dyspnea (i.e., shortness of breath). Despite efforts to treat children for specific symptoms, treatments were successful in only 27% of children with pain and 16% with dyspnea (Wolfe, Grier, et al., 2000).

Similar findings have been found in geriatric studies of end-of-life care. Foley (1995), for example, found that a third of elderly patients were in unnecessary pain during the 24 hours prior to death, and two thirds had pain in the last month of their lives. Such findings support a widely held belief that dying patients receive less relief from symptoms during end-of-life care than they should, and that this is even more pronounced when dying patients are children (IOM, 2003; Schechter, 1989; Sirkia, Saarinen, Ahlgren, & Hovi, 1997; Walco, Cassidy, & Schechter, 1994; Zeltzer, 1994; see also chapter 7, this volume). A more recent survey, however, found that "81% of parents reported that the amount of pain medication their children received at the end of life was usually or always enough" (E. C. Meyer, Burns, Griffith, & Truog, 2002, p. 227).

A large part of the problem is that medical staff in tertiary care hospitals do not recognize the extent of children's suffering at end of life because they are trained to focus too much on cure as a goal of aggressive treatment, and they have too little training and clinical experience in caring for dying children. For example, 75% of children and adolescents with cancer today are cured, and children and adolescents account for only 4% of all deaths each year (IOM, 2003).

There is growing consensus that physicians are inadequately trained about death and dying during their preclinical and clinical years of medical school and then into their residency training (Khaneja & Milrod, 1998; Mermann et al., 1991; Rappaport & Witzke, 1993; Sahler, Frager, Levetown, Cohn, & Lipson, 2000; Von Gunten,

Ferris, & Emanuel, 2000). A survey of pediatric oncologists in 1998 by the American Society of Clinical Oncology found a serious lack of training in end-of-life care and a strikingly high reliance on trial and error in learning to care for dying children. "Ninety-two percent of doctors said that they had learned about end of life care by unguided trial and error" (Hilden et al., 2001, p. 206).

The study also reported that pediatric oncologists generally were anxious about discussing the likelihood of death with children and their parents; for example, "47% of pediatric oncologists do not initiate a discussion of advance directives; instead they leave this to the family to initiate" (Hilden et al, 2001, p. 207). On the other hand, 55% of parents whose children had died in intensive care units after forgoing life-sustaining treatment believed that they had little or no control of situations during their child's final days. Despite this, 76% agreed with staff regarding the decision to discontinue life support (E. C. Meyer et al., 2002). The American Society of Clinical Oncology concluded that there are substantial challenges to overcome barriers among caregivers to integrate curative intent, symptom control, psychosocial support, and palliative care in routine care of seriously ill children. According to Morgan and Murphy (2000), barriers to effective palliation reflect the overall perception of pediatricians, other caregivers, and families that discontinuing aggressive care means that they are giving up and, in effect, failing.

At a meeting of the Supportive Care Committee of the Children's Oncology Group (COG), it was reported that parents claimed that they were not adequately informed that the purpose of allowing their children to participate in Phase I cancer treatment protocols was for experimental research rather than finding a cure for their child's cancer. Reticence to so advise parents (and patients) of the transition from curative to palliative care reflects a more general disinclination among providers to deal with end-of-life issues and palliative care options in pediatrics. To help overcome this, COG is preparing a paragraph to be included in all Phase I informed consent documents to remind providers to discuss end-of-life issues when enrolling patients. Part of this paragraph (in draft) states, "At this time, as Phase I therapy is being offered, the possibility of a cure of the child's underlying disease is quite small. While not giving up all hope, the patient/family must be informed that the balance of primary approach needs now to be moved to the goal of providing for comfort" (COG, 2001).

## Palliative Care

### Geriatric Medicine

The emergent and expanding interest in palliative care today has been a response to the aging of the "baby boomer" generation, which also has fostered the development of geriatrics as an important medical subspecialty. Issues of palliative care in geriatric medicine have led to innovative ways to consider myriad options about how to handle death, dying, and end-of-life decisions. They have raised heretofore unthought-of bioethical questions about the uses and abuses of advancing medical protocols, technologies, and genetic engineering. Current debates about physician-assisted suicide and euthanasia laws are dramatic illustrations of end-of-life care bioethical concerns (American Psychological Association Working Group, 2000; New York State Task Force, 2000). Among geriatricians, decisions about end of life are coming to be considered moral and bioethical imperatives of how medicine cares for those for whom it can no longer promise a cure (IOM, 1997). As an aging baby boomer myself, I welcome this growing interest in how we die, how we might be comforted when facing death, and how we might be empowered to make our own decisions about ways of dying when we are terminally ill.

However, unlike geriatrics, in pediatrics dying is still considered very much a failure of medicine, and palliative care options are not as easy to approach, discuss, or resolve. End-of-life decisions regarding children are different from those involving adults (particularly the elderly) and therefore require their own sets of standards apart from geriatric medicine. Some of the issues that distinguish geriatric from pediatric end-of-life care involve the course of disease in children versus adults, decisions about withdrawing or withholding care, means of introducing advance directives, and guardianship over the best interests of children. Therefore, palliative care for children can never be a simple extension (or dumbing down) of adult palliative care.

The continuation of aggressive medical procedures, even when there is little realistic hope of a cure, is much more likely to occur for children than it is for adults (Morgan & Murphy, 2000). However, the stronger push to continue aggressive care means that too often less attention is given to controlling children's painful symptoms, and there is less time for patients, family, and caregivers to address emotions about death and grieving. Along these same lines, in our culture there is a greater sense of the failure of medicine when it involves the death of a child compared to the death of an adult. This also creates a stronger push to continue aggressive treatments. Having to face the failure of hope for a cure for a child has been described as the greatest ordeal of any pediatrician and the reason why so many primary care pediatricians choose not to pursue pediatric subspecialties such as oncology, cardiology, and transplantation (Wiener, 1970).

## Defining Palliative Care

Like any emerging inquiry, there are different definitions of palliative care. They have to do with questions about when, in the course of care from a potentially life-threatening diagnosis to the time when end-of-life decisions are considered, should the idea of palliative care fit. In this regard, there are broader and narrower definitions of palliative care. The IOM's Committee on Palliative and End-of-Life Care for Children and Their Families, for example, adopts a broad view. They define palliative care as "care that seeks to prevent, relieve, reduce, or soothe the symptoms produced by serious medical conditions or their treatment and to maintain patients' quality of life" (IOM, 2001, p. 30). It follows from this kind of definition that the benefits of palliative care need not be limited to people who are thought to be (or have a high probability of) dying.

In contrast, the World Health Organization (1990), for example, supports a narrower view of palliative care. They define palliative care as "the active total care of patients whose disease is not responsive to curative treatment... [when] control of pain, of other symptoms, and of psychological, social, and spiritual problems are paramount" (p. 11). Without the involvement of psychosocial members of a treatment team, the idea of palliative care likely will be understood in terms of the narrow definition and, accordingly, as the entry of the "grim reapers."

The American Academy of Pediatrics (2000) seeks to promote a more integrated model of palliative and curative treatment such that physicians and families do not have to exhaust all curative options to reverse the disease process before considering palliative interventions to relieve symptoms, regardless of their impact on the underlying disease. They further recognize that, at times,

> It may be difficult to define individual therapies as either curative or palliative. For example, mechanical ventilation often is viewed as a life-prolonging or curative therapy.... However, such support... may provide symptomatic relief from dyspnea and significantly improve a child's quality of life. (p. 352)

Cystic fibrosis is another example for which aggressive treatment without curative intent but to improve quality of life has prolonged children's life expectancies from several years to decades.

While fully recognizing that the concern for effective pain management, symptom relief, and maintaining quality of life are integral components of medicine at all stages of treatment, from diagnosis to death, interest here is in palliative care at the end of life. Then, the need to monitor the relative balance between comfort and quality of life with hopes of extending life becomes overwhelming and paramount. But, ways of defining and assessing quality of life in palliative care at the end-of-life are controversial and difficult. The American Academy of Pediatrics (1994) cautioned that quality of life must be determined according to a patient's subjective experience of life and not according to how parents or health care providers perceive the experience. Hence, there is not necessarily a direct relationship among a patient's medical condition, the treatment he or she is receiving, and his or her quality of life (Casarett, 2003; Cohen, 2003).

Specialty and subspecialty areas in medicine evolve when we recognize that other fields of medicine have not adequately addressed the needs of special classes of patients. In this regard, we might question the need for yet another medical subspecialty in palliative end-of-life care. In other words, if all physicians were trained to provide palliative care as a basic component of medical practice, do we need such a subspecialty? We probably do because progressively fatal end-of-life care presents unique sets of scenarios that transcend the initiating diagnosis.

At its best, palliative care always is multidisciplinary, including physicians, nurses, social workers, psychologists, chaplains, and child life specialists (Lloyd-Williams, 2003). Comprehensive palliative care encompasses the following kinds of clinical skills: (a) communicating, (b) decision making, (c) management of complications of treatment and disease, (d) symptom control, (e) psychosocial care of patient and family, and (f) care of the dying (Foley & Gelband, 2001).

## Research in Pediatric Palliative Care

Reflecting its early stage of inquiry, there is relatively little research in pediatric palliative care (Davies, Steele, Stajduhar, & Bruce, 2003). Although to date most palliative care studies have been in the field of nursing, a review of 50 leading textbooks in pediatric nursing found only 2% of their contents discussed end-of-life care (Ferrell, 2003). Most of the literature rests on case studies from clinical practice rather than controlled studies using quantitative data. Most studies are retrospective and cross sectional (rather than longitudinal or based across a sequence of events).

The two primary areas of palliative care research reflect the physical and psychological aspects of end-of-life issues: (a) pain and symptom management and (b) psychosocial support and quality of life. There is very little research directly involving children as active or direct participants at the end of their lives. Findings rest more on the perspectives of parents and care providers. Given who dies in pediatric hospitals, most of the research on end-of-life care is shaped by the disciplinary needs and concerns of pediatric oncology.

Barriers to quantitative research on end-of-care of children include (a) diversity, both within and beyond oncology, of different kinds of illnesses and medical conditions at end of life; (b) small number of participants at any one institution, which therefore requires complicated multicenter trials; (c) lack of developmentally appropriate assessment tools; (d) the sense that it is an intrusive and risky topic to study; (e) bioethical concerns; and (f) regulatory constraints imposed by institutional review boards on studies of end-of-life care in children.

Third-year pediatric residents were surveyed in 1984 about their experiences in end-of-life care. Those findings led the authors to conclude that end-of life care in pediatrics "continues to have a shadowy subterranean existence" (Sack, Fritz, Krener, & Sprunger, 1984, p. 681). Although insufficient attention has been devoted to end-of-life issues for children and their families, there is clear and compelling evidence to believe that this is changing in significant ways relative to emergent questions in practice, research, training, and policy (American Psychological Association's Task Force, 2003).

## When Does End-of-Life Care Begin?

Children dying in hospitals challenge caregivers' relationships with parents in myriad ways. Families and medical staff become increasingly entwined. It becomes particularly dramatic when questions arise concerning the futility of attempting to continue heroic and life-sustaining treatments. Although it remains the responsibility of the attending physician to clearly explain, when appropriate, to parents and their children the futility of further treatments, it is never clear how decisions to continue or to withhold curative care are ultimately made.

Often, physicians' explanations of what is medically happening unwittingly carry the decision to either suspend or prolong aggressive interventions for cure despite their professed (or not-so-professed) obligation to adhere to the principle of patient autonomy. Sometimes, our perceptions of children's suffering pushes the decision to suspend care. Alternatively, it is more likely that there are times when, because of their denial or inability to accept their child's death, parents insist on treatments that physicians and other caregivers perceive as tragically prolonging the child's dying process and suffering. There also are times when decisions to prolong aggressive curative care are seen by hospital administrators as poor uses of institutional resources. Further problems arise when there are conflicting concerns, biases, and theoretical ideologies among different medical subspecialists (often between pediatric intensivists in the intensive care units and specialists treating the presenting diagnoses) as well as among the differing professional roles assumed by the range of caregivers: residents, attendings, fellows, social workers, psychologists, and nurses.

Our sense of the onset of end-of-life care typically begins when an attending physician concludes that there is no realistic chance of cure. This usually is documented in the medical chart and sometimes with reference to DNR (do not resuscitate) status, when consent for such has been obtained from parents. When and how this conclusion is communicated to patients and families and how it impacts decision making about end-of-life issues and palliative care are concerns in medicine. There are many studies that document the myriad problems that medical caregivers have in discussing with patients and their families issues about palliative care and the growing need for better education, training, and professional development across all disciplines in this area and at all stages of professional experience (Heaven & Maquire, 2003; von Gunten et al., 2000; Ptacek & Eberhardt, 1996; Tulsky, Fischer, Rose, & Arnold, 1998). Parents often have reported that communications with caregivers at their children's end of life were vague and confusing (J. M. Hilden et al., 2001; Whittam, 1993). Oncologists, on the other hand, reported that their most troublesome problem in end-of-life care were unrealistic expectations for cure on the part of families (Hilden et al., 2000).

Caregivers need to learn how to overcome a variety of fears when communicating bad news in end-of-life care: (a) fear of being blamed for the outcome; (b) fear of not knowing the outcome; (c) fear of releasing an uncontrollable reaction in the other; (d) fear of expressing and controlling one's own emotions; and (e) fear of not having the answers (Browning & Meyer, 2003; Sahler, McAnarney, & Friedman, 1981). When breaking bad news, they have to arrive at a reasonable balance between the offer of hope and the reality of end-of-life decisions (Buckman, 1992; Fallowfield, 1993; Larson & Tobin, 2000; Ptacek & Eberhardt, 1996).

Caregivers in end-of-life pediatric care need training in the following areas: (a) engaging with children and families; (b) relieving pain and other symptoms; (c) analyzing ethical challenges in end-of-life decision making; (d) responding to suffering and bereavement; (e) improving communication and relationships; (f) establishing continuity of care; (g) providing staff support; and (h) being sensitive to culturally diverse beliefs and values about death and dying. Among psychologists, training in basic pediatric medicine and awareness of the cultural milieu of a hospital is essential, if for no other reason than to know which questions to ask in the press of practice to learn more about such things as causes of death and the dying process; nature of trauma; children's understanding of their condition and understanding of death; adherence and compliance issues; and ways to commemorate children's lives. An excellent example of this kind of training in pediatric palliative care for all caregivers can be found in the work of Browning (2002).

## End-of-Life Decisions

There always is, in hospitals, a fine line between dying and death. How, when, and why this line becomes either tauter or looser typically is in the hands of senior attending physicians making end-of-life medical decisions. The further they move from struggling to sustain life for hope of a cure toward the interminable biological degradation of dying, the less their decisions become matters of what is scientifically correct or wrong. Instead, there remain only questions about what means there are to what ends. If the end is curative, then certain things will be done, and these things might preclude opportunities to fully provide patients with palliative care. If there is no hope for cure, then other things will be done to provide the patient with as much as can be done to relieve pain, manage symptoms, and provide a decent quality of life. There even is broad agreement that "analgesics may be ethically administered to terminally ill patients at doses risking death due to respiratory depression, provided that lower doses and other means have proven inadequate, that the intention is to relieve pain and not to induce death, and that permission has been obtained with full disclosure of the risk of death" (Freyer, 1992, p. 141; see also Tadmor, Postovsky, Elhasid, Barak, & Arush, 2003).

When the attending physician finds that treatment no longer benefits the patient and should be forgone, the patient and parents need to be so notified. Parents cannot compel a physician to provide any treatment that a physician judges as unlikely to benefit the patient, and parents cannot withhold treatment from a child if a physician thinks it will substantially benefit the child (Council on Ethical and Judicial Affairs, 1991). The latter case requires invoking the intervention of child protective services to contravene parental authority. However, laws and judicial decisions in some states allow parents to exercise broad discretion when acting on their child's behalf (Armstrong, 1988).

Particularly difficult questions in pediatrics regarding end-of-life care occur when child patients (typically adolescents) choose end-of-life treatment options that go against what their parents or siblings prefer. In such cases, physicians, along with the rest of the medical staff, are put in a particularly difficult situation in which they have to negotiate between conflicting interests to consider the best interests of the patient. Although this hardly ever was the case in the 1980s (Nitschke et al., 1982), the increasing end-of-life care options today make it more likely to have conflicting interests between patients and their families. There is a compelling need for further studies of this.

## Right or Wrong?

End-of-life decisions about caring for children in hospitals never are simply right or wrong. They stretch the limits of medical practice that we like to think of as orderly and utterly rational. There is a dearth of reliable empirical evidence to guide us in considering end-of-life decisions (IOM, 2001). At the point when life-and-death decisions have to be made about how to proceed with clinical care, medicine struggles to adapt new ways of understanding the relation of illness to humanity.

There is a continuing debate about the appropriateness of applying life-sustaining medical technologies to all critically ill children (American Academy of Pediatrics, 1994; Weir, 1992). The greatest controversy has surrounded decisions about the treatment of newborns with readily identifiable medical problems, including genetic disorders, malformations, and deformations (Anspach, 1993; Bosk, 1992). Although medicine is an applied science, it becomes increasingly imperfect and scientifically uncertain as it moves toward end-of-life decisions in individual cases. As scientific uncertainties regarding outcomes escalate, physicians find that they have only a range of noncontingent statistical probabilities on which to rely.

A major problem in considering kinds of palliative care is that we do not know what outcomes are desirable. In the literal sense, the outcome is clear—the child is going to die—but, to what extent can it be shown that palliative care has a positive impact on the welfare of a dying child and his or her family, and how can we measure this? The scientific community, often with a disdaining nod to the contingencies of practice, describe this as a process of moving from nomothetic to ideographic science. This breach between the science of medicine and clinical practice inevitably expands as we move toward end-of-life decisions; ultimately, it pushes medicine to its limits to reveal its best and worst aspects.

There can be no theory of dying if, by a theory, we mean a set of principles and standards that apply across individuals and situations, even if not across times and cultures. There are no natural and few empirically based answers to most of the questions that arise at end-of-life care, particularly when they involve children. Hence, answers to end-of-life care ultimately rest on bioethics that, in the most profound sense, capture the cultural and moral lessons by which we live. Accordingly, there can never be a correct or incorrect way of dying. Those who promulgate such a coercive orthodoxy about dying are at best misled or, worse, imperious. From my experience with end-of-life issues in pediatrics, all standards of practice boil down to somehow finding ways to respect and honor what patients, within the purview of family-based practice, find is best for them.

While advance medical directives, power-of-attorney documents, and DNR orders address the clinical management of dying in a legal sense, they say little about dying in the biological, psychosocial, and cultural senses. Questions about how, from whom, by whom, and particularly when to solicit a DNR order are some of the most difficult in pediatrics. How DNR directives are elicited raises questions about whether the DNR (a) is more caregiver centered than patient centered; (b) reflects a natural process of dying or the medically technological means that can circumvent a sense of a natural process; and (c) is veiled in language that is more negative than positive. Questions of this kind have led some to advocate substituting the DNR order with a different kind of directive—an AND (i.e., allow natural death) order (C. Meyer, 2003).

### Discontinuing Life-Sustaining Treatments

The purpose of discontinuing life-sustaining treatments is to allow incurably ill patients to die free from needless suffering. There is consensus among philosophers, theologians, physicians, and attorneys that it is ethically permissible to withdraw or withhold treatment or even forgo extensive, invasive, and burdensome diagnostic procedures if the burdens of continuing them exceed their benefits as judged from the patient's point of view (Council on Ethical and Judicial Affairs, 1986). However, special considerations arise when the discontinuation of life-sustaining treatment involves children. Like adults, when children fail primary therapy or develop life-threatening complications, their chances for survival decrease along with their tolerance for continued treatment. The continuation of life-sustaining treatment risks seriously impairing the quality of their remaining lives. For example, continuing chemotherapeutic agents entails substantial side effects, such as severe immunosuppression, infections, nausea and vomiting, mucositis, and profound malaise.

Although withholding treatment and discontinuing treatment at the end of life have the same intent and are morally equivalent, decisions to discontinue treatment are tougher than those to withhold treatment (Council on Ethical and Judicial Affairs, 1986). It is hardly ever clear when to discontinue treatment and much more so in the care of children than adults because

> each child's case, while sharing some similarities with others, represents a unique composite of medical, developmental, psychosocial, and familial factors integral to making such determinations. The evaluation of these factors is complicated by clinical scenarios that are often technically complex and always emotionally charged. (Freyer, 1992, p. 136)

Some find that, when there is a reasonable option to initiate life-sustaining treatment, it is ethically advisable to provisionally start a time-limited trial using clearly defined and well-adhered-to criteria for stopping should treatment prove ineffective or unacceptably burdensome (Freyer, 1992). Having said as much, during the last month of life the majority of children who die from chronic conditions receive some kind of therapies for the purpose of cure or prolonging life.

## Patient Autonomy in Pediatrics

The idea of autonomy in medicine refers to a patient's right to choose or refuse treatment. It is ethically ensured by the practice of informed consent. In the case of children, it requires that they be informed in a developmentally appropriate way of the nature and consequences of treatment, discontinuing treatment, and palliative care. However, it is not clear at what stage of development and under which conditions children are functionally competent to (a) rationally consider multiple factors in predicting future consequences; (b) comprehend medical information regarding relations among treatment, symptoms, and outcome probabilities; (c) be free from the coercion of others to make a medical decision; and (d) fully appreciate the immediacy and permanence of their choices.

Even adults are confused by subtle yet complex distinctions between being incurably ill and imminently dying. A study found that 43 of 44 parents of children with end-stage cancer agreed that children older than 5 years have the capacity to make decisions about experimental treatments and ought to be included in final-stage conferences with physicians (Nitschke et al., 1982). Even though we like to think that children in these situations have a seemingly precocious understanding of what is going on, we know very little about what it means for children to consent to initiate or withdraw heroic and life-sustaining measures and therefore how much autonomy they ought to be given in such cases.

We like to assume that parents will make judgments and take actions that advance the interests of their children. Yet, there are biases inherent in the nature of parent-child relations that preclude the idea of a necessarily common regard of autonomy between a child and his or her parents. Parents have some interests that are separate from those of their children. Sometimes, they involve their own needs and desires; other times, they involve those of their spouses, the siblings of the child patient, and other family members. Therefore, pediatricians, more so than parents, are ethically and legally obligated to function as agents in the best interests of children in medical situations. There is consensus in medicine that life-sustaining treatment should be forgone if the competent child patient does not wish it; on the other hand, it should not be withheld if the child patient believes it will benefit him or her, even when parents refuse it. Medical ethicists have proposed the following:

> If a minor has experienced an illness for some time, understands it and the benefits and

> burdens of its treatment, has the ability to reason about it, has previously been involved in decision making about it, and has a comprehension of death that recognizes its personal significance and finality, then that person, irrespective of age, is competent to consent to forgoing life-sustaining treatment. (Leikin, 1989, p. 21)

A study of adult patients with advanced cancer found that most wanted an active role in medical decision making, but a substantial minority (28%) chose a passive role (Rothenbacher, Lutz, & Porzsolt, 1997). However, other ethicists consider the premise of patient autonomy a bioethical paradox that places unwanted and debilitating burdens on patients (children or adults) who want to place their hopes in the hands of physicians they find competent and who they trust (Schneider, 1998). On the other hand, some pediatric subspecialists find it awkward to be asked by parents such kinds of questions as, "What would you do if this were your child?"

## Principles and Practices

There often is a world of difference between practice guidelines derived from abstract conceptual frameworks and how they are applied in practice. No other decision in medicine has greater consequences, emotional biases, and ethical concerns than decisions about whether to withhold or withdraw treatment. Guidelines concerning such decisions have long been clearly and consistently stated (Fleischman et al., 1994). Decisions to withhold or withdraw treatment need to consider the benefits of treatment against levels of harm (e.g., pain, suffering, and quality of life) to the patient.

In practice, however, the boundaries between what is clearly beneficial and is not beneficial are blurred and produce scenarios in which the benefits are marginal or uncertain. Likewise, the boundaries between levels of harm are not easily dichotomized in simple high/low (yes/no) terms. Levels of pain and suffering are subjective, culturally understood, and very difficult to measure.

Hence, providers and families are faced with decisions when beneficial outcomes are uncertain and possibilities of harm are considerable. Parents have reported that the three principle factors, in descending order of importance, guiding their end-of-life decisions about withholding care from their children were (a) their sense of their child's quality of life; (b) chances of their child getting better; and (c) their amount of pain or discomfort. Factors such as "What I believe my child would have wanted," religious/spiritual beliefs, advice of hospital staff, and financial costs were not critical factors for them (E. C. Meyer, Burns, Griffith, & Truog, 2002).

### When to Stop

A survey questioned what percentage benefit would be needed for someone to agree to chemotherapy as a treatment for cancer. The difference between cancer patients and oncologists, respectively, was dramatic: 10% and 50%. Even for the relief of symptoms (not cure), patients were willing to accept a 10% chance of improvement compared to 50% for oncologists (Slevin et al., 1990). Is it because oncologists are more aware of the toxicities of chemotherapy and have seen too many suffering patients being treated for too long for too little benefit, or does it reflect the overwhelming fear that adults have of dying? What about children?

There is such a profound sense of the failure of medicine when it involves the death of a child compared to an adult that there is a substantially greater momentum to continue aggressive treatments, even when they provide little realistic hope of a cure and often impose barriers to adequate palliation for children (Morgan & Murphy, 2000; Whittam, 1993). For example, one study in a major medical center found that 56% of children with cancer were receiving cancer-directed therapy in the last month of their lives (Wolfe, Klar, et al., 2000). Increasing toxicities of curative treatments at end-of-life create conditions by which children's quality of life often is compromised. In these situations, parents are forced to face the gruesome question of whether it is better to hang on to a glimmer of hope and have their child live a little longer, even though he or she is suffering, or die sooner but in relative comfort (McCallum, Byrne, & Bruera, 2000; van der Wal, Renfurm, van Vught, & Gemke, 1999).

Wolfe, Klar, et al. (2000) found that parents of children who died of cancer first recognized that their child had no realistic chance for cure 106 days prior to their death, while pediatric oncologists came to such conclusions 206 days prior. They reported that "as their children's cancer advanced, parents' understanding that their child no longer had a realistic chance for cure was delayed, lagging behind the explicit documentation of this fact by the primary oncologist by more than 3 months" (p. 2473). In addition, parents in this study recalled having had a discussion at some time with a caregiver about their child not having a realistic chance for cure, but only 49% of them understood that this meant that their child was terminally ill. These findings speak to the difficulty that pediatric oncologists have in breaking bad news and openly and honestly discussing end-of-life issues. However, just as important, the findings reflect parents' reluctance to consider the probability that their child is likely to die.

For many physicians who deal with life-threatening diseases, decisions to continue aggressive and invasive treatments in the hope of a cure simply is a win-win situation. It is so difficult for them to accept the idea of children dying in their care that they pursue procedures (e.g., complex microneurosurgeries, bone marrow transplants) that may hold little hope for recovery but because, by doing so, there is a chance for hope. A pediatric neurosurgeon put it this way: "Standing by and doing nothing while a child dies was not an option for me. I resolved never to give up on a kid without fighting for as long and hard as the child and his parents were willing" (Epstein, 2003, p. 54). It also is not uncommon for them to believe that, even if they lose a child to the procedure, they will have learned things that will benefit other patients down the road.

As much as we might hear that the aim of palliative care is to comfort patients by providing adequate pain management and maintaining quality of life, this is not so obvious in tertiary care pediatric practices, in which aggressive and invasive treatment protocols are pursued in the hope of a cure. This is a sensitive issue that health care providers often are reluctant to discuss. Those who care for children in such critical ways are less able to bring themselves to the point of knowing when to relinquish hope of curative treatment and when to provide the palliative means for children to have calm and comfortable deaths. This is as much the case for the medical staff as it is for the parents. The interpersonal dynamics between medical staff and parents around this issue become a veiled dance back and forth that is tragic when, in the end, the child dies.

*Acknowledgments.* Preparation of this chapter was supported partly by a grant from the W. T. Grant Foundation, for which the author is extremely grateful. Membership on the Task Force on End-of-Life Issues for Children and Adolescents of the American Psychological Association was a significant contributory factor in preparing this chapter, as was being a Rockefeller Foundation Resident Scholar at the Villa Serbelloni in Bellagio, Italy.

Parts of this chapter have been adapted from D. Bearison's book, *When Treatment Fails: How Medicine Cares for Dying Children* (Oxford University Press, 2005).

## References

Allumbaugh, D. L., & Hoyt, W. T. (1999). Effectiveness of grief therapy: A meta-analysis. *Journal of Consulting Pyschology, 46*, 370–380.

American Academy of Pediatrics. (1994). Guidelines on forgoing life-sustaining medical treatment. *Pediatrics, 93*, 532–536.

American Academy of Pediatrics, Committee on Bioethics. (1996). Ethics and the care of critically ill infants and children. *Pediatrics, 93*, 149–152.

American Academy of Pediatrics, Committee on Bioethics and Committee on Hospital Care. (2000). Palliative care for children. *Pediatrics, 106*, 351–357.

American Psychological Association Task Force on End-of-Life Issues for Children. (2003, November). *Unpublished proceedings of the task force*. Washington, DC: American Psychological Association.

American Psychological Association Working Group on Assisted Suicide and End-of-Life Decisions. (2000, May). *Report to the Board of Directors of the American Psychological Association*. Washington, DC: American Psychological Association.

Anspach, R. R. (1993). *Who lives: Fateful choices in the intensive-care nursery*. Berkeley, CA: University of California Press.

Armstrong, C. J. (1988). Judicial involvement in treatment decisions: The emerging consensus. In J. Civetta, R. W. Taylor, & R. R. Karby (Eds.), *Critical care*. Philadelphia: Lippincott.

Bearison, D., & Pacifici, C. (1989). Children's event knowledge of cancer treatment. *Journal of Applied Developmental Psychology, 10*, 469–486.

Bearison, D. J. (1991). *"They never want to tell you"—Children talk about cancer*. Cambridge, MA: Harvard University Press.

Bearison, D. J. (2005). *When treatment fails: How medicine cares for dying children*. New York: Oxford University Press.

Benfield, D. G., Leib, S. A., & Reuter, J. (1976). Grief responses of parents after referral of the critically ill newborn to a regional center. *New England Journal of Medicine, 294*, 975–978.

Binger, C., Ablin, A., Feuerstein, R., Kushner, J., Zoger, S., & Mikkelen, C. (1969). Childhood leukemia: Emotional impact on the family. *New England Journal of Medicine, 280*, 414–418.

Bluebond-Langner, M. (1978). *The private worlds of dying children*. Princeton, NJ: Princeton University Press.

Bohannon, J. (1991). Religiosity related to grief levels of bereaved mothers and fathers. *Omega, 23*, 153–159.

Bonanno, G. A. (2004). Loss, trauma, and human resilience. *American Psychologist, 59*, 20–28.

Bosk, C. L. (1992). *All God mistakes: Genetic counseling in a pediatric hospital*. Chicago: University of Chicago Press.

Browning, D. (2002). *What matters to families?* Videotape series. The Initiative for Pediatric Palliative Care Curriculum. Newton, MA: Education Development Center. Retrieved December 12, 2003, from http://www.ippcweb.org

Browning, D., & Meyer, E. (2003, November). *Difficult conversations with children and families in palliative care*. Paper presented at the meeting of the Initiative for Pediatric Palliative Care, New York.

Buckman, R. (1992). *How to break bad news: A guide for health care professionals*. Baltimore, MD: Johns Hopkins University Press.

Casarett, D. J. (2003). Assessing decision-making capacity in the setting of palliative care research. In R. K. Portenoy & E. Bruera (Eds.), *Issues in palliative care research* (pp. 243–258). New York: Oxford University Press.

Children's Oncology Group, Task Force on End-of-Life Care. (2001, October). Semi-annual Meeting, San Antonio, TX.

Cohen, S. R. (2003). Assessing quality of life in palliative care. In R. K. Portenoy & E. Bruera (Eds.), *Issues in palliative care research* (pp. 231–241). New York: Oxford University Press.

Council on Ethical and Judicial Affairs of the American Medical Association. (1986). *Withholding or withdrawing life-prolonging treatment*. Chicago: American Medical Association.

Council on Ethical and Judicial Affairs of the American Medical Association. (1991). Pediatrics and the patient self-determination act. *Pediatrics, 1265*, 1868–1871.

Davies, B., Steele, R., Stajduhar, K., & Bruce, A. (2003). Research in pediatric palliative care. In R. K. Portenoy & E. Bruera (Eds.), *Issues in palliative care research* (pp. 355–370). New York: Oxford University Press.

Epstein, E. (2003). *If I get to five: What children can teach us about courage and character*. New York: Holt.

Fallowfield, L. (1993). Giving sad and bad news. *Lancet, 341*, 476–478.

Faulkner, K. W. (2001). Children understanding of death. In A. Armstrong-Dailey & S. Zarbock (Eds.), *Hospice care for children* (2nd. ed., pp. 9–22). New York: Oxford University Press.

Ferrell, B. (2003, November). End of Life Nursing Education Consortium (ELNEC): National efforts to improve pediatric palliative care. Paper presented at the meeting of the Initiative for Pediatric Palliative Care, New York, NY.

Finkbeiner, A. K. (1996). *After the death of a child: Living with loss through the years*. New York: Free Press.

Fleischman, A. R., Nolan, K., Dubler, N. N., Epstein, M. F., Gerben, M. A., Jellinek, M. S., et al. (1994). Caring for gravely ill children. *Pediatrics, 94*, 433–439.

Foley, K. M. (1995). Pain, physician assisted dying and euthanasia. *Pain, 4*, 163–178.

Foley, K. M., & Gelband, H. (Eds.). (2001). *Improving palliative care for cancer: Summary and recommendations*. Report of the National Cancer Policy Board of the Institute of Medicine and the Commission on Life Sciences of the National Research Council. Washington, DC: National Academy Press.

Frager, G. (1996). Pediatric palliative care: Building the model, bridging the gap. *Journal of Palliative Care, 12*, 9–12.

Freyer, D. R. (1992). Children with cancer: Special considerations in the discontinuation of life-sustaining treatment. *Medical and Pediatric Oncology, 20*, 136–142.

Friedman, S. B., Chodoff, P., Mason, J. W., & Hamburg, D. A. (1963). Behavioral observations on parents anticipating the death of a child. *Pediatrics, 32*, 610–625.

Galli, R. (2000). *Rescuing Jeffrey: A memoir*. New York: St. Martins.

Gawande, A. (2002). *Complications: A surgeon notes on an imperfect science*. New York: Henry Holt.

Heaven, C. M., & Maquire, P. (2003). Communication issues. In M. Lloyd-Williams (Ed.), *Psychosocial issues in palliative care* (pp. 13–34). New York: Oxford University Press.

Hilden, J., & Tobin, D. R. (2003). *Shelter from the storm: Caring for a child with a life-threatening condition*. Cambridge, MA: Persues.

Hilden, J. M., Emmanuel, E. J., Fairclough, D. L., Link, M. P., Foley, K. M., Clarridge, B. C., et al. (2001). Attitudes and practices among pediatric oncologists regarding end-of-life care: Results of the 1998 American Society of Clinical Oncology Survey. *Journal of Clinical Oncology*, 19, 205–212.

Hilden J. M., Waterson, J., & Chrastek, J. (2003). Tell the children. *Journal of Clinical Oncology Supplement (The art of oncology: When the tumor is not the target), 21*, 37s–39s.

Huijier, H. A. (2003, November). *Cultural challenges in family centered care*. Paper presented at the Initiative for Pediatric Palliative Care National Symposium, New York, NY.

Institute of Medicine. (1997). *Approaching death: Improving care at the end of life*. Washington, DC: National Academy Press.

Institute of Medicine. (2001). *Improving palliative care for cancer*. Washington, DC: National Academy of Sciences.

Institute of Medicine of the National Academies. (2003). *When children die: Improving palliative and end-of-life care for children and their families*. Washington, DC: National Academies Press.

Jordan, J. R., & Neimeyer, R. A. (2003). Does grief counseling work? *Death Studies, 27*, 765–786.

Kato, P. M., & Mann, T. (1999). A synthesis of psychological interventions for the bereaved. *Clinical Psychology Review, 19*, 275–296.

Khaneja, S., & Milrod, B. (1998). Educational needs among pediatricians regarding caring for terminally ill children. *Archives of Pediatric and Adolescent Medicine, 152*, 909–914.

Klass, D. (1988). *Parental grief: Solace and resolution*. New York: Springer.

Kubler-Ross, E. (1983). *On children and death*. New York: Macmillan.

Lansdown, R., & Benjamin, G. (1985). The development of the concept of death in children aged 5–9 years. *Child Care Health and Development, 11*, 13–20.

Larson, D., & Tobin (2000). End-of-life conversations: Evolving practice and theory. *Journal of the American Medical Association, 284*, 1573–1578.

Lauer, M., & Camitta, B. (1980). Home care for dying children: A nursing model. *Journal of Pediatrics, 997*, 1032–1035.

Leikin, S. (1989). A proposal concerning decisions to forgo life-sustaining treatment for young people *Journal of Pediatrics, 115*, 17–22.

Levetown, M. (1996). Ethical aspects of pediatric palliative care. *Journal of Palliative Care, 12*, 35–39.

Lloyd-Williams, M. (Ed.). (2003). *Psychosocial issues in palliative care*. New York: Oxford University Press.

Martinson, I. (1993). Hospice care for children: Past, present, and future. *Journal of Pediatric Oncology Nursing, 10*, 93–98.

Martinson, I. M., & Papadatou, D. (1994). Care of the dying child and the bereaved. In D. J. Bearison & R. K. Mulhern (Eds.). *Pediatric psychooncology: Psychological perspectives on children with cancer* (pp. 193–214). New York: Oxford University Press.

Masera, G., Spinetta, J. J., Jankovic, M., Ablin, A. R., D'Angio, G. J., Van Dongen-Melman, J., et al. (1999). Guidelines for assistance to terminally ill children with cancer: A report of the SIOP working committee on psychological issues in pediatric oncology. *Medical Pediatric Oncology, 32*, 44–48.

McCallum, D. E., Byrne, P., & Bruera, E. (2000). How children die in hospital. *Journal of Pain and Symptom Management, 20*, 417–423.

Mermann, A. C., Gunn, D. B., & Dickinson, G. E. (1991). Learning to care for the dying: A survey of medical schools and a model course. *Academy of Medicine, 66*, 35–38.

Meyer, C. (2003). Allow natural death: An alternative to DNR? Rockford, MI: Hospice Patients Alliance. http://www.hospicepatients.org/and.html December 14, 2003.

Meyer, E. C., Burns, J. P., Griffith, J., & Truog, R. D. (2002). Parental perspectives on end-of-life care in the pediatric intensive care unit. *Critical Care Medicine, 30*, 226–231.

Miles, M. S., & Demi, A. S. (1986). Guilt in bereaved parents. In T. A. Rando (Ed.), *Parental loss of a child* (pp. 97–118). Champaign, IL: Research Press.

Miller, W. R., & Thoresen, C. E. (2003). Spirituality, religion, and health: An emerging research field. *American Psychologist, 58*, 24–35.

Morgan, E. R., & Murphy, S. B. (2000). Care of children who are dying of cancer. *New England Journal of Medicine, 342*, 347–348.

Murphy, S. A., Johnson, C., Cain, K. C., Gupta, A. D., Diamond, M., Lohan, J., et al. (1998). Broad-spectrum group treatment for parents bereaved by the violent death of their 12 to 28 year-old children: A randomized controlled trial. *Death Studies, 22*, 209–235.

New York State Task Force on Life and Law. (2000) *When death is sought: Assisted suicide and euthanasia in the medical context* (2nd ed.). Albany, NY: NYS Department of Health.

Nitschke, R., Humphrey, G. B., Sexauer, C. L., Catron, B., Wunder, S., & Jay, S. (1982). Therapeutic choices made by patients with end-stage cancer. *Behavioral Pediatrics, 101*, 471–476.

Nuland, S.(1994). *How we die: Reflections on life final chapter*. New York: Knopf.

Portenoy, R. K., & Bruera, E. (Eds.) (2003). *Issues in palliative care research*. New York: Oxford University Press.

Ptacek, J. T., & Eberhardt, T. L. (1996). Breading bad news: A review of the literature. *Journal of the American Medical Association, 276*, 496–502.

Rando, T. (1983). An investigation of grief and adaptation in parents whose children have died from cancer. *Journal of Pediatric Psychology, 8*, 3–20.

Rappaport, W., & Witzke, D. (1993). Education about death and dying during the clinical years of medical school. *Surgery, 113*, 163–165.

Rosof, B. (1994). *The worst loss: How families heal from the death of a child.* New York: Henry Holt.

Rothenbacher, D., Lutz, M., Porzsolt, F. (1997). Treatment decisions in palliative cancer care: Patients preferences for involvement and doctors' knowledge about it. *European Journal of Cancer, 33*, 1184–1189.

Rubin, S. (1993). The death of a child is forever: The life course impact of child loss. In M. S. Stroebe, W. Stroebe, & R. O. Hansson (Eds.), *Handbook of bereavement* (pp. 285–299). Cambridge: Cambridge University Press.

Sack, W. H., Fritz, G., Krener, P. G., & Sprunger, L. (1984). Death and the pediatric house officer revisited. *Pediatrics, 73*, 676–681.

Sahler, O. J., Z., Frager, G., Levetown, M., Cohn, F. G., & Lipson, M. A. (2000). Medical education about end-of-life care in the pediatric setting: Principles, challenges, and opportunities. *Pediatrics, 105*, 575–584.

Sahler, O. J., Z, McAnarney, E. R., & Friedman, S. B. (1981). Factors influencing pediatric interns relationships with dying children and their parents. *Pediatrics, 67*, 207–215.

Schechter, N. L. (1989). The undertreatment of pain in children: An overview. *Pediatric Clinics of North America, 36*, 781–794.

Schneider, C. E. (1998). *The practice of autonomy: Patients, doctors, and medical decisions.* New York: Oxford University Press.

Sirkia, K., Saarinen, U. M., Ahlgren, B., & Hovi, L. (1997). Terminal care of the child with cancer at home. *Acta Pediatrics, 86*, 1125–1130.

Slevin, M. L., Stubbs, L., Plant, H. J., Wilson, P., Gregory, W. M., Ames, P. J., et al. (1990) Attitudes to chemotherapy: Comparing views of patients with cancer with those of doctors, nurses, and general public. *British Medical Journal, 300*, 1458–1460.

Sourkes, B. (1996). The broken heart: Anticipatory grief in the child facing death. *Journal of Palliative Care, 12*, 56–59.

Spinetta, J. J. (1974). The dying child's awareness of death: A review. *Psychological Bulletin, 81*, 256–260.

Spinetta, J. J. & Maloney, L. (1975). Death anxiety in the outpatient leukemic child. *Pediatrics, 56*, 1034–1037.

Spinetta, J. J., Swarner, J. A., & Sheposh, J. P. (1981). Effective parental coping following the death of a child from cancer. *Journal of Pediatric Psychology, 6*, 251–263.

Stajduhar, K., & Davies, B. (1998). Death at home: Challenges for families and directions for the future. *Journal of Palliative Care, 14*, 8–14.

Tadmor, C. S., Postovsky, S., Elhasid, R., Barak, A. B., & Arush, M. W. (2003). Policies designed to enhance the quality of life of children with cancer at the end-of-life. *Pediatric Hematology and Oncology, 20*, 43–54.

Tulsky, J. A., Fischer, G. S., Rose, M. R., & Arnold, R. M. (1998). Opening the black box: How do physicians communicate about advance directives. *Annals of Internal Medicine, 129*, 441–449.

van der Wal, M. E., Renfurm, L. N., van Vught, A. J., & Gemke, R. J. (1999). Circumstances of dying in hospitalized children. *European Journal of Pediatrics, 158*, 560–565.

Von Gunten, C. F., Ferris, F. D., & Emanuel, L. L. (2000). Ensuring competency in end-of-life care: Communication and relational skills. *Journal of the American Medical Assoc., 284*, 3051–3057.

Waechter, E. H. (1987). Children reactions to fatal illness. In T. Krulik, B. Holaday, & I. M. Martinson (Eds.), *The child and family facing life-threatening illness* (pp. 293–312). Philadelphia: Lippincott.

Walco, G. A., Cassidy, R. C., & Schechter, N. L. (1994). Pain, hurt, and harm: The ethics of pain control in infants and children. *New England Journal of Medicine, 331*, 541–544.

Weir, R. F. (1992). *Selective nontreatment of handicapped newborns: Moral dilemmas in neonatal medicine.* New York: Oxford University Press.

Whittam, E. H. (1993). Terminal care of the dying child: Psychosocial implications of care. *Cancer, 71*, Suppl., 3450–3462.

Wiener, J. M. (1970) Attitudes of pediatricians toward the care of fatally ill children. *Journal of Pediatrics, 76*, 700–705.

Wolfe, J., Grier, H. E., Klar, N., Levin, S. B., Ellenbogen, J. M., Salem-Schatz, S., et al. (2000). Symptoms and suffering at the end of life in children with cancer. *New England Journal of Medicine, 342*, 326–333.

Wolfe, J., Klar, N., Grier, H. E., Duncan, J., Salem-Schatz, S., Emanuel, E. J., et al. (2000). Understanding of prognosis among parents of children who died of cancer: Impact on treatment goals and integration of palliative care. *Journal of the American Medical Assoc., 284,* 2469–2475.

World Health Organization. (1990). *Cancer pain relief and palliative care.* WHO Technical Report Series 804. Geneva: Author.

Zeltzer, L. (1994). Pain and symptom management. In D. J. Bearison & R. K. Mulhern (Eds.), *Pediatric psychooncology: Psychological perspectives on children with cancer* (pp. 61–83). New York: Oxford University Press.

Joanna Breyer, Aurora Sanfeliz, Cori E. Cieurzo, and Eugene A. Meyer

# Loss and Grief

## Introduction

There are many types of loss, but in most Western cultures, the death of a child is considered the most difficult loss because of the symbolic meaning and value associated with having children (Rubin & Malkinson, 2001). In such cultures, the death of a child is considered "out of order" and shatters basic expectations regarding the sequence and predictability of events (Rando, 1983; Schmidt, 1987). The loss of a child challenges the evolutionary role of the parent as "protector" and may result in feelings of despair, isolation, and guilt (Finkbeiner, 1996). This reaction to losing a child is perhaps related to the lower mortality rate experienced in many Western cultures. Cultures with higher infant mortality rates may view the significance of a child's death differently (Eisenbruch, 1984a). There are also differences in how people of various ethnic backgrounds experience the loss of a child within the United States (Kalish & Reynolds, 1976).

Despite the extensive history of research and writings on loss and bereavement, there is a dearth of controlled studies specific to bereavement in the pediatric oncology population. Ethical and methodological challenges may account for the limited research in this area. In addition, the increase in the survival rate for pediatric oncology patients over the past several decades has resulted in an emphasis on the study of coping and adjustment of survivors. In the United States, mortality rates associated with pediatric cancers have been declining for over a quarter century. Between 1975 and 1995, the overall decline in mortality was nearly 40% (Ries, 1999). Still, an estimated 1,500 deaths were expected in 2003 among children diagnosed with cancer between the ages of birth and 14 years, indicating that clinicians in this field are still frequently confronted with anticipatory grief and subsequent bereavement issues for patients and families (American Cancer Society, 2003).

The current chapter provides a brief overview of relevant bereavement literature in the context of describing bereavement in pediatric oncology and introduces a model of coping with bereavement suited to describing the range of reactions to the loss of a child. Anticipatory grief, acute and long-term grief, and complicated grief are discussed as they relate to parents, siblings, and health care providers. Clinical vignettes and parent quotes are used to illustrate some of the clinical issues raised. For a more

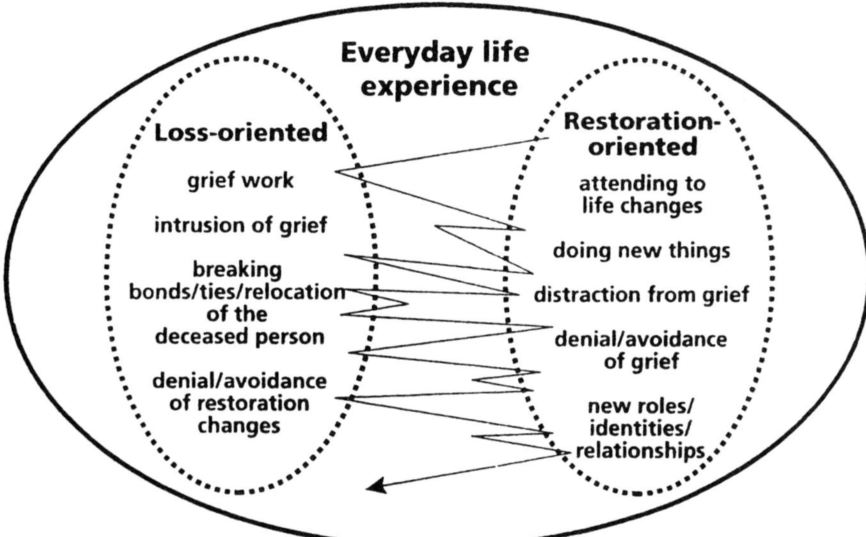


**Figure 19-1.** A dual-process model of coping with bereavement. From *Handbook of Bereavement Research: Consequences, Coping, and Care*, by M. S. Stroebe, R. O. Hansson, W. Stroebe, & H. Schut, H. (Eds.), 2001, p. 396, American Psychological Association, Washington, DC. Copyright 2001 Stroebe and Schut. Reprinted with permission.

comprehensive review of research on grief and bereavement, refer to the *Handbook of Bereavement Research: Consequences, Coping, and Care* (Stroebe, Hansson, Stroebe, & Schut, 2001).

In this chapter, *bereavement* is defined as the loss of a significant relationship through death; *grief* is the natural emotional response to the loss, potentially affecting the cognitive, spiritual, and social functioning of the individual. The term *health care providers* refers to the people providing medical or psychosocial care for the child and family.

## Dual-Process Model of Coping

Various theories were proposed throughout the 20th century regarding bereavement and what constitutes adaptive coping. Stroebe and Schut (2001) suggested that existing bereavement theories can be classified into four categories: (a) general stress and trauma theories (Horowitz, 1986; Lazarus & Folkman, 1984); (b) general theories of grief (Bowlby, 1980; Freud, 1953; Rubin, 1981); (c) models of coping specific to bereavement (Janoff-Bulman, 1992; Worden, 2002); and (d) integrative models (Bonanno & Kaltman, 1999; Stroebe & Schut, 1999). In the current chapter, an integrative model known as the dual-process model of coping (DPMC; Stroebe & Schut, 1999, 2001) is reviewed, and its applicability to the loss of a child because of cancer is considered.

Most current grief theories conceptualize grieving as a fluid and dynamic process, deemphasizing fixed "stages" of grief (Bowlby & Parkes, 1970; Parkes & Weiss, 1983). A credible model of bereavement coping must allow for a wide range of coping styles while explaining both positive and negative outcomes. The DPMC is sufficiently flexible to account for individual differences in the grieving process encountered in the field of pediatric oncology (see figure 19-1). This model allows for the consideration of gender differences in grieving as well as cultural differences in coping with grief (Stroebe & Schut, 2001).

### Loss-Oriented Versus Restoration-Oriented Stressors

The DPMC describes two general categories of stressors and coping experienced in response to a life-changing loss. These categories are described as loss oriented and restoration oriented. Loss-oriented stressors and coping behaviors are associated with an individual's negative and positive appraisals of some aspect of the loss itself, for instance, crying over the loss, ruminating over aspects of the death, laughing at happy memories of the loved one, or imagining how different life would be if the loved one were still alive. Loss-oriented coping includes ways in which bereaved individuals continue a connection with the deceased.

Restoration-oriented stressors and coping behaviors are associated with the need to maintain functioning in the world in the absence of the loved one. When an individual sustains a significant loss, he or she is faced with new roles, responsibilities, and life changes that need to be managed. For instance, when a child dies, a parent may need to continue to care for surviving siblings and continue working to provide income for the family. The restoration-oriented stressors outlined in the DPMC mirror some of the "tasks of grief" that have been highlighted by other authors (Worden, 2002). The DPMC also allows for major changes in the bereaved person's world, roles, and identity. For example, the death of an only child would deprive the mother and father of their identities as parents.

In addition to the two categories of bereavement processes specified by the DPMC, the theory also suggests that "periodic withdrawal" or "time off" from one's grief facilitates healing. The activities that serve this purpose will vary by individual. For some individuals, focusing on projects at work or school may provide this respite. The DPMC does not suggest that effective coping requires that an individual focus on one type of coping activity versus another. Indeed, this model differs from other theories of bereavement in hypothesizing that effective coping requires oscillation between loss-oriented and restoration-oriented activity.

## Oscillation

The DPMC postulates that bereaved individuals will move back and forth between confronting and avoiding loss-oriented and restoration-oriented stress and that this oscillation is necessary to cope adaptively with the loss. The model does not speculate about how this process is regulated but merely emphasizes that it needs to occur. The oscillations are seen as a process as opposed to a static state or trait. In addition, adaptive coping as described by the DPMC requires balancing these oscillations between negative and positive emotion and between confrontation and avoidance of one's grief. It is hypothesized that the experiences of positive emotions and thoughts and time off from one's grief serve a restorative function for the griever and in turn allow the griever to return to dealing with the loss.

This balancing depends on the individual's needs, beliefs, and culture and does not imply an equal distribution of time or energy spent confronting, avoiding, or taking time out from one's grief. Hence, this model allows for the individual differences in preferred coping styles likely to exist within a family. Over time, it is hypothesized that individuals will repeatedly confront aspects of their loss through the oscillation process, but they are likely to experience changes in the intensity of their reactions to the loss. The diminishing intensity allows them to integrate better the loss into their life as they maintain daily functioning.

## Individual Differences and the Model

The DPMC model is sensitive to individual differences in adaptive coping with loss based on culture, gender, and interpersonal differences. Rosenblatt (2001) pointed out that theoretical and clinical models are always built on cultural assumptions. The DPMC postulates that, to some extent, variation in an individual's ability to move back and forth between loss and restoration-oriented stressors may be accounted for by cultural values. For example, as families experience anticipatory grief, religious beliefs may enhance a family's tendency to avoid thoughts about the child's dying while they pray for a miracle. At the same time, religious beliefs, particularly those related to life after death, may foster the family's ability to confront the loss.

Cultural norms will also likely influence emotional expression during the acute grief phase and the setting in which emotional expression is considered appropriate. For instance, in Bali the cultural norm is to express happiness at funeral ceremonies to facilitate the release of the spirits of the deceased (Wikan, 1990); among bereaved Latinos, *ataque de nervios* (an intense emotional and physiological reaction) is a common expression of grief at the time of burial (Guarnaccia, Delacancela, & Carrillo, 1989).

In addition to cultural variations in coping responses to bereavement, gender differences have been noted throughout the literature as well. Research and clinical experience suggest that women may be more likely than men to be focused on loss-oriented responses to grief and so may spend more time processing and focusing on the loss (Stroebe & Schut, 2001). In Western societies, men are often encouraged to be more stoic and therefore may tend to exhibit more restoration-oriented responses than women. Indeed, extreme interpersonal differences in focus on loss-oriented or restoration-oriented stressors can be a potential long-term complication for grieving couples; it is discussed in the Complicated Grief section of this chapter.

## Anticipatory Grief

Anticipatory grief is a multidimensional and subjective experience that relates to the emotional, physical, cognitive, and behavioral responses associated with the anticipation of a loved one's death (Corr & Corr, 2000; Fulton & Gottesman, 1980; Rando, 1986). Research on anticipatory grief has focused primarily on women experiencing the death of their spouses (Marris, 1958; Parkes, 1970; Parkes & Weiss, 1983) and the experiences of parents with terminally ill children (Bozeman, Orbach, & Sutherland, 1955; Natterson & Knudson, 1960; Richmond & Waisman, 1955).

There have been conflicting results regarding the role of anticipatory grief in an individual's overall ability to cope during and after the death. Rando (1986) suggested that not all families or individuals will be able to (or choose to) start grieving simply because they have been forewarned of the impending death of a loved one. An individual's manner of coping with such devastating information will dictate his or her ability to engage in anticipatory grieving. Personal styles may range from actively engaging in anticipatory grieving, acknowledging the information but choosing to focus on the hope that it will not happen, or denying the accuracy of the information.

There are important cultural and developmental factors that may affect the disclosure and processing of information about the impending loss and therefore shape the nature and course of anticipatory grieving (Die-Trill & Holland, 1993; Mitchell, 1998). The developmental stage in the life cycle of the family and the ages of its individual members interact with the stage and nature of the illness in shaping the overall experience of the family (Rolland, 1994). The process of anticipatory grieving for families facing the death of young child is likely to be different from that for families of adolescents or young adults. Family members are more likely to allow adolescents or young adults to play a more active role in their end-of-life care because of perceived emotional and cognitive maturity.

Some studies suggested that there may be negative effects associated with severe anticipatory grieving as it sometimes leads to premature emotional detachment from the dying person (Lindemann, 1944). It can also minimize expected grief reactions at the time of actual death, exposing the mourner to social disapproval or leading the mourner to dispense with traditional rites that may have individual and social value (Fulton & Fulton, 1971). Rosenblatt (1983) suggested that as death approaches, family members may invest more time and energy in the physical caretaking of the dying family member. The increased focus on this relationship can make it more difficult for family members to engage in anticipatory grief and more painful to subsequently disengage from memories and emotional experiences related to the loved one. Other studies have suggested that a period of anticipatory grief is unrelated to or marginally related to the actual grief or mourning experience following the death of a loved one (Benfield, Leib, & Reuter, 1976).

The majority of the clinical research, however, suggests that there are some potentially positive effects associated with the opportunity to experience a moderate amount of anticipatory grief (Binger et al., 1969; Burton, 1974; Futterman, Hoffman, & Sabshin, 1972; Rando, 1983). Anticipating the death of a loved one can provide individuals with opportunities for completing "unfinished business" with the dying person and for helping the dying person have a dignified, pain-free death, which in turn results in a "healthier" grieving process for the caretaking relatives (Byock, 1997; Corr, 1992; Doka, 1993; Nuland, 1994).

The DPMC, originally used to describe the bereavement process, may also be helpful in understanding the grieving that occurs prior to the death of a child. Some families are able to confront the strong emotions associated with the awareness of the imminent death of their child while fulfilling many other responsibilities, such as taking care of other children and work. Among those daily responsibilities, parents need to take care of their dying child, a challenging task that relates to both their loss and their ability to remain engaged in the world. This makes the distinction between loss-oriented and restoration-oriented stress less clear than at other times in the grieving process.

The model captures the dynamic interaction between different kinds of stress typically faced by families during the anticipatory grief period in pediatric oncology. The anticipated death of child to cancer entails a unique set of psychological challenges for parents. When facing the loss of a child to cancer, parents grieve over their dreams for a healthy child, the loss of the child's abilities (i.e., to run and play, to attend school regularly), the child's ongoing physical deterioration, and the losses that the death of the child will bring to the entire family (Rando, 1986). At the same time, there may be an increased focus and intensity on the relationship between the parents/siblings and the dying child. Particularly if the child is cared for at home, one or both of the parents' routines may revolve around the care of the child and result in the intensification of the emotional bond with the child.

There are some circumstances when families have no warning about the imminent death of a child, such as incurable, advanced disease at the time of diagnosis or sudden complications related to disease progression or subsequent medical treatment. More often than not, however, there is a period of time between diagnosis, treatment, and death when families become aware of the child's imminent death and may engage in anticipatory grieving. The terminal phase of the illness can last for months or even years.

Depending on the chosen modality of medical treatment or palliative care, the family may face different challenges (Martinson & Papadatou, 1994). Shanfield, Swain, and Benjamin (1987) found that bereaved parents who had lost their child to cancer had fewer psychiatric and physical complaints than those whose children had died in accidents. This difference may be partially accounted for by the former group having had an opportunity to engage in anticipatory mourning (Dijkstra & Stroebe, 1998), which may ease the course of bereavement and reduce postdeath symptoms (Sanders, 1993).

During the time period when parents are forewarned of their child's impending death, they may be faced with multiple internal and external struggles that are not always easily reconciled but may facilitate oscillation between stressors. For example, parents may be struggling internally to come to terms with the realization that their child is dying, yet externally they must continue to negotiate the world that includes their relationship with the dying child, significant family members, friends, and the medical team. Clearly, the emotional valence attached to these different stressors can vary. Financial responsibilities may require that a parent return to work, leading to a restoration-oriented focus that may be viewed positively or negatively depending on the parent's appraisal (relief from having to focus on the child's impending death or frustration about having to "abandon" the child during this time). Similarly, siblings are also likely to experience oscillations between loss-oriented and restoration-oriented stressors as they balance and negotiate their relationship to and feelings about their dying sibling with the demands of school, relationship with other family members, and relationship with peers (who may be playing a more prominent role in their life because of their parent's preoccupation with their dying sibling).

Both a family's cultural identity and the "culture" of the medical unit can influence a family's course of anticipatory grief. At some point during the critical stage of the child's illness, when standard treatments have failed, parents may face the difficult decision about trying a novel/experimental agent (sometimes referred to as a Phase I clinical trial) versus symptom management. The parents must struggle to balance trying every reasonable effort to extend or save the child's life with sustaining the best possible quality of life. Some parents may experience a need to feel that they have "tried everything" to save their child's life. This may lead parents to avoid anticipatory grief for fear that this will be perceived by the child, medical team, or other family members as having "given up" on the child. In contrast, when medical care is focused on symptom management, parents may be more likely to engage in anticipatory grief. The medical culture of the hospital may influence these decisions for parents as they look to health care providers for guidance.

Parents often voice the difficulties associated with acknowledging their sadness about their impending loss while at the same time managing to take care of their dying child, other children, and daily responsibilities: "How can I be there for Jane when I feel so devastated that I can't even look at her without crying?" "I don't want to be so sad that I cannot enjoy whatever time I have left with him."

"I can't think about him dying right now, I want to be fully present and available for him." "How can I begin to think about her dying when I need to care for my other three children?" Some families, recognizing that they may feel too devastated when the death occurs, choose to make arrangements ahead of time: "I can't believe that I have planned his funeral already . . . but I had to do it now. I know I won't be able to do it when the time comes." For others, making arrangements prior to the loss is discrepant with their wish to maintain hope: "I cannot even consider having hospice involved because that would mean that I have given up on her." Some parents may acknowledge the probability of death but deliberately decide to postpone grieving: "I am not going to grieve one second longer than I have to, or before I have to." They may also be trying to balance their reactions with the wishes and attitude of their child (see clinical vignette 1).

### *Clinical Vignette 1*

Fourteen-year-old Marilyn was diagnosed with osteosarcoma and relapsed after arm surgery and completion of initial medical treatment. Marilyn and her parents were told by the medical team at a family meeting that, given her relapse, there was no curative treatment. Marilyn became hysterical and ordered her oncologist to explore different options. She stated that she was "not ready to die," and that she was not going to die. She subsequently refused to talk with her oncologist about do not resuscitate (DNR) status or her declining health situation. Marilyn's parents, who had supported her active participation in all major treatment decisions, were at first unwilling to have any discussions with the medical team without Marilyn present and appeared to share her attitude. However, the medical team was finally able to explain that, although the team wanted to honor Marilyn's wishes, it was necessary for some decisions to be thought about in advance of a medical crisis. Marilyn's parents were then able to discuss options for DNR and end-of-life treatment. Marilyn remained at home for the last 2.5 weeks of her life with assistance from a visiting home nurse. She refused hospice services. The last night before she died, her parents and Marilyn were able to acknowledge to each other that she was going to die, how sad they were, how much they loved each other, and how she would still be part of their lives. The priest was called and Marilyn was able to tell him the kind of funeral service she wanted.

In addition, it is often the case in the pediatric oncology setting that a child may have been close to dying several times prior to the actual death. This seesaw success in cheating death may interfere with the family's ability to be emotionally prepared for the actual death and may deplete their emotional and physical resources. Some family members may experience feelings of guilt associated with their wish that the child's suffering come to an end (Sourkes, 1991). Overall, the DPMC would suggest that parents who are able to achieve a balance in the anticipatory grief phase between some acknowledgment of the impending loss and maximizing the quality of time they have left with their child may be the parents who are better able to shift between focusing on the loss and functioning in the world after the child's death, resulting in normal rather than complicated grief.

## The Dying Child

The first studies of dying children were conducted in the 1950s and raised many questions regarding children's conceptual understanding of death and dying and how to talk to children regarding their medical illness and potential or anticipated death (Martinson & Papadatou, 1994). Although it is recognized that there is no definitive developmental or chronological age by which a child develops an understanding of the concept of death, some developmental guidelines have been offered in the literature to provide a frame of reference for understanding the evolution of the concept of death through childhood and adolescence (Lefrancois, 1993; Reynolds, Miller, Jelalian, & Spirito, 1995). Such frameworks are helpful to health care providers in pediatric oncology when working with the dying child, parents, and siblings.

Although long-term bereavement outcome information on predeath interventions is limited, there are impressive descriptive clinical accounts of the beneficial effects of individual therapy with dying children (Sourkes, 1996) and useful guidelines on how to talk to children of different ages about death and dying (Greenham & Lohmann, 1982; Grollman, 1990; Schonfeld, 1993; Spinetta, 1974). Despite the emotional challenge of these conversations with dying children and their siblings, health care providers may find it reassuring to know that children seem able to monitor how much information they need or can "take in" at one time (Sourkes, 1996).

In general, it is recommended that parents and health care providers follow the child's lead in determining how much information the child receives regarding his or her medical condition. This may be a difficult task for parents or health care providers, who feel the need to say goodbye to the child and feel motivated by their own anxiety and grief to inform the child of his or her medical status. On the other extreme, some parents may resist giving their child any medical information even when the child is actively seeking such information because they do not want to "remove hope" from the child. When a child asks a question about his or her medical status, an honest, developmentally appropriate answer is desirable, in keeping with the child's coping ability, preference of parents, and family cultural values.

Children's reactions to their impending death or to the fact that their medical status is very serious will vary. Some may not want to talk about it at all; others may express their concerns or need to talk about it in symbolic and indirect ways. Still other children, particularly adolescents, may want to be more directly involved in planning for the end of their life, saying their good-byes to people they love, giving away their possessions, and thinking about their funeral. Children may worry that they will be left alone or forgotten, that they will be in pain, and how their parents will manage without them. It is important for health care providers working with children at the end of life to address these worries and be aware of the child and family's religious and cultural values, which can be a significant source of support and comfort.

## Parents

Parents struggle with issues on multiple dimensions during this time, oscillating between accepting and denying the inevitability of their child's death and managing their own inner turmoil while negotiating relationships and responsibilities with the child, family members, and medical team. Parents may appear to have assimilated the information that their child is going to die at one point in time and at another point focus on their hope for the child's cure. Parents may focus solely on their grief during one clinic visit and then at the very next clinic visit focus on day-to-day issues without acknowledging the child's impending death. Occasionally, the parents (or primary caregivers) become so focused on their anticipatory grief that they are unable to pay attention to the child. The challenge for health care providers may be to know how to acknowledge respectfully the parents' emotional state while conveying necessary information and encouraging an ongoing connection with the child (see clinical vignette 2).

### *Clinical Vignette 2*

A 12-year-old girl, Jane, diagnosed with an incurable cancer, required treatment and pain management in the hospital for most of her end-of-life care. Previously, she had lived with her grandmother, grandfather, and younger brother in a town many hours away. Her grandfather was a stone mason, not very talkative, who strongly disliked coming to the hospital. He stayed with Jane's brother at home during Jane's final hospital admission. Jane's grandmother (a strong advocate for her) took a leave of absence from her job and stayed with Jane throughout hospital stays. The grandmother was angry with her husband for not coming to the hospital more and for participating so little in Jane's end-of-life care. As Jane's medical status deteriorated, she began asking to see her grandfather. In a telephone conversation with the family's psychosocial clinician, Jane's grandfather indicated that he loved his granddaughter very much and felt that his granddaughter "knew" that she was loved even though her grandfather was not at the hospital with her. Jane's grandfather also said that he needed to finish carving Jane's tombstone, just as he had made other things from stone for her throughout her life. With encouragement from the psychosocial clinician, Jane's grandfather began calling daily to remind his granddaughter that he loved her. During the final days of Jane's life, her grandfather was able to come to the hospital to be near her, even though this was very difficult for him.

Parents with a prior or current psychiatric diagnosis or those who have expressed suicidal ideation related to the possibility of losing a child need to be followed particularly closely. If outside therapists are involved, close communication (with consent of the parent) about the child's condition and parents' coping needs to be maintained. It is important to distinguish temporary expressions of despair and sadness from more concerning statements or attitudes in which guilt and sense of identity and purpose are related to the survival of the child. Of clinical significance are increasing levels of denial of the child's impending death, limited face-to-face contact with medical health care providers, increasing use of alternative approaches, decreasing capacity to hear contrary viewpoints, and indication of complete physical exhaustion. If significant risk factors for suicide are present, a formal safety assessment is needed, including the evaluation of a suicide plan, availability and means, seriousness of intent, restraining influences, impulsivity, and level of depression.

As the child's condition deteriorates, health care providers may need to consider a psychopharmacological evaluation for very distressed parents, a safety plan for when the child actually dies if concerns exist for the safety (i.e., potential to harm self) of any family member, and a plan for transitioning family members from the hospital-based mental health provider to a community-based provider. As Worden (2002) suggested, medications may be helpful for modulating physiological arousal, alleviating specific symptoms of distress (such as difficulty sleeping), maintaining appropriate level of alertness, and managing clinical anxiety and depression during anticipatory grief (see clinical vignette 3).

### *Clinical Vignette 3*

John was a 16-year-old boy who had been diagnosed with rhabdomyosarcoma. He had serious initial medical complications and almost died several times during the course of his treatment. During an admission to the intensive care unit for treatment-related complications, it was discovered that his cancer had metastasized to other parts of his body. He was given experimental chemotherapy for symptom control and to delay disease progression. The oncologist was surprised by the excellent response the disease had to this treatment as the tumors shrank, and John was able to return to school. During this respite, John also enjoyed staying out late with friends and took pleasure in engaging in his normal life activities. His parents had very different coping styles. John's father was emotionally overwhelmed by the initial diagnosis, exhibiting anxiety symptoms and having difficulty sleeping. He benefited from a consultation for psychopharmacological intervention. Despite having lost her own mother to cancer at a young age, John's mother had coped with her distress about her son's medical condition by focusing on supporting John and her husband through the ordeal of treatment and the subsequent spread of disease. When John's disease showed some response to treatment and allowed him to return to normal life activities for a time, his mother began anticipating his death and experienced unbearable grief, with difficulty sleeping, eating, and functioning in general. She was unable to enjoy time with him because she was always thinking to herself, "This will be the last time he is able to do these things," and experiencing memories of her mother's death. The family's psychosocial clinician pointed out that she had been in "overdrive" trying to take care of John and her husband and had not allowed herself to truly integrate what was happening to their family throughout the crisis. Now that John was "acting like himself" again, she had a respite from providing such intensive care and was experiencing all of the emotion she had kept at bay and was reminded of her mother's death. The psychosocial clinician recommended a psychopharmacological consultation. Subsequently, John's mother started a trial of antidepressants and received weekly therapy to help manage her justifiably intense emotions. These interventions allowed her to continue to be present and to care for her son and husband without having to neglect her own emotional and psychological well-being.

Medications can enable parents to make better use of individual psychotherapy, which in turn may provide a safe space for parents to express and process strong feelings, particularly sadness, anger, guilt, and fear. Parents may also need support finding strategies to balance these intense emotions with their desire to be strong, to take care of their dying child, and to manage relationships with their spouses, other family members, and individuals in the community. Relaxation, hypnosis, biofeedback, and other behavioral techniques may help modulate the physiological arousal often generated by the stress related to anticipatory grieving. Clinical interventions should support individuals and families as they attempt to manage the anticipatory grief and the daily demands of taking care of their dying child. This is a challenging time in a family's life that may have an impact on how parents later cope with their acute grief and how they make meaning of the death of their child.

## Siblings

Research has generated mixed results related to siblings' adjustment during anticipatory grieving. Some studies have identified siblings as being "at risk" for school, peer, and family problems; other studies have suggested an increase in self-esteem, resilience, and closeness to other family members (Stoneman & Berma, 1993). Clinical reports suggest that it is important to involve siblings in the care of the terminally ill child, to promote closeness and expression of feelings (love, sadness, guilt, anger, etc.) in the family context, and to provide opportunities for children to express their grief separately from their parents (Daniels, Miller, Billings, & Moos, 1986; Robinson & Mahon, 1997; Rolland, 1994). Family therapy may also be useful in helping all family members to acknowledge differences in their individual coping styles and to find a way to share their intense emotions and make meaning of their anticipated loss.

Siblings will develop important memories of the dying brother or sister during this time. Items such as photographs or handprints made together may have significant meaning to the sibling after the death. If the sibling does not want to visit his brother or sister as the time of death approaches, the sibling can be encouraged to send a picture, small gift, or a message to continue to feel involved. When a sibling chooses to visit his brother or sister in the hospital, to minimize the potential for shock and the formation of traumatic memories, the sibling needs to be prepared in advance, using age-appropriate explanations, for changes that may be found in his brother or sister, such as the presence of a breathing tube, an inability to communicate verbally, or significant changes in weight or appearance.

How and when siblings are informed of their brother or sister's likely death is also important. Parents may or may not choose to discuss with health care providers the timing and content of such conversations or may even request the presence of health care providers when they inform the siblings. The information provided to the sibling and how it is provided may influence how included the sibling feels in the potential death of a brother or sister. The more gradually the sibling absorbs the news, the less devastating the shock of the death is likely to be.

Thus, the sibling may benefit from receiving honest, developmentally appropriate information on a regular basis regarding the brother or sister's medical status throughout the illness, including information regarding the success or lack of success of the medical treatment. The quantity of information provided to the sibling should be based on the sibling's coping style (i.e., adjusts better with more information versus adjusts better with minimal, necessary information). Conversely, some siblings will deny the information regarding the possible death of a brother or sister despite how clearly they have been informed. Regardless of the siblings' response at the time they are informed of the impending death, they should be reassured that they can ask their parents any time they have a question about their ill brother or sister.

## Implications for Health care Providers

Health care providers may find themselves in a variety of supporting roles while parents experience anticipatory grief. They will usually be required to provide a range of care, from gentle guidance and support to clinical interventions targeting grief symptom management and psychiatric symptoms. It is important to maintain the delicate balance between supporting family members in holding on to some hope and helping them prepare in appropriate ways to face the loss of their child. In pediatric oncology, health care providers are more likely to be involved with the family's coping efforts during anticipatory grieving rather than after the child's death. The health care provider's sensitivity during conversations on end-of-life care (i.e., DNR orders, pain management, comfort care measures, withdrawal of support, autopsy) may facilitate the family's decision-making process and minimize later feelings of guilt and self-blame. Health care providers' support during this phase may help family members make the transition from hoping for the child's recovery to hoping for a peaceful and pain-free death.

What happens during the anticipatory grief phase will provide the raw material from which survivors will be forming their "stories" about the death and, it is hoped, will give meaning or form to their experience. Sometimes, to preserve a particular story, parents may engage in behavior that looks like denial (see clinical vignette 4). Health care providers may use different therapeutic modalities (individual/family therapy, art therapy, play therapy, etc.) to support the dying child and the family in ways that suit their style of coping. Adequate pain and symptom management as well as facilitation of the creation of family memories and narratives are central goals of pediatric end-of-life-care (Wolfe et al., 2000).

*Clinical Vignette 4*

Anne was a 7-year-old girl who had been diagnosed with Stage 4 neuroblastoma at 3 years of age. She had a bone marrow transplant at age 4 and then relapsed at 6 years of age. There was no curative medical treatment given this relapse, although chemotherapy to control tumor growth was utilized. Despite the chemotherapy, Anne became increasingly symptomatic, with prominent tumor growth on her face and neck. Her oncologist felt Anne had, at most, a few weeks to live. Anne's mother had been consistently positive and upbeat throughout Anne's initial treatment and relapse, never acknowledging the likelihood that Anne would die. The medical team was very concerned about her apparent denial. However, as Anne's medical status continued to deteriorate, her mother began talking to team members about other families at the clinic whose child had died from cancer. During Anne's last clinic visit, her mother referred to Anne's lethargy as likely caused by the flu. Anne died at home a week later. Several months later, when speaking to members of the medical team, Anne's mother stated that the one thing she could not have tolerated was if Anne had been scared during her final weeks of life. She had been determined that Anne would live a normal and happy life for as long as possible. Anne was a well-adjusted, lovable, and engaging child who continued going to school until about 2 weeks before she died. The medical team felt that, as Anne's death approached, her mother was indirectly preparing herself by reminding herself that other families had undergone and survived the death of their child.

The hospice movement has made it possible for many children to have the choice to die at home, which may enhance quality of life and family adjustment (Martinson & Papadatou, 1994). However, sometimes death in the hospital may be preferable because the hospital team can provide more comprehensive management of pain and complicated symptoms while providing extensive professional support for the family. This can especially be true for families experiencing internal conflict (divorce or separation of parents, etc.) or when safety for a family member is a concern (suicidal/homicidal ideation, compromised judgment, etc.). The medical team often faces the challenge of balancing the sedative effects of pain medication with the family's need to interact with the child. Integrative therapies (hypnosis, imagery, relaxation, Reiki, massage, and therapeutic touch) may also be considered for symptom management.

## Acute and Long-Term Grief

When the child dies, the parents and siblings must begin to deal with actual grief and make the transition from "loving in presence" to "loving in absence" (Attig, 2000). As the DPMC emphasizes, they will need to adjust to the loss of the child and to reengage in the world. If some oscillation between these areas occurs, with varying negative and positive assessments and reassessments, gradually the intensity and frequency of the acute grief reactions will reduce and healing will begin.

### Parents

Regardless of the coping style used in the period of anticipatory grief, the actual event of the child's death leaves parents faced with the reality of their tragic loss. The moment and manner of a child's death can greatly influence parents' transition from anticipatory grief to acute grief and is likely to be permanently engraved in the parents' memory (Rosenthal, 2000). Many factors influence a parent's experience of the loss of a child, such as being absent or present at the time of the child's death, whether the child dies in the hospital or at home, if the child's death is perceived as painless and peaceful or difficult, or whether the actual death was sudden or more gradual. Each individual (parent, sibling, grandparent, friend) may experience and react to the moment of death differently.

At the time of a child's death, parents experience an extreme sense of loss, yet at the same time are asked to make important postdeath decisions. Depending on the extent to which parents engaged in anticipatory grieving and planned for postdeath arrangements, at the time of death they may need to decide what to do with the child's body (burial, cremation); how to acknowledge the child's death (funeral notice, wake, burial service); how to remember and celebrate the child's life (burial service, memorial ideas); and how to tell family members, friends, and coworkers. These expectations placed on families at such a difficult time may foster the oscillations between "processing the loss" and "functioning in the real world" or may serve to create further stress. If parents have the assistance of friends, extended family, religious mentors, or health care providers to make postdeath arrangements, they may feel more "free" to focus on the loss.

The loss of a child affects parents in many ways. Studies focusing on bereaved parents have resulted in mixed reports regarding the prevalence of health and psychiatric problems (Birenbaum, Stewart, & Phillips, 1996; Martinson, Davies, & McClowry, 1991; Moore, Gilliss, & Martinson, 1988); recovery from the loss (Lehman, Wortman, & Williams, 1987; Rando, 1983); divorce rates and effects on marital closeness (Kaplan, Smith, Grobstein, & Fischman, 1973; Lansky, Cairns, Hussanein, Wehr, & Lowman, 1978; Rando, 1986); and increased mortality rates (Clerico et al., 1995; Levav, Friedlander, Kark, & Peritz, 1988). Similarly, inconclusive outcomes have been reported in the literature regarding the bereavement of siblings (Oltjenbruns, 2001).

Limitations in the various methodologies used for studies of grief and bereavement may warrant cautious interpretation of results. Even in studies that have relied on more rigorous methodology, a variety of outcomes have been reported (Dijkstra & Stroebe, 1998). Despite variability in the research findings, general themes relating to the diverse presentation and resolution of grief symptoms, gender and cultural differences in grief expression, and factors affecting coping (i.e., the role of continuing bonds, attachment and family dynamics, emotional regulation, expression of negative and positive emotions) have implications for parental coping after the loss of a child to cancer.

There is tremendous variability in the range and intensity of the biopsychosocial grief symptoms experienced by individuals (see table 19-1). As noted by Worden (2002):

> For some, grief is a very intense experience, whereas for others it is rather mild. For some, grief begins at the time they hear of the loss, while for others it is a delayed experience. In some cases grief goes on for a relatively brief period of time, while in others it seems to go on forever. (p. 38)

Individual characteristics within a cultural and family context will influence the types of symptoms expressed, intensity of symptoms expressed, and duration of grieving (Eisenbruch, 1984a, 1984b). Hofer (1984) described some symptoms as lasting minutes to hours (i.e., crying spells) and others lasting days to weeks or months (i.e., fatigue, difficulty concentrating). Some chronic symptoms of bereavement representing the more severe biological changes include decreased body weight, sleep disturbance, cardiovascular changes, endocrine changes, and immunological changes. Parents may have a primary mode for experiencing their acute grief; they may experience acute grief affectively, cognitively, behaviorally, somatically, or in a blend of these ways (Martin & Doka, 2000).

**Table 19-1.** Biopsychosocial Symptoms of Acute Grief

| *Affective* | *Behavioral* | *Cognitive* | *Physiological* |
|---|---|---|---|
| Depression | Agitation | Preoccupation with deceased | Changes in appetite |
| Despair | Crying | Helplessness | Changes in sleep |
| Anxiety | Fatigue | Hopelessness | Somatic complaints |
| Anhedonia | Social withdrawal | Memory problems | Heightened arousal |
| Guilt | Hypervigilence | Concentration problems | Susceptibility to illness |
| Anger | | Self reproach | Energy loss |
| Loneliness | | Sense of unreality | |
| Numbness | | | |

Factors that may influence how a parent expresses and experiences acute grief include prior experience with loss, temperament, and personal meaning of the loss. Not everyone will have recurring, intense emotional reactions as part of their grief experience. Different coping strategies may be more or less helpful depending on the way in which a parent experiences acute grief (i.e., more affectively, cognitively/behaviorally, somatically, or a combination). Parents who tend to experience acute grief more affectively (often mothers) are likely to be helped by expressing feelings and seeking support from others. Parents experiencing more cognitive/behavioral symptoms (often fathers) may have less-intense affect and may be helped by cognitively processing their grief and immersing themselves in activities, sometimes directly or indirectly related to the loss (Martin & Doka, 2000). Problems may occur when the support available does not "fit" an individual's coping style (Cook & Oltjenbruns, 1998). The problems that result from this lack of fit are discussed in the Complicated Grief section. Adaptive coping with the loss of a child can best be understood as an accommodation that changes over time and that includes a different focus, emphasis, and understanding of the loss than had previously existed.

Studies have shown great variability among individuals and cultures regarding the resolution of grief symptoms over time (Eisenbruch, 1984a). For example, some cultures practice a "second burial," usually 2–3 years after the death (Pardo, 1982; Watson, 1982). As part of the cultural script of grieving, these transitional rites set expectations about emotional expression, somatic symptoms, social participation, the relationship with the deceased, and the survivor's ability to reassume daily responsibilities (Woodrick, 1995). Results from studies to date suggest that for many parents of children who have died, a "1-year mark" is too early to speak of "recovery" (Martinson, 1991; Rando, 1983). Indeed, it seems that parents learn to "accommodate" the loss of their child as opposed to "recovering" from such a loss. Some parents still feel intense grief 2–3 years after the death of their child, and most will continue to experience brief, and potentially intense, grief reactions (i.e., at the anniversary of the child's death or on the child's birth date) for years to come (Malkinson & Bar-Tur, 1999; Rando, 1983).

However, except for those experiencing complicated grief, most parents will find that the waves of intense feelings, thoughts, or somatic symptoms gradually lessen in intensity and frequency as time passes after the child's death. As noted, in the DPMC the back-and-forth process between focus on the loss (burial, memorial, sharing memories with family and friends, finding meaning to the loss) and the gradual refocus on current tasks and demands (other siblings, allowing support from family and friends, returning to work, appreciating relationships) over time is hypothesized to help the parent accommodate the loss of the child.

Feeling connected in some fashion to the deceased child is a frequent phenomenon in many cultures (Eisenbruch, 1984a). The extent to which it occurs in Western cultures has been highlighted (Klass & Walter, 2001). In one pediatric oncology study of 43 bereaved parents, 88% of these parents experienced feelings of continued connection with their deceased child, with primarily positive psychological benefits (Sormanti & August, 1997). Many parents will find satisfaction in tasks or challenges connected in some way to their deceased child. Thus, the loss of a child to cancer continues to have an impact on and to shape family life long after the death. Clinically, it appears that making some positive meaning, not out of the loss itself but out of the consequences of the loss, is a striking element in the personal stories of bereaved parents and appears to contribute to personal healing (Finkbeiner, 1996; B. Schatz, 1986; W. Schatz, 1986; Schiff, 1978).

Family-based research has investigated the impact of prior attachments, multigenerational history of loss, and family coping styles and communication patterns on adjustment of family members after loss (Walsh & McGoldrick, 1991). Kissane et al. (1996) found that families less able to provide emotional support, to tolerate emotional expression, or to resolve differences were at higher risk for more postbereavement complications than those families with more positive patterns of coping. Early postbereavement interventions to facilitate family interactions and shared coping were proposed for these high-risk families.

The role of expressing negative emotions (often labeled *grief work*) may have been overemphasized (Wortman & Silver, 2001), while the role of positive emotions is underemphasized in effective coping with grief (Folkman, 2001).

Although the sole expression of either negative or positive emotion does not appear to be associated with better adjustment, some suppression in the expression of negative emotions has been associated with better longer-term adjustment (Bonanno, 2001). It also has been suggested that the outcome of the expression of emotion, whether it leads to reappraisals or a shift in perspective rather than to repetitive ruminations, is associated with adjustment (Pennebaker, Zech, & Rime, 2001).

Research has identified some protective factors related to uncomplicated grieving, including (a) moderate levels of anticipatory grieving, (b) the experience of a pain-free death for the loved one, and (c) understanding the cause of death (Worden, 2002). In pediatric oncology, there is some evidence to suggest that having the child die at home (Martinson & Papadatou, 1994), involving the parents and other siblings in the care of their terminally ill child (Davies, 1999; Rolland, 1994), enhancing the quality of life of the dying child, and providing effective pain control (Wolfe et al., 2000) often help the family's subsequent overall adjustment.

## Siblings

Reviews have provided an overview of the response of a sibling to the loss of a brother or sister (Davies, 1999; Oltjenbruns, 2001) and have emphasized that the developmental context in which a loss occurs informs the sibling's reaction. A sibling's understanding of death, previous experience with loss, personality, coping style, bond with the deceased, and family dynamics will all have an impact on the sibling's adjustment after the death (Davies, 1999). Specifically, when the loss is caused by cancer, it has been hypothesized that the type of treatment received, the length of treatment, and the degree of suffering experienced by the dying child might influence sibling bereavement (Davies, 1999). It has also been suggested that having the child die at home and including the sibling in the illness experience and death-related events may have a positive impact on future adjustment (Davies, 1988a; Lauer, Mulhern, Bohne, & Camitta, 1985; Martinson & Campos, 1991; Mulhern, Lauer, & Hoffman, 1983).

After the death of a child to cancer, siblings may be experiencing a double loss: the loss of a brother or sister and the loss of the parents' normal affection and support because of their own grief experience. The sibling bereavement experience will, to some extent, be dictated by the parents' and family's coping. Family communication styles and cohesiveness have been stressed as important factors in sibling bereavement. Studies have suggested that greater family cohesiveness is related to fewer behavior problems for siblings during the years following the loss of their brother or sister, and that limited communication among family members, suppression of grief, avoidance of change, and rejection of support may lead to less-adaptive behavior (Davies, 1988a, 1988b; Davies, Spinetta, Martinson, McClowry, & Kulenkamp, 1986). Depending on the family's style, the sibling may or may not be given a choice regarding participation in the loss-focused activities (wake, funeral) or with subsequent restoration-oriented activities (back to school, extracurricular activities, etc.). The lack of choice between confrontation and avoidance of these activities may be further complicated by the sibling's relationship with and observations of the parents' behavior and attitudes. These experiences will likely occur in the context of the sibling confronting a new and complicated mix of emotions (sadness, anger, confusion, a wish to protect and comfort and to be protected and comforted).

The bereaved sibling may have such questions as "Is it all right to talk about my brother? To play with his toys? To go into his room? To express feelings about his death?" Such questions may need to be negotiated by parents or primary caregivers, and how they are answered may serve to facilitate the child's healing journey. As noted for adults, bereaved siblings may express a range of biopsychosocial symptoms. In addition to the symptoms listed in table 19-1, a bereaved sibling may exhibit more behavioral signs of distress, such as acting-out behaviors, showing off, disobedience, or a decline in school performance. They may also present with somatic complaints similar to those of the deceased or somatic symptoms such as enuresis. School-aged siblings may also feel isolated from their peers or confused regarding how much information to share regarding their brother or sister's illness and death. Simultaneously, peer interaction may provide the sibling with welcome respite from his or her intense grief experience and that of other family members (the time-out concept as noted by the DPMC). Over time, as the child matures cognitively and emotionally and the parents become more emotionally available, new opportunities will often emerge to reassess (or "regrieve") the death and its impact on the sibling and the family (Davies, 1999; Oltjenbruns, 2001).

## Implications for Health Care Providers

Health care providers in pediatric oncology need to proceed cautiously in their interventions and in making outside referrals, particularly near the time of the child's death. Reviews of the efficacy of bereavement interventions have challenged traditional thoughts regarding bereavement counseling, indicating that bereavement counseling may have negative or positive effects depending on the individual, the external circumstances, and the timing and type of the intervention (Kato & Mann, 1999; Litterer Allumbaugh & Hoyt, 1999; Schneiderman, Winders, Tallett, & Feldman, 1994; Schut, Stroebe, van den Bout, & Terheggen, 2001).

The review by Schut et al. (2001) highlighted the complexity of evaluating the existing bereavement intervention literature because of the variety of interventions and populations studied as well as the range in quality of research methodology employed and the different outcomes measured. In that review, interventions were categorized as primary preventive interventions (interventions general in nature, with open recruitment of individuals experiencing "normal" bereavement), secondary preventive interventions (interventions specifically targeting at-risk individuals), and tertiary preventive interventions (interventions targeting individuals experiencing complicated grief).

Schut et al. (2001) found little empirical evidence to support the use of primary preventive interventions for grieving adults and even noted that the earlier the intervention, the more likely some individuals would show adverse consequences. In contrast, some studies did show positive results from primary interventions for bereaved children. Because parental bereavement is considered a high-risk factor, interventions for bereaved parents were only considered in reviewing studies regarding secondary preventive interventions. Schut et al. concluded that, overall, modest effects of secondary interventions were present, with some indication that such effects were temporary and may be gender specific. Differential effects found for parents by gender and symptom severity (Murphy, Chung, & Johnson, 2002) have prompted the suggestion that perhaps parental bereavement is too broad a criterion for high-risk grief and should be further differentiated (Schut et al.).

Although the characteristics of the sample population were less clear, studies reviewed regarding tertiary preventive interventions appeared to have moderate, lasting effects for individuals experiencing complicated grief. As noted, methodological limitations were noted for practically every study, thus limiting the interpretation of results. Specifically, individuals in these studies who were looking for help or referred specifically for intervention (i.e., tertiary preventive intervention studies) may have been more committed to the idea of intervention and had greater need for intervention, resulting in what would appear to be a "stronger effect." Despite methodological limitations of most studies reviewed, Schut et al. (2001) concluded that "the more complicated the grief process appears to be or to become, the better the chances of interventions leading to positive results" (p. 731). Clinical reports also documented long-term effective treatment of individuals with complicated grief, often combining individual or group therapy with medication (Jacobs, 1993).

At the time of the child's death, in pediatric oncology the health care provider's role has changed from facilitating the anticipatory grieving process to supporting the family through the moment of intense grief (loss oriented) and easing their transition into the world outside the hospital without their child (restoration oriented). Health care providers need to be aware of cultural and family traditions to ensure that other hospital/medical staff respect these differences (Walsh & McGoldrick, 1991), including the family's wishes about washing, dressing, and staying with the body. Although health care providers may be unable to relieve the emotional pain of family members at the time of death, they can offer emotional support, reframe potentially negative perceptions, and perhaps help to create memories that will, over time, encourage healing. For example, if a parent is distressed by having been out of the room when the child died, a health care provider might gently suggest that perhaps the child needed the parent to be out of the room in order to "let go," or a sibling might be hugged and told what a wonderful brother he has been.

Many medical professionals will have provided care to the child during the illness and palliative care and are likely to experience grief reactions to the loss. In addition, in the hospital, other patients and families are likely to be aware when a death has occurred, and health care providers may need to consider how to continue caring for patients, acknowledging their own grief and protecting the privacy of the family that sustained the loss. In some situations, nursing or resident support groups may be appropriate and well received, depending on the intensity of the relationship shared with the child and the child's family. Regular multidisciplinary bereavement rounds for those involved in the care of the child who died can also provide a forum for health care providers to share their thoughts, feelings, and experiences regarding the death as well as facilitate coordination of follow-up with the family.

After the child's death, during the acute grief period, health care providers' knowledge of and connection to the family will help them determine their role with the family (i.e., attending versus not attending the wake or funeral service, phone call versus card versus visit to the home). Although some families want to maintain contact with hospital-based health care providers for support, others may prefer to avoid anyone or anything that reminds them of their child's recent medical experience and death. Therefore, some parents may want to return to the hospital to meet with members of the medical team; other parents may not. Overall, the role of members of the medical team at the time of and after the child's death will be influenced by numerous factors, including whether the child dies at home or in the hospital, whether support services from hospice have become involved, the relationship between the hospital/medical team and the family, the proximity of the family's home to the medical center, and the degree of support services determined to be needed or desired by the family.

Although bereavement follow-up services are important, hospital-based health care providers in pediatric oncology are typically less actively involved once the postdeath arrangements have been made and carried out. Care for the parents and siblings after the child's death may often be provided by professionals in the community. In some instances, professionals in the community (i.e., religious leaders, therapists, etc.) may already have been involved prior to the child's death. Therefore, although it is not essential that all hospital-based health care providers be skilled providers of bereavement interventions, it is important that they understand the varied course of grief and styles of grieving, be aware of potential risk factors for complicated grieving, be able to recognize complicated grieving, and be familiar with appropriate resources in the community to facilitate the long-term care of the surviving family members.[1]

The purpose of contact with the families during this early acute stage of grief is to provide emotional support; facilitate normal grief; offer psychoeducation about the grief process; give some therapeutic suggestions if appropriate; monitor individual and family grief patterns, particularly with high-risk families; and make appropriate outside referrals. A priority for health care providers at this point is to "do no harm" and not interfere with a normal grieving process, for example, by making an early referral to a parent support group for a parent who may not be an "affective" griever. At this point, it may be difficult to judge if a parent or sibling is suffering from an extreme acute grief reaction that will ease over several months or whether the parent or sibling is developing a form of complicated grief. Time and regular contact over several months may be needed to make that clinical judgment. The intensity and unrelenting quality of the distress; the parents' level of concern about their own, their spouse's, or their surviving children's reactions; and the level of discord in the family are all relevant factors to consider in deciding whether additional professional help is needed.

## Complicated Grief

It has been suggested that the distinction between normal and complicated grief is based on the intensity, degree, and duration of grief symptoms (Worden, 2002). Thus, individuals who experience grief symptoms that appear more intense, extreme, or extended than expected given the social and cultural context are considered to be experiencing complicated grief. Divergence from normal grief is recognized within each culture. For example, among the Toraja of Indonesia, bereaved individuals often report dreams in which the deceased provides advice. Dreams with significantly different content (i.e., the deceased inviting the dreamer to join him or her) would be seen as indicative of complicated grief (Holland, 1995). Diagnosis of psychiatric disorders in the presence of bereavement requires caution. Some grievers may present with symptoms characteristic of a disorder (i.e., major depressive episode) yet may be experiencing normal grief. In the general bereavement literature, complications in the grieving process have been associated with deterioration in the bereaved individual's physical health, increased risk for psychiatric disorders, and increased mortality rates (Hofer, 1984; Kaprio, Kosenvuo, & Rita, 1987; McHorney & Mor, 1988; Schaefer, Quesenberry, & Wi, 1995). It is therefore important to recognize individuals who may be at risk for developing complicated grief.

### Parents

Research and clinical experience suggest that there are individual, experiential, and environmental factors associated with increased risk for complicated grief (Reynolds et al., 1995; Worden, 2002) and should be noted by pediatric oncology health care providers. Individual risk factors include a history of prior psychiatric difficulties, past history of loss, complicated attachment history, and a dependent/enmeshed/ambivalent relationship with the deceased. Individuals who show strong acute and chronic physiological responses and somatic symptoms may be at increased risk for health complications (Hofer, 1984). Experiential characteristics such as the type of death (i.e., traumatic/unexpected death) may also be risk factors. It has also been proposed that the loss of a child is so devastating that it should be considered, in and of itself, a risk factor for complicated grief (Rando, 1991). Environmental characteristics such as few social, family, or community supports as well as other environmental stressors at the time of or shortly after the loss (i.e., significant marital conflict, other losses, significant financial problems) may also increase the risk of complicated grief.

Not only is the quantity of the support available to the individual important, but also how well the available support fits with the bereaved individual's coping style. Different experiences of grief, ways of expressing grief, and expectations regarding mourning behavior can be a source of confusion, tension, and potential long-term conflict between parents (Cook & Oltjenbruns, 1998). Sometimes, the pace and preferred mode of emotional expression of one parent may be criticized or challenged by the other, perhaps creating friction in the relationship and a situation in which that individual feels constrained, pressured, or further isolated. This may trigger further adverse intrapersonal and interpersonal reactions. For example, a wife who has found attending a bereaved parents support group helpful may insist that her husband attend as well, which may not be helpful to him given his mode of coping. The husband may prefer to engage in some distracting activity (i.e., play golf or talk to a friend).

In addition, it is possible for a parent to become "stuck" in an extreme mode of coping or functioning and therefore not experience the oscillations or temporary respite from grief hypothesized by the DPMC to facilitate healing. It may take a longer period of time for that parent to adjust to the loss of the child. A parent heavily focused on the negative thoughts, memories, and experiences associated with the loss may have difficulty managing the restoration-oriented tasks that could help shift attention and emotion. Conversely, if a parent is stuck avoiding thoughts and emotions about the loss, the parent will have a constricted focus in daily functioning and spend significant energy avoiding internal or external cues that may trigger associations with the deceased child. The biopsychosocial toll such reactions can have on an individual will likely cause additional stress not only for him or her, but also for the partner and may create conflict in the relationship.

### Siblings

Siblings have the potential to reassess grief in different ways as they get older. The DPMC would suggest that, as siblings age, they will have greater capacity to determine their own confrontation/avoidance of the loss, reappraise the meaning and effect of the loss, and make greater use of outside supports and resources to help further adjustment. The risk factors listed for parents also apply for siblings. Just as with parents, the frequency, duration, and intensity of worrisome thoughts, feelings, and behaviors should help guide identification of complicated grief in siblings.

### Implications for Health Care Providers

The importance of health care providers knowing the risk factors and appropriate treatment for different types of complicated grief has been mentioned. In addition, high-risk families who are not well connected to local supports or mental health clinics may initially need the hospital-based health care providers to remain in regular contact to provide some care and support and to monitor safety until adequate community supports are in place.

When incompatible grieving styles exist and are causing increasing tension between family members or within the bereaved individual's support network, referral to a professionally led or self-help group might be appropriate. Because gender is often associated with particular grieving styles (Martin & Doka, 2000), health care providers might consider gender-specific referrals. Sibling groups may provide an opportunity for interaction with similarly aged bereaved siblings and opportunities to share feelings of isolation, sadness, anger, guilt, and helplessness or simply to hear how other siblings are managing the myriad emotions and changes in family life since the loss.

When bereaved individuals present with posttraumatic stress disorder (PTSD) or traumatic grief (Prigerson & Jacobs, 2001), it has been noted that treatment for the trauma needs to occur before other issues about the loss can be addressed. For this reason, a referral should be made to a therapist experienced in trauma as well as bereavement (Foa, Keane, & Friedman, 2000; Jacobs, 1993; Rando, 2000). Some symptoms such as intrusive thoughts and flashbacks are common for parents after their child dies. For most parents, the intensity and frequency of these thoughts and images will decrease over time without meeting criteria for PTSD. Care must be taken not to "retraumatize" or delay the recovery of those who are beginning to recover on their own from a traumatic loss. This may account for the negative effects found for some parents who join support groups soon after bereavement (Murphy et al., 2002).

Major depression and generalized anxiety disorder are some of the other psychiatric problems that parents or siblings may develop following bereavement. Just as with PTSD, a referral needs to be made to an appropriate community therapist familiar with treating psychiatric disorders in the presence of grief. Parents who experience strong physiological grief responses and somatic symptoms may benefit from referrals to clinicians who teach stress management interventions (e.g., biofeedback, meditation, self-hypnosis, cognitive behavioral strategies) that attempt to modulate those extreme reactions and facilitate a return to homeostasis. Parents who have prior psychiatric histories or histories of loss or abuse or whose child's death was drawn out, appeared painful, or was hard to witness (bleeding, choking) may be at particular risk for PTSD symptoms as part of their bereavement and may require intensive psychotherapy (see clinical vignette 5).

### *Clinical Vignette 5*

Elaine, the mother of 18-year-old Jake, had a history of physical and sexual abuse in childhood and early adulthood. Jake died following complications from a bone marrow transplant. Jake's death, although expected, was traumatic. Although Elaine had other children, she was closest to Jake. Elaine experienced Jake's death as traumatic, overwhelming, and all embracing, affecting every aspect of her life (experienced emotionally, cognitively, spiritually, behaviorally, and physiologically). She continued to experience intrusive memories and flashbacks and would feel drawn to return to the medical setting and to talk with medical staff connected with her son despite the fact that these visits were traumatizing. She was angry at her husband for grieving differently. She focused on relationships that were connected to Jake and had difficulty with relationships that were not. She had many somatic symptoms and missed much time at work. Despite a social context in which her emotional distress was understood and supported, her distress increased over time. One year after Jake's death, she began working with an individual counselor and shortly after was hospitalized for suicidal thoughts and self-destructive behavior. She was diagnosed with major depression and PTSD. Subsequent therapeutic work had both a loss and a restoration-oriented emphasis. Therapy focused on tolerating other styles of grieving; on helping her shift back and forth more easily between her thoughts and feelings about Jake and the demands of her current life; on reframing the meaning of the loss; and on helping her understand how guilt, low self-esteem, and reluctance to accept treatment that might ease the traumatic memories were barriers to recovery. She needed help to understand that recovery was not a betrayal of Jake and to discover what else in her current life gave it meaning, including positive ways to honor Jake's memory. Still, some years later, incidents, memories, and anniversaries continued to trigger negative cycles that took considerable work to reverse.

Parents who denied or avoided acknowledging the certainty of their child's death or whose child passed away abruptly from medical/disease complications (stroke, overwhelming infection) will have to cope with the shock of the loss as well as with the loss itself. This experience may place them at particular risk for delayed grief (see clinical vignette 6). Health care providers should use caution when assessing for the presence of delayed grief. Some individuals may be designated as experiencing delayed grief when they are actually coping well within a particular grief response mode that works for them but involves minimal expression of negative emotion. Other instances of delayed grief may require interventions. Parents may consistently avoid thoughts, feelings, people, and places associated with their child's death, which may have a negative impact on their functioning and relationships, as indicated in clinical vignette 6. Some parents may increase use of alcohol, illicit drugs, or even prescription drugs in an effort to avoid physiological, cognitive, and emotional reactions to the death of their child. The use of such substances may interfere with the natural grieving process, family relationships, and general functioning and threaten the immediate and long-term safety of the parent. These parents will need professional help and support in gradually experiencing feelings and thoughts associated with their loss or further disruption in their life may occur.

### *Clinical Vignette 6*

The mother of a 7-year-old boy, Mark, an only child who died from relapsed neuroblastoma, was emotionally available, loving, and devoted throughout the extended terminal phase of his illness. She took a leave of absence from her work to be with him. Despite repeated attempts by the medical staff, she avoided discussions of the seriousness of his condition and always maintained a positive attitude. In fact, she became angry with her husband if he showed any "pessimism" regarding Mark's chances for survival. After Mark's death, the psychosocial clinician remained in regular telephone contact with the parents for over a year. Mark's mother initially commented on how she had not believed Mark was going to die. She had heard people say it but had not believed it. Her emotional pain was terrible, and she described Mark's death as "losing part of myself." Over the several months after Mark's death, she returned to work, began going out in the evenings with people from work, and spent less and less time at home with her husband. She said it was too painful, and that they were both so sad they could not comfort each other. A referral for couples counseling was made locally, and they met sometimes individually and sometimes together with the counselor for many months. Finally, they separated. She attributed the separation to long-standing differences in their marriage that their son's illness had kept masked. He attributed it to her unresolved sadness at their son's death, triggered by associations with him and their surroundings.

## Conclusion

This chapter integrates clinical experience and previous research findings to describe the unique challenges associated with losing a child to cancer and to offer suggestions for health care providers. The multiple paths that parents may take, before and after the death of a child to cancer, as related to individual, gender, family, and cultural factors have been stressed.

Death from childhood cancer can often be foreseen, allowing the family the possibility of engaging in anticipatory grief. During this complex time, families may be faced with the sadness of the child's imminent death, the desire to provide the best quality of life, the hope that more treatment may still work, and other responsibilities. We have provided suggestions for clinical interventions that may help some families balance their experience of grief with making the most of the time left with their child, creating memories, and negotiating a complex medical system. Given the intense emotions experienced at the time of the death, events surrounding it can play a significant role in the family's experience of acute and long-term grief. They will provide the raw material from which families will create memories and narratives of their child's life and death. After the child's death, families who may have been mainly focused on taking care of their dying child need to reengage in daily routines altered throughout the illness. At this time, families may experience a significant change in their relationship with the medical team, which may add to their sense of loss. We have summarized relevant findings from research evaluating clinical interventions with bereaved individuals and stressed important considerations when working with grieving families in pediatric oncology.

There are individual and cultural differences in how families cope with the death of a child to cancer. Parents who are able to engage in anticipatory grief at the same time as they maximize the quality of life of their dying child are likely to negotiate satisfactorily the multiple challenges of later bereavement. Others who cannot, or choose not to, grieve their loss prior to the death may also be able to negotiate the mourning process with much sadness but without serious complications. However, a small proportion of bereaved parents are at risk for complicated grief. Past experiences with loss, mental health history, perception of events around the death, inability to engage in anticipatory grief, difficulty modulating their grief prior to the death, or lack of support and additional life stressors are factors that may lead to a more difficult bereavement process. Over time, most parents seem to be able, without professional interventions, to integrate their feelings and thoughts about the loss with the demands of daily life. Other parents, however, will benefit from appropriate and timely professional help. Many bereaved parents may, at some point, find it helpful to share their experiences with other bereaved families.

Throughout this chapter, we demonstrated the face validity of the DPMC as a powerful framework to describe the process of anticipatory, acute, and long-term grief in pediatric oncology. We analyzed, based on the DPMC, clinical interventions that may be helpful in facilitating the grieving process. Systematic research is needed to assess the applicability of the DPMC to pediatric oncology. Qualitative longitudinal studies could explore families' grief trajectories and the importance of individual characteristics (attachment styles, biological markers, gender); family interaction patterns; cultural differences; and environmental stressors in identifying individuals and families at risk for complicated grief. Findings could further guide health care providers in the design and effective use of clinical interventions and programs to support bereaved families. Research could also expand the use the DPMC to explore how families, survivors, and their health care providers cope with the multiple losses associated with childhood cancer (i.e., the loss of a limb or physical and cognitive functioning; changes in appearance; lengthy school absences; missed developmental milestones; long-term effects of treatment; etc.).

Human beings have a unique capacity to form close bonds and, consequently, a unique capacity to experience intense grief when those bonds are severed. Parents and siblings of children who die from cancer take many different paths, over many years, to incorporate the loss and continue with their lives. Often, they find the necessary internal and external resources to cope on their own. However, sometimes they need professional help at particular moments in their journey. Many parents and siblings find meaning in giving to others as a way to honor and remember their loved one. Indeed, there is no greater testimony to the resilience of the human spirit than the capacity to surmount the loss and, in some cases, use it as an impetus to make inner transformations and constructive life changes.

## Note

1. Additional information regarding bereavement follow-up programs, some available support services/bereavement literature, and concepts for health care providers to consider in their clinical work with bereaved pediatric oncology families is available from the authors on request.

## References

American Cancer Society. (2003). *Facts and figures 2003*. Retrieved December 3, 2003, from http://www.cancer.org/downloads/STT/CAFF2003PWSecured.pdf

Attig, T. (2000). Anticipatory mourning and the transition to loving in absence. In T. A. Rando (Ed.), *Clinical dimensions of anticipatory mourning* (pp. 115–134). Champaign, IL: Research Press.

Benfield, D., Leib, S., & Reuter, J. (1976). Grief response of parents after referral of the critically ill newborn to a regional center. *New England Journal of Medicine, 294*, 975–978.

Binger, C., Ablin, A., Feuerstein, R., Kushner, J., Zoger, S., & Mikkelsen, C. (1969). Childhood leukemia: Emotional impact on patient and family. *New England Journal of Medicine, 280*, 414–418.

Birenbaum, L. K., Stewart, B. J., & Phillips, D. S. (1996). Health status of bereaved parents. *Nursing Research, 45*, 105–109.

Bonanno, G. (2001). Grief and emotion: A social-functional perspective. In M. S. Stroebe, R. O. Hansson, W. Stroebe, & H. Schut (Eds.), *Handbook of bereavement research: Consequences, coping, and care* (pp. 493–516). Washington, DC: American Psychological Association.

Bonanno, G., & Kaltman, S. (1999). Toward an integrative perspective on bereavement. *Psychological Bulletin, 125*, 760–776.

Bowlby, J. (1980). *Attachment and loss. Vol. 3. Loss: Sadness and depression*. London: Hogarth.

Bowlby, J., & Parkes, C. M. (1970). Separation and loss within the family. In E. J. Anthony (Ed.), *The child in his family* (pp. 197–216). New York: Wiley.

Bozeman, M. F., Orbach, C. E., & Sutherland, A. M. (1955). Psychological impact of cancer and its treatment. *Cancer, 8*, 1–19.

Burton, L. (1974). Tolerating the intolerable: The problems facing parents and children following diagnosis. In L. Burton (Ed.), *Care of the child facing death*. London: Routledge and Kegan Paul.

Byock, I. R. (1997). *Dying well: The prospect for growth at the end of life*. New York: Riverhead Books.

Clerico, A., Ragni, G., Antimi, A., Minori, A., Juraga, A., & Castello, M. A. (1995). Behaviour after cancer death in offspring: Coping attitude and replacement dynamics. *New Trends in Experimental and Clinical Psychology, 11*, 87–89.

Cook, A., & Oltjenbruns, K. (1998). *Dying and grieving: Lifespan and family perspectives*. Fort Worth, TX: Harcourt Brace.

Corr, C. A. (1992). A task-based approach to coping with dying. *Omega, 24*, 81–94.

Corr, C. A., & Corr, D. M. (2000). Anticipatory mourning and coping with dying: Similarities, differences, and suggested guidelines for helpers. In T. A. Rando (Ed.), *Clinical dimensions of anticipatory mourning* (pp. 223–252). Champaign, IL: Research Press.

Daniels, D., Miller, J. J., Billings, A. G., & Moos, R. H. (1986). Psychological functioning of children with rheumatic disease. *Journal of Pediatrics, 109*, 279–383.

Davies, B. (1988a). The family environment in bereaved families and its relationship to surviving sibling behavior. *Children's Health Care, 17*, 22–32.

Davies, B. (1988b). Shared life space and sibling bereavement responses. *Cancer Nursing, 11*, 339–347.

Davies, B. (1999). *Shadows in the sun: The experiences of sibling bereavement in childhood*. Philadelphia: Brunner/Mazel.

Davies, B., Spinetta, J., Martinson, I., McClowry, S., & Kulenkamp, E. (1986). Manifestations of levels of functioning in grieving families. *Journal of Family Issues, 7*, 297–313.

Die-Trill, M., & Holland, J. (1993). Cross-cultural differences in the care of patients with cancer: A review. *General Hospital Psychiatry, 15*, 21–30.

Dijkstra, I., & Stroebe, M. S. (1998). The impact of a child's death on parents: A myth (not yet) disproved? *Journal of Family Studies, 4*, 159–185.

Doka, K. (1993). *Living with life-threatening illness: A guide for patients, their families, and caregivers*. Lexington, MA: Lexington Books.

Eisenbruch, M. (1984a). Cross-cultural aspects of bereavement I: A conceptual framework for comparative analysis. *Culture, Medicine, and Psychiatry, 8*, 283–309.

Eisenbruch, M. (1984b). Cross-cultural aspects of bereavement. II: Ethnic and cultural variations in the development of bereavement practices. *Culture, Medicine, and Psychiatry, 8*, 315–347.

Finkbeiner, A. (1996). *After the death of a child: Living with loss through the years*. New York: Free Press.

Foa, E. B., Keane, T. M., & Friedman, M. J. (Eds.). (2000). *Effective treatment for PTSD*. New York: Guilford Press.

Folkman, S. (2001). Revised coping theory and the process of bereavement. In M. S. Stroebe, R. O. Hansson, W. Stroebe, & H. Schut (Eds.), *Handbook of bereavement research: Consequences, coping, and care* (pp. 563–584). Washington, DC: American Psychological Association.

Freud, S. (1953). Mourning and melancholia (J. Strachey, Trans.). In J. Strachey (Ed.), *Standard edition of the complete psychological works of Sigmund Freud*. London: Hogarth.

Fulton, R., & Fulton, J. (1971). A psychosocial aspect of terminal care: Anticipatory grief. *Omega, 2*, 91–100.

Fulton, R., & Gottesman, D. J. (1980). Anticipatory grief: A psychosocial concept reconsidered. *British Journal of Psychiatry, 137*, 45–54.

Futterman, E., Hoffman, I., & Sabshin, M. (1972). Parental anticipatory mourning. In B. Shoenberg, A. Carr, D. Peretz, & A. H. Kutscher (Eds.), *Psychosocial aspects of terminal care*. New York: Columbia University Press.

Greenham, D. E., & Lohmann, R. A. (1982). Children facing death: Recurring patterns of adaptation. *Health Social Work, 7*, 89–94.

Grollman, E. A. (1990). *Talking about death: A dialogue between parent and child* (3rd ed.). Boston: Beacon.

Guarnaccia, P. J., Delacancela, V., & Carrillo, E. (1989). The multiple meanings of *ataques de nervios* in the Latino community. *Medical Anthropology, 11*, 47–62.

Hofer, M. A. (1984). Relationships as regulators: A psychobiological perspective on bereavement. *Psychosomatic Medicine, 46*, 183–197.

Holland, D. (1995). To the afterworld and back: Mourning and dreams of the dead among the Toraja. *Ethos, 23*, 424.

Horowitz, M. (1986). *Stress response syndromes*. Northvale, NJ: Aronson.

Jacobs, S. (1993). *Pathologic grief: Maladaption to loss*. Washington, DC: American Psychiatric Press.

Janoff-Bulman, R. (1992). *Shattered assumptions: Towards a new psychology of trauma*. New York: Free Press.

Kalish, R. A., & Reynolds, D. K. (1976). *Death and ethnicity: A psychocultural study*. Los Angeles: University of Southern California Press.

Kaplan, D., Smith, A., Grobstein, R., & Fischman, S. (1973). Family mediation of stress. *Social Casework, 18*, 60–69.

Kaprio, J., Kosenvuo, M., & Rita, H. (1987). Mortality after bereavement: A prospective study of 95,647 widowed persons. *American Journal of Public Health, 77*, 283–287.

Kato, P. M., & Mann, T. (1999). A synthesis of psychological interventions for the bereaved. *Clinical Psychology Review, 19*, 275–296.

Kissane, D. W., Bloch, S., Dowe, D. L., Snyder, R. M., Onghena, P., McKenzie, D. P., et al. (1996). The Melbourne family grief study. I: Perceptions of family functioning in bereavement. *The American Journal of Psychiatry, 153*, 650–658.

Klass, D., & Walter, T. (2001). Processes of grieving: How bonds are continued. In M. S. Stroebe, R. O. Hansson, W. Stroebe, & H. Schut (Eds.), *Handbook of bereavement research: Consequences, coping, and care*. Washington, DC: American Psychological Association.

Lansky, S., Cairns, N., Hussanein, R., Wehr, B., & Lowman, J. (1978). Childhood cancer: Parental discord and divorce. *Pediatrics, 62*, 184–188.

Lauer, M. E., Mulhern, R. K., Bohne, J. B., & Camitta, B. M. (1985). Children's perceptions of their sibling's death at home or hospital: The precursors of differential adjustment. *Cancer Nursing, 8*, 21–27.

Lazarus, R., & Folkman, S. (1984). *Stress, appraisal and coping*. New York: Springer.

Lefrancois, G. R. (1993). *The Lifespan* (4th ed.). Belmont, CA: Wadsworth.

Lehman, D. R., Wortman, C. B., & Williams, A. F. (1987). Long-term effects of losing a spouse or child in a motor vehicle crash. *Journal of Personality and Social Psychology, 52*, 218–231.

Levav, I., Friedlander, Y., Kark, J. D., & Peritz, E. (1988). An epidemiological study of mortality of among bereaved parents. *The New England Journal of Medicine, 319*, 457–461.

Lindemann, E. (1944). Symptomatology and management of acute grief. *American Journal of Psychiatry, 101*, 141–148.

Litterer Allumbaugh, D., & Hoyt, W. T. (1999). Effectiveness of grief therapy: A meta-analysis. *Journal of Counseling Psychology, 46*, 370–380.

Malkinson, R., & Bar-Tur, L. (1999). The aging of grief in Israel: A perspective of bereaved parents. *Death Studies, 23*, 413–431.

Marris, P. (1958). *Widows and their families*. London: Routledge.

Martin, T., & Doka, K. (2000). *Men don't cry . . . Women do: Transcending gender stereotypes of grief*. Philadelphia: Brunner/Mazel.

Martinson, I. (1991). Grief is an individual journey: Follow-up of families postdeath of a child with cancer. In D. Papadatou & C. Papadatos (Eds.), *Children and death* (pp. 255–265). New York: Hemisphere Publishing.

Martinson, I., & Campos, R. G. (1991). Adolescent bereavement: Long-term responses to a sibling's death from cancer. *Journal of Adolescent Research, 6*, 54–69.

Martinson, I., Davies, B., & McClowry, S. (1991). Parental depression following the death of a child. *Death Studies, 15*, 259–267.

Martinson, I., & Papadatou, D. (1994). Care of the dying child and the bereaved. In D. J. Bearison & R. K. Mulhern (Eds.), *Pediatric psychooncology: Psychological perspectives on children with cancer* (pp. 193–214). New York: Oxford University Press.

McHorney, C. A., & Mor, V. (1988). Predictors of bereavement depression and its health services consequences. *Medical Care, 26*, 882–893.

Mitchell, J. L. (1998). Cross cultural issues in the disclosure of cancer. *Cancer Practice, 3*, 153–160.

Moore, I. M., Gilliss, C. L., & Martinson, I. (1988). Psychosomatic symptoms in parents 2 years after the death of a child with cancer. *Nursing Research, 37*, 104–107.

Mulhern, R. K., Lauer, M. E., & Hoffman, R. G. (1983). Death of a child at home or in the hospital: Subsequent psychological adjustment of the family. *Pediatrics, 71*, 743–747.

Murphy, S. A., Chung, I. J., & Johnson, L. C. (2002). Patterns of mental distress following the violent death of a child and predictors of change over time. *Research in Nursing and Health, 25*, 425–437.

Natterson, J. M., & Knudson, A. G. (1960). Observations concerning fear of death in fatally ill children and their mothers. *Psychosomatic Medicine, 22*, 456–465.

Nuland, S. B. (1994). *How we die*. New York: Alfred Knopf.

Oltjenbruns, K. A. (2001). Developmental context of childhood: Grief and regrief phenomena. In M. S. Stroebe, R. O. Hansson, W. Stroebe, & H. Schut (Eds.), *Handbook of bereavement research: Consequences, coping, and care* (pp. 169–197). Washington, DC: American Psychological Association.

Pardo, I. (1982). The elaboration of mourning in a traditional area of Naples. *Rassegna Italiana di Sociologia, 23*, 535–569.

Parkes, C. M. (1970). The first year of bereavement: A longitudinal study of the reaction of London widows to the death of their husbands. *Psychiatry, 33*, 442–467.

Parkes, C. M., & Weiss, R. S. (1983). *Recovery from bereavement*. New York: Basic.

Pennebaker, J. W., Zech, E., & Rime, B. (2001). Disclosing and sharing emotion: Psychological, social, and health consequences. In M. S. Stroebe, R. O. Hansson, W. Stroebe, & H. Schut (Eds.), *Handbook of bereavement research: Consequences, coping, and care* (pp. 517–544). Washington, DC: American Psychological Association.

Prigerson, H. G., & Jacobs, S. C. (2001). Traumatic grief as a distinct disorder: A rationale, consensus criteria, and a preliminary empirical test. In M. S. Stroebe, R. O. Hansson, W. Stroebe, & H. Schut (Eds.), *Handbook of bereavement research: Consequences, coping, and care* (pp. 613–646). Washington, DC: American Psychological Association.

Rando, T. A. (1983). An investigation of grief and adaptation in parents whose children have died of cancer. *Journal of Pediatric Psychology, 8*, 3–20.

Rando, T. A. (1986). *Parental loss of a child*. Champaign, IL: Research Press.

Rando, T. A. (1991). Parental adjustment to the loss of a child. In D. Papadatou & C. Papadatos (Eds.), *Children and death* (pp. 233–253). New York: Hemisphere.

Rando, T. A. (2000). On the experience of traumatic stress in anticipatory and post-death mourning. In T. A. Rando (Ed.), *Clinical dimensions of anticipatory mourning. Theory and practice working with the dying, their loved ones, and their caregivers* (pp. 155–221). Champaign, IL: Research Press.

Reynolds, L. A., Miller, D. L., Jelalian, E., & Spirito, A. (1995). Anticipatory grief and bereavement. In M. C. Roberts (Ed.), *Handbook of pediatric psychology* (2nd ed.). New York: Guilford Press.

Richmond, J. B., & Waisman, H. D. (1955). Psychological aspects of management of children with malignant diseases. *American Journal of Diseases in Children, 88*, 42–47.

Ries, L. A. G. (1999). Childhood cancer mortality. In L. A. G. Ries, M. A. Smith, J. G. Gurney, M. Linet, T. Tamra, J. L. Young, & G. R. Bunin (Eds.), *Cancer incidence and survival among children and adolescents: United States SEER program 1975–1995* (NIH Publication No. 99-4649, pp. 165–168). Bethesda, MD: National Cancer Institute, SEER Program.

Robinson, L., & Mahon, M. M. (1997). Sibling bereavement: A concept analysis. *Death Studies, 21*, 477–499.

Rolland, J. (1994). *Families, illness, and disability: An integrative treatment model*. New York: Basic.

Rosenblatt, P. (1983). *Bitter, bitter tears: 19th century diarists and 20th century grief theories*. Minneapolis: University of Minnesota Press.

Rosenblatt, P. (2001). A social constructionist perspective on cultural differences in grief. In M. S. Stroebe, R. O. Hansson, W. Stroebe, & H. Schut (Eds.), *Handbook of bereavement research: Consequences, coping, and care* (pp. 285–300). Washington, DC: American Psychological Association.

Rosenthal, P. (2000). *Parent grief: Narratives of loss and relationship*. Philadelphia: Brunner/Mazel.

Rubin, S. (1981). A two-track model of bereavement: Theory and application in research. *American Journal of Orthopsychiatry, 51*, 101–119.

Rubin, S., & Malkinson, R. (2001). Parental response to child loss across the life cycle: Clinical and research perspectives. In M. S. Stroebe, R. O. Hansson, W. Stroebe, & H. Schut (Eds.), *Handbook of bereavement research: Consequences, coping, and care* (pp. 219–240). Washington, DC: American Psychological Association.

Sanders, C. M. (1993). Risk factors in bereavement outcome. In M. S. Stroebe, R. O. Hansson, & W. Stroebe (Eds.), *Handbook of bereavement: Theory, research, and intervention* (pp. 255–267). Cambridge, MA: Cambridge University Press.

Schaefer, C., Quesenberry, C. P., & Wi, S. (1995). Mortality following conjugal bereavement and the effects of a shared environment. *American Journal of Epidemiology, 141*, 1142–1152.

Schatz, B. (1986). Grief of mothers. In T. A. Rando (Ed.), *Parental loss of a child* (pp. 303–314). Champaign, IL: Research Press.

Schatz, W. (1986). Grief of fathers. In T. A. Rando (Ed.), *Parental loss and grief* (pp. 293–302). Champaign, IL: Research Press.

Schiff, H. S. (1978). *The bereaved parent*. New York: Penguin Books.

Schmidt, L. (1987). Working with bereaved parents. In T. Krulik, B. Holaday, & I. M. Martinson (Eds.),

*The child and family facing life-threatening illness* (pp. 327–344). Philadelphia: Lippincott.

Schneiderman, G., Winders, P., Tallett, S., & Feldman, W. (1994). Do child and/or parent bereavement programs work? *Canadian Journal of Psychiatry, 39*, 215–217.

Schonfeld, D. J. (1993). Talking to children about death. *Journal of Pediatric Health Care, 7*, 269–274.

Schut, H., Stroebe, M. S., van den Bout, J., & Terheggen, M. (2001). The efficacy of bereavement interventions: Determining who benefits. In M. S. Stroebe, R. O. Hansson, W. Stroebe, & H. Schut (Eds.), *Handbook of bereavement research: Consequences, coping, and care* (pp. 705–737). Washington, DC: American Psychological Association.

Shanfield, S., Swain, B., & Benjamin, G. (1987). Parents' responses to the death of adult children from accidents and cancer: A comparison. *Omega, 17*, 289–297.

Sormanti, M., & August, J. (1997). Parental bereavement: Spiritual connections with deceased children. *American Journal of Orthopsychiatry, 67*, 460–469.

Sourkes, B. (1991). Truth of life: Art therapy with pediatric oncology patients and their siblings. *Journal of Psychosocial Oncology, 9*, 81–96.

Sourkes, B. (1996). The broken heart: Anticipatory grief in children facing death. *Journal of Palliative Care, 12*, 56–59.

Spinetta, J. (1974). The dying child's awareness of death: A review. *Psychological Bulletin, 81*, 256–260.

Stoneman, Z., & Berma, P. W. (1993). *The effects of mental retardation, disability, and illness on sibling relationships*. Baltimore, MD: Brookes.

Stroebe, M. S., Hansson, R. O., Stroebe, W., & Schut, H. (2001). *Handbook of bereavement research: Consequences, coping, and care*. Washington, DC: American Psychological Association.

Stroebe, M. S., & Schut, H. (1999). The dual process model of coping with bereavement: Rationale and description. *Death Studies, 23*, 197–224.

Stroebe, M. S., & Schut, H. (2001). Models of coping with bereavement: A review. In M. S. Stroebe, R. O. Hansson, W. Stroebe, & H. Schut (Eds.), *Handbook of bereavement research: Consequences, coping, and care* (pp. 375–404). Washington, DC: American Psychological Association.

Walsh, F., & McGoldrick, M. (Eds.). (1991). *Living beyond loss: Death in the family*. New York: Norton.

Watson, J. L. (1982). Of flesh and bones: The management of death pollution in Cantonese society. In J. P. M. Bloch (Ed.), *Death and regeneration of life*. Cambridge, MA: Cambridge University Press.

Wikan, U. (1990). *Managing turbulent hearts: A Balinese formula for living*. Chicago: University of Chicago Press.

Wolfe, J., Grier, H. E., Klar, N., Levin, S. B., Ellenbogen, J. M., Salem-Schatz, S., et al. (2000). Symptoms and suffering at the end of life in children with cancer. *New England Journal of Medicine, 342*, 226–233.

Woodrick, A. C. (1995). A lifetime of mourning: Grief work among Yucatec Maya women. *Ethos, 23*, 401–423.

Worden, W. (2002). *Grief counseling and grief therapy: A handbook for the mental health practitioner* (3rd ed.). New York: Springer.

Wortman, C. B., & Silver, R. C. (2001). The myths of coping with loss revisited. In M. S. Stroebe, R. O. Hansson, W. Stroebe, & H. Schut (Eds.), *Handbook of bereavement research: Consequences, coping, and care* (pp. 405–430). Washington, DC: American Psychological Association.

# V

# Prevention of Primary and Secondary Malignancies

Andrea Farkas Patenaude

and Katherine A. Schneider

# Genetic Issues

The hallmark of genetic medicine is that medical concerns of one individual are germane not only for that person, but also for their offspring and future generations. Pediatric cancer patients, survivors of childhood cancers, their parents, and their siblings all have concerns that are likely to be increasingly affected by advances in genetics.

It has been estimated that between 10% and 15% of pediatric cancers are either hereditary or familial in origin (Quesnel & Malkin, 1997). Advances in genetics will help identify pediatric cancers that have a hereditary origin as well as genetic syndromes, identified by other phenotypic features, which put the mutation carrier at increased risk for some types of cancer. Knowledge about hereditary cancer syndromes will help determine the risk of a second malignancy in pediatric survivors, risks of cancer in siblings, and of course, cancer risk for future offspring. To accurately estimate the risk of second primary malignancy in survivors, it is crucial to be able to identify and separate those survivors who do and do not have cancer of hereditary origin because the latter group typically faces excess risk for developing other cancers that are part of the inherited cancer syndrome.

Genetic testing is currently available for several cancer syndromes that occur in childhood, most of which are relatively rare. In individual cases, predictive genetic testing may improve the likelihood that a cancer may be discovered in its early and most treatable stages. Reproductive technologies that involve genetic analysis may be important for some survivors who wish to avoid having a child with an inherited predisposition to cancer. Also, pharmacogenomics, the matching of pharmacologic treatments to patients based on genetic analysis of likely efficacy or susceptibility to adverse side effects, will likely become an important way in which genetic medicine affects pediatric cancer patients through reducing the burdens of cancer treatment. The ultimate goal of the translation of genetic findings into pediatric oncology practice is the development of targeted strategies to prevent the development of cancer.

With genetic advances come questions about the ethical application of genetic technology. The confluence of these concerns has been recognized by the creation within the Human Genome Project of the Ethical, Legal, and Social Implications Program, which provides funding for the study of how the social integration of the new genetics will affect individuals, families, and societies. The Ethical, Legal, and Social Implications Program also has as its goals the identification and reduction of disparities in access to genetic knowledge and technology. Testing children for hereditary cancer risk raises important and difficult questions. Ethical concerns are reduced if there is demonstrated medical benefit, but there are nonetheless questions about how best to counsel parents and children and how to resolve ethical conflicts within families related to genetic testing. While genetic testing of children for adult-onset cancers has been generally discouraged, there is a vocal minority of researchers who espouse the belief that adolescents should have access to genetic testing despite being minors (Michie & Marteau, 1995; Michie, McDonald, Bobrow, McKeown, & Marteau, 1996). There is, however, very little empirical research to support or refute their position. This is an area likely to be much explored in the future.

This chapter discusses the concerns of survivors and their parents about genetics and illustrates how knowledge about hereditary cancers modifies information of interest to all survivors about associated risks for secondary malignancy or cancer in offspring. It provides an overview of which pediatric cancers are known to have hereditary etiologies and how genetic counseling may be a useful adjunct service in pediatric oncology. We also discuss the literature on children and genetic testing as it relates to issues that may arise in families of pediatric cancer survivors and some ways the future treatment of pediatric cancer and the quality of life of survivors may be influenced by genetic technology.

## First, an Important Distinction

All cancers are genetic (Ganjavi & Malkin, 2002; Lynch, 1998). This means that it is changes in the genetic programming of cells that causes the cascade of cellular events that results in malignancy. Most of these deoxyribonucleic acid (DNA) errors are what are termed *sporadic* errors in the gene that have occurred in a single cell. These sporadic changes occur during a person's lifetime (often caused by carcinogens). These sporadic DNA errors are not carried in the germline and thus are not passed on to future generations. Therefore, most cancer is not "inherited" even though it is genetic. Cancer genetic counseling is largely concerned with genetic changes in the germline and are therefore passed from generation to generation. Although this does not necessarily mean that each person inheriting the genetic mutation or error goes on to develop cancer, it does mean that each carrier will have an increased susceptibility to getting cancer.

## Concerns About the Inheritance of Increased Cancer Susceptibility Among Parents of Pediatric Survivors

The diagnosis of cancer in a child raises critical existential questions for many parents about how or why their child was chosen for such a catastrophic and unexpected twist of fate. Parents of children with cancer are haunted by fears that something they did or conveyed to their child was responsible for causing the child's cancer. A survey of 47 mothers of pediatric oncology patients revealed that although the majority understood from their physicians that there is no known etiology for most childhood cancers, 83% harbored their own theories about why their child developed cancer (Patenaude, Basili, Fairclough, & Li, 1996). More than 70% of the mothers in this study reported reading about genetics and cancer. Nearly a third of the mothers reported being moderately worried about whether cancer in their family was an inherited disease; 26% said they worried "quite a bit" or "to an extreme" about hereditary cancer. Only 17% of the mothers had discussed their concerns about hereditary cancer with their child's pediatric oncologist. Nearly the same percentage had discussed their concerns about hereditary cancer with their children.

Mothers in that study (Patenaude, Basili, et al., 1996) were asked hypothetically if there was a genetic test available to determine whether their child's cancer was caused by inherited alterations whether they would test themselves and their healthy children under age 18 years (the siblings of the patient). Over one half of the mothers said they would be tested themselves, even if there were no anticipated medical benefits of testing. Of the mothers, 60% believed that finding out if they were mutation carriers would influence future childbearing plans. Regarding the hypothetical genetic testing of their healthy children, about half would test their child only if knowing about a mutation would reduce the risk of developing or dying from cancer. An additional 42% stated they would test their healthy children in the absence of any potential medical benefit just to know if they were mutation carriers. Actual family history of cancer did not significantly influence mothers' beliefs about seeking genetic testing for themselves and their children. Mothers believed that knowing the genetic status of their children would influence their own emotional well-being and would also affect how rapidly and frequently they sought medical advice for their currently healthy children.

## Fertility and Cancer Risk to Offspring of Pediatric Survivors

As pediatric cancers have become increasingly curable and both the number of survivors and their average age has increased, greater attention has been focused on long-term effects, including the survivors' fertility, and on the health of survivors' offspring. Survivors and their parents worried first about whether they would be able to conceive children and then about whether those children would have increased cancer risks themselves because of either the effects of cancer treatments or possible hereditary predisposition.

Studies have shown that radiation therapy and alkylating agents in many chemotherapy protocols diminish or eliminate fertility. Male patients are more affected by alkylating agent chemotherapy than female patients, although the fertility of females who receive abdominal radiation is also adversely affected (Byrne, 1999; Levy & Stillman, 1991; Nicholson & Byrne, 1993). Sperm banking has become an option considered essential to offer to adolescent males with cancer prior to the onset of treatment (Wallace & Thomson, 2003). The preservation of oocytes of female patients is much more difficult and has not proven to be effective. The potential for use of donor eggs, however, offers female survivors some hope of carrying a pregnancy, even if their fertility is impaired by treatment.

Many childhood cancer survivors do, however, retain their fertility and go on to have children. Reports from the Childhood Cancer Survivor Study showed lower birth weights in babies whose survivor mothers had experienced radiation to or near the ovaries (Green et al., 2002) and, for male patients, fewer live births resulting from pregnancies in their partners compared to live births to partners of their male siblings (Green et al., 2003).

Concerns also have been raised about risk of cancer in the children of pediatric cancer survivors. A number of studies have shown that, although most fertile survivors have normal, healthy children, there is some increased risk of cancer in the offspring of pediatric cancer survivors (Hawkins, Draper, & Winter, 1995; Mulvihill et al., 1987). Most of these studies included relatively few patients.

The presence of nationwide cancer registries in the Scandinavian countries facilitated a population-based study of the cancer rates among survivors of pediatric cancer (Sankila et al., 1998). That study followed 5,847 offspring of 14,652 Scandinavian and Icelandic pediatric cancer survivors for a total of 86,780 person-years. It initially yielded standardized incident rates of 1.6, indicating that survivors had 1.6 times the risk of having a child with cancer compared to the standard of 1.0 among parents who did not have cancer in childhood (Sankila et al., 1998). With greater knowledge about hereditary cancer syndromes, this study was able to more effectively separate out cases of hereditary cancer syndromes such as Li-Fraumeni syndrome (LFS), von Hippel-Lindau (VHL) syndrome, neurofibromatosis, and hereditary retinoblastoma. When the hereditary cancer cases were removed, the final standardized incident rate was only 1.3, or less than 1 case of excess cancer per 1,000 survivor offspring.

Such studies serve to further relieve the concerns of most pediatric cancer survivors about their risk of having children who will develop cancer in childhood. This relief is not relevant, however, for the minority of pediatric cancer patients whose illness is attributable to an inherited cancer syndrome.

## Cancer Risk for Siblings of Pediatric Cancer Patients

Parents of children with cancer also are concerned about whether their other, currently healthy, children are at any increased risk of cancer. Given the range of parents' personal theories for the etiology of their child's cancer, this question likely includes both parental concerns about possible inherited predisposition and concerns about environmental effects that might have triggered cancer in one of their children.

Studies in this area have been reassuring and suggest that, other than in families with inherited cancer syndromes, siblings are not at increased risk for cancer. Another study utilizing the Nordic registries followed 42,195 siblings of 25,687 children with cancer for a median of 16.7 years (range 0–40 years) or 694,625 person-years of follow-up. An initial excess of cancers was found in the number of observed versus expected sibling cancers (353 vs. 284.2), for a standardized incident ratio of 1.24. However, when the 34 sibling cancers occurring before age 20 years that were assumed to be hereditary were removed from the analysis, the standardized incident ratio was reduced to 1.0, indicating no increase over expectation in siblings of pediatric cancer patients. Similarly, the standardized incident ratio for adult siblings was close to 1.0 (Winther et al., 2001).

## Risk of Second Malignancies Among Pediatric Survivors

The most concerning late effect of childhood cancer is the development of a second primary malignancy. Several large-scale studies in the general population at 20–25 years postdiagnosis have shown that the cumulative incidence of secondary malignancy is between three- and sixfold increased risk compared to the background incidence of cancer (Neglia et al., 2001; Olsen et al., 1993). The most common types of secondary malignancy were bone, breast, central nervous system, and endocrine cancers (Bhatia & Sklar, 2002; Neglia et al., 2001). Particular types of second malignancies were strongly associated with certain primary malignancies, but there was no type of primary malignancy that was free of the risk that a second malignancy could occur. The primary pediatric malignancies most commonly associated with second cancers were retinoblastoma, soft tissue sarcomas, and Hodgkin's disease. Although second cancers do occur after acute lymphoblastic leukemia (ALL) and central nervous system tumors, the most common pediatric cancers, pediatric survivors of these cancers tend to have lower rates of secondary malignancy. Younger age at diagnosis is also correlated with a greater risk of secondary malignancy (Bhatia & Sklar, 2002), as are higher doses of radiation therapy and certain forms of chemotherapy.

In a U.S. study of 13,581 pediatric survivors a median of 15 years from diagnosis, only 1.88 excess cancers occurred per 1,000 patient-years of follow-up (Neglia et al., 2001). The actual rates of secondary malignancy are not high enough to overshadow the successes of treatment for pediatric cancer. There is, however, a marked contrast between the very low risk of second cancers in children with sporadic forms of cancer and the higher rates of secondary malignancy that children with hereditary cancer face. One of the hallmarks of cancer predisposition syndromes is that they tend to convey predisposition to multiple cancers, resulting in second, third, and even fourth malignancies in some patients (Hisada, Garber, Fung, Fraumeni, & Li, 1998).

When calculating second malignancy rates, complex analysis of the data is needed to factor out age-, gender- and treatment-related effects and the influence of hereditary cancers (Friedrich, 2001). In turn, care must be taken in planning appropriate follow-up surveillance strategies for individual patients based on their risk factors. It is also necessary to consider the interaction effect of hereditary predisposition and treatment variables because individuals with some cancer predisposition syndromes like LFS and hereditary retinoblastoma appear to be particularly sensitive to radiation exposure (Boyle et al., 2002; Wong et al., 1997). This, of course, has serious implications both for the therapeutic use of radiation and for the continuing use of screening procedures, such as mammography, that involve low levels of radiation exposure (Friedrich, 2001).

## Inherited Cancer Syndromes in Pediatrics

Recognition of hereditary cancer syndromes in the pediatric oncology clinic necessitates an awareness of the general and specific characteristics of hereditary cancer syndromes. We provide an overview of the clinical features of hereditary cancer syndromes and then briefly discuss specific hereditary syndromes that can cause cancers in children. We also discuss some other pediatric conditions associated with increased cancer risk in family members. Finally, we discuss the psychological issues that are unique or heightened in members of families of childhood cancer patients who are known or suspected of having a hereditary cancer syndrome.

## Characteristics of Hereditary Cancer Syndromes

Hereditary cancers are typically marked by (a) three or more family members with similar or related cancers; (b) earlier-than-usual age of onset; (c) predisposition to multiple cancers, leading to multifocal or bilateral cancers or multiple primary cancers in one individual; (d) increased rate of bilaterality in bilateral organ sites such as eyes, breasts, kidneys; and (e) in dominantly inherited syndromes, the presence of related cancers through multiple generations (although features may be subtle). Although these characteristics are not present in all cases of hereditary cancers, they can serve as a template to alert practitioners to the possible presence of a hereditary cancer syndrome.

The *earlier age of onset* refers to disease development at younger than typical ages. For example, women with mutations in breast/ovarian cancer predisposition genes, like *BRCA1* and *BRCA2*, develop breast cancers more typically in their 30s and 40s as opposed to women in the general population, whose breast cancers more frequently occur when the women are in their 50s, 60s, or older. The earlier age of onset characteristic holds true for a number of hereditary pediatric cancers as well. The median age of diagnosis of Wilms' tumor, a kidney tumor with both sporadic and hereditary forms, is 40 months. However, hereditary Wilms' tumors develop at a median of 30 months of age and are more likely to occur in both kidneys (bilateral) (Breslow, Beckwith, Ciol, & Sharples, 1988). Another example is hereditary retinoblastoma, which occurs on average at 12 months of age, while sporadic retinoblastoma occurs at 2.1 years of age on average (Knudson, 1975).

## Hereditary Syndromes That Predispose to Pediatric Malignancies

### Retinoblastoma

Retinoblastoma is the most common tumor of the eye in children. About 10% of cases of retinoblastoma are from families with a known family history of retinoblastoma. In addition, about 25% occur bilaterally and are assumed to be inherited. An additional 10% of the unilateral cases that occur in families without a family history are found to be caused by mutations in the *RB1* gene, the tumor suppressor gene that, when altered, causes retinoblastoma. *RB1* was the first tumor suppressor gene to be found and is often said to be the paradigm for cancers caused by such genes.

Retinoblastoma occurs very early in the lifespan, often in the first year of life, and very few cases are diagnosed after the age of 5 years. The tendency of hereditary cases of retinoblastoma to be bilateral means that there is a greater chance that children with hereditary retinoblastoma will lose vision in at least one eye. Children with hereditary retinoblastoma also have very high rates of second malignancies. Risk estimates range from 26% (Eng et al., 1993) to 68% (Abrahamson et al., 1984). The most common second cancers for patients with hereditary retinoblastoma are osteosarcomas, particularly if the patient received radiation as part of treatment. Children with hereditary retinoblastoma also have increased rates of developing leukemia and osteosarcoma (Wong et al., 1997).

### Li-Fraumeni Syndrome

LFS is a rare cancer syndrome that was discovered by careful observations of excess cancers in families of sarcoma patients. The classic definition of LFS is a proband (patient who brings the family to medical attention) diagnosed before age 45 years with sarcoma who has a first-degree relative who was diagnosed with cancer before age 45 years and another first- or second-degree relative with any cancer diagnosed younger than age 45 years or with a sarcoma at any age. Cancers most frequently found in LFS are soft tissue sarcomas, osteosarcoma, adrenocortical carcinomas, breast cancer, brain tumors, and acute leukemias. Beyond this classic definition, there are Li-Fraumeni-like families who may have fewer component cancers in individuals under age 60 years (Quesnel & Malkin, 1997).

In 60%–80% of the cases of classic LFS, a mutation in the *p53* gene, another tumor suppressor gene, can be identified. Members of LFS families who have *p53* mutations have a 90% lifetime risk of developing cancer and a 40% chance of cancer in childhood (Williams & Strong, 1985). Genetic testing is available for alterations in *p53* for individuals suspected of having LFS.

Unfortunately, there are no effective detection or prevention strategies for most LFS-associated cancers. LFS family histories are often devastatingly sad, with parents and children both ill with cancer simultaneously or with unusual patterns of diagnoses, such as one family with three adolescents who have all died from osteogenic sarcoma. Patients with LFS are sensitive to radiation, and alternate treatments should be considered when possible because of the high risk of secondary malignancies within the radiation field.

All children with adrenocortical carcinoma should be evaluated for *p53* mutations because their risk of being a mutation carrier may be 50%, even in the absence of a significant family history (Ribeiro et al., 2001). Children with other LFS-associated malignancies (brain tumor, sarcoma, leukemia) should be referred for genetic counseling and consideration of genetic testing if they have a first- or second-degree relative with cancer under age 60 years. Early detection improves the chances that a cancer is diagnosed at a more curable stage. Female mutation carriers (or suspected carriers) should have regular breast surveillance, including at least clinical examinations and mammograms beginning at around age 25 years. Men and women who are *p53* mutation carriers should have regular checkups with a well-informed physician and should become familiar with the early warning signs of cancer.

LFS is a dominantly inherited condition, meaning that offspring of *p53* mutation carriers have a 50/50 chance of inheriting the deleterious mutation. Many centers have been reluctant to test healthy, minor siblings of pediatric oncology patients who are *p53* mutation carriers because of the lack of immediate medical benefit. However, some centers have offered genetic testing to minors at 50% risk of being mutation carriers, sometimes under significant parental pressure (D. G. R. Evans, Maher, Macleod, Davies, & Craufurd, 1997; Malkin, Australie, Shuman, Barrerra, & Weksberg, 1996).

### *Wilms' Tumor*

The genetics of Wilms' tumor are more complicated than those of the dominantly inherited, high-penetrance genes discussed. Wilms' tumor is of the kidney and is the most common solid tumor of children (Breslow et al., 1988). About 10% of Wilms' tumors run in families. *WT1* is a gene that has been found to be mutated in a high proportion of hereditary Wilms' tumor cases. It is also, however, mutated in 5%–15% of cases that are not familial.

Increased risk for Wilms' tumor occurs as part of several congenital syndromes, including WAGR (which stands for Wilms' tumor, aniridia or absence of the iris, G for ambiguous genitalia, and R for mental retardation); Denys-Drash syndrome, which is characterized by urogenital malformations; and Beckwith-Weidemann syndrome, which can include hemihypertrophy, macroglossia (enlarged tongue), and macrosomia or gigantism. Different mutations of the *WT1* gene are associated with WAGR and Denys-Drash syndrome. It is believed that there may need to be other conditions present besides a mutation in *WT1* to cause Wilms' tumor to develop. Therefore, although genetic testing for *WT1* is possible, it is sometimes difficult to interpret the findings in terms of associated cancer risk. It is also believed that there are several other genes that convey predisposition to Wilms' tumor, but this is yet to be established.

### *Familial Adenomatous Polyposis*

Familial adenomatous polyposis (FAP) is a rare hereditary syndrome characterized by the development of at least 100 (but typically hundreds or thousands) polyps in the colon that, if left unattended, give the individual a 100% risk of developing colon cancer (Offit, 1998). Without removal of the colon (total colectomy), 37% of patients with FAP will develop colon cancer by age 40 years. Screening of the colon with annual colonoscopies is typically initiated in children thought or known to be at risk around age 10 years. Surgery can usually be delayed until 16 years of age or later, depending on the number of polyps found on colonoscopy. There is also a milder form of FAP called attenuated FAP that leads to fewer than 100 polyps at somewhat older ages. In families with attenuated FAP, a negative colonoscopy in a teenager or young adult does not rule out the possibility that the person is at risk.

The underlying cause of FAP is a mutation in the *APC* gene, another tumor suppressor gene. *APC* is a dominantly inherited gene. Offspring of an affected parent have a 50% chance of having FAP. Predictive genetic testing in children with an affected sibling or parent and a known *APC* mutation is recommended because children with true negative results could be spared the unpleasant annual screenings. Because there is a clear medical benefit to testing children at risk for carrying *APC* mutations, it is a circumstance in which the genetic testing of children has been encouraged by medical organizations and professionals. As a result, there are several psychological studies of the impact of genetic testing for *APC* on children and adolescents (see section the Children and Genetic Testing for Cancer Genes: What Do We Know? section).

### *Von Hippel-Lindau Disease*

VHL disease is a rare hereditary cancer syndrome characterized by tumors of the central nervous system (cerebellum, spine, and brain stem) and retina; by increased rates of renal cell carcinoma and pheochromocytomas (tumors of the adrenal glands); and by other related tumors and benign cysts (Maher & Kaelin, 1997). Diagnosis often occurs in the second or third decade (Schneider, 2002). Because of the complex and varied presentation of VHL syndrome, multidisciplinary medical surveillance is recommended, with some aspects beginning in childhood (Maher et al., 1990). Patients with known VHL disease and at-risk relatives are told to undergo annual physical examination, urine cytology, indirect ophthalmologic exam (from age 5 years), angiography (from age 10 years), brain magnetic resonance imaging (from age 15 years), annual renal ultrasound, and annual 24-hour urine collection.

The cloning of the tumor suppressor gene *VHL* in 1993 led to identification of mutations in the *VHL* gene in more than 80% of VHL families (Couch, Lindor, Karnes, & Michels, 2000). This enables close relatives of mutation carriers to learn if they are at risk for VHL. In families with an identified mutation, those with true negative test results can abandon the extensive and expensive annual screening. Individuals who carry a *VHL* mutation and those in classic VHL families in which a mutation has not been detected are advised to continue to pursue surveillance and screening as they are associated with significant improvement in the length of life for patients with VHL syndrome (Maher & Kaelin, 1997). Correlations between genotype (what genetic analysis shows) and phenotype (symptoms visible in the patient) offer indications of whether some symptoms, notably pheochromocytomas, are likely to be part of the syndrome for particular individuals (Couch et al., 2000). Because at least some aspects of the extensive screening for VHL are recommended for children, genetic testing of children for mutations in their *VHL* gene are considered in most centers as having medical benefit.

### *Multiple Endocrine Neoplasia Type II*

Multiple endocrine neoplasia Type II (MEN2) is an autosomally dominant inherited condition attributable to mutations in the *RET* gene; individuals (including sometimes very young children) develop, among other symptoms, a rare form of thyroid cancer called medullary thyroid carcinoma. There are two subtypes of MEN2: MEN 2A typically has onset in early adulthood; MEN2B has onset in early childhood (PDQ Cancer Genetics Summary, 2001). Other features of MEN2B include parathyroid tumors and tumors of the adrenal gland called pheochromocytomas.

People with *RET* mutations are at high risk of developing cancer, estimated to be a 70% risk by age 70 years. It had been customary to use physiological indicators to determine who was recommended for thyroidectomy and when it occurred. This requires ongoing measurement of a variety of indicators. However, even in some cases of asymptomatic individuals in MEN2 families, advanced medullary thyroid cancer (MTC) was found when surgery occurred, often leading to fatal outcomes.

Genetic testing has allowed for clearer and earlier identification of those at risk of MTC and surveillance only of those who are found to be mutation carriers (van Heurn et al., 1999). Genetic testing of young children is recommended in families with *RET* mutations. Children found to be mutation carriers typically undergo prophylactic thyroidectomy. There is some difference of opinion about just how early thyroidectomy should occur (Lips, 1998) because MTC has been found as early as 2 years of age in a child with MEN2A and as early as 1 year of age in a child with MEN2B (vanHeurn et al., 1999). There are some data on the emotional reactions of children undergoing genetic testing for MEN2 (Grosfeld et al., 1996, 2000) (see section on emotional issues).

### *Associated Hereditary Conditions With Increased Risks for Childhood Cancer*

There are a number of syndromes that predispose individuals to increased cancer risks. These conditions are characterized by defects in DNA repair. Patients with xeroderma pigmentosa are highly sensitive to sun exposure and have more than 1,000 times greater risk than normal of developing skin cancer in exposed areas (Kraemer, 1997). Beginning in infancy, patients have greatly increased chances of developing a range of skin cancers.

Patients with Fanconi's anemia have higher-than-usual risks of developing acute leukemia (Ganjavi & Malkin, 2002). Ataxia-telangiectasia is a progressively debilitating disease involving cerebellar ataxia and degenerate spinal musculature atrophy that is usually fatal before 45 years of age. It is associated with higher-than-average rates of leukemias and lymphomas, which can occur in adolescence or early adulthood (Schneider, 2002). Interesting links to breast cancer predisposition have been found in mothers of patients with ataxia-telangiectasia (i.e., heterozygous carriers of the *AT* gene mutation).

Neurofibromatosis, Type 1 (NF1), is a common genetic disorder (1 in 3,000 people) (Offit, 1998) that includes a 2%–5% increased risk of developing malignancies (Schneider, 2002). The gene, *NF1*, responsible for NF1 was cloned in 1990, but the large size of the gene and the variety of mutations have complicated interpretation of genetic testing. NF1 has highly variable effects that can be present from childhood and can include increased risk for astrocytomas, sarcomas, optic gliomas, and juvenile chronic myelogenous leukemia (Offit, 1998).

Neurofibromatosis, Type 2 (NF2), is a much rarer genetic condition attributable to a different gene, *NF2*. It is characterized by usually benign tumors of the spine and skin. Deafness can result from compression of the acoustic nerve. Opacity of the lens of the eye may also occur.

Both NF1 and NF2 patients typically have café-au-lait spots in unusual numbers on their skin. Genetic testing of relatives of individuals found to have neurofibromatosis can spare those who are found not to be mutation carriers the extensive medical follow-up that would otherwise occur.

## Psychological Issues for Hereditary Cancer Patients and Their Families

### At Diagnosis

The possibility that a child recently diagnosed with cancer could have an inherited condition adds a great burden to the already considerable worry of the child's parents. It is very common for parents of newly diagnosed patients to ask about the cancer risks to their other, healthy children. In contrast to the majority of parents who can be reassured that their other, healthy children are not likely to develop cancer, parents who learn their child's cancer is hereditary may be told that each of their other children has a 50/50 chance of being a carrier of the altered gene. Because most cancer gene mutations are inherited from a parent, there also may be immediate fear that the parent is at high risk to develop cancer. Although not the typical scenario, there are cases in which the increased hereditary cancer risk to the currently healthy parent is recognized only after the diagnosis of the child with cancer (Lynch, Katz, Bogard, & Lynch, 1985).

The question of whether to pursue genetic testing for the patient, parent, or the siblings in hereditary cancer families must be considered, raising both hopes and fears. In families in which there was no previous knowledge of the hereditary cancer syndrome, there also may be a need to inform other relatives (aunts, uncles, and cousins) about the risk that they or their offspring might have. It is a challenge for parents of a child newly diagnosed with cancer to absorb the full meaning of the hereditary risks that affect both the ill child and others in the family at the same time that they receive all of the information about the child's illness and treatment options.

Tensions between parents may increase as differences in focus, guilt, or blame for the hereditary condition surface. At a time when concerns about health insurance are paramount, worry multiplies about the future health of the parent and the continued access to health insurance, should that parent become ill. Parents who considered or needed to change jobs may be particularly worried about discrimination based on genetic risk status and may instead stay with unsatisfying work environments to ensure continued access to health insurance. Legislation that allows for the portability of health insurance should greatly lessen concern about parental "job lock." Worry about financial matters or the health of so many family members may increase the distress of the ill child, who may feel guilty that the illness is making his or her parents so upset. Younger children may also fear more directly that their parents will not be able to care for them, because of either illness in the parent or preoccupation about other matters.

Even when the hereditary condition in the family has been previously established, the diagnosis of cancer in a child is a very difficult blow. The parent who has a mutation (and who may or may not have had cancer) may harbor guilt about the child's illness. Despite the intellectual awareness that the parent did not choose to pass this "bad gene" along, the feelings of helplessness and guilt can be quite powerful. This circumstance will arise more frequently in future years as hereditary cancer syndromes are identified in more individuals, many of whom are likely to go on to have children. In hereditary cancer families, there are frequently multiple deaths from cancer, often of quite young people. It is more difficult in these families to encourage hope in the child by differentiating their cancer from cancer in older people. An ill parent's cancer treatment may occur concurrently with the newly diagnosed child's treatment. Although this may encourage camaraderie between parent and child, it increases the burden on the other spouse and siblings. Practical issues such as the greater number of doctor visits that may be necessary to deal with the medical issues relevant to all family members may further strain parents' coping abilities.

## Long-Term Emotional Issues and Concerns in Hereditary Cancer Families

Because of the increased risk of second primary malignancies among cancer patients with hereditary forms of cancer, fear about cancer remains high even after the initial cancer is brought into remission and appears cured. Surveillance for other possible cancers may necessitate medical visits to a variety of specialists, adding to the family illness burden and to concerns about the medicalization of the ill child. It may be difficult for some children to understand why they must be monitored for so long by so many doctors. Also, because there are no specific screening tests for some of the pediatric inherited cancers, parents of children who are carriers may have even more heightened reactions to minor symptoms, such as fever, than do parents of childhood cancer survivors generally. Unless siblings have had genetic testing (which is rarely the case), parents of children in a hereditary cancer family are likely to overreact to symptoms in any of their children.

In families in which it is known which children are mutation carriers, it may be difficult for children not to misinterpret differential parental attention to the medical issues of those children who carry the mutated gene. In addition, the continuing threat of hereditary cancer can complicate the developmental separation that is already difficult for pediatric cancer survivors and their parents when the children reach adolescence and young adulthood.

When children with a hereditary cancer syndrome reach adulthood, their consideration of whether to have children of their own is even more complex than for other pediatric cancer survivors. Genetic counseling may help to educate the patient and spouse about the possible risks to offspring. Couples in which one person has a diagnosed hereditary cancer syndrome can consider the use of reproductive technologies. One option is preimplantation diagnosis, the testing of an embryo that has been fertilized in vitro for the specific gene mutation prior to implantation into the uterus of the mother. Other options include prenatal testing of a normally conceived embryo or the use of donor sperm or donor eggs. Those couples unwilling to take the risk of passing on the deleterious mutation and unwilling to utilize reproductive technology may decide to adopt a child or to remain childless.

These are emotionally very complex issues that encompass ethical, religious, financial, and family considerations. Individuals with a cancer-predisposing mutation often feel that the decision they make about having children who might carry a cancer-predisposing mutation reflects on the question of whether their own life has been worth living. Some conclude that to purposely avoid having such a child would imply, erroneously, that their own life has not been a valuable one. Spouses may have different reactions to these issues and may come to different conclusions about using advanced reproductive methods or about adopting a child. It may be unclear how the decision to proceed should be made and whose feelings should be given the most weight. Parents of this now-adult survivor making such a decision may also have different feelings from their son or daughter. They may wish strongly that their child and that child's spouse could be spared the sadness and worry of having a child with an increased risk of cancer; the survivor may feel strongly that having a biological child is critical evidence of some aspects of "normalcy."

Another issue in families for whom hereditary cancer syndromes exist is that of unresolved grief. It seems to occur because of the proximity of multiple deaths over several generations of a family. The loss of a parent at an early age is more common in these families with hereditary cancers because cancer occurs at earlier-than-expected ages. The increased cancer risk to the children makes it more difficult for the children to differentiate themselves from their dead parents or grandparents, an important step in mourning. Also, recurrent grief in older relatives may leave them with few emotional resources to help those in the younger generations experience their own sadness, fear, and anger. Financial burdens are heightened by the early death of adults because of cancer, which may in turn limit access to outside sources of therapeutic assistance.

In some cases, the cancer diagnosis of a parent was not explained to a child, leading to unresolved feelings of anger and betrayal that can compound reactions of grief. Some parents find it difficult to share information with their children out of wanting to protect them. Others, conversely, may share too many details with the children, unduly frightening them.

## Ethical and Social Issues Regarding the Genetic Testing of Children

In making decisions about the genetic testing of children, the first consideration is whether there is immediate medical benefit to the child from the information gained through testing. In the case of FAP, genetic test results can have an immediate impact on the screening recommendations for children, either freeing them from annual colonoscopies beginning at around the age of 10 years or further supporting the need for such procedures. Testing for MEN2B is another good example of a genetic test that would alter medical care depending on the result. With a hereditary cancer syndrome, however, such as LFS, the determination of medical benefit from genetic testing is much less clear. The absence of early detection strategies for most of the LFS-associated cancers makes at least some specialists conclude that there is little medical benefit to be gained from testing children.

The decision to test a child is made by the parents of the child. This proxy determination eliminates the possibility that the individual might choose not to be tested as an adult, a decision that many adults in hereditary cancer families have made (Patenaude, Schneider, et al., 1996). There are many concerns about the familial impact of knowing whether particular children are mutation carriers. Parental communication to children of different ages about their hereditary risk is subject to the parents' interpretation of the meaning of the test result. Some parents insist that the child not be informed. When children are told, developmental concerns and preoccupation with illness may make it difficult for a child to take in accurate knowledge about their hereditary cancer risk and its implications.

Although pediatric oncologists have been pioneers in the direct discussion with children of difficult issues such as diagnosis with cancer, treatment recurrence, or impending death, like most health professionals, they have little experience discussing genetic cancer predisposition with children. We know relatively little about how such discussions are experienced by the children who participate in them.

Another issue related to the testing of children is that genetic knowledge is rapidly changing, and with these changes, knowledge about the risks for cancers or associated conditions associated with a particular mutation is likely to change. This places some burden on health care providers to provide updated genetic information to survivors, but this is logistically very difficult to accomplish (Patenaude, 1996).

In addition, there remains concern about whether information about inherited cancer risk will be used by insurers to discriminate against mutation carriers. Because hereditary cancer syndromes increase risk for second malignancies, survivors of pediatric cancers and their parents may worry about future insurability or employability. Healthy siblings who are found to be mutation carriers might also be concerned about these issues despite being asymptomatic. Forty-one states now have legislation protecting the privacy of genetic information, which contributes to the near-nonexistence of cases of discrimination in health insurance against mutation carriers.

Research is needed on the family impact of genetic information regarding hereditary cancer risk, on the ways in which children learn about cancer and genetics within cancer families and how they view genetic testing, and on the short- and long-term impacts of testing. We review the limited research that does exist on children who have been tested. We also briefly discuss research to date on how children in families in which a parent has been tested for an adult-onset cancer have been informed or not informed about the genetic testing.

## Children and Genetic Testing for Cancer Genes: What Do We Know?

### Research on the Genetic Testing of Children

Research on the psychosocial outcomes of the genetic testing of children has been largely conducted on patients with two diseases, MEN2B and FAP, conditions for which the medical benefits of testing for children are well accepted. A study from the United Kingdom and Australia of 60 children, aged 10–16 years, who had undergone *APC* testing because they were from families with FAP found that the children had mean depression, anxiety, and behavioral symptom scores in the normative range (Michie, Bobrow, & Marteau, 2001). Thirty-one children were mutation carriers; 29 were mutation negative, meaning that they could avoid the repeated annual colonoscopies recommended for mutation carriers. The children appeared able to understand the implications of their test results. Most of the children rated themselves as healthy, and there were no self-esteem differences between mutation-positive and mutation-negative children.

Of the mutation carriers, 10%, however, expressed regret about knowing their mutation status. Although this was a small study, this is an interesting and intriguing finding because relatively few adults undergoing genetic testing express overt regret that they have been tested. It is not clear if this represents a true difference in how children and adults feel about genetic testing or if it represents what pediatric psycho-oncologists often observe: Children are simply more direct in their communication about difficult topics than adults. More qualitative investigation of the responses of tested children may evoke a better understanding of what the underlying issues are when children tested for medical benefit experience adverse emotional outcomes.

In the United States, Codori and colleagues at Johns Hopkins University studied a group of 43 children tested for mutations in the *APC* gene because they had a parent with FAP (Codori, Petersen, Boyd, Brandt, & Giardiello, 1996). About half of the children were mutation carriers. Findings from this study revealed that the emotional outcomes of testing were not aligned solely with mutation status. Three children who had scored below clinical levels prior to result disclosure, two of whom were mutation negative, scored in the clinical range on an anxiety measure after testing. Mutation carriers who had an ill mother (vs. father) obtained higher depression scores. Both mutation-positive and mutation-negative children with ill mothers were more anxious than children whose father was the ill parent. Parents who were not ill seemed to report depressive symptoms more readily following findings that their children had positive or mixed (some positive, some negative) genetic test results.

In a later study, a 28- to 55-month follow-up of children tested for *APC* mutations at Johns Hopkins, the mean scores on an anxiety measure for both children with APC mutations and children who were negative were in the average range and did not differ by mutation status (Codori et al., 2003). The children's emotional outcomes, however, did appear to be highly influenced by the mutation status of their siblings. Having a test result that differed from one's siblings appeared to be more highly correlated with clinically significant anxiety or depression than being from a family for whom all the tested children were positive. These results appear similar to the findings by Smith, West, Croyle, and Botkin (1999) who studied adults tested for *BRCA1* in Utah. They found that an individual's psychological response to genetic testing was a factor not only of their own test result, but also of the mutation status of their other tested relatives, especially siblings. In the Johns Hopkins study, parents whose children had mixed results evidenced the most depressive symptoms after genetic testing, especially the healthy parent. The guilt of the parent who conveys the deleterious mutation to one or more children apparently modifies the parent's ability to focus on or express their own sadness about their child's status. It also may be more difficult for the ill parent to express disappointment at having a child who shares their own characteristics, even if those characteristics are ones that the adult would prefer not to have. Again, it is clear from the complexity of the findings that there is still much to be investigated and understood about emotional reactions to genetic testing in children and their parents.

In the Netherlands, genetic testing for MEN2 is available from the age of 5 years. One Dutch study investigated the emotional status of 90 individuals over the age of 16 years (which is the age of consent for genetic testing in the Netherlands) who were requesting MEN2 testing for themselves and the partners of these individuals and 26 couples requesting MEN2 testing for their young children. Findings revealed that levels of distress on multiple standard measures of anxiety and depression in most applicants were not different from population means. Distress was higher (within the clinical ranges), however, in those under age 25 years applying for testing themselves and in those in this age group who were not married. Within this subgroup, the highest baseline distress scores were among individual applicants who were 15–20 years old, who were at high risk of being a mutation carrier, and who tended to deal with problems by avoidance. It is of interest that because those applying for testing themselves were generally above the age at which thyroid cancer would have been found, they were generally able to anticipate that they would not be carriers, which may explain their reduced anxiety. The younger applicants had higher likelihoods that they could be carriers and were thus confronted with issues of mortality during the vulnerable period of their adolescence. Home interviews showed that there also was considerable ambivalence about testing in a third of the young applicants. Overall, 30% of individuals applying for themselves and 39% of parents applying had expressed ambivalence about genetic testing.

Posttest knowledge of the genetics of MEN2 was low even after genetic counseling in many individuals and parents applying for testing (Grosfeld et al., 2000). Parents expressed the belief that testing would help ensure that carrier children received potentially life-saving surveillance. About one half of the parents, though, were sufficiently skeptical of the accuracy of the test result to state that they would want their children who tested negative to receive further clinical screening. The investigators believed that many of the individuals applying for testing had been encouraged by physicians shortly after testing became available, and that some (12%) felt pressured to be tested, a factor that has been associated negatively with satisfaction about testing (Bloch, 1992). The researchers also cautioned that, when participation in testing is encouraged for medical reasons, a subset of more vulnerable individuals, especially young people, may agree to be tested without fully exploring the possible ramifications. They suggested increased counseling and attention to any ambivalence or other concerns of the young participant. They worried that, because pre- and posttest distress are correlated (Croyle, 1997), these individuals in comparison to other participants may have more difficult adjustment after receiving their test result.

It is clear that these are early studies, but they do suggest that, even when there are obvious medical benefits to being tested, there are deep emotional issues that interact with the "logic" of learning one's test result. Ambivalence and vulnerability because of young age or premorbid depression (not uncommon in families in which parents and others may have been sick or died) should be evaluated in those seeking genetic counseling and testing. It may be necessary to counsel individuals, especially young people, several times to convey all of the necessary factual information regarding genetic disease. The difficulty may be not only the breadth of information to be conveyed (basics of genetics; implications of the family history; information about possible test results; implications of the result for other relatives, especially offspring; risks and benefits of testing; testing cost and logistics; etc.), but also the fact that the information may have heavy emotional overlays related to past family events or fears for the future.

### Research on Communication of Parental Genetic Test Results to Children

A number of professional organizations have weighed in with the view that children themselves should not be tested for adult-onset hereditary conditions when there is no medical benefit to the child of knowing his or her mutation status (American Medical Association, 1995; American Society of Human Genetics, 1995; Clinical Genetics Society, 1994). In clinical practice, providers typically do not offer genetic testing for adult-onset conditions to children, although there are reports in the literature of unusual circumstances, such as both parents being terminally ill, under which some children have been tested (Evans et al., 1997).

Opinion is divided about whether testing children in families with known hereditary predisposition to adult-onset cancer syndromes is advisable or whether it represents a form of paternalism (Michie & Marteau, 1998). Children in families in which cancer has been linked to a hereditary predisposition, however, are often quite sensitive to the possible hereditary nature of cancer in their family. This awareness is likely only to increase with more coverage of scientific findings about cancer and genetics in the popular media and greater integration of such knowledge into high school science curricula.

We do not know much about how children react to actually learning that a parent has undergone genetic testing and received a positive test result or how children at risk feel about being tested themselves. The available data come mainly from research on family communication in families with hereditary breast cancer with *BRCA1/2* mutations. Even that data are mostly from parental report or discussion of hypothetical outcomes with adolescents. There are difficult ethical and methodological concerns about approaching children directly to inquire about their knowledge of parental mutation status. It is obviously not ethical to raise topics with children that their parents wish not to discuss with them, so it may be particularly difficult to learn about the psychosocial concerns of children whose parents have not disclosed the familial genetic test results. Because many of the parents who are tested for cancer genes also have had cancer, it is difficult (although not theoretically impossible) methodologically to separate out the effects of having a parent with cancer from specific concerns about the parent's hereditary mutation status and implications of that status.

A small study of 20 children, aged 11–17 years, whose mothers were tested for *BRCA1/2* mutations at Georgetown University demonstrated that the children worried quite a bit about family members developing cancer. Ninety percent indicated they would be interested in learning their own mutation status. Qualitative interviews demonstrated that children who had been informed of their mother's test result were particularly distressed to learn that their mother had increased risks not only for another breast cancer, but also for other cancers, especially ovarian cancer (Tercyak, Peshkin, Streisand, & Lerman, 2001).

A study of how 133 parents of children aged 11–17 years communicated their *BRCA1/2* test result to their children demonstrated that the decision to inform children appeared to reflect general family patterns regarding the openness of communication rather than the test result itself (Tercyak, Hughes, et al., 2001). In most families, all of the children were told despite differences in their ages. Higher general anxiety in the parent was associated with the decision to communicate the result to children. In general, parental anxiety did not subside after informing children of the parent's test result.

It is obvious that how and what children are informed will influence their response to learning that they or their parent may be at increased hereditary risk for cancer. In the future, it is likely that there will be considerable research on the important issues of how children respond, what children of different ages comprehend about what they have been told, and how knowledge of documented hereditary risk for cancer in their family influences long-term planning and well-being. Pediatric psychologists, who have the methodological and interpersonal skills to approach and evaluate children, will be ideal candidates to conduct such research. Important ethical and methodological concerns will need to be addressed. Also, it will be of interest to respond to practical clinical questions about how to contact and communicate to children changing information about cancer risk relevant to their family's genetic status. Pediatric providers face particular challenges in thinking about how and when to bring new genetic information to the attention of their pediatric at-risk or potentially at-risk patients.

## Future Implications of Genetic Advances for Pediatric Oncology Patients and Survivors

### Treatment Effects

Pharmacogenomics represents a very important implication of advancing genetic knowledge. Pharmacogenomics is the targeting of medication choice and dosage to patients based on individual genetic analysis of the genes responsible for drug metabolism. A startling pharmacogenomic success story concerns the *TPMT* gene and the metabolism of two chemotherapy agents, mercaptopurine (MP) and azathioprine (AZA) (W. E. Evans, 2001).

Deficiencies in TMPT enzyme activity can be determined on the basis of the individual's genotype. Deficiencies in TMPT activity have been linked to serious hematopoietic, dose-limiting toxicities in about 10% of patients with pediatric ALL undergoing chemotherapies that include MP and AZA (Relling et al., 1999). When these patients receive full doses of MP and AZA, they have such severe reactions that they are forced to miss or delay receiving many doses of their chemotherapy and are more prone to infection because of the hematopoietic toxicities that develop. This represents a severe, potentially life-threatening complication.

Before the genetic molecular basis for TMPT activity was discovered, it was likely that such a reaction in patients would result in a dose reduction for the entire chemotherapy regimen. The finding that a 90% dose reduction in MP or AZA for these patients eliminates the adverse hematopoietic toxicity in patients with TPMT deficiencies has greatly improved the outlook for the success of chemotherapy in treating them. "The TPMT genetic polymorphism illustrates the potential utility of pharmacogenomics to optimize ALL therapy on the basis of each patient's inherited ability to metabolize and respond to antileukemic agents" (W. E. Evans et al., 2001, p. 2300). Furthermore, differences in underlying genetic genotypes that affect drug metabolism may be responsible for differences in survival of children from different ethnic and cultural backgrounds. This knowledge offers new hope for improving the efficacy of chemotherapy and for reducing the burden of adverse side effects experienced by pediatric oncology patients.

Ultimately, gene therapies may be available to correct defects in genetic alterations responsible for the underlying disease mechanisms that are etiological in pediatric (and other) cancers (Rubnitz & Crist, 1997). These goals are still far off and will require lengthy and difficult testing of novel therapies. Informing patients and parents about the risks and benefits of such novel treatments will require the education of health care professionals about both specific and general advances in genetics.

As awareness grows in the general public, parents of newly diagnosed pediatric cancer patients will more frequently ask their child's health care providers questions related to the genetics of their child's disease (Nichols, Li, Haber, & Diller, 1998). It will be important not only for pediatric oncologists and oncology nurses to be informed about such advances, but also for pediatric psychologists to understand enough about these matters to help patients and their parents understand what is clinically available now and what may be decades away. This understanding may aid mental health professionals in supporting patients and parents who may be frustrated that genetic science cannot immediately improve the outlook for preventing or curing cancer in their family.

## Genetic Counseling Needs

Although the number of identified hereditary cancer syndromes that affect children and the total number of affected patients may be small, increasing knowledge is raising greater concern about genetics among parents and pediatric cancer survivors. Genetic counselors can address concerns about genetic etiologies of the cancer, concern about the heritability of cancer predisposition for the children of survivors, and concern about hereditary factors in the treatment of the cancer.

Genetic counseling provides a useful service not only when a hereditary condition has been identified and genetic testing is available, but also when families can be reassured that the cancer in their family is unlikely to be caused by inherited factors. The presence of genetic counselors in pediatric oncology or childhood cancer survivor clinics offers the opportunity for these questions to be considered at length and for carefully researched and constructed answers based on extensive family history taking and, in some cases, genetic test results (Schneider, 2002). The counseling interaction allows for discussion of how genetic information should be conveyed to the patient, siblings, grandparents, and other at-risk relatives. It also allows for consideration of the extent of psychological distress this genetic information engenders and whether referral for longer-term psychological counseling is warranted. It permits discussion of the privacy concerns and of the current protections available for genetic information in the particular state where the patient resides. Finally, the genetic counselor and pediatric oncologist can work together to determine which, if any, surveillance strategies are recommended to detect as early as possible any related cancers or other conditions for which the patient is at increased hereditary risk. Although currently rare, it is likely that the presence of genetic counselors within the pediatric oncology setting will increase in coming decades.

## Conclusion

The impact of advances in genetic knowledge transcends far beyond the identification of a number of hereditary cancer syndromes that increase risks of childhood cancer. Separation of sporadic and hereditary cases influences data on risk for secondary malignancies, risks of cancer to siblings and future offspring, and survival statistics. Treatment of present and especially future pediatric oncology patients is likely to be highly influenced by advances in pharmacogenomics, which should also reduce the personal burdens of adverse side effects of chemotherapies on pediatric cancer patients. For at least some patients who have cancers with hereditary origins, genetic testing can help to identify and clarify their diagnosis and assist with treatment decisions and lifelong surveillance. Siblings and even parents of these patients may also benefit from genetic testing if knowledge of mutation status can lead to early detection or prevention of the related cancers or other conditions. Ultimately, genetic information may be used to tailor prevention strategies or gene therapy treatments.

All of these uses of genetics will have a profound psychological impact on pediatric cancer patients, long-term survivors, and their parents and other family members. Pediatric psycho-oncologists are among those health professionals who should include genetic education in their training in order to offer patients the kind of understanding that allows them to share the emotional impact of receiving such complex and personal information. Psychologists can listen empathically, can help refer patients appropriately for genetic counseling or other genetic services, and can assist patients and family members in coping with the communication and integration of this far-reaching and often-unexpected information.

## References


Abramson, D. H., Ellsworth, R. M., Kitchin, F. D., & Tung, G. (1984). Second non-ocular tumors in retinoblastoma survivors. Are they radiation-induced? *Ophthalmology, 91*, 1351–1355.

American Medical Association Council on Ethical and Judicial Affairs. (1995). Testing children for genetic status. *Code of Medical Ethics*. Report 66.

American Society of Human Genetics Board of Directors and the American College of Medical Genetics Board of Directors. (1995). Points to consider: Ethical, legal, and psychosocial implications of genetic testing in children and adolescents. *American Journal of Human Genetics, 57*, 1233–1241.

Bhatia, S., & Sklar, C. (2002). Second cancers in survivors of childhood cancer. *Nature.com, 2*, 124–132.

Bloch, M., Adams, S., Wiggins, S., Huggins, M., & Hayden, M. R. (1992). Predictive testing for Huntington disease in Canada: The experience of those receiving an increased risk. *American Journal of Medical Genetics, 42*, 499–507.

Boyle, J. M., Spreadborough, A. R., Greaves, M. J., Birch, J. M., Varley, J. M., & Scott, D. (2002). Delayed chromosome changes in gamma-irradiated normal and Li-Fraumeni fibroblasts. *Radiation Research, 157*, 158–165.

Breslow, N., Beckwith, J. B., Ciol, M., & Sharples K. (1988). Age distribution of Wilm's tumor: Report from the National Wilm's Tumor Study. *Cancer Research, 48*, 1653–1657.

Byrne, J. (1999). Infertility and premature menopause in childhood cancer survivors. *Medical and Pediatric Oncology, 33*, 24–28.

Codori, A.-M., Petersen, G. M., Boyd, P. A., Brandt, J., & Giardello, F. M. (1996). Genetic testing for cancer in children: Short term psychological effects. *Archives of Pediatric and Adolescent Medicine, 150*, 1131–1138.

Codori, A.-M., Zawacki, K. L., Petersen, G. M., Miglioretti, D. L., Bacon, J. A., Trimbath, J. D., et al. (2003). Genetic testing for hereditary colorectal cancer in children: Long-term psychological effects. *American Journal of Medical Genetics, 116A*, 117–128.

Clinical Genetics Society (1994). Report of the Working Party on the genetic testing of children. *Journal of Medical Genetics, 31*, 785–797.

Couch, V., Lindor, N., Karnes, P., & Michels, V. V. (2000). von Hippel-Lindau disease. *Mayo Clinic Proceedings, 75*, 265–272.

Croyle, R., Smith, K. R., Botkin, J. R., Baty, B., & Nash, J. (1997). Psychological responses to

BRCA1 mutation testing: preliminary findings. *Health Psychology, 16*, 63–72.

Eng, C., Li, F. P., Abramson, D. H., Ellsworth, R M., Wong, F. L., Goldman, M. B., et al. (1993). Mortality from second tumors among long-term survivors of retinoblastoma. *Journal of the National Cancer Institute, 85*, 1121–1128.

Evans, D. G. R., Maher, E. R., Macleod, R., Davies, D. R., & Craufurd, D. (1997). Uptake of genetic testing for cancer predisposition. *Journal of Medical Genetics, 34*, 746–748.

Evans, W. E. (2001). Pharmacogenomics: marshalling the human genome to individualise drug therapy. *Gut 2003, 52*, Suppl 2 ii 8–10.

Evans, W. E., Hon, Y. Y., Bomgaars, L., Coutre, S., Holdsworth, M., Janco, R., et al. (2001). Preponderance of thiopurine S-methyltransferase and heterozygosity among patients intolerant to mercaptopurine or Azathioprine. *Journal of Clinical Oncology, 19*, 2293–2301.

Friedrich, M. J. (2001). Lowering the risk of second malignancy in survivors of childhood cancer. *Journal of the American Medical Association, 285*, 2435–2437.

Ganjavi, H., & Malkin, D. (2002). Genetics of childhood cancer. *Clinical Orthopaedics and Related Research, 401*, 75–87.

Green, D. M., Whitton, J. A., Stovall, M., Merteus, A. C., Donaldson, S. S., Ruymann, F. B., Pendergrass, T. W., & Robison, L. L. (2002). Pregnancy outcomes of female survivors of childhood cancer: A report from the Childhood Cancer Survivor Study. *American Journal of Obstetrics and Gynecology, 187*, 1070–1080.

Green, D. M., Whitton, J. A., Stovall, M., Merteus, A. C., Donaldson, S. S., Ruymann, F. B., Pendergrass, T. W., & Robison, L. L. (2003). Pregnancy outcome of partners of male survivors of childhood cancer: A report from the Childhood Cancer Survivor Study. *Journal of Clinical Oncology, 21*, 716–721.

Grosfeld, F. J. M., Lips, C. J. M., Beemer, F. A., Blijham, G. H., Quirijnen, J. M. S. P., Mastenbroek, P. L., et al. (2000). Distress in MEN 2 family members and partners prior to DNA test disclosure. *American Journal of Medical Genetics, 91*, 1–7.

Grosfeld, F. J. M., Lips, C. J. M., Ten Kroode, H. F. J., Beemer, F. A., Van Spijker, H. G., & Brouwers-Smalbraak, G. J. (1996). Psychosocial consequences of DNA analysis for MEN type 2. *Oncology, 10*, 141–157.

Hawkins, M. M., Draper, G. J., & Winter, D. L. (1995). Cancer in the offspring of survivors of childhood leukaemia and non-Hodgkin lymphomas. *British Journal of Cancer, 71*, 1335–1339.

Hisada, M., Garber, J. E., Fung, C. Y., Fraumeni, J. F., Jr., & Li, F. P. (1998). Multiple primary cancers in families with Li-Fraumeni syndrome. *Journal of the National Cancer Institute, 90*, 606–611.

Knudson, A. (1975). Mutation and childhood cancer: A probabilistic model for the incidence of retinoblastoma. *Proceedings of the National Academy of Sciences of the United States of America, 72*, 5116–5120.

Kraemer, K. H. (1997). Sunlight and skin cancer: Another link revealed. *Proceedings of the National Academy of Sciences of the United States of America, 94*, 11–14.

Levy, M. J., & Stillman, R. J. (1991). Reproductive potential in survivors of childhood malignancies. *Pediatrician, 18*, 61–70.

Lips, C. J. M. (1998). Clinical management of the multiple endocrine neoplasia syndromes: Results of a computerized opinion poll at the Sixth International Workshop on Multiple Endocrine Neoplasia and von Hippel-Lindau disease. *Journal of Internal Medicine, 24*, 589–594.

Lynch, H. T. (1998) Introduction to *Clinical cancer genetics* by K. Offit. New York: Wiley-Liss.

Lynch, H. T., Katz, D. A., Bogard, P. J., & Lynch, J. F. (1985). The sarcoma, breast cancer, lung cancer, and adrenocortical carcinoma syndrome revisited: Childhood cancer. *American Journal of Diseases of Children, 139*, 134–146.

Maher, E. R., & Kaelin, W. G., Jr. (1997). von Hippel-Lindau disease. *Medicine (Baltimore), 76*, 381–391.

Maher, E. R., Yates, J. R. W., Harries, R., Benjamin, C., Harris, R., Moore, A. T., et al. (1990). Clinical features and natural history of von Hippel-Lindau disease. *Quarterly Journal of Medicine, 77*, 1153–1170.

Malkin, D., Australie, K., Shuman, C., Barrerra, M., & Weksberg, R. (1996). Parental attitudes to genetic counseling and predictive testing for childhood cancer. *American Journal of Human Genetics, 59*, A7.

Michie, S., Bobrow, M., Marteau, T. M., on behalf of the *FAP* Collaborative Research Group. (2001). Predictive genetic testing in children and adults: A study of emotional impact. *Journal of Medical Genetics 38*, 519–526.

Michie, S., & Marteau, T. M. (1995). Response to GIG's response to the U.K. Clinical Genetics Society report, "The Genetic Testing of Children." *Journal of Medical Genetics, 32*, 838.

Michie, S., & Marteau, T. M. (1998). Predictive genetic testing in children: The need for psychological research. In A. Clarke (Ed.), *The genetic testing of children.* Oxford: Bios Scientific Publishers, 169–179.

Michie, S., McDonald, V., Bobrow, M., McKeown, C., & Marteau, T. (1996). Parents' responses to predictive genetic testing in their children: Report of a single case study. *Journal of Medical Genetics, 33,* 313–318.

Mulvihill, J. J., Myers, M. H., Connelly, R. R., Byrne, J., Austin, D. F., Bragg, K., et al. (1987). Cancer in the offspring of long-term survivors of childhood cancer. *International Journal of Cancer, 43,* 975–978.

Neglia, J. P., Friedman, D. L., Yasui, Y., Mertens, A. C., Hammond, S., Stovall, M., et al. (2001). Second malignant neoplasms in 5-year survivors of childhood cancer: Childhood cancer survivor study. *Journal of the National Cancer Institute, 93,* 618–629.

Nichols, K., Li, F. P., Haber, D., & Diller, L. (1998). Childhood cancer predisposition: Application of molecular testing and future implications. *The Journal of Pediatrics, 132,* 389–397.

Nicholson, H. S., & Byrne, J. (1993). Fertility and pregnancy after treatment for cancer during childhood or adolescence. *Cancer, 71,* 3392–3399.

Offit, K. (1998). *Clinical Cancer Genetics: Risk counseling and management.* New York: Wiley and Liss, p. 129.

Olsen, J. H., Garwicz, S., Hertz, H., Jonmundsson, G., Langmark, F., Lanning, M., Lie, S. O., et al. (1993). Second malignant neoplasms after cancer in childhood or adolescence. *British Medical Journal, 307,* 1030–1036.

Patenaude, A. F. (1996). The genetic testing of children for cancer susceptibility: Ethical, legal, and social issues. *Behavioral Sciences and the Law, 14,* 393–410.

Patenaude, A. F., Basili, L., Fairclough, D. L., & Li, F. P. (1996). Attitudes of 47 mothers of pediatric oncology patients towards genetic testing for cancer predisposition. *Journal of Clinical Oncology, 14,* 415–421.

Patenaude, A. F., Schneider, K. A., Kieffer, S. A., Calzone, K. A., Stopfer, J. E., Basili, L. A., et al. (1996). Acceptance of invitations for p53 and BRCA1 predisposition testing: Factors influencing potential utilization of cancer genetic testing. *Psycho-oncology, 5,* 241–250.

*PDQ NIH Cancer Genetics summary.* Retrieved March 8, 2001, from the NIH PDQ Cancer Genetics Web site: http://www.nci.nih.gov/cancer_information/pdq/

Quesnel, S., & Malkin, D. (1997). Genetic predisposition to cancer and familial cancer syndromes. *Pediatric Clinics of North America, 44,* 791–808.

Relling, M. V., Hancock, M. L., Rivera, G. K, Sandlund, J. T., Ribeiro, R. C., Krynetski, E. Y., et al. (1999). Mercaptopurine therapy intolerance and heterozygosity at the thiopurine S-methyltransferase gene locus. *Journal of the National Cancer Institute, 91,* 2001–2008.

Ribeiro, R. C., Sandrini, F., Figueiredo, B., Zambetti, G. P., Michalkiewicz, E., Lafferty, A. R., et al. (2001). An inherited p53 mutation that contributes in a tissue-specific manner to pediatric adrenal cortical carcinoma. *Proceedings of the National Academy of Sciences of the United States of America, 98,* 9330–9335.

Rubnitz, J., & Crist, W. M. (1997). Molecular genetics of childhood cancer: Implications for pathogenesis, diagnosis, and treatment. *Pediatrics, 100,* 101–108.

Sankila, R., Olsen, J. H., Anderson, H., Garwiecz, S., Glattre, E., Hertz, H., et al. (1998). Risk of cancer among the offspring of childhood cancer survivors. *The New England Journal of Medicine, 338,* 1339–1344.

Schneider, K. (2002). *Counseling about cancer: Strategies for genetic counseling* (2nd ed.) New York: Wiley-Liss.

Smith, K. R., West, J. A., Croyle, R. T., & Botkin, J. R. (1999). Familial context of genetic testing for cancer susceptibility: Moderating effect of siblings' test results on psychological distress 1 to 2 weeks after *BRCA1* mutation testing. *Cancer, Epidemiology, Biomarkers, and Prevention, 8,* 385–392.

Tercyak, K. P., Hughes, C., Main, D., Snyder, C., Lynch, J. F., Lynch, H. T. R., et al. (2001). Parental communication of *BRCA1/2* genetic test results to children. *Patient Education and Counseling, 42,* 213–224.

Tercyak, K. P, Peshkin, B. N., Streisand, R., & Lerman, C. (2001). Psychological issues among children of hereditary breast cancer gene (*BRCA1/2*) testing participants. *Psycho-oncology, 10,* 336–346.

Wallace, W. H., & Thomson, A. B. (2003). Preservation of fertility in children treated for cancer. *Archives of Disease in Childhood, 88,* 493–496.

Winther, J. F., Boice, J. D., Jr., Hrafn, T., Bautz, A., Barlow, L., Eystein, G., et al. (2001). Cancer in siblings of children with cancer in the Nordic countries: A population–based cohort study. *Lancet, 358,* 711–717.

Williams, W. C., & Strong, L. C. (1985). Genetic epidemiology of soft tissue sarcomas in children. In H. R. Muller and W. Weber (Eds.), *Familial cancer* (pp. 151–153). Basel, Switzerland: Karger.

Wong, F. L., Boice, J. D., Jr., Abramson, D. H., Tarone, R. E., Kleinerman, R. A., Stovall, M. A., et al. (1997). Cancer incidence after retinoblastoma: Radiation dose and sarcoma risk. *Journal of the American Medical Association, 278,* 1262–1267.

van Heurn, L. W. E., Schaap, C., Sie, G., Haagen, A. A. M., Gerver, W. J., Freling, G., et al. (1999). Predictive DNA testing for multiple endocrine neoplasia 2: A therapeutic challenge of prophylactic thyroidectomy in very young children. *Journal of Pediatric Surgery, 34,* 568–571.

Vida L. Tyc

# Prevention and Cessation of Tobacco Use and Exposure to Environmental Tobacco Smoke

## Introduction

Tobacco use remains the single most important preventable cause of premature death and disability in the United States and is a critical health issue for our nation's youths. Cigarette smoking is the most common form of tobacco use among adolescents (Centers for Disease Control and Prevention, 2001), with over 90% of adult smokers initiating smoking at or before age 19 years (Mowery, Brick, & Farrelly, 2000). Consequently, reduction of tobacco use during adolescence is especially critical before lifelong smoking habits are established. Current national health objectives for children and adolescents focus on reducing health risks related to tobacco use and exposure to secondhand smoke (U.S. Department of Health and Human Services, 2000). Specific objectives include reducing the initiation of tobacco use among children and adolescents, reducing their average age of first use of tobacco products, increasing cessation attempts by current smokers, and reducing the proportion of children who are regularly exposed to tobacco smoke in the home.

These health objectives are especially important for children and adolescents with cancer, who may be at even greater risk than their healthy peers for tobacco-related health problems because of their compromised health status (Hollen & Hobbie, 1996). Exposure to environmental tobacco smoke (ETS) has similar serious consequences for the child with cancer (Alligne & Stoddard, 1997; Cook & Strachan, 1999). Interventions that attempt to prevent, reduce, or terminate tobacco use and ETS exposure could therefore contribute to a decrease in the morbidity and mortality of patients treated for cancer.

This chapter reviews the prevalence of tobacco use, the magnified health effects associated with tobacco use, and some of the correlates associated with tobacco use among young patients treated for cancer. We also describe tobacco interventions that have been conducted with this population and discuss how health care providers involved in the treatment or long-term care of childhood cancer patients can assist their high-risk patients in making healthy lifestyle choices, including the decision to abstain from, reduce, or quit smoking and to avoid environmental tobacco exposures.

## Tobacco-Related Health Risks

Tobacco use is a significant behavioral health problem that poses serious health risks for young patients treated for cancer. There are a number of antineoplastic therapies commonly used in the treatment of pediatric cancer patients that are associated with cardiopulmonary toxicities and organ compromise that can be potentiated by tobacco use. Selected subgroups of patients treated with cardiopulmonary toxic agents or thoracic radiation therapy may be most susceptible to the detrimental long-term consequences of tobacco use. For example, patients treated with carmustine and bleomycin (O'Driscoll et al., 1990) or pulmonary radiation therapy (Benoist, Lemerle, & Jean, 1982) may develop serious respiratory problems and restrictive lung disease if they smoke. Likewise, long-term tobacco use may also increase the risk of congestive heart failure and related cardiac problems in patients treated with anthracyclines (Lipshultz et al., 1991). More acute complications of tobacco use include damage to the patient's protective airway cilia, which can predispose the immunosuppressed patient to respiratory infections because of compromised mucosal defenses. Tobacco use may also aggravate the physical symptoms of young cancer patients, particularly those with respiratory problems and acute radiation mucositis.

Adult studies have shown that cigarette smoking and radiation therapy have a multiplicative effect on the risk of subsequent lung cancer in survivors of Hodgkin's disease (Boivin, 1995). Similarly, increased rate and duration of symptoms (Des Rochers, Dische, & Saunders, 1992), diminished efficacy of radiation therapy (Cinciripini, Gritz, Tsoh, & Skaar, 1998), reduced survival time (Goodman, Kolonel, Wilkens, Yoshizawa, & Le Marchand, 1990), and greater risk of disease recurrence or a second primary tumor (Day et al., 1994) have been reported in head and neck cancer patients who continue to smoke when compared to patients who quit smoking on learning their diagnosis. Pediatric cancer patients are already at risk for developing second cancers because of treatment-induced (Hawkins & Stevens, 1996; Marina, 1997) and genetic predispositions (Malkin et al., 1992), and tobacco use may exacerbate these vulnerabilities. The potential effect of tobacco use on treatment efficacy among pediatric cancer patients deserves further study.

Despite the lack of definitive empirical data on the relationship between ETS exposure and cancer treatment-related morbidity, the pediatric oncology community clearly recognizes the deleterious effects of ETS exposure in young cancer patients (Tyc, Hudson, Hadley, & Throckmorton-Belzer, 2001). As is the case with primary tobacco use, exposure to ETS may exacerbate the physical symptoms of young cancer patients, and long-term exposure to high levels of ETS may increase their risk of treatment-related cardiovascular and pulmonary disease (Environmental Protection Agency, 1992). There is overwhelming evidence of the noxious impact of exposure to tobacco smoke on children's health, including increased incidence of pneumonia and bronchitis; higher rates of respiratory illness, wheezing, middle ear effusions, and otitis media (Environmental Protection Agency, 1992; Etzel, 1994); and development of asthma or exacerbation of existing asthmatic symptoms (Cook & Strachan, 1999). Children whose caregivers smoke have a disproportionate number of these and similar medical conditions, and their incidence increases with higher levels of exposure (DiFranza & Lew, 1996). Therefore, patients who come from smoking households, particularly those with compromised respiratory and pulmonary status (e.g., reactive airway disease/asthma/allergies), are likely to be at elevated risk for treatment-related complications if continually exposed to ETS. In addition to the health risks associated with ETS exposure, children who are exposed to parent smokers are more likely to start smoking themselves (Biglan, Duncan, Ary, & Smolkowski, 1995), thereby increasing their risk for primary tobacco-related health problems in the future.

## Prevalence of Adolescent Smoking

Although the prevalence of cigarette smoking among middle and high school students in the United States has gradually declined since the mid-1990s (Johnston, O'Malley, & Bachman, 2002), a substantial number of youngsters continue to engage in this unhealthy habit. According to the 2000 National Household Survey on Drug Abuse, more than 2,000 youngsters become smokers each day and join nearly 3 million of their peers who smoke (Office of Applied Studies, 2002). Data from the 2000 National Youth Tobacco Survey showed that 28% of high school students and 11% of middle school students were current smokers (Centers for Disease Control and Prevention,

2001). Males, white and Hispanic students, and those in higher grades were most likely to smoke. Nationally, 6.7% and 8.4% of high school and middle school students, respectively, reported that they first smoked a cigarette before the age of 11 years. Once having started, 61.0% of current adolescent smokers desired to quit smoking, and approximately 59% had tried to quit smoking cigarettes during the previous year. However, studies estimated that only 4% of adolescent smokers successfully quit in a given year (Engels, Knibbe, deVries, & Drop, 1998; Zhu, Sun, Billings, Choi, & Malarcher, 1999).

One might expect that youngsters who have been treated for cancer would avoid carcinogens, especially if their health care provider counseled them about tobacco-related health risks during their treatment. The bulk of published studies reported the prevalence of smoking among adolescent cancer survivors and showed that smoking rates among survivors are somewhat lower than those reported for healthy adolescents. Estimates of smoking rates reported in individual studies should, however, be interpreted with caution as they are based on small sample sizes and employed differing definitions of current smoking/tobacco use.

Mulhern et al. (1995) reported that less than 10% of survivors 11–17 years of age used tobacco, although this estimate was based on parents' report of their children's behavior. Other studies based on adolescent self-reports reported that between 5% and 15% of teen survivors aged 10–19 years of age engaged in cigarette smoking (Hollen & Hobbie, 1993; Hollen, Hobbie, & Finley, 1999; Tyc, Hadley, & Crockett, 2001a; Tyc, Rai, et al., 2003). Limited data are available regarding the smoking rates among youngsters undergoing treatment for cancer. In a study conducted at a large pediatric oncology institution, data from 104 children over 10 years of age who were consecutively admitted during a 1-year period indicated that 6.7% of patients were current smokers based on their self-report (Tyc, Throckmorton-Belzer, et al. 2003). However, these results were limited to families who completed an institutional psychosocial history assessment and provided information about tobacco use at the time of admission. No data regarding the number of cessation attempts among current adolescent smokers were available.

Rates of smoking among older patients who have completed and survived their cancer treatment are generally higher than those obtained from younger survivors. Previous American and Canadian studies reported that between 17% and 20% of young adult survivors were current smokers, with higher percentages of survivors having experimented with tobacco in the past (Larcombe, Mott, & Hunt, 2002; Mulhern et al., 1995; Tao et al., 1998). Results from the Childhood Cancer Survivor Study, the largest research cohort of cancer survivors ever assembled in the United States, demonstrated that 17% of 5-year survivors at least 18 years of age were identified as current smokers, with another 10% identified as former smokers (K. Emmons et al., 2002). Older age at diagnosis, lower household income, less education, and not having had pulmonary-related cancer treatment or brain irradiation were associated with a statistically significant relative risk of smoking initiation among survivors. Consistent with national trends, African Americans were significantly less likely to initiate smoking than non-blacks. Although these collective results showed that survivors smoke at rates below the general population, these rates are still alarming in that survivors are exposed to treatments that are known to compromise their cardiac, vascular, and pulmonary functioning. Moreover, the reported smoking cessation rate among cancer survivors was only modestly greater than that in the general population (K. Emmons et al., 2002), demonstrating the persistence of their established smoking habits.

It is possible that the use of tobacco is greater than that reported across studies because of patient reluctance to admit their smoking behaviors to health care providers in a medical setting. Nonetheless, the lower smoking rates in young cancer patients and childhood cancer survivors, relative to their healthy peers, may be attributed to a less-active social life and subsequently less exposure to smoking models because of the restrictions of their disease or treatment-related late effects (Larcombe et al., 2000). The reduction in risk of smoking onset among survivors with more severe treatment-related neurological or neuropsychological deficits secondary to radiation treatment to the brain may be explained by their residence in environments where opportunities to start smoking are restricted (K. Emmons et al., 2002). The experience of pediatric cancer and specifically the age at diagnosis, treatment-related adverse side effects, and the positive impact of supportive care services traditionally offered to young patients as they undergo cancer therapy may also serve to disrupt or delay future tobacco use (Larcombe et al., 2000). Further research is needed to better investigate these hypotheses and examine other factors that may influence adolescent smoking behaviors.

## Prevalence of Adolescent Exposure to Tobacco Smoke

Exposure to ETS has also been examined in pediatric cancer patients, although this is a relatively untapped area of research in this population. The presence of smokers in the home has typically been employed as a gross estimate of youngsters who are at risk for exposure to ETS. Data from the National Health Nutrition Examination Survey III indicated that almost 40% of children younger than 5 years of age in the United States live with a smoker (Gergen, Fowler, Maurer, Davis, & Overpeck, 1998). Approximately 44% of youths aged 12–18 years who were sampled in the 1999 National Youth Tobacco survey lived in a household with at least one smoker, and 6.2 million youths were estimated to be directly exposed to ETS in the home (Farrelly, Chen, Thomas, & Healton, 2001). Parental smoke was a primary source of exposure in these households (Brownson, Eriksen, Davis, & Warner, 1997). Children with cancer spend a significant proportion of their time indoors and are likely to spend more time with their parents because of the restrictions of their disease.

In the only study to date to examine ETS in a sample of 303 pediatric cancer patients (age <20 years) consecutively admitted to a large pediatric oncology institution during a 12-month period, Tyc, Throckmorton-Belzer, et al. (2003) found that approximately 45% of newly diagnosed patients lived in households with at least one current parent smoker. In 10 households, the identified smoker was another family member. Of current nonsmoking parents, 20% reported past tobacco use. These findings are consistent with national surveys that reported comparable percentages of children living in smoking households (Farrelly et al., 2001; Gergen et al., 1998).

In a smaller but related study that asked 47 smoking parents of youngsters treated for cancer about their child's exposure, approximately 72% of parents reported smoking in the presence of their child, and almost 58% of parents smoked inside the home (Tyc, Klosky, Throckmorton-Belzer, Lensing, & Rai, in press). The majority of parents (76.6%) smoked in their cars, and nearly 70% of parents allowed others to smoke in the child's presence. Combined results from these two studies demonstrated that a significant number of pediatric cancer patients are at risk for exposure to ETS during their treatment, and many are directly exposed to their parent's cigarettes on a regular basis. The threshold for adverse health effects associated with continued exposure to ETS is lowered and the risks are magnified in children treated for cancer, particularly if a parent continues to smoke throughout their cancer therapy.

## Behavioral Risk Factors and Psychosocial Correlates of Youth Tobacco Use

Despite the volume of research on the correlates of adolescent tobacco use, factors that influence tobacco use among pediatric cancer patients have received little attention. Whereas actual tobacco use is the ideal outcome measure in adolescent smoking research, smoking behaviors may not be readily apparent for years. Although not a substitute for behavioral measures, self-reported intention to use tobacco has consistently been used as a proximal outcome measure in adolescent smoking studies because prospective studies have demonstrated intentions to be a strong predictor of future smoking behavior (Conrad, Flay, & Hill, 1992; Eckhardt, Woodruff, & Elder, 1994).

A longitudinal study of a nationally representative sample of 4,500 adolescents who had never puffed on a cigarette at baseline found that susceptibility to smoking, defined as the absence of clear intentions not to smoke, was a strong predictor of experimentation with cigarettes 4 years later (Pierce, Choi, Gilpin, Farkas, & Merritt, 1996). Although it is not clear if intentions to smoke can similarly predict later smoking behaviors among young cancer patients, self-reported intentions to smoke have been used as a primary outcome measure in smoking studies conducted with pediatric patients treated for cancer.

In the few studies that have examined future smoking intentions, young cancer patients and survivors have consistently reported low intentions to smoke (Tyc et al., 2001a; Tyc, Rai, et al., 2003; Tyc, Lensing, Klosky, & Rai, 2003). In one study, adolescent patients undergoing treatment for cancer were one third as likely as their healthy peers to report some intention to smoke in the future (Tyc, Lensing, Klosky, & Rai, 2003). Older age, less tobacco-related knowledge, greater perceived value of smoking, and past tobacco use have been found to be predictors of greater intentions to use tobacco among preadolescent and adolescent cancer survivors (Tyc et al., 2001a; Tyc, Lensing, Rai, et al., 2003). These same variables have been found to influence tobacco use among healthy adolescents (Caravajal, Wiatrek, Evans, Knee, & Nash, 2000; Flay, Ockene, & Tager, 1992; Landrine, Richardson, Klonoff, & Flay, 1994; Moss, Allen, & Giovino, 1995; Robinson & Klesges, 1997; Robinson, Klesges, Zbikowski, & Glaser, 1997).

The low intention scores obtained by cancer patients across studies should not be interpreted to suggest that they are not at risk for later tobacco use, but rather that they would be good candidates for preventive tobacco interventions given their lack of a firm decision to abstain from future tobacco use. However, low baseline intention scores and limited variability of the intention measures employed could also limit one's ability to detect intervention effects for programs designed to further reduce intentions to smoke (Tyc et al., 2001a). Therefore, more sensitive measures of intentions need to be developed for this patient group.

Perceived vulnerability (PV) to health risks is a well-recognized component of current cognitive-motivational models of health behavior (Weinstein, 1993) that has been examined in relation to tobacco use among adolescent cancer survivors. Tyc and colleagues (2001a; Tyc, Rai, et al., 2003) reported that preadolescent and adolescent cancer survivors have heightened perceptions of PV to tobacco-related health risks. Compared to their healthy peers, adolescent patients undergoing cancer treatment were also observed to report greater PV to tobacco-related as well as general health risks (Tyc, Lensing, Klosky, et al., 2003). These findings are consistent with the suggestion of earlier work that young cancer patients appear to have a generalized notion that their health is vulnerable because of their cancer treatment experience (Mulhern et al., 1995).

Although an inverse relationship between PV to risks and the practice of some risky behaviors has been noted for healthy adolescents (Gerrard, Gibbons, Benthin, & Hessling, 1996; Gerrard, Gibbons, & Bushman, 1996, Tyas & Pederson, 1998), PV has not been found to be a significant predictor of future intentions to use tobacco (Tyc et al., 2001a; Tyc, Lensing, Rai, et al., 2003) or more global health behavior outcomes (Tyc, Hadley, & Crockett, 2001b) among pediatric cancer survivors. PV, however, has been shown to predict readiness to quit smoking and confidence in one's ability to quit (e.g., self-efficacy) among childhood cancer survivors 18 years of age and older (K. M. Emmons et al., 2003). In one study, young adult cancer survivors who perceived themselves as highly vulnerable to smoking-related illnesses were 1.2 times more likely to report readiness to quit smoking and believed they were more confident in their ability to quit compared to survivors with lower PV (K. M. Emmons et al., 2003).

Perceptions of vulnerability may be necessary, therefore, but not sufficient to motivate avoidance or cessation of tobacco use in this vulnerable patient population. It may be that the PV-behavior link among survivors is moderated by or related to additional variables that have not been examined. Alternatively, it may be that dimensions of perceived risk other than the cognitive representation of likelihood, characteristic of the PV measure typically employed in these studies (e.g., salience of the threat of affective response), are more critical in assessing future tobacco abstinence among adolescent cancer survivors.

A number of other attitudinal and psychosocial factors that have been associated with adolescent smoking include perceived social support (Pederson, Kovall, McGrady, & Tyas, 1998), low self-esteem (Jackson, Bee-Gates, & Henriksen, 1994; Pederson et al., 1998), and a less-optimistic attitude (Caravajal et al., 2000). Caravajal and colleagues found that multiethnic middle school students who were low in self-esteem and higher in social assertiveness appeared to be most at risk for the onset of smoking, whereas those low in optimism appeared to be most at risk for escalation of smoking.

Some of these same factors may increase the likelihood of tobacco use among adolescent cancer survivors. Hollen and Hobbie (1993, 1996) reported that nonresilient teen survivors (those with a less-even temperament, lower self-esteem, lower social support, and lower resistance to social pressure) with poor quality decision-making skills were more likely to engage in substance use, including cigarette smoking. The authors concluded that interventions aimed at enhancing survivors' decision-making skills as a means of reducing risk behaviors may provide a promising approach for adolescent cancer survivors.

Additional factors that have not been adequately studied in the context of tobacco use among young cancer patients but have been found to contribute to tobacco use among healthy adolescents include depression and anxiety (Koval, Pederson, Mills, McGrady, & Caravajal, 2000); social influences, including peer's, best friend's, and parents; smoking status (Biglan et al., 1995; Johnson et al., 2002; Wang, Fitzhugh, Westerfield & Eddy, 1995); and other sociodemographic variables (Robinson et al., 1997). A long-term prospective study of personality factors found that rebelliousness and risk taking measured among healthy fifth graders were the most significant predictors of daily smoking 7 years later (Burt, Dinh, Peterson, & Sarason, 2000). Many of these same variables that influence smoking onset and its progression have been important in adolescents' attempts to quit smoking (Sussman, 2002; Zhu et al., 1999). Whether these factors similarly affect the cancer patient's decision to initiate and continue to use tobacco certainly warrants further study.

In the only study to date to examine factors associated with smoking behaviors and mediators of cessation among cancer survivors who smoke, it was reported that older and less-educated survivors and those with a higher percentage of smokers in their social networks smoked more often (K. M. Emmons et al., 2003). The sample was composed of 796 childhood cancer survivors who were diagnosed with cancer before the age of 21 years, had survived at least 5 years, and were at least 18 years of age. Approximately 53% of smoking survivors were nicotine dependent, and 82% expressed an interest in quitting. Despite greater motivation to quit smoking among childhood cancer survivors compared to the general population, survivors were not highly confident in their ability to quit. More than half of the survivors reported making at least one unsuccessful quit attempt in the past year. Male survivors, those who were diagnosed with cancer at an older age, those who believed that their cancer history put them at increased risk for smoking-related illness, and those who received more encouragement from family and friends to quit were more confident in their ability to quit and more ready to change their smoking behaviors. Overall, results suggested that childhood cancer survivors may be highly receptive to smoking cessation interventions. Smoking programs that target psychosocial factors, such as perceptions of disease risk and social support, may be most effective.

## Factors Associated With Environmental Tobacco Smoke Exposure

To our knowledge, only one published study to date has investigated patient demographic, medical, and smoking status variables that are associated with ETS exposure among pediatric cancer patients. This study involved children aged 10–18 years who were undergoing cancer treatment or who had completed treatment (Tyc et al., in press). Although the sample size was small and the study was largely exploratory, older children and Caucasian children were reported to be at greater risk for ETS exposure based on cumulative ETS exposure scores that accounted for exposures from various sources and different settings. The racial differences in ETS exposure were not surprising in light of previous research that found that observed parental smoking is less common for African American children than European children (Robinson & Klesges, 1997) in addition to increased household smoking restrictions noted among African American families (Koepke, Flay, & Johnson, 1990). Similar cumulative ETS scores were obtained for children currently undergoing treatment and those who completed treatment such that treatment status did not affect the child's risk of exposure.

Interestingly, children who had smoked in the past or who were current smokers had higher ETS exposure scores than children who had never used tobacco. These results are consistent with previously reported national findings for high school students (Farrelly et al., 2001). Although the direction of the relationship between ETS exposure and the child's smoking status could not be determined in this study, it is likely that increased exposure to tobacco smoke was associated with greater opportunity to be exposed to smoking models. However, it should be noted that ETS estimates were based on parental report and provided only a gross estimate of ETS exposure, which was likely underestimated because of parents' limited sensitivity in observing and estimating exposure as well as the potential demand characteristics associated with reporting exposure. In addition, the data were not weighted for exposure time spent in various locations.

## Smoking Interventions

### Adult Studies

A limited number of studies have evaluated the efficacy of smoking treatment approaches with adult cancer patient populations, including those with lung, breast, prostate, cervical, or head and neck cancer (Cox et al., 2002; Pinto, Eakin, & Maruyama, 2000). Short-term (e.g., 4–6 weeks postintervention) smoking abstinence rates have been found to range from 21% to 75% in these studies (Griebel, Wewers, & Baker, 1998; Stanislaw & Wewers, 1994; Wewers, Bowen, Stanislaw, & Desimone, 1994). In a study examining long-term tobacco abstinence rates, Schnoll and colleagues (2003) found no significant difference in quit rates at a 6- or 12-month follow-up between adult cancer patients randomly assigned to receive either usual care or a National Institutes of Health physician-based smoking intervention. Patients were more likely to quit smoking at 12 months if they smoked 15 or fewer cigarettes per day, had head and neck or lung cancer, tried a group cessation program, and showed greater baseline desire to quit. These findings were consistent with an earlier study that also reported no significant difference in the quit rates between patients provided with a physician-based cessation treatment and those randomly assigned to a control comparison group (Gritz et al., 1993). Although training physicians to provide smoking cessation treatment to cancer patients failed to yield significant gains in long-term patient quit rates, physician adherence to the National Institutes of Health clinical practice guidelines was enhanced among physicians of patients in the intervention group. These findings suggest that higher intensity interventions (e.g., physician-based intervention plus adjunctive behavioral and pharmacological treatment) may be necessary for patients who continue to smoke despite a diagnosis of cancer.

In a study focused exclusively on lung cancer patients, Cox et al. (2002) found that lung cancer patients who were treated clinically for nicotine dependence were significantly more likely to achieve 6-month tobacco abstinence compared with controls matched for date of treatment. After receiving an intervention that consisted of consultation with a trained nicotine dependence counselor and an individualized treatment plan incorporating behavioral, pharmacological, and relapse prevention approaches, the 7-day point prevalence tobacco abstinence rate at 6 months was 22% for lung cancer patients and 14% for controls. No significant difference was detected between lung cancer patients and controls on tobacco abstinence rates after adjusting for chronological age, gender, baseline cigarettes smoked per day, and stage of readiness to quit. The findings provided some support for early intervention close in time to the initial diagnosis. Patients whose diagnosis of lung cancer occurred within 3 months of the intervention were more likely to be abstinent from tobacco at 6-month follow-up compared with lung cancer patients who received their diagnosis at an earlier time point.

Although the components implemented in these collective adult studies may be adapted for use and influence the development of smoking cessation interventions for pediatric oncology patients, there are a number of limitations that should be considered. First, the studies have been conducted with relatively small sample sizes with limited ethnic diversity. They also have limited generalizability to the cancer population at large because of referral biases, rely on self-reported tobacco use without biochemical verification of smoking status, and are unable to employ "true" control groups that receive no active treatment that can undermine the study's internal validity. Further, outcome measures have typically employed 7-day point prevalence abstinence rates with no data on interval tobacco use status to determine continuous abstinence rates. As observed in the general population of smokers, interventions for cancer patients may need to be tailored to the person's level of readiness to quit and incorporate a social support component including the treatment team as well as family members to enhance treatment outcomes (Gritz et al., 1993; Schnoll et al., 2003).

## Adolescent Studies

To date, few empirical studies on smoking interventions for adolescents with cancer have been published, and even fewer have employed randomized, experimental designs. Unlike the adult studies that have focused on cessation, much of the effort to reduce tobacco use in this population has focused primarily on preventing the initiation of tobacco use, particularly among survivors. Working from the perspective that quality decision-making skills are critical for teens confronting risk behaviors such as smoking, Hollen and associates (1999) tested the effects of a tailored decision-making program aimed at reducing risk behaviors among a convenience sample of adolescents, aged 13–21 years, who survived cancer. This 1-day, 5-hour camp intervention, which focused on alcohol and illicit drug use in addition to tobacco use, was evaluated using a quasi-experimental pretest/posttest design with repeated measures. At 12 months postintervention, the effect of the intervention for improving decision making was statistically significant, although risk motivation for smoking and self-reported smoking behavior were not affected. Despite the modest intervention effects, a clinician-delivered approach that teaches adolescents treated for cancer to weigh the consequences of tobacco use within the context of their individual treatment histories and provides essential health content related to survivorship offers promise for adolescents making tobacco-related choices.

In the first prospective randomized health promotion trial conducted with 272 adolescent cancer survivors attending a long-term follow-up clinic, Hudson et al. (2002) evaluated the efficacy of a late effects counseling and behavioral intervention on survivors' health knowledge, health perceptions, and practice of health behaviors. In this study, adolescents were randomly assigned to receive either standard care or standard care plus a late effects counseling/behavioral intervention at their annual medical visit. Standard care consisted of breast or testicular examination taught by a nurse using a breast/testicular model, late effects screening based on clinical history and treatment exposures, a thorough clinical assessment by a clinician, and late effects counseling. The intervention group received the standard care plus discussion of a written treatment and late effects summary, health behavior training in one of five health goals selected by the survivor, commitment to practicing the selected health behavior, and telephone follow-up to reinforce the behavioral training. In addition to smoking cessation, targeted health behaviors included sun protection, dietary fat and weight reduction, and regular exercise.

The intervention was based on the health belief model, which relates an increased likelihood of behavioral change to greater perceptions of vulnerability to health risks. This approach failed to produce significant changes in knowledge, perceptions, and health behaviors, including tobacco use, at the 12-month follow-up visit. However, a major limitation of the study was that health goals were selected by survivors rather than assigned by the clinician using standardized objective risk criteria. Although this allowed adolescents to have a sense of control regarding their health goal activities, they may have selected the health goal about which they were most knowledgeable or one to which they could easily commit and that required less effort to practice rather than selecting the behavior that was most relevant to reducing their specific health risks. According to the investigators, differences in the survivors' subjective biases and perceived salience of their selected health goals may have masked important intervention effects.

Working from the same conceptual model employed in the Hudson et al. (2002) study but focusing only on tobacco use, Tyc, Rai, et al. (2003) demonstrated the efficacy of a brief tobacco risk counseling intervention for cancer survivors aged 10–18 years. Compared to survivors who received standard advice about tobacco-related health risks, survivors who were randomly assigned to receive late effects counseling in addition to an educational video, goal setting, written physician feedback, smoking literature, and follow-up telephone counseling obtained higher tobacco knowledge scores and reported greater PV to tobacco-related diseases as well as lower intentions to smoke at 12 months postintervention. Self-reported intention to use tobacco has consistently been used as a proximal outcome measure in adolescent smoking research and has been demonstrated to be a strong predictor of future smoking behavior (Conrad et al., 1992; Eckhardt et al., 1994).

Similar to the program developed by Hudson and colleagues (2002), this intervention was conducted by health care professionals in a single session within the patient's routine medical visits with periodic telephone follow-up. However, these findings suggest that a greater intensity of intervention-based contact (e.g., higher intervention dosage) and booster sessions may be necessary to promote more lasting effects on knowledge, health perceptions, and future tobacco practices. As with the above-mentioned studies conducted with adolescent survivors of cancer, this study was limited by reliance on self-report of smoking behaviors, a small sample size with few minority participants, and the use of nonstandardized, user-developed instruments with limited psychometric data that may have contributed to measurement problems and restricted variability on some of the outcomes assessed.

## Environmental Tobacco Smoke Studies

To date, there are no published studies of clinician-delivered interventions to reduce the young cancer patient's exposure to ETS. We are currently examining the efficacy of a clinician-delivered intervention to reduce ETS exposure among children with cancer, as measured by parent report and urinary cotinine (a metabolite of nicotine) levels. This randomized trial will involve an ETS experimental group and a standard care control group who are followed longitudinally and measured over 12 months. The proposed six-session intervention is a parent-based risk counseling program that is built on components of the health belief model (Weinstein, 1993) and social learning theory (Bandura, 1977) and incorporates behavioral shaping methods that have been effective with parents of children with asthma (Meltzer, Hovell, Meltzer, Atkins, & dePeyster, 1993). This approach will be tailored to meet the demands of the parents of a child with cancer within the context of the child's ongoing treatment. We also plan to evaluate the impact of the ETS intervention on acute toxicities and relevant health outcomes in pediatric cancer patients.

## Implications for Clinician-Delivered Smoking Interventions

It is crucial that health care providers involved in the diagnosis, treatment, or long-term care of childhood cancer patients take a primary role in counseling patients about the dangers of tobacco use and encourage tobacco abstinence as a lifestyle choice. In addition to clinicians providing care during cancer therapy, pediatricians, internists, family practice physicians, and others who manage the long-term care of patients as they age should also assume responsibility for tobacco counseling. It is well documented that even brief physician-delivered counseling has a beneficial impact on the smoking behaviors of adults (Fiore, Bailey, & Cohen, 1996). However, health care providers do not routinely engage in tobacco control screening and counseling (Frankowski, Weaver, & Secker-Walker, 1993; Gregario, 1994) because of time constraints, lack of compensation by third-party payers for smoking cessation counseling, and limited training in how to deliver antitobacco messages.

At a minimum, practice guidelines (Epps & Manley, 1993; Glynn & Manley, 1993) suggest that health care providers should routinely incorporate the following activities into the patient's routine medical care: (a) anticipate tobacco use and risk factors for tobacco use; (b) ask all patients about their smoking status; (c) advise about tobacco-related health risks and encourage smokers to stop and nonsmokers to continue to abstain from tobacco use; (d) assist patients who are ready to quit by providing self-help smoking cessation materials and suggesting a quit date; and (e) arrange for routine follow-up support. The nature of these activities will vary according to the child's age, developmental status, and smoking habits of family members (Epps & Manley, 1993; Glynn & Manley, 1993). These same steps should be taken to counsel caregivers who smoke in their child's presence. For youngsters treated for cancer and their families, health care professionals can deliver powerful messages regarding the health risks of tobacco use and exposure to tobacco smoke because of their credibility, medical expertise, and often long-term relationship and regular contact with patients.

Application of the available research findings to the development of smoking prevention interventions for young cancer patients would require emphasis on the specific factors that have been demonstrated to influence their intentions to use tobacco to be maximally effective. Health care providers who counsel young patients should thoroughly assess their past as well as current tobacco habits and discuss the patient's perceptions of the personal benefits and value associated with tobacco use. Providing information about tobacco-related health risks, addressing factors that prompted early experimentation with tobacco, and modifying misperceptions of the positive value associated with tobacco use may be especially beneficial to the cancer patients who express intentions to use tobacco in the future. Assisting the adolescent in identifying alternative strategies to achieve similar benefits thought to be associated with tobacco use should also be emphasized. For example, if the patient perceives tobacco use as important to stress reduction, more appropriate stress management strategies should be encouraged. Likewise, for patients who perceive tobacco as socially enhancing, teaching alternative health-enhancing strategies to elicit positive social responses should be considered.

Additional factors should be considered when delivering smoking interventions to young cancer patients to enhance the impact of more traditional approaches borrowed from adolescent school-based programs (see Table 21-1). Although the behavioral goals of smoking prevention and cessation interventions are similarly applicable to both the healthy adolescent and the young patient treated for cancer, revisions to the content and the manner in which the intervention is delivered may be necessary. Reliance on the supportive and motivational aspects of the treatment setting may also be important in promoting behavioral change in the young cancer patient. Promoting accurate perceptions of disease risk related to smoking should be a priority intervention objective. Previous research has demonstrated that, although survivors may be aware of the general health risks associated with smoking, they may not be sufficiently aware of how these risks are impacted by prior treatment-related exposures (Emmons et al., 2002). Therefore, personalized risk information that is framed in the context of the patient's specific treatment history, current clinical condition, organs most vulnerable to treatment effects, and other psychosocial risk factors should be conveyed to patients to increase their understanding of why they are at particular risk for certain health problems (Tyc, Hudson, Hinds, Elliott, & Kibby, 1997). For example, patients with Hodgkin's disease who receive high-dose mantle radiation therapy and whose family members smoke may be at greater risk than the patient diagnosed with

**Table 21-1.** Steps for Health Care Provider–Delivered Smoking Prevention and Cessation Interventions With Pediatric Cancer Patients

| *Basic Steps* |
|---|
| Ask about past and current tobacco use at each medical visit |
| Advise about health risks associated with tobacco use |
| Emphasize short-term negative social consequences of smoking |
| Encourage abstinence/cessation |
| Establish signed agreement for abstinence/cessation |
| Discuss resistance/refusal skills or provide self-help literature, discuss behavioral smoking cessation strategies, and establish quit dates |
| Arrange follow-up telephone contact or return visit |
| *Additional Steps* |
| Inform of acute complications of tobacco use during therapy |
| Inform of chronic complications of tobacco use after therapy |
| Explain increased risk of adverse health effects relative to healthy peers |
| Provide personalized risk information relative to treatment history |
| Address accuracy of perceived health risks |
| Discuss smoking behaviors of family members and social networks or social support for quitting |

leukemia and treated with chemotherapy alone (see Table 21-1).

Unlike traditional approaches, interventions that capitalize on the young cancer patient's concerns about health protection and their heightened perceptions of vulnerability (Tyc, Rai, et al., 2003) may be highly effective. Likewise, ETS interventions that capitalize on caregivers' perceptions of their child's health vulnerability secondary to their cancer experience may motivate caregivers to stop smoking around their child. Emphasizing the cancer patients' risk for tobacco-related health problems as greater than their healthy peers who have never been treated for cancer may be especially significant in motivating patients to take action in responsibly protecting their health. However, it is important to first frame the smoking behavior as a risk for any adolescent and then explain the additional risks of the synergistic effects of smoking and cytotoxic therapies for the young cancer patient. This offers a more "normalizing" approach (Hollen & Hobbie, 1996) that recognizes the patients' needs to identify with their peers and does not produce unnecessary anxiety and hypervigilance. Although provision of risk behavior information may not by itself be sufficient in preventing smoking onset or impacting smoking cessation, it is critical to provide this risk information as a component of an effective counseling intervention.

Results from studies with young adult survivors suggest that those who are less educated and have lower incomes are a group at greater risk for future smoking onset and should be targeted for intervention (Emmons et al. 2002). Among smoking survivors, cessation interventions that capitalize on the survivors' increased motivation to quit smoking and focus on increasing self-efficacy and skill building are encouraged (Emmons et al., 2003). Addressing the high rate of smoking in the survivors' social network and obtaining support from survivors' family and friends during the quitting process are also important (Emmons et al., 2003). Many of these same factors may also be significant but have never been explored in adolescents with cancer who want to stop smoking. Given the high rate of nicotine dependence and unsuccessful quit attempts reported by young adult survivors, pharmacotherapies should be considered for this population. Bupropion and nicotine replacement therapy have been previously shown to increase quit rates in adults (Jorenby, 2001).

## Conclusion and Future Directions

Understanding why pediatric patients with cancer smoke and identifying effective ways to prevent smoking onset and to stop patients from smoking or exposing themselves to dangerous levels of ETS is a daunting and challenging task for health care professionals. As this chapter suggests, the areas of smoking prevention and cessation as well as ETS reduction among pediatric cancer patients are relatively unexplored. Longitudinal prevention and cessation trials are necessary to investigate strategies that effectively deter smoking in this vulnerable population as well as resolve several outstanding research questions.

First, the optimal timing for implementing tobacco risk education for pediatric cancer patients has not been adequately studied. Patients may be more sensitized to their health at diagnosis or during treatment and therefore more receptive to health risk counseling at that time. Alternatively, the physician and emotional stressors associated with diagnosis and eradication of their disease may prevent the patient from focusing on less acute health concerns. Tobacco-based health education may have greater impact after patients have completed their therapy when remission is assured and their medical care is focused on surveillance of treatment-related health problems. Clarification of these issues in future studies is necessary to determine when cancer patients are most receptive to tobacco counseling.

In addition, development of smoking programs tailored to preadolescent cancer patients should be a priority in order to direct prevention efforts before the prime age of smoking initiation, usually 12–14 years (Swan, Creeser, & Murray, 2000). Additional research addressing method of presentation of risk information (e.g., health care provider vs. peer, group vs. individual, computer vs. provider delivered) is warranted to identify the most effective mechanism for delivery of the antismoking message. K. M. Emmons and colleagues (2003) are beginning to address these issues in a study currently conducted with young adult cancer survivors that will test the effectiveness of a peer-based counseling approach to smoking cessation. Their approach is guided by several health behavior theories and attempts to match the content and message of behavior change to the participants' level of readiness to quit smoking.

Last, development of smoking prevention and cessation programs that involve parent participation and are directed at families of cancer patients are critical. Parental attention to their own smoking habits, particularly in the presence of their child, as well as their ability to effectively communicate their disapproval of their child's smoking habits and enforce smoking restrictions in the home should be issues that are addressed in future research. Likewise, interventions that address the effects of direct tobacco use and exposure to secondary tobacco smoke simultaneously will provide a comprehensive approach to tobacco control in this population.

## References


Alligne, C. W., & Stoddard, J. J. (1997). Tobacco and children: an economic evaluation of the medical effects of parental smoking. *Archives of Pediatric and Adolescent Medicine, 151*, 648–653.

Bandura, A. (1977). *Social learning theory*. Englewood Cliffs, NJ: Prentice-Hall.

Benoist, M. R., Lemerle, J., & Jean, R. (1982). Effects on pulmonary function of whole lung irradiation for Wilm's tumor in children. *Thorax, 37*, 175–180.

Biglan, A., Duncan, T. E., Ary, D. V., & Smolkowski, K. (1995). Peer and parental influences on adolescent tobacco use. *Journal of Behavioral Medicine, 18*, 315–330.

Boivin, J. (1995). Smoking, treatment for Hodgkin's disease, and subsequent lung cancer risk. *Journal of the National Cancer Institute, 87*, 1502–1503.

Brownson, R. C., Eriksen, R. M., Davis, R. M., & Warner, K. E. (1997). Environmental tobacco smoke: Health effects and policies to reduce exposure. *Annual Review of Public Health, 18*, 163–185.

Burt, R. D., Dinh, K. T., Peterson, A. V., & Sarason, I. (2000). Predicting adolescent smoking: A prospective study of personality variables. *Preventive Medicine, 30*, 115–125.

Caravajal, S. C., Wiatrek, D. E., Evans, R. I., Knee, C. R., & Nash, S. G. (2000). Psychosocial determinants of the onset and escalation of smoking: Cross-sectional and prospective findings in multiethnic middle school samples. *Journal of Adolescent Health, 27*, 255–265.

Centers for Disease Control and Prevention. (2001). CDC Surveillance Summaries, November 2, 2001. *Morbidity and Mortality Weekly Report*, 50(No. SS-4).

Cinciripini, P. M., Gritz, E. R., Tsoh, J. Y., & Skaar, K. L. (1998). Smoking cessation and cancer prevention. In J. C. Holland (Ed.), *Psycho-oncology* (pp. 27–44). New York: Oxford University Press.

Conrad, K. M., Flay, B. R., & Hill, D. (1992). Why children start smoking cigarettes: Predictors of onset. *British Journal of Addiction, 87*, 1711–1724.

Cook, D. G., & Strachan, D. P. (1999). Health effects of passive smoking: Summary of effects of parental smoking on the respiratory health of children and implications for research. *Thorax, 54*, 357–366.

Cox, L. S., Patten, C. A., Ebbert, J. O., Drews, A. A., Croghan, G. A., Clark, M. M., et al. (2002). Tobacco use outcomes among patients with lung cancer treated for nicotine dependence. *Journal of Clinical Oncology, 20*, 3461–3469.

Day, G. L., Blot, W. J., Shore, R. E., McLaughlin, J. K., Austin, D. F., Greenberg, R. S., et al. (1994). Second cancers following oral and pharyngeal cancers: role of tobacco and alcohol. *Journal of the National Cancer Institute, 86*, 131–137.

Des Rochers, C., Dische, S., & Sanders, M.I. (1992). The problem of cigarette smoking in radiotherapy for cancer in the head and neck. *Clinical Oncology, 4*, 214–216.

DiFranza, J. R., & Lew, R. A. (1996). Morbidity and mortality in children associated with the use of tobacco products by other people. *Pediatrics, 97*, 560–568.

Eckhardt, L., Woodruff, S. I., & Elder, J. P. (1994). A longitudinal analysis of adolescent smoking and its correlates. *Journal of School Health, 64*, 767–772.

Emmons, K., Li, F., Whitton, J., Mertens, A. C., Hutchinson, R., Diller, L., et al. (2002). Predictors of smoking initiation and cessation among childhood cancer survivors: a report from the Childhood Cancer Survivor Study. *Journal of Clinical Oncology, 20*, 1608–1616.

Emmons, K. M., Butterfield, R. M., Puleo, E., Park, E. R., Mertens, A., Gritz, E. R., et al. (2003). Smoking among participants in the childhood cancer survivors cohort: The Partnership for Health Study. *Journal of Clinical Oncology, 21*, 189–196.

Engels, R., Knibbe, H., deVries, H., & Drop, M. J. (1998). Antecedents of smoking cessation among adolescents: Who is motivated to change? *Preventive Medicine, 27*, 348–357.

Environmental Protection Agency, Office of Research and Development, Office of Air and Radiation.

(1992). *Respiratory health effects of passive smoking: Lung cancer and other disorders* (Publication EPA/600/6-90/006F). Washington, DC: Environmental Protection Agency.

Epps, R. P., & Manley, M. W. (1993). Prevention of tobacco use during childhood and adolescence. *Cancer, 72*, 1002–1004.

Etzel, R. A. (1994). Environmental tobacco smoke. *Immunology and Allergy Clinics of North America, 14*, 621–633.

Farrelly, M. C., Chen, J., Thomas, K. Y., & Healton, C. G. (2001). Youth exposure to environmental tobacco smoke. *American Legacy Foundation First Look Report, 6*, 6–24.

Fiore, M. C., Bailey, W. C., & Cohen, S. F. (1996). *Smoking cessation: Clinical practice guideline No. 18*. Washington, DC: Department of Health and Human Services, Public Health Service, Agency for Health Care Policy and Research, and Centers for Disease Control.

Flay, B. R., Ockene, J., & Tager, I. B. (1992). Smoking: epidemiology, cessation, and prevention. *Chest, 102*, 2775–3015.

Frankowski, B. L., Weaver, S. O., & Secker-Walker, R. H. (1993). Advising parents to stop smoking: Pediatricians' and parents' attitudes. *Pediatrics, 91*, 296–300.

Gergen, P. J., Fowler, J. A., Maurer, K. R., Davis, W. W., & Overpeck, M. D. (1998). The burden of environmental smoke exposure on the respiratory health of children 2 months of age through 5 years of age in the United States: Third National Health and Nutrition Examination Survey, 1988 to 1994. *Pediatrics, 101*. Retrieved September 15, 2003 from http://www.pediatrics.org/cgi/content/full/101/2/e8

Gerrard, M., Gibbons, F. X., Benthin, A. C., & Hessling, R. M. (1996). A longitudinal study of the reciprocal nature of risk behaviors and cognitions in adolescents: What you do shapes what you think and vice versa. *Health Psychology, 15*, 344–354.

Gerrard, M., Gibbons, F. X., & Bushman, B. J. (1996). Relation between perceived vulnerability to HIV and precautionary sexual behavior. *Psychological Bulletin, 119*, 390–409.

Glynn, T. J., & Manley, M. W. (1993). *How to help your patients stop smoking: A National Cancer Institute manual for physicians* (DHHS Publication No. 93-3064). Bethesda, MD: Smoking and Tobacco Program, Division of Cancer Prevention and Control, National Institutes of Health, pp. 1–77.

Goodman, M. T., Kolonel, L. N., Wilkens, L. R., Yoshizawa, C. N., & Le Marchand, L. (1990). Smoking history and survival among lung cancer patients. *Cancer Causes Control, 1*, 155–163.

Gregario, D. I. (1994). Counseling adolescents for smoking prevention: A survey of primary care physicians and dentists. *American Journal of Public Health, 84*, 1151–1153.

Griebel, B., Wewers, M. E., & Baker, C. A. (1998). The effectiveness of a nurse-managed minimal smoking cessation intervention among hospitalized patients with cancer. *Oncology Nursing Forum, 25*, 897–902.

Gritz, E. R., Carr, C. R., Rapkin, D., Abemayor, E., Chang, L. J., Wong, W. K., et al. (1993). Predictors of long-term smoking cessation in head and neck cancer patients. *Cancer Epidemiology Biomarkers and Prevention, 2*, 261–270.

Hawkins, M. M., & Stevens, M. C. G. (1996). The long term survivors. *British Medical Bulletin, 52*, 898–923.

Hollen, P. J., & Hobbie, W. L. (1993). Risk taking and decision making of adolescent long-term survivors of cancer. *Oncology Nursing Forum, 20*, 769–776.

Hollen, P. J., & Hobbie, W. L. (1996). Decision-making and risk behaviors of cancer-surviving adolescents and their peers. *Journal of Pediatric Oncology Nursing, 13*, 121–134.

Hollen, P. J., Hobbie, W. L., & Finley, S. M. (1999). Testing the effects of a decision-making and risk-reduction program for cancer-surviving adolescents. *Oncology Nursing Forum, 26*, 1475–1486.

Hudson, M. M., Tyc, V. L., Srivastava, D. K., Gattuso, J., Quargnenti, A., Crom, D. B., et al. (2002). Multi-component behavioral interventions to promote health protective behaviors in childhood cancer survivors: The Protect Study. *Medical and Pediatric Oncology, 39*, 2–11.

Jackson, C., Bee-Gates, D. J., & Henriksen, L. (1994). Authoritative parenting, child competencies, and initiation of cigarette smoking. *Health Education Quarterly, 21*, 103–116.

Johnson, C. C., Li, D., Perry, C. L., Elder, J. P., Feldman, H. A., Kelder, S. H., et al. (2002). Fifth through eighth grade longitudinal predictors of tobacco use among a racially diverse cohort: CATCH. *Journal of School Health, 72*, 58–64.

Johnston, L. D., O'Malley, P. M., & Bachman, J. G. (2002). *Monitoring the future national survey results on drug use, 1975–2001. Vol. 1: Secondary school students* (NIH Publication No. 02-5106). Bethesda, MD: National Institute on Drug Abuse.

Jorenby, D. E. (2001). Smoking cessation strategies for the 21st century. *Circulation, 104*, e51–e52.

Koepke, D., Flay, B. R. & Johnson, C. A. (1990). Health behaviors in minority families: The case of cigarette smoking. *Family and Community Health, 13*, 34–43.

Koval, J. J., Pederson, L. L., Mills, C. A., McGrady, G. A., & Caravajal, S. C. (2000). Models of the relationship of stress, depression, and other psychosocial factors to smoking behavior: A comparison of a cohort of students in Grades 6 and 8. *Preventive Medicine, 30*, 463–477.

Landrine, H., Richardson, J. L., Klonoff, E. A., & Flay, B. (1994). Cultural diversity in the predictors of adolescent cigarette smoking: The relative influence of peers. *Journal of Behavioral Medicine, 17*, 331–336.

Larcombe, I., Mott, M., & Hunt, L. (2002). Lifestyle behaviors of young adult survivors of childhood cancer. *British Journal of Cancer, 87*, 1204–1209.

Lipshultz, S. E., Colan, S. D., Gelbar, R. D., Perez-Atayde, A. R., Sallan, S. E., & Sanders, S. P. (1991). Late cardiac effects of doxorubicin therapy for acute lymphoblastic leukemia in childhood. *New England Journal of Medicine, 324*, 808–815.

Malkin, D., Jolly, K. W., Barbier, N., Look, A. T., Friend, S. H., Gebhart, N. C., et al. (1992). Germline mutations of the p53 tumor-suppressor gene in children and young adults with second malignant neoplasms. *New England Journal of Medicine, 326*, 1309–1315.

Marina, N. (1997). Long-term survivors of childhood cancer. *Pediatric Clinics of North America, 44*, 1021–1042.

Meltzer, S. B., Hovell, M. F., Meltzer, E. O., Atkins, C. J., & de Peyster, A. (1993). Reduction of secondary smoke exposure to asthmatic children: Parent counseling. *Journal of Asthma, 30*, 391–400.

Moss, A. J., Allen, K. F., & Giovino, C. A. (1995). *Recurrent trends in adolescent smoking, smoking uptake correlates, and expectations about the future: advance data.* Hyattsville, MD: U.S. Department of Health and Human Services, Public Health Service, Centers for Disease Control and Prevention, National Center for Health Statistics.

Mowery, P. D., Brick, P. D., & Farrelly, M. C. (2000). *Legacy first look report 3. Pathways to established smoking: Results from the 1999 National Youth Tobacco Survey.* Washington, DC: American Legacy Foundation.

Mulhern, R. K., Tyc, V. L., Phipps, S., Crom, D., Barclay, D., Greenwald, C., et al. (1995). Health-related behaviors of survivors of childhood cancer. *Medical and Pediatric Oncology, 25*, 159–165.

O'Driscoll, B. R., Hasleton, P. S., Taylor, P. M., Poulter, L. W., Gattamaneni, H. R., & Woodcock, A. H. (1990). Active lung fibrosis up to 17 years after chemotherapy with carmustine (BCNU) in childhood. *New England Journal of Medicine, 323*, 378–382.

Office of Applied Studies. (2002). *Results from the 2001 National Household Survey on Drug Abuse: Vol. 3. Detailed tables.* Rockville, MD: Substance Abuse and mental Health Services Administration.

Pederson, L. L., Kovall, J. J., McGrady, G. A., & Tyas, S. L. (1998). The degree and type of relationship between psychosocial variables and smoking status for students in Grade 8: Is there a dose-response relationship? *Preventive Medicine, 27*, 337–347.

Pierce, J. P., Choi, W. S., Gilpin, E. A., Farkas, A. J., & Merritt, R. K. (1996). Validation of susceptibility as a predictor of which adolescents take up smoking in the United States. *Health Psychology, 15*, 355–361.

Pinto, B. M., Eakin, E., & Maruyama, N. C. (2000). Health behavior changes after a cancer diagnosis: What do we know and where do we go from here? *Annals of Behavior Medicine, 22*, 38–52.

Robinson, L. A., & Klesges, R. C. (1997). Ethnic and gender differences in risk factors for smoking onset. *Health Psychology, 16*, 499–505.

Robinson, L. A., Klesges, R. C., Zbikowski, S. M., & Glaser, R. (1997). Predictors of adolescent smoking in a biracial sample. *Journal of Consulting and Clinical Psychology, 65*, 653–662.

Schnoll, R. A., Zhang, B., Rue, M., Krook, J. E., Spears, W. T., Marcus, A. C., et al. (2003). Brief physician-initiated quit smoking strategies for clinical oncology settings: a trial coordinated by the Eastern Cooperative Oncology Group. *Journal of Clinical Oncology, 21*, 355–365.

Stanislaw, A. E., & Wewers, M. E. (1994). A smoking cessation intervention with hospitalized surgical cancer patients: A pilot study. *Cancer Nursing, 17*, 81–86.

Sussman, S. (2002). Effects of 66 adolescent tobacco use cessation trials and 17 prospective studies of self-initiated quitting. *Tobacco Induced Diseases, 1*, 35–81.

Swan, A. V., Creeser, R., & Murray, M. (1990). When and why children first start to smoke. *International Journal of Epidemiology, 19*, 323–330.

Tao, M. L., Guo, M. D., Weiss, R., Byrne, J., Mills, J. L., Robison, L. L., et al. (1998). Smoking in adult survivors of childhood acute lymphoblastic leukemia. *Journal of the National Cancer Institute, 90*, 219–225.

Tyas, S. L., & Pederson, L. L. (1998). Psychosocial factors related to adolescent smoking: A critical review of the literature. *Tobacco Control, 7*, 409–420.

Tyc, V. L., Hadley, W., & Crockett, G. (2001a). Brief report: Predictors of intentions to use tobacco among adolescent survivors of cancer. *Journal of Pediatric Psychology, 26*, 117–121.

Tyc, V. L, Hadley, W., & Crockett, G. (2001b). Prediction of health behaviors in pediatric cancer survivors. *Medical and Pediatric Oncology, 37*, 42–46.

Tyc, V. L., Hudson, M. M., Hadley, W., & Throckmorton-Belzer, L. (2001). Pediatric cancer patients and parents who smoke: Counseling guidelines. *Primary Care and Cancer, 21*, 9–16.

Tyc, V. L., Hudson, M. M., Hinds, P., Elliott, V., & Kibby, M. Y. (1997). Tobacco use among pediatric cancer patients: Recommendations for developing clinical smoking interventions. *Journal of Clinical Oncology, 15*, 2194–2204.

Tyc, V. L., Klosky, J., Throckmorton-Belzer, L., Lensing, S., & Rai, S. (2004). Parent-reported environmental tobacco smoke exposure among preadolescents and adolescents treated for cancer. *Psycho-Oncology., 13*, 537–546.

Tyc, V. L., Lensing, S., Klosky, J., Rai, S., & Robinson, L. (2005). A comparison of tobacco-related risk factors between adolescents with and without cancer. *Journal of Pediatric Psychology, 30*, 359–370.

Tyc, V. L., Lensing, S., Rai, S., Klosky, J., Stewart, D., & Gattuso, J. (in press). Predicting perceived vulnerability to tobacco-related health risks and future intentions to use tobacco among pediatric cancer survivors. *Patient Education and Counseling.*

Tyc, V. L., Rai, S. N., Lensing, S., Klosky, J. K., Stewart, D. B., & Gattuso, J. (2003). Intervention to reduce intentions to use tobacco among pediatric cancer survivors. *Journal of Clinical Oncology, 21*, 1366–1372.

Tyc, V. L., Throckmorton-Belzer, L., Klosky, J. L., Greeson, F. L., Lensing, S., Rai, S., et al. (2004). Smoking among parents of pediatric cancer patients and children's exposure to environmental tobacco smoke. *Journal of Child Health Care, 8*, 286–298.

U.S. Department of Health and Human Services. (2000, November). *Healthy People 2010: Understanding and improving health* (2nd ed.). Washington, DC: U.S. Government Printing Office.

Wang, M. Q., Fitzhugh, E. C., Westerfield, R. C., & Eddy, J. M. (1995). Family and peer influences on smoking behavior among American adolescents: An age trend. *Journal of Adolescent Health, 16*, 200–203.

Weinstein, N. D. (1993). Testing four competing theories of health-protective behavior. *Health Psychology, 12*, 324–333.

Wewers, M. E., Bowen, J. M., Stanislaw, A. E., & Desimone, V. B. (1994). A nurse-delivered smoking cessation intervention among hospitalized postoperative patients-influence of a smoking-related diagnosis: A pilot study. *Heart and Lung, 23*, 151–156.

Zhu, S. H., Sun, J., Billings, S. C., Choi, W. S., & Malarcher, A. (1999). Predictors of smoking cessation in U.S. adolescents. *American Journal of Preventive Medicine, 16*, 202–207.

Dawn K. Wilson and Sarah F. Griffin

# Health Promotion and Primary Prevention of Cancer

## Introduction

There are a number of important preventable risk factors that have been associated with the prevalence and incidence of various types of cancers. These risk factors include sedentary lifestyle, poor diet, obesity, sun exposure, and tobacco use (Friedenreich & Orenstein, 2002; Healthy People 2010, 1998; Pappo, 2003; Slattery, Schumacher, West, Robison, & French, 1990). These risk factors are modifiable, and early prevention in childhood may reduce the likelihood of developing cancers such as melanoma and lung, colon, breast, prostate, and endometrial cancers (IARC Working Group, 2002). For example, according to the International Agency for Research on Cancer, between one fourth and one third of cancer cases may be attributed to the combined effects of obesity and physical inactivity (IARC Working Group, 2002), thus promoting both weight control and physical activity in youths may be beneficial for preventing cancer. Therefore, the identification of multiple risk factors that may be linked to cancer prevention that could be incorporated into prevention programs may be an effective approach for cancer prevention in youth.

A social ecological model is presented in this chapter as a framework for understanding multilevel strategies for promoting healthy lifestyles to prevent cancer in youths (Bronfenbrenner, 1979, 1992; Wilson & Evans, 2003). According to the ecological model, health behavior is affected by intrapersonal, social, cultural, and physical environmental variables. A social ecological framework (McLeroy, Bibeau, Steckler, & Glanz, 1988) conceptualizes health behavior (e.g., physical activity) as affected by multiple levels of influence (see figure 22-1).

Based on this social ecological model, five levels of influence are specified: (a) individual influences (e.g., biological and psychosocial); (b) interpersonal influences (e.g., family, peers); (c) institutional factors (e.g., school, work sites); (d) community factors (e.g., relationship among organizations, institutions, and social networks); and (e) public policy (e.g., laws and policies at the local, state, national, and international levels). In this model, health behaviors such as physical activity, nutrition, sun exposure, and tobacco use are conceptualized as a function of the interaction of individual, family, and peer influences and school, community, mass media, and public policy

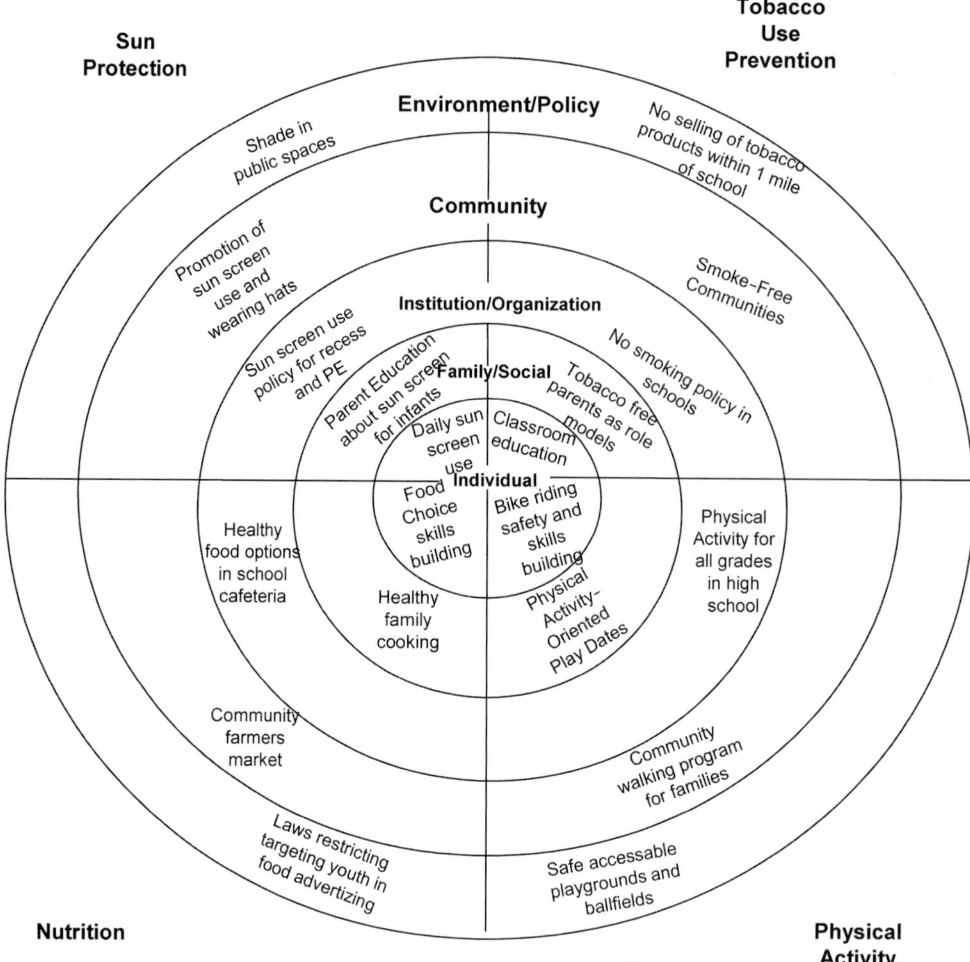


**Figure 22-1.** Ecological model representing multiple levels of interventions for nutrition, physical activity, sun protection, and tobacco prevention.

influences. This model highlights intervention activities that could be implemented at each level of the model pertaining to the four health behaviors covered in this chapter. This model suggests that health-related lifestyle behaviors are multifaceted and dynamic and are developed in a social context through personal, interpersonal, and environmental interactions. In this chapter, we highlight the promotion of positive health behaviors in youths within the context of this ecological framework.

We review the evidence suggesting an association between lifestyle risk factors and cancer. Next, we present the national guidelines for promoting physical activity, nutrition, sun exposure prevention, and tobacco use prevention. For an extensive look at smoking prevention, see also chapter 21 in this volume. Finally, we present an ecological perspective of health promotion strategies that are appropriate for children and adolescents for increasing physical activity, healthy diet, skin cancer protection, and tobacco use prevention.

## Risk Factors Associated With Cancer

This section reviews the epidemiological evidence that demonstrates the associations between health behaviors such as physical activity, nutrition, sun exposure, and tobacco use and various forms of cancer. This evidence should assist health care providers and health professionals in understanding the rationale for educating and encouraging children, parents, and family members about the importance of engaging in healthy lifestyle habits that may reduce the risk of developing cancer in early adulthood.

## Epidemiological Studies of Physical Activity

Several reviews of the literature indicated that over 170 observational epidemiological studies have been conducted examining the relationship between physical activity and cancer (Friedenreich & Orenstein, 2002; Lee, 2003; Thune & Furberg, 2001). The strongest evidence for a protective effect of physical activity on cancer has been shown for colon and breast cancers. In addition, the research on physical activity and these types of cancers have shown dose response relationships (i.e., the more physically active, the lower the risk), providing further evidence of the benefits of physical activity on cancer prevention. A total of 46 of 51 of these studies demonstrated a reduction in colon cancer risk for men and women who engaged in high levels of occupational or recreational physical activity (independent of diet and body mass index). Average risk reduction from physical activity ranged from 40% to 50% and was as high as 70% across studies. A total of 25 of 29 studies found a dose response relationship suggesting that incremental increases in levels of physical activity were associated with corresponding decreasing levels of colon cancer risk. Of 40 studies, 32 demonstrated a reduction in risk of breast cancer for the women who were more physically active. The risk reduction average for all studies was 30%–40%, although there was a wide range in risk reduction levels across studies. Evidence for a dose response relationship between physical activity and cancer was found in 20 of the 32 studies.

Some epidemiological studies have also shown that regular physical activity may reduce the risk of prostate, endometrial, and lung cancers. A total of 15 of 30 studies demonstrated reduced rates of prostate cancer for men who were more physically active. The average risk reduction across all 15 studies was between 10% and 30%. Two studies found a decreased risk only for a subset of physically active men. No association was found in 9 studies, and 4 studies actually showed increased risk associated physical activity. A total of 9 of 13 endometrial cancer studies showed an inverse association between cancer risk and increased physical activity, with an average risk reduction between 30% and 40%. Finally, a total of 8 of 11 lung cancer studies demonstrated an inverse association between lung cancer and physical activity, with an average risk reduction ranging from 30% to 40% (Friedenreich & Orenstein, 2002; Lee, 2003; Thune & Furberg, 2001).

In summary, substantial epidemiological evidence exists indicating a moderate-to-strong inverse relationship between physical activity and specific types of cancer, such as colon and breast cancers. However, not enough evidence exists that clearly defines the relationship between physical activity and other types of cancer, including dose response and possible threshold effects. In addition, it is important to note that physical activity has been measured inconsistently (method and time frame for recall assessment) and not always objectively (often used self-assessment tools) or comprehensively (infrequently measured physical activity type, frequency, duration, and intensity). Future research is needed, including controlled randomized clinical trials, to evaluate the effects of increasing physical activity on cancer prevention in a prospective design.

There have been a relatively large number of studies examining the prevalence of physical activity in children. In a review, Taylor and Sallis (1997) reported that only one half of youths were meeting the national guidelines for physical activity. Ethnic minority adolescents were less physically active than white adolescents were. Sallis, Zakarian, Hovell, and Hofstetter (1996) have also reported that, in a multiethnic sample, adolescents who were classified in the lower socioeconomic level reported engaging in less physical activity lessons after school, having lower frequency of physical education classes, and being involved in less vigorous activity when in physical education classes. In general, a substantial number of children and adolescents are not engaging in regular physical activity, and this may increase the likelihood that they are inactive as adults.

## Epidemiological Studies of Childhood Nutrition

Intake of dietary fruits and vegetables, fat, cholesterol, and sodium has been associated with major risk factors such as incidence of cancer, elevated blood cholesterol, obesity, and high blood pressure (American Heart Association, 1988; Maynard, Gunnell, Emmett, Frankel, & Smith, 2003). These risk factors have been detected among children (Newman, Freedman, & Berenson, 1986) and have been shown to track from childhood into the adult years (Kelder, Perry, Klepp, & Lytle, 1994; Maynard et al., 2003; Nicklas, Webber, Johnson, Srinivasan, & Berenson, 1995).

Maynard et al. (2003) conducted a 60-year follow-up of a large cohort of men and women in rural and urban areas of England and Scotland. Increased childhood fruit intake was associated with a significant reduced risk of incidence of cancer. This association was somewhat weaker for cancer mortality. The researchers suggested that antioxidant constituents in fruits and vegetables protect against free radical–mediated damage to deoxyribonucleic acid (DNA), and that this may provide a protective effect of early diet on adult cancer risk. A number of investigators have also documented that insufficient intake of dietary fiber may be associated with increased risk of colon cancer (Burkitt, Walker, & Painter, 1972; Gurr & Asp, 1994). Other investigators, such as Pryor, Slattery, Robison, and Egger (1989), have shown that the relationship between dietary fat and fiber intake in adolescence and breast cancer in adulthood is inconclusive. However, both laboratory and epidemiological studies have provided evidence that dietary fat intake may be associated with prostate, ovary, and colorectal cancer (Metlin, 1993). Slattery et al. (1990) showed that men who consume higher levels of saturated fatty acids are at slightly increased risk for developing prostate cancer after adjusting for adolescent dietary factors. These epidemiological studies provided moderate-to-strong evidence for the role of healthy diet in preventing the development of certain types of cancer in early adulthood.

The prevalence of dietary practices in children and adolescents has been reported by a number of investigators. Several investigators have reported that fruit and vegetable intake among adolescent populations does not meet the national guidelines (see National Guidelines for Health Behaviors section). Cullen et al. (1999) studied 5,881 adolescents and young adults (aged 14–21 years) who completed a Survey on Youth Risk Behavior. In particular, fruit intake was decreased for males and females during the high school years. Consistent with this finding, Neumark-Sztainer, Story, Resnick, and Blum (1998) reported that among 30,000 adolescents who completed the Minnesota Health Survey, 28% had inadequate fruit intake, and 36% had inadequate vegetable intake. In general, the data on adolescent populations suggest that a substantial number of these youths are not eating an adequate amount of fruits and vegetables.

## Epidemiological Studies of Tobacco Use

A substantial number of studies have demonstrated a strong positive association between tobacco use and lung cancer (Jemal, Cokkinides, Shafey, & Thun, 2003). These data also indicate a dose response relationship. Adolescent smoking cessation prevalence decreased in the United States between 1991 and 2000 (Johnston, O'Malley, & Bachman, 2002; Nelson et al., 1995). In 1999 and 2000, 48.6% of adolescents in the United States had experimented with tobacco use, and 7.8% were established smokers (Mowery, Farrelly, Haviland, Gable, & Wells, 2004).

National surveys have shown that adolescent smoking behavior is higher among whites and Hispanics than among African Americans (Centers for Disease Control and Prevention, 1998). The literature on smoking initiation and ethnicity, however, has been inconsistent. Although some national studies have shown that smoking initiation begins sooner in whites and Hispanics than among African Americans (Centers for Disease Control and Prevention, 1998; Mowery et al., 2004), a study of over 6,000 youths in California and Oregon reported that African Americans started smoking sooner and showed greater lifetime smoking than did whites (Ellickson, Orlando, Tucker, & Klein, 2004).

## Epidemiological Studies of Skin Cancers

Epidemiological studies indicated that skin cancer is the most common form of cancer in the United States, and the incidences of melanoma in developed counties have risen steadily for the past century (Glanz, Lew, Song, & Cook 1999). There are two classifications of skin cancers, melanoma and nonmelanoma. Melanoma cancer is more strongly genetically determined, and nonmelanoma cancer is more strongly related to sun exposure during childhood. However, previous research has shown that sun exposure is associated with both types of skin cancers (Dulon et al., 2002; Pappo, 2003). Lifetime sun exposure, intense sun exposure during childhood, and intermittent sun exposure also have been more strongly associated with the later development of both melanoma and nonmelanoma cancers (Pappo, 2003). Several investigators have documented that the presence of melanocytic nevi (large brown spots) during childhood are positively associated with malignant melanoma (Dulon et al., 2002; Gallagher & McLean, 1990; Kelly et al., 1994). Melanocytic nevi are correlated with painful sunburns and sun exposure, especially during childhood years (Dulon et al., 2002). One of the most comprehensive studies indicating that regular sun exposure is an important risk factor for developing nevi in adolescence was conducted in Queensland, Australia, by Darlington, Siskind, Green, and Green (2002). This was a longitudinal study that followed adolescents for 5 years, demonstrating positive associations between sun exposure and rates of nevi. Taken together, the studies on sun exposure and skin cancer during the first 19 years of life showed a positive association with an increased incidence of skin cancer, thus, prevention of sun exposure and protective behaviors should begin in childhood.

## National Guidelines for Health Behaviors

### *Physical Activity Guidelines*

The guidelines for physical activity standards in adolescents were published by Sallis and Patrick (1994). The guidelines suggest that adolescents should engage in 60 minutes of moderate-to-vigorous activity every day of the week.

### *Nutrition Guidelines*

The year 2010 health objectives outlined in 2000 by the U.S. Department of Health and Human Services (USDHHS) advocate specific recommendations for adolescents. They recommend that children and adolescents limit their intake of dietary fat to 30% and saturated fat to 10% of their total calories. Children and adolescents should also eat daily at least three servings of vegetables (one third dark green or deep yellow), two servings of fruits, six or more servings of grains, and three servings of calcium-enriched foods and should reduce their sodium intake to no more than 2,400 mg/daily by eliminating the use of table salt, preparing foods without salt, and purchasing more low-sodium foods. Note all of these guidelines are primarily focused on restricting foods by eliminating high-fat and high-salt intake. Thus, these guidelines promote foods that are less tasty and perhaps not appealing especially to children and adolescents.

### *Sun Protection Guidelines*

National guidelines include recommendations that children and adolescents do not expose themselves to sun without protection for more than 30 minutes per day between the hours of 10 a.m. and 4 p.m. (Robinson, Rademaker, Sylvester, & Cook, 1997).

### *Tobacco Use*

The surgeon general recommends that children and adults not initiate smoking (USDHHS, 2000). National policies for reducing secondhand smoke among children have become increasingly present in the United States given the negative health effects of secondhand smoke (Sandler, Everson, Wilcox, & Browder, 1985; Woodward & Laugesen, 2001). It is recommended that young children and adolescents not be exposed to prolonged secondhand smoke in the home as well as in public settings such as schools, recreational facilities, and daycare centers.

## Ecological Strategies for Promoting Healthy Lifestyles

Health care providers and health professional have become increasing interested in understanding and developing new approaches for promoting long-term health habits among children and adolescents. For health professionals to be effective at changing health behaviors among youths, it is important to understand the complexity of their social and environmental surroundings. Figure 22-1 presents an integrated model for understanding factors that affect health-promoting behaviors in children and adolescents. This integrated model is derived from ecologically based models (Bronfenbrenner, 1979,

1992; McLeroy et al., 1988; Wilson & Evans, 2003) that consider the interactions between individuals and their environments. According to the ecological model, health behavior is affected by intrapersonal, social, cultural, and physical environmental variables. A basic tenet of the ecological perspective is reciprocal determinism (Bandura, 1986, 1989; Glanz, Lewis, & Rimer, 1997), which suggests that behavior and the environment influence each other.

The integrated model in figure 22-1 emphasizes the need to consider multiple levels of behaviors across multiple levels of social, cultural, and physical environments. These variables include the child's individual perspective, family/social influences, school, community, work site, mass media, and public policy. The environmental influences may be divided into proximal and distal contexts. The proximal ones are embedded within the distal ones (Bronfenbrenner, 1979, 1992). For example, local no smoking zoning or policies prohibiting smoking in public places are influenced by national tobacco policies. Consistent with McLeroy et al.'s (1988) model, we specify five levels of influence: (a) intrapersonal influences, (b) interpersonal influences, (c) institutional factors, (d) community factors, and (e) public policy.

The model presented in figure 22-1 shows specifically the convergence of individual, social, and environmental factors from an ecological perspective in addressing physical activity, nutrition, sun protection, and tobacco use behaviors. For example, although all levels of the ecological model are important, policy interventions have been most commonly used in reducing tobacco use in children. In contrast, behaviors most frequently addressed at the individual level include nutrition and physical activity. Although all of the behaviors in figure 22-1 involve parents, sun protection interventions have focused their social marketing approaches primarily toward parents of children. In summary, this figure shows important strategies that need further investigation and illustrates that the strategies can be linked across multiple levels of the model and across multiple health behaviors.

### *Physical Activity Interventions*

There are a number of health benefits resulting from engaging in regular physical activity. For example, previous research has shown that engaging in regular physical activity is associated with improvements in circulation, ventilation, bowel transit time, energy balance, immune function, insulin and insulinlike growth factors, metabolic hormones, and increased capacity to repair DNA (Friedenreich & Orenstein, 2002; Thune & Furberg, 2001). It has been suggested that regular physical activity may help to reduce the risk of cancer through decreasing abdominal fat mass, which is highly metabolic and associated with cancer risk (Lee, 2003; Matsuzawa et al., 1995). Problems with insulin metabolism have been associated with both obesity and physical inactivity (McTiernan, Ulrich, Slate, & Potter, 1998; Ma et al., 1999). Furthermore, some research indicated that engaging in regular physical activity may also reduce the amount of adipose tissue, which may in turn reduce the risk of developing certain cancers such as postmenopausal breast cancer and colon cancer (IARC Working Group, 2002).

The literature on behavioral school-based physical activity interventions has demonstrated inconsistent effects on increasing physical activity in children and adolescents. In general, school-based intervention studies have utilized a social cognitive theory perspective that focuses on individual and institution levels of the model presented in figure 22-1. The majority of the studies have demonstrated only modest changes in students' physical activity during physical education class time and little change in overall physical activity outside school class time (Baranowski, Anderson, & Carmack, 1998). Few of the studies have examined or demonstrated that behavioral or psychosocial factors mediate the changes in the physical activity because of the intervention (Baranowski et al., 1998).

Several large intervention trials have specifically targeted adolescents. For example, the Planet Health project (Gortmaker et al., 1999) evaluated a school-based social cognitive theory and behavioral choice intervention in 1,295 sixth and seventh graders over 2 years. The intervention was a physical education curriculum-based program to decrease consumption of high-fat foods and television watching and to increase fruit and vegetable intake and moderate-to-vigorous physical activity. Although overall the intervention did reduce the prevalence of obesity in girls (especially among African Americans), there were no significant changes in physical activity because of the intervention, and only television viewing predicted changes in obesity prevalence in this study.

The Minnesota Heart Health Program was a quasi-experimental school-based study in which 2,376 sixth graders participated in a social cognitive theory intervention or no intervention (Kelder, Perry, & Klepp, 1993) designed to increase physical activity outside school physical education classes. After 7 years, the study demonstrated that girls were more likely to show an increase in physical activity than boys were. The Stanford Adolescent Heart Health Program (Killen et al., 1988) was a social cognitive theory school-based randomized trial that involved 1,447 tenth graders in a classroom-based instruction intervention designed to increase levels of aerobic physical activity. After 7 weeks of intervention and at a 2-month follow-up, there was an increase in the percentage of adolescents who engaged in regular physical activity as compared to the control schools (30.2% vs. 20.0%). Physical activity and knowledge scores increased.

Several large-scale school-based trials also have shown modest results for increasing physical activity in elementary children, such as the Child and Adolescent Trial on Cardiovascular Health (CATCH) trial (Edmundson et al., 1996; Luepker et al., 1996; McKenzie, Sallis, Faucette, Roby, & Kolody, 1993; McKenzie et al., 1996; Sallis et al., 1997).

In summary, school-based behavioral interventions in children and adolescents have resulted in modest to no change in physical activity levels outside class time (Baranowski et al., 1998; Stone, McKenzie, Welk, & Booth, 1998). In addition, behavioral and psychosocial theories have only accounted for a relatively small amount of the variability in physical activity behaviors (~30%), and most intervention studies have not measured mediating variables (Baranowski et al., 1998). To increase the effectiveness of physical activity interventions, more research is needed that focuses on better understanding the theoretical predictors of physical activity, and more interventions are needed that specifically effect change in the hypothesized mediators.

### *Nutrition Interventions*

Dietary modification may reduce the risk and incidence of chronic illnesses such as cancer and cardiovascular disease in children and adolescents (Berenson, Srinivasan, Weber, & Wattigney, 1991; Gliksman, Lazarus, & Wilson, 1993; Maynard et al., 2003; USDHHS, 2000). Several large-scale clinical trials have demonstrated that establishing healthy eating habits during childhood is feasible. For example, CATCH is one of the largest clinical trials to examine the effects of a social cognitive theory intervention on promoting healthy eating in children (Edmondson et al., 1996; Luepker et al., 1996; Stone et al., 1996). A total of 96 elementary schools across four study sites were randomly assigned to either a cognitive behavioral intervention that promoted low-fat and low-sodium foods or to a no treatment control condition. The findings indicated sustained significant effects at 3-year follow-up for improvement in self-reported dietary knowledge, intentions, self-efficacy (self-confidence), dietary behavior, and perceived social reinforcement for healthy food choices for the intervention children.

In another large trial, the Dietary Intervention Study in Children (DISC), 663 preadolescent children with elevated lipids were randomly assigned to either a cognitive behavioral intervention or a usual care group (DISC Collaborative Research Group, 1994). After 3 years, the intervention children showed significant reductions in total calories from saturated fat compared to the usual care group.

Both of these studies provided evidence that establishing long-term healthy dietary habits in children and adolescents is possible. These studies also provided good examples of utilizing multiple levels of the ecological model by targeting nutrition changes at the child's individual level, parent level, and school level.

### *Skin Cancer Prevention Interventions*

Social marketing strategies have been used to reduce sun exposure and increase sunscreen use (Graffunder et al., 1999). These strategies have been targeted at children, parents, and caregivers. In a randomized study by Buller, Goldberg, and Buller (1997), fourth graders ($N = 2{,}032$) participated in a school-based intervention involving classroom instruction and interactive health fairs. The results demonstrated that intervention students showed greater increases in knowledge of sun protective behaviors posttreatment than did students in the control schools. In another study, Vitols and Oats (1997) also examined the effects of school-based intervention on increasing sun protective behaviors. The intervention included educational and behavior skills components. The results showed an increase in knowledge for increasing sun protective behaviors.

A community-based intervention by Miller, Geller, Wood, Lew, and Koh (1999) examined the effects of a multidimensional program combining community activism, publicity campaigns, and behavioral interventions. The goals of the program were to increase knowledge, attitudes of parent/caregiver and children, and sun protection behavior. There was a decrease in sunburns of children and an increase in role modeling of sun protection factors and sunscreen use as a result of the program.

In a randomized trial, Glanz, Geller, Shigaki, Maddock, and Isnec (2002) examined the effectiveness of the Pool Cool Sun-Protection Intervention that was implemented at 28 pools in two geographical regions, Massachusetts and Hawaii. The intervention program was provided to children (mean age = 6.6 years, standard deviation [*SD*] = 1.5), parents, and pool staff and emphasized using sunscreen, wearing hats and shirts, wearing sunglasses, and avoiding sunburns. The key elements of the intervention focused on improving skills training and appeal (social norms) of practicing sun protective behaviors. A total of eight sun safety sessions was presented as part of a swimming class at local pools over a 2- to 4-week period. Environmental elements of the program included offering free sunscreen, sun safety signs, and posters and providing adequate shading to prevent sunburn. The results demonstrated a significant increase in sunscreen use, shade seeking, and total sunscreen protection habits and reduced numbers of sunburns compared to the control group. A substantial improvement also was shown for sun protection policies and environmental supports. The Glanz et al. study illustrated the importance of using a multilevel ecological approach for influencing sun protection behavior in children.

### *Tobacco Use Prevention Programs*

Chapter 21 of this book is devoted to smoking cessation in youths. Although many tobacco use interventions in youths target individual-level change, more broadly defined intervention studies have targeted policy and environmental changes. For example, in a study by Biglan, Koehn, et al. (1996), an intervention aimed at increasing reinforcements for not selling tobacco products among commercial vendors (e.g., grocery stores, markets, gas stations, etc.), included five levels: mobilized community support for not selling tobacco products, merchant education, changing consequences for clerks selling or refusing to sell tobacco, publicity about clerks' refusal to sell tobacco products, and provision of feedback to store owners and managers about the prevalence of sales to adolescents. The results of this intervention demonstrated that tobacco sales were reduced by 55% over the course of a 1-year intervention. Other similar studies using multilevel approaches to tobacco cessation also have been effective (Biglan, Ary, et al., 1996).

## Multilevel and Multibehavior Interventions

Table 22-1 highlights seminal studies using multilevel and multibehavioral interventions aimed at the four health behaviors addressed in this chapter. These studies helped to advance our understanding of the value of multilevel, multibehavioral interventions. All of the studies functioned on at least three of the five levels of the model. For example, all of the interventions listed included an individual-level component that addressed individual-level change through education or skills-building efforts, and many of the interventions included institutional- or organization-level efforts that focused on making changes in organizations that serve youths, such as schools or recreation facilities. The complexity of using a multilevel design in conducting intervention programs makes it harder to discern the underlying mechanism of the effect. Practitioners, however, often function at all five levels of the ecological model in addressing health behaviors as outlined in figure 22-1. It is also important to highlight the notion that certain levels of the ecological model may be more appropriate, feasible, and effective for different health behaviors and different target populations.

## Conclusions

This chapter outlines the key behaviors that are important to cancer prevention in children and

**Table 22-1.** Studies Testing Ecological Multilevel Interventions

| *Topic* | *Study Design* | *Individual* | *Family/Social* | *Institution/ Organization* | *Community* | *Environment/Policy* | *Outcome* |
|---|---|---|---|---|---|---|---|
| Nutrition | Give Me 5 Fruits and Vegetables a Day (Barnowski et al., 2000): Based on social cognitive theory; implemented in schools; intervention to increase fourth and fifth graders to eat more fruits and vegetables | 12-session classroom curriculum | Parent newsletters with information about increasing fruit and vegetable intake. Videotape paralleling classroom curriculum Family nights | Teacher training through 1-day workshop | | | Positive impact on fruit and vegetable consumption |
| Nutrition and physical activity | CATCH (Perry et al., 1997): Based on social cognitive theory; implemented in schools to elementary age children to increase physical activity and fruit and vegetable consumption and decrease fat intake | Classroom curricula: Hearty Heart and Friends, FACTS for 5, Go for Health | Family Fun Night: games, fitness-related activities, and healthy snacks | Eat Smart: To get schools to incorporate dietary guidelines into food services CATCH PE: increase time spent wi | | | Positive changes in school food service, physical education programs, and youth nutrition and physical activity behaviors |
| Physical activity | Minnesota Heart Health Program (Kelder et al., 1993): Based on social learning theory; designed to increase physical activity outside school classes | Classroom curriculum to increase knowledge, behavioral skills, and self-efficacy in monitoring, choosing activities, and safety | Peer social support for physical activity outside physical education classes | School-level change | Communitywide competitions to exercise outside school | | After 7 years, girls more likely to show increase in physical activity than boys, but there was slight increase for boys |

(*continued*)

**Table 22-1.** *(continued)*

| *Topic* | *Study Design* | *Individual* | *Family/Social* | *Institution/ Organization* | *Community* | *Environment/Policy* | *Outcome* |
|---|---|---|---|---|---|---|---|
| Tobacco use | Massachusetts Comprehensive Tobacco Control Program | School programs to raise awareness of harmful effects and engage in positive antitobacco efforts | | | Antitobacco media campaign | Enforcement of youth access to tobacco laws | Significant decreases in lifetime and current cigarette, smokeless tobacco use and current cigar use |
| Sun safety | Pool Cool (Glanz et al., 2002): Based on social cognitive theory; implemented at community pools; aimed to increase sun protection behaviors | Sun safety educational lessons with youths Skills-building session with youths | | Training for lifeguards on sun safety and incorporating sun safety activities | | Provision of sunscreen and shade at pools Posters and signs with sun safe messages Consultation on policy changes | Modest but significant increases in youths' sunscreen use, shade seeking, and total sun protection habits; reduced sunburns in fair skin; and increase in pool sun protection policies |

adolescents. Although not all behaviors that are linked to cancer are included in this chapter, the key behaviors that have the most potential in having an impact on preventing cancer are presented. A major emphasis of this chapter is on highlighting the importance of using interventions at multiple levels of the ecological model. More work also needs to be conducted on targeting multiple behaviors in the model proposed in figure 22-1. Longitudinal studies will be important to show how behavioral changes can reduce the prevalence of certain types of cancers. In addition, focusing on multiple risk behaviors will be important because many of these behaviors coexist. For example, increasing physical activity that might include outdoor sports will also require using sunscreen protection. If performance in physically active sports is a priority for youths, both good nutrition and tobacco use prevention will be necessary to obtain their goals. A better understanding of how to maintain these behavioral skills over the life span should be the goal of future research.

## References


American Heart Association. (1988). Dietary guidelines for healthy American adults. *Circulation, 77,* 721–724.

Bandura, A. (1986). *Social foundations of thought and action*. Englewood Cliffs, NJ: Prentice-Hall.

Bandura, A. (1989). Perceived self-efficacy in the exercise of personal agency. *The Psychologist: Bulletin of the British Psychological Society, 10,* 411–424.

Baranowski, T., Anderson, C., & Carmack, C. (1998). Mediating variable framework in physical activity interventions: How are we doing? How might we do better? *American Journal of Preventive Medicine, 15,* 266–297.

Baranowski, T., Davis, M., Resnicow, K., Baranwoski, J., Doyle, C., Lin, L. S., et al. (2000). Gimme 5 fruit, juice, and vegetable for fun and health: Outcome evaluation. *Health Education and Behavior, 27,* 96–111.

Berenson, G., Srinivasan, S., Webber, L., & Wattigney, W. (1991). Coronary heart disease as a pediatric disorder. *Progress in Cardiology, 4,* 127–139.

Biglan, A., Ary, D., Yudelson, H., Duncan, T. E., Hood, D., James, L., et al. (1996). Experimental evaluation of a modular approach to mobilizing anti-tobacco influences of peers and parents. *American Journal of Community Psychology, 24,* 311–339.

Biglan, A., Koehn, A. D., Levings, D., Smith, S., Wright, Z, James, L., et al. (1996). Mobilizing positive reinforcement in communities to reduce youth access to tobacco. *American Journal of Community Psychology, 24,* 625–638.

Bronfenbrenner, U. (1979). *The ecology of human development: Experiments by nature and design.* Cambridge, MA: Harvard University Press.

Bronfenbrenner, U. (1992). Ecological systems theory. In R. Vasta (Ed.), *Six theories of child development* (pp. 187–250). London: Kingsley.

Buller, M. K., Goldberg, G., & Buller, D. B. (1997). Sun Smart Day: A pilot program for photoprotection education. *Pediatric Dermatology, 14,* 257–263.

Burkitt, D. P., Walker, A. R. P., & Painter, N. S. (1972). Effect of dietary fibre on stools and transit times and its role in the causation of disease. *Lancet, 2,* 1408–1412.

Centers for Disease Control and Prevention. (1998). Tobacco use among U.S. racial/ethnic minority groups—African Americans, American Indians and Alaska Natives, Asian Americans and Pacific Islanders, and Hispanics: A report of the surgeon general. *MMWR Morbidity and Mortality Weekly Report, 47*(RR-18), 2.

Cullen, K. W., Koehly, L. M., Anderson, C., Baranowski, T., Prokhorov, A., Basen-Engquist, K., et al. (1999). Gender differences in chronic disease risk behaviors through the transition out of high school. *American Journal of Preventive Medicine, 17,* 1–7.

Darlington, S., Siskind, V., Green, L., & Green, A. (2002). Longitudinal study of melanocytic nevi in adolescents. *Journal of the American Academy of Dermatology, 46,* 715–722.

DISC Collaborative Research Group. (1994). Cholesterol-lowering diet is effective and safe in children with elevated LDL-cholesterol: Three-year results of the Dietary Intervention Study in Children (DISC). *Circulation, 90,* I-8, 39A.

Dulon, M., Weichenthal, M., Blettner, M., Breitbart, M., Hetzer, M., Greinert, R., et al. (2002). Sun exposure and number of nevi in 5- to 6 year-old European children. *Journal of Clinical Epidemiology, 55,* 1075–1081.

Edmundson, E., Parcel, G. S., Feleman, H. A., Elder, J., Perry, C. L., Johnson, C. C., et al. (1996). The effects of the Child and Adolescent Trial for Cardiovascular Health upon psychosocial determinants on diet and physical activity behavior. *Preventive Medicine, 25,* 442–454.

Ellickson, P. L., Orlando, M., Tucker, J. S., & Klein, D. (2004). From adolescence to young adulthood: Racial/ethnic disparities in smoking. *American Journal of Public Health, 94,* 293–299.

Friedenreich, C. M., & Orenstein, M. R. (2002). Physical activity and cancer prevention: Etiologic evidence and biological mechanisms. *The Journal of Nutrition, 132*, 3456S–3464S.

Gallagher, R. P., & McLean, D. I. (1990). Suntan, sunburn, and pigmentation factors and the frequency of acquired melanocytic nevi in children. *Archives of Dermatology, 126*, 770–776.

Glanz, K., Geller, A. C., Shigaki, D., Maddock, J. E., & Isnec, M. R. (2002). A randomized trial of skin cancer prevention in aquatics settings: The Pool Cool program. *Health Psychology, 21*, 579–587.

Glanz, K., Lew, R. A., Song, V., & Cook, V. A. (1999). Factors associated with skin cancer prevention practices in a multiethnic population. *Health Education and Behavior, 26*, 344–349.

Glanz, K., Lewis, F. M., & Rimer, B. (1997). *Health behavior and health education.* San Francisco: Jossey-Bass.

Gliksman, M. D., Lazarus, R., & Wilson, A. (1993). Differences in serum lipids in Australian children. Is diet responsible? *International Journal of Epidemiology, 22*, 247–254.

Gortmaker, S. L., Peterson, K., Wiecha, J., Sobol, A. M., Dixit, S., Fox, M. K., et al. (1999). Reducing obesity via a school-based interdisciplinary intervention among youth. *Archives of Pediatric and Adolescent Medicine, 153*, 409–418.

Graffunder, C. M., Wyatt, S. W., Bewerse, B. Hall, I., Reilley, B., & Lee-Pethal, R. (1999). Skin cancer prevention: The problem, responses, and lessons learned. *Health Education and Behavior, 26*, 308–316.

Gurr, M. I., & Asp, N. G. (1994). *Dietary fibre.* Washington, DC: International Life Science Press.

Healthy People 2010. (1998). Priority health behaviors: Tobacco use. www.healthpeople.gov/hpscript/keyword. Key word: Tobbacco. November 2004.

IARC Working Group. (2002). *IARC handbook of cancer prevention. Vol. 6: Weight control and physical activity*. Lyon: France.

Jemal, A., Cokkinides, V. E., Shafey, O., & Thun, M. J. (2003). Lung cancer trends in young adults: An early indicator of progress in tobacco control (United States). *Cancer Causes Control, 14*, 579–585.

Johntson, L. D., O'Malley, P. M., & Bachman, J. G. (2002). *Teen smoking declines sharply in 2002, more than offsetting large increases in the early 1990s.* Retrieved December 2002 from the University of Michigan News and Information Services Web site: http://www.monitoringthefuture.org.

Kelder, S. D., Perry, C. L., Klepp, K. I., & Lytle, L. L. (1994). Longitudinal tracking of adolescent smoking, physical activity, and food choice behaviors. *American Journal of Public Health, 84*, 1121–1126.

Kelder, S. H., Perry, C. L., & Klepp, K. I. (1993). Community wide youth exercise promotion: Long-term outcomes of the Minnesota Heart Health Program and the Class of 1989 Study. *Journal of School Health, 63*, 218–223.

Kelly, J. W., River, J. K., MacLennon, R., Harrison, S., Lewis, A. E., & Tate, B. J. (1994). Sunlight: A major factor associated with the development of melanocytic nevi in Australian schoolchildren. *Journal of the American Academy of Dermatology, 30*, 40–48.

Killen, J. D., Telch, M. J., Robinson, T. N., Maccoby, N., Taylor, C. B., & Farquhar, J. W. (1988). Cardiovascular disease risk reduction for 10th graders: A multiple-factor school-based approach. *Journal of the American Medical Association, 260*, 1728–1733.

Lee, I. M. (2003). Physical activity and cancer prevention: Data from epidemiologic studies. *Medicine and Science in Sports and Medicine, 35*, 1823–1827.

Luepker, R. V., Perry, C. L., McKinlay, S. M., Nader, P. R., Parcel, G. S., Stone, E. J., et al. (1996). Outcomes of a field trial to improve children's dietary patterns and physical activity: The Child and Adolescent Trial for Cardiovascular Health (CATCH). *Journal of the American Medical Association, 275*, 768–776.

Ma, J., Pollak, M. N., Giovannucci, E., Chan, J. M., Tao, Y., Hennekens, C. H., et al. (1999). Prospective study of colorectal cancer risk in men and plasma levels of insulin-like growth factor (IGF)-I and IGF-binding protein-3. *Journal of the National Cancer Institute, 91*, 620–625.

Matsuzawa, Y., Shimomura, I., Nakamura, T., Keno, Y., Kotari, K., & Tokunaga, K. (1995). Pathophysiology and pathogenesis of visceral fat obesity. *Obesity Research, 3*, 187S–194S.

Maynard, M., Gunnell, D., Emmett, P., Frankel, S., & Smith, D. (2003). Fruit, vegetables, and antioxidants in childhood and risk of adult cancer: The Blood Orr cohort. *Journal of Epidemiology and Community Health, 57*, 218–237.

McKenzie, T. L., Nader, P. R., Strikmiller, P. K., Yang, M., Stone, E. J., Perry, C. L., et al. (1996). School physical education: Effect of the child and adolescent trial for cardiovascular health. *Preventive Medicine, 25*, 423–431.

McKenzie, T. L., Sallis, J. F., Faucette, N., Roby, J. J., & Kolody, B. (1993). Effects of a curriculum and inservice program on the quality of elementary physical education classes. *Research Quarterly for Exercise and Sport, 64*, 178–189.

McLeroy, K. R., Bibeau, D., Steckler, A., & Glanz, K. (1988). An ecological perspective on health promotion programs. *Health Education Quarterly, 15*, 351–378.

McTiernan, A., Ulrich, C., Slate, S., & Potter, J. (1998). Physical activity and cancer etiology: Associations and mechanisms. *Cancer Causes and Control: CCC, 9*, 487–509.

Mettlin, C. (1993). Dietary cancer prevention in children. *Cancer, 71*, 3367–3369.

Miller, D. R., Geller, A. C., Wood, M. C., Lew, R. A., & Koh, H. K. (1999). The Famouth Safe Skin Project: Evaluation of a community program to promote sun protection in youth. *Health Education and Behavior, 26*, 369–384.

Mowery, P. D., Farrelly, M. C., Haviland, L., Gable, J. M., & Wells, H. E. (2004). Progression to established smoking among US youth. *American Journal of Public Health, 94*, 331–337.

Nelson, D. E., Giovino, G. A., Shopland, D. R., Mowery, P. D., Mills, S. L., & Eriksen, M. P. (1995). Trends in cigarette smoking among U.S. adolescents, 1974–1991. *American Journal of Public Health, 85*, 34–40.

Neumark-Sztainer, D., Story, M., Resnick, M. D., & Blum, R. W. (1998). Lessons learned about adolescent nutrition from the Minnesota Adolescent Health Survey. *Journal of the American Dietetic Association, 98*, 1449–1456.

Newman, W. P., Freedman, D. S., & Berenson, G. (1986). Relation of serum lipoprotein levels and systolic blood pressure to early atherosclerosis: The Bogalusa Heart Study. *New England Journal of Medicine, 314*, 138–144.

Nicklas, T. A., Webber, L. S., Johnson, C. C., Srinivasan, S. R., & Berenson, G. S. (1995). Foundations for health promotion with youth: A review of observations from the Bogalusa Heart Study. *Journal of Health Education, 26*(Suppl. 2), 18–26.

Pappo, A. S. (2003). Melanoma in children and adolescents. *European Journal of Cancer, 39*, 2651–61.

Perry, C. L., Sellers, D. E., Johnson, C., Pedersen, S., Bachman, K. J., Parcel G. S., et al. (1997). The Child and Adolescent Trial for Cardiovascular Health (CATCH): Intervention, implementation, and feasibility for elementary schools in the United States. *Health Education and Behavior, 24*, 716–735.

Pryor, M., Slattery, M. L., Robison, L. M., & Egger, M. (1989). Adolescent diet and breast cancer in Utah. *Cancer Research, 49*, 2161–2167.

Robinson, J. K, Rademaker, A. W., Sylvester, M. A., & Cook, B. (1997). Summer sun exposure: Knowledge, attitudes, and behaviors of Midwest adolescents. *Preventive Medicine, 26*, 364–372.

Sallis, J. F., McKenzie, T. L., Alcaraz, J. E., Kolody, B., Faucette, N., & Hovell, M. F. (1997). The effects of a 2-year physical education program (SPARK) on physical activity and fitness in elementary school students. *American Journal of Public Health, 87*, 1328–1334.

Sallis, J. F., & Patrick, K. (1994). Physical activity guidelines for adolescents: Consensus statement. *Pediatric Exercise Science, 6*, 302–314.

Sallis, J. F., Zakarian, J. M., Hovell, M. F., & Hofstetter. (1996). Ethnic, socioeconomic, and sex differences in physical activity among adolescents. *Journal of Clinical Epidemiology, 49*, 125–134.

Sandler, D. P., Everson, R. B., Wilcox, A. J., & Browder, J. P. (1985). Cancer risk in adulthood from early life exposure to parents' smoking. *American Journal of Public Health, 75*, 487–492.

Slattery, M. L., Schumacher, M. C., West, D. W., Robison, L. M., & French, T. K. (1990). Food-consumption trends between adolescent and adult years and subsequent risk of prostate cancer. *The American Journal of Clinical Nutrition, 52*, 752–757.

Stone, E. J., McKenzie, T. L., Welk, G. J., & Booth, M. L. (1998). Effects of physical activity interventions in youth: Review and synthesis. *American Journal of Preventive Medicine, 15*, 298–315.

Stone, E. J., Osganian, S. K., Mckinlay, S., Wu, M. C., Webber, L. S., Luepker, R. V., et al. (1996). Operational design and quality control in the CATCH Multicenter Trial. *Preventive Medicine, 25*, 384–399.

Taylor, W. C., & Sallis, J. F. (1997). Determinants of physical activity in children. In A. P. Simopoulos and K. N. Pavlou (Ed.), *Nutrition and fitness: Metabolic and behavioral aspects in health and disease* (pp. 159–167). Washington, DC: American Psychological Association.

Thune, I., & Furberg, A. (2001). Physical activity and cancer risk: Dose-response and cancer, all sites and site-specific. *Medicine and Science in Sports and Exercise, 33*, S530–S550.

U.S. Department of Health and Human Services. (2000). *Healthy People 2010: Understanding and improving health*. Washington, DC: U.S. Government Printing Office.

Vitols, P., & Oates, R. K. (1997). Teaching children about skin cancer prevention: Why wait for adolescence? *Australia New Zealand Public Health Journal, 21*, 602–605.

Wilson, D. K., & Evans, A. E. (2003). Health promotion in children and adolescents: An integration of psychosocial and environmental approaches. In M. C. Roberts (Ed.), *Handbook of pediatric psychology* (3rd ed., pp. 161–178). New York: Guilford.

Woodward, A., & Laugesen, M. (2001). How many deaths are caused by second hand cigarette smoke? *Tobacco Control, 10*, 383–388.

# Sickle Cell Disease

Kathryn E. Gustafson, Melanie J. Bonner, Kristina K. Hardy, and Robert J. Thompson, Jr.

# Biopsychosocial and Developmental Issues in Sickle Cell Disease

As advances in health care have prolonged and improved the quality of life of children with chronic illnesses such as sickle cell disease (SCD), psychologists have sought to understand the impact of the illnesses on children and their families and to formulate effective interventions to enhance adaptation. These efforts have been informed by a biopsychosocial conceptual approach such that the biomedical, psychological, and social-ecological processes associated with successful adaptation and effective intervention have been explored (Thompson & Gustafson, 1996). Moreover, it has been recognized that chronic childhood illness occurs within the ongoing context of the child's cognitive and socioemotional development. Development occurs as a consequence of the transactions between the innate qualities of the biological organism and life experiences occurring in a psychosocial context (Thompson, 1985). There is a continuous and mutual influence of the child and the child's environment, and the implications of the chronic illness for the child's cognitive, social and emotional development will vary depending on the impact of the disease at each stage of development (Perrin & Gerrity, 1984).

The child's interactions with the environment can be affected by SCD or other chronic illness both directly and indirectly (Thompson & Gustafson, 1996). There can be a direct effect in terms of the biological processes of the disease on systems of the body that result in cognitive, motor, sensory, or other functional impairments. SCD, for example, is a hematological disorder but poses a risk to cognitive processes through central nervous system (CNS) stroke. There can also be an indirect effect of the chronic illness in terms of the effects of the disease on the child's attainment of normative psychosocial developmental tasks that arise during phases of the life course. The pain crises that are associated with SCD, for example, may interfere with a child's developmental tasks, including gaining autonomy, participating fully in school, interacting with peers, and forming an integrated sense of self-identity (e.g., Robinson, 1999; Sexson & Dingle, 1997).

This chapter reviews the biopsychosocial and developmental issues that are relevant to SCD. Because subsequent chapters in this volume also review the neuropsychological and psychosocial issues in detail, this review is not meant to be exhaustive. Instead, this chapter provides an understanding of relevant biopsychosocial and developmental issues in adaptation and outcome in children with SCD and their families by reviewing (a) the biomedical aspects of the disease itself; (b) the biopsychosocial conceptual models that have been promulgated in an effort to understand risk and resistance factors in adaptation to SCD; (c) what is known about the contribution of biopsychosocial risk and resistance factors to psychological adjustment in children with SCD and their parents; and (d) biopsychosocial issues in neurocognitive and developmental outcomes in these children.

## Biomedical Aspects of Sickle Cell Disease

SCD is a group of inherited disorders affecting approximately 1 in every 400–500 African American newborns in the United States (Tarnowski & Brown, 2000), thereby representing a significant public health concern (Thompson, Gustafson, & Ware, 1998). Although most common in persons of African descent, SCD also affects other ethnic groups, including persons of Mediterranean, Caribbean, South and Central American, Arabian, and East Indian descent.

SCD results from an autosomal recessive genetic deficit and is classified by genotype. Persons affected with SCD demonstrate abnormal genes for hemoglobin (Hb) S, which produces a change in the shape of red blood cells from their normal disk shape to a sickle shape. These abnormally shaped cells obstruct normal blood flow and production of new red blood cells, resulting in chronic anemia. The most common type of SCD is the homozygous condition, sickle cell anemia (Hb SS), which is caused by two abnormal genes for hemoglobin S and is associated with earlier and more frequent and severe symptoms than other types (Charache, Lubin, & Reid, 1989). Other common types include sickle cell hemoglobin C (Hb SC) and sickle $\beta$-thalassemia (Hb S $\beta$-thalassemia). Persons who inherit only one abnormal gene have the sickle cell trait, which is associated with a predominance of normal hemoglobin and is not a disease.

In addition to anemia, common symptoms associated with SCD include vasoocclusions that contribute to tissue and organ damage and pain crises. Vasoocclusions that occur in the brain put children with SCD at increased risk for neurological diseases, including stroke. Cerebrovascular accidents occur in 5%–10% of children with SCD, and "silent" strokes occur in 11%–20% of children with SCD (Balkaran et al., 1992; Hindmarsh, Brozovic, Brook, & Davies, 1987; Pavlakis et al., 1988; Powars, Wilson, Imbus, Pegelow, & Allen, 1978). Silent strokes are not clinically detectable on routine physical examination but reflect microvascular accidents that are detectable by radiographic techniques (Hindmarsh et al., 1987; Pavalakis et al., 1988). Both types of stroke contribute to morbidity.

Although SCD continues to be associated with a reduced life expectancy (median age of survival is 42 years for males and 48 years for females) (Charache, 1994; Platt et al., 1994), treatment for the disease has improved significantly (A. R. Cohen, 1998; Ris & Grueneich, 2000). These treatment advances reflect findings from clinical, molecular, and genetic studies (Hagar & Vichinsky, 2000) and use of new tools, including transcranial Doppler ultrasonography to evaluate patients for stroke risk (Adams, 2000; Adams et al., 1998).

In addition, new therapies are currently under investigation, including hydroxyurea, an antineoplastic drug that stimulates the production of fetal hemoglobin (Hb F), which is a determinant in the clinical severity of patients with SCD. The clinical trials completed to date have demonstrated encouraging findings (Hoppe et al., 2000; Kinney et al., 1999; Rogers, 1997; Vichinsky, 1997; Ware, Zimmerman, & Schultz, 1999). Finally, use of bone marrow transplantation holds promise for some patients with SCD (Hoppe & Walters, 2001; Nietert, Abboud, Silverstein, & Jackson, 2000; Walters et al., 2000).

## Biopsychosocial Models of Adaptation to Chronic Illness

Concurrent with the advances in the biomedical sciences, there have been advances in behavioral science. First, information technology has advanced such that increasingly sophisticated data analytic methods are possible that allow consideration of multiple variables. Second, conceptual models have been promulgated that address the complexity and multiple determinants of human behavior (Thompson & Gustafson, 1996). Underlying these conceptual models has been the biopsychosocial approach that includes consideration of psychosocial factors in addition to biomedical factors. Examples of these models are described next.

The social-ecological systems theory perspective formulated by Bronfenbrenner (1977, 1979) has had the most impact on our understanding of adaptation to chronic childhood illness. Social ecology has been defined as "the study of the relation between the developing human being and the settings and contexts in which the person is actively involved" (Kazak, 1989, p. 26). The social ecological theory proposes that the child is in the center of a series of concentric rings, and that the rings represent the settings that have bidirectional influences on the child. The concentric rings that are closest to the child represent the family and settings, such as school, whereas the more distant rings represent societal values and culture. There are several major tenets of the social ecological theory. First, not only does the environment affect the child, but also the child affects the environment. Second, there are interconnections between the settings that influence the child's development. Third, there are transitions or successive shifts in roles and settings across the life span that have developmental significance for the child (Bronfenbrenner, 1979).

The transactional model of development (Sameroff & Chandler, 1975) also has been influential in terms of the focus on the effect that children have on the environment through their specific characteristics and on the bidirectional influence between the child and the parents over time. Children are seen as active participants in shaping their environment rather than as passive participants in the socialization process of the family and larger social environment.

Also relevant to understanding the impact of chronic illness on children and the family has been the impact of parents' child-rearing behaviors, or parenting processes, on child development (Thompson & Gustafson, 1996). Processes that have been considered important include the effect on parenting behaviors of maternal cognitions, such as beliefs, appraisals, expectations, and attributions, which in turn affect children's development. Maternal cognitions about children's development reflect the influence of the sociocultural environment (Miller, 1988) and guide mothers' responses to their children's behavior (Mills & Rubin, 1990; Rubin, Mills, & Rose-Krasnor, 1989). Maternal stress and distress also influence maternal appraisals and expectations of children's behavior and development (Crnic & Greenberg, 1990) and mothers' behavioral interactions with their children (Webster-Stratton, 1990). Indeed, lower social and cognitive competencies in children have been associated with daily parenting stress and maternal depression (Crnic & Greenberg, 1990; Lyons-Ruth, Zoll, Connell, & Grunebaum, 1986).

Chronic childhood illness has been conceptualized as a potential stressor to which the child and family systems endeavor to adapt (Thompson & Gustafson, 1996). Drawing from the body of literature on stress and coping processes, stress is conceptualized as not inherent in the situation itself but as arising from person-environment transactions (Lazarus & Folkman, 1984). Stress is associated with the person's appraisal of the degree of threat in a situation relative to the available environmental resources and individual coping skills. Adjustment has been associated with cognitive appraisals (Lazarus & Folkman, 1984) and with expectations of self-efficacy (Bandura, 1977) and of control (Strickland, 1978). Social support has been shown to mitigate the effects of stress (Haggerty, 1980).

## Biopsychosocial Models of Adaptation to Sickle Cell Disease

There have been two biopsychosocial models of adaptation to illness that have been evaluated in the specific situation of adaptation to SCD: the transactional stress and coping model of Thompson and colleagues (Thompson, Gil, Burbach, Keith, & Kinney, 1993; 1993b; Thompson, Gustafson, George, & Spock, 1994; Thompson & Gustafson, 1996) and the risk-resistance adaptation model developed by Wallander and colleagues (Wallander & Varni, 1992; Wallander, Varni, Babani, Banis, & Wilcox, 1988, 1989).

The transactional stress and coping model has sought to understand the independent and combined influence of biomedical and psychosocial processes in understanding adaptation in children and adolescents with SCD and their mothers (Thompson & Gustafson, 1996). This model utilizes a social-ecological systems theory perspective (Bronfenbrenner, 1977). In this model, shown in

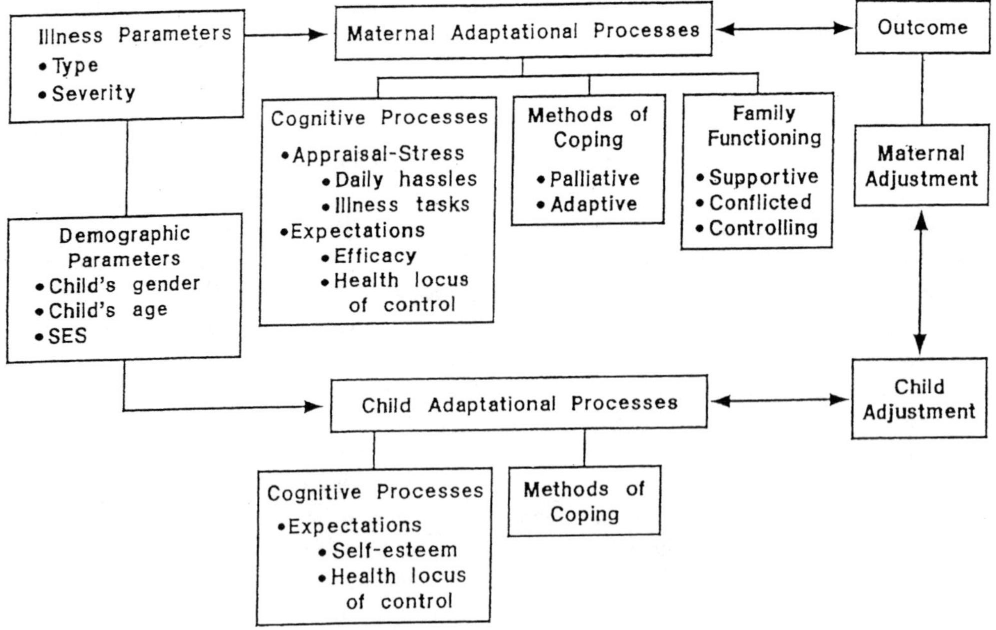


**Figure 23-1.** Transactional stress and coping model of adjustment to chronic illness. SES, socioeconomic status. From "Change Over a 12-Month Period in the Psychological Adjustment of Children and Adolescents With Cystic Fibrosis," by R. J. Thompson, Jr., K. E. Gustafson, L. K. George, and A. Spock, 1994, *Journal of Pediatric Psychology, 19*, 189–203. Reprinted with permission.

figure 23-1, chronic illness is viewed as a potential stressor to which the individual child and family system endeavor to adapt. The illness-outcome relationship is hypothesized to be a function of the transactions among biomedical, developmental, and psychosocial processes. The focus of the model is on the child and family processes hypothesized to further mediate the illness-outcome relationship over and above the contributions of the illness and demographic parameters (Thompson & Gustafson, 1996).

The psychosocial mediational processes that were chosen to be included in this model were processes that (a) had empirical evidence that the process served to reduce the impact of stress and (b) were salient as potential intervention targets. Utilizing the ecological-systems theory perspective, it was hypothesized that the psychological adjustment of children was influenced by the levels of stress and distress experienced by other family members, and that the adjustment of other family members was influenced by child adjustment. Thus, adjustment was considered in terms of child adjustment, maternal adjustment, and their interrelationship.

The psychosocial mediational processes of the model that were examined in relationship to psychological adjustment of children with SCD were the cognitive processes of expectations about self-esteem and health locus of control and methods of coping, specifically pain-coping strategies. For maternal adjustment, the psychosocial mediational processes that were included in the model were (a) the cognitive processes of appraisal of daily stress and illness stress, expectations of efficacy regarding managing illness tasks, and health locus of control; (b) coping methods; and (c) social support in terms of family functioning.

Also stemming from the stress and coping tradition is the risk-resistance adaptation model developed by Wallander and colleagues (Wallander & Varni, 1992; Wallander et al., 1988, 1989). This model has also been used to examine adjustment in children with SCD and their caregivers (Brown, Lambert, et al., 2000) as well as in adolescents with SCD (Burlew, Telfair, Colangelo, & Wright, 2000). In this model, shown in figure 23-2, factors that are hypothesized as related to adaptation are organized into a risk-resistance framework. Adaptation is multidimensional and includes mental

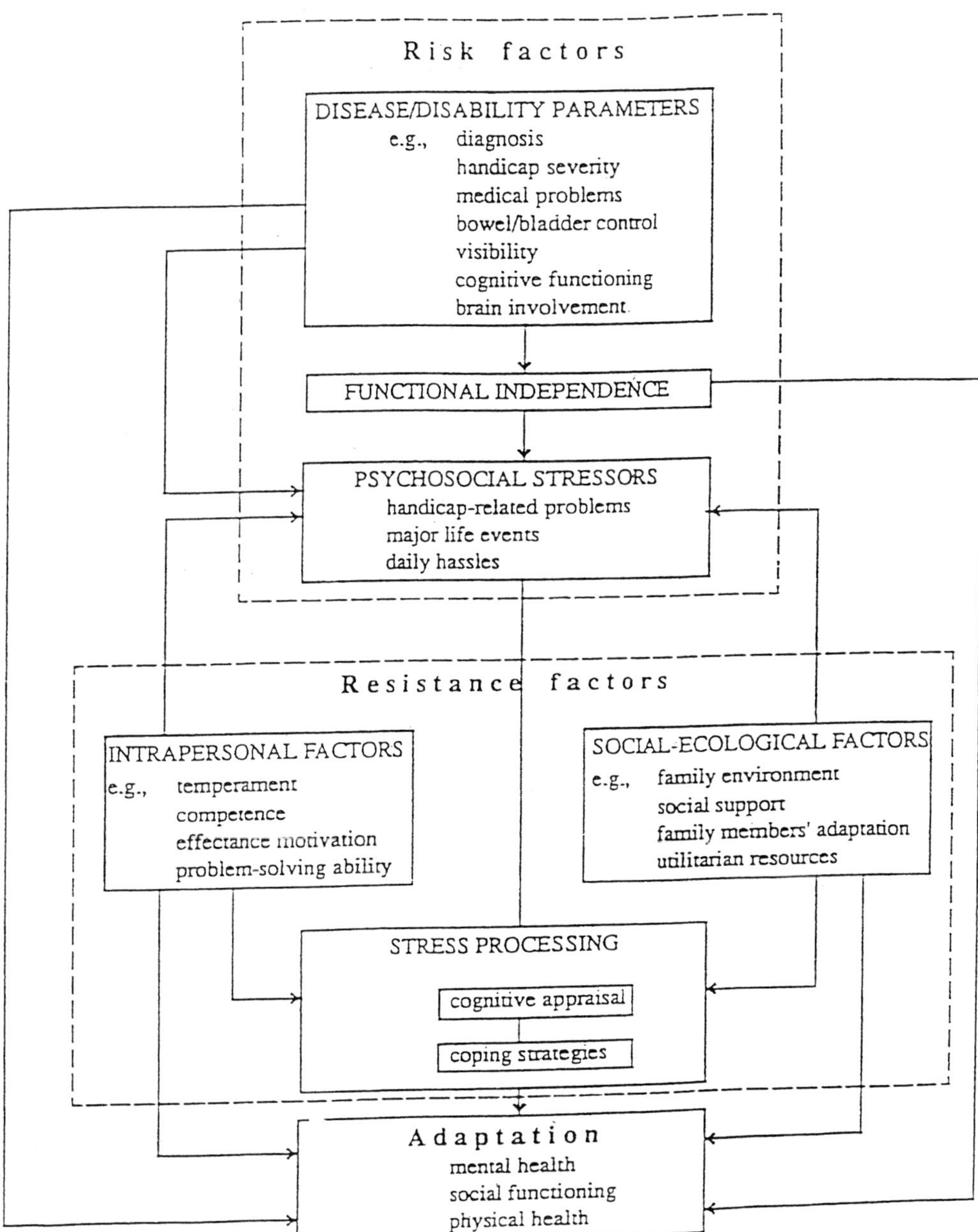


**Figure 23-2.** Disability-stress-coping model of adjustment to chronic illness. From "Children With Chronic Physical Disorders: Maternal Reports of Their Psychological Adjustment," by J. L. Wallander, J. W. Varni, L. Babani, H. T. Banis, and K. T. Wilcox, 1989, *Journal of Pediatric Psychology, 13*, 197–212. Reprinted with permission.

health, social functioning, and physical functioning. There are several stress factors that are hypothesized to increase risk for developing psychosocial problems in children and caregivers. The risk factors include disease/disability parameters such as diagnosis, brain involvement, visibility; functional limitations from the disease; and psychosocial stressors such as major life events, daily hassles, or transitions. Also included in the model are three broad types of resistance factors considered coping resources. First, intrapersonal factors are relatively stable factors, such as temperament, competence, effectance motivation, and problem-solving ability. Second, stress-processing factors include cognitive appraisal and coping behaviors. Third, social ecological factors include family environment, social support, family members' adaptation, and utilitarian resources.

## Model-Driven Studies of Adaptation in Children with Sickle Cell Disease

Studies of adaptation in children with SCD have suggested that these children are at greater risk for emotional adjustment problems than are their non-ill peers; however, good adjustment in these children is also possible. Informed primarily by parent and child report data, investigations have found estimates of psychological problems occurring in one third to almost two thirds of samples (Barbarin, Whitten, & Bond, 1994; Cepeda, Yang, Price, & Shah, 1997; Thompson et al., 1993; Thompson, Gustafson, & Gil, 1995), with internalizing problems (particularly anxiety-based disorders) occurring more frequently than externalizing problems. Barbarin (1999), however, argued that adjustment problems in some children with SCD may reflect the difficulties faced by African American children from financially disadvantaged communities. As such, poverty may be a separate factor contributing to emotional adjustment problems in children with SCD (Barbarin, Whitten, Bond, & Conner-Warren, 1999). In general, studies of adjustment of children with SCD have suggested that there is considerable variability in adaptation, and that biomedical and psychosocial factors should be explored as a means of understanding this variability in outcome.

Most studies of adaptation to SCD have not been driven by biopsychosocial models of adaptation to illness. However, recent studies have attempted to understand the variability in adjustment outcome by employing biopsychosocial models to guide the research.

The transactional stress and coping model (Thompson & Gustafson, 1996) has been used in several studies of adaptation in children and adolescents with SCD and their mothers. In a study of 50 children and adolescents (aged 7 to 14 years) with SCD (Thompson et al., 1993), 50% of children met criteria for one or more diagnoses on a structured diagnostic interview based on the *Diagnostic and Statistical Manual of Mental Disorders*, third edition (*DSM-III*; American Psychiatric Association, 1980). Internalizing diagnoses, including anxiety and phobic and obsessive-compulsive disorders, were the most frequent (38%), whereas externalizing problems, including conduct disorder and oppositional disorder, were infrequent. In terms of mothers' report of child adjustment problems, 36% were reported to be problem free or sociable on the Missouri Children's Behavior Checklist (MCBC) (Sines, Pauker, Sines, & Owen, 1969), whereas 64% were rated as having a behavior problem profile. The most frequent behavior problem profile was the internal behavior problem profile, whereas the external, mixed internal and external, undifferentiated disturbance, and low social skills profiles were infrequent.

In terms of the psychosocial mediational processes of the transactional stress and coping model, with illness and demographic parameters controlled, parental anxiety accounted for 16% and 33% of the variance in mother-reported internalizing and externalizing behavior problems, respectively. Maternal distress did not account for a significant increment in child-reported symptoms on the diagnostic interview. Children's pain-coping strategies, specifically negative thinking strategies, accounted for a 20% increment in variance in child-reported symptoms. The variables of the transactional stress and coping model accounted for 30% of the variance in child-reported symptoms and 45%–49% of the variance in mother-reported behavior problems, respectively (Thompson et al., 1993a).

In a sample of 35 adolescents (13–17 years old) with SCD, 51% of the adolescents reported symptoms that yielded at least one *DSM-III* diagnosis on the diagnostic interview (Thompson et al., 1995). The most frequent diagnoses were anxiety disorders (26%), phobic disorder (23%), and oppositional disorder (14%). Relative to adolescents with good adjustment, adolescents with poor adjustment had significantly lower expectations of efficacy regarding illness tasks, higher levels of palliative coping, and pain-coping strategies characterized by negative thinking and passive adherence. Negative thinking pain-coping strategies and palliative illness coping accounted for 52% of the variance in adjustment.

Given the importance of a developmental perspective to understanding adjustment in children and adolescents with SCD, the participants in these studies were followed longitudinally to examine patterns of adjustment over time. In 35 children (aged 7 to 14 years at study entry) who completed the initial and follow-up protocols (average of 10 months later), adjustment was again assessed using the children's reports on the diagnostic interview and mother's reports on the MCBC (Thompson, Gil, Burbach et al., 1994). Of the children, 29% had stable poor adjustment (*DSM-III* diagnosis at both times), and 31% of the children had stable good adjustment (no diagnosis at either time). There were 40% of the children who changed classification on the diagnostic interview over the 10-month period. Anxiety diagnoses were the most common at the initial and follow-up assessment points. There was little congruence, however, in specific diagnoses on the diagnostic interview across the initial and follow-up assessment points.

On the MCBC, 60% of the children at the initial assessment and 69% of the children at the follow-up assessment obtained a behavior problem profile. A behavior problem profile was obtained at both assessment points for 49% of the children, and a problem-free profile was obtained at both points for 20% of the children. The internal behavior problem profile was the most frequent at both assessment points, but there was little congruence in specific behavior patterns at entry into the study and at follow-up. Thus, although the group data reflect consistency in rate of adjustment problems based on child and mother report, there were changes in the adjustment classification of individual children and in specific diagnoses and behavior patterns (Thompson, Gil, Burbach, et al., 1994).

In terms of the variables of the transactional stress and coping model, with initial levels of child adjustment controlled, children's pain-coping strategies accounted for a significant increment in child-reported symptoms (19%) and mother-reported internalizing symptoms (8%). These findings suggest that decreasing pain-coping strategies characterized by negative thinking and increasing coping attempts strategies may be helpful in efforts to enhance adjustment in children with SCD (Thompson et al., 1994). Indeed, researchers have demonstrated that children and adolescents with high levels of coping attempts maintained greater levels of social, school, and home activities than those with "negative thinking" or "passive adherence" coping styles (Gil, Williams, Thompson, & Kinney, 1991; Gil et al., 1993, 1997).

Thompson and colleagues also extended the longitudinal investigation of children and adolescents with SCD and their mothers to a third assessment point approximately 2 years after study entry (Thompson, Gustafson, Gil, Kinney & Spock, 1999). Included in this second follow-up investigation were 50 children with SCD and their mothers who had data at all three assessment points. Child-reported total symptom scores declined over time. Consistently good adjustment was reported by 17% of the children, and consistently poor adjustment was reported by 15% of the children. There was a very low level of consistency in classification across time based on child report of symptoms.

Rates of mother-reported behavior problems also declined over time (Thompson, Gustafson, et al., 1999). Consistently good adjustment was reported for 19% and consistently poor adjustment was reported for 47% of the children based on mother report, with a moderate level of stability in classification. Mothers who reported their children as consistently demonstrating behavior problems had higher levels of self-reported anxiety, depression, and overall distress than mothers who consistently reported their children as demonstrating good adjustment. Child pain coping characterized by use of negative thinking and fewer coping attempts at baseline was associated with higher levels of child-reported symptoms at the 2-year follow-up. Lower child self-worth and higher maternal anxiety at baseline accounted for significant increments in variance in mother-reported child behavior problems at follow-up.

The Cooperative Study of Sickle Cell Disease examined family functioning and behavior problems in a large sample of children with SCD. In the initial cross-sectional study of 289 children, 30% evidenced a mother-reported behavior problem (Thompson, Armstrong et al., 1999). Demographic and biomedical variables only accounted for 4% of the variance in child behavior problems, whereas family functioning characterized by high levels of conflict and a lack of organization and support accounted for an additional 19% of the variance. A prospective, longitudinal study of 222 children who had two complete sets of data over the 9-year study period (Thompson et al., 2003) revealed that 9% of the children demonstrated stable behavior problems over time. Stable behavior problems over time were associated with higher initial levels of family conflict, and an increase in behavior problems was associated with an increase in family conflict. Thus, maternal appraisal of family functioning characterized by conflict appears to be a significant risk factor for behavior problems in children with SCD.

The risk-resistance model (Wallander & Varni, 1992; Wallander et al., 1988, 1989) has been used in a study to examine adjustment in 55 children aged 5 to 16 years with SCD and their primary caregivers (Brown, Lambert, et al., 2000). Consistent with the risk-resistance model, risk factors were examined, including disease parameters (disease severity, diagnosis, symptom frequency); functional independence (adaptive behavior, activities of daily living); and caregiver's psychosocial stressors (income, social class, family stress). Resistance factors were also examined, including the children's intrapersonal resources (competence, self-esteem, health locus of control); caregivers' social ecological factors (family functioning, family social support and resources); and caregivers' stress processing (coping strategies). Child adjustment was assessed using parent report on the CBCL (Achenbach, 1991).

In terms of parent report of child adjustment, 20% met criteria for poor adjustment in terms of internalizing problems (e.g., symptoms of anxiety, depression), and 35% met criteria for poor adjustment in terms of externalizing problems (e.g., acting-out behaviors). Using the risk-resistance model, only child health locus of control emerged as a significant predictor of child internalizing and externalizing problems. Children's reports of a cognitive processing style characterized by internal beliefs of expectation of control over their health were associated with better child adjustment. There were trends toward risk factors, including adaptive behavior and self-esteem, in predicting child adjustment (Brown et al., 2000).

The risk-resistance model was also employed in a national sample of 90 adolescents with SCD aged 14 to 19 years who had participated in the Cooperative Study of Sickle Cell Disease (Burlew et al., 2000). Adjustment was assessed using measures of state and trait anxiety and depressive symptoms. Intrapersonal factors included social assertion, self-esteem, and positive outlook. The stress-processing variables were coping style and general knowledge of SCD. The social-ecological variable was family environment. Of the sample, 26% reported mild-to-severe levels of depressive symptoms, whereas state and trait anxiety scores were generally below the mean scores of the normative sample. Regression analysis revealed that social assertiveness and social support coping contributed significantly to state anxiety. Medical severity did not make a significant contribution to the model. Social assertiveness, self-esteem, social support coping, and family relations all contributed significantly to trait anxiety, whereas medical severity did not contribute significantly to the model. Self-esteem and family relations contributed significantly to the variability in depressive symptoms, whereas medical severity did not contribute significantly.

In summary, these model-driven studies of adaptation in children and adolescents with SCD have provided some support for variables of the biopsychosocial models. Findings from both the risk-resistance model and the transactional stress and coping model suggest that psychosocial factors contribute significantly more to adjustment than do biomedical factors. Factors associated with better adjustment in children and adolescents with SCD include intrapersonal factors such as having an internal health locus of control or positive self-esteem, stress-processing factors such as pain-coping strategies that deemphasize negative thinking, and social ecological factors such as family relationships and functioning. These factors suggest that interventions that target cognitive processes such as self-esteem and health locus of control, stress processes such as pain coping, and social-ecological factors such as family functioning may be important for enhancing adaptation to the stressor of SCD.

## Model-Driven Studies of Adaptation in Caregivers of Children With Sickle Cell Disease

Caregiver adjustment to SCD has also been examined using the transactional stress and coping model to guide the research. The psychological adjustment of 78 mothers of children and adolescents (aged 7 to 17 years) was assessed in a cross-sectional study (Thompson et al., 1993). Good adjustment was reported by 64% and poor adjustment was reported by 36% of the mothers on the Symptom Checklist-90-R (Derogatis, 1983), which is a self-report measure of psychological distress. Good and poor adjustment subgroups did not differ significantly on any of the illness or demographic variables. However, compared to mothers with poor adjustment, mothers with good adjustment had significantly lower levels of daily stress, less use of palliative coping, a lower ratio of palliative to adaptive coping, and higher levels of family supportiveness. Significant increments in variance in maternal distress was accounted for over and above that accounted for by the illness and demographic variables by ratio of palliative to adaptive coping, stress of daily hassles, and family functioning emphasizing control. Together, the variables of the model accounted for 55% of the variance in maternal distress, with 46% accounted for by the psychosocial adaptation processes (Thompson et al., 1993).

In a subsequent longitudinal study, 60 mothers of the original cohort completed a follow-up assessment 8–16 months later (Thompson et al., 1994). Maternal adjustment did not change significantly over time. However, the rate of poor adjustment decreased from 37% initially to 28% at follow-up. Twenty percent of mothers reported poor adjustment at both assessment points, and 55% of mothers reported good adjustment at both assessment points. Compared with mothers with stable poor adjustment, mothers with stable good adjustment had significantly lower levels of daily stress and illness stress, less use of palliative coping methods overall and in relation to adaptive coping methods, and higher levels of family supportiveness.

In the second follow-up study, approximately 2 years after study entry, there was an increase in the rate of poor adjustment over time from 30% to 41% of mothers of children with SCD (Thompson, Gustafson, Gil, Kinney, & Spock, 1999). Consistently good adjustment was demonstrated by 43% of the mothers, and consistently poor adjustment was demonstrated by 13% of the mothers. Markers of stable good and poor adjustment subgroups were examined. Mothers with stable good adjustment differed significantly from those with stable poor adjustment in terms of lower levels of daily stress and illness stress and lower levels of palliative coping methods in relation to adaptive methods. More daily stress, higher use of palliative coping, lower use of adaptive coping, and higher levels of family control at baseline were associated with higher maternal distress at the 2-year follow-up assessment.

In the sample of mothers of adolescents with SCD (Thompson et al., 1995), 33% of mothers met criteria for poor adjustment. However, maternal distress was not related to adolescent SCD illness severity measures, but maternal distress was associated with illness-related stress, daily hassles, and palliative coping. Of the variance in maternal depression, 57% was accounted for by the stress of daily hassles and stress regarding illness tasks. Thirty-four percent of the variance in maternal anxiety was accounted for by the stress of daily hassles.

Brown and colleagues (2000) also assessed caregiver adjustment using the risk-resistance model to guide their research. As with the Thompson et al. studies, caregiver adjustment was assessed using the Symptom Checklist-90-R (Deragotis, 1983). Findings revealed that 35% of caregivers met criteria for poor adjustment on this measure. Caregiver adjustment was associated primarily with stress-processing variables in terms of caregiver coping strategies. Greater use of disengagement coping strategies was associated with poorer adjustment. The risk factors of the model, including disease severity and caregiver psychosocial stress, were not associated with caregiver adjustment. Moreover, other than stress processing, the resistance factors (family functioning, family social support) were not associated with caregiver adjustment (Brown et al., 2000).

Thus, these studies support the role of several of the processes of the biopsychosocial models that have been promulgated for understanding the variability in maternal adjustment in mothers of children and adolescents with SCD. As with the studies of adjustment in children and adolescents, the biomedical factors did not contribute significantly to adjustment. Factors associated with better caregiver adjustment included coping strategies that deemphasize disengagement and palliative methods and that are more active and adaptive; lower perceptions of daily and illness stress; and more functional family relationships. Thus, interventions that enhance coping, address stress management, and improve family relationships are likely to enhance adaptation in the situation of the stressor of SCD. Nonetheless, a considerable amount of variance in maternal adjustment has not been accounted for, which suggests the need for assessment of other psychosocial variables that are salient to adjustment in mothers of children with SCD. For example, processes of care taking and child rearing (i.e., parenting processes) could affect not only the parent's and the child's psychological adjustment but also the cognitive and social-emotional development of the child.

Thompson and colleagues examined these factors in a subsequent study that looked at adjustment in mothers of infants and toddlers diagnosed with SCD (Thompson, Gustafson, Bonner, & Ware, 2002). The contributions of biomedical risk, parent cognitive processes of daily stress and attributional style, and family functioning to parent psychological adjustment were examined in this study. However, it was further hypothesized that these parents would be at risk for a learned helplessness attributional style given the uncontrollability of events associated with SCD. A learned helplessness attributional style would negatively affect parenting and influence parental adaptation. Cognitions about and knowledge of child development were also deemed relevant to parenting processes and were included as variables that affect parenting.

Consistent with studies of parents of older children, 24% of parents of young children evidenced clinical levels of psychological distress. Regression analyses revealed that parent distress was associated with the Hb SC phenotype, higher levels of daily stress, lower parent expectations of efficacy, and less knowledge of child development. These variables accounted for 49% of the variance in parent distress. Thus, findings of the role of daily stress and parent efficacy expectations appear quite robust across studies of parents with a wide age range of children with SCD. Family functioning appears important in adjustment in parents of children and adolescents but did not emerge as a salient factor in adjustment of these parents of young children. Cognitions about and knowledge of child development, but not attributions of learned helplessness, are important parenting processes associated with parent adjustment. It also is important to understand the role of these processes in child neurocognitive development and outcome, described next. Thompson and colleagues (2002) did investigate these processes in terms of child neurodevelopmental outcome as well.

## Neurodevelopmental Considerations in Sickle Cell Disease

A relatively large body of research has examined neurocognitive and academic performance of children with SCD. Most studies have not been driven by biopsychosocial frameworks and have not considered risk factors beyond the biomedical risk of the illness itself to neurocognitive functioning. Sociodemographic factors have largely been ignored (Brown, Armstrong, & Eckman, 1993), as have important socioenvironmental variables such as parenting process variables (Thompson et al., 2002).

The available evidence has suggested that children with SCD are at increased risk for neurocognitive impairment, with lower intellectual functioning and greater neuropsychological deficits in patients with SCD compared with sibling controls (Brown, Buchanan et al., 1993; Swift et al., 1989; Wasserman et al., 1991). Deficits have been seen primarily in the areas of visual motor integration, attention and concentration, memory (Fowler et al., 1988; Wasserman, Wilimas, Fairclough, Mulhern, & Wang, 1991), mathematics (Wasserman et al., 1991), and reading and spelling (Fowler et al., 1988).

The nature and severity of the neurocognitive deficits seen in children with SCD vary as a function of several variables, including the presence of cerebral infarction. Studies investigating the impact of overt clinical stroke on cognitive functioning in children with SCD have demonstrated expected findings, with the location and pattern of the stroke affecting the pattern of neuropsychological deficits. Left hemisphere stroke results in expected impairments in language functions, including verbal intelligence, language, and immediate verbal/auditory memory, whereas right hemisphere stroke results in relative difficulties with nonverbal/spatial functions (M. J. Cohen, Branch, McKie, & Adams, 1997). Anterior strokes have been associated with deficits in attention, executive functioning, and verbal working memory (Craft, Schatz, Glauser, Lee, & DeBaun, 1993; Schatz et al., 1999; White, Salorio, Schatz, & DeBaun, 2000).

Although children with overt evidence of stroke have more significant neuropsychological impairment than children with silent stroke, children with silent stroke do demonstrate a pattern of neuropsychological difficulties that are greater than that of children with no magnetic resonance imaging abnormalities (Armstrong et al., 1996). Children with silent stroke perform more poorly than children without silent stroke on tests of arithmetic, vocabulary, and visual-motor speed (Armstrong et al., 1996) and on tasks requiring sustained attention (Brown, Davis, et al., 2000). Moreover, magnetic resonance imaging abnormalities without evidence of clinical stroke have been associated with greater variability in neuropsychological performance in terms of subtest scatter and score discrepancies, although not with IQ or composite scores (Ris, Grueneich, & Kalinyak, 1995). Finally, 60% of a sample of children with silent strokes had been retained in school or required special education services compared with 27% of children without silent stroke and 6% of sibling controls (Schatz, Brown, Pascual, Hsu, & De Baun, 2001). By the end of the third year of follow-up, 74% of children with silent stroke were demonstrating such academic attainment problems.

Variability in neurocognitive functioning of children with SCD may reflect, at least partly, their disproportionately low socioeconomic status (Brown, Buchanan, et al., 1993). Indeed, research has suggested that in general children who are raised in low-income homes demonstrate average cognitive functioning on standardized tests in infancy and demonstrate gradual declines in neurocognitive functioning during the preschool period. By kindergarten, a disproportionate number of children are functioning one or more standard deviations below the mean (Burchinal, Campbell, Bryant, Wasik, & Ramey, 1997). Moreover, cognitive performance is associated with mothers' cognitive functioning, democratic or nonauthoritarian parental attitudes, responsiveness of the infant, and responsiveness and stimulation in the family environment. Given that many children with SCD reside in low-income homes, the cognitive deficits that are seen in some children with SCD occur within the context of early declines in functioning associated with economic disadvantage.

Understanding of factors that are associated with the neurocognitive development of children with SCD is especially important given the large body of literature that supports the high proportion of neurocognitive problems in these children. It is important to determine at what point in children's development the deficits in neurocognitive functioning are initially manifested. Moreover, a biopsychosocial framework is important in understanding the variability in child neurocognitive outcome. This would allow an understanding of the independent and combined contributions of biomedical and psychosocial processes to child cognitive functioning and suggest those factors that could serve as salient intervention targets.

Given that many studies of neurocognitive outcome in school-aged children and adolescents have been completed, Thompson and colleagues (Thompson et al., 2002) sought to extend the assessment of neurocognitive functioning to children with SCD who were preschool aged or younger. This study was guided by the cognitive and stress-processing model of parenting influences on child development (Thompson & Gustafson, 1996), which reflects an integration of the transactional stress and coping model of adaptation to chronic childhood illness (Thompson & Gustafson, 1996) with Belsky's (1984) process model of parenting. Using this model, parenting is affected by parental stress and distress and child characteristics, which in turn affects child developmental outcome. In this study of child neurocognitive outcome, SCD severity variables are considered biomedical risk, and parent cognitive processes, distress, knowledge of child development, and family functioning constitute parenting risk.

This study included 89 young children with SCD and their parents. Measures of child development were obtained at 6, 12, 24, and 36 months of age, and parents completed measures of the cognitive processes of daily stress and attributional style, psychological adjustment, and family functioning. Consistent with that reported in older children, this longitudinal study of early neurocognitive functioning in young children with SCD found that neurocognitive impairment is evident in early childhood, and that there is a significant decline in neurocognitive functioning during the first 36 months of life. By 24 months of age, 29% of the children had mental development scores and 24% of the children had motor development scores that were more than one standard deviation below the mean for the normative group. Mental development, but not motor development, declined over time, with this decline occurring between 12 and 24 months of age. This pattern of decline is consistent with the cognitive declines seen in studies of poor and African American children without chronic illness (Burchinal et al., 1997).

Multiple regression analyses were used to examine the independent and combined contributions of biomedical and parenting risk factors to developmental outcome at 24 months of age. In terms of motor development outcome, only SCD phenotype made a significant contribution. In terms of mental development outcome, however, learned helplessness attributional style by mothers and SCD phenotype both contributed significantly and accounted for 42% of the variance in mental development. Thus, poorer mental and motor developmental outcome was associated with Hb SS phenotype, and poorer mental development was also associated with a learned helplessness attributional style.

## Developmental Issues in Social and School Functioning

Major developmental tasks of childhood are to function adaptively within the school environment and to enjoy positive social relationships with same-age peers. Yet, children with SCD confront challenges in progressing through important normative developmental experiences, including social relationships and school attendance and performance. SCD-related symptoms may interfere with several aspects of children's school and social functioning (Bonner, Gustafson, Schumacher, & Thompson, 1999). If pain is experienced during school hours, children's attention, concentration, and motivation may be adversely affected. Because medications used to manage SCD pain often cause children to feel drowsy or lethargic, children receiving such treatment may have less energy and mental alertness for academic tasks. In addition, as analgesics do not completely control pain in the majority of patients (Beyer, 2000), painful crises may disrupt school attendance for academic or extracurricular activities (Eaton, Haye, Armstrong, Pegelow, & Thomas, 1995; Gil et al., 2000; Shapiro et al., 1995).

Despite the increased risk for challenges to social functioning and peer relationships in children with chronic illness, relatively few studies in this important area have been conducted (LaGreca, 1990, 1992), and fewer still pertain to children with SCD. Numerous factors associated with the direct and indirect affects of SCD on physical, cognitive, and psychosocial functioning may put children with SCD at increased risk for problematic peer relations. Children may be at increased risk for social adjustment problems because of factors associated with functional limitations, medical compliance, and school absenteeism. Indeed, investigators have found that children with SCD spend less time with peers participating in social activities, have fewer friends than non-ill peers (Lemanek, Buckloh, Woods, & Butler, 1995; Schuman, Armstrong, Pegelow, & Routh, 1993), are less well accepted by their peers (Noll et al., 1996), and are rated as less socially competent (Barbarin, 1999).

Moreover, Nassau and Drotar (1997) noted that the cognitive difficulties exhibited by some children with SCD secondary to stroke or other disease processes also interfere with competency in the social domain. Specifically, nonverbal skill deficits may make it difficult for children to perceive or comprehend important subtle features of many social interactions. Indeed, children with SCD with CNS involvement have been found to exhibit more difficulties with social information processing and emotional functioning than children with SCD without CNS involvement or children with milder forms of SCD (Boni, Brown, Davis, Hsu, & Hopkins, 2001). These groups of children did not differ in routine social situations, whereas situations that were more complex or ambiguous posed a more significant problem for children with SCD with CNS involvement. Furthermore, problems associated with inattention and impulsivity may make children less desirable as playmates because of their inability to follow the rules or organization of group activities. Finally, poor academic functioning has been associated in the developmental literature with peer rejection (see Asher & Parker, 1989; Wentzel & Asher, 1995).

## Conclusion

Advances in medical care have resulted in improved medical management and a more favorable long-term prognosis for children with SCD. Early diagnosis through newborn screening programs has enabled initiation of prophylactic treatment and entry into comprehensive care programs that have reduced mortality and morbidity. Nonetheless, SCD can disrupt the normal processes of children's development and family functioning, as well as the transactions between the child and his or her environment. Children and their caregivers are at increased risk for poor adaptation when confronting this disease. However, biopsychosocial conceptual frameworks have enhanced our understanding of the correlates of risk status in terms of processes that mediate cognitive and psychosocial outcome.

Adaptation to SCD has been assessed in terms of psychosocial adjustment, particularly in terms of whether a child's functioning is age appropriate, normative, and following a trajectory toward positive adult functioning (Wallander & Thompson, 1995). Adjustment is multidimensional and involves behavioral and emotional adjustment, self-esteem, social functioning, and school performance. Children and adolescents with SCD are at increased risk primarily for internalizing, anxiety-based problems, with externalizing problems much less frequent. These children are also at risk for neurocognitive problems associated with both clinical and silent stroke, and these problems in turn can affect school and social functioning. Despite this risk, good adjustment is possible and is the most likely outcome. Psychosocial factors that are associated with risk and resistance in the face of the threat of this illness have been delineated and include self-esteem; health locus of control; coping methods, particularly pain coping; and family functioning.

Consistent with a systems theory perspective, parental and family functioning also have been considered important both in terms of independent outcomes and in terms of the impact on child functioning. Assessments of caregiver adjustment have also revealed a greater risk for poor outcome, with caregivers reporting elevated levels of psychological distress. Factors associated with risk and resiliency have included daily and illness stress, coping methods, family functioning, and knowledge of child development. Studies of adjustment in caregivers have predominantly assessed adjustment in mothers, with few studies examining adjustment in fathers or other caregivers. Studies of siblings have also been underrepresented in the literature.

Moreover, studies have primarily employed cross-sectional designs, with only a few extant longitudinal studies. Those longitudinal studies that have been completed have shown that there is considerable variability in adjustment at the level of the individual. Markers of stable poor adjustment in children include more use of pain-coping strategies characterized by negative thinking and higher levels of conflictual family functioning. Markers of stable poor adjustment in mothers include more daily stress and illness stress, higher use of palliative coping, and lower levels of family supportiveness. These initial longitudinal studies are beginning to provide important information about adjustment as a function of illness course and developmental transitions.

These investigations of the biopsychosocial models have demonstrated that psychosocial processes appear much more significant to the variability in outcome of children and caregivers than are biomedical parameters. However, the findings of these studies only account for approximately 30–55% of the variance in adjustment in children and caregivers. Considerable variance remains unaccounted for, which attests to the need to incorporate additional relevant psychosocial processes into these models.

Nonetheless, the enhanced understanding offered by biopsychosocial research provides an opportunity to delineate salient intervention targets and to develop effective prevention and treatment programs that will improve the quality of life of children and families affected by this disease. First, improved coping methods, both general coping methods and pain-coping methods, would be important to improving adjustment in children with SCD and their caregivers. Indeed, interventions to promote effective pain coping have been investigated with promising results (Gil et al., 2001). Second, enhancement of family functioning through family systems-based interventions would also likely serve to improve outcome in these families. Third, parenting processes could also serve as salient intervention targets. Interventions could be designed to reduce parental stress and distress and to promote parenting knowledge and skills that are conducive to child cognitive and socioemotional development. Interventions with parents could also help parents support their children's efforts in dealing effectively with the tasks of the illness as well as the tasks of maintaining normative, age-appropriate interactions and functioning across their developmental course.

Although our current knowledge base is still incomplete and demonstrates many areas for continued inquiry, the research is sufficient to warrant moving to systematic intervention studies. Such experimental-level research will allow further refinement of the biopsychosocial models and provide us with more effective intervention methods for enhancing the quality of life of individuals with SCD through fostering optimal cognitive and psychosocial development in these children and more positive adaptation in caregivers and family members.

## References


Achenbach, T. M. (1991). *Manual for the Child Behavior Checklist and Revised Child Behavior Profile.* Burlington, VT: University of Vermont.

Adams, R. J. (2000). Lessons from the Stroke Prevention Trial in Sickle Cell Anemia (STOP) study. *Journal of Child Neurology, 15*, 344–349.

Adams, R. J., McKie, V.C., Brambilla, D., Carl, E., Gallagher, D., Nichols, F.T., et al. (1998). Stroke prevention trial in sickle cell anemia. *Controlled Clinical Trials, 19*, 110–129.

American Psychiatric Association. (1980). *Diagnostic and statistical manual of mental disorders* (3rd ed.). Washington, DC: Author.

Armstrong, F. D., Thompson, R. J., Jr., Wang, W., Zimmerman, R. A., Pegelow, C. H., Miller, S., et al. (1996). Cognitive functioning and brain magnetic resonance imaging in children with sickle cell disease. *Pediatrics, 97*, 864–870.

Asher, S. R., & Parker, J. G. (1989). Significance of peer relationship problems in childhood. In B. H. Schneider & G. Attili, G. (Eds.), *Social competence in developmental perspective* (NATO Advanced Science Institutes Series, Series D: Behavioural and Social Sciences, Vol. 51, pp. 5–23). Dordrecht, The Netherlands: Kluwer.

Balkaran, B., Char, G., Morris, J. S., Thomas, P. W., Serjeant, B. E., & Sergeant, G. R. (1992). Stroke in a cohort of patients with homozygous sickle cell disease. *Journal of Pediatrics, 120*, 360–366.

Bandura, A. (1977). Self-efficacy: Toward a unifying theory of behavioral change. *Psychological Review, 84*, 191–215.

Barbarin, O. A. (1999). Do parental coping, involvement, religiosity, and racial identity mediate children's psychological adjustment to sickle cell disease. *Journal of Black Psychology, 25*, 391–426.

Barbarin, O. A., Whitten, C. F., & Bond, S. (1994). Estimating rates of psychosocial problems in urban and poor children with sickle cell anemia. *Health and Social Work, 19*, 112–119.

Barbarin, O. A., Whitten, C. F., Bond, S., & Conner-Warren, R. (1999). The social and cultural context of coping with sickle cell disease: II. The role of financial hardship in adjustment to sickle cell disease. *Journal of Black Psychology, 25*, 294–315.

Belsky, J. (1984). The determinants of parenting: A process model. *Child Development, 55*, 83–96.

Beyer, J. E. (2000). Judging the effectiveness of analgesia for children and adolescents during vaso-occlusive events of sickle cell disease. *Journal of Pain and Symptom Management, 19*, 63–72.

Boni, L. C., Brown, R. T., Davis, P. C., Hsu, L., & Hopkins, K. (2001). Social information processing and magnetic resonance imaging in children with sickle cell disease. *Journal of Pediatric Psychology, 26*, 309–319.

Bonner, M. J., Gustafson, K. E., Schumacher, E., & Thompson, R. J., Jr. (1999). The impact of sickle cell disease on cognitive functioning and learning. *School Psychology Review, 28*, 182–193.

Bronfenbrenner, U. (1977). Toward an experimental ecology of human development. *American Psychologist, 32*, 513–531.

Bronfenbrenner, U. (1979). *The ecology of human development.* Cambridge, MA: Harvard University Press.

Brown, R. T., Armstrong, F. D., & Eckman, J. R. (1993). Neurocognitive aspects of pediatric sickle cell disease. *Journal of Learning Disabilities, 26*, 33–45.

Brown, R. T., Buchanan, I., Doepke, K., Eckman, J. R., Baldwin, K., Goonan, B., et al. (1993). Cognitive and academic functioning in children with sickle cell disease. *Journal of Clinical Child Psychology, 22*, 207–218.

Brown, R. T., Davis, P. C., Lambert, R., Hsu, L., Hopkins, K., & Eckman, J. (2000). Neurocognitive functioning and magnetic resonance imaging in children with sickle cell disease. *Journal of Pediatric Psychology, 25*, 503–513.

Brown, R. T., Lambert, R., Devine, D., Baldwin, K., Casey, R., Doepke, K., et al. (2000). Risk-resistance adaptation model for caregivers and their children with sickle cell syndromes. *Annals of Behavioral Medicine, 22,* 158–169.

Burchinal, M. R., Campbell, F. A., Bryant, D. M., Wasik, B. H., & Ramey, C. T. (1997). Early intervention and mediating processes in cognitive performance of children of low-income African-American families. *Child Development, 68,* 935–954.

Burlew, K., Telfair, J., Colangelo, L., & Wright, E. C. (2000). Factors that influence adolescent adaptation to sickle cell disease. *Journal of Pediatric Psychology, 25,* 287–299.

Cepeda, M. L., Yang, Y., Price, C., & Shah, A. (1997). Mental disorders in children and adolescents with sickle cell disease. Sout*hern Medical Journal, 90,* 284–287.

Charache, S. (1994). Natural history of disease: Adults. In S. H., Embury, R. P. Hebbel, N. Mohandas, & M. H. Steinberg (Eds.), *Sickle cell disease: Basic principles and clinical practice* (pp. 413–421). New York: Raven Press.

Charache, S., Lubin, B., & Reid, C. D. (1989). *Management and therapy of sickle cell disease* (NIH Publication No. 89-2117). Washington, DC: National Institutes of Health.

Cohen, A. R. (1998). Sickle cell disease: New treatments, new questions [Editorial]. *The New England Journal of Medicine, 339,* 42–44.

Cohen, M. J., Branch, W. B., McKie, V. C., & Adams, R. J. (1997). Neuropsychological impairment in children with sickle cell anemia and cerebrovascular accidents. *Clinical Pediatrics, 33,* 517–524.

Craft, S., Schatz, J., Glauser, T., Lee, B., & DeBaun, M. (1993). Neuropsychological effects of stroke in children with sickle cell anemia. *Journal of Pediatrics, 123,* 712–717.

Crnic, K. A., & Greenberg, M. T. (1990). Minor parenting stress with young children. *Child Development, 61,* 1628–1637.

Derogatis, L. R. (1983). *SCL-90-R: Administration, scoring, and procedures manual II.* Baltimore, MD: Clinical Psychometrics Research.

Eaton, M. L., Haye, J. S., Armstrong, F. D., Pegelow, C. H., & Thomas, M. (1995). Hospitalizations for painful episodes: Association with school absenteeism and academic performance in children and adolescents with sickle cell anemia. *Issues in Comprehensive Pediatric Nursing, 18,* 1–9.

Fowler, M. G., Whitt, J. K., Lallinger, R. R., Nash, K. B., Atkinson, S. S., Wells, R. J., et al. (1988). Neuropsychologic and academic functioning of children with sickle cell anemia. *Developmental and Behavioral Pediatrics, 9,* 213–220.

Gil, K. M., Anthony, K. K., Carson, J. W., Redding-Lallinger, R., Daeschner, C. W., & Ware, R. E. (2001). Daily coping practice predicts treatment effects in children with sickle cell disease. *Journal of Pediatric Psychology, 26,* 163–173.

Gil, K. M., Porter, L. S., Ready, J., Workman, E., Sedway, J., & Anthony, K. K. (2000). Pain in children and adolescents with sickle-cell disease: An analysis of daily pain diaries. *Children's Health Care, 29,* 225–241.

Gil, K. M., Thompson, R. J., Jr., Keith, B. R., Tota-Faucette, M., Noll, S., & Kinney, T.R. (1993). Sickle cell disease pain in children and adolescents: Change in pain frequency and coping strategies over time. *Journal of Pediatric Psychology, 18,* 621–637.

Gil, K. M., Williams, D. A., Thompson, R. J., Jr., & Kinney, T. R. (1991). Sickle cell disease in children and adolescents: The relation of child and parent pain coping strategies to adjustment. *Journal of Pediatric Psychology, 16,* 643–663.

Gil, K. M., Wilson, J. J., Edens, J. L., Workman, E., Ready, J., Sedway, J., et al. (1997). Cognitive coping skills training in children with sickle cell disease. *International Journal of Behavioral Medicine, 4,* 365–378.

Hagar, R. W., & Vichinsky, E. P. (2000). Major changes in sickle cell disease. *Advances in Pediatrics, 47,* 249–272.

Haggerty, R. J. (1980). Life stress, illness, and social supports. *Developmental Medicine and Child Neurology, 22,* 391–400.

Hindmarsh, P. C., Brozovic, M., Brook C. G., & Davies, S. C. (1987). Incidence of overt and covert neurological damage in children with sickle cell disease. *Postgraduate Medical Journal, 63,* 751–753.

Hoppe, C., Vichinsky, E., Quirolo, K., van Warmerdam, J., Allen, K., & Styles, L. (2000). Use of hydroxyurea in children 2–5 with sickle cell disease. *Journal of Pediatric Hematology/Oncology, 22,* 330–334.

Hoppe, C. C., & Walters, M. C. (2001). Bone marrow transplantation in sickle cell anemia. *Current Opinion in Oncology, 13,* 85–90.

Kazak, A. E. (1989). Families of chronically ill children: A systems and social-ecological model of adaptation and challenge. *Journal of Consulting and Clinical Psychology, 57,* 25–30.

Kinney, T. R., Sleeper, L. A., Wang, W. C., Zimmerman, R. A., Pegelow, C. H., Ohene-Frempong, K., et al. (1999). Silent cerebral infarcts in sickle cell anemia: A risk factor analysis. *Pediatrics, 103,* 640–645.

LaGreca, A. M. (1990). Social consequences of pediatric conditions: Fertile area for future investigation and intervention. *Journal of Pediatric Psychology, 15,* 285–307.

LaGreca, A. M. (1992). Peer influences in pediatric chronic illness: An update. *Journal of Pediatric Psychology, 17,* 775–784.

Lazarus, R. S., & Folkman, S. (1984). *Stress, appraisal, and coping.* New York: Springer.

Lemanek, K. L., Buckloh, L., Woods, G., & Butler, R. (1995). Diseases of the circulatory system: Sickle cell disease and hemophilia. In M. Roberts (Ed.), *Handbook of pediatric psychology* (pp. 286–309). New York: Guilford Press.

Lyons-Ruth, K., Zoll, D., Connell, D., & Grunebaum, H. V. (1986). The depressed mother and her one-year-old infant: Environment, interaction, attachment, and infant development. In T. Field & E. Tronick (Eds.), *Maternal depression and infant disturbance* (pp. 61–82). San Francisco: Jossey-Bass.

Miller, S. A. (1988). Parents' beliefs about children's cognitive development. *Child Development, 59,* 259–285.

Mills, R. S. L., & Rubin, K. H. (1990). Parental beliefs about problematic social behaviors in early childhood. *Child Development, 61,* 138–151.

Nassau, J. H., & Drotar, D. (1997). Social competence among children with central nervous system-related chronic health conditions: A review. *Journal of Pediatric Psychology, 22,* 771–793.

Nietert, P. J., Abboud, M. R., Silverstein, M. D., & Jackson, S. M. (2000). Bone marrow transplantation versus periodic prophylactic blood transfusions in sickle cell patients with high risk for ischemic stroke: A decision analysis. *Blood, 95,* 3057–3064.

Noll, R. B., Vannatta, K., Koontz, K., Kalinyak, K., Bukowski, W. M., & Davies, W.H. (1996). Peer relationships and emotional well-being of youngsters with sickle cell disease. *Child Development, 67,* 423–436.

Pavlakis, S. G., Bello, J., Prohovnik, I., Sutton, M., Ince, C., Mohr, J. P., et al. (1988). Brain infarction in sickle cell anemia: Magnetic resonance imaging correlates. *Annals of Neurology, 23,* 125–130.

Perrin, E. C., & Gerrity, P. S. (1984). Development of children with a chronic illness. *Pediatric Clinics of North America, 31,* 19–32.

Platt, O., Brambilla, D. J., Rosse, W. F., Milner, P. F., Castro, O., Steinberg, M. H., et al. (1994). Mortality in sickle cell disease: Life expectancy and risk factors for early death. *New England Journal of Medicine, 339,* 1639–1644.

Powars, D., Wilson, B., Imbus, C., Pegelow, C. H., & Allen, J. (1978). The natural history of stoke in sickle cell disease. *America Journal of Medicine, 65,* 461–471.

Ris, M. D., & Grueneich, R., (2000). Sickle cell disease. In K. O. Yeates, M. D. Ris, & H. G. Taylor (Eds.), *Pediatric neuropsychology* (pp. 320–335). New York: Guilford Press.

Ris, M.D., Grueneich, R., & Kalinyak, K. (1995). Neuropsychological risk in children with sickle cell disease [Abstract]. *Journal of the International Neuropsychological Society, 1,* 360.

Robinson, M. R. (1999). There is no shame in pain: Coping and functional ability in adolescents with sickle cell disease. *Journal of Black Psychology, 25,* 336–355.

Rogers, Z. R. (1997). Hydroxyurea therapy for diverse pediatric populations with sickle cell disease. *Seminars in Hematology, 34,* 42–47.

Rubin, K. H., Mills, R. S. L., & Rose-Krasnor, L. (1989). Maternal beliefs and children's social competence. In B. H. Schneider, G. Attili, J. Nadel, & R. P. Weissberg (Eds.), *Social competence in developmental perspective* (pp. 313–331). Dordrecht, The Netherlands: Kluwer.

Sameroff, A. J., & Chandler, M. J. (1975). Reproductive risk and the continuum of caretaking causality. In F. D. Horowitz, M. Hetherington, S. Scarr-Salapatek, & G. Siegel (Eds.), *Review of child development* (Vol. 4, pp. 187–244). Chicago: University of Chicago Press.

Schatz, J., Brown, R. T., Pascaul, J. M., Hsu, L., & DeBaun, M. R. (2001). Poor school and cognitive functioning with silent cerebral infarcts and sickle cell disease. *Neurology, 56,* 1109–1111.

Schatz, J., Craft, S., Koby, M., Siegel, M. J., Resar, L., Lee, R., et al. (1999). Neuropsychologic deficits in children with sickle cell disease and cerebral infarction: The role of lesion location and volume. *Child Neuropsychology, 5,* 92–103.

Schuman, W., Armstrong, S., Pegelow, C., & Routh, D. (1993). Enhanced parenting knowledge and skills in mothers of preschool children with sickle cell disease. *Journal of Pediatric Psychology, 18,* 575–591.

Sexson, S. B., & Dingle, A. D. (1997). Medical problems that might present with academic difficulties. *Child and Adolescent Psychiatric Clinics of North America, 63,* 509–522.

Shapiro, B. S., Dinges, D. F., Orne, E. C., Bauer, N., Reilly, L. B., Whitehouse, W. G., et al. (1995). Home management of sickle cell-related pain in children and adolescents: Natural history and impact on school attendance. *Pain, 61,* 139–144.

Sines, J. O., Pauker, J. D., Sines, L. K., & Owen, D. R. (1969). Identification of clinically relevant dimensions of children's behavior. *Journal of Consulting and Clinical Psychology, 33*, 728–734.

Strickland, B. R. (1978). Internal-external expectancies and health-related behaviors. *Journal of Consulting and Clinical Psychology, 46*, 1192–1211.

Swift, A. V., Cohen, M. J., Hynd, G. W., Wisenbaker, J. M., McKie, K. M., Makari, G., et al. (1989). Neuropsychological impairment in children with sickle cell anemia. *Pediatrics, 84*, 1077–1085.

Tarnowski, K., & Brown, R. T. (2000). Psychological aspects of pediatric disorders. In M. Hersen & R. Ammerman (Eds.), *Advanced abnormal child psychology* (2nd ed., pp. 131–152). Hillsdale, NJ: Erlbaum.

Thompson, R. J., Jr. (1985). Coping with the stress of chronic childhood illness. In A. N. O'Quinn (Ed.), *Management of chronic disorders of childhood* (pp. 11–41). Boston: Hall.

Thompson, R. J., Jr., Armstrong, F. D., Kronenberger, W. G., Scott, D., McCabe, M. A., et al. (1999). Family functioning, neurocognitive functioning, and behavior problems in children with sickle cell disease. *Journal of Pediatric Psychology, 24*, 491–498.

Thompson, R. J., Jr., Armstrong, F. D., Link, C. L., Pegelow, C. H., Moser, F., & Wang, W. C. (2003). A prospective study of the relationship over time of behavior problems, intellectual functioning, and family functioning in children with sickle cell disease: A report from the Cooperative Study of Sickle Cell Disease. *Journal of Pediatric Psychology, 28*, 59–65.

Thompson, R. J., Jr., Gil, K. M., Burbach, D. J., Keith, B. R., Gustafson, K. E., George, L. K., et al. (1994). Psychological adjustment of children with sickle cell disease: Stability and change over a 10-month period. *Journal of Consulting and Clinical Psychology, 62*, 856–860.

Thompson, R. J., Jr., Gil, K. M., Burbach, D. J., Keith, B. R., & Kinney, T. R. (1993). Role of child and maternal processes in the psychological adjustment of children with sickle cell disease. *Journal of Consulting and Clinical Psychology, 61*, 468–474.

Thompson, R. J., Gil, K. M., Gustafson, K. E., George, L. K., Keith, B. R., Spock, A., et al. (1994). Stability and change in the psychological adjustment of mothers of children and adolescents with cystic fibrosis and sickle cell disease. *Journal of Pediatric Psychology, 19*, 171–188.

Thompson, R. J., Jr., & Gustafson, K. (1996). *Adaptation to chronic childhood illness.* Washington, DC: American Psychological Association.

Thompson, R. J., Jr., Gustafson, K., Bonner, M. J., & Ware, R. E. (2002). Neurocognitive development of young children with sickle cell disease through 3 years of age. *Journal of Pediatric Psychology, 27*, 235–244.

Thompson, R. J., Jr., Gustafson, K. E., George, L. K., & Spock, A. (1994). Change over a 12-month period in the psychological adjustment of children and adolescents with cystic fibrosis. *Journal of Pediatric Psychology, 19*, 189–203.

Thompson, R. J., Jr., Gustafson, K., & Gil, K. M. (1995). Psychological adjustment of adolescents with cystic fibrosis or sickle cell disease and their mothers. In J. Wallander & L. Siegal (Eds.), *Advances in pediatric psychology: II. Behavioral perspectives on adolescent health* (pp. 232–247). New York: Guilford.

Thompson, R. J., Jr., Gustafson, K. E., Gil, K. M., Kinney, T. R., & Spock, A. (1999). Change in the psychological adjustment of children with cystic fibrosis or sickle cell disease and their mothers. *Journal of Clinical Psychology in Medical Settings, 6*, 373–392.

Thompson, R. J., Gustafson, K. E., & Ware, R. E. (1998). Hematologic disorders. In R. T. Ammerman & J. V. Campo (Eds.), *Handbook of pediatric psychology and psychiatry. Vol. 2: Disease, injury, and illness* (pp. 298–312). Boston: Allyn and Bacon.

Vichinsky, E. P. (1997). Hydroxyurea in children: Present and future. *Seminars in Hematology, 34*, 22–29.

Wallander, J. L., & Thompson, R. J., Jr. (1995). Psychosocial adjustment of children with chronic physical conditions. In M. C. Roberts (Ed.), *Handbook of pediatric psychology* (2nd ed., pp. 124–141). New York: Guilford Press.

Wallander, J. L., & Varni, J. W. (1992). Adjustment in children with chronic physical disorders: Programmatic research on a disability-stress-coping model. In A. M. LaGreca, L. Siegal, J. L. Wallander, & C. E. Walker (Eds.), *Stress and coping with pediatric conditions* (pp. 279–298). New York: Guilford Press.

Wallander, J. L., Varni, J. W., Babani, L., Banis, H. T., & Wilcox, K. T. (1988). Children with chronic physical disorders: Maternal reports of their psychological adjustment. *Journal of Pediatric Psychology, 13*, 197–212.

Wallander, J. L., Varni, J. W., Babani, L. Banis, H. T., & Wilcox, K. T. (1989). Family resources as resistance factors for psychological maladjustment in chronically ill and handicapped children. *Journal of Pediatric Psychology, 14*, 157–173.

Walters, M. C., Storb, R., Patience, M., Leisenring, W., Taylor, T., Sanders, J. E., et al. (2000). Impact of bone marrow transplantation for symptomatic sickle cell disease: An interim report. *Blood, 95*, 1918–1924.

Ware, R. E., Zimmerman, S. A., & Schultz, W. H. (1999). Hydroxyurea as an alternative to blood transfusions for the prevention of recurrent stroke in children with sickle cell disease. *Blood, 94*, 3022–3066.

Wasserman, A. L., Wilimas, J. A., Fairclough, D. L., Mulhern, R. K. & Wang, W. (1991). Subtler neuropsychological deficits in children with sickle cell disease. *American Journal of Pediatric Hematology/Oncology, 13*, 14–20.

Webster-Stratton, C. (1990). Stress: A potential description of parent perceptions and family interactions. *Journal of Clinical Child Psychology, 19*, 302–312.

Wentzel, K. R., & Asher, S. R. (1995). The academic lives of neglected, rejected, popular, and controversial children. *Child Development, 66*, 754–763.

White, D. A., Salorio, C. F., Schatz, J., & DeBaun, M. (2000). Preliminary study of working memory in children with stroke related to sickle cell disease. *Journal of Clinical and Experimental Neuropsychology, 22*, 257–264.

Jeffrey Schatz and Eve S. Puffer

# Neuropsychological Aspects of Sickle Cell Disease

The purpose of this chapter is to summarize current knowledge about the brain bases of the psychological effects of sickle cell disease (SCD). For the purpose of this chapter, we categorize two broad approaches commonly used to identify the behavioral correlates of brain function. Psychological or behavioral models are used that have been developed *independent of* the study of the nervous system. A common example of this approach is psychoeducational assessment, which focuses on constructs relevant to functional outcomes such as IQ scores and academic skills. Psychological models are also used for assessments that have been derived more directly from neuroscience. This approach typically involves assessing specific neurocognitive domains derived from theories of brain organization, such as language, visual-spatial, and executive functions.

## Sources of Neurological Effects in Sickle Cell Disease

SCD offers a challenge to neuropsychologists because of the multiple factors to consider for understanding brain function. Because SCD is a genetic condition present from birth, the disease is likely to interact with developmental factors in infancy or early childhood. Because of social-historical factors, individuals with SCD are more likely than the general population to grow up in difficult social and economic conditions that place them at higher risk for some adverse brain effects. The disease itself also has specific effects on the brain that may lead to acquired brain injury during childhood or later in life. This context creates a challenge; there are multiple potential routes for brain effects that could have an impact on psychological functioning throughout the life span. We discuss research to date on a number of these factors, including pregnancy and birth risks, social and environmental factors in early childhood, and more direct effects of the disease on the brain. These factors are discussed in their likely order of impact based on current research, with direct effects of SCD on the brain having the most robust and well-established effects on neuropsychological functioning. An overview is presented in table 24-1.

## Pregnancy and Birth Risks

Mothers of children born with SCD either have SCD or trait. Data on pregnancy outcomes of

**Table 24-1.** Overview of Potential Neurological Causes of Psychological Effects of Sickle Cell Disease

| *Potential Mechanism of Brain Effects* | *Status of Research* | *Overall Risk* | *Relative Risk* | *Possible Brain Effects From Mechanism* | *Typical Psychological Impact If Brain Effects Are Present* |
|---|---|---|---|---|---|
| Perinatal insults | Higher perinatal risks in SCD; risks have not been directly linked to neurocognitive outcomes | 22% rate of preterm birth with maternal SCD; rate of insults unknown | Perinatal risks 2–4 times more likely than pregnancies without maternal SCD | Increased risk of periventricular leukomalacia or hemorrhage, leukoencephalopathy | Small impact on IQ; small-to-medium effect on visual-spatial and visual-motor skills |
| Nutritional deficits | Nutrition deficiencies documented; no direct linkage shown to neurocognitive outcomes | Not well documented | Up to 20% higher energy needs; depends on dietary compensation | With protein-energy malnutrition: Fewer synapses, less myelin, reduced brain weight | Incremental effects: Decreased IQ scores, verbal ability, and processing speed; weak visual memory |
| Overt stroke | Well-established effect on neurocognitive functioning | 4%–7% risk | ~200 times the general population risk in children | Focal regions of cerebral infarction frequently occurring in frontal and parietal lobes | Depends on location and extent of cerebral infarction; often medium-to-large effect on IQ; attention and executive skills deficits are often pronounced |
| Silent stroke | Established effect on neurocognitive functioning | 15%–27% risk depending on MRI methods | 4–5 times higher than the general population rate | Focal regions of cerebral infarction frequently occurring in the deep white matter and striatum | Depends on location and extent of cerebral infarction; small impact on IQ and math achievement; medium-size effect on verbal skills, attention, and executive skills |
| Localized perfusion problems | Limited correlational data with neurocognitive functioning | 10%–40% in small *n* studies | Unknown | Potentially reversible disruption of normal brain function because of insufficient oxygen and/or glucose delivery | Specific cognitive deficits depending on region and extent of tissue affected |
| Anemia-related diffuse hypoxia | Strong correlational data between anemia severity and neurocognitive effects | Unknown; may be an incremental effect with anemia severity | Unknown | Diffuse hypoxic disruption or damage to neurons; diffuse microinfarction | Incremental effect on IQ; specific areas of cognitive deficit not well established |

mothers with SCD or trait indicate that most of these pregnancies are successful and without serious complications (Koshy, 1995; Sun, Wilburn, Raynor, & Jamieson, 2001). Despite the overall success of these pregnancies, they are higher risk compared to those of similar mothers without sickle cell trait or disease. For mothers with SCD, there appears to be a somewhat higher risk for intrauterine growth restriction, antepartum hospital admission of the child, and postpartum infection for the child (Sun et al., 2001). In addition, mothers with sickle cell anemia have been shown to be more likely to have preterm births, infants with low birth weight, or premature rupture of membranes that increases the risk of infection for the child (Koshy, 1995; J. A. Smith et al., 1996; Sun et al., 2001). The potential impact of these higher-risk pregnancies on neurocognitive development has not typically been considered in research studies of SCD.

The data assessing if there are increased perinatal complications in mothers with sickle cell *trait* have been less clear. One report of birth complications among mothers with sickle cell trait indicated fewer complications relative to mothers with SCD; however, some negative outcomes were reported to be more likely for mothers with sickle cell trait relative to those without the trait (Balgir, Dash, & Das, 1997). Subtle effects on the fetus that are not clear-cut birth complications may also be present. Manzar (2000) reported that births with mothers who have sickle cell trait were associated with elevated amounts of circulating nucleated red blood cells in the cord blood, an index of intrauterine fetal hypoxia. This finding suggests that fetal hypoxia may be occurring at or before the time of birth (Ferber, Grassi, Akyol, O'Reilly-Green, & Divon, 2003; Hanlon-Lundberg & Kirby, 1999; Saracoglu, Sahin, Eser, Gol, & Turkkani, 2000). It is not known if this finding is important for subsequent brain development in children with SCD, but the finding raises important questions regarding potential prenatal risk factors in SCD.

Overall, these data indicate that, as a group, children with SCD are more likely to have had perinatal risks for brain injury, such as preterm birth, low birth weight, and possible mild fetal hypoxia. Potential brain effects from these complications include white matter injury and decreased volume of cortical tissue later in childhood (Forfar et al., 1994; Inder et al., 1999; Peterson, 2003). Although these brain effects from perinatal injury would not be expected in most children with SCD, when present, subtle long-term behavioral effects on the child would be most evident in the areas of fine motor control, visual-spatial functions, and mathematical abilities (Picard, Del Dotto, & Breslau, 1999; Taylor, Klein, Minich, & Hack, 2000).

In the neuropsychological literature on SCD, it has been rare for researchers to report the frequency or severity of birth risks for the children with SCD and the comparison groups. Although these birth risks may exert only a small influence on study outcomes, failure to account for this factor may cause researchers to overestimate the effect of other factors, such as direct disease effects on the brain. Likewise, when assessing an individual child with SCD, one should conduct a careful examination of pregnancy and birth risks so that these factors are not ignored when considering the potential causes of neuropsychological assessment results.

## Social and Environmental Factors in Early Childhood

Social and environmental factors early in child development can have a large impact on brain development and subsequent behavioral patterns (for reviews, see Georgieff & Rao, 2001; Gunnar, 2001; Mendola, Selevan, Gutter, & Rice, 2002). A significant percentage of children with SCD grow up in families living below or near the poverty level; this increases the risk for a range of negative influences, including inadequate nutrition, suboptimal cognitive stimulation, and harmful environmental exposures (e.g., lead) (Evans, 2004; McLoyd, 1998). Hence, it is not surprising that socioeconomic status is a significant predictor of a range of cognitive and behavioral outcomes for children with SCD (e.g., Brown et al., 1993; Devine, Brown, Lambert, Donegan, & Eckman, 1998; Lemanek, Moore, Gresham, Williamson, & Kelley, 1986).

Among the environmental factors described above, there has been increased attention paid to undernutrition among children with SCD. Children with SCD show nutritional deficiencies compared to demographically matched, healthy control groups, including deficits in protein-energy, zinc, riboflavin, and vitamins A, E, C, $B_{12}$, $B_6$, and folic acid (Chiu, Vichinsky, Ho, Liu, & Lubin, 1990; Kennedy et al., 2001; Nelson et al., 2002; Sindel, Dishuck, Baliga, & Mankad, 1990). Iron deficiencies have also been identified in some cases, but results are not consistent (Stettler, Zemel, Kawchak, Ohene-Frempong, & Stallings, 2001). Several potential explanations for these deficits have emerged, but the most likely causes are increased metabolic demands and the effects of acute illness that are not compensated for through increased dietary intake.

One study reported that diets of families of children with SCD did not include adequate nutrients based on recommended dietary intake for children (Williams, George, & Wang, 1997). However, most studies that directly studied dietary intake have shown that children with SCD typically eat the same amount of calories, protein, and nutrients as matched comparison children. Despite this similar intake, nutritional differences are evident between the groups, suggesting a lack of compensation in dietary intake for the higher nutritional needs of children with SCD.

Several studies have found that children with SCD have up to 20% higher resting energy expenditure and resting metabolic rate than other children (Gray et al., 1992; Singhal, Parker, Linsell, & Serjeant, 2002). Thus, they are metabolizing energy more quickly than it is replenished, creating an energy deficit. In some studies, children with SCD also showed a decrease in active energy expenditure, suggesting that some children compensate for their energy deficit by decreasing their physical activity (Barden et al., 2000; Singhal, Davies, Wierenga, Thomas, & Serjeant, 1997). Other physiological factors, such as nonspecific intestinal malabsorption or overexcretion of nutrients, may further impact nutritional deficiencies in these children, but these factors have not been examined in detail to date (Kennedy et al., 2001).

Acute periods of illness and hospitalizations related to SCD also may play an important role in maintaining low nutritional status in children with SCD. Studies showed that energy and micronutrient intake is lower during acute illness, perhaps because of pain-related anorexia (Fung et al., 2001; Malinauskas et al., 2000). Lower dietary intake in these circumstances exacerbates the energy deficit during times when metabolic demands are likely to be high.

Nutritional deficits in protein-energy requirements and zinc are particularly relevant to neuropsychology because of their established link to brain and cognitive development. Protein-energy deficiencies can result in decreases in neurotransmitter production, synaptic formation, myelination of axons, and total brain weight (Winick & Noble, 1966; Winick & Rosso, 1969a, 1969b). Children with protein-energy undernutrition show decreases in general intellectual functioning, visual-spatial processing, verbal ability, and speed of information processing that are related to the nutritional deficits (Pollitt & Gorman, 1994; Pollitt, Gorman, Engle, Rivera, & Martorell, 1995; Pollitt, Watkins, & Husaini, 1997). These and other studies of cognitive effects of nutrition deficits have suggested that protein-energy malnutrition may also exacerbate the effects of other neurological factors present during development (Georgieff & Rao, 2001; Rao et al., 1999). Thus, malnutrition could be a direct or interactive cause of neurocognitive deficits.

Zinc deficiency is another particularly important area of concern for brain development. Zinc deficiency during early development has been linked to decreases in the arborization of dendrites and decreases in regional brain mass in the cerebellum, limbic system, and cerebral cortex (Frederickson & Danscher, 1990). Behavioral effects of zinc deficiency are believed to include less spontaneous motor activity, poorer short-term visual memory, and poorer concept formation and abstract reasoning abilities (Golub et al., 1994; Sandstead et al., 1998). It is notable, however, that unlike the effects of protein-energy malnutrition, the brain effects of zinc deficiency have sometimes been reversible with treatment (Sandstead et al., 1998).

Researchers have yet to establish the extent that undernutrition has an impact on cognitive or brain development among children with SCD. Given the extent of nutritional deficiencies reported, it seems reasonable to believe that neurocognitive development is negatively impacted by inadequate nutrition, at least some children with SCD. Nutritional deficits can be thought of on a continuum from optimal nutrition, to temporary disequilibrium between needs and intake, to functional changes in response to more chronic deficits, and finally to noticeable negative effects on body organs and composition. The precise threshold at which undernutrition begins to have an impact on neurocognitive functioning in children is not well established. Research is needed to determine whether malnutrition is a narrow issue affecting brain development in relatively few children or a more widespread issue for children with SCD.

## Direct Effects of Sickle Cell Disease on the Brain

SCD produces two major types of complications that can affect organs, including the brain. First, vessels can become blocked, cutting off blood flow to part of the organ. This event may be caused by the viscosity changes and clumping of red blood cells that accompanies sickling (the most recognized mechanism) or thrombocytosis, a result of high platelet levels. The development of stenosis in large vessels is another source of blockage. The microscopic changes that accompany large-vessel stenosis have been described, but the fundamental processes that lead to large-vessel disease are not well understood (Oyesiku, Barrow, & Eckman, 1991). The second major type of complication is a reduction in the oxygen-carrying capacity of the blood supply to the organs. This reduction can be caused by the decreased oxygen-carrying capacity of hemoglobin S red blood cells (particularly when they polymerize into the sickled state) and the increased loss of red blood cells that results in hemolytic anemia. Other research has suggested that oxygen regulation factors during sleep (e.g., in the case of sleep apnea) may also create transient oxygen delivery problems (Brooks, Koziol, Chiarucci, & Berman, 1996; Kirkham et al., 2001; Robertson, Aldrich, Hanash, & Goldstein, 1988; Wali, Al-Lamki, Soliman, & Al-Okbi, 2000).

The direct effects of SCD can include both focal and diffuse effects on brain function that are discussed in detail in the following sections. These include two types of cerebrovascular accidents, overt stroke and silent cerebral infarction, as well as other direct effects of SCD, including localized metabolic and perfusion deficits, and diffuse effects on neurons.

### Overt Stroke

*Definition and Prevalence.* The most widely recognized cause of brain injury in SCD is overt stroke. Overt stroke is typically defined as the presence of characteristic neurological signs of a cerebral vascular accident (e.g., acute onset of motor weakness) that persist for at least 24 hours. Usually, the onset of these symptoms is followed by neuroimaging exams that show the expected vascular or brain tissue changes. This is distinct from a transient ischemic attack, in which symptoms remit in less than 24 hours and do not result in abnormalities on neuroimaging, or a silent stroke, a cerebral infarction that is evident on neuroimaging exams but has no accompanying neurological symptoms. Examples of neuroimaging exams in overt and silent stroke are shown in figure 24-1.

Overt stroke typically involves large-vessel disease. The most frequent brain regions affected are those supplied by the middle or anterior cerebral arteries, such as the middle and superior frontal gyri and the parietal cortex (Pavlakis, Prohovnik, Piomelli, & DeVivo, 1989). However, lesions may occur in a wide variety of forebrain regions, and the volume of tissue affected varies greatly. We have typically found that overt stroke affects more than 40 cubic centimeters of brain tissue as viewed on traditional T2-weighted magnetic resonance imaging (MRI) images. When a smaller volume of tissue has been affected, the lesion is more likely to result from a silent cerebral infarct (see figure 24-2).

The association of SCD and overt stroke has been noted in the published scientific literature since 1923 (Sydenstricker, Mulherin, & Houseal, 1923). Risk for overt stroke varies across genotypes in SCD, with highest risk associated with the homozygous form (SS). Other genetic factors also appear to affect stroke risk (Adekile et al., 2002; Hoppe et al., 2004). In the United States, the Cooperative Study of Sickle Cell Disease (CSSCD) data from 1978 to 1988 placed the prevalence rate of stroke across forms of SCD at 4%, with a 5% prevalence rate for those with SS disease (Ohene-Frempong et al., 1998). Other reports from larger studies have indicated prevalence rates of 5%–7% (Balkaran et al., 1992; Bernaudin et al., 2000; Powars, Wilson, Imbus, Pegelow, & Allen, 1978). Therefore, SCD is associated with an approximate 200-fold increase in risk for childhood stroke compared to the general population (Earley et al., 1998).

Strokes can occur throughout childhood, although the highest incidence of first stroke appears to be between 2 and 5 years of age

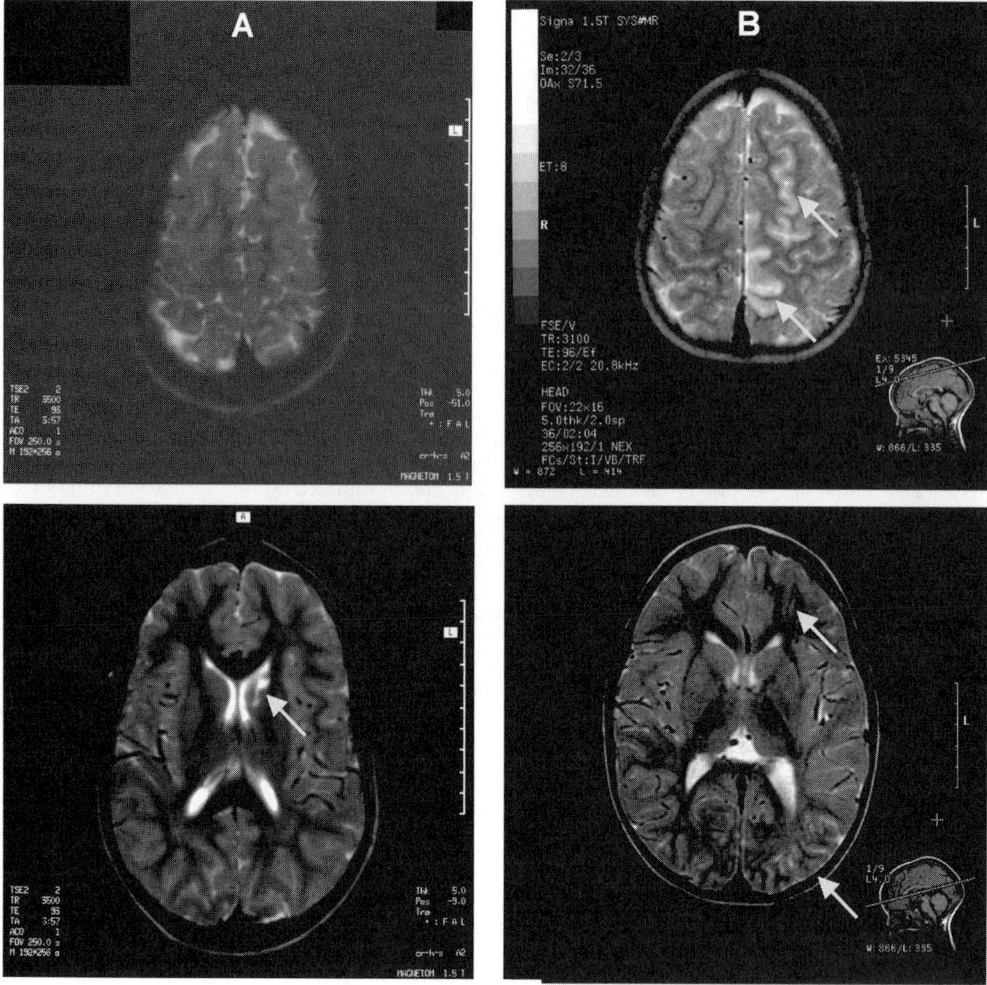


**Figure 24-1.** Sample T2-weighted MRI scans in the axial plane showing a silent cerebral infarct in the head of the caudate nucleus (Panel A, left) and the infarcts from an overt stroke in the frontal cortex, parietal cortex, and frontal white matter (Panel B, right).

(Ohene-Frempong et al., 1998). The rate of stroke recurrence is approximately 70% over a 3-year period if prophylactic blood transfusion therapy is not conducted (Powars et al., 1978; Wilimas, Goff, Anderson, Langston, & Thompson, 1980). With chronic transfusion therapy, the rate of recurrent stroke is approximately 10% (Pegelow et al., 1995). This research is particularly important for psychological outcomes given the significant impact of stroke on cognitive and academic functioning.

*Psychoeducational Outcomes.* Studies that have emphasized psychoeducational approaches to measurement have indicated that overt stroke is associated with a medium-to-large effect on general intellectual functioning and academic achievement. Published studies comparing general intellectual ability (IQ scores) of children with overt stroke to those with SCD and normal neuroimaging exams have reported IQ scores approximately 14 standard score points lower for children with stroke (see table 24-2). Because of variability in location and amount of damage that can result from strokes, there is large variability across studies in the magnitude of the effect of stroke on general intellectual functioning. Several studies using the Wechsler scales have reported somewhat larger deficits for Performance IQ than for Verbal IQ among children with overt stroke (Armstrong et al., 1996; Bernaudin et al., 2000; Wang et al., 2001); this

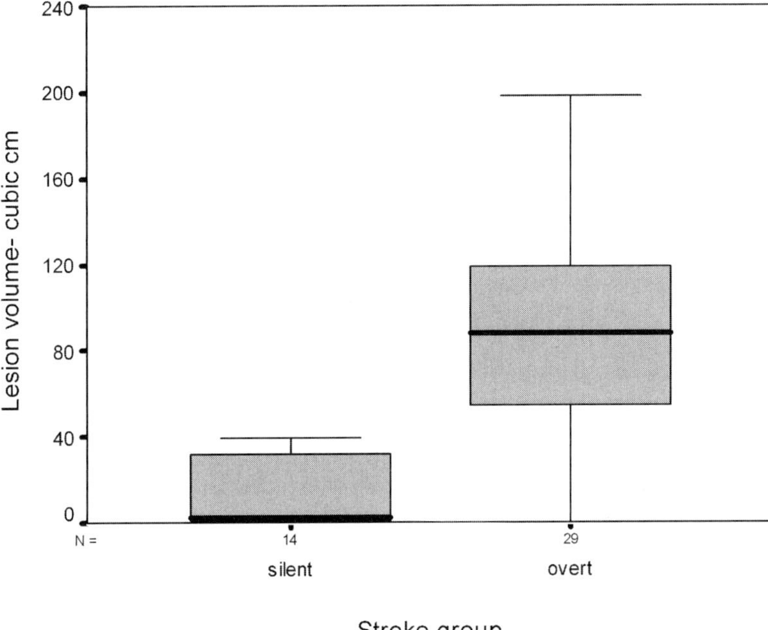


**Figure 24-2.** Boxplot showing the median, quartile, and 95% confidence interval for lesion volume. The 95% confidence interval lies between 0 and 200 cubic centimeters for the overt stroke cases with a relatively normal distribution. Children with silent cerebral infarcts showed a positively skewed distribution and never had more than 40 cubic centimeters of tissue injury in this sample. Data compiled from Schatz et al. (1999, 2000).

pattern suggests that stroke affects the expression of visual-motor cognitive abilities more severely than auditory-verbal abilities. This issue is addressed in the next section on more specific brain-behavior relationships.

Children with SCD and overt stroke also show poorer performance on standardized measures of academic achievement skills than children without cerebral infarction, particularly in mathematics. Wang et al. (2001) described academic achievement data for a relatively large sample of children with SCD and overt stroke compared to those with normal MRI. Mean scores were in the low-average range for the Broad Reading scale of the

**Table 24-2.** Studies of General Intellectual Functioning Following Overt Stroke

| *Study* | *SCD With Stroke (n)* | *SCD With Normal MRI (n)* | *IQ, Stroke* | *IQ, Controls* | *Difference* |
|---|---|---|---|---|---|
| Hariman, Griffith, Hurtig, & Keehn, 1991 | 14 | 14 | 68.4 | 91.4 | −23.0 |
| Armstrong et al., 1996 | 9 | 161 | 70.8 | 90.0 | −19.2 |
| Steen et al., 1998 | 13 | 17 | 70.6 | 78.9 | −8.3 |
| Bernaudin et al., 2000 | 11 | 143 | 82.7 | 90.9 | −8.2 |
| Brown et al., 2000 | 22 | 30 | 75.0 | 81.7 | −6.7 |
| Wang et al., 2001 | 20 | 122 | 76.9 | 84.8 | −7.9 |
| Mean weighted by study *n* | | | 74.3 | 88.1 | −13.8 |

Woodcock-Johnson Psycho-Educational Battery–Revised (WJ-R) for children with stroke ($M = 84.6$) compared with mean scores in the average range for children with SCD and normal MRI ($M = 93.9$). For the WJ-R Broad Mathematics scale, children with stroke showed mean performance in the borderline range ($M = 77.3$) compared with performance in the average range for children with normal MRI ($M = 90.7$). In this and other studies, the decrements in academic skills for children with overt stroke are as large as, or larger than, the decrement in general intellectual functioning (Armstrong et al., 1996; Brown et al., 2000; Wang et al., 2001).

*Brain-Behavior Relationships.* Studies that have incorporated a more traditional neuropsychological framework for assessing cognitive abilities have indicated that the psychological effects of stroke are dependent on the location and volume of cerebral infarction. Of particular importance, damage to the anterior portions of the forebrain occurs frequently and results in characteristic deficits in attention, memory, and executive skills. Cortical injury to watershed regions of the vascular distribution is common with overt stroke, and it is not unusual for more than one lobe of the cortex to be affected. Despite this pattern, there tends to be a preponderance of frontal and subcortical frontal injury. For example, Brown et al. (2000) reported that 96% of children with overt stroke had injury to frontal regions, and in a mixed sample of children with overt and silent stroke, Schatz et al. (1999) found that 86% of the cases with cerebral infarction had frontal injury. In this study by Schatz et al., cerebral infarction limited to frontal regions occurred approximately twice as often (7 of 28 cases) as infarction limited to posterior regions (4 of 28 cases). The report by Brown et al. (2000) also indicated a high proportion of stroke cases that included parietal lobe injury (77%).

The typical pattern of injury from stroke in SCD appears to result in some converging areas of cognitive deficit. Attention regulation and executive skills are frequently impacted; these domains include abilities such as selectively attending to important information in the environment, maintaining attention over time, flexibly shifting the focus of attention, organizing thoughts and behavior in support of adaptive functioning (e.g., planning), and monitoring one's behavior for errors. DeBaun et al. (1998) examined the frequency of statistically deficient test scores from neuropsychological testing in children with strokes and siblings without SCD; measures of attention and executive skills yielded the most robust sensitivity and specificity data (see table 24-3).

Similarly, Brown et al. (2000) examined performance of children with SCD and overt, silent, or no stroke in three specific cognitive domains (attention and executive functioning, language functioning, visual-spatial functioning) and found that group differences emerged only on the attention and executive functioning domain. Within the attention and executive skills domain, children with overt stroke performed worse than both comparison groups on a measure of selective and sustained attention, whereas differences were less evident on a measure of sequencing and mental flexibility.

Difficulties with attention and executive skills appear to have a relatively specific relationship with injury to frontal regions and can occur with even a relatively small volume of injury (Craft, Schatz, Glauser, Lee, & DeBaun, 1993; Schatz et al., 1999; Watkins et al., 1998). This can have a serious impact on a child because attention and executive skills are closely related to memory and learning abilities. Frontal brain injury in SCD has been related to reduced efficiency in rehearsing verbal information in working memory, difficulties with manipulating verbal information in working memory, and poorer retrieval of verbal information on memory recall trials (Brandling-Bennett, White, Armstrong, Christ, & DeBaun, 2003; White, Saloria, Schatz, & DeBaun, 2000). These data suggest specific learning mechanisms associated with frontal injury that would have an impact on academic learning and other functional outcomes for most children with stroke.

Somewhat less research has focused on differences in neuropsychological functioning related to the hemisphere sustaining injury. Two studies that have directly compared children with left versus right hemisphere injury have demonstrated relative sparing of language functions with right hemisphere injury, whereas as visual-spatial deficits occur more ubiquitously (Cohen, Branch, McKie, & Adams, 1994; Schatz, Craft, Koby, & DeBaun, 2004). Visual-spatial deficits appear to be related to both the presence of injury in posterior parietal-temporal regions and the total volume of injury (Craft et al., 1993; Schatz et al., 1999). More subtle patterns of visual-spatial deficits may differ

**Table 24-3.** Sensitivity and Specificity Data for Selected Measures Based on Scoring >1.5 Standard Deviations From Age-Based Norms

| *Test (Construct or Constructs Measured)* | *Sensitivity to Stroke (n = 28)* | *Specificity Based on Siblings Without SCD (n = 17)* |
|---|---|---|
| DAS Word Definitions (expressive vocabulary) | 39% | 100% |
| WJ-R Picture Vocabulary (confrontational naming, one-word vocabulary) | 46% | 76% |
| DAS Pattern Construction (visual-spatial analysis and construction) | 43% | 82% |
| Benton's Judgment of Line Orientation (visual-spatial analysis) | 46% | 76% |
| Wisconsin Card Sorting Test (concept formation, set shifting) | 64% | 71% |
| Test of Variables of Attention (selective and sustained attention) | 89% | 88% |
| Tower of Hanoi (planning, sequencing, impulsivity) | 86% | 82% |

*Note:* The sample consisted of 21 children with overt stroke and 7 children with silent stroke; data did not differ significantly between overt and silent stroke groups. DAS, Differential Abilities Scale; WJ-R, Woodcock-Johnson Psycho-Educational Battery–Revised. Data from DeBaun et al. (1998).

across left and right hemisphere injury (Schatz, Craft, et al., 2004), but the behavioral significance of these subtle processing differences is not clear. Both language and visual-spatial domains appear to be strongly related to the overall volume of injury, although the visual-spatial domain shows the most robust correlation (Schatz et al., 1999). Overall, it appears that the anterior-posterior gradient is a more robust factor to consider in terms of understanding the cognitive effects of stroke in children with SCD, but additional information may be obtained from considering hemispheric differences as well. Limitations are discussed in the Intervention section regarding the use of structural imaging alone to establish the hemisphere affected as functional neuroimaging studies have suggested unilateral structural injury can sometimes result in bilateral problems with brain function.

The processing of social and emotional information is a relatively complex type of information processing that can also be affected by overt stroke, especially in the case of injury to prefrontal cortical regions. Boni, Brown, Davis, Hsu, and Hopkins (2001) examined measures of nonverbal emotional decoding skills in 21 children with cerebral vascular accidents as compared to 20 children with SCD and normal structural MRI. Children with stroke demonstrated significantly poorer ability to accurately read facial expressions and decode emotional information from voices. These processing deficits likely have an impact on social behavior, particularly as the complexity of social relationships increases from childhood into adolescence.

Despite the high prevalence of cognitive and academic skills deficits following stroke, emotional and behavioral disorders do not appear to be strongly related to the presence of overt stroke. The majority of these data have been based on maternal reported behavior symptoms as measured with Achenbach's Child Behavior Checklist (Armstrong et al., 1996; Brown et al., 2000; R. J. Thompson et al., 1999, 2003). However, the Child Behavior Checklist was designed to assess traditional patterns of childhood psychopathology that may not map well onto the behavioral or emotional effects of brain injury. The use of more recently developed tools such as the Behavioral Report Inventory of Executive Functions (Gioia, Isquith, Guy, & Kenworthy, 2000), which was designed to capture the behavioral effects of central nervous system dysfunction, may better capture the day-to-day behavioral impact of stroke in children. Also, internalizing symptoms may be difficult to measure strictly through parent report (Meade, Lumley, & Casey, 2001), and additional child-reported measures would be useful to support the data from the existing studies. Despite these caveats, it appears that the impact of stroke on psychological functioning is largely in terms of cognitive dysfunction and academic skill deficits rather than internalizing or externalizing behavior problems.

### *Silent Cerebral Infarcts*

*Definition and Prevalence.* Silent cerebral infarcts are a more recently identified condition than overt stroke. As stated, silent cerebral infarcts (also known as silent strokes) are defined as abnormal neuroimaging results that look like cerebral vascular injury despite no history of an overt clinical event (e.g., loss of speech or motor abilities) to indicate a stroke. Many issues regarding silent strokes remain unclear, including their full impact on children with SCD and the best methods of identification, prevention, and treatment.

Silent cerebral infarcts were first identified in the published literature in 1987 (Hindmarsh, Brozovic, Brook, & Davies, 1987). The physical or psychological effects of these lesions were unclear to the authors of the 1987 report. Two subsequent lines of information have helped to highlight the importance of understanding this phenomenon in relation to SCD. First, silent cerebral infarcts appear on neuroimaging exams for a high percentage of children with SCD. Second, the lesions are related to deficits in cognitive functioning and poorer functional outcomes in school.

The first major epidemiological report of the prevalence of silent cerebral infarcts was conducted as part of the CSSCD. Armstrong et al. (1996) reported an overall 12% prevalence rate of silent cerebral infarcts among children with SCD and a 16% prevalence rate among children with the SS form of SCD. The study examined children 6–12 years of age using standard T1, T2, and proton density-weighted brain MRI on 0.6T to 1.5T machines. A comparably large multisite study using similar sequences and 1.0T or 1.5T machines indicated a 15% prevalence rate for silent cerebral infarcts for both the overall group and the SS subtype (Bernaudin et al., 2000).

More recent data have suggested that the consistent use of a 1.5T imaging machine and the inclusion of newer imaging techniques demonstrate an even higher rate of silent cerebral infarcts. Steen, Emudianughe, et al. (2003) examined 185 children with SCD at a single site using a 1.5T MRI machine for all participants and higher-resolution sequences in approximately one third of the sample (i.e., thin-slice T1- and T2-weighted sequences and a fluid-attenuated inversion recovery sequence [FLAIR]). The ages of the children were comparable to the study of Bernaudin et al. (2000). Steen, Emudianughe, et al. (2003) found a 35% rate of silent cerebral infarcts in this sample. The use of thin-slice and FLAIR imaging was associated with a 23% higher rate of damage evident to brain parenchyma, suggesting that many cases of silent cerebral infarction may be missed without the use of more current imaging methods.

*Psychoeducational Outcomes.* The second reason for increased interest in silent cerebral infarcts has been the documentation of cognitive decrements associated with the condition. Silent cerebral infarcts appear to have an impact on cognitive functioning and are associated with decrements in verbal skills, selective and sustained attention, and executive skills. These areas of cognitive deficit are also accompanied by poorer achievement in mathematics (Armstrong et al., 1996; Wang et al., 2001) and more functional problems with academic attainment (Schatz, Brown, Pascual, Hsu, & DeBaun, 2001).

Armstrong et al. (1996) were the first to report intelligence test results for a relatively large sample of children with silent cerebral infarcts ($n = 24$). The authors also statistically covaried hematocrit levels and demographic variables when comparing cognitive scores among children with overt stroke, silent stroke, and normal MRI. This statistical control is important because children with cerebral vascular injury may have more severe courses of the disease in general. Armstrong et al. found that children with silent infarcts scored approximately 7 standard score points lower on the Wechsler Scale (Wisconsin Intelligence Scale for Children–Revised, WISC-R) Full-Scale IQ and 9 standard score points lower on Verbal IQ than children with normal MRI (after controlling for other variables). Specific subtest differences were found for the WISC-R Vocabulary, Arithmetic, and Coding subtests. Subsequent data from the CSSCD with the third edition of the WISC (WISC-III) found very similar results with slight differences in the specific IQ subtests that reached statistical significance (Wang et al., 2001).

Bernaudin et al. (2000) also showed the most robust differences between children with silent infarcts and those with normal MRI on the Verbal Comprehension factor of the WISC-III (approximately 14 standard score points difference). The distribution of scores for the children with silent cerebral infarcts in this study appeared to be bimodal, suggesting important differences between subgroups of children with silent infarcts. It appeared to Bernaudin et al. that cognitive decrements were only evident among children with both silent cerebral infarcts *and* low hematocrit levels. However, silent cerebral infarcts have been associated with poorer cognitive functioning independent of hematocrit levels in several studies (Armstrong et al., 1996; Steen, Miles, et al., 2003). Another potential reason for a bimodal distribution has been suggested by studies of lesion volume in silent cerebral infarcts. Schatz, White, Moinuddin, Armstrong, and DeBaun (2002) reported what appeared to be a threshold effect among children with silent cerebral infarcts; those with a small volume of injury on T2-weighted scans (<6.7 cubic centimeters) had IQ scores similar to children with SCD and normal MRI, whereas children with a large volume of injury (>6.8 cubic centimeters) showed lower Full-Scale IQ scores than the other two groups.

*Brain-Behavior Relationships.* A similar pattern of brain-behavior relationships appears to occur for children with silent stroke as for overt stroke. It is important to keep in mind, however, that silent cerebral infarcts typically involve disruption of the blood supply from smaller arteries. Therefore, the injury with silent stroke is more likely to involve smaller and more localized areas of cortical tissue and subcortical structures, including deep white matter regions (Moser et al., 1996). Studies to date have examined somewhat crude lesion categories, such as anterior versus posterior brain injury, which may not detect more subtle differences between the locations of lesions. Typical neuropsychological test batteries in studies of SCD have also not been designed to differentiate between factors such as cortical versus subcortical injury.

Studies of silent stroke that have focused on neuropsychological domains have reported a preponderance of cognitive effects on tests of vigilance, selective attention, and executive skills (Brown et al., 2000; Craft et al., 1993; DeBaun et al., 1998). These areas of deficit appear to be related to injury in frontal brain regions (Brown et al., 2000; Craft et al., 1993; Schatz et al., 1999). One study that examined school performance of children with silent cerebral infarction indicated that over half of these children had either been retained in school or required special academic services (Schatz et al., 2001). This was more than twice the rate of school difficulties of children with SCD and normal MRI. Although math achievement scores have been shown to be affected among children with silent cerebral infarcts (Armstrong et al., 1996; Wang et al., 2001), the rate of delays in basic academic skills appears to be much lower than the rate of attainment problems (Schatz et al., 2001). This discrepancy between classroom performance and scores on tests of academic skills has been attributed to the prevalence of specific attention and executive skill deficits, which may be an insidious problem for school performance. Traditional psychoeducational evaluations may not be well suited to detect these areas of deficit.

### *Other Sources of Cognitive Effects From Sickle Cell Disease*

Previously, researchers have speculated that older studies reporting cognitive deficits among children with SCD and no clinical history of stroke may have found these results because of the failure to account for silent cerebral infarction (Craft et al., 1993; White & DeBaun, 1998). Although the cognitive effects of silent stroke may have partly accounted for these previous findings, it appears that there are additional cognitive effects of SCD for some children with normal structural MRI (Schatz, Finke, Kellett, & Kramer, 2002; Steen et al., 2005; Steen, Miles, et al., 2003). On average, this decrement appears to be approximately 5 standard score points for measures of general intellectual functioning (Schatz, Finke, et al., 2002; Steen, Miles, et al., 2003). This small effect for the group average on IQ testing, however, may be misleading for two reasons: (a) There appear to be larger deficits on specific measures of cognitive functioning, and (b) it is likely that subgroups of children with SCD and normal MRI are completely unaffected, which pulls up the group average (Schatz, Finke, et al., 2002; Steen, Miles, et al., 2003).

One source of data that strongly implicate disease-related causes of these cognitive effects is the relationship between anemia severity (typically measured by hematocrit or hemoglobin levels) and cognitive functioning. Although some early studies did not find this relationship (Fowler et al., 1988;

Swift et al., 1989), studies have shown a moderate-to-large correlation between anemia severity and cognitive functioning in children with SCD and normal MRI (Bernaudin et al., 2000; Brown et al., 1993; Steen, Xiong, Mulhern, Langston, & Wang, 1999; Steen, Miles, et al., 2003). Correlations between anemia severity and cognition have been reported for general intellectual functioning (Bernaudin et al., 2000; Brown et al., 1993; Schatz, Finke, & Roberts, 2004; Steen et al., 1999; Steen, Miles, et al., 2003); verbal ability (Schatz et al., 2004; Steen, Miles, et al., 2003); and specific measures of attention and working memory (Brown et al., 1993; Schatz et al., 2004; Steen, Miles, et al., 2003). A similar relationship appears between cognitive functioning and cerebral blood flow velocity on transcranial Doppler (TCD) ultrasonography: Higher blood flow velocities in the middle cerebral artery are associated with deficits in verbal ability, sustained attention, and executive skills (Kral et al., 2003).

The markers of more severe disease (i.e., severe anemia, abnormal TCD) are likely associated with processes that affect brain function, at least partly independent of silent cerebral infarction. Two likely sources of these cognitive effects are (a) focal regions of tissue dysfunction that are still structurally intact and (b) diffuse structural effects on the brain that are not evident on standard visual inspection of MRI scans.

*Localized Metabolic and Perfusion Problems.* Brain function can be disrupted in SCD through inadequate supply of glucose or oxygen without necessarily resulting in visible cerebral infarction on structural MRI (Rodgers et al., 1988). Studies using positron emission tomography (PET) or perfusion MRI in children with SCD, although not conducted with large population-based samples, have reported a relatively high prevalence of these abnormalities. The two major types of studies used to examine these effects in children with SCD are glucose metabolism studies using PET (Powars et al., 1999; Reed, Jagust, Al-Mateen, & Vichinsky, 1999) and perfusion studies of the microvascular blood supply using either PET or MRI (Kirkham et al., 2001; Oguz et al., 2003; Powars et al., 1999). The degree to which these functional effects on the brain have an impact on cognitive functioning has not been well established, but there are data to suggest these effects on the brain may be partly responsible for cognitive deficits.

Powars et al. (1999) described interrelationships among traditional structural MRI, PET metabolism and perfusion studies, and neuropsychological testing in a group of 49 children with SCD who were primarily selected on the basis of previous signs of neurological disease. Among these children, 20 had only soft neurological signs such as subtle motor incoordination or a history of an acute hypoxic event without stroke symptoms (termed by the authors as category II), and 10 were asymptomatic by clinical history and neurological exam (category III). Of the 10 of the category II children, 7 had normal structural MRI and abnormal PET scans; 4 of the 10 category III children had normal MRI and abnormal PET scans. IQ scores for the 11 children with normal structural MRI and abnormal PET scans were noted to be approximately one standard deviation below the population average ($M = 86$), whereas category III children with normal MRI and PET typically had IQ scores near or above 100. Direct statistical comparisons between these two small subgroups, however, were not reported.

Similar high rates of functional neuroimaging deficits have been noted using perfusion MRI. Kirkham et al. (2001) reported on perfusion MRI and structural MRI including FLAIR in 48 children with SCD. Of the children whose only neurological symptom was a history of headache ($n = 9$), 2 were found to have normal structural MRI but abnormal regional perfusion. Among 10 completely asymptomatic children with SCD, 1 child had normal MRI but abnormal regional perfusion. A second study using very similar methods reported 4 of 14 children without any significant neurological history or symptoms had normal structural MRI but abnormal regional cerebral perfusion (Oguz et al., 2003). Other notable findings from the functional neuroimaging studies described are that (a) many children with structural lesions show more extensive brain regions affected on functional neuroimaging, (b) unilateral structural lesions frequently cause bilateral deficits as seen on functional neuroimaging, and (c) the structural lesions from silent cerebral infarction often can occur without functional lesions appearing on neuroimaging.

The functional neuroimaging studies to date have typically focused on recruiting children with SCD who are likely to have neurological involvement, so the precise base rate of these perfusion problems in the general pediatric SCD population is difficult to ascertain from these data. Continued use of these functional neuroimaging tools in conjunction with structural MRI will be important for a more complete characterization of the brain effects of SCD. More studies are needed that incorporate psychological assessment with these neuroimaging tools to better understand how well perfusion deficits explain the cognitive deficits found in children with no visible cerebral infarction.

*Diffuse Brain Effects.* In addition to the more localized sources of brain effects described, some researchers have posited that there are diffuse effects of SCD on the brain. Much of the data in support of this view have come from quantitative neuroimaging studies of brain structure. The major source of data in this area has been studies of the inherent T1 tissue values on MRI. T1 values are the rate at which tissue loses energy following the radio-frequency pulse during MRI exams (also called the spin lattice relaxation time of the tissue). The molecular makeup of the tissue is one factor that affects T1 values, and it therefore can provide an index of subtle differences in the composition of tissue. Steen et al. (1998, 1999, 2004; Steen, Emudianughe, et al., 2003) have reported T1 differences in normal appearing gray matter in regions such as the thalamus, caudate, and cortex for children with SCD compared to age-matched controls. The changes in T1 values appear to be relatively consistent across gray matter regions; this type of brain effect is distinctly different from the more localized brain changes described in the previous sections. In younger children, these changes appear as elevated T1 values before 2 years of age and rapidly shift to decreased T1 values after age 4 years (Steen et al., 2004). The size of the decrease in T1 in older children correlates robustly with both anemia severity (hematocrit) and general cognitive ability scores among children with SCD (Steen et al., 1999).

T1 values of otherwise healthy-appearing tissue can differ from typical values for a variety of reasons; however, the most likely explanation for these changes in children with SCD is that decreased T1 is a sign of neuronal changes (Steen et al., 1998, 1999; Steen, Emudianughe, et al., 2003). Steen and colleagues attributed this diffuse effect on brain tissue to anemia-induced hypoxic changes, which presumably are occurring in a relatively diffuse manner throughout gray matter. The brain is typically protected from oxygen deprivation more than other organs through autoregulatory mechanisms (Fan, Chen, Schuessler, & Chien, 1980; Kamitomo, Alonso, Okai, Longo, & Gilbert, 1993), but there is some evidence that this autoregulation does not fully occur in SCD; this could lead to a chronic oxygen shortage in the brain (Kennan, Suzaka, Nagel, & Fabry, 2004; Nahavandi, Tavakkoli, Hasan, Wyche, & Castro, 2004).

The major limitation of this work on diffuse brain effects has been the reliance on purely cross-sectional and correlational data. The data presented are consistent with the hypothesis of diffuse hypoxic damage, but additional data to rule out competing causal explanations are needed. Longitudinal studies to document any progression of the presumed hypoxic damage would help to strengthen the support for this view, particularly if changes in hypoxic risk over time could be shown to vary with changes in T1 values and cognition over time. In addition, this hypothesis could be better investigated by evaluating T1 changes over time in children receiving interventions that might decrease the rate of hypoxic damage.

## Intervention

Intervention efforts toward preventing or mitigating neurocognitive effects from SCD can be divided into primary, secondary, and tertiary prevention. Although primary and secondary prevention tools are most desirable, much of our knowledge about treatment for neurocognitive deficits lies in the areas of tertiary prevention. That is, we have techniques to mitigate the impact of these neurocognitive effects on quality of life or functional outcomes. Nonetheless, there are primary and secondary prevention techniques to consider.

### Primary and Secondary Prevention

Primary prevention efforts for the entire population of children with SCD can be developed to support brain resilience, optimize nutrition, and prevent stroke. It has been recognized for many decades that optimal environmental stimulation and parenting early in life promote greater resistance to the behavioral effects of brain insults. This finding is supported by research both with nonhuman animals (Donovick, Burright, & Swidler, 1973; Hughes, 1965; C. J. Smith, 1959) and with children (Greenberg & Crnic, 1988; Kilbride, Thorstad, & Daily, 2004; Koeppen-Schomerus, Eley, Wolke, Gringras, & Plomin, 2000; Landry, Smith, Miller-Loncar, & Swank, 1997; J. A. Smith et al., 1996). Thus, an optimal early social environment can play a protective role for children with SCD by increasing brain resilience. This approach could be particularly important for the more mild or subtle forms of brain insults that can occur with SCD. Psychosocial programs oriented toward education and support of positive parenting practices, reducing family stress, and optimizing cognitive stimulation (e.g., literacy programs for early childhood) should be considered for their potential impact on both psychological and brain health.

There also appears to be renewed interest in nutritional research in SCD, and this research needs to be translated into better nutritional education or support programs to optimize nutritional intake. It is important to note that studies of children living in low socioeconomic circumstances have found that nutritional supplementation can remove most of the association between socioeconomic status and cognitive test scores in early adolescence (Pollitt & Gorman, 1994; Pollitt et al., 1995, 1997). Analogous studies have not yet been conducted for pediatric SCD, but this work suggests a potential route for improving psychological outcomes.

An important new development in primary prevention is the established predictive power of TCD ultrasound of the large cerebral vessels to detect children likely to have an overt stroke (Adams et al., 1998). The use of TCD monitoring, along with prophylactic blood transfusions for those at high risk, has been shown to prevent approximately 90% of first strokes in children with SCD (Adams et al., 1998). The National Heart, Lung, and Blood Institute has therefore recommended that all children with SCD aged 2–16 years receive TCD screening, although there are several limitations to this recommendation.

First, the optimal time between screenings is not known and likely depends on the age of the child and prior TCD results (Adams et al., 2004). Second, the Stroke Prevention Trial in Sickle Cell Anemia protocol developed by Adams and colleagues requires special training for TCD technicians in specific methods, and most individuals outside a few major medical centers do not yet have access to this TCD screening method. Thus, important dissemination issues still need to be addressed. A final issue of concern is the management of blood transfusions to prevent stroke in children identified with the TCD screenings because it is unclear how long a patient must stay on this protocol to prevent stroke. Chronic transfusion therapy is a significant burden to families, and taking on this burden to prevent an unseen future complication requires a leap of faith. Given the extensive morbidity and risk of death associated with stroke, however, TCD monitoring and preventive transfusion therapy are vital tools to preventing morbidity and mortality. Individuals with psychosocial expertise could play a role in supporting family education, facilitating clinician-family communication, and addressing organizational systems issues that may impede the dissemination of this prevention tool.

The delivery of transfusion therapy to prevent stroke is a secondary prevention effort in that it targets high-risk individuals to prevent morbidity from stroke. Bone marrow transplant and oral hydroxyurea treatment have also been used as secondary prevention tools to reduce the risk of recurrent stroke in some children (Walters et al., 1996; Ware, Zimmerman, & Schultz, 1999). At present, there are no established methods for primary or secondary preventive intervention to address the morbidity from silent cerebral infarcts or possible diffuse brain effects. It has been noted in several studies that blood transfusions may reverse local perfusion problems or improve cognitive functioning (Herold et al., 1986; Kral et al., 2003; Powars et al., 1999). Current Phase III trials funded by the National Institutes of Health are under way to evaluate the impact of chronic transfusion therapy to prevent progressive silent cerebral infarcts and associated cognitive deficits (Silent Cerebral Infarct Multicenter Clinical Trial) and the impact of oral hydroxyurea on developmental and clinical outcomes in young children (Pediatric Hydroxyurea in Sickle Cell Anemia). Information on both of these trials can be found at http://clinicaltrials.gov/ct. Given the potential health risks of chronic transfusion therapy, bone marrow transplant, and oral hydroxyurea treatments, the risk-to-benefit ratio of these interventions to prevent morbidity from silent cerebral infarcts or other disease-related processes requires careful analysis, and the necessary data have not yet been collected.

### Tertiary Prevention

Interventions to reduce the effects of neurocognitive deficits on quality-of-life outcomes need to target the child, the family, and the school environment. Much of the available information on intervention strategies comes from more general rehabilitation strategies in pediatric psychology rather than strategies specifically developed for SCD.

Techniques for child-level intervention include cognitive remediation strategies and possible pharmacological interventions. Cognitive remediation typically involves strategy training and extensive practice of weaker skills. Although research studies to date have shown mixed outcomes, the use of cognitive rehabilitation to support recovery after a brain injury is still recommended (National Institutes of Health, 1998). Preliminary study of rehabilitation for children with stroke and cognitive deficits appears encouraging (Yerys et al., 2003) and is consistent with other studies highlighting the potential role of strategy training for improving functioning following brain injury (Brett & Laatsch, 1998).

Pharmacological treatments such as methylphenidate, a stimulant medication frequently used to manage attentional problems, have also been suggested as techniques to address attention deficits following brain injury. Stimulant drugs appear to reduce depression and improve motor recovery following stroke, but their role in improving cognitive functioning after a stroke is less clear (Challman & Lipsky, 2000). Several reports have indicated a potential role of methylphenidate in treating chronic attention deficits in children with central nervous system effects from cancer (Meyers, Weitzner, Valentine, & Levin, 1998; Thompson et al., 2001), but no published reports have examined this approach in children with attention problems related to SCD.

Education of family members and teachers about the type of neurocognitive deficits and how these may reveal themselves in day-to-day behavior is an important and sometimes overlooked method for reducing secondary adjustment problems. Teachers and other educators often do not have adequate information on the specific classroom needs that accompany a chronic health condition (Robinson, Kellett, Schatz, Carroll, & McRedmond, 2001). Many hospitals and schools are relatively well prepared for transitions from acute hospitalization to school, but after the initial transition, there is insufficient expertise in the more persistent issues for a child with a chronic health condition. This is particularly evident when children transition from classroom to classroom or school to school. It is not unusual to find a teacher who is unaware that a child has SCD or even that the child has had a stroke in the past. This is a matter for concern given that these children may need special learning strategies and that teachers may need to detect fever or other disease symptoms that have serious consequences for children with SCD.

It is relatively easy to see physical disabilities and to appreciate the disease-related challenges for someone with hemiparesis or similar sensorimotor difficulties. Cognitive deficits, particularly attention and executive skill deficits, however, can be subtle and are sometimes mistaken for a lack of motivation, low effort, or even passive aggressive behavior. Such misattributions can contribute to inaccurate labeling of the child, negative adult-child interactions that create problematic behavior, and inappropriate behavioral intervention plans. An extreme example of this is a child we have worked with who was routinely being suspended from school because of "oppositional" behavior. The child had sustained a stroke with significant injury to prefrontal areas of the brain. Despite IQ scores in the average range, the child exhibited executive skill deficits on neuropsychological evaluations that suggested significant impulsivity and poor frustration tolerance secondary to the brain injury. Education about reasonable expectations and alternative strategies for the child (given the brain injury) helped most of the educators to set more realistic goals and redirect the child's behavior rather than engaging in negative confrontations that exacerbated the child's limited frustration tolerance.

In addition, more extensive advocacy and environmental changes are often appropriate for a child with cognitive deficits related to SCD. We have found that, without outside advocacy from hospital staff, fewer than half of children with SCD who may qualify for accommodations actually

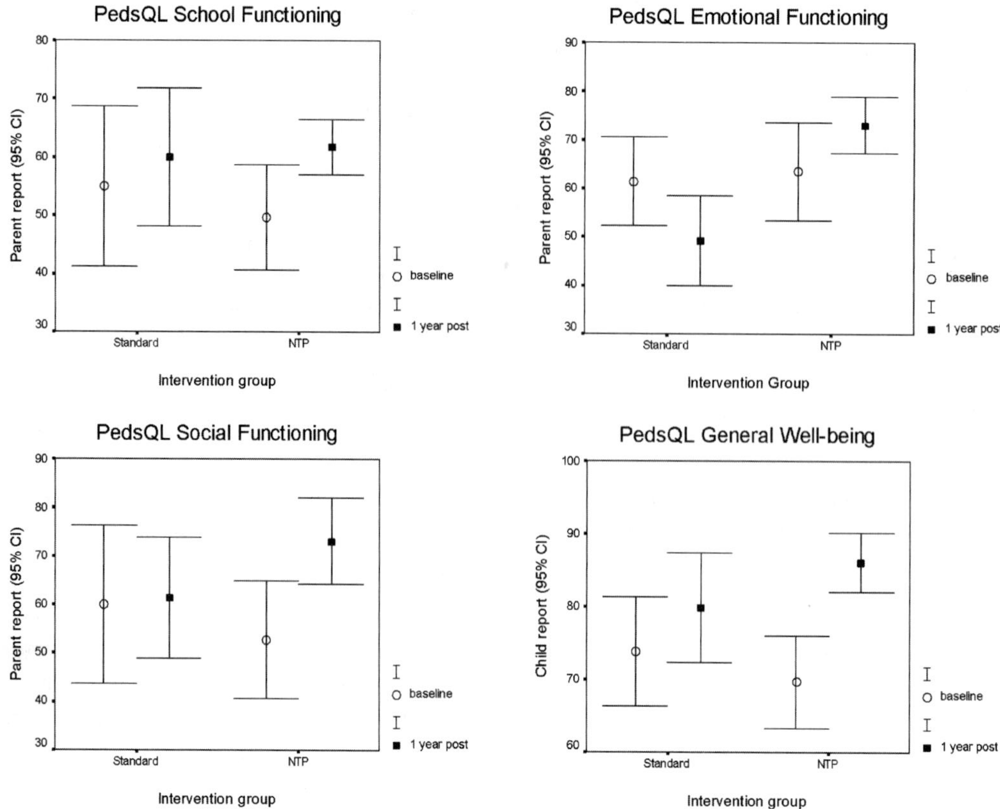


**Figure 24-3.** Pediatric quality-of-life (*PedsQL* version 3.0) data at baseline and 1 year after school interventions for children with brain injuries from SCD with stroke or brain tumors. Group 1 received school plans supplemented by information from hospital records and neuropsychological evaluation reports (termed standard care). Group 2 received the same external information but also had consultation time at the school with a pediatric neuropsychologist and an education specialist (termed neuropsychologically-informed team planning (NTP)). Both groups showed improvement in the School Functioning scale, but Group 2 showed better outcomes for the Emotional Functioning, Social Functioning, and General Well-Being scales. CI, confidence interval.

receive a 504 plan or individualized education plan (IEP). A 504 plan is for children who are fully capable of functioning in a regular classroom but need minor modifications in the classroom structure. This may include increased access to water and the bathroom (to maintain hydration), increased time to complete in-class exams or worksheets (because of attention difficulties), or similar adjustments to typical classroom procedures. Parents, when attempting to pursue these plans on their own, often report frustration and a lack of responsiveness by many schools unaware of the seriousness of SCD.

We have also found that students with more extensive educational needs who qualify for an IEP face difficulties because of some of the unique needs of children with unusual health conditions. Most special education programs are largely equipped to deal with mental retardation, specific learning disabilities (e.g., dyslexia), and severe emotional/behavioral problems. Children with stroke from SCD typically do not fit well into any of these categories, and the school staff may not have the expertise to devise a high-quality individualized plan. Preliminary data from an intervention study suggest that there is an important role for hospital-based professionals in supporting children's school adjustment (Schatz, Robinson, & Puffer, 2004).

We have compared psychosocial outcomes for children with educational plans developed by parents and school teams ($n = 21$) to children for whom a pediatric neuropsychologist and education expert in chronic health conditions worked directly with the parents and school team to develop an IEP ($n = 34$). The children included both those with SCD and stroke and children with brain tumors, but there were no differences in the study outcomes based on diagnosis. Baseline quality-of-life ratings by parents and the children before intervention did not differ between the groups, but after 1 year, the children whose school team received additional consultation showed improvements in social adjustment, emotional adjustment, and general sense of well-being that were not found in the other group (Schatz, Robinson, et al., 2004). School adjustment improved for both groups but appeared to be more robust for the group receiving additional expert consultation (see figure 24-3). Given the time and financial pressures that most hospital-based professionals face, the additional time required to conduct direct observations of child and teacher behavior at a school, consult with teachers, and attend school IEP meetings is a significant burden. Our experience and data, however, suggest that such consultation efforts can yield a meaningful difference in children's adjustment to stroke and other forms of brain injury.

## Summary and Conclusions

This chapter provides a review of the brain bases of psychological effects in SCD. SCD is a complex disorder that can affect brain function throughout the life span. The mechanisms of neurological effects of SCD, as well as neurocognitive outcomes, vary greatly across individuals. Overt stroke is the most recognized cause of neurocognitive deficits in SCD, but a number of other risk factors for neurological functioning may occur, such as perinatal brain injury, nutritional deficiencies, and other direct effects of SCD on the brain (e.g., silent cerebral infarcts). These other sources of neurological effects are more prevalent than overt stroke, but typically are associated with less-severe cognitive effects.

Significant progress has been made to develop the technology to prevent most cases of overt stroke from SCD. Although more work in overt stroke prevention remains to be done, interventions are needed to prevent or remediate the more prevalent, subtle brain effects such as silent cerebral infarcts or perfusion deficits. Additional research clarifying the relative importance of these other sources of neurocognitive deficits is also needed. The extent to which these factors create cognitive deficits and have an impact on quality of life is not fully understood, and such knowledge would be helpful to prioritize these factors for intervention research. Until additional intervention strategies are developed, the best practices for supporting children with SCD involve optimizing the early social and physical environment, educating people to recognize the psychological effects of SCD, and advocating for supportive services to minimize the impact of disease effects on functional outcomes.

## References


Adams, R. J., Brambilla, D. J., Granger, S., Gallagher, D., Vichinsky, E., Abboud, M. R., et al. (2004). Stroke and conversion to high risk in children screened with transcranial Doppler ultrasound during the STOP study. *Blood, 103,* 3689–3694.

Adams, R. J., McKie, V. C., Hsu, L., Files, B., Vichinsky, E., Pegelow, C., et al. (1998). Stroke prevention trial in sickle cell anemia. *New England Journal of Medicine, 339,* 5–11.

Adekile, A. D., Yacoub, F., Gupta, R., Sinan, T., Haider, M. Z., Habeeb, Y., et al. (2002). Silent brain infarcts are rare in Kuwaiti children with sickle cell disease and high HbF. *American Journal of Hematology, 70,* 228–231.

Armstrong, F. D., Thompson, R. J., Wang, W. C., Zimmerman, R., Pegelow, C. H., Miller, S., et al. (1996). Cognitive functioning and brain magnetic resonance imaging in children with sickle cell disease. *Pediatrics, 97,* 864–870.

Balgir, R. S., Dash, B. P., & Das, R. K. (1997). Fetal outcome and childhood mortality in offspring of mothers with sickle cell trait and disease. *Indian Journal of Pediatrics, 64,* 79–84.

Balkaran, B., Char, G., Morris, J. S., Thomas, P. W., Serjeant, B. E., & Serjeant, G. R. (1992). Stroke in a cohort of patients with homozygous sickle cell disease. *Journal of Pediatrics, 120,* 360–366.

Barden, E. M., Zemel, B. S., Kawchak, D. A., Goran, M. I., Ohene-Frempong, K., & Stallings, V. A. (2000). Total and resting energy expenditure in children with sickle cell disease. *Journal of Pediatrics, 136,* 73–79.

Bernaudin, F., Verlhac, S., Freard, F., Roudot-Thoraval, F., Benkerrou, M., Thuret, I., et al. (2000). Multicenter prospective study of children with sickle cell disease: Radiographic and psychometric correlation. *Journal of Child Neurology, 15,* 333–343.

Boni, L. C., Brown, R. T., Davis, P. C., Hsu, L., & Hopkins, K. (2001). Social information processing and magnetic resonance imaging in children with sickle cell disease. *Journal of Pediatric Psychology, 26*, 309–319.

Brandling-Bennett, E. M., White, D. A., Armstrong, M. M., Christ, S. E., & DeBaun, M. R. (2003). Patterns of verbal long-term and working memory performance reveal deficits in strategic processing in children with frontal infarcts related to sickle cell disease. *Developmental Neuropsychology, 24*, 423–434.

Brett, A. W., & Laatsch, L. (1998). Cognitive rehabilitation therapy of brain-injured students in a public high school setting. *Pediatric Rehabilitation, 2*, 27–31.

Brooks, L. J., Koziol, S. M., Chiarucci, K. M., & Berman, B. W. (1996). Does sleep-disordered breathing contribute to the clinical severity of sickle cell anemia? *Journal of Pediatric Hematology/Oncology, 18*, 135–139.

Brown, R. T., Buchanan, I., Doepke, K., Eckman, J. R., Baldwin, K., Goonan, B., et al. (1993). Cognitive and academic functioning in children with sickle cell disease. *Journal of Clinical Child Psychology, 22*, 207–218.

Brown, R. T., Davis, P. C., Lambert, R., Hsu, L., Hopkins, K., & Eckman, J. (2000). Neurocognitive functioning and magnetic resonance imaging in children with sickle cell disease. *Journal of Pediatric Psychology, 25*, 503–513.

Challman, T. D., & Lipsky, J. J. (2000). Methylphenidate: its pharmacology and uses. *Mayo Clinical Procedures, 75*, 711–721.

Chiu, D., Vichinsky, E., Ho, S. L., Liu, T., & Lubin, B. H. (1990). Vitamin C deficiency in patients with sickle cell anemia. *American Journal of Pediatric Hematology/Oncology, 12*, 262–267.

Cohen, M. J., Branch, W. B., McKie, V. C., & Adams, R. J. (1994). Neuropsychological impairment in children with sickle cell anemia and cerebrovascular accidents. *Clinical Pediatrics, 33*, 517–524.

Craft, S., Schatz, J., Glauser, T. A., Lee, B., & DeBaun, M. R. (1993). Neuropsychologic effects of stroke in children with sickle cell anemia. *Journal of Pediatrics, 123*, 712–717.

DeBaun, M. R., Schatz, J., Siegel, M. J., Koby, M., Craft, S., Resar, L., et al. (1998). Cognitive screening examinations for silent cerebral infarcts in sickle cell disease. *Neurology, 50*, 1678–1682.

Devine, D., Brown, R. T., Lambert, R., Donegan, J. E., & Eckman, J. (1998). Predictors of psychosocial and cognitive adaptation in children with sickle cell syndromes. *Journal of Clinical Psychology in Medical Settings, 5*, 295–313.

Donovick, P. J., Burright, R. G., & Swidler, M. A. (1973). Presurgical rearing environment alters exploration, fluid consumption, and learning of septal lesioned and control rats. *Physiology and Behavior, 11*, 543–553.

Earley, C. J., Kittner, S. J., Feeser, B. R., Epstein, A., Wozniak, M. A., Wityk, R., et al. (1998). Stroke in children and sickle-cell disease: Baltimore-Washington Cooperative Young Stroke Study. *Neurology, 51*, 169–176.

Evans, G. W. (2004). The environment of childhood poverty. *American Psychologist, 59*, 77–92.

Fan, F. C., Chen, R. Y., Schuessler, G. B., & Chien, S. (1980). Effects of hematocrit variations on regional hemodynamics and oxygen transport in the dog. *American Journal of Physiology, 238*, H545–H522.

Ferber, A., Grassi, A., Akyol, D., O'Reilly-Green, C., & Divon, M. Y. (2003). The association of fetal heart rate patterns with nucleated red blood cell counts at birth. *American Journal of Obstetrics and Gynecology, 188*, 1228–1230.

Forfar, J. O., Hume, R., McPhail, F. M., Maxwell, S. M., Wilkinson, E. M., Lin, J. P., et al. (1994). Low birthweight: A 10-year outcome study of the continuum of reproductive casualty. *Developmental Medicine and Child Neurology, 36*, 1037–1048.

Fowler, M. G., Whitt, J. K., Redding-Lallinger, R., Nash, K. B., Atkinson, S. S., Wells, R. J., et al. (1988). Neuropsychologic and academic functioning of children with sickle cell anemia. *Journal of Developmental and Behavioral Pediatrics, 9*, 213–220.

Frederickson, C. J., & Danscher, G. (1990). Zinc-containing neurons in hippocampus and related CNS structures. *Progress in Brain Research, 83*, 71–84.

Fung, E. B., Malinauskas, B. M., Kawchak, D. A., Koh, B. Y., Zemel, B. S., Gropper, S. S., et al. (2001). Energy expenditure and intake in children with sickle cell disease during acute illness. *Clinical Nutrition, 20*, 131–138.

Georgieff, M. K., & Rao, R. (2001). The role of nutrition in cognitive development. In C. A. Nelson & M. Luciana (Eds.), *Handbook of developmental cognitive neuroscience* (pp. 491–504). Cambridge, MA: MIT Press.

Gioia, G. A., Isquith, P. K., Guy, S. C., & Kenworthy, L. (2000). *Behavior Rating Inventory of Executive Function™ (BRIEF™)*. Lutz, FL: Psychological Assessment Resources.

Golub, M. S., Takeuchi, P. T., Keen, C. L., Gershwin, M. E., Hendrickx, A. G., & Lonnerdal, B. (1994). Modulation of behavioral performance of prepubertal monkeys by moderate dietary zinc deprivation. *American Journal of Clinical Nutrition, 60,* 238–243.

Gray, N. T., Bartlett, J. M., Kolasa, K. M., Marcuard, S. P., Holbrook, C. T., & Horner, R. D. (1992). Nutritional status and dietary intake of children with sickle cell anemia. *American Journal of Pediatric Hematology/Oncology, 14,* 57–61.

Greenberg, M. T., & Crnic, K. A. (1988). Longitudinal predictors of developmental status and social interaction in premature and full-term infants at age two. *Child Development, 59,* 554–570.

Gunnar, M. R. (2001). Effects of early deprivation: Findings from orphanage-reared infants and children. In C. A. Nelson and M. Luciana (Eds.), *Handbook of developmental cognitive neuroscience* (pp. 617–630). Cambridge, MA: MIT Press.

Hanlon-Lundberg, K. M., & Kirby, R. S. (1999). Nucleated red blood cell as a marker of acidemia in term neonates. *American Journal of Obstetrics and Gynecology, 181,* 196–201.

Hariman, L. M., Griffith, E. R., Hurtig, A. L., & Keehn, M. T. (1991). Functional outcomes of children with sickle-cell disease affected by stroke. *Archives of Physical and Medical Rehabilitation, 72,* 498–502.

Herold, S., Brozovic, M., Gibbs, J., Lammertsma, A. A., Leenders, K. L., Carr, D., et al. (1986). Measurement of regional cerebral blood flow, blood volume and oxygen metabolism in patients with sickle cell disease using positron emission tomography. *Stroke, 17,* 692.

Hindmarsh, P. C., Brozovic, M., Brook, C. G., & Davies, S. C. (1987). Incidence of overt and covert neurological damage in children with sickle cell disease. *Postgraduate Medical Journal, 63,* 751–753.

Hoppe, C., Klitz, W., Cheng, S., Apple, R., Steiner, L., Robles, L., et al. (2004). Gene interactions and stroke risk in children with sickle cell anemia. *Blood, 103,* 2391–2396.

Hughes, K. R. (1965). Dorsal and ventral hippocampus lesions and maze learning: Influence of preoperative environment. *Canadian Journal of Psychology, 19,* 325–332.

Inder, T. E., Huppi, P. S., Warfield, S., Kikinis, R., Zientara, G. P., Barnes, P. D., et al. (1999). Periventricular white matter injury in the premature infant is followed by reduced cerebral cortical gray matter volume at term. *Annals of Neurology, 46,* 755–760.

Kamitomo, M., Alonso, J. G., Okai, T., Longo, L. D., & Gilbert, R. D. (1993). Effects of long-term, high-altitude hypoxemia on bovine fetal cardiac output and blood flow distribution. *American Journal of Obstetrics and Gynecology, 169,* 701–707.

Kennan, R. P., Suzaka, S. M., Nagel, R. L., & Fabry, M. E. (2004). Decreased cerebral perfusion correlates with increased BOLD hyperoxia response in transgenic models of sickle cell disease. *Magnetic Resonance in Medicine, 51,* 525–532.

Kennedy, T. S., Fung, E. B., Kawchak, D. A., Zemel, B. S., Ohene-Frempong, K., & Stallings, V. A. (2001). Red blood cell folate and serum vitamin B12 status in children with sickle cell disease. *Journal of Pediatric Hematology/Oncology, 23,* 165–169.

Kilbride, H. W., Thorstad, K., & Daily, D. K. (2004). Preschool outcome of less than 801-gram preterm infants compared with full-term siblings. *Pediatrics, 113,* 742–747.

Kirkham, F. J., Hewes, D. K., Prengler, M., Wade, A., Lane, R., & Evans, J. P. (2001). Nocturnal hypoxaemia and central-nervous-system events in sickle-cell disease. *Lancet, 357,* 1656–1659.

Koeppen-Schomerus, G., Eley, T. C., Wolke, D., Gringras, P., & Plomin, R. (2000). The interaction of prematurity with genetic and environmental influences on cognitive development in twins. *Journal of Pediatrics, 137,* 527–533.

Koshy, M. (1995). Sickle cell disease and pregnancy. *Blood Reviews, 9,* 157–164.

Kral, M. C., Brown, R. T., Nietert, P. J., Abboud, M. R., Jackson, S. M., & Hynd, G. W. (2003). Transcranial Doppler ultrasonography and neurocognitive functioning in children with sickle cell disease. *Pediatrics, 112,* 324–331.

Landry, S. H., Smith, K. E., Miller-Loncar, C. L., & Swank, P. R. (1997). Predicting cognitive-language and social growth curves from early maternal behaviors in children at varying degrees of biological risk. *Developmental Psychology, 33,* 1040–1053.

Lemanek, K. L., Moore, S. L., Gresham, F. M., Williamson, D. A., & Kelley, M. L. (1986). Psychological adjustment of children with sickle cell anemia. *Journal of Pediatric Psychology, 11,* 397–409.

Malinauskas, B. M., Gropper, S. S., Kawchak, D. A., Zemel, B. S., Ohene-Frempong, K., & Stallings, V. A. (2000). Impact of acute illness on nutritional status of infants and young children with sickle cell disease. *Journal of the American Dietetic Association, 100,* 330–334.

Manzar, S. (2000). Maternal sickle cell trait and fetal hypoxia. *American Journal of Perinatology, 17,* 367–370.

McLoyd, V. C. (1998). Socioeconomic disadvantage and child development. *American Psychologist, 53,* 185–204.

Meade, J. A., Lumley, M. A., & Casey, R. J. (2001). Stress, emotional skill, and illness in children: The importance of distinguishing between children's and parents' reports of illness. *Journal of Child Psychology and Psychiatry, 42,* 405–412.

Mendola, P., Selevan, S. G., Gutter, S., & Rice, D. (2002). Environmental factors associated with a spectrum of neurodevelopmental deficits. *Mental Retardation and Developmental Disabilities Research Review, 8,* 188–197.

Meyers, C. A., Weitzner, M. A., Valentine, A. D., & Levin, V. A. (1998). Methylphenidate therapy improves cognition, mood, and function of brain tumor patients. *Journal of Clinical Oncology, 16,* 2522–2527.

Moser, F. G., Miller, S. T., Bello, J. A., Pegelow, C. H., Zimmerman, R. A., Wang, W. C., et al. (1996). The spectrum of brain MR abnormalities in sickle-cell disease: A report from the Cooperative Study of Sickle Cell Disease. *American Journal of Neuroradiology, 17,* 965–972.

Nahavandi, M., Tavakkoli, F., Hasan, S. P., Wyche, M. Q., & Castro, O. (2004). Cerebral oximetry in patients with sickle cell disease. *European Journal of Clinical Investigation, 34,* 143–148.

National Institutes of Health. (1998). *Rehabilitation of persons with traumatic brain injury. NIH Consensus Statement, 26–28* (pp. 1–41). Kensington, MD: U.S. Government Printing Office.

Nelson, M. C., Zemel, B. S., Kawchak, D. A., Barden, E. M., Fongillo, E. A., Jr., Coburn, S. P., et al. (2002). Vitamin B-6 status of children with sickle cell disease. *Journal of Pediatric Hematology/ Oncology, 24,* 463–469.

Oguz, K. K., Golay, X., Pizzini, F. B., Freer, C. A., Winrow, N., Ichord, R., et al. (2003). Sickle cell disease: continuous arterial spin-labeling perfusion MR imaging in children. *Radiology, 227,* 567–574.

Ohene-Frempong, K., Weiner, S. J., Sleeper, L. A., Miller, S. T., Embury, S., Moohr, J. W., et al. (1998). Cerebrovascular accidents in sickle cell disease: Rates and risk factors. *Blood, 91,* 288–294.

Oyesiku, N. M., Barrow, D. L., & Eckman, J. R. (1991). Intracranial aneurysms in sickle-cell anemia: Clinical features and pathogenesis. *Journal of Neurosurgery, 75,* 356–363.

Pavlakis, S. G., Prohovnik, I., Piomelli, S., & DeVivo, D. C. (1989). Neurologic complications of sickle cell disease. *Advances in Pediatrics, 36,* 247–276.

Pegelow, C. H., Adams, R. J., McKie, V., Abboud, M., Berman, B., Miller, S. T., et al. (1995). Risk of recurrent stroke in patients with sickle cell disease treated with erythrocyte transfusions. *Journal of Pediatrics, 126,* 896–899.

Peterson, B. S. (2003). Brain imaging studies of the anatomical and functional consequences of preterm birth for human brain development. *Annals of the New York Academy of Sciences, 1008,* 219–237.

Picard, E. M., Del Dotto, J. E., & Breslau, N. (1999). Prematurity and low birthweight. In M. D. Ris, K. O. Yeates, & H. G. Taylor (Eds.), *Pediatric neuropsychology: Research, theory, and practice* (pp. 237–251). New York: Guilford Publications.

Pollitt, E., & Gorman, K. S. (1994). Nutritional deficiencies as developmental risk factors. In C. A. Nelson (Ed.), *Threats to optimal development: The Minnesota symposium on child psychology* (pp. 121–144). Hillsdale, NJ: Erlbaum.

Pollitt, E., Gorman, K. S., Engle, P. L, Rivera, J. A., & Martorell, R. (1995). Nutrition in early life and the fulfillment of intellectual potential. *Journal of Nutrition, 125,* 111S–1118S.

Pollitt, E., Watkins, W. E., & Husaini, M. A. (1997). Three-month nutritional supplementation in Indonesian infants and toddlers benefits memory function 8 years later. *American Journal of Clinical Nutrition, 66,* 1357–1363.

Powars, D. R., Conti, P. S., Wong, W. Y, Groncy, P., Hyman, C., Smith, E., et al. (1999). Cerebral vasculopathy in sickle cell anemia: diagnostic contribution of positron emission tomography. *Blood, 93,* 71–79.

Powars, D., Wilson, B., Imbus, C., Pegelow, C., & Allen, J. (1978). The natural history of stroke in sickle cell disease. *American Journal of Medicine, 65,* 461–471.

Rao, R., DeUngria, M., Sullivan, D., Wu, P., Wobken, J. D., Nelson, C. A., et al. (1999). Perinatal brain iron deficiency increases the vulnerability of rat hippocampus to hypoxic ischemic insult. *Journal of Nutrition, 129,* 199–206.

Reed, W., Jagust, W., Al-Mateen, M., & Vichinsky, E. (1999). Role of positron emission tomography in determining the extent of CNS ischemia in patients with sickle cell disease. *American Journal of Hematology, 60,* 268–272.

Robertson, P. L., Aldrich, M. S., Hanash, S. M., & Goldstein, G. W. (1988). Stroke associated with obstructive sleep apnea in a child with sickle cell anemia. *Annals of Neurology, 23,* 614–616.

Robinson, J. S., Kellett, J. M., Schatz, J., Carroll, B., & McRedmond, K. (2001, November). *Faculty needs assessment for the educational management of youth with chronic health conditions.* Paper presented at the annual meeting of the National Hemophilia Foundation, Nashville, TN.

Rodgers, G. P., Clark, C. M., Larson, S. M., Rapoport, S. I., Nienhuis, A. W., & Schechter, A. N. (1988). Brain glucose metabolism in neurologically normal patients with sickle cell disease. *Archives of Neurology, 45,* 78–82.

Sanstead, H. H., Penland, J. G., Alcock, N. W., Dayal, H. H., Cen, X. C., Li, J. S., et al. (1998). Effects of repletion with zinc and other micronutrients on neuropsychologic performance and growth of Chinese children. *American Journal of Clinical Nutrition, 68,* 470S–475S.

Saracoglu, F., Sahin, I., Eser, E., Gol, K., & Turkkani, B. (2000). Nucleated red blood cells as a marker in acute and chronic fetal asphyxia. *International Journal of Gynaecology and Obstetrics, 71,* 113–118.

Schatz, J., Brown, R. T., Pascual, J. M., Hsu, L., & DeBaun, M. R. (2001). Poor school and cognitive functioning with silent cerebral infarcts and sickle cell disease. *Neurology, 56,* 1109–1111.

Schatz, J., Craft, S., Koby, M., & DeBaun, M. R. (2000). A lesion analysis of visual orienting performance in children with cerebral vascular injury. *Developmental Neuropsychology, 17,* 49–61.

Schatz, J., Craft, S., Koby, M., & DeBaun, M. R. (2004). Asymmetries in visual-spatial processing following childhood stroke. *Neuropsychology, 18,* 340–52.

Schatz, J., Craft, S., Koby, M., Siegel, M. J., Resar, L., Lee, R. R., et al. (1999). Neuropsychologic deficits in children with sickle cell disease and cerebral infarction: Role of lesion site and volume. *Child Neuropsychology, 5,* 92–103.

Schatz, J., Finke, R. L., Kellett, J. M., & Kramer, J. H. (2002). Cognitive functioning in children with sickle cell disease: A meta-analysis. *Journal of Pediatric Psychology, 8,* 739–748.

Schatz J., Finke, R. L., & Roberts, C. W. (2004). Interactions among biomedical and environmental factors in cognitive development: A preliminary study of sickle cell disease. *Journal of Developmental and Behavioral Pediatrics, 25,* 303–310.

Schatz, J., Robinson, J. S., & Puffer, E. S. (2004, September). *Promoting school success following childhood stroke: Standard school advocacy versus a neuropsychologically-informed team planning approach.* Paper presented at the 27th annual meeting of the National Sickle Cell Disease Program, Los Angeles, CA.

Schatz, J., White, D. A., Moinuddin, A., Armstrong, M., & DeBaun, M. R. (2002). Lesion burden and cognitive morbidity in children with sickle cell disease. *Journal of Child Neurology, 17,* 891–895.

Sindel, L. J., Dishuck, J. F., Baliga, B. S., & Mankad, V. N. (1990). Micronutrient deficiency and neutrophil function in sickle cell disease. *Annals of the New York Academy of Sciences, 587,* 70–77.

Singhal, A., Davies, P., Wierenga, K. J., Thomas, P., & Serjeant, G. (1997). Is there an energy deficiency in homozygous sickle cell disease? *American Journal of Clinical Nutrition, 66,* 386–390.

Singhal, A., Parker, S., Linsell, L., & Serjeant, G. (2002). Energy intake and resting metabolic rate in preschool Jamaican children with homozygous sickle cell disease. *American Journal of Clinical Nutrition, 75,* 1093–1097.

Smith, C. J. (1959). Mass action and early environment in the rat. *Journal of Comparative Physiological Psychology, 52,* 154–156.

Smith, J. A., Espeland, M., Bellevue, R., Bonds, D., Brown, A. K., & Koshy, M. (1996). Pregnancy in sickle cell disease: experience of the Cooperative Study of Sickle Cell Disease. *American Journal of Obstetrics and Gynecology, 87,* 199–204.

Steen, R. G., Emudianughe, T., Hankins, G. M., Wynn, L. W., Wang, W. C., Xiong, X., et al. (2003). Brain imaging findings in pediatric patients with sickle cell disease. *Radiology, 228,* 216–225.

Steen, R. G., Fineberg-Buchner, C., Hankins, G., Weiss, L., Prifitera, A., & Mulhern, R. K. (2005). Neurocognitive deficits in children with sickle cell disease. *Journal of Child Neurology, 20,* 102–107.

Steen, R. G., Hunte, M., Traipe, E., Hurh, P., Wu, S., Bilaniuk, L., et al. (2004). Brain T(1) in young children with sickle cell disease: Evidence of early abnormalities in brain development. *Magnetic Resonance Imaging, 22,* 299–306.

Steen, R. G., Miles, M. A., Helton, K. J., Strawn, S., Wang, W. C., Xiong, X., et al. (2003). Cognitive impairment in children with hemoglobin SS sickle cell disease: Relationship to MR imaging findings and hematocrit. *American Journal of Neuroradiology, 24,* 382–389.

Steen, R. G., Reddick, W. E., Mulhern, R. K., Langston, J. W., Ogg, R. J., Bieberich, A. A., et al. (1998). Quantitative MRI of the brain in children with sickle cell disease reveals abnormalities unseen by conventional MRI. *Journal of Magnetic Resonance Imaging, 8,* 535–543.

Steen, R. G., Xiong, X., Mulhern, R. K., Langston, J. W., & Wang, W. C. (1999). Subtle brain abnormalities in children with sickle cell disease: Relationship with blood hematocrit. *Annals of Neurology, 45,* 279–286.

Stettler, N., Zemel, B. S., Kawchak, D. A., Ohene-Frempong, K., & Stallings, V. A. (2001). Iron status of children with sickle cell disease. *Journal of Parenteral Enteral Nutrition, 25,* 36–38.

Sun, P. M., Wilburn, W., Raynor, B. D., & Jamieson, D. (2001). Sickle cell disease in pregnancy: 20 years of experience at Grady Memorial Hospital, Atlanta, Georgia. *American Journal of Obstetrics and Gynecology, 184,* 1127–1130.

Swift, A. V., Cohen, M. J., Hynd, G. W., Wisenbaker, J. M., McKie, K. M., Makari, G., et al. (1989).

Neuropsychological impairment in children with sickle cell anemia. *Pediatrics, 84,* 1077–1085.

Sydenstricker, V. P., Mulherin, W. A., & Houseal, R. W. (1923). Sickle cell anemia. *American Journal of Diseases of Children, 26,* 132–154.

Taylor, H. G., Klein, N., Minich, N. M., & Hack, M. (2000). Middle-school-age outcomes in children with very low birth weight. *Child Development, 71,* 1495–1511.

Thompson, R. J., Armstrong, F. D., Kronenberger, W. G., Scott, D., McCabe, M. A., Smith, B., et al. (1999). Family functioning, neurocognitive functioning, and behavior problems in children with sickle cell disease. *Journal of Pediatric Psychology, 24,* 491–498.

Thompson, R. J., Armstrong, F. D., Link, C. L., Pegelow, C. H., Moser, F., & Wang, W. C. (2003). A prospective study of the relationship over time of behavior problems, intellectual functioning, and family functioning in children with sickle cell disease: A report from the Cooperative Study of Sickle Cell Disease. *Journal of Pediatric Psychology, 28,* 59–65.

Thompson, S. J., Leigh, L., Christensen, R., Xiong, X., Kun, L. E., Heideman, R. L., et al. (2001). Immediate neurocognitive effects of methylphenidate on learning-impaired survivors of childhood cancer. *Journal of Clinical Oncology, 19,* 1802–1808.

Wali, Y. A., Al-Lamki, Z., Soliman, H., & Al-Okbi, H. (2000). Adenotonsillar hypertrophy: A precipitating factor of cerebrovascular accident in a child with sickle cell anemia. *Journal of Tropical Pediatrics, 46,* 246–248.

Walters, M. C., Patience, M., Leisenring, W., Eckman, J. R., Scott, J. P., Mentzer, W. C., et al. (1996). Bone marrow transplantation for sickle cell disease. *New England Journal of Medicine, 335,* 369–376.

Wang, W., Enos, L., Gallagher, D., Thompson, R., Guarini, L., Vichinsky, E., et al. (2001). Neuropsychologic performance in school-aged children with sickle cell disease: A report from the Cooperative Study of Sickle Cell Disease. *Journal of Pediatrics, 139,* 391–397.

Ware, R. E., Zimmerman, S. A., & Schultz, W. H. (1999). Hydroxyurea as an alternative to blood transfusions for the prevention of recurrent stroke in children with sickle cell disease. *Blood, 94,* 3022–3026.

Watkins, K. E., Hewes, D. K., Connelly, A., Kendall, B. E., Kingsley, D. P., Evans, J. E., et al. (1998). Cognitive deficits associated with frontal lobe infarction in children with sickle cell disease. *Developmental Medicine and Child Neurology, 40,* 536–543.

White, D. A., & DeBaun, M. R. (1998). Cognitive and behavioral function in children with sickle cell disease: A review and discussion of methodological issues. *Journal of Pediatric Hematology Oncology, 20,* 458–462.

White, D. A., Saloria, C. F., Schatz, J., & DeBaun, M. R. (2000). Preliminary study of working memory in children with stroke related to sickle cell disease. *Journal of Clinical and Experimental Neuropsychology, 22,* 257–264.

Wilimas, J., Goff, J. R., Anderson, H. R., Langston, J. W., & Thompson, E. (1980). Efficacy of transfusion therapy for one to two years in patients with sickle cell disease and cerebrovascular accidents. *Journal of Pediatrics, 96,* 205–208.

Williams, R., George, E. O., & Wang, W. (1997). Nutrition assessment in children with sickle cell disease. *Journal of the Association of Academic Minority Physiologists, 8,* 44–48.

Winick, M., & Noble, A. (1966). Cellular responses in rats during malnutrition at various ages. *Journal of Nutrition, 89,* 300–306.

Winick, M., & Rosso, P. (1969a). The effects of severe early malnutrition on cellular growth of human brain. *Pediatric Research, 3,* 181–184.

Winick, M., & Rosso, P. (1969b). Head circumference and cellular growth of the brain in normal and marasmic children. *Journal of Pediatrics, 74,* 774–778.

Yerys, B. E., White, D. A., Salorio, C. F., McKinstry, R., Moinuddin, A., & DeBaun, M. R. (2003). Memory strategy training in children with cerebral infarcts related to sickle cell disease. *Journal of Pediatric Hematology/Oncology, 25,* 495–498.

Lamia P. Barakat, Laurie A. Lash, Meredith J. Lutz, and D. Colette Nicolaou

# Psychosocial Adaptation of Children and Adolescents With Sickle Cell Disease

Sickle Cell has brought me both pain and joy
My school friends make fun of my yellow eyes
And along with the sickle cell pain, my friends make it worst
I have to learn to cope with my sickness
Because it is one for life

I have to be strong for myself and especially for my mom
She brings the joyful part of sickle cell to me.

Shernel Grant
(www.sicklecellsociety.org/sicklescene/poets.htm)

Sickle cell disease (SCD), a chronic genetic disorder, can produce a host of potentially life-threatening complications that may have an impact on the physical integrity and psychosocial adaptation of the affected child or adolescent. The nature of SCD presents many risk factors, particularly for those children with the most severe form, sickle cell anemia (hemoglobin [Hb] SS). Most common and significant is that SCD involves recurrent, unpredictable pain that can interfere with daily functioning, including social activities and school attendance.

Treatment for SCD varies in intensity and invasiveness depending on severity of complications. It may involve daily management (i.e., hydration, restrictions on activities, prophylactic antibiotics, and pain management) as well as preventive follow-up care. Regular blood transfusions are required for children who have had stroke, are at risk for stroke, or experience severe pain crises. Alternative solutions for those with the most severe disease include hydroxyurea and bone marrow transplant.

Children with SCD experience pain episodes that vary in severity, duration, and frequency (Brown, Doepke, & Kaslow, 1993). In children with SCD, intense pain episodes often result in repeated hospitalizations and absences from school (Brown, Doepke, et al., 1993). In addition, some forms of pain management, including limitation of physical activity, may interfere with children's ability to participate in sport activities or to engage in peer relations when they are experiencing a pain crisis. Moreover, the occurrence of cerebrovascular accidents (CVAs) or stroke can have an impact on academic achievement and long-term occupational outcomes (Lemanek, Buckloh, Woods, & Butler, 1995).

Although comparisons to other pediatric populations may be useful for understanding processes involved in adaptation, there are aspects of the lives of children and adolescents with SCD, and of their disease, that require a specifically modified approach to the investigation of psychosocial adaptation and application of the current pediatric literature. These issues include the genetic nature of this life-threatening and life-shortening disease, the high prevalence of the disease in African American individuals in the United States, and the multiple stressors faced by children and adolescents with SCD. In addition to health-related stressors, children and adolescents with SCD are faced with challenges related to ethnic minority status and the associated experiences of prejudice, discrimination, decreased access to health care, urban environmental stressors, and barriers related to socioeconomic status (SES) that may have an impact on their health status and psychosocial adaptation (Barbarin & Christian, 1999; Baskin et al., 1998; Johnson et al., 1995).

To demonstrate the interrelation of these factors, caregivers may not divulge the diagnosis of their child to school staff out of concern for stigmatization surrounding SCD and discrimination against their child. In addition, families of children and adolescents with SCD may not seek health care services when needed because of distrust of the medical community and its institutions, and when coupled with a lack of access to services, medical complications may be exacerbated (Baskin et al., 1998). Moreover, the demands of treatment for SCD may seem onerous in the context of the multiple requirements and stressors associated with struggles to meet the family's basic needs (Barbarin & Christian, 1999). In addition to formulating understanding of risk factors in children and adolescents with SCD, unique aspects require a broader consideration of resources that support adaptation, including the role of religion and spirituality as part of adaptive coping and variations on two-parent family structures that incorporate adults other than parents to provide support to the child (as discussed in this volume's chapter 26 on family systems issues).

Careful consideration of these factors compels one to adopt a culturally sensitive and competent approach to empirical investigation of psychosocial adaptation of children and adolescents with SCD, to interpretation of current research findings, and to development of culturally competent, potentially effective interventions (S. Y. Lewis, 1992). A culturally sensitive approach suggests that strategies and measures used with other pediatric groups may not be completely relevant or appropriate for use with children and adolescents with SCD. In addition, methods that fail to account for the multiple stressors these children and their families experience will fall short of the goals of prediction and development of effective interventions (Airhihenbuwa, 1990; Boyd-Franklin, Steiner, & Boland, 1995).

With these caveats in mind, two types of models focus this discussion of psychosocial adaptation of children and adolescents with SCD: the social ecological model as applied to children with chronic illness (Kazak, 1989) and risk-and-resistance models for explaining variations in adaptation across children and disease groups (Wallander & Thompson, 1995; Wallander & Varni, 1998) (see figure 25-1). Risk-and-resistance models provide a useful structure for organizing and understanding the findings regarding psychosocial adaptation of children and adolescents with SCD while offering flexibility in capturing the unique aspects of this population that may guide subsequent investigations and intervention development. Because risk-and-resistance models do not explicitly articulate the complex roles that sociocultural factors and psychosocial stressors may play in adaptation, the social ecological model, with its emphasis on interactions among various systems in which the child functions, is noted here. This model, by articulating the important roles of family relationships and societal-level influences, including culture, guided the expansion of risk-and-resistance models in this review. Not all aspects of risk-and-resistance models have been studied, and all variables that have been studied are not included in this review. The focus herein is on factors with theoretical or empirical relevance to the adaptation of children and adolescents with SCD (and these are highlighted on the figure 25-1).

In comparison with demographically matched comparison groups, children and adolescents with SCD are at risk for the development of psychological distress and problems in the areas of internalizing disorders, self-esteem, and general quality of life as well as neurocognitive functioning and school achievement. Thompson and colleagues (2003) found that 30% of children enrolled in the Cooperative Study of Sickle Cell Disease displayed some type of internalizing or externalizing behavior problems. Findings also pointed to the remarkable resilience of many children and adolescents with SCD in that problems noted are often not at a level of psychopathology, and that the majority of youths with SCD function adaptively. This provides a reminder that strength can be developed while facing difficult stressors, and that children and families can thrive in the face of such challenges.

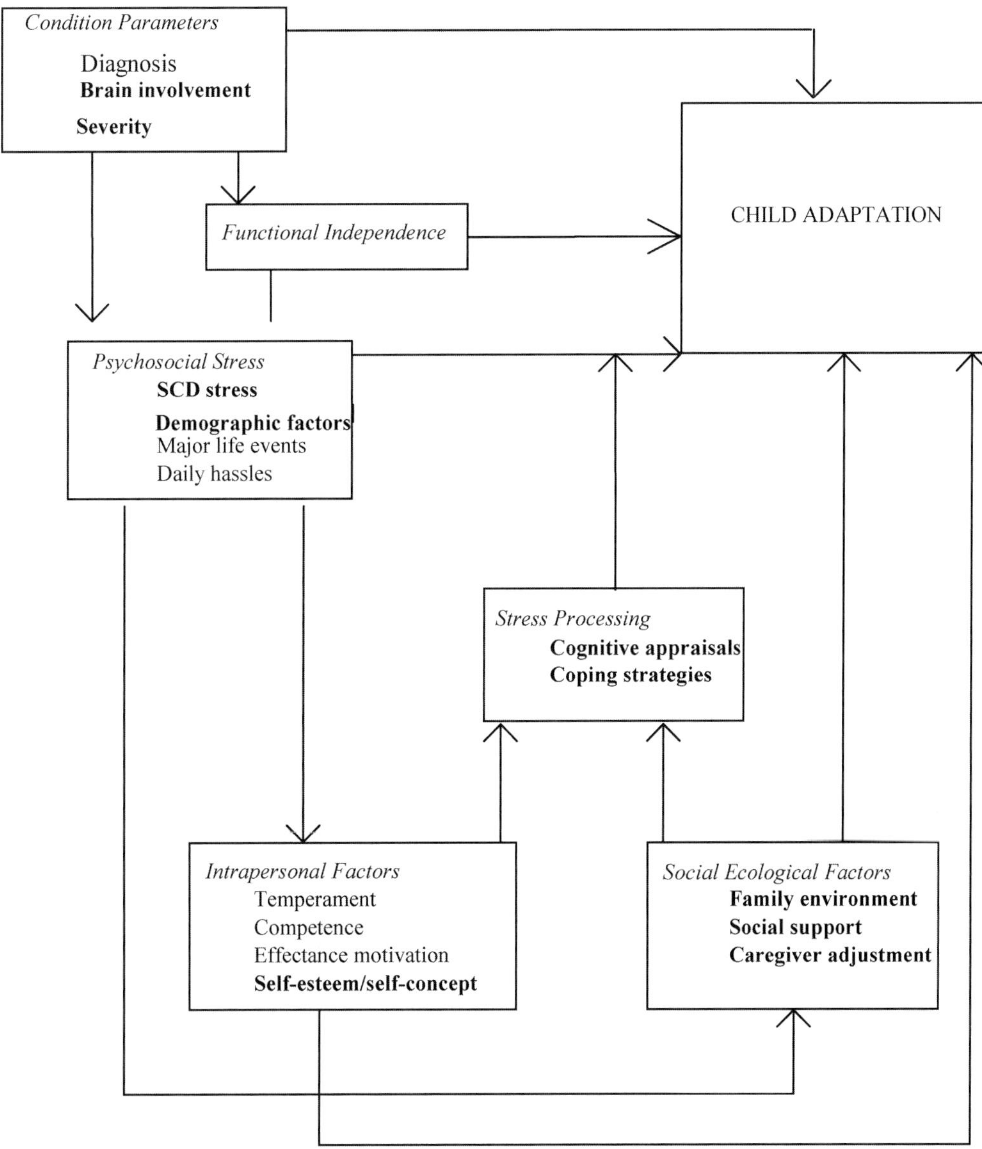


**Figure 25-1.** Risk-and-resistance model (Wallander & Thompson, 1995).

## Psychosocial Adaptation in Pediatric Sickle Cell Disease

Increased attention to pediatric adaptation outcomes within chronically ill pediatric populations has led to a systematic descriptive investigation into the measurement of adaptation for specific disease, child, and socioecological parameters and has allowed for the description of adaptational processes potentially responsible for detected variances in adaptation. Psychosocial adaptation addresses a broad range of potential behavioral and psychosocial outcome variables relevant within a pediatric framework and should be viewed through a developmental perspective to capture age-appropriate, normative, and healthy movement toward adulthood. However, a clear delineation of psychosocial adaptation has been difficult to operationalize because of its encompassing nature. Nevertheless, the construct of psychosocial adaptation has been conceptualized by three principal categories: behavior problems or externalizing disorders, emotional behavior problems or internalizing disorders, and social competence variables.

Psychosocial adaptation has been viewed within the context of one's overall quality of life, including physical, psychological, and social health as a function of one's perceptions, appraisals, and coping processes (Testa & Simonson, 1996). Physical symptoms, such as disability of functioning, psychological affect, emotional stability, social interpersonal relations, and work or school performance, are all targeted quality of life variables measured through objective health outcomes as well as through subjective evaluations such as the Pediatric Quality of Life Inventory™ (PedsQL) (Varni et al., 1998) and the Miami Quality of Life Questionnaire (QOL) (Armstrong et al., 1999). Quality of life measures address a variety of relevant adaptation dimensions, and research is just beginning to assess the deleterious impact of SCD on quality of life as it relates to adaptation (Palermo, Schwartz, Drotar, & McGowan, 2002; Thomas & Taylor, 2002).

Although several other factors are often associated with adaptation, such as self-esteem and personality functioning, it is helpful to examine the employment of externalizing behaviors, internalizing behaviors, and social competence within the literature, as well as the assessment tools and research designs used to document psychosocial adaptation. The most widely used measurement of psychosocial adaptation in children and adolescents with SCD is the Child Behavior Checklist (CBCL) (Achenbach, 1991; Achenbach & Edelbrock, 1983, 1986, 1987), which is a multiaxial, empirically based assessment that aims to obtain data from multiple sources across several informants to create a more comprehensive profile of an individual's functioning. It was designed to detect variations in child behaviors across different settings by appraising cognitive and physical domains through parent and teacher reports, as well as though direct assessment of the child (Maruish, 1999).

All three forms of the CBCL are composed of an internalizing dimension, which includes the following subscales: withdrawal, somatic complaints, and anxious/depressed mood. In addition, there is an externalizing dimension, which assesses delinquent and aggressive behaviors, and there are three other subscales within the CBCL that measure social problems, thought problems, and attention problems. Furthermore, the parent report form assesses social competence through an activity subscale, a social subscale, and a school subscale. The child self-report form addresses social competence through the measurement of activities and social functioning.

The CBCL is a well-validated measure that offers several advantages in the assessment of psychosocial adaptation because of its multimodal sensitivities and perspectives. Unfortunately, however, concordance rates among parent, teacher, and child reports have been found to be quite low (Achenbach, McConaughy, & Howell, 1987), yet several factors have been identified that may account for various discrepancies. The reliability of structured interviews for younger children is relatively low (Edelbrock, Costello, Dulcan, Conover, & Kalas, 1986; Edelbrock, Costello, Dulcan, Kalas, & Conover, 1985), and the types of symptoms a child experiences are differentially reported by parents, who tend to describe more externalizing behaviors compared to children, who account more internalizing problems (Hodges, Gordon, & Lennon, 1990; Thompson, Merritt, Keith, Murphy, & Johndrow, 1993). Gender and age also facilitate variations in parent and child reports of symptoms (Thompson, Gil, Burbach, Keith, & Kinney, 1993).

In light of the frequent use of normative samples as the comparison, it is important to recognize the limitations of the CBCL within a primarily African American SCD population and to be aware that cultural and content validity may be questionable for these children (Lambert, Rowan, Lyubansky, & Russ, 2002). Similar problems may arise for other measures of adaptation that are less well validated and have been standardized on primarily Caucasian samples. Furthermore, because the CBCL has not been specifically designed for use among chronically ill populations, one must be aware of possible erroneous biases and conclusions. For example, physical complaints, detected by the somatic scale, often provide evidence of an internalizing disorder. Perrin, Stein, and Drotar (1991) also noted that the potential to overlook mild adaptation problems often experienced among these populations as well as ambiguous social competence estimates, which emphasize unique methodological issues associated with the assessment of chronically ill children.

There is a lack of consistency within the current literature regarding the use and type of comparison groups most appropriate for pediatric sickle cell populations. As noted, several studies did not use comparison groups when assessing psychosocial adaptation, but rather used normative data from the general population as a means of comparison (Brown, Eckman, Baldwin, Buchanan, & Dingle, 1995). However, one must be aware of the limitations of using measures not specifically normed for African American populations (Molock & Belgrave, 1994). Alternatively, siblings of patients with SCD (Lee, Phoenix, Brown, & Jackson, 1997), other pediatric populations (Thompson, Gustafson, Gil, Godfry, & Murphy, 1998), and randomly selected healthy children have been used as reference groups for SCD samples (Midence, McManus, Fuggle, & Davies, 1996). More precise comparison groups can be compiled by matching children and adolescents with SCD with healthy comparisons on a number of variables, including age, sex, SES, and IQ scores (Lemanek, Moore, Gresham, Williamson, & Kelley, 1986; Noll et al., 1996), an approach that is strongly recommended. The selection of appropriate comparison groups is crucial to understanding the implications of results by allowing the untangling of variables that may directly or indirectly have an impact on the relationship between SCD and psychosocial adaptation.

Three primary areas of investigation among children and adolescents with SCD serve to provide a comprehensive assessment of psychosocial adaptation: externalizing behavior problems, internalizing behavior problems, and social competence. A thorough review of the current literature on these outcomes is essential to provide a foundation for understanding the psychosocial adaptation of children and adolescents with SCD and the accompanying underlying processes.

### Externalizing Behavior Problems

Although externalizing behavior problems often have been associated with pediatric populations, research has yielded primarily unsupportive results in terms of SCD samples. Lemanek and colleagues (1986) found that children diagnosed with SCD demonstrated conduct-related behavior problems in a variety of settings, including at home, at school, and among their peers. However, scores on the externalizing behavior problem scale were not significantly different from normative samples and remained within the normal range of functioning on the CBCL. The authors suggested that low SES might be a more likely explanation for higher levels of symptoms when detected in this population rather than specific SCD-related characteristics.

Thompson and colleagues (1998) assessed psychosocial adaptation in children and adolescents with SCD to determine the prevalence of problems in adaptation as well as underlying adaptational processes. Their study, involving 49 children between the ages of 7 and 12 years, revealed that 7.5% of the sample experienced externalizing disorders, including conduct and oppositional defiant disorder, suggesting moderately low prevalence of these diagnoses in youths with SCD compared to a sample of children with cystic fibrosis, of whom 35% were detected to have externalizing disorders.

In addition, Kell, Kliewer, Erickson, and Ohene-Frempong (1998) found that, on both parent and child report measures, adolescents with SCD did not have an increased risk of externalizing behavior problems compared to normative samples. Moreover, Barbarin (1999) reported lower levels of externalizing behavior problems among youths with SCD compared to a demographically matched comparison group. A further investigation into the complexity of psychosocial adaptation by Hurtig and White (1986) suggested an interaction between developmental and gender variables in adaptation outcome. They found differences among boys and girls across age groups; older boys consistently displayed more behavior problems than their younger counterparts.

Findings from research on externalizing behavior problems varies, but overall suggest no increased risk. Based on studies using normative samples, children and adolescents with SCD may exhibit more externalizing behavior problems while remaining within the nonclinical range; however, no difference or better functioning was found when demographically matched comparison groups were employed. Subsequently, findings suggest an interaction between age and gender in which older adolescent males display the highest degree of externalizing problems among the pediatric SCD population. These results highlight the need for further research with demographically matched comparison groups and suggest looking at demographic factors when evaluating children and adolescents with SCD.

### Internalizing Behavior Problems

Internalizing disorders, including anxiety and depression, are the most frequently identified problems in adaptation experienced by children and adolescents with SCD (Thompson et al., 2003). In an initial study of adaptation among 24 adolescents with SCD, Morgan and Jackson (1986) found significantly higher rates of depressive symptoms as well as lower satisfaction with their bodies when compared to matched, healthy controls. Furthermore, Barbarin, Whitten, and Bonds (1994) found that 25% of their sample experienced internalizing symptoms in the form of depression or anxiety.

Similar to the age effects seen for externalizing behavior problems, adolescents with SCD have been found to exhibit increased internalizing behavior problems compared to school-aged children (Brown, Kaslow, et al., 1993; Hurtig, Koepke, & Park, 1989; Hurtig & White, 1986; Midence, Fuggle, & Davies, 1993). In addition, male adolescents showed higher rates of internalizing behavior problems than females (Hurtig & Park, 1989; Kell et al., 1998), who nevertheless scored significantly higher on somatic complaints, schizoid, depressed withdrawal, and delinquent behavior domains than normative samples (Hurtig & Park, 1989).

As noted, the frequency of internalizing disorder diagnoses among children and adolescents with SCD has been estimated as approximately 37.5% (Thompson et al., 1998). Anxiety disorders were the most prevalent diagnosis (27.5%) among the sample; however, instability over time and poor congruence between mother- and child-reported behavior problems beckon for more thorough longitudinal investigations of changes in adaptation for individual children as they develop (Thompson, Gil, Keith, et al., 1994; Thompson, Gustafson, Gil, Kinney, & Spock, 1999).

Despite this support for the increased prevalence of internalizing behavior problems among children and adolescents with SCD relative to their healthy peers, an early study by Lemanek et al. (1986) did not find elevated rates of internalizing behavior problems among children and adolescents as compared to normative data or normal controls. In a more recent study, 14 youths with SCD scored lower on a self-report measure of depression compared to their healthy siblings (Lee et al., 1997). Conversely, Brown, Kaslow, and colleagues (1993) found that 61 children and adolescents reported higher levels of symptoms of depression, and their mothers reported more internalizing behavior problems compared with healthy sibling controls. These contradictory findings suggest the need for further study of internalizing behavior problems with careful attention to the use of demographically matched comparison groups that are independent of SCD participants.

### Social Competence

Taking into account the high rate of absenteeism, limited peer contact, delayed physical maturation, and restricted activity associated with SCD, it is not surprising that children and adolescents may show problematic social development (Clark, Striefel, Bedlington, & Naiman, 1989) and have been found to be at greater risk for inadequate social competence (Brown, Kaslow, et al., 1993; Kumar, Powars, Allen, & Haywood, 1976). Moreover, when compared to healthy comparisons, adolescents with SCD have been found to participate in fewer social and nonsocial activities, to be less successful academically, and to be more likely to have repeated a grade in school (Morgan & Jackson, 1986).

Conversely, Lemanek, Horwitz, and Ohene-Frempong (1994) did not find significantly lower social competence among children aged 4–8 years with SCD as assessed by self-, parent, and teacher reports; however, these findings may be caused by age effects. For example, younger children have difficulty making realistic judgments about themselves (Harter & Pike, 1984). Also, the effects of delayed puberty on peer relationships (which seem to be important in an adolescent sample) would not be apparent in this age group. In another exception to these findings, significant differences compared to demographically matched, healthy peers in social competence were not observed by Rodrigue and colleagues as assessed through parent and teacher reports (Rodrigue, Streisand, Banko, Kedar, & Pitel, 1996). However, mean scores were one standard deviation below the

CBCL normative mean, and adolescents within the sample did indeed view themselves as significantly socially impaired based on self-reports.

Hurtig and White (1986), in a cross-sectional study of 50 children with SCD, found an age-and-sex interaction in terms of social adaptation. They reported that although boys experience a distinct and robust drop in self-reported social competence, including nonacademic activities, peer relationships, and social functioning, both boys and girls with SCD undergo decreased social competence as they progress through adolescence. A subsequent study revealed similar significant differences between pediatric patients with SCD and normative samples in three domains: activities, social functioning, and school functioning (Hurtig & Park, 1989). In both studies, adolescent boys had the poorest rates of social competence compared to their younger male counterparts as well as to all age groups of females in the sample.

Additional gender differences were found among peer-rated evaluations of social relationships compared to same-classroom comparison peers (Noll et al., 1996). Females with SCD, aged 8–14 years, were perceived by matched classroom comparison peers as having significantly lower sociability/leadership qualities and fewer reciprocated friendships; they received fewer best friend nominations and were deemed less well liked. Males in the sample had significantly lower aggressive/disruptive scores, which may be a result of avoidance of physical confrontations because of the physical limitations associated with SCD.

Clearly, complications of SCD can have a significant impact on social relationships and the development of social competence. Noll et al. (1996) asserted the importance of social interactions for acceptance and prestige among young females; however, chronic fatigue and reduced participation in activities limit opportunities for females with SCD to hone their social skills and to develop the confidence to use them. On the other hand, some studies suggested that males are more at risk for social problems because of the unique impact of the illness on functional skills and opportunities necessary to build social competence (Hurtig & White, 1986).

In addition to clarifying the role of gender in the development of social competence in youths with SCD, family aspects should be addressed. Parents of chronically ill children may be overprotective, which may lead to further insufficiencies in social maturity (Rodrigue et al., 1996). Finally, there are significant implications of these findings into adulthood as inadequate social competence in childhood has been associated with elevated risk for developing psychological, academic, and family problems (Cicchetti, Toth, & Bush, 1988).

## Risk-and-Resistance Models Applied to Sickle Cell Disease

Findings regarding externalizing behavior problems, internalizing behavior problems, and social competence among children and adolescents with SCD suggest that, although at risk, particularly in the area of social competence, most youths show resilience in response to SCD and other life stressors. Whether children and adolescents adapt successfully to chronic illness relies on a combination of external and internal factors (e.g., coping behaviors, temperament, family functioning, appraisal of illness severity, functional impairment, disease severity). Various risk-and-resistance models have been proposed to integrate these psychosocial variables (Thompson, Gil, et al., 1993; Wallander & Varni, 1998; Wallander, Varni, Babani, Banis, & Wilcox, 1989). The disability-stress-coping model indicates the importance of disease- and non-disease-related stressors on children's adaptation to a chronic medical condition and relies on a series of risk-and-resistance factors that Wallander et al. (1989) hypothesized as having an impact on adaptation. Figure 25-1 presents the model, with variables studied in children and adolescents with SCD highlighted.

### Risk Factors

Within the model, risk factors, labeled as disability stress, include "disease parameters" that are suggested to place children at an increased risk for developing problems in adaptation. Specifically, the severity of the physical condition, the visibility of the condition, the presence of neurological impairment, and the functional independence of the child are mentioned. Additional risk factors include psychosocial stress, as measured by daily hassles and major life events.

Wallander et al. (1989) discussed how children with a chronic illness are at increased risk for maladaptation because they are exposed to events that healthy peers typically do not encounter. In addition to the stress of the illness itself, children might have to cope with painful medical procedures, changes in the severity of the illness, medical protocols, and physical impairment (L. Peterson, 1989; Wallander et al., 1989). Children with a chronic illness must also cope with changes within their social and family context, including alterations in school functioning, social relationships, and family environment. Families who have a child with a chronic illness may be under increased financial strain, emotional burden, and time limitations. Not only do events specific to illness cause concern, but also the additional disease-related stressors can cause normal life events to be more difficult for a child with chronic illness.

### Disease Parameters

*Disease Severity.* Disease parameters mentioned in the model, specifically disease severity, have not been found to have a significant impact on psychological adaptation to SCD. Across studies, results suggested that disease severity, as measured by variables like SCD genotype, pain frequency, number of days hospitalized, and other information gained from medical indicators of illness severity, has a minimal effect on psychological adaptation to SCD, as indicated by internalizing and externalizing behavior problems and adherence to treatment recommendations (Barakat, Smith-Whitley, & Ohene-Frempong, 2002; Brown, Kaslow, et al., 1993; Burlew, Telfair, Colangelo, & Wright, 2000; Devine, Brown, Lambert, Donegan, & Eckman, 1998; Lutz, Barakat, Smith-Whitley, & Ohene-Frempong, 2004). For example, Burlew et al. (2000) reported on a sample of 90 adolescents with SCD, comparing the role of psychosocial and biomedical factors in predicting adaptation. Psychosocial variables contributed significantly to the prediction of state and trait anxiety as well as depression, but biomedical risk (measured as a severity index based on SCD complications over the 5 years prior to study participation) did not. Similarly, Lutz and colleagues (2004) reported that disease severity, an additive score of disease complications in the year prior to participation, was not significantly associated with internalizing and externalizing behavior problems and quality of life in 73 children and adolescents with SCD.

Other researchers have found a link between disease severity and measures of stress experienced by families and children as a result of SCD (Casey, Brown, & Bakeman, 2000). Also, Barbarin et al. (1994) reported that in their sample, children who experienced severe bouts of pain were more likely to suffer from depressive symptoms; 25% of the sample experienced internalizing symptoms in the form of depression or anxiety.

Although additional research to explore the association among illness severity, disease-related stress, and adaptation is necessary, studies evaluating different ways to define and measure disease severity are also essential. There is no direct and agreed-on measure of disease severity in SCD (Hurtig et al., 1989). Although commonly used, SCD genotype gathered through file review may not be an adequate measure of disease severity (with HbSS considered most severe), as children with HbSC and Hbβ-thalassemia also present with severe disease-related complications (Casey et al., 2000). Significant variability in severity within SCD types has resulted in formulations with SCD complications used to reflect severity and with ratings of severity by health providers. Nonetheless, improvement in measurement has not led to findings of a role for disease severity. Direct physiological measures, including hemoglobin levels or organ damage (e.g., CVAs), may have merit but are not often used (Hurtig et al., 1989). Other work in pediatric samples suggests that perceived illness severity is associated with adaptation; parent and child report of disease severity may be more indicative of the intensity of the child's disease than objective measures (Barakat et al., 1997; Stuber et al., 1997; Thompson, Gil, Gustafson, et al., 1994).

*Neuropsychological Functioning.* Included as a risk factor in the model, neuropsychological functioning is of particular importance when discussing SCD. Deficits in neuropsychological functioning serve as significant risks to healthy psychological adaptation in SCD because neuropsychological impairments that occur as a result of stroke, chronic anemia, and ischemia may significantly impair functioning in these children. In studies assessing neuropsychological functioning in children with SCD without stroke history, results have indicated differences on measures of academic achievement and neuropsychological tests; however, others have suggested that when compared to children matched on SES status and ethnicity, these differences are not apparent (F. D. Armstrong et al., 1996; Brown, Doepke, et al., 1993; Fowler et al., 1988; Noll et al., 1987; Swift et al., 1989).

Children with SCD who have experienced CVAs or other types of neurological impairment have shown difficulty on measures of neuropsychological functioning even in comparison to matched controls (Wasserman, Williams, Fairclough, Mulher, & Wang, 1991). Medical or disease risk factors that have an impact on brain functioning can also affect adaptation because children with brain impairment may need increased financial resources and increased help in daily living skills, which may result in increased family stress. In addition, studies have suggested that decreased adaptive behavior or functional independence, which can occur as a result of neuropsychological impairment, has significant negative impact on psychological adaptation (Casey et al., 2000).

### *Psychosocial Stress*

There is a dearth of research examining psychosocial stress beyond disease severity despite the many potential stressors that children and adolescents with SCD are likely to experience. Moreover, findings for disease severity are inconsistent and weak, suggesting that other psychosocial stress, including life events, functional status, and poverty, require further attention. Although not discussed within the risk-and-resistance model proposed by Wallander and colleagues (1989), demographic factors, such as age, gender, SES/perceived financial hardship, and race may pose as potential "risks" in a child's adaptation to chronic illness and are particularly essential to address in the case of SCD.

***Age.*** As noted, adolescents with SCD generally experience more problems in adaptation than their younger counterparts (Brown et al., 1995; Hurtig et al., 1989; Scott & Scott, 1999), although these findings have not been consistently reported (Lutz et al., 2004; Thompson et al., 2003). Whether these symptoms develop over time, perhaps caused by increased symptoms of SCD often experienced in adolescence and increased developmental pressures (Baskin et al., 1998; Lutz et al., 2004), is not totally clear because of a lack of prospective studies.

Adolescence is a critical time developmentally in terms of separation from the family, the formation of one's identity, the centrality of social relationships, and the development of future plans in terms of education and vocation. SCD, in combination with risk factors associated with lower SES and minority racial status, presents adolescents with SCD with an additional set of challenges that can impede one's ability to gain independence from the family and to find acceptance from peers—both essential to the process of successfully traversing adolescence (Baskin et al., 1998). Although many meet these challenges with success, the strains of adapting to a chronic, unpredictable illness in the face of other obstacles puts the adolescent with SCD at particular risk for problematic adaptation.

Adolescents with SCD report more problems with peer relationships, greater behavior problems, and poorer self-esteem compared with healthy peers and with younger children with SCD (Scott & Scott, 1999). Moreover, nonadherence to treatment recommendations increases during adolescence partly because of more adaptation problems, increased responsibilities for medical care, and developmental demands particular to adolescence (Barakat et al., 2002; Baskin et al., 1998).

There appears to be continuity in problematic adaptation from adolescence into adulthood. Not only do adults with SCD report continued problems with social relationships and academic and employment attainment, but it appears that the poor self-esteem as well as difficult and reduced social relationships found for adolescents potentially contribute to the high level of internalizing symptoms, namely, anxiety and depression, reported by adults with SCD (Farber, Koshy, & Kinney, 1985). In addition, adolescents and young adults with SCD may need more support as their health care providers change during this time. Adolescents and young adults with SCD, who were surveyed regarding responses to transitioning from pediatric to adult health care facilities, worried whether adult care providers would be responsive to reports of pain and other aspects of provision of health care services. Many believed that more support and guidance during this time would facilitate a smoother transition (Telfair, Myers, & Drezner, 1994).

*Gender.* Males with SCD, particularly in adolescence, experience greater problems than females in adaptation, including internalizing symptoms, externalizing symptoms, social relations, and low self-esteem (Brown et al., 1995; Brown, Kaslow, et al., 1993; Hurtig et al., 1989; also see Baskin et al., 1998, for a review and see Thompson et al., 2003, for an exception). For example, older adolescent boys were particularly vulnerable to somatic, immature, and hyperactive behaviors (Hurtig & Park, 1989). Conversely, older girls were less likely to exhibit behavioral problems compared to younger girls. However, female adolescents appeared more resistant to externalizing behavior problems overall than males in the sample.

These findings may be attributed to higher SCD complications in males (Barakat et al., 2002; Lutz et al., 2004) and the impact that SCD complications can have on separation and individuation from the family, identity development, and social acceptance and support (Scott & Scott, 1999); males with SCD reported poorer family functioning than females, thus supporting this interpretation (Lutz et al., 2004). For example, short stature, delayed puberty, and decreased physical stamina are more likely to have a negative impact on male adolescents' successful transition through adolescence than that of females because of the more central role that physical prowess plays in adaptation of male adolescents (Berk, 2002). In addition, the cultural emphasis on male strength and physical activity place adolescent males with SCD at an increased risk for maladaptation (Hurtig et al., 1989; Hurtig & White, 1986).

*Socioeconomic Status and Perceived Financial Hardship.* It is imperative that the role of SES and associated conditions of poverty in outcomes for children and adolescents with SCD be examined more closely. The psychosocial problems identified for youths with SCD may be explained by SES over and above illness factors because of the prevalence of poverty among African American children (some estimate up to 46%) (Barbarin, Whitten, Bond, & Conner-Warren, 1999; Garfinkel, 1996). Review of the extant literature shows few studies that examined the role of SES as a major goal of the study. Those studies that did examine the independent impact of SES and related factors on adaptation have shown positive findings (Barbarin & Christian, 1999; Devine et al., 1998; Lemanek et al., 1986).

Barbarin and colleagues (1999) conducted interviews with 327 children with SCD and their parents and found that perceived financial hardship may be more important than objective measures of economic status and contributes to adaptation independent of disease-related variables. Perceived financial hardship was defined as the caregiver's perceived inability to meet basic needs or "subjective poverty." Furthermore, these authors suggested that subjective poverty may magnify consequences of SCD on health and psychosocial adaptation as a significant interaction was found between poverty and illness severity ratings.

Devine et al. (1998) reported on a study of 74 children and adolescents with SCD in which SES made an independent contribution to the prediction of internalizing and externalizing behavior problems and adaptive behaviors. SES in this study also was the only variable to predict intellectual abilities and academic achievement.

*Race.* Discussion of racial and cultural influences on adaptation has not been undertaken in the SCD literature and may focus on several aspects, including identity development, disparities in health service delivery, and beliefs about SCD (Sterling, Peterson, & Weekes, 1997). A historical lack of acknowledgment of disparities in service delivery in health systems based on racial/ethnic background has been associated with limited research to address the impact of race/ethnicity and its social context on adaptation of children and adolescents with SCD (Barbarin & Christian, 1999). Furthermore, any attempt to assess the impact of race and culture must disentangle culture from SES, make an effort to understand variations among African Americans in their approach to SCD, and avoid making interpretations of findings based on a majority cultural context (Sterling et al., 1997).

Studies of racial and cultural impact must take into account its bearing on the family, how the family responds and adapts to SCD, and how different family structures may interact with outcome. For example, as Barbarin and Christian (1999) suggested, beliefs about SCD, such as those related to it as a disease more prevalent among African

Americans in the United States, must be studied as they guide the manner in which families address SCD symptoms, communicate with others about their children's needs, and interact with health care systems. As noted, families may not reveal the child's diagnosis to school staff or may be reluctant to seek health care services when required.

A related issue is that, although increasing, the limited funding for comprehensive sickle cell centers in the United States has resulted in a lack of access to comprehensive health services for many children with SCD, particularly those in rural regions. This lack of access can result in increased and protracted symptomatology (i.e., pain) and has secondary effects, including missed school days and reduced engagement in activities (Scott & Scott, 1999).

Researchers have begun to address psychosocial stress, but explicit consideration of racial/ethnic issues remains sparse. As noted, the strongest research designs have used demographically matched, healthy comparison groups to untangle the roles of SCD, race/ethnicity, and SES.

## Resistance Factors

Resistance factors are thought to influence the impact of risk factors (disability stress) on child adaptation. Unlike risk factors that can directly influence adaptation, moderator and mediator variables, labeled in Wallander et al.'s (1989) model as resistance factors, are able to influence adaptation directly or through an association with risk factors like disease severity. Wallander et al. (1989) hypothesized that a child's personal characteristics, including temperament, competence, effectance motivation, and social problem-solving abilities, have an impact on social-ecological variables like psychosocial environment, adaptation of family members, availability of family resources, and social support (Frank et al., 1998), thereby influencing adaptation. In addition, "stress-processing" variables, such as appraisals of SCD and coping, play a significant role in adaptation, as is emphasized within the model (Wallander et al., 1989).

Wallander et al.'s (1989) disability-stress-coping model has been applied in a number of studies to organize the approach to evaluating the effect that various factors have on adaptation of children with SCD and their families. In this section, the focus is on studies that have evaluated the indirect role of multiple resistance factors on adaptation, whereas in subsequent sections the role of specific factors is addressed.

Most prominent in this effort, Brown et al. (2000) used the risk-resistance model to examine adaptation using standard measures in 55 children with SCD and their primary caregivers during a routine clinic visit. Children from families of low SES and with SCD genotype Hb SS were prevalent within the sample. Disability stress was calculated as a composite score that included the number of pain episodes, the number of emergency room visits, and the number of hospitalizations experienced by the child in the past 12 months. Findings regarding the caregivers of children with SCD were similar to previous studies. Approximately 35% of caregivers in this sample reported levels of general parental maladaptation with no differences seen between caregivers regarding child's gender or genotype (Brown et al., 2000). In addition, caregivers' adaptation was associated with coping strategies used, indicating partial support for the stress-processing variables as hypothesized in the Wallander et al. (1989) model. Primary caregivers' use of disengagement coping strategies was related to caregiver adaptation when other disease (i.e., disease severity) and psychosocial stressors (i.e., life events and primary caregivers' income) were adjusted for within the analyses. Results supported that caregivers who reported less use of disengagement coping strategies had better adaptation (Brown et al., 2000).

Although caregiver coping style was related to caregiver adaptation, parental coping style was not related to child adaptation. Caregiver adaptation was related to child adaptation, suggesting that caregiver coping style may indirectly affect child adaptation. The risk-and-resistance factors proposed in the disability-stress-coping model accounted for approximately one fifth of the variance in caregiver adaptation, while 8% of the variance predicted by the model was attributed to stress-processing variables (Brown et al., 2000).

In analyses conducted with the child data, trends suggested that risk factors, specifically functional stressors (adaptive behavior and self-esteem of the child), were associated with child adaptation as rated by the caregivers. Overall, the results did not support a relationship between family functioning variables and adaptation of caregivers or children with SCD. Brown et al.

(2000) found that risk-and-resistance factors accounted for less than 25% of the variance associated with child adaptation. In addition, children's report of internal locus of control over their health was associated with child adaptation (as rated by the caregivers), accounting for 17% of the variance discussed here. Brown and others (2000) suggested that children's belief that they have control over their own health may result in more adaptive, problem-solving coping mechanisms. Brown et al. (2000) noted that future studies need to be conducted using larger samples, and across illnesses, before definitive statements regarding the direction of the effect between child adaptation and caregiver coping mechanisms can be made.

A subsequent study by Casey et al. (2000) specifically focused on the use of the disability-stress-coping model in understanding psychological adaptation in 118 children and adolescents with SCD. No significant relationship was found between disease severity and adaptation, although results indicated that severity was associated with stress. Casey and colleagues attributed increases in daily hassles associated with a more severe pattern of the disease to be the cause of increased stress. The model hypothesized that the child's functional independence and disability stress level will mediate the relationship between child adaptation and disease severity (Casey et al., 2000). Results showed a significant association between children's adaptation and their functional level of independence, with functional independence accounting for more than 18% of the variance in child adaptation. Family functioning, as measured by family cohesion, child competence, and family adaptability, approached, but did not reach, significance in determining variance in child adaptation. In addition, the relationship between coping and adaptation was evaluated. Results indicated that both disengagement and engagement coping did not moderate the impact of stress on adaptation.

In another study of risk-and-resistance factors, Burlew and colleagues (2000) explored whether intrapersonal factors (self-esteem, social assertiveness), stress-processing variables (use of social support), and family relations moderated the association between biomedical risk factors and adaptation to SCD as measured by depression and anxiety. The study evaluated 90 adolescents with SCD-SS. Overall results did not support hypotheses that resistance factors (intrapersonal, stress processing, or family relations) moderated the association between biomedical risk variables and adaptation; however, resistance factors did significantly contribute to adaptation. Increased levels of social assertiveness and social support were associated with decreased anxiety, and all resistance factors significantly contributed to anxiety scores in the expected direction. Similarly, all of the resistance factors significantly contributed to depression scores, with better self-esteem and more cohesive family relations associated with decreased scores on the depression measure. Although biomedical risk factors were included, these factors did not make significant contributions to either anxiety or depression scores. Results of this study emphasize the importance of evaluating resistance factors when examining adaptation to SCD, although moderation hypotheses were not supported, and biomedical risk factors played a nonsignificant role in analyses (Burlew et al., 2000).

In studies evaluating the model with children experiencing acute pain crisis or fever and infection as a result of SCD, the role of risk-and-resistance factors has been explored. Using a sample of children being treated in a hematology acute care unit (HACU) for pain or infection-related symptoms, Barakat et al. (2002) measured risk (SCD genotype to reflect severity and a summary variable for SCD complications) and resistance (child and parent coping; family functioning) factors. Adaptation measures in the current study included total behavior problems in the child and treatment adherence. Although treatment adherence has not been widely used in research of risk-and-resistance models as an outcome measure representing adaptation, it has been used throughout the pediatric literature to reflect the family and child's level of adaptation to the medical regimen.

In the current study (Barakat et al., 2002), treatment adherence was measured in multiple ways: (a) a nurse practitioner rating of treatment adherence; (b) number of SCD-related care and treatment activities engaged in by families as reported by primary caregiver; (c) percentage of agreement between primary caregivers' report of SCD-related treatment activities and medical staff report of recommendations for SCD treatment; and finally (d) family/child attendance at follow-up clinic in the past year.

Results suggested that although disease severity was not significantly related to treatment adherence, disease-related stress, especially the frequency of HACU admissions, was associated with treatment adherence, such that as individuals experienced more HACU admissions they showed increased treatment adherence. Psychosocial variables, including increased family problem solving and decreased reliance on passive coping strategies by caregivers were associated with greater treatment adherence. However, other factors (child report variables, child and parent active coping, child and parent general functioning) were not associated with adherence to treatment regimen.

Using the same sample as discussed in the Barakat et al. (2002) study, additional analyses were conducted to evaluate the impact of risk-and-resistance factors on child quality of life and total behavior problems (Lutz et al., 2004). Of children sampled for the study, 9.3% were found to fall into the clinical range and 9.3% in the borderline-to-clinical range based on their CBCL total behavior problem scores. Demographic variables played a significant role in the analyses as child age and gender had an impact on the level of disability stress (a measure of the amount of stress a family experienced as a result of SCD), quality of life, and family functioning, such that older children showed higher disability stress and increased parent-reported quality of life. Male children showed decreased scores on family functioning and quality of life.

To explore if resistance factors (caregiver coping and family functioning) moderated the association between disability stress and child adaptation, a series of hierarchical regressions was conducted (Lutz et al., 2004). Initial results revealed that child active coping moderated the association between disability stress and adaptation (parent rated QOL); however, post hoc analyses did not support moderation. No other resistance factors served as moderator variables, but child age, child gender, and caregiver-reported active coping approached significance in accounting for the variance in parent-reported QOL. Correlational analyses suggested that increased family functioning was associated with increased child active coping.

The results (Lutz et al., 2004) evidenced are similar to those in other studies (Brown et al., 2000; Casey et al., 2000) that evaluated risk-and-resistance factors because disease severity was not found to impact adaptation. In addition, this study indicated that disability stress also did not play an important role in determining the level of adaptation to SCD. Results provide evidence as to the importance of demographic factors (gender and age) in determining children's risk for experiencing problems with family functioning and maladaptation.

In sum, findings regarding the role of resistance factors in the adaptation of children and adolescents with SCD are inconsistent, with some studies reporting the expected moderation effects, some studies reporting direct effects, and still other studies reporting no effects. Moreover, when significant associations have been found, the effects have been moderate to small. Certainly, problems related to sample size and limited power may limit findings in studies that attempt to evaluate a number of risk-and-resistance factors. In addition, the lack of attention to the use of measures developed and standardized with African American samples may obscure existing effects. Finally, the studies reported here were all cross sectional and therefore did not allow for the exploration of the development of adaptation over time and in response to the interactions of multiple risk-and-resistance factors. What follows is a discussion of findings regarding specific resistance factors.

### *Intrapersonal Factors: Self-Esteem and Self-Concept*

According to risk-and-resistance models (Thompson, Gil, et al., 1993; Wallander et al., 1989), fairly stable intrapersonal factors such as self-esteem and self-concept serve as significant variables that have an impact on child adaptation. Wallander et al. (1989) asserted that intrapersonal characteristics serve as resistance factors that, when enmeshed with other resistance factors as well as delineated risk factors, will account for overall psychosocial adaptation of a child. Similarly, Thompson, Gil, and colleagues (1993) advocated that self-esteem influences an individual's expectations and in turn affects the individual's stress processing and adaptation.

Consequently, it has been suggested that beliefs about self-worth and efficacy are a vital component for adaptation in the face of a chronic illness. Indeed, self-concept is modified as a result of physical and cognitive developmental changes associated with the progression through childhood, adolescence, and young adulthood. The subsequent illness-related and environmental stressors that accompany SCD may exacerbate the developmental changes seen among healthy populations during this time.

Kumar et al. (1976) first revealed that adolescents with SCD had a diminished sense of self-concept compared to matched normal controls. These findings have been extended to suggest that adolescents with SCD display greater dissatisfaction with body image (Morgan & Jackson, 1986). However, much variability has been found among studies investigating intrapersonal factors. Several studies found no significant differences in self-concept among children and adolescents with SCD compared to healthy controls (Lemanek et al., 1986), same-classroom comparison peers (Noll et al., 1996), adolescents with other chronic diseases (Kellerman, Zeltzer, Ellenberg, Dash, & Rigler, 1980), or national norms among diverse age categories (Hurtig & White, 1986). In fact, elevated self-concept has been observed among preschool children with SCD, who may, however, not be able to appropriately assess their abilities and skills (Lemanek et al., 1994).

As noted, lower levels of intrapersonal variables, such as self-esteem and social assertion, have been found to contribute significantly to anxiety and depression among adolescents (Burlew et al., 2000), and higher levels of self-concept have been associated with overall adaptive outcomes (Moise, Drotar, Doershuk, & Stern, 1987). In addition, low levels of perceived self-worth are associated with higher self-reported illness symptoms. Consequently, a significant degree of variance in adaptation can be accounted for by self-worth among children with SCD (Thompson et al., 1998). It seems that problems with self-esteem and self-concept may arise during adolescence; therefore, understanding the role that SCD plays in the achievement of important developmental tasks of this stage is essential.

### *Stress-Processing Variables*

*Appraisals.* Stress-processing variables include cognitive appraisals and coping methods. When a child or adolescent encounters a situation that may potentially cause stress, he or she makes a series of judgments, also known as appraisals, to assess the impending risk to self and to loved ones. Lazarus and Launier (1978) suggested that there are two types of appraisals, primary and secondary. Primary appraisals are subjective appraisals of an event. Secondary appraisals are appraisals of one's resources, which require an individual to evaluate the cause of the event, whether the individual will be effective in dealing with the event, and if so, possible coping strategies that may be used (Lazarus & Folkman, 1984).

In evaluating whether the individual will be effective in dealing with the event, an individual engages in several different types of secondary appraisals (Lazarus & Launier, 1978). In determining a personal explanation about the cause of the stressful event, an individual engages in causal attributions, which may be internal (caused by self) or external (caused by another object or person); stable (consistent) or unstable (transient over time); and specific (only happens in a certain situation) or global (happening in any situation) (C. Peterson & Seligman, 1984). Once a cause is determined, the individual evaluates personal resources that may be used to deal with the event. A hopeful individual foresees that he or she has the personal resources required to achieve a goal and then actively applies those resources (Snyder et al., 1997).

Research has indicated support for the role of appraisals (appraisals of stress, attributions, hope) in psychological adaptation to SCD (Brown, Kaslow, et al., 1993; H. A. Lewis & Kliewer, 1996; Thompson et al., 1998). Thompson and colleagues (1998) examined the association between appraisals of stress and adaptation in 49 children with SCD and 43 children with cystic fibrosis. Results indicated that appraisal of stress was significantly associated with psychological adaptation in children with SCD. In particular, high levels of appraised stress were associated with higher levels of child maladaptation. In children with SCD, stress appraisals accounted for 6% of the variance in psychological adaptation.

Lewis and Kliewer (1996) examined the effect of hope on physical and psychological adaptation of children and adolescents with SCD. Results indicated that higher levels of hope were associated with lower anxiety symptoms, lower physical anxiety symptoms, and higher concentration. However, hope was not associated with depression or physical adaptation, perhaps because of low statistical power.

Furthermore, Brown, Kaslow, and colleagues (1993) studied differences in the attributional style and psychological adaptation of 61 children with SCD and 15 healthy siblings. Similar to findings in other studies, the data suggested that children with SCD endorsed more negative attributions or a depressive attributional style and depressive symptoms in comparison to their healthy siblings.

In sum, research has indicated that appraisals may be impacted by SCD in children and adolescents. Moreover, appraisals seem to be associated with psychological adaptation. In particular, higher levels of stress appraisals, an internal attributional style, and lower levels of hope are associated with poorer psychological adaptation. More research is necessary to understand how appraisals may be shaped over time by the process of responding to a chronic illness as well as elucidating the role of race and culture in the development of adaptive or maladaptive appraisals.

*Coping.* Lazarus and Folkman (1984) defined the coping process as "constantly changing cognitive and behavioral efforts to manage specific external and/or internal demands that are appraised as taxing or exceeding the resources of the person" (p. 141). Compas, Connor-Smith, Saltzman, Thomsen, and Wadsworth (2001) defined coping as "conscious volitional efforts to regulate emotion, cognition, behavior, physiology, and the environment in response to stressful events or circumstances" (p. 91). The commonality between definitions is that coping is a response to a situation that the individual perceives to be producing undue stress.

As with coping definitions, dimensions of coping also vary in how they are conceptualized and measured. Child coping dimensions include problem- and emotion-focused coping; primary and secondary control coping; cognitive and behavioral coping; active and passive coping; approach and avoidance coping; and engagement and disengagement coping (Compas et al., 2001). A main criticism of coping dimensions is that they are too broad and often overlap. Therefore, in addressing these concerns, various categories of coping factors have been suggested. Ryan-Wenger (1992) identified 15 categories of child coping strategies commonly used: aggressive activities, behavioral avoidance, behavioral distraction, cognitive avoidance, cognitive distraction, cognitive problem solving, cognitive restructuring, emotional expression, endurance, information seeking, isolating activities, self-controlling activities, social support, spiritual support, and stressor modification.

Assessment of coping strategies varies among youths with SCD and their primary caregivers. SCD studies focusing on the measurement of coping have used a number of coping measures with the most common coping measure used the Coping Strategies Questionnaire (CSQ) (Rosentiel & Keefe, 1983), modified by Gil, Abrams, Phillips, and Keefe (1989) to be SCD specific. The CSQ for children with SCD is comprised of three subscales: coping attempts, negative thinking, and passive adherence. The coping attempts subscale includes the following items: diverting attention, reinterpreting pain, ignoring painful sensations, using calming self-statements, and increasing behavior activity. The negative thinking subscale entails four items: catastrophizing, using fearful self-statements, using anger self-statements, and isolation. Finally, the passive adherence subscale is made up of 6 items: resting, taking fluids, praying and hoping, heat/cold/massage, control, and decreasing pain. Another subscale used less often, the illness-focused subscale, was derived from the heat/cold/massage, resting, praying and hoping, and taking fluids items. The CSQ for primary caregivers of youths with SCD is comprised of the same three subscales.

Demographic (age, gender) and situational factors (parental coping, family functioning) may influence the development and use of particular coping strategies. Coping strategies used by youths with SCD have been examined to determine whether there is a difference according to age. Research has indicated that in comparison to children, adolescents tended to use coping strategies such as negative thinking and passive adherence more frequently (Gil et al., 1993; Gil, Williams, Thompson, & Kinney, 1991; Gil, Wilson, & Edens, 1997). In addition, Gil et al. (1997) found that children and adolescents did not differ on coping attempts; however, adolescents did use more illness-focused coping strategies.

Spirito and colleagues examined coping strategies in 177 children and adolescents with chronic illness, including SCD (Spirito, Stark, Gil, & Tyc, 1995). Results indicated that adolescents used strategies such as blaming others and wishful thinking less than children; however, adolescents engaged in higher levels of resignation. In contrast to the above findings, Kliewer and Lewis (1995) reported that although age was not related to either active or avoidance coping, support-seeking coping strategies were positively associated with age.

Research has also examined whether coping strategies remain stable as youths develop. Gil et al. (1997) investigated the stability of coping strategies in a sample of 93 children and adolescents with SCD over an 18-month period and found instability in adolescents' use of coping attempts, negative thinking, and illness-focused coping strategies. For children, results suggested stability in the use of negative thinking. In contrast, in an earlier report, Gil and colleagues (1993) found, over a 9-month period, that the use of coping attempts, negative thinking, and passive adherence was stable for children with SCD. Adolescents were consistent in their use of coping attempts but not negative thinking and passive adherence.

Only a few studies have investigated whether gender has a significant effect on the types of coping strategies employed by children and adolescents with SCD, with inconsistent and mostly nonsignificant results. For example, Gil et al. (1997) reported that over an 18-month period, girls increased their use of coping attempts while boys used less active cognitive and behavioral pain-coping strategies. However, an earlier study by Gil and colleagues (1991) found that girls and boys exhibited no significant difference in coping attempts, negative thinking, and passive adherence. Similarly, Kliewer and Lewis (1995) indicated that gender had no effect on use of active or avoidance coping.

It has been suggested that children model the coping strategies of those around them (Band, 1990). Mixed findings have been reported by several studies investigating whether coping strategies of children with SCD are associated with coping strategies employed by their caregivers. Although significant associations are found, correlations between similar coping strategies used by parent and child are not consistently significant, and varied coping categories measured across studies make comparisons of results difficult.

For example, in a sample of 39 children and adolescents with SCD and their caregivers, Kliewer and Lewis (1995) found that greater reliance on avoidance coping by children was related to greater use of active coping strategies by primary caregivers. The authors suggested that this finding might be the result of children's response to the knowledge that their caregivers will provide for their SCD-related needs. Gil and colleagues (1991) also indicated that parental coping strategies were associated with child coping strategies. Sharpe and colleagues reported that child coping was not significantly associated with maternal coping strategies in a sample of 55 children with SCD and their mothers (Sharpe, Brown, Thompson, & Eckman, 1994).

Family factors have been linked to children's use of particular coping strategies. Kliewer and Lewis (1995) investigated the effect of family cohesion on children's use of active and avoidance coping strategies. Findings suggested that greater family cohesion was associated with more active coping strategies in children; however, avoidance coping was not related to family cohesion. Consistent with these findings, Sharpe and colleagues (1994) found, for children with SCD, there was a relationship between less reliance on disengagement coping and greater family adaptability.

For children and adolescents with SCD, coping strategies have been related to the extent of health care utilization in that active coping has been associated with reduced health utilization, including emergency room visits (Gil et al., 1991; H. A. Lewis & Kliewer, 1996). In addition, higher levels of negative thinking and passive adherence have been related to more visits to the emergency room (Gil et al., 1989, 1991), greater number of hospital stays (Gil et al., 1989), and increased contact with health care professionals (Gil et al., 1993).

It has been suggested that there is an association between coping strategies and psychological outcome. In particular, research by H. A. Lewis and Kliewer (1996) indicated that greater use of active coping was related to lower levels of physiological anxiety symptoms, while increased distraction coping was associated with more symptoms of depression. Finally, more reliance on avoidance coping was associated with difficulties with concentration and anxiety symptoms.

Similarly, Thompson, Gil, and colleagues (1993) and Thompson, Gil, Keith, and coworkers (1994) indicated that higher use of negative thinking coping strategies was associated with more internalizing and externalizing behavior symptoms as reported by mothers of children with SCD. Moreover, Gil et al. (1991) examined pain-coping strategies and psychological adaptation in children and adolescents with SCD. Results indicated that coping strategies were associated with psychological adaptation. Specifically, children who used more negative thinking coping strategies evidenced poorer psychological adaptation. However, coping attempts and passive adherence were not associated with psychological maladaptation.

In an earlier study, Gil et al. (1989) found that higher levels of both negative thinking and passive adherence were associated with higher levels of maladaptation in children and adolescents with SCD. In contrast, Sharpe and colleagues (1994) found that engagement and disengagement coping were not significantly associated with internalizing and externalizing behavior problems. However, a trend for an association between disengagement coping and internalizing behavior problems was noted.

In fully understanding the role of coping in child adaptation, pediatric research (Casey et al., 2000; H. A. Lewis & Kliewer, 1996; Lutz et al., 2004) has begun to investigate mediation and moderation effects of coping methods implored by children and adolescents. H. A. Lewis and Kliewer (1996) examined the association of appraisals (hope), coping, and adaptation, using mediator and moderator models, in children with SCD. Findings indicated that the relationship of hope with anxiety, depression, and health care utilization was not mediated by coping factors. Instead, active, support, and distraction coping acted as moderators in the relationship between hope and anxiety. Children who reported greater levels of hope and of active, support, and distraction coping strategies reported fewer anxiety symptoms.

In sum, from a handful of well-conducted studies, higher levels of engagement coping (i.e., active/approach) have been related to better medical, physical, and psychological adaptation in children and adolescents with SCD, whereas higher levels of disengagement coping (i.e., passive/avoidance) have been associated with poorer medical, physical, and psychological adaptation in children and adolescents with SCD. The current coping literature lacks prospective research, incorporation of risk factors including race and culture, and examination of situation specificity (e.g., coping in response to pain, coping in response to other illness-related stressors), thereby limiting understanding of how these coping processes influence adaptation over time.

### *Social/ecological variables*

*Caregiver Psychological Functioning.* Examination of social/ecological variables focuses on the impact of caregiver adaptation and family environment. Although it is clear that caregivers of children and adolescents with SCD experience a host of disease-related caregiving demands (Ievers-Landis et al., 2001) and psychosocial stressors (McLoyd, 1990) that have the potential to impact their parenting and their adaptation, implications for caregivers' psychosocial functioning are less clear. Research on caregiver psychological functioning is inconsistent and has been found to be similar to (Brown, Kaslow, et al., 1993) and better than (Barbarin, 1999) normative samples and matched controls. The key to understanding the differences in findings seems to be the use of comparison groups that are matched on demographic variables, leading to conclusions that caregivers are resilient in the face of both SCD-related and psychosocial stress.

Just as with children and adolescents with SCD, if distress occurs, it seldom reaches the level of psychopathology; however, the role of psychosocial stress, in addition to SCD-related demands, must be taken into account. For example, Barbarin (1999) reported that primary caregivers did not differ from matched controls; in fact, fathers showed better adaptation on some measures, but caregiver psychological adaptation was predictive of child adaptation, as was parents' religiosity and racial attributions.

Furthermore, similar to findings across chronic pediatric conditions (Drotar, 1997), variations in caregiver adaptation do impact the adaptation of children and adolescents with SCD. Devine et al. (1998) found that caregiver psychological adaptation was associated with externalizing behavior problems in their children and adolescents with SCD, and Brown, Kaslow, et al. (1993) reported an association of maternal psychological functioning with child internalizing behavior problems. These findings have been confirmed in other samples using comparison groups (Midence et al., 1996). However, because of a lack of prospective designs, the direction of effect is unclear; it may be that child and adolescent difficulties in adaptation lead to poorer maternal adjustment over time. Furthermore, the mechanisms of effect have not been investigated. For example, it may be that distressed caregivers parent in ways that are harsh and inconsistent, leading to conflict within the family and resulting in poorer adaptation among their children and adolescents (McLoyd, 1990).

*Family Functioning.* Well-established (Barakat & Kazak, 1999) findings supportive of a link between family functioning and psychosocial adaptation in pediatric samples have been reported since the role of family functioning in risk-and-resistance models was first articulated (Wallander et al., 1989). Wallander and colleagues examined the influence of family environment on behavior problems in a sample of 153 children with various chronic illnesses and physical disabilities. They reported that family functioning was linked to children's outcomes with consistent findings for family conflict; however, cohesion, organization, and control also had a role in influencing adaptation.

Barbarin (1999) put forward a model of family functioning and its mediational role in adaptation specific to African American families of children and adolescents with SCD. He proposed that life stressors, SCD, and SES are stressors that have an impact on parental adaptation and, in turn, family functioning. Moreover, the model explicitly articulates that the sociocultural context of the family will influence how the family functions. Using a series of semistructured interviews of 77 children with SCD, 28 of their siblings, and 74 healthy, demographically matched comparisons, Barbarin found some support for the model. Families of children with SCD were functioning moderately well and showed higher scores on scales measuring organization than comparison families, with caregivers highly involved in everyday decision making in their children's lives. Barbarin also reported that children whose caregivers felt supported by their extended family and who had strong emotional ties to their family had better functioning. The finding of better family functioning was reported also in a sample of British children with SCD, with families showing more cohesion and less conflict than a comparison group (Midence et al., 1996).

For SCD, the findings regarding a direct association of family functioning with adaptation are strongest; however, there are reports of family functioning acting as a moderator of the impact of stress on adaptation, with some inconsistencies across studies (perhaps because of differences in measures of family functioning and their subscales). Family conflict has been particularly associated with poorer adaptation among children and adolescents with SCD; conversely, family cohesion, flexibility, and expressiveness have been less consistently associated with better adaptation. In cross-sectional and prospective studies involving the same sample of children from the Cooperative Study of Sickle Cell Disease, Thompson and associates reported that family conflict predicted total behavior problems on the CBCL concurrently and longitudinally over and above the contribution of demographic risk factors (Thompson, Armstrong, et al., 1999; Thompson et al., 2003).

A number of other studies with smaller samples and cross-sectional research designs have led to similar results. Burlew and colleagues (2000), in their sample of adolescents with SCD, found that family environment (based on a measure of family cohesion, expressiveness, and conflict) accounted for a significant portion of the variance in trait anxiety and cognitive symptoms of depression over and above the contribution of biomedical risk and other psychosocial resistance factors.

Kell and associates (1998) reported a negative association of family competence with behavior problems in 80 adolescents with SCD. The standard measure of family functioning used in this study assessed competence as reflecting cohesion, emotional expressiveness, and conflict. In addition, Brown, Kaslow, and colleagues (1993) found that lower family cohesion was associated with greater self-reports of depression, maternal reports of externalizing behavior problems, and teacher reports of problems in social competence.

Moreover, family functioning has been associated with outcomes other than behavior problems and social competence. Barakat et al. (2002), in a sample of 73 primary caregivers of children and adolescents with SCD, found that family flexibility was significantly associated with treatment adherence, suggesting active problem solving within the family in response to illness-specific and general stress supports adherence to recommendations for medical interventions.

Regarding moderation, Ievers, Brown, Lambert, Hsu, and Eckman (1998), with a sample of 67 caregivers of children and adolescents with SCD, using standard caregiver report measures assessed family functioning as well as child and caregiver psychosocial functioning. Findings supported the hypothesis that family functioning would serve as a moderator of the association of child-related stress (in this case, child externalizing symptoms reported by caregivers) and caregiver psychosocial adaptation (hostility). Family functioning variables reflecting cohesion and adaptability were significant. Although this study suggested a role for family functioning in the adaptation of caregivers and its complex relationship to child functioning, it did not address whether family functioning moderates the impact of disease-related stress on the adaptation of youth with SCD.

In contrast, Devine et al. (1998) reported that family functioning, using a standard measure of caregiver report of family adaptability and cohesion, was not associated with behavior problems or adaptive behavior of their children with SCD. Brown et al. (1995) reported similar findings using a standard measure of family functioning, noting that family cohesion showed a moderate association with adaptive behavior, but no correlations were significant in a sample of 61 children and adolescents with SCD. In another study, contrary to expectation, greater family flexibility was associated with more internalizing behavior problems among children with SCD (Brown, Kaslow, et al., 1993).

A report by Brown and Lambert (1999) may shed light on these discrepancies. They provided data to support the need to use multiple informants in studies assessing family functioning and its role in adaptational outcomes. In their sample of 38 children with SCD, children and primary caregivers each completed a standard measure of family functioning and psychosocial functioning. Findings indicated low reliability between child and caregiver reports of family functioning. Moreover, low family cohesiveness was associated with depressive symptoms for children only when both child and caregiver reports were consistent in identifying problems with family functioning.

Furthermore, inconsistencies in the findings on family functioning may be caused by problems with the measures used to reflect family environment and to a lack of accounting for the various family structures present for children and adolescents with SCD. Regarding measures of family functioning, many of the assessment procedures used have not been conceptualized explicitly with African American families, and although minority families are included as part of a larger normative sample, examination of reliability and validity of measures specifically for this population has not been undertaken. Measures that are developed and standardized with African American families are rarely reported in the literature. Moreover, families define "family" in many different ways, so that studies tapping only the perspective of a primary caregiver cannot adequately assess the way families work and the support available to youths with SCD. Thus, examination of family functioning using culturally sensitive measurement approaches and designs that allow identification of processes as they unfold over time are needed (Brown & Lambert, 1999; Drotar, 1997).

## Future Directions and Implications

Children and adolescents with SCD face a host of risks in responding to the challenges of their illness and in meeting the stressors inherent in their external social environment. Many of these youths adapt well and show a resilience that is not completely understood, although some children and adolescents are at risk for the development of psychological distress, particularly in the area of social competence. Based in risk-and-resistance models, poorer outcomes have been found for males, particularly those in adolescence, and those with neurocognitive dysfunction. Whereas healthier, more resilient outcomes have been associated with youths who have positive self-concepts, function within cohesive and flexible families with low conflict, and use (and have caregivers that use) engagement coping strategies. Caregiver adaptation, and the availability of supports to caregivers and their children with SCD, is also an important aspect of adaptation.

However, more attention needs to be devoted to several areas of investigation, with a particular eye to maintaining research designs that are culturally sensitive and competent, allowing researchers to disentangle the effect of SCD and the impact of the sociocultural context in contributing to SCD outcomes. This may be accomplished through the use of measures that are developed and normed with African American youths, inclusion of demographically matched comparison groups that can include siblings, but more important, can be drawn from the communities in which children and adolescents with SCD live and investigation of direct and indirect effects of resistance factors from the viewpoints of multiple informants (youths with SCD, primary caregivers, and teachers) and multiple family members (youths with SCD, all caregivers, healthy siblings). Furthermore, collaboration across health care sites may be necessary to increase sample sizes sufficiently to support adequate power in studies addressing numerous risk-and-resistance factors. Prospective studies will allow for conclusions regarding change in the adaptation process and potential risk-and-resistance variables over developmental stages for children and adolescents.

Finally, an effort must be made to operationalize the role of sociocultural and psychosocial risk and (possibly) resistance factors, including race and culture. Careful forethought will allow researchers to ask the types of questions that will give the information needed to understand these effects and must be completed within heterogeneous samples of youths with SCD to identify variations in effect across patients. The work of Kazak and colleagues (Kazak, 1989) in delineating multisystems interactions among children with chronic illness can help guide this approach.

Findings regarding the role of resistance factors highlight the need for intervention research that targets appraisals and coping within a family context (Drotar, 1997). In particular, because adolescents are at the greatest risk for developing problems in psychosocial adaptation, intervention programs specifically targeted toward the successful transition between childhood and adolescence may serve to better equip and prepare patients with SCD for the developmental challenges ahead and potentially prevent future maladaptation.

Intervention research in pediatric SCD is scarce and that published is focused on pain management. Kaslow and colleagues (1997, 2000), in a pilot study of a psychoeducational intervention for families of youths with SCD targeting psychosocial outcomes, reported only limited findings of improved knowledge compared with a standard treatment group. They suggested that interventions targeting families can be successful if efforts are made to recruit and maintain participation of significant family members within communities and across treatment centers, short-term and targeted interventions are considered, use of culturally sensitive assessment measures and culturally competent treatment approaches, and modifications are made to the design based on age of the patient with SCD. Moreover, the need for such work to improve the quality of life of youths with SCD and the functioning of their families is underscored.

## References


Achenbach, T. M. (1991). *Integrative guide for the 1991 CBCL/-18, YSR, and TRF profiles*. Burlington: University of Vermont.

Achenbach, T. M., & Edelbrock, C. (1983). *Manual for the Child Behavior Checklist 14-18 and Revised Child Behavior Profile*. Burlington: University of Vermont.

Achenbach, T. M., & Edelbrock, C. (1986). *Manual for the Teacher's Report Form and Teacher Version of the Child Behavior Profile*. Burlington: University of Vermont.

Achenbach, T. M., & Edelbrock, C. (1987). *Manual for the Youth Self-Report and Profile*. Burlington: University of Vermont, Department of Psychiatry.

Achenbach, T. M., McConaughy, S. H., & Howell, C. T. (1987). Child/adolescent behavioral and emotional problems: Implications of cross-informant correlations for situational specificity. *Psychological Bulletin, 101*, 213–232.

Airhihenbuwa, C. (1990). Health promotion and disease prevention strategies for African Americans: A conceptual model. In R. Braithwaite & S. Taylor (Eds.), *Health issues in the black community* (pp. 267–280). San Francisco: Jossey-Bass.

Armstrong, F. D., Thompson, R. J., Wang, W., Zimmerman, R., Pegelow, C. H., Miller, S., et al. (1996). Cognitive functioning and brain magnetic resonance imaging in children with sickle cell disease. *Pediatrics, 96*, 864–870.

Armstrong, F. D., Toledano, S. R., Miloslavich, K., Lackman-Zeman, L., Levy, J. D., Gay, C. L., et al. (1999). The Miami Pediatric Quality of Life Questionnaire: Parent Scale. *Journal of Cancer*, Suppl. 12, 11–17.

Band, E. B. (1990). Children's coping with diabetes: Understanding the role of cognitive development. *Journal of Pediatric Psychology, 15*, 27–41.

Barakat, L. P., & Kazak, A. E. (1999). Family issues related to cognitive aspects of chronic illness in children. In R. T. Brown (Ed.), *Cognitive aspects of chronic illness in children* (pp. 333–354). New York: Guilford.

Barakat, L. P., Kazak, A. E., Meadows, A. T., Casey, R., Meeske, K., & Stuber, M. L. (1997). Families surviving childhood cancer: A comparison of posttraumatic stress syndromes with families of healthy children. *Journal of Pediatric Psychology, 22*, 843–859.

Barakat, L. P., Smith-Whitley, K., & Ohene-Frempong, K. (2002). Treatment adherence in children with sickle cell disease: Disease-related risk and psychosocial resistance factors. *Journal of Clinical Psychology in Medical Settings, 9*, 201–505.

Barbarin, O. A. (1999). Do parental coping, involvement, religiosity, and racial identity mediate children's psychological adaptation to sickle cell disease? *Journal of Black Psychology, 25*, 391–426.

Barbarin, O. A., & Christian, M. (1999). The social and cultural context of coping with sickle cell disease: I. A review of biomedical and psychosocial issues. *Journal of Black Psychology, 25*, 277–293.

Barbarin, O. A., Whitten, C. F., & Bonds, S. M. (1994). Estimating rates of psychosocial problems in urban and poor children with sickle cell anemia. *Health and Social Work*, 19, 112–119.

Barbarin, O. A., Whitten, C. F., Bond, S., & Conner-Warren, R. (1999). The social and cultural context of coping with sickle cell disease: II. The role of financial hardship in adaptation to sickle cell disease. *Journal of Black Psychology, 25*, 294–315.

Baskin, M. L., Collins, M. H., Brown, F., Griffith, J. R., Samuels, D., Moody, A., et al. (1998). Psychosocial considerations in sickle cell disease (SCD): The transition from adolescence to young adulthood. *Journal of Clinical Psychology in Medical Settings, 5*, 315–341.

Berk, L. E. (2002). *Infants, children, and adolescents* (4th ed.). Boston: Allyn and Bacon.

Boyd-Franklin, N., Steiner, G. L., & Boland, M. G. (Eds.) (1995). *Children, families, and HIV/AIDS: Psychosocial and therapeutic issues*. New York: Guilford.

Brown, R. T., Doepke, K. J., & Kaslow, N. J. (1993). Risk-resistance-adaptation model for pediatric chronic illness: Sickle cell syndrome as an example. *Clinical Psychology Review, 13*, 119–132.

Brown, R. T., Eckman, J., Baldwin, K., Buchanan, I., & Dingle, A. D. (1995). Protective aspects of adaptive behavior in children with sickle cell syndromes. *Children's Health Care, 24*, 205–222.

Brown, R. T., Kaslow, N. J., Doepke, K., Buchanan, I., Eckman, J., Baldwin, K., et al. (1993). Psychosocial and family functioning in children with sickle cell syndrome and their mothers. *Journal of the American Academy of Child and Adolescent Psychiatry, 32*, 545–553.

Brown, R. T., & Lambert, R. (1999). Family functioning and children's adaptation in the presence of a chronic illness: Concordance between children with sickle cell disease and caretakers. *Families, Systems and Health, 17*, 165.

Brown, R. T., Lambert, R., Devine, D., Baldwin, K., Casey, R., Doepke, K., et al. (2000). Risk-resistance adaptation model for caregivers and their children with sickle cell syndromes. *Annals of Behavioral Medicine, 22* , 158–169.

Burlew, K., Telfair, J., Colangelo, L., & Wright, E. C. (2000). Factors that influence adolescent adaptation to sickle cell disease. *Journal of Pediatric Psychology, 25*, 287–299.

Casey, R., Brown, R. T., & Bakeman, R. (2000). Predicting adaptation in children and adolescents with sickle cell disease: A test of the risk-resistance-adaptation model. *Rehabilitation Psychology, 45*, 155–178.

Cicchetti, D., Toth, S., & Bush, M. (1988). Developmental psychopathology and incompetence in childhood: Suggestions for intervention. In B. B. Lahey & A. E. Kazdin (Eds.), *Advances in clinical child psychology*, vol. II, (pp. 1–71). New York, NY: Plenum Press.

Clark, H. B., Striefel, S., Bedlington, M. M., & Naiman, D. E. (1989). A social skills development model: Coping strategies for children with chronic illness. *Children's Health Care, 18*, 19–29.

Compas, B. E., Connor-Smith, J. K., Saltzman, H., Thomsen, A. H., & Wadsworth, M. E. (2001). Coping with stress during childhood and adolescence: problems, progress, and potential theory and research. *Psychological Bulletin, 127*, 87–127.

Devine, D., Brown, R. T., Lambert, R., Donegan, J. E., & Eckman, J. (1998). Predictors of psychosocial and cognitive adaptation in children with sickle cell syndromes. *Journal of Clinical Psychology in Medical Settings, 5*, 295–313.

Drotar, D. (1997). Relating parent and family functioning to the psychological adaptation of children with chronic health conditions: What have we learned? What do we need to know? *Journal of Pediatric Psychology, 22*, 149–165.

Edelbrock, C., Costello, A. J., Dulcan, M. K., Conover, N. C., & Kalas, R. (1986). Parent-child agreement on child psychiatric symptoms assessed via structured interview. *Journal of Child Psychology and Psychiatry and Allied Discipline, 27*, 181–190.

Edelbrock, C., Costello, A. J., Dulcan, M. K., Kalas, R., &Conover, N. C. (1985). Age differences in the reliability of the psychiatric interview of the child. *Child Development, 56*, 265–275.

Farber, M. D., Koshy, M., & Kinney, T. R. (1985). Cooperative study of sickle cell disease:

Demographic and socioeconomic characteristics of patients and families with sickle cell disease. *Journal of Chronic Disease, 38*, 495–505.

Fowler, M. G., Whitt, J. K., Lallinger, R. R., Nash, K. B., Atkinson, S. S., Wells, R. J., et al. (1988). Neuropsychological and academic functioning of children with sickle cell anemia. *Journal of Developmental and Behavioral Pediatrics, 9*, 213–220.

Frank, R. G., Thayer, J. F., Hagglund, K. J., Vieth, A. Z., Schop, L. H., Beck, N. C., et al. (1998). Trajectories of adaptation in pediatric chronic illness: The importance of the individual. *Journal of Consulting and Clinical Psychology, 66*, 521–532.

Garfinkel, I. (1996). *Social policies for children.* Washington, DC: Brookings Institution.

Gil, K. M., Abrams, M. R., Phillips, G., & Keefe, F. J. (1989). Sickle cell disease pain: Relation of coping strategies to adjustment. *Journal of Consulting and Clinical Psychology, 57*, 725–731.

Gil, K. M., Thompson, R. J., Keith, B. R., Tota-Faucette, M., Noll, S., & Kinney, T. R. (1993). Sickle cell disease pain in children and adolescents: Change in pain frequency and coping strategies over time. *Journal of Pediatric Psychology, 18*, 621–637.

Gil, K. M., Williams, D. A., Thompson, R. J., & Kinney, T. R. (1991). Sickle cell disease in children and adolescents: The relation of child and parent pain coping strategies to adjustment. *Journal of Pediatric Psychology, 16*, 643–663.

Gil, K. M., Wilson, J. J., & Edens, J. L. (1997). The stability of pain coping strategies in young children, adolescents, and adults with sickle cell disease over an 18-month period. *Clinical Journal of Pain, 13*, 110–115.

Harter, S., & Pike, R. (1984). The pictorial scale of perceived competence and social acceptance for young children. *Child Development, 55*, 1969–1982.

Hodges, K., Gordon, Y., & Lennon, M. P. (1990). Parent-child agreement on symptoms assessed via a clinical research interview for children: The Child Assessment Schedule (CAS). *Journal of Child Psychology and Psychiatry and Allied Disciplines, 31*, 427–436.

Hurtig, A. L., Koepke, D., & Park, K. B. (1989). Relation between severity of chronic illness and adaptation in children and adolescents with sickle cell disease. *Journal of Pediatric Psychology, 14*, 117–132.

Hurtig, A. L., & Park, K. B. (1989). Adaptation and coping in adolescents with sickle cell disease. *Annals of the New York Academy of Sciences, 565*, 172–182.

Hurtig, A. L., & White, L. S. (1986). Psychosocial adaptation in children and adolescents with sickle cell disease. *Journal of Pediatric Psychology, 11*, 411–27.

Ievers, C. E., Brown, R. T., Lambert, R. G., Hsu, L., & Eckman, J. R. (1998). Family functioning and social support in the adaptation of caregivers of children with sickle cell syndromes. *Journal of Pediatric Psychology, 23*, 377–388.

Ievers-Landis, C. E., Brown, R. T., Drotar, D., Bunke, V., Lambert, R., & Walker, A. A. (2001). Situational analysis of parenting problems for caregivers of children with sickle cell syndromes. *Journal of Developmental and Behavioral Pediatrics, 22*, 169–178.

Johnson, K. W., Anderson, N. B., Bastida, E., Kramer, B. J., Williams, D., & Wong, M. (1995). Panel II: Macrosocial and environmental influences on minority health. *Health Psychology, 14*, 601–612.

Kaslow, N. J., Collins, M. H., Loundy, M. R., Brown, F., Hollins, L. D., & Eckman, J. (1997). Empirically validated family interventions for pediatric psychology: Sickle cell disease as an exemplar. *Journal of Pediatric Psychology, 22*, 213–227.

Kaslow, N. J., Collins, M. H., Rashid, F. L., Baskin, M. L., Griffith, J. R., Hollins, L., et al. (2000). The efficacy of a pilot family psychoeducational intervention for pediatric sickle cell disease. *Families, Systems and Health, 18*, 381.

Kazak, A. E. (1989). Families of chronically ill children: A systems and social-ecological model of adaptation and challenge. *Journal of Consulting and Clinical Psychology, 57*, 25–30.

Kell, R. S., Kliewer, W., Erickson, M. T., & Ohene-Frempong, K. (1998). Psychological adaptation of adolescents with sickle cell disease: relations with demographic, medical, and family competence variables. *Journal of Pediatric Psychology, 23*, 301–312.

Kellerman, J., Zeltzer, L., Ellenberg, L., Dash, J., & Rigler, D. (1980). Psychological effects of illness in adolescence. I. Anxiety, self-esteem, and perception of control. *Journal of Pediatrics, 97*, 126–131.

Kliewer, W., & Lewis, H. (1995). Family influences on coping processes in children and adolescents with sickle cell disease. *Journal of Pediatric Psychology, 20*, 511–525.

Kumar, S., Powars, D., Allen, J., & Haywood, L. J. (1976). Anxiety, self-concept, and personal and social adaptations in children with sickle cell anemia. *Journal of Pediatrics, 88*, 859–863.

Lambert, M. C., Rowan, G. T., Lyubansky, M., & Russ, C. M. (2002). Do problems of clinic-referred

African-American children overlap with the Child Behavior Checklist? *Journal of Child and Family Studies, 11*, 271–285.

Lazarus, R. S., & Folkman, S. (1984). *Stress, appraisal, and coping.* New York: Springer.

Lazarus, R. S., & Launier, R. (1978). Stress-related transactions between persons and environment. In L. A. Pervin & M. Lewis (Eds.), *Perspectives in interactional psychology* (pp. 287–327). New York: Plenum.

Lee, E. J., Phoenix, D., Brown, W., & Jackson, B. S. (1997). A comparison study of children with sickle cell disease and their non-diseased siblings on hopelessness, depression, and perceived competence. *Journal of Advanced Nursing, 25*, 79–86.

Lemanek, K. L., Buckloh, L. M., Woods, G., & Butler, R. (1995). Diseases of the circulatory system: Sickle cell disease and hemophilia. In M. C. Robers (Ed.), *Handbook of pediatric psychology* (2nd ed.) (pp. 286–309). New York: Guilford Press.

Lemanek, K. L., Horwitz, W., & Ohene-Frempong, K. (1994). A multiperspective investigation of social competence in children with sickle cell disease. *Journal of Pediatric Psychology, 19*, 443–56.

Lemanek, K. L., Moore, S. L., Gresham, F. M., Williamson, D. A., & Kelley, M. L. (1986). Psychological adaptation of children with sickle cell anemia. *Journal of Pediatric Psychology, 11*, 397–410.

Lewis, H. A., & Kliewer, W. (1996). Hope, coping, and adjustment among children with sickle cell disease: Tests of mediator and moderator models. *Journal of Pediatric Psychology, 21*, 25–41.

Lewis, S. Y. (July, 1992). *Cultural competency model.* Presentation at the National Pediatric HIV Resource Center Core Curriculum.

Lutz, M. J., Barakat, L. P., Smith-Whitley, K., & Ohene-Frempong, K. (2004). Psychological children with sickle cell disease: Family functioning and coping. *Rehabilitation Psychology, 49*, 224–232.

Maruish, M. E. (Ed.). (1999). *The use of psychological testing for treatment planning and outcomes assessment* (2nd ed.). Mahwah, NJ: Erlbaum.

McLoyd, V. C. (1990). The impact of economic hardship on black families and children: Psychological distress, parenting, and socioemotional development. *Child Development, 61*, 311–346.

Midence, K., Fuggle, P., & Davies, S. C. (1993). Psychosocial aspects of sickle cell disease (SCD) in childhood and adolescence: a review. *British Journal of Clinical Psychology, 32*, 271–280.

Midence, K., McManus, C., Fuggle, P., & Davies, S. (1996). Psychological adaptation and family functioning in a group of British children with sickle cell disease: Preliminary empirical findings and a meta-analysis. *British Journal of Clinical Psychology, 35*, 439–450.

Moise, J. R., Drotar, D., Doershuk, C. F., & Stern, R. C. (1987). Correlates of psychosocial adjustment among young adults with cystic fibrosis. *Journal of Developmental and Behavioral Pediatrics, 8*, 141–148.

Molock, S. D., & Belgrave, F. Z. (1994). Depression and anxiety in patients with sickle cell disease: conceptual and methodological considerations. *Journal of Health and Social Policy, 5*, 39–53.

Morgan, S. A., & Jackson, J. (1986). Psychological and social concomitants of sickle cell anemia in adolescents. *Journal of Pediatric Psychology, 11*, 429–440.

Noll, R. B., Stith, L., Gartstein, M. A., Ris, M. D., Grueneich, R., Vannatta, K., et al. (1987). Correlates of psychosocial adaptation among young adults with cystic fibrosis. *Journal of Developmental and Behavioral Pediatrics, 8*, 141–148.

Noll, R. B., Vannatta, K., Koontz, K., Kalinyak, K., Bukowski, W. M., & Davies, W. H. (1996). Peer relationships and emotional well-being of youngsters with sickle cell disease. *Child Development, 67*, 423–436.

Palermo, T. M., Schwartz, L., Drotar, D., & McGowan, K. (2002). Parental report of health related quality of life in children with sickle cell disease. *Journal of Behavioral Medicine, 25*, 269–283.

Perrin, E. C., Stein, R. E., & Drotar, D. (1991). Cautions in using the Child Behavior Checklist: Observations based on research about children with a chronic illness. *Journal of Pediatric Psychology, 16*, 411–421.

Peterson, C., & Seligman, M. E. P. (1984). Causal explanations as a risk factor for depression: Theory and evidence. *Psychological Review, 91*, 347–374.

Peterson, L. (1989). Coping by children undergoing stressful medical procedures: Some conceptual, methodological, and therapeutic issues. *Journal of Consulting and Clinical Psychology, 57*, 380–387.

Rodrigue, J. R., Streisand, R., Banko, C., Kedar, A., & Pitel, P. A. (1996). Social functioning, peer relations, and internalizing and externalizing problems among youths with sickle cell disease. *Children's Health Care, 25*, 37–52.

Rosential, A. K., & Keefe, F. J. (1983). The use of coping strategies in chronic low back pain patients: Relationship to patient characteristics and current adjustment. *Pain, 17*, 33–44.

Ryan-Wenger, N. M. (1992). A taxonomy of children's coping strategies: A step toward theory development. *American Journal of Orthopsychiatry, 62,* 256–263.

Scott, K. D., & Scott, A. A. (1999). Cultural therapeutic awareness and sickle cell anemia. *Journal of Black Psychology, 25,* 316–335.

Sharpe, J. N., Brown, R. T., Thompson, N. J., & Eckman, J. (1994). Predictors of coping with pain in mothers and their children with sickle cell syndrome. *Journal of the American Academy of Child and Adolescent Psychiatry, 33,* 1246–1255.

Snyder, C. R., Hoza, B., Pelhaam, W. E., Rapoff, M., Ware, L., Danovsky, M., et al. (1997). The development and validation of the Children's Hope Scale. *Journal of Pediatric Psychology, 22,* 399–421.

Spirito, A., Stark, L. J., Gil, K. M., & Tyc, V. L. (1995). Coping with everyday and disease-related stressors by chronically ill children and adolescents. *Journal of the American Academy of Child and Adolescent Psychiatry, 34,* 283–290.

Sterling, Y. M., Peterson, J., & Weekes, D. P. (1997). African-American families with chronically ill children: Oversights and insights. *Journal of Pediatric Nursing, 12,* 292–300.

Stuber, M. L., Kazak, A. E., Meeske, K., Barakat, L., Guthrie, D., Garnier, H., et al. (1997). Predictors of posttraumatic stress symptoms in childhood cancer survivors. *Pediatrics, 100,* 958–964.

Swift, A. V., Cohen, M. J., Hynd, G. W., Wisenbaker, J. M., McKie, K. M., Makari, G., et al. (1989). Neuropsychologic impairment in children with sickle cell anemia. *Pediatrics, 84,* 1077–1085.

Telfair, J., Myers, J., & Drezner, S. (1994). Transfer as a component of the transition of adolescents with sickle cell disease to adult care: Adolescent, adult, and parent perspectives. *Journal of Adolescent Health, 15,* 558–565.

Testa, M. A., & Simonson, D. C. (1996). Current concepts: Assessment of quality of life. *The New England Journal of Medicine, 334,* 835–840.

Thomas, V. J., & Taylor, L. M. (2002). The psychosocial experience of people with sickle cell disease and its impact on quality of life: Qualitative findings from focus groups. *British Journal of Health Psychology, 7,* 835–840.

Thompson, R. J., Armstrong, F. D., Kronenberger, W. G., Scott, D., McCabe, M. A., Smith, B., et al. (1999). Family functioning, neurocognitive functioning, and behavior problems in children with sickle cell disease. *Journal of Pediatric Psychology, 24,* 491–498.

Thompson, R. J., Armstrong, F. D., Link, C. L., Pegelow, C. H., Moser, F., & Wang, W. C. (2003). A prospective study of the relationship over time of behavior problems, intellectual functioning, and family functioning in children with sickle cell disease: A report from the Cooperative Study of Sickle Cell Disease. *Journal of Pediatric Psychology, 28,* 59–65.

Thompson, R. J., Gil, K. M., Burbach, D. J., Keith, B. R., & Kinney, T. R. (1993). Psychological adaptation of mothers of children and adolescents with sickle cell disease: The role of stress, coping methods, and family functioning. *Journal of Pediatric Psychology, 18,* 549–559.

Thompson, R. J., Gil, K. M., Gustafson, K. E., George, L. K., Keith, B. R., Spock, A., et al. (1994). Stability and change in the psychological adjustment of mother of children and adolescents with cystic fibrosis and sickle cell disease. *Journal of Pediatric Psychology, 19,* 171–188.

Thompson, R. J., Gil, K. M., Keith, B. R., Gustafson, K. E., George, L. K., & Kinney, T. R. (1994). Psychological adaptation of children with sickle cell disease: Stability and change over a 10-month period. *Journal of Consulting and Clinical Psychology, 62,* 856–8566.

Thompson, R. J., Gustafson, K. E., Gil, K. M., Godfrey, J., & Murphy, L. M. (1998). Illness specific patterns of psychological adaptation and cognitive adaptational processes in children with cystic fibrosis and sickle cell disease. *Journal of Clinical Psychology, 54,* 121–128.

Thompson, R. J., Gustafson, K. E., Gil, K. M., Kinney, T. R., & Spock, A. (1999). Change in the psychological adjustment of children with cystic fibrosis or sickle cell disease and their mothers. *Journal of Clinical Psychology in Medical Settings, 6,* 373–392.

Thompson, R. J., Merritt, K. A., Keith, B. R., Murphy, L. B., & Johndrow, D. A. (1993). Mother-child agreement on the child assessment schedule with nonreferred children: A research note. *Journal of Child Psychology and Psychiatry and Allied Disciplines, 34,* 813–20.

Varni, J. W., Katz, E. R., Seid, M., Quiggins, D. J. L., Friedman-Bender, A., & Castro, C. M. (1998). The Pediatric Cancer Quality of Life Inventory (PCQL). I. Instrument development, descriptive statistics, and cross-informant variance. *Journal of Behavioral Medicine, 21,* 179–204.

Wallander, J. L., & Thompson, R. J. (1995). Psychosocial adaptation of children with chronic physical conditions. In M. C. Roberts (Ed.), *Handbook of pediatric psychology* (2nd ed., pp. 124–141). New York: Guilford Press.

Wallander, J. L., & Varni, J. W. (1998). Effects of pediatric chronic physical disorders on child and family adaptation. *Journal of Child Psychology and Psychiatry, 39,* 29–46.

Wallander, J. L., Varni, J. W., Babani, L., Banis, H. T., & Wilcox, K. T. (1989). Family resources as resistance factors for psychological maladjustment in chronically ill and handicapped children. *Journal of Pediatric Psychology, 14,* 157–173.

Wasserman, A. L., Wilimas, J. A., Fairclough, D. L., Mulher, R. K., & Wang, W. (1991). Subtle neuropsychological deficits in children with sickle cell disease. *The American Journal of Pediatric Hematology/Oncology, 13,* 14–20.

Jerilynn Radcliffe, Lamia P. Barakat, and Rhonda C. Boyd

# Family Systems Issues in Pediatric Sickle Cell Disease

Because sickle cell disease (SCD) largely affects individuals of African descent, throughout this chapter the importance of a culturally sensitive and competent family systems approach to understanding family issues in SCD is advocated. After African American families are described in some depth, including their strengths, unique features, and special concerns, frameworks for understanding how SCD may have an impact on family functioning are presented with emphasis on the developmental-ecological model of family functioning (Kazak, 1989). This model is used to characterize family systems issues associated with SCD, and specific elements are examined. Developmental changes in family adaptation over the course of the illness are considered, as are efforts to intervene in family adaptation. Broad sociocultural systems issues with an impact on families of African descent are described, and the need for culturally sensitive and respectful approaches to families affected by SCD is underscored. Finally, unexamined areas in family systems issues for pediatric SCD are considered, with suggestions for further research. Understanding family systems issues in pediatric SCD is critical to providing effective care and to facilitating optimal adaptation in the context of the disease and its treatment.

A discussion of family issues pertinent to SCD must start by acknowledging that sociocultural factors, including race, ethnicity, and culture, are central because African Americans are the primary group diagnosed with SCD in the United States, and that family functioning is impacted by SCD and its treatment demands almost immediately following the birth of a child. There are a host of sociocultural factors that have an impact on African Americans that may increase resilience or risk to overall family adaptation to a child's disease. Therefore, it is imperative to understand families of children with SCD in the context of the immediate conditions in which they live and the larger sociopolitical context in which they function (Johnson et al., 1995; Sterling, Peterson, & Weekes, 1997).

Families of children and adolescents with SCD have a number of characteristics that may influence their responses to SCD (Boyd-Franklin, 2003; S. A. Hill, 1996), including having a higher likelihood of single-parent structure, relying on extended family support and flexible family roles, stress related to low socioeconomic status (i.e., perceived poverty, lack of employment opportunities, reduced access to health care, and living in stressful urban environments), and factors associated with ethnic minority status, including the experience of prejudice and discrimination.

Although these characteristics may be perceived as risk factors, and indeed poverty has been linked to poorer psychological outcomes particularly for African American families in which highly stressed parents engage in less-effective parenting practices (McLoyd, 1990; Mistry, Vandewater, Huston, & McLoyd, 2002), they also bring a set of strengths, strategies, values, and capabilities that can support resilience (Boyd-Franklin, 2003; Boyd-Franklin, Aleman, Steiner, Drelich, & Norford, 1995; Johnson et al., 1995; Murry, Bynum, Brody, Willert, & Stephens, 2001; Young, 1995). Significant strengths of African American families include strong work orientation, strong and consistent extended kin networks and adaptability of family roles, high achievement orientation, resourcefulness, and strong religious orientation (Gary, Beatty, Berry, & Price, 1983; R. Hill, 1972, 1999; U.S. Department of Health and Human Services, 2001).

Consideration of the interactions of race, ethnicity, and culture with other important factors in the lives of families of children and adolescents with SCD leads to clearer understanding of the variations among families of youths with SCD and elucidation of differences from other chronic illness groups. Use of both qualitative and quantitative approaches to family research has proven to be the most fruitful in defining family functioning and associated factors, and both are reported in this chapter.

SCD profoundly affects the lives of children and their families from birth and throughout life. Although universal newborn screening for SCD was recommended by the American Medical Association in 1987 to reduce morbidity and mortality, only 40 states have adopted newborn screening. Furthermore, programs are underfunded in many states, and information provided is often inadequate, provided through form letter, and delayed (S. A. Hill, 1996; Rao & Kramer, 1993). Although H. A. Williams (1993) reported that discrimination in the health care system was not perceived in a small sample of black caregivers of children with either hematological or oncological diseases, African Americans may be wary of newborn screening programs for a genetic disorder, fearing further prejudice and discrimination for their children based on the diagnosis of SCD. Moreover, new parents are faced with a multitude of information requirements regarding their responsibilities for the care of their infant with SCD before they are fully able to process the diagnosis itself, increasing initial uncertainty, stress, and fear (Rao & Kramer, 1993).

SCD permeates the family biologically as well as psychosocially, economically, and systemically. Because SCD is hereditary, biological parents are trait bearers or themselves affected, several siblings in a family may be affected, and even healthy siblings may be trait bearers. SCD includes a number of medical complications, including recurrent pain, pulmonary and cardiac complications, cerebral vascular accidents (stroke), growth failure and delayed puberty, susceptibility to infections, and hepatobiliary and genitourinary complications (Lemanek, Ranalli, Green, Biega, & Lupia, 2003). Caring for a child with SCD involves multiple clinic visits, hospitalizations, and constant attention to managing the medical complications and their treatments, which may extend beyond medications to more intensive or invasive treatments such as transfusion, hydroxyurea, or even bone marrow transplantation. Providing this care often challenges even the most resilient family because parents may overly focus on the ill child, press healthy siblings into service as adjunctive caregivers, or simply struggle to attend to basic needs of all family members, including themselves.

Prominent models and supportive empirical research of psychosocial adaptation place the family at the center of socioecological factors that serve a resistance role, buffering the impact of stress related to chronic illness on outcome (Drotar, 1997; Perrin, Ayoub, & Willett, 1993; Wallander & Varni, 1998). Family functioning is an important component in understanding parent and child adaptation to SCD. Studies regarding the functioning of families of children with SCD have had mixed outcomes; some families show better functioning than controls, some show deleterious effects, and others suggest no differences from controls (Burlew, Evans, & Oler, 1989; Hurtig, 1994; Midence, McManus, Fuggle, & Davies, 1996; Noll et al., 1994; Schuman, Armstrong, Pegelow, & Routh, 1993).

For example, Schuman and colleagues reported on a sample of 25 mothers of preschool children with SCD compared to demographically matched mothers of healthy children. Mothers completed standard scales of parenting knowledge and skills and were observed in interaction with their children. They reported that mothers of children with SCD had more knowledge of appropriate parenting approaches and were more positive in their interactions with their children in comparison to the control mothers. Similarly, Noll and colleagues (1994) showed that reports of family conflict did not differ between 32 caregivers of children and adolescents with SCD and matched comparison caregivers.

Family functioning has been shown to have a direct effect on the adaptation of children and their caregivers as well as an indirect or mediating role (Brown & Lambert, 1999; Burlew, Telfair, Colangelo, & Wright, 2000; Drotar, 1997; Ievers, Brown, Lambert, Hsu, & Eckman, 1998; Kell, Kliewer, Erickson, & Ohene-Frempong, 1998; Thompson, Gil, Burbach, Keith, & Kinney, 1993). As an example of this research, Kell and colleagues (1993), using standard scales, reported that family competence was associated with better psychosocial adaptation in 80 adolescents with SCD. Similarly, Burlew et al. (2000) found family functioning predicted a significant amount of the variance in the psychological adjustment of 90 adolescents with SCD. For caregivers, Thompson and colleagues (1993) found better adaptation among 78 mothers of children and adolescents with SCD, who reported more supportive family relationships on a standardized scale. Moreover, from the National Collaborative Study of Sickle Cell Disease, in a prospective data set with 222 children with SCD, Thompson and colleagues (2003) found that family conflict predicted significant behavior problems over time. It should be noted that there are exceptions to these findings (Devine, Brown, Lambert, Donegan, & Eckman, 1998), and this issue is discussed in greater detail elsewhere in this volume (chapter 25).

## Relevant Models Addressing Family and Chronic Illness in Childhood

Pediatric psychology has attempted to characterize patterns of family functioning among children with chronic illness by way of theoretical models supported by empirical research to verify proposed associations and causal paths. The role of the family is increasingly recognized as foreground, not background, and critically important in managing chronic illness in children (Kazak, Rourke, & Krump, 2003). The family is seen as the key to promoting adherence to recommended treatment regimens and psychosocial outcomes among children and adolescents with chronic illness; at the same time, the chronic condition is thought to reciprocally impact the functioning of family members and the family as a whole.

Kazak's social-ecological model (Kazak, 1989) offers a helpful framework for understanding family functioning in the context of chronic illness in childhood. Adapted from Bronfenbrenner's model (1979) of systems that progress from the smallest social units to the largest, most inclusive social units, Kazak's model begins with a focus on the child, the disease, parents, siblings, and the family as the primary unit and then includes nested, interacting systems at successively greater distances from this central unit. The systems are viewed as reciprocally interacting with one another; ultimately, all systems affect the child with chronic illness. The microsystem includes the child, the illness and its treatment, siblings, parents, and the family; the mesosystem includes peers, school, hospital, hospital staff, and neighborhoods; and the exosystem includes religion, law, technology, parents' social networks, social class, and culture. An additional dimension is time, incorporating developmental processes of all elements within systems into the model. Although not descriptive of specific process mechanisms, Kazak's model is helpful in conceptualizing the levels of systems that have an impact on a child and family with SCD and the complex transactions among the systems (see figure 26-1).

Rolland (1994) offered a model for conceptualizing microsystemic, disease-specific influences on family functioning, depending on the nature of the disease or condition. For example, in Rolland's model, SCD would be characterized as having an acute onset, a relapsing course, a life-shortening prognosis in the case of SCD hemoglobin (Hb), and a nonincapacitating course. This set of conditions is expected to have an impact on the family uniquely compared to childhood diseases with conditions that vary from those described for SCD. However, Rolland's model is limited in that it focuses only on disease conditions and does not take into account ecological variables that may have significant impact on the family, such as, in the case of SCD, racism or poverty.

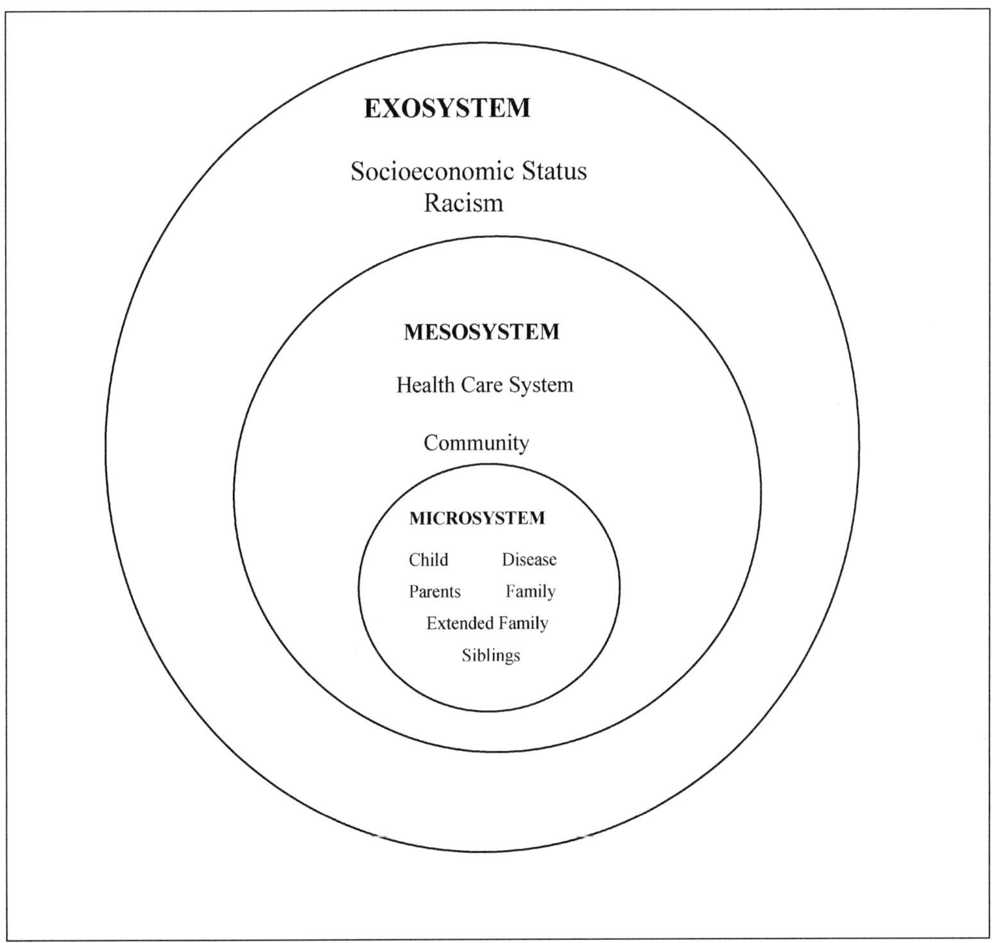


**Figure 26-1.** Adaptation of Kazak's (1989) model of ecological factors with an impact on family adaptation to chronic disease to relevant issues in pediatric sickle cell disease.

Wallander and Varni (1992, 1998) and Thompson, Gustafson, Hamlett, & Spock (1992) proposed models in which risk and resistance factors are linked with disease adaptation. These "noncategorical" models of chronic illness emphasize commonalities among families in confronting the stress of the child's condition and providing care to the child, while at the same time maintaining the family as an economic, social, and emotional unit that provides for the developmental and psychosocial needs of all its members. Brown et al. (2000) found support for a risk-and-resilience model for children with SCD. Thompson's model views maternal adjustment as a key element in child psychological outcome and uses the maternal-child unit as the central lens through which to examine the family. For example, in a longitudinal study examining adjustment processes, Thompson, Gustafson, Gil, Kinney, and Spock (1999) contrasted mother and child adjustment between two disease groups (cystic fibrosis and SCD) to highlight both similarities and differences in adaptational processes. However, because of the importance of the extended family within the African American community, a model primarily focusing on maternal-child processes may overlook the important transactional contributions of other family and community members.

A complete examination of all types of systems that have an impact on children and families with SCD is beyond the scope of this discussion, which focuses primarily on elements of the microsystem, as described by Kazak (1989). However, several elements within the mesosytem and exosystem are especially pertinent to African and African American families and are discussed as well.

## Microsystem

As noted in Kazak's (1989) model of family systems, elements within the microsystem are the child, disease, parents, siblings, and family. When discussing microsystem-level interactions, the focus is on how particular factors have an impact on the way the family functions around SCD. In doing this, it is important to differentiate what has been assumed about family functioning and SCD, what is known about family functioning, and what is yet to be documented. Although there is some literature related to aspects of family functioning and factors that influence family functioning, it is clear that the ways family members relate to one another and how SCD has an impact on those relationships over time has not yet been fully delineated in a culturally appropriate manner.

Researchers often use family functioning, coping, and social support measures developed on and standardized with primarily majority (white and middle class points of reference) samples, leading to conceptualizations and conclusions that may not fit well with the ways in which families function over time in the African American community with SCD (Boyd-Franklin, 2003). Professionals working with children with SCD and their families may have inaccurate perceptions of these relationships based on conclusions reached only from observations during admissions and clinic visits but not from day-to-day observations of family interaction. Such misperceptions may pose a problem for alliance with the family for the purpose of encouraging adherence to recommended treatments.

Moreover, both researchers and clinicians often define family as members of the child's household; however, it is imperative that what is considered as family be clearly defined by patients themselves because it has been suggested that household structure and perceived family do not correspond in African American samples (Reeb et al., 1986), and often secondary caregivers do not live in the same household with the child (S. A. Hill, 1996). That is, family can be found in a number of households and can incorporate extended kin and nonblood relatives, yet the contributions made by these extended kin networks are central to the psychosocial functioning of children with SCD and their primary caregivers.

In a unique study of assumptions, Noll, McKellop, Vannatta, and Kalinyak (1999) asked 48 caregivers of children with SCD, 48 matched caregivers of healthy classroom peers, and 12 professionals in the area of pediatric SCD to complete a standard measure of child-rearing practices. Although professionals were consistent in viewing protectiveness, parental worry, and discipline as areas of difference between caregivers of children with SCD and comparison caregivers, the actual findings based on caregiver ratings showed few differences between the groups. Noll et al. (1999) found that caregivers of children with SCD had higher scores for only two items, one that reflected worry about the health of the child and one that indicated a concern that the child would be viewed differently from other children. Also, illness severity was not highly associated with reports of child-rearing practices. The finding regarding concern about health was viewed as typical of caregivers of children with chronic illness because others have reported that caregivers' wishes and expectations for their children with chronic illnesses focus on the chronic condition (e.g., improvement in symptoms and treatment) (Wolman, Garwick, Kohrman, & Blum, 2001). The second finding was understood as reflecting the concern that African American caregivers hold for issues that may lead to increased discrimination for their children, with other studies supporting that caregivers of children of minority and low socioeconomic status worry about the impact of these conditions of living on their children's adjustment (Wolman et al., 2001).

### Gender and Age

Across studies, girls with SCD report better family functioning than do boys. Hurtig (1994), using structured interviews and standard scales with 70 families of children and adolescents with SCD, found that caregivers and their children reported good-to-excellent family functioning, with better functioning reported in families of girls with SCD. Similar findings were reported by Lutz, Barakat, Smith-Whitley, and Ohene-Frempong (2003) in a study involving 73 caregivers and 23 children and adolescents with SCD who were administered standard scales during an admission to an acute care unit for pain or fever.

Results showed that females reported higher levels of family functioning. The association of gender and family functioning may partly be explained by the findings of poorer psychological adjustment in males with SCD compared to females, particularly in adolescence (Barbarin, 1999). Whether family dysfunction has an impact on or is the result of problems in psychological adjustment in males is not clear because of a lack of prospective studies. However, Thompson and colleagues (2003) noted consistency in reported level of family functioning over a 9-year period, suggesting that there may not be age effects on family functioning.

## Disease Severity

Although disease severity has been hypothesized as a factor influencing overall adaptation among families, including those with SCD, illness severity per se seems to pose little risk to family functioning in families of children with chronic illness (Barakat & Kazak, 1999), including those with SCD (Hurtig, 1994; Noll et al., 1999). In contrast, Barbarin, Whitten, Bond, and Conner-Warren (1999) reported that, among families with a family member with SCD, illness severity did have an impact on family adjustment, but less so than financial hardship.

Related to disease severity is adherence to treatment because this is also affected by family variables. Treatment adherence has received little attention in sickle cell research because of a number of challenges in operationalizing and measuring adherence across various ages and treatment regimens (Barakat, Smith-Whitley, & Ohene-Frempong, 2002). Risk-and-resistance models have been used to explain treatment adherence in pediatric samples (Christiaanse, Lavigne, & Lerner, 1989) and in a SCD sample. Barakat and colleagues (2002) found that a number of risk-and-resistance factors, including family flexibility, accounted for a significant portion of the variance in treatment adherence in a sample of 73 families of children and adolescents with SCD who were interviewed using standard measures during an admission to an acute care unit for pain or fever.

## Psychosocial and Caregiving Stress

Families of children and adolescents with SCD are especially stressed (Burlew et al., 1989; Rao & Kramer, 1993), although level of stress may be consistent across children at varying levels of disease severity along with their families. Burlew and colleagues suggested that chronic illness has an impact on the family on three levels: cognitive (education in terms of illness care), emotional responses to the illness, and behavioral requirements of illness management. In their literature review, they confirmed that caregivers of children and adolescents with SCD experience high levels of stress related to the management of SCD.

Caregivers of children with SCD have reported caregiving problems specific to SCD in addition to the typical problems associated with raising children in challenging circumstances. Mothers of infants with SCD have been reported to experience stressors related to concern about their child being in pain, in response to the diagnosis of their infant with SCD, and related to ongoing care for their child (Rao & Kramer, 1993). Moreover, in comparison to mothers of infants with sickle cell trait, the mothers of infants with SCD in this sample reported more stress in response to the diagnosis and management of SCD, although the identified stressors were quite similar.

Ievers-Landis and colleagues (2001), using a semistructured interview with 37 caregivers of school-aged children with SCD, found that the areas of nutrition, minimizing pain episodes, and children conveying negative feelings about having SCD were the most frequently endorsed problematic aspects of raising a child with SCD—with more caregiving problems reported for boys than for girls and with the most difficult and upsetting problem related to the management of pain episodes. In a small sample of caregivers of school-aged children with SCD, in a prospective series of structured interviews, Northington (2000) also found that caregivers experienced high demands related to responsibilities for preventing and managing pain, infections, and other symptoms of SCD. These caregiver demands were exacerbated by the unpredictable nature of the symptoms and the caregivers' experience of chronic sorrow or sadness over losses for the child and themselves that were associated with their child's diagnosis. This chronic sorrow was experienced again in the presence of SCD symptoms that served as reminders of the child's illness.

S. A. Hill (1996), in an interview with 32 mothers of children with SCD, described family responses to a diagnosis of SCD in a child as beginning with a foundation of disbelief over the diagnosis (because mothers did not know they carried sickle cell trait or understand how SCD could be transmitted based on who their partner was) and subsequent guilt over having given the child this genetic disease. In addition, mothers faced fathers who often did not readily acknowledge their contribution to the diagnosis because they did not know of their sickle cell status. However, these mothers reported that, with time, they developed competent caregiving strategies that worked to prevent painful episodes and reduce the intensity of painful crises. Although caregiving stress in these families is high (because of limited resources and the addition of the demands of an unpredictable, chronic condition), mothers did not complain about this stress and instead focused on their strengths in addressing SCD issues and the availability of extended family and friendship supports, including other parents of children with SCD. Northington (2000) confirmed that caregivers in her sample believed they were able to face the demands of SCD care realistically and competently and "move on" in spite of periodic feelings of sadness (p. 141). Furthermore, many families reported that SCD does not have an adverse impact on family relations (Hurtig, 1994; Thompson et al., 1993).

## What Is Family?

*Family*, once used primarily to describe biological parents living together with their biological children, has become a multireferential term in the current social environment. Broader, more diverse, and more fluid definitions of family are now accepted. Although the extended family is not unique to the African American community, the extended family remains an important cultural component based on its persistence and prevalence in the context of African American family life (Wilson, 1989). The extended family, which includes relatives and fictive kin, is important not only for single-mother households, but also for two-parent families within its structure (Hunter, Pearson, Ialongo, & Kellam, 1998; Pearson, Hunter, Cook, Ialongo, & Kellam, 1997).

Although the presence of an extended family can be a source of family conflict and increased stress in the lives of its members (Chase-Landsdale, Gordon, Coley, Walkschlag, & Brooks-Gunn, 1999; Murry et al., 2001), an extended family network can facilitate children's social adjustment (Kellam, Adams, Brown, & Ensminger, 1982; Kellam, Ensminger, & Turner, 1977), offer emotional and instrumental support, increase interaction among adults, and promote positive parenting behaviors (Jarrett, 2000; Taylor & Roberts, 1995; Wilson, 1989). A critical function of African American families is to buffer the effects of racism and promote a sense of cultural pride and well-being within their children (Billingsley, 1992; Stevenson, Reed, & Bodison, 1996). In addition, extended family support has been shown to serve as a protective factor for ethnic minority youths with high levels of stressors and disadvantaged neighborhoods (Dubow, Edwards, & Ippolito, 1997; Stevenson, 1998).

An important function of the African American family is racial socialization, which is the process by which messages and behaviors about racial issues are communicated to children in an effort to help them cope with the adverse effects of discrimination in racially stressful environments. Families are the primary socializing agents for African American children, especially regarding racial matters (Bowman & Howard, 1985; Thorton, Chatters, Taylor, & Allen, 1990). This socialization includes buffering against the effects of racism and promoting a sense of competence, cultural pride, and well-being within their children (Billingsley, 1992; Stevenson et al., 1996) despite racist practices, negative media images, and stereotypes (Thomas & Speight, 1999).

Hughes and Chen (1997) identified the most frequently communicated messages from parents to their children aged 4–14 years as (a) cultural socialization; (b) preparation for bias; and (c) promotion of mistrust. For example, families may convey messages of racial pride, acceptance of race, and limited opportunities because of race (Thornton et al., 1990). The results of racial socialization include cultural pride and the development of coping mechanisms that allow individuals to better anticipate, identify, and negotiate racist encounters (Stevenson et al., 1996).

Parents differ in their emphasis on race in raising their children (Thorton et al., 1990). For example, African American families can be classified into three categories based on the types of socialization messages: (a) mainstream socialization is focused on Eurocentric values and beliefs;

(b) minority socialization emphasizes trying to work within a racist society with a degree of passive acceptance of racism; and (c) black cultural socialization transmits Afrocentric values, such as harmony, communalism, movement, and spirituality (Boykin & Toms, 1985). However, it appears as though racial socialization fosters protective factors and competence in African American children and thus promotes social competence. Racial socialization may be especially necessary for African American children and families with SCD to interact effectively with the health care system and other larger social organizations such as schools.

The importance of extended family members, particularly grandparents, in such family functions of child care, mutual support, and economic interrelatedness is now more widely acknowledged, as are the instrumental roles of other family members. Similarly, the assistance and support of other adults can diminish the stress and burden of illness for families caring for a youth with SCD. In caring for a child with SCD, a number of extended family members may play some role in providing care for the affected child, especially because of the widespread impact of the disease on home, school, social, and community functioning.

As noted, the extended family has been linked with positive outcomes for both parents and children and can buffer children from poor outcomes. The literature on family issues in SCD has begun to reflect a broader definition of family than simply biological mother or mother and father with biological children. Although some studies included only mother or mother and father as "primary caregiver" respondents (Casey, Brown, & Bakeman, 2000), other family studies included grandparents, aunts, and other care providers (Barakat et al., 2002; Dilworth-Anderson, 1994). Against this background of strengths, stressors, and concerns, families of African descent face the challenges of SCD among their children.

Family structure is often described in the SCD literature regarding family composition and household head. However, regardless of type of family structure, maternal adjustment has been found to strongly influence the whole family. For example, Sharpe, Brown, Thompson, and Eckman (1994) found that families' overall adaptation to SCD was heavily associated with the effectiveness of the mother's coping strategies to manage pain in the child with SCD. This same study also found that, conversely, mothers' use of a disengagement coping style was strongly associated with internalizing behaviors, pessimism, and negative thinking in affected children.

### *Two-Parent Families*

Two-parent family structures including both biological parents are a less-common family structure in SCD. Thus, there is a dearth of research examining the impact of SCD on the relationship between parents. In one study, Evans, Burlew, and Oler (1988) requested 78 parents of children with SCD living in two-parent families and 72 demographically matched parents of healthy children to complete a standard measure of marital satisfaction among parents. Findings revealed that parents of children with SCD reported less marital satisfaction than parents of healthy children. Findings from other samples of families of children with chronic conditions suggest that caregiving demands associated with illness may improve satisfaction or decrease satisfaction, and that this impact is not necessarily stable over time (Barakat & Kazak, 1999; Bashe & Kirby, 2001). Further research is required with families of children and adolescents with SCD, keeping in mind that the marital dyad may not involve both biological parents and may encompass two partners who are long-term cohabitants but not legally married (Boyd-Franklin, 2003).

### *Single-Mother Families*

Hurtig (1994) reported no effect of family structure on family relations as reported by caregivers and children and adolescents with SCD. In contrast, Evans and colleagues (1988) did find that single mothers reported less-satisfactory parent-child relationships compared to mothers in two-parent families. McLoyd (1990) suggested that risks associated with single-mother family status to the parent-child relationship are not direct or consistent across African American families, further clarifying that risk emanates from parental distress and low levels of social support and its impact on parenting style instead of merely single-parent family status.

### *Fathers*

Because fathers are less often the primary or secondary caregivers in African American families of children and adolescents with SCD (H. A. Williams, 1993) and because they seldom are successfully recruited for participation in family research, an inaccurate assumption might be made that fathers are not involved in the lives of their children with SCD (Boyd-Franklin, 2003). Contrary to this perception, there is evidence to suggest that when fathers do act as caregivers, they are very involved in the care of their child with SCD (H. A. Williams, 1993). In addition, the mental health of fathers of children with SCD has been found to contribute importantly to adjustment among their children (Barbarin, 1999). Barbarin also found that fathers of children with SCD showed higher levels of overall mental health when compared with the fathers of matched community controls and lower anxiety, loss of control, and distress than the matched controls. In addition to biological fathers, father figures also may play an important role in family adjustment to a child's SCD.

Clearly, improved efforts are needed to identify and include fathers in family research in pediatric SCD. Furthermore, because many families of children and adolescents with SCD are headed by single mothers, the mother's partner may serve as a father figure and must be included in future research designs (Murry et al., 2001).

### *Siblings*

Although just beginning to receive attention, the well-being of siblings of children with SCD also plays some role in influencing the psychological functioning of the child with SCD as well as overall family functioning. It has been speculated that the development of healthy siblings may be compromised in some way by having a sibling with chronic illness (Burlew et al., 1989). Barbarin (1999) reported that siblings of children with SCD had higher self-report scores of depressive symptoms and parent report scores of behavior problems than found for the children with SCD or children in the healthy comparison group. Gender effects were found as well because brothers of a child with SCD appeared to have more difficulties in psychological functioning than sisters of affected children.

In contrast, a study comparing siblings with demographically matched peers found no differences among siblings of children with SCD in objectively determined peer ratings and social acceptance or in the children's views of their own peer relationships or social acceptance (Noll, Yosua, Vannatta, & Kalinyak, 1995). However, because so little study has been made of siblings of children with SCD and their contribution to the adjustment of the ill child and the family (and vice versa), further study of these relationships is warranted.

### *Extended Family Networks*

Outside of studies that included extended family as primary caregivers, few studies have examined the role of extended family networks in the functioning of families of children with SCD. African American families are proud of the integral role of extended kin in their lives, and grandparents can play an extensive role in caregiving for their grandchildren, especially in times of crisis or need (Boyd-Franklin, 2003; Boyd-Franklin, Aleman, Jean-Gilles, & Lewis, 1995). Thus, the role of kin is expanded in families with children with SCD, and children with SCD and their mothers may show more competence in the presence of supportive extended family networks (Dilworth-Anderson, 1994).

Dilworth-Anderson (1994) reported, using semistructured interviews, on a study of grandparent involvement in caregiving for 34 school-aged children with SCD. Grandparents made up the majority of secondary caregivers in this sample, with very few mothers reporting reliance on supports outside the family. In addition to fathers, mothers reported that they most relied on maternal grandmothers (their own mothers) and maternal aunts following the diagnosis of their children, maternal grandmother support was the most consistent over time (compared with other secondary caregivers), and all mothers were satisfied with the support provided by their mothers. Furthermore, mothers' self-esteem and coping were bolstered by the presence of the maternal grandmother as secondary caregiver, and children's self-esteem and competence was higher in the presence of father and extended family support as opposed to support from outside the family.

Extended family networks may provide ongoing, consistent, and particularly instrumental or tangible support to African American caregivers of children with SCD. H. A. Williams (1993) reported on a pilot study using structured interviews to compare the social support of 17 Caucasian caregivers and 20 African American caregivers recruited through a pediatric hematology/oncology unit. Results suggested that both sets of caregivers experienced satisfaction with the support they received, although African American caregivers reported greater satisfaction. African American caregivers reported receiving and relying on more instrumental support, whereas Caucasian caregivers reported receiving and relying on more emotional support. Furthermore, black caregivers had smaller networks made up primarily of family members and received far less spontaneous support than their Caucasian counterparts. H. A. Williams suggested that these differences may have resulted from the higher incidence of single-parent household, lower socioeconomic status, and more urban dwelling status of the African American families in the sample.

In the Hurtig (1994) study, social support was associated with better family relations, indicating that availability of a support network and satisfaction with support received may enhance positive family functioning in families of children with SCD. This finding has been confirmed in a number of studies (see Burlew et al., 1989, for a review), with some exceptions (Noll et al., 1994).

In their review of the literature regarding African American single-mother families and child adjustment, Murry and colleagues (2001) provided confirmation for the protective role that involvement of extended kin, particularly grandmothers, can bring to families. The mechanism of effect on children's outcomes seems to be in bolstering the well-being of the mother or primary caregiver so that she can engage in more adaptive interactions with her child. Thompson and colleagues (1993) provided evidence in mothers of children and adolescents that would support this interpretation in that, for these mothers, family supportiveness was associated with better adjustment.

## Caregiver Coping and the Role of Beliefs About Illness and Spirituality

According to Garwick, Kohrman, Titus, Wolman, and Blum (1999), families construct beliefs or explanations about chronic conditions that are shaped by cultural beliefs about illness. These cognitions affect how they respond to stressful aspects of caregiving and interact with health care systems (Garwick et al., 1999). Family functioning has been associated with coping strategies used by children with SCD and their caregivers to address SCD-related stress (Lutz et al., 2003). In this study, child-reported family functioning was associated with greater reliance on active coping strategies by the child; conversely, parent-reported family functioning was associated with increased use of passive coping strategies on the part of caregivers. The unexpected finding may have been caused by a low level of coping reported by families during an acute care admission for pain or fever at the time of data collection.

Although some studies suggest that spirituality can be a burden in coping with stressors, including chronic illness (Boyd-Franklin, Aleman, Jean-Gilles, & Lewis, 1995), among African American families spirituality is viewed as a strength and resource, and many report praying as a primary coping strategy (Boyd-Franklin, 2003). This is well summarized in a quote of an African American grandmother of a child with a chronic illness, "God never gives you more than you can bear, and I do all things through God, who strengthens me" (Boyd-Franklin, Aleman, Steiner, Drelich, & Norford, 1995, p. 125).

## Mesosystem

Significant mesosystem factors that have an impact on families with SCD are the school, community, and health care system. Because children and adolescents and school functioning are discussed elsewhere in this volume (chapter 25), this discussion addresses the health care system and its impact on family functioning and the impact of community as these relate to families' adaptation to SCD.

### The Health Care System

The health care system significantly influences families of children with SCD. However, discussion of many important aspects of the complex interplay of political, economic, entitlement, and socioeconomic factors with health care system access and availability for children with SCD and their families is well beyond the scope of this chapter. More immediately relevant to the care of children with SCD, however, are the relationships among families affected by SCD, health care providers, and health service utilization.

Relationships between parents and health care providers have long been recognized as important. Relationships among parents, children, and health care providers in pediatric settings have many tasks to accomplish in the course of caring for children with SCD, and these relationships do change over time as well (Nobile & Drotar, 2003). Parents' relationships with their child's health care provider are key in their access to information, services, and treatments necessary for their child's health. However, there may be particular issues unique to caregivers of children with SCD that have an impact on their dealings with health care providers.

The reciprocal relationships of children with SCD, their families, and health care providers are just beginning to be studied. Applegate et al. (2003) studied the effects of a brief intervention in which parents of children with SCD and parents of children with cystic fibrosis were encouraged write down their questions for a medical care provider just prior to the actual visit. Although this intervention proved effective in terms of increasing the number of questions asked during the visit among those parents whose children had cystic fibrosis, this was not the case for the families of children with SCD. Applegate and colleagues speculated that the amount of time spent by the families of children with SCD with nonphysician health care providers (i.e., nurses while the children were receiving transfusion therapy) may have reduced the number of questions that these families wished to ask physicians. As the two samples were studied separately, systematic study of other factors with an impact on family–health care provider relationships, such as the race/ethnicity of both groups of families or the concordance between race/ethnicity of families and care providers, were not examined.

Health care service utilization, and its relationship to family characteristics, is another emerging area of study. A study of adolescents with SCD and their families examined relationships among disease knowledge, adolescent adjustment, and health care service utilization (Logan, Radcliffe, & Smith-Whitley, 2002). In this sample of 70 adolescents and their parents, both parent characteristics and disease severity were associated with patterns of health care service use. Parents' increased knowledge of SCD was associated with higher frequency of routine health care service use; disease severity was associated with frequency of urgent service use. Significant life events and clinical maladjustment of adolescents or families were not predictive of urgent service use. However, more frequent illness-related stress was associated with greater use of all types of medical services, including routine and urgent types. Both illness and family variables were jointly linked to the utilization of health services among families with SCD. These studies of parent-provider relations and factors influencing health care service utilization represent just a beginning in the understanding of how to effectively reduce barriers to health care utilization for children and families impacted by SCD and, ultimately, how to provide optimal care.

### Community

Community, especially community safety, is another significant mesosystem-level issue that affects many children. Many African American individuals are concerned about violence in their communities and the safety of their children, especially their sons (Boyd-Franklin, Franklin, & Toussaint, 2001). Youths, especially urban children, are chronically exposed to violence as victims and even more so as witnesses of violence (Osofsky, Wewers, Hann, & Fick, 1993; Richters & Martinez, 1993). African American children are disproportionately affected by exposure to community violence (Bell & Jenkins, 1993; Selner-O'Hagan, Kindlon, Buka, Raudenbush, & Earls, 1998). Many urban children are continuously exposed to violence throughout their lives (DuRant, Cadenhead, Pendergrast, Slavens, & Linder, 1994) and have experienced multiple losses as a result (Farrell & Bruce, 1997). Exposure to community violence has been associated with a host of maladaptive outcomes in youths, such as symptoms of general distress, anxiety, posttraumatic stress, depression, school difficulties, aggression, and externalizing behaviors (Cooley-Quille, Boyd, Frantz, & Walsch, 2001; Fitzpatrick, 1993; Margolin & Gordis, 2000). Children with SCD, especially those living in urban contexts, may experience stress from exposure to community violence, which exacerbates disease symptoms.

## Exosystem

Kazak's model (1989) includes a number of exosystem elements. Two of these, socioeconomic status and the effects of culture, are particularly relevant to family systems impacted by SCD.

### Socioeconomic Status

Relationships between socioeconomic status and adjustment outcomes for children and families with SCD have been variable. As much as socioeconomic status may include psychosocial stressors, socioeconomic status has not been associated with family relations, as studied through reports by caregivers and their children with SCD (Hurtig, 1994). However, others have suggested that psychosocial stress unrelated to SCD is associated with family adjustment outcome (Thompson et al., 1993). More complex relationships between financial and socioeconomic status and family adjustment outcomes are indicated in other studies.

For example, Barbarin et al. (1999) found through hierarchical multiple regression of factors influencing outcomes in child and family functioning that financial hardship contributed independently to impaired child and family functioning among those families with a child with SCD. However, when basic needs were met, poverty did not contribute significantly to poor outcome in family adjustment. In fact, those parents with the lowest incomes were less angry and anxious and reported higher academic expectations for their children with SCD than those families with higher incomes.

### Culture and the Effects of Racism

Exposure to racism is a pervasive and common stressor in the lives of African American individuals living in the United States. Racism is defined as beliefs, attitudes, institutional arrangements, and acts that tend to denigrate individuals or groups because of phenotypic characteristics or ethnic group affiliation (Clark, Anderson, Clark, & Williams, 1999). There are limited empirical data available concerning the effects of racism on African Americans; however, research studies indicated negative psychological outcomes. For example, being a victim of racial discrimination has been associated with elevated depressive symptoms and poorer well-being among African American youths and adults (e.g., Simons et al., 2002; D. R. Williams, Neighbors, & Jackson, 2003).

Psychological responses to perceptions of racism in adults include anger, paranoia, anxiety, helplessness-hopelessness, frustration, resentment, and fear (Armstead, Lawler, Gorden, Cross, & Gibbons, 1989; Bullock & Houston, 1987; Kessler, Mickelson, & Williams, 1999). Similarly, slurs, false accusations, or exclusion from activities based on race are likely to undermine a child's sense of worth and control (Simons et al., 2002). Institutional racism and personal experiences with racism have been shown to be associated with hopelessness as well as internalizing and externalizing problems in African American boys (Nyborg & Curry, 2003). In addition, caregivers' report of racial discrimination is related to children's depressive symptoms, suggesting that ethnic minority children are distressed by witnessing racial discrimination against those of their ethnic group and can be negatively affected by living in a racist environment although they are not necessarily a direct target of discrimination (Simons et al., 2002). For children with SCD, exposure to racism may be an additional stressor that can negatively affect their psychological outcomes (Barbarin & Christian, 1999).

### Change in Family Functioning Over Time

The significance of developmental processes in adaptation to chronic illness has been noted (Holmbeck, 2002; Wallander & Varni, 1998), but only limited longitudinal work has been conducted on the developmental processes of families affected by SCD. Changes in the psychological adjustment of children with SCD and their mothers were studied over 2 years by researchers at Duke University (Thompson et al., 1999). Although only 32% of children with SCD showed consistency in adjustment classification over 2 years based on their self-reports, 77% of mothers of children with SCD reported their own adjustment within the same classification. Interestingly, despite the relatively low temporal consistency in child reports of their own adjustment, 66% of mothers showed continuity in classification of behavior problems among their children over the 2-year study period. Daily hassles, illness-related stress, and the use of active, rather than palliative, coping strategies contributed significantly to maternal adaptation.

The largest longitudinal investigation to date has been through the National Cooperative Study of Sickle Cell Disease, in which family variables and child adjustment problems were studied prospectively in the context of a larger study of neuropsychological outcomes and magnetic resonance imaging findings (Thompson et al., 2003). In this study, a subset of 222 children who had at least two assessments at least 2 years apart over the study period of 9 years were evaluated for intellectual ability, child behavior problems, and family functioning. The children ranged in age from 5 to 15 years at time of first evaluation and 7 to 17 years of age at the time of the final evaluation. Only mother-completed measures of child adjustment (Child Behavior Checklist) (Achenbach & Edelbrock, 1983) and family function (Family Environment Scale) (Moos & Moos, 1981) were used. No significant overall changes in reported behavior problems or scores of family function were found over time, although a decrease in intellectual ability over time was found. The rate of behavior problems in children was significantly increased with a higher baseline level of family conflict. Interestingly, the risk of behavior problems was not significantly related to magnetic resonance imaging classification, gender, educational level of the mother, or child's age. An increase in behavior problems over time was significantly associated with increases in family conflict over time. Of interest is the finding that the risk of having increased behavior problems over time decreased among those children with higher levels of intellectual functioning at baseline, even though there might be some subsequent decline in cognitive ability among the children.

## Family/Systems Interventions in Sickle Cell Disease

Structured interventions for families around adjustment to and management of SCD are emerging in the literature. These interventions vary in the breadth of their focus, from management of specific aspects of SCD to those with an impact on more general disease management. A unique and broadly focused approach to family intervention for SCD is that of Kaslow and coworkers (Kaslow & Brown, 1995; Kaslow et al., 2000); their group developed a family psychoeducational intervention for pediatric SCD with the goal of increasing disease knowledge, level of family functioning, and levels of family support, with the purpose of influencing overall adjustment to SCD.

The guiding principles for this intervention were comprehensive. To intervene effectively with families affected by SCD, the therapist was viewed as needing to be (a) familiar with SCD, including genetics, physical symptoms, disease processes, and interventions; (b) aware of the impact of the disease on the child's functioning; (c) knowledgeable about the social context of the child and family impacted by SCD; (d) informed about characteristics of African American families; and (e) trained in adapting family therapy approaches to African American families. The intervention program was a brief, manualized, developmentally and culturally sensitive treatment that was individualized for each child and family in terms of unique needs and competencies. The intervention incorporated a risk-resistance-adaptation perspective and a transactional stress and coping model.

Empowerment of the family system was viewed as the key feature of therapeutic change for these families, consistent with Boyd-Franklin (2003). This intervention facilitated the development of a solid working alliance among family members and between the family, health care providers, and the medical community. A multisystems approach was employed because effective intervention was viewed as including and impacting multiple levels of functioning, including the child, family, extended family, church, community networks, and the health care system.

Kaslow's model included a relatively brief (6–12 session) course of family therapy instituted in response to an acute condition or when problems were noted around disease management. The frequency and duration of sessions were variable, depending on the intensity of the individual situation. Although the ideal setting for family therapy included all persons involved in the family, in reality the most common session membership included the primary caregiver and the child or adolescent with SCD. Other family members were included as they were able to participate, as were siblings or other children living in the home. The rationale was to simplify the family's involvement (eliminate the need for babysitting) and to promote involvement. The sessions included (a) developmentally tailored disease education and introduction to family therapy; (b) prevention, including preventive health care strategies that can serve as resistance factors in successful disease management; (c) stress processing and coping, including pain management strategies and general coping strategies; (d) enhancing intrapersonal variables, such as the ability to share feelings; (e) promoting positive friendship patterns and good family relations; and finally (f) review of information, treatment termination, and follow-up plans.

Thirty-nine children and adolescents were randomly assigned either to the treatment condition ($n = 20$) or a standard care condition ($n = 19$). Those in the treatment condition completed the six-session manualized psychoeducational program. A 6-month follow-up was included to assess long-term effects of the treatment. The family intervention group demonstrated significantly greater gains in disease knowledge among both caregivers and children than the standard treatment group, and children in the treatment group maintained their disease knowledge at the 6-month follow-up, although rated levels of anxiety among the children in the treatment group were significantly greater as well. Kaslow noted that both children and caregivers increased their knowledge of SCD and hypothesized that, as children become more knowledgeable about their disease and as caregivers become more cognizant of the disease process as well, there is an overall increase in the family's sense of empowerment and control. This greater sense of empowerment is thought to have a positive impact on the family's ability to manage the child's illness and navigate the health care system. This type of clinical intervention serves as an important prototype of systematic, family-oriented disease adaptation intervention in SCD.

## Summary and Final Thoughts

Families negotiating the stressors and challenges of a lifelong, life-threatening illness in a child, at the same time conducting all the tasks necessary to maintain a family and promote the development of all family members, in the larger context of experiencing the many daily stressors associated with membership in an ethnic minority group. Although families of children with SCD have been found to be largely successful in promoting adaptation among children with SCD, healthy siblings, and the extended family of caregivers, this has been accomplished despite their own challenges in many cases and limited understanding of how best to work with African American families on the part of the health care community. Pain management, adherence to treatment, and appropriate use of health care resources remain significant concerns in the management of SCD, and there is currently little understanding of how health care professionals can best empower families to accomplish these important tasks. Further research pertaining to family systems issues in SCD should continue to discover risk and resilience factors among these families while at the same time take into account such important and unique variables as extended definitions of family and the effect of ethnic minority status in family–care provider interactions. This information will allow for the development of more effective family-centered interventions to support at-risk families in the management of SCD. Elucidating the nature of family interactions around important areas of disease management, such as pain intervention, has yet to be defined and is another potentially fruitful and important line of research. Finally, further research needs to address how respect and cultural sensitivity can be developed among health care providers and how these variables influence health care outcomes among children and adolescents with SCD.

*Acknowledgment.* The work described in this chapter was supported by a grant from the National Institutes of Health (5 U54 HL70596J-2).

## References

Achenbach, T. M., & Edelbrock, C. S. (1983). *Manual for the Child Behavior Checklist and Child Behavior Profile*. Burlington: University of Vermont.

Applegate, H., Webb, P. M., Elkin, T. D., Neul, S. K. T., Drabman, R. S., Moll, G. W., et al. (2003). Improving parent participation at pediatric diabetes and sickle cell appointments using a brief intervention. *Children's Health Care, 32*, 125–136.

Armstead, C. A., Lawler, K. A., Gorden, G., Cross, J., & Gibbons, J. (1989). Relationship of racial stressors to blood pressure responses and anger expression in black college students. *Health Psychology, 8*, 541–556.

Barakat, L. P., & Kazak, A. E. (1999). Family issues. In R. T. Brown (Ed.), *Cognitive aspects of chronic illness in children* (pp. 333–354). New York: Guilford.

Barakat, L. P., Smith-Whitley, K., & Ohene-Frempong, K. (2002). Treatment adherence in children with sickle cell disease: Disease-related risk and psychosocial resistance factors. *Journal of Clinical Psychology in Medical Settings, 9*, 201–209.

Barbarin, O. A. (1999). Do parental coping, involvement, religiosity, and racial identity mediate children's psychological adjustment to sickle cell disease? *Journal of Black Psychology, 25*, 391–426.

Barbarin, O. A., & Christian, M. (1999). The social and cultural context of coping with sickle cell disease: I. A review of biological and psychosocial issues. *Journal of Black Psychology, 25*, 277–293.

Barbarin, O. A., Whitten, C. F., Bond, S., & Conner-Warren, R. (1999). The social and cultural context of coping with sickle cell disease: II. The role of financial hardship in adjustment to sickle cell disease. *Journal of Black Psychology, 25*, 294–315.

Bashe, P. B., & Kirby, B. L. (2001). *The oasis guide to Asperger syndrome*. New York: Crown.

Bell, C. C., & Jenkins, E. J. (1993). Community violence and children on Chicago's southside. *Psychiatry, 56*, 46–54.

Billingsley, A. (1992). *Climbing Jacob's ladder*. New York: Simon and Schuster.

Bowman, P. J., & Howard, C. S. (1985). Race-related socialization, motivation, and academic achievement: A study of black youth in three-generation families. *Journal of the American Academy of Child Psychiatry, 24*, 134–141.

Boyd-Franklin, N. (2003). *Black families in therapy: Understanding the African American experience* (3rd ed.). New York: Guilford Press.

Boyd-Franklin, N., Aleman, J. C., Jean-Gilles, M. M., & Lewis, S. Y. (1995). Cultural sensitivity and competence. In N. Boyd-Franklin, G. L. Steiner, & M. G. Boland (Eds.), *Children, families and HIV/AIDS: Psychosocial and therapeutic issues* (pp. 53–77). New York: Guilford.

Boyd-Franklin, N., Aleman, J. C., Steiner, G. L., Drelich, E. W., & Norford, B. C. (1995). Family systems interventions and family therapy. In N. Boyd-Franklin, G. L. Steiner, & M. G. Boland (Eds.), *Children, families and HIV/AIDS: Psychosocial and therapeutic issues* (pp. 115–126). New York: Guilford.

Boyd-Franklin, N., Franklin, A. J., & Toussaint, P. (2001). *Boys into men: Raising our African American teenage sons*. New York: Plume.

Boykin, A. W., & Toms, F.D. (1985). Black child socialization: A conceptual framework. In H. P. McAdoo & J. L. McAdoo (Eds.), *Black children: Social, educational, and parental environments* (pp. 33–51). Newbury Park, CA: Sage.

Bronfenbrenner, U. (1979). *The ecology of human development*. Cambridge, MA: Harvard University Press.

Brown, R. T., & Lambert, R. (1999). Family functioning and children's adjustment in the presence of a chronic illness: Concordance between children with sickle cell disease and caretakers. *Families, Systems, and Health, 17*, 165–179.

Brown, R. T., Lambert, R., Devine, D., Baldwin, K., Casey, R., Doepke, K., et al. (2000). Risk-resistance adaptation model for caregivers and their children with sickle cell disease. *Annals of Behavioral Medicine, 22*, 158–169.

Bullock, S. C., & Houston, E. (1987). Perceptions of racism by black medical students attending white medical schools. *Journal of the National Medical Association, 79*, 601–608.

Burlew, A. K., Evans, R., & Oler, C. (1989). The impact of a child with sickle cell disease on family dynamics. *Annals of the New York Academy of Sciences, 565*, 161–171.

Burlew, A. K., Telfair, J., Colangelo, L., & Wright, E. C. (2000). Factors that influence adolescent adaptation to sickle cell disease. *Journal of Pediatric Psychology, 25*, 287–299.

Casey, R., Brown, R. T., & Bakeman, R. (2000). Predicting adjustment in children and adolescents with sickle cell disease: A test of the risk-resistance-adaptation model. *Rehabilitation Psychology, 45*, 155–178.

Chase-Lansdale, P. L., Gordon, R. A., Coley, R. L., Walkschlag, L. S., & Brooks-Gunn, J. (1999). Young African American multigenerational families in poverty: The contexts, exchanges, and processes of lives. In M. E. Hetherington, *Coping with divorce, single parenting, and remarriage: A risk and resiliency perspective* (pp. 165–191). Mahwah, NJ: Erlbaum.

Christiaanse, M. E., Lavigne, J. V., & Lerner, C. V. (1989). Psychosocial aspects of compliance in children and adolescents with asthma. *Journal of Developmental and Behavioral Pediatrics, 10*, 75–80.

Clark, R., Anderson, N. B., Clark, V. A., & Williams, D. R. (1999). Racism as a stressor for African Americans: A biopsychosocial model. *American Psychologist, 54*, 805–816.

Cooley-Quille, M., Boyd, R. C., Frantz, E., & Walsch, J. (2001). Emotional and behavioral impact of exposure to community violence in inner-city adolescents. *Journal of Child Clinical Psychology, 30*, 199–206.

Devine, D., Brown, R. T., Lambert, R., Donegan, J. E., & Eckman, J. (1998). Predictors of psychosocial and cognitive adaptation in children with sickle cell syndromes. *Journal of Clinical Psychology in Medical Settings, 5*, 295–313.

Dilworth-Anderson, P. (1994). The importance of grandparents in extended-kin caregiving to black children with sickle cell disease. *Journal of Health and Social Policy, 5*, 185–202.

Drotar, D. (1997). Relating parent and family functioning to the psychological adjustment of children with chronic health conditions: What have we learned? What do we need to know? *Journal of Pediatric Psychology, 22*, 149–165.

Dubow, E. F., Edwards, S., & Ippolito, M. F. (1997). Life stressors, neighborhood disadvantage, and resources: A focus on inner-city children's adjustment. *Journal of Clinical Child Psychology, 26*, 130–144.

DuRant, R. H., Cadenhead, C., Pendergrast, R. A., Slavens, G., & Linder, C. W. (1994). Factors associated with the use of violence among urban black adolescents. *American Journal of Public Health, 84*, 612–617.

Evans, R., Burlew, A. K., & Oler, C. (1988). Children with sickle cell anemia: Parental relations, parent-child relations, and child behavior. *Social Work, 33*, 127–130.

Farrell, A. D., & Bruce, S. E. (1997). The role of exposure to community violence and developmental problems among inner-city youth. *Journal of Clinical Child Psychology, 26*, 2–14.

Fitzpatrick, K. M. (1993). Exposure to violence and presence of depression among low-income African-American youth. *Journal of Consulting and Clinical Psychology, 61*, 528–531.

Garwick, A., Kohrman, C., Titus, J., Wolman, C., & Blum, R. (1999). Variations in families' explanations of childhood chronic conditions: A cross-cultural perspective. In H. I. McCubbin, E. A. Thompson, A. Thompson, & J. A. Futrell (Eds.), *The dynamics of resilient families* (pp. 165–202). Thousand Oaks, CA: Sage.

Gary, L. E., Beatty, L. A., Berry, G. I., & Price, M. D. (1983). *Stable black families: Final report*. Washington, DC: Institute for Urban Affairs and Research, Howard University.

Hill, R. (1972). *The strengths of black families*. New York: Emerson-Hall.

Hill, R. (1999). *The strengths of black families: 25 years later*. Lanham, MD: University Press of America.

Hill, S. A. (1996). Caregiving in African American families: Caring for children with sickle cell disease. In S. D. Logan (Ed.), *The black family: Strengths, self-help, and positive change* (pp. 39–52). Boulder, CO: Westview Press.

Holmbeck, G. N. (2002). A developmental perspective on adolescent health and illness: An introduction to the special issues. *Journal of Pediatric Psychology, 27*, 409–416.

Hughes, D., & Chen, L. (1997). When and what parents tell children about race: An examination of race-related socialization among African American mothers. *Applied Developmental Science, 1*, 200–214.

Hunter, A. G., Pearson, J. L., Ialongo, N. S., & Kellam, S. G. (1998). Parenting alone to multiple caregivers: Child care and parenting arrangements in black and white urban families. *Family Relations, 47*, 343–353.

Hurtig, A. L. (1994). Relationships in families of children and adolescents with sickle cell disease. *Journal of Health and Social Policy, 5*, 161–183.

Ievers, C. E., Brown, R. T., Lambert, R. G., Hsu, L., & Eckman, J. R. (1998). Family functioning and social support in the adaptation of caregivers of children with sickle cell syndromes. *Journal of Pediatric Psychology, 23*, 377–388.

Ievers-Landis, C. E., Brown, R. T., Drotar, D., Bunke, V., Lambert, R. G., & Walker, A. A. (2001). Situational analysis of parenting problems for caregivers of children with sickle cell syndromes. *Journal of Developmental and Behavioral Pediatrics, 22*, 169–178.

Jarrett, R. L. (2000). Voices from below: The use of ethnographic research for informing a public policy. In J. M. Mercier, S. Garasky, & M. C. Shelly (Eds.), *Redefining family policy: Implications for the 21st century* (pp. 67–84). Ames: Iowa State University Press.

Johnson, K. W., Anderson, N. B., Bastida, E., Kramer, B. J., Williams, D., & Wong, M. (1995). Panel II: Macrosocial and environmental influences on minority health. *Health Psychology, 14*, 601–612.

Kaslow, N. J., & Brown, F. (1995). Culturally sensitive family interventions for chronically ill youth: Sickle cell disease as an example. *Family Systems Medicine, 13*, 201–213.

Kaslow, N. J., Collins, M. H., Rashid, F. L., Baskin, M. L., Griffith, J. R., Hollins, L., et al. (2000). The efficacy of a pilot family psychoeducational intervention for pediatric sickle cell disease (SCD). *Families, Systems and Health, 8*, 381–404.

Kazak, A. E. (1989). Families of chronically ill children: A systems and social ecological model of adaptation and challenge. *Journal of Consulting and Clinical Psychology, 57*, 25–30.

Kazak, A. E., Rourke, M. T., & Krump, T. A. (2003). Family and other systems in pediatric psychology. In M. C. Roberts (Ed.), *Handbook of pediatric psychology* (3rd ed., pp. 159–175). New York: Guilford Press.

Kell, R. S., Kliewer, W., Erickson, M. T., & Ohene-Frempong, K. (1998). Psychological adjustment of adolescents with sickle cell disease: Relations with demographic, medical, and family competence variables. *Journal of Pediatric Psychology, 23*, 301–312.

Kellam, S. G., Adams, R. G., Brown, C. H., & Ensminger, M. E. (1982). The long-term evolution of the family structure of teenage and older mothers. *Journal of Marriage and the Family, 46*, 539–554.

Kellam, S. G., Ensminger, M. E., & Turner, J. T. (1977). Family structure and the mental health of children. *Archives of General Psychiatry, 34*, 1012–1022.

Kessler, R. C., Mickelson, K. D., & Williams, D. R. (1999). The prevalence, distribution, and mental health correlates of perceived discrimination in the United States. *Journal of Health and Social Behavior, 40*, 208–230.

Lemanek, K. L., Ranalli, M. A., Green, K., Biega, C., & Lupia, C. (2003). Diseases of the blood: Sickle cell disease and hemophilia. In M. C. Roberts (Ed.), *Handbook of pediatric psychology* (3rd ed., pp. 321–341). New York: Guilford.

Logan, D. E., Radcliffe, J., & Smith-Whitley, K. (2002). Parent factors and adolescent sickle cell disease: Associations with patterns of health service use. *Journal of Pediatric Psychology, 27*, 475–484.

Lutz, M. J., Barakat, L. P., Smith-Whitley, K., & Ohene-Frempong, K. (in press). Psychological adjustment of children with sickle cell disease: Family functioning and coping. *Rehabilitation Psychology, 49*(3), 224–232.

Margolin, G., & Gordis, E. B. (2000). The effects of family and community violence on children. *Annual Review of Psychology, 51*, 445–479.

McLoyd, V. C. (1990). The impact of economic hardship on black families and children: Psychological distress, parenting, and socioemotional development. *Child Development, 61*, 311–346.

Midence, K., McManus, C., Fuggle, P., & Davies, S. (1996). Psychological adjustment and family functioning in a group of British children with sickle cell disease: Preliminary empirical findings and a meta-analysis. *British Journal of Clinical Psychology, 35*, 439–450.

Mistry, R. S., Vandewater, E. A., Huston, A. C., & McLoyd, V. C. (2002). Economic well-being and children's social adjustment: The role of family process in an ethnically diverse low-income sample. *Child Development, 73*, 935–951.

Moos, R. H., & Moos, R. H. (1981). *Family Environment Scale manual*. Palo Alto, CA: Consulting Psychologists Press.

Murry, V. M., Bynum, M. S., Brody, G. H., Willert, A., & Stephens, D. (2001). African American single mothers and children in context: A review of studies on risk and resilience. *Clinical Child and Family Psychology Review, 4*, 133–155.

Nobile, C., & Drotar, D. (2003). Research on the quality of parent-provider communication in pediatric care: Implications and recommendations. *Developmental and Behavioral Pediatrics, 24*, 279–290.

Noll, R. B., McKellop, J. M., Vannatta, K., & Kalinyak, K. (1999). Child-rearing practices of primary caregivers of children with sickle cell disease: The perspective of professionals and caregivers. *Journal of Pediatric Psychology, 23*, 131–140.

Noll, R. B., Swiecki, E., Garstein, M., Vannatta, K., Kalinyak, K., Davies, W. H., et al. (1994). Parental distress, family conflict, and role of social support for caregivers with or without a child with sickle cell disease. *Family Systems Medicine, 12*, 281–294.

Noll, R. B., Yosua, L. A., Vannatta, K., & Kalinyak, K. (1995). Social competence of siblings of children with sickle cell anemia. *Journal of Pediatric Psychology, 20*, 165–172.

Northington, L. (2000). Chronic sorrow in caregivers of school age children with sickle cell disease: A grounded theory approach. *Issues in Comprehensive Pediatric Nursing, 23*, 141–154.

Nyborg, V. M., & Curry, J. F. (2003). The impact of perceived racism: Psychological symptoms among African American boys. *Journal of the Clinical Child and Adolescent Psychology, 32*, 258–266.

Osofsky, J. D., Wewers, S., Hann, D. M., & Fick, A. C. (1993). Chronic community violence: What is happening to our children? *Psychiatry, 56*, 36–45.

Pearson, J. L., Hunter, A. G., Cook, J. M., Ialongo, N. S., & Kellam, S. G. (1997). Grandmother involvement in child caregiving in an urban community. *Gerontologist, 37*, 650–657.

Perrin, E. C., Ayoub, C. C., & Willett, J. B. (1993). In the eyes of the beholder: Family and maternal influences on perceptions of adjustment of children with a chronic illness. *Developmental and Behavioral Pediatrics, 14*, 94–105.

Rao, R. P., & Kramer, L. (1993). Stress and coping among mothers of infants with a sickle cell condition. *Children's Health Care, 22*, 169–188.

Reeb, K. G., Graham, A. V., Kitson, G. C., Zyzanski, S. J., Weber, M. A., & Engel, A. (1986). Defining family in family medicine: Perceived family versus household structure in an urban black population. *The Journal of Family Practice, 23*, 351–355.

Richters, J. E., & Martinez, P. (1993). The NIMH community violence project: I. Children as victims of and witnesses to violence. *Psychiatry, 56*, 7–21.

Rolland, J. S. (1994). *Family, illness and disability: An integrative treatment model*. New York: Basic Books.

Schuman, W. B., Armstrong, F. D., Pegelow, C. H., & Routh, D. K. (1993). Enhanced parenting knowledge and skills in mothers of preschool children with sickle cell disease. *Journal of Pediatric Psychology, 18*, 575–591.

Selner-O'Hagan, M. B., Kindlon, D. J., Buka, S. L., Raudenbush, S. W., & Earls, F. J. (1998). Assessing exposure to violence in urban youth. *Journal of Child Psychology and Psychiatry and Allied Disciplines, 39*, 215–229.

Sharpe, J. N., Brown, R. T., Thompson, N. J., & Eckman, J. (1994). Predictors of coping with pain in mothers and their children with sickle cell syndrome. *Journal of the American Academy of Child and Adolescent Psychiatry, 33*, 1246–1255.

Simons, R. L., Murry, V., McLoyd, V., Lin, K., Cutrona, C., & Conger, R. D. (2002). Discrimination, crime, ethnicity, and parenting as correlates of depressive symptoms among African American children: A multilevel analysis. *Development and Psychopathology, 14*, 371–393.

Sterling, Y. M., Peterson, J., & Weekes, D. P. (1997). African-American families with chronically ill children: Oversights and insights. *Journal of Pediatric Nursing, 12*, 292–300.

Stevenson, H. C. (1998). Raising safe villages: Cultural-ecological factors that influence the emotional adjustment of adolescents. *Journal of Black Psychology, 24*, 44–59.

Stevenson, H. C., Reed, J., & Bodison, P. (1996). Kinship social support and adolescent racial socialization beliefs: Extending the self to family. *Journal of Black Psychology, 22*, 498–508.

Taylor, R. D., & Roberts, D. (1995). Kinship support and maternal and adolescent well-being in economically disadvantaged African American families. *Child Development, 66*, 1585–1597.

Thomas, A. J., & Speight, S. L. (1999). Racial identity and racial socialization attitudes of African American parents. *Journal of Black Psychology, 25*, 152–170.

Thompson, R. J., Jr., Armstrong, F. D., Link, C. L., Pegelow, C. H., Moser, F., & Wang, W. C. (2003). A prospective study of the relationship over time of behavior problems, intellectual functioning, and family functioning in children with sickle cell disease: A report from the Cooperative Study of Sickle Cell Disease. *Journal of Pediatric Psychology, 28*, 59–65.

Thompson, R. J., Jr., Gil, K. M., Burbach, D. J., Keith, B. R., & Kinney, T. R. (1993). Psychological adjustment of mothers of children and adolescents with sickle cell disease: The role of stress, coping methods, and family functioning. *Journal of Pediatric Psychology, 18*, 549–559.

Thompson, R. J., Jr., Gil, K. M., Keith, B. R., Gustafson, K. E., George, L. K., & Kinney, T. R. (1994). Psychological adjustment of children with sickle cell disease: Stability and change over a 10-month period. *Journal of Consulting and Clinical Psychology, 62*, 856–860.

Thompson, R. L., Jr., Gustafson, K. E., Hamlett, K. W., & Spock, A. (1992). Stress, coping, and family functioning in the psychological adjustment of mothers of children with cystic fibrosis. *Journal of Pediatric Psychology, 17*, 573–585.

Thompson, R. J., Jr., Gustafson, K. E., Gil, K. M., Kinney, T. R., & Spock, A. (1999). Change in the psychological adjustment of children with cystic fibrosis or sickle cell disease and their mothers. *Journal of Clinical Psychology in Medical Settings, 6*, 373–392.

Thorton, M., Chatters, L. M., Taylor, R. J., & Allen, W. A. (1990). Socio-demographic and environmental correlates of racial socialization by black parents. *Child Development, 61*, 401–409.

U.S. Department of Health and Human Services (2001). *Mental health: Culture, race, and ethnicity—A supplement to mental health: A report of the Surgeon General.* Rockville, MD: U.S. Department of Health and Human Services, Substance Abuse and Mental Health Services Administration, Center for Mental Health Services.

Wallander, J. L., & Varni, J. W. (1992). Adjustment in children with chronic physical disorders: Programmatic research on a disability-stress-coping model. In A. M. La Greca, L. Siegel, J. L. Wallander, & C. E. Walker (Eds.), *Stress and coping in child health* (pp. 279–298). New York: Guilford Press.

Wallander, J. L., & Varni, J. W. (1998). Effects of pediatric chronic physical disorders on child and family adjustment. *Journal of Child Psychology and Psychiatry, 39*, 29–46.

Williams, H. A. (1993). A comparison of social support and social networks of black parents and white parents with chronically ill children. *Social Science and Medicine, 37*, 1509–1520.

Williams, D. R., Neighbors, H. W., & Jackson, J. S. (2003). Racial/ethnic discrimination and health: Findings from community studies. *American Journal of Public Health, 93*, 200–208.

Wilson, M. N. (1989). Child development in the context of the black extended family. *American Psychologist, 44*, 380–385.

Wolman, C., Garwick, A., Kohrman, C., & Blum, R. (2001). Parents' wishes and expectations for children with chronic conditions. *Journal of Developmental and Physical Disabilities, 13*, 261–277.

Young, J. B. (1995). Black families with a chronically disabled family member: A framework for study. *The Association of Black Nursing Faculty Journal, 6*, 68–73.

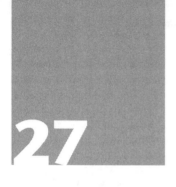

Nicole F. Swain, Monica J. Mitchell, and Scott W. Powers

# Pain Management of Sickle Cell Disease

Acute and chronic pain episodes are common experiences for many individuals living with sickle cell disease (SCD). The management of pain related to SCD is primary palliative and includes pharmacological, nonpharmacological, and preventive therapies (Ballas, 2002). This chapter focuses on issues relevant to the assessment and treatment of sickle cell pain in primarily pediatric populations, although some of the adult literature is reviewed, particularly as it relates to children and adolescents.

## Characteristics of Sickle Cell Disease

SCD is a hereditary disorder. The disorder primarily affects people of Caribbean and African origin in addition to a small percentage of people of Indian, Mediterranean and Middle Eastern descent (National Association of Health Authorities and Trusts–NAHAT, 1991). SCD is also prevalent in Hispanic and Latino populations. Red blood cells containing sickle hemoglobin become rigid. These cells then become elongated and "sickled" in shape, which makes it very difficult for the sickle cells to move smoothly and flow through microcirculation (Morrison & Vedro, 1989).

Symptoms of SCD include chronic anemia, susceptibility to infection, and vaso-occlusive crises or vaso-occlusive episodes (VOEs), resulting in severe pain that can last hours to weeks (Wang, George, & Wilimas, 1988). This vaso-occlusion is caused when sickle cells are unable to flow through arteries, capillaries, arterioles, and other blood vessels and as a result obstruct blood flow. This sickling can occur anywhere in the body, including fingers, arms, ribs, abdomen, and organs such as the brain and eyes (Morrison & Vedro, 1989), but it most commonly occurs in the spleen, bones, and joints (Elander & Midence, 1996). These restrictions in blood flow result in severe pain.

In addition, other major clinical problems arise from SCD, including stroke, acute chest syndrome, aseptic necrosis of the hips and shoulders, infections, anemia, leg ulcers, and priapism (Serjeant, 1992). Acute chest syndrome is a significant concern and is the leading cause of mortality in both children and adults with SCD (Platt et al., 1994). Stroke tends to be the most disabling condition and is also a significant cause of death. Stroke in SCD patients accounts for approximately 6% of deaths related to sickle cell disease (Platt et al., 1994).

The course of SCD during the life span is highly variable. The course of the disease for one person can change over time and can be quite different from that of another person. Severe pain can be experienced as early as 6 months of age, and the frequency of VOEs in patients and between patients is highly variable; one patient may have only a few VOEs every few years, and another may have painful episodes much more frequently (Platt et al., 1991). In addition, VOEs may be preceded by certain events such as illness, dehydration, trauma, exposure to cold, or emotional upset or may not be preceded by any specific event (Morrison & Vedro, 1989).

Over the past decade, newer advances in the treatment of SCD include hydroxyurea and bone marrow transplantations. Hydroxyurea is a newer therapy that was approved by the U.S. Food and Drug Administration in 1998 for SCD (Benjamin et al., 1999; Charache et al., 1995). It appears to be an effective prophylactic agent that reduces the frequency of painful episodes and acute chest syndrome in adults. Charache et al. (1995) reported that hydroxyurea has had a significant impact on the frequency and intensity of pain experienced by some patients. In a review, Amrolia, Almeida, Davies, and Roberts (2003) reported that hydroxyurea has been demonstrated to reduce the frequency of painful crises in children as well.

Bone marrow transplantation remains the only cure for SCD (Amrolia et al., 2003). With strict criteria for inclusion and the need for a sibling donor with identically matched human leukocyte antigen, it is estimated that fewer than 10% of children with SCD fulfill the inclusion criteria, and among this 10%, only 1 in 5 will have a matched donor to qualify for a bone marrow transplant (Davies & Roberts, 1996). However, among those who have undergone transplants, results show an overall survival rate of 92%–94% and event-free survival of 75%–84% at 6–11 years posttreatment (Amrolia et al., 2003). Research continues to examine prospective new treatment modalities such as stem cell transplantation, short-chain fatty acids, membrane-active drugs, and gene therapy (Amrolia et al., 2003).

Current treatment continues to focus significantly on management of the chronic and repetitive vaso-occlusive episodes, or painful crises, which tend to be unpredictable and alternate between symptom-free periods. These severe pain episodes and the general chronic pain sickle cell patients endure have been the focus of pain management strategies. Pain management in SCD includes pharmacological approaches, nonpharmacological approaches, and a combination of the two. Sickle cell pain is complex and is strongly affected by multiple factors, including pathophysiological, psychological, social, cultural, and spiritual factors (Ballas, 2002).

## Assessment of Sickle Cell Pain

Assessment of type, location, and intensity of pain is crucial in determining the best pain management strategy for pharmacological and nonpharmacological treatment. Obtaining baseline information regarding the experience of pain during initial pain assessment is critical for measuring the effectiveness of analgesics that are delivered. In addition, it is important to determine the patient's subjective pain experience and how the patient is reporting the pain experience. Subsequent assessments then allow appropriate dosing of analgesics to provide the best relief of pain and allow the identification of adverse effects or complications (Ballas, 2002). Also, subsequent assessments allow information about the efficacy of other nonpharmacological treatments that may have been used.

Because pain is a subjective experience, pain assessment is primarily based on patient self-report, especially in adult patients. As the initiative of adequate pain assessment is put forth, assessment of pain in children has been a significant focus for health care professionals. It had been thought years ago that children were unreliable in self-report of their pain. However, research supported that children can provide accurate reports and descriptions of their pain experience (McGrath, 1990; Ross & Ross, 1984a, 1984b). In addition, children's reports of pain with SCD can be measured reliably (Graumlich et al., 2001; Walco & Dampier, 1990). Recommendations have been made that a comprehensive, multidimensional assessment strategy be implemented as a critical first step toward developing effective clinical interventions in pediatric populations (Graumlich et al., 2001; Varni & Thompson, 1985; Walco & Dampier, 1990).

In a study by Graumlich et al. (2001), pain was assessed in a sample of children with SCD from a multidimensional approach. Both parents and children were interviewed. Information obtained included pain intensity (using a visual analog scale); pain location (using a body diagram); descriptors of pain representing the sensory, affective, and evaluative qualities of pain; interference of daily functioning because of pain; children's and parents' perceptions of pain (knowledge of SCD and strategies to manage pain at home); and beliefs about pain, including perceptions of seriousness, severity, barriers to pain management, benefits of pain management, and perceptions of self-efficacy to perform pain management. Overall results of this work concluded that, on many variables, parent and child report were not significantly different from each other. Yet, in some areas, children reported information of which parents were not aware (i.e., more frequent chest pain, which is significant in light of acute chest syndrome that many patients with SCD encounter). The importance of acquiring the child's self-report was noted in addition to the significance of other findings being instrumental in providing directions for future research in SCD pain assessment and treatment (i.e., impact on daily functioning and perceptions of seriousness and severity of pediatric SCD).

However, adequate pain assessment continues to remain problematic at times because of such instances as clinicians' limited knowledge of SCD; pain and its management; disbelief of patients' report of pain intensity and medication needed; variability and unpredictability of pain episodes; and racial, ethnic, and socioeconomic factors that can affect communication between health care professionals and families (Benjamin et al., 1999). In the hospital setting, pain assessment and management of painful episodes can vary quite a bit (Masi & Woods, 1993), although the American Pain Society (1999) has published guidelines in assessing both acute pain during a painful episode and recurring or chronic pain with a comprehensive pain assessment that is multidimensional and is focused toward treatment planning.

In addition, medical personnel have varying beliefs in the efficacy of certain analgesics such as opioids. Also, the fear of dependence can be a factor in the administration of opioids. Ballas (1998) reported that tolerance and physical dependence do occur in some patients, but addiction to opioids is rare. Still, reports of attitudes and perceptions of medical practitioners have shown that beliefs of frequent addiction in patients with SCD can be more common than not.

In a descriptive study examining the perceptions and attitudes of emergency medicine physicians and hematologists regarding pain management for patients with SCD, over one half (53%) of the emergency department physicians believed that more than one fifth of patients they treated were addicted to pain medications as compared to 23% of the hematologists believing that more than 20% of their patients were addicted. Both physician groups thought the frequency of addiction in children and adolescents with SCD was less than for adults but still perceived a relatively high percentage of addiction (46% of emergency department physicians and 4% of hematologists believed that more than 10% of the children and adolescents were addicted) (Shapiro, Benjamin, Payne, & Heidrich, 1997).

Further still, some physicians in certain geographic areas and countries in the world, such as in Africa and the Caribbean, rarely use opiates for the treatment of SCD. Other treating professionals worry about adverse effects such as severe respiratory depression and in turn do not administer opioids for pain control (Elander & Midence, 1996). These beliefs, perceptions, and attitudes can potentially lead to inadequate treatment of pain that in turn leaves patients asking for more pain medication and exaggerating their pain behavior to obtain analgesics. This pseudoaddiction (Weissman & Haddox, 1989) situation then reinforces the physician's underlying suspicion of substance abuse, leading to a cycle of miscommunication and inadequate pain control.

Even with continued research in the area of pain assessment, there continues to be controversy regarding how to effectively and adequately assess the pain experience. In addition, there are patient variables (i.e., age of patient) and health professional variables (i.e., physician/nurse practitioner beliefs of the efficacy or adverse side effects of administering opioids) to take into consideration. Further research and implementation of practice guidelines for pain assessment in SCD is needed.

## Pharmacological Treatment for SCD Pain

### Opioids

As reported in the literature, the standard treatment protocol for a painful episode has not changed much in the last few years and includes rest, rehydration, treatment of infections or other complications, and use of analgesics (Morrison & Vedro, 1989). Most mild-to-moderate pain is managed at home; severe painful episodes usually require hospitalization. Parenteral opiates are commonly used in hospital emergency departments to manage severe SCD pain (Elander & Midence, 1996).

In the United States and the United Kingdom, some of the most commonly used opioid agonists include pethidine (meperidine/Demerol) for short-lasting, acute pain (Kotila, 2005; Pegelow, 1992); morphine, especially for new patients and children (Johnson, 2003); and hydromorphone (Dilaudid) (Ballas, 2002). However, the use of pethidine is becoming more controversial both in the United Kingdom and in the United States because of the problems related to its use (i.e., it is metabolized to norpethidine, which is a renally excreted cerebral irritant causing such symptoms as dysphoria and seizures) (Benjamin et al., 1999; Rees et al., 2003). Longer-acting opioids such as oxycodone controlled release and morphine controlled release are typically used for managing chronic pain and are often employed in combination with other shorter-acting opioids for breakthrough pain (Ballas, 2002).

The adverse effects of opioid agonists include itching, nausea, vomiting, sedation, respiratory depression, and seizures. Severe sedation and significant respiratory depression are the most important and are potentially fatal effects of the use of opiates (Ballas, 2002). Opioid antagonists have been traditionally used to counteract the depressive effects of opioid agonists. However, there is some preliminary data to support the use of opioid antagonists in conjunction with opioid agonists. These data suggest that the combination may enhance the analgesic effect and possibly prevent or delay tolerance to opioid agonists (Crain & Shen, 2000). This finding is still preliminary but is novel and thought provoking in the use of opioids in the management.

Different routes of administration of opioids are available to patients suffering severe pain episodes requiring hospitalization. The research thus far has examined more traditional methods of opioid administration (i.e., nurse-administered injections and continuous intravenous infusions) in contrast to newer patient-controlled analgesia (PCA) pumps. The current literature has produced both pros and cons regarding each type of administration and has not heavily favored any one way of administration of opiates. In a study by Jacob et al. (2003), children with SCD who were utilizing PCA during hospitalization were found to self-administer only 35% of the analgesic medications that were prescribed. Not surprisingly, these children also reported little pain relief. These findings supported an earlier study by Shapiro and Cohen (1993), who reported that patients (both children and young adults) only used 37% of pain medications available to them. These findings are in contrast to the beliefs of some clinicians and health professionals that SCD patients are likely to be drug seeking.

Despite easy access to opioids (Schechter, Berrien, & Katz, 1988), children only choose to use opioid medication when their pain is intolerable. In addition, this usage tends to decrease as their painful episodes subside. However, there is debate as to whether patients with SCD obtain adequate pain control using PCA. As noted by Jacob et al. (2003), children reported minimal pain relief, which could be attributed to them not using the full medication available. One hypothesis is that these children did not know how to titrate PCA administration for optimal pain control. Thus, it is recommended that clinicians need to monitor and assist children more closely with this type of self-administration process (Jacob et al., 2003). In addition, children might share the same fears of dependence or addiction that their parents or caregivers do, which could influence how much they self-administer or whether they are allowed to engage in PCA at all (Graumlich et al., 2001; Shapiro & Cohen, 1993). These fears are still very prevalent even though there is research to support that patients on a similar self-administered regimen for several weeks do not appear to develop clinically significant opioid dependence (Hill & Mather, 1993).

However, there is research to support that children can self-administer adequate amounts of analgesics through PCA. A study by Holbrook (1990) concluded that children in the PCA group used greater quantities of meperidine than the children in the non-PCA, conventional group. Half of the children in the PCA group experienced pain relief within 6 hours compared to less than 20% obtaining pain relief within 6 hours in the non-PCA group. Patients, families, and staff expressed satisfaction and preference for PCA when given a choice for pain management. Furthermore, in adult studies, the main benefit reported in using PCA is that it assists patients to establish more control over their pain relief and allows more independence from hospital staff (Johnson, 2003). However, disadvantages included ineffective analgesic regimens, pump malfunctions, and increased risk of skin infections (Johnson, 2003).

## Nonopioids

In a review by Ballas (2002), additional pharmacological agents commonly used to manage SCD pain include nonopioids such as paracetamol (acetaminophen), nonsteroidal anti-inflammatory drugs (NSAIDs), topical agents, and corticosteroids. Adverse side effects can be significant with the use of these medications. Paracetamol can damage the liver when given in high doses and must be monitored and the dosage reduced in patients with liver disease. NSAIDs are generally contraindicated for patients with renal disease or peptic ulcer disease. There are other potentially serious systematic adverse effects of NSAIDs, including gastropathy and hemostatic effects. However, Ketorolac, an NSAID, used concomitantly with opioids has been reported to provide an additional analgesic effect and to decrease the amount of opioids consumed during longer periods of treatment (i.e., 5 or more days of treatment of an acute painful episode) (Perlin et al., 1994). Also, in a controlled trial of continuous infusion Tordal, another NSAID, children with SCD have been shown to benefit, with improved pain scores and shortened hospital stays (Perlin et al., 1994).

Corticosteroids such as dexamethasone and hydrocortisone have been supported in uncontrolled observations (Araujo & Comerlatti, 1990; Robinson, 1979). In addition, methylprednisolone has been shown in a placebo-controlled trial to reduce conventional analgesics among hospitalized children and adolescents. However, these children and adolescents were found to suffer recurrent episodes of pain after treatment terminated (Griffin, McIntire, & Buchanan, 1994).

Adjuvants that are typically used for the management of SCD pain include antihistamines, antidepressants, benzodiazepines, and anticonvulsants. The role of selective serotonin reuptake inhibitors in sickle cell pain is unknown at this time. Adjuvants as a group tend to enhance the analgesic effect of opioids, improve their adverse effects, and maintain their own mild analgesic effect (Ballas, 2002). Understanding the effectiveness of antidepressants on SCD pain would be particularly important given the dynamic relationship between pain and depression and the fact that pain and depression share neurotransmitters and transpire via shared biological pathways (Bair, Robinson Katon, & Kroenke, 2003). Several studies showed that tricyclic antidepressants may be particularly effective in managing chronic and recurrent pain (Vu, 2004), perhaps given the sleep-enhancing and muscle-relaxing effects of this medication.

## Home Management

Although the majority of SCD hospital admissions (approximately 90% of all SCD-related emergency admissions) (Davies, 1994) are because of VOEs, by far the majority of painful episodes, nearly 90% in one study of children and adolescents with SCD, are treated and managed in the home environment (Shapiro et al., 1995). Most often, only severe painful episodes require hospitalization; therefore, mild-to-moderate painful episodes and chronic SCD pain are subject to home management (Ballas, 2002).

The World Health Organization (1990) has proposed a three-step analgesic ladder for the home treatment of pain (not specific to SCD pain but applicable to this patient group) by which mild pain is usually treated with nonpharmacological agents alone (i.e., bed rest, hydration, massage, relaxation, heating pads, baths, self-hypnosis) (Jacob et al., 2003) or in combination with a nonopioid. Moderate pain may require the addition of an opioid with or without an adjuvant, and significant pain usually requires hospitalization.

Although much of SCD pain is managed at home, home management of sickle cell-related pain is an area of research that is not well developed, and little exists to clarify the impact of SCD on families and home life. Investigations and descriptive studies have targeted examining the home life of patients with SCD in the hopes of filling this gap in the literature. Investigations have included examining pain frequency and intensity in the home environment, assessing common pain management strategies used by individuals with SCD and their families, investigating the impact on school attendance, and discussing the issues related to devising and implementing empirically validated family interventions.

In a study by Conner-Warren (1996), pain intensity and home pain management strategies were assessed in a group of children with SCD. Through the use of the African American Oucher Scale (Denyes & Villarruel, 1990) and pain diaries, results showed that at the onset of a VOE at home the majority of the children (60%) reported pain comparable to that from a minor accident or injury; the remaining children reported more severe pain comparable to that resulting from a major accident or injury. In addition, the investigator reported an age difference by which the older children in the sample tended to report higher levels of pain than the younger children. Results also revealed that the most frequently used pain management strategies employed at home were Tylenol with codeine, fluid, ibuprofen, sleeping, reading, watching television, exercising, and the application of heat. Those children who used either dry or moist heat reported higher pain intensity prior to the application of heat than those who did not.

In another study, Dampier, Ely, Brodecki, and O'Neal (2002) investigated the incidence of pain and types of home pain management techniques used in children and adolescents with SCD. From daily diaries, results demonstrated a wide range of pain frequency. In addition, a gender difference was found; girls reported more frequent pain than boys. There was no gender difference regarding pain intensity. The older adolescent group reported more frequent days of medication use and more use with potent opioids than did the younger children. Single analgesics were used on more than half of all pain days and included acetaminophen, ibuprofen, and acetaminophen and codeine; more potent opioids such as meperidine and morphine were used less frequently as single agents. On some days, multiple analgesics were administered, and it was found that these analgesic combinations tended to provide better pain relief than single agents. However, pain still went untreated on a modest number of days. The researchers suggested that parental beliefs and attitudes about pain medication may play a role in whether children receive medication for pain, how much medication they receive, and what kind of medication is administered. The possibility of widespread negative concerns about the use of opioids may have contributed to the substantial use of nonopioid analgesics alone, even on days with severe pain.

Shapiro et al. (1995) not only examined sickle cell-related pain in children and adolescents in the home environment but also investigated the impact on school attendance. Again through pain diaries, these investigators also found an age difference by which older patients reported longer painful episodes, but there was no relationship found between age and the frequency or intensity of pain or the number of painful episodes. School attendance data demonstrated that patients missed school on 41% of the days on which they reported pain. Of these school days missed, 65% were missed when pain was managed at home, and 35% were missed when pain was managed in the hospital. The children in this study missed an average of 6–8 weeks of school per year, but only missed on average 2.7 consecutive school days. The researchers cautioned that, because the sample was small, these results should be interpreted cautiously and are not necessarily representative of all children with SCD. Even so, a significant discussion point about school absenteeism was made. These children over the course of a school year miss a tremendous amount of class. However, they are not missing an abundance of *consecutive* school days that would potentially qualify them for homebound tutoring in many states. Thus, these children may be missed or not eligible for academic help and support that would facilitate their success in school and help keep them from falling behind in their academic work.

Mitchell et al. (2003) conducted eight focus groups across three major medical centers (i.e., Cincinnati, Columbus, and Cleveland) with 54 parents of 48 children aged 7 to 13 years with SCD to better understand the complex social, cultural, and economic issues that have an impact on pain experiences, treatment decisions, and coping. Questions were developed in meetings by clinicians and researchers who work with children with SCD and their families and with two researchers with extensive experience in conducting focus group studies. Questions were developed to examine areas important to intervention research: (a) the barriers and facilitators to pain management, particularly at home, where the majority of pain episodes occur; and (b) the impact of pain and related sequelae on patient and family coping.

All transcripts were coded, using standardized coding procedures, for major and minor themes that emerged during group discussion (Krueger,

1998). Transcripts were further coded for within-site and cross-site consensus of themes (Krueger, 1998). A summary of the pain-related questions posed and cross-site consensus findings are presented below.

Transcripts were further coded for within-site and cross-site consensus of themes (Krueger, 1998). Responses/themes that were rated by three coders as having within-site and cross-site consensus, *consensus responses/themes*, were included in the final summary:

1. How do you manage your child's pain at home? Consensus responses revealed that parents often provide encouragement, apply heat, massage pain site, administer medication, provide encouragement and support, and encourage/support relaxation in their children.
2. How do you make decisions about when to manage your child's pain at home versus the hospital? Consensus responses included parents opting for the hospital when their child has a high fever/temperature, when their plan does not work, or when their eyes were yellow. Many parents reported that they left it up to the child regarding when to go to the hospital, or they waited for their child to indicate when it was time to go. At all three sites, a fear of challenges/hassles in the emergency room also factored into their weighing of options.
3. How are your family activities affected when your child is having pain? Parents reported that they often have to compromise on the original plan or terminate activities early, and that preparation for activities is more difficult.
4. How does pain affect your child's social life? Many parents reported that friendships and social activities are normal/not affected; others stated that activities were limited (e.g., sports), that their child was self-conscious about appearance and delayed development, and that their child's anxiety/concern about illness and mortality limited participation. Parents overwhelmingly agreed that their child frequently missed school because of SCD, a consequence that may further impact academic and social functioning.

Consensus ratings across all of the questions revealed that parents primarily deferred to children's verbal and nonverbal cues in encouraging home management strategies, including medication, distraction, and relaxation, and for deciding when to go to the emergency room. Understanding how parents identify the early warning signs of pain and illness and how they make decisions regarding these signs is critically important to maximizing intervention and educational services. Other factors, such as intuition and spirituality, previous experiences, day/timing, staff training issues, and physician recommendations, also have an impact on parent decision making. Families also rely on support and prayer in coping with pain and related consequences. At all three sites and in all of the focus groups, parents suggested that staff training around cultural and disease impact would foster sensitivity in care. Enhancing support and educational services for patients and families and furthering school and community education are recommended by parents as areas for future intervention.

Identification of characteristics of individuals with SCD and their primary support people or caregivers is important for understanding the influence on the management of pain. Understanding the cultural and familial environment is also crucial in trying to devise and implement sensitive and appropriate interventions for this chronically ill group. Interventions need to be sensitive to such factors as health beliefs, level of knowledge and understanding of SCD, attitudes about pain management strategies, coping styles, relationship and attitudes toward the health care team, socioeconomic issues, psychological or psychiatric comorbidity, family composition, family issues, cultural factors, and parenting skills, to name a few (Benjamin et al., 1999; Graumlich et al., 2001; Kaslow et al., 1997). It is undoubtedly clear that the need for more research regarding family experience of SCD and empirically validated family intervention exists and is becoming a significant focus in the zeitgeist for providing optimal and multidimensional care for patients with SCD.

## The Impact of Individual Coping Styles and Strategies on Pain Management

One area of research that is better developed and well documented in the literature is the impact of individual coping styles on adjustment and functioning. Coping strategies have been found to be related to psychosocial adjustment and functioning (Gil et al., 1993; Thompson et al., 1994). Specifically, negative coping strategies and thought patterns significantly influence pain reported by patients with SCD (Benjamin et al., 1999). Much research on coping strategies in children with SCD has been undertaken by Gil and colleagues.

In Gil, Williams, Thompson, and Kinney (1991), pain-coping strategies and adjustment (i.e., psychological distress and health care utilization) were reliably assessed among children with SCD and their parents at a clinic visit. In this study, results demonstrated that the coping strategies that children with SCD report using to cope with pain predict adjustment to SCD. The coping strategies that parents of children with SCD use also predict the child's adjustment to SCD (Gil et al., 1991). Further, parental pain-coping strategies are related to pain-coping strategies in their children (Gil et al., 1991. Children high on negative thinking and passive adherence were less active in school and social activities, required more health care services, and were more psychologically distressed (i.e., had higher levels of depressive symptoms, anxiety, and behavioral problems) during painful episodes (Gil et al., 1993). In addition, the investigators noted their older sample was higher on passive adherence and negative thinking than their younger counterparts. It was noted that adolescence may be a developmental period when ineffective coping strategies may become more entrenched, thus leading to higher risk in developing problems in coping with pain and poor psychosocial adjustment in adulthood. Children high on coping attempts were more active and required less-frequent health care services. In addition, parents high on coping attempts and low on passive adherence had children who were more active.

In a 9-month follow-up study of Gil et al. (1991), Gil et al. (1993) found baseline coping attempts were associated with higher levels of school, household, and social activity during painful episodes. Baseline passive adherence and increases in negative thinking over time were associated with more frequent health care contacts during the subsequent 9 months. Baseline and follow-up coping strategies remained relatively stable for younger children; however, in adolescents, pain-coping strategies appeared to change. This change tended to be toward increased negative thinking and passive adherence. Gil et al. posited that, in comparison to adults, there is more potential for change in young children and adolescents. Pain-coping strategies were highly stable in adults (Gil, Wilson, & Edens, 1997), especially for negative thinking and illness-focused strategies (formerly passive adherence). Adults who are negative in their thinking and passive in their attempts to cope seem to persist with this ineffective coping pattern over time. Thus, targeting interventions in children and young adolescents may facilitate learning of effective coping strategies before noneffective coping strategies become entrenched in adulthood.

## Nonpharmacological Treatment for Sickle Cell Disease Pain

Research in both the United States and Great Britain strongly support pain management strategies that incorporate psychological intervention. Patients with sickle cell disease frequently experience feelings of helplessness, loss of control, depression, and anxiety symptoms during painful episodes, which can exacerbate their pain and influence the pain presentation (Pallister, 1992). The majority of hospitalized patients with SCD in Waters and Thomas's (1995) study reported that they wanted to be more involved in the management and control of their pain. Descriptive studies have revealed that approximately one third of children with SCD have significant symptoms of depression (Barbarin, Whitten, & Bonds, 1994; Yang, Cepeda, Price, Shah, & Mankad, 1994). Adults with SCD also show a high prevalence for depression and other mental health problems (Barrett et al., 1988; Thompson, Gil, Abrams, & Phillips, 1992).

However, the literature has not been completely consistent, especially regarding children. In a classroom study comparing children with SCD and same-classroom comparison peers, children with SCD were quite similar to the matched comparison group on various psychosocial variables (Noll et al., 1996). Differences in methodological approaches, including use of different comparison groups may attribute to diverse findings between studies. However among individuals with SCD who struggle with mood issues, pain, school difficulties, social problems, and decreased adaptive functioning, psychological intervention has been effective in significantly reducing psychological distress, improving self-efficacy, and reducing hospital admissions and health care contact (Gil et al., 2001; V. Thomas, 2000; V. N. Thomas, Wilson-Barnett, & Goodhart, 1998).

Examining the association between daily stress and mood with pain, health care use, and school activity in a sample of adolescents with SCD, Gil et al. (2003) found that greater frequencies in daily stress and negative mood were significantly associated with increases in same-day pain, health care use, and reductions in both school and social activity. Conversely, increases in positive mood were significantly associated with fewer reports of pain, reduced health care use, and increased participation in activities. These associations do not speak to any causal relationships but do support pain management approaches that are more comprehensive in nature, including stress and mood management strategies as part of a cognitive behavioral pain management program (Gil et al., 2001; Gil, Wilson, Edens, & Workman, 1997).

There is growing empirical support for the efficacy of cognitive behavioral interventions in adults with disease-related pain (Compas, Haaga, Keefe, Leitenberg, & Williams, 1998; Wilson & Gil, 1996). However, psychological intervention research focused on disease-related pain in children lags behind that of the adult literature (Walco, Sterling, Conte, & Engel, 1999). Amid the literature on SCD intervention and outcome, much of the research consists of case studies, uncontrolled observations, and pilot studies that may or may not include a control group for comparison. From these efforts, there is compelling evidence to support further larger sample, controlled clinical trials in the area of SCD intervention.

## Cognitive Behavioral Therapy

Interventions that include components of cognition (i.e., thoughts, beliefs and expectations), affect (emotion), and behavior have been shown to be effective in a range of acute and chronic pain syndromes (Powers, 1999; V. N. Thomas et al., 1998; Walco, Varni, & Ilowite, 1992). Efforts have turned to examining the efficacy of cognitive behavioral therapy (CBT) in patients with SCD (Gil et al., 1996; Gil, Wilson, Edens, Workman, et al., 1997; Powers, Mitchell, Graumlich, Byars, & Kalinyak, 2002; V. Thomas, 2000; V. N. Thomas et al., 1998). As research has shown, coping strategies are related to psychosocial adjustment, pain report, and health care use in children and adults with SCD. Gil et al. (1993) suggested that cognitive behavioral treatment programs especially include the training of children and adolescents with SCD to modify their negative thinking and passive coping patterns and in turn to take an active approach to coping. Results to date have been promising and generally concluded that CBT can be beneficial in the management of sickle cell-related pain in both children and adults.

In an adult study, Gil et al. (1996) examined the effects of a cognitive coping skills training program among 64 African Americans with SCD. Patients were randomly assigned into either a coping skills condition or an education control condition. Before and after treatment, cognitive coping strategies, clinical pain, and health behaviors were measured. In addition, pain sensitivity to a noxious stimulus presented in a standardized fashion (i.e., finger pressure stimulator) both before and after treatment was measured. Also, during treatment, patients practiced the finger pressure stimulator in both groups. Results at posttest (approximately 1 month) demonstrated that patients in the coping skills group had a significantly lower tendency to report pain during noxious stimulation, demonstrated an enhanced ability to discriminate stimuli of various intensities, and evidenced higher levels of coping attempts and lower levels of negative thinking than did patients in the education control group. In a 3-month follow-up of this study, Gil et al. (2000) reviewed daily diaries of pain, health care contacts, and coping practice in addition to the other measures administered at pre- and posttreatment. Daily diary review showed that, on pain days, participants were more likely to practice their coping strategies. In addition, they had less major health care contacts on days that they used their strategies than on days when they did not use their strategies. Follow-up on cognitive coping strategies, clinical pain, and pain sensitivity to a noxious stimulus revealed that participants in the coping group still reported significantly lower laboratory pain and greater coping attempts in comparison to the control group. However, the ability to sharply discriminate stimuli of various intensities was no longer significant. In addition, the lower levels of negative thinking were no longer significant. The investigators noted that these findings are again consistent with previous findings that negative thinking patterns are likely to become more entrenched and less amenable to change in adulthood (Gil, Wilson, & Edens, 1997).

Gil, Wilson, Edens, Workman, et al. (1997) also implemented the same methodology in a sample of children with SCD. Following only one session of coping skills training and 1 review session 1 week later, children in the coping skills group compared to those in the standard medical care group reported lowered negative thinking scores. At posttest, children in the coping skills group also reported less pain during low levels of laboratory pain stimulation compared to the control group. These results suggest that brief coping skills training may result in lower levels of negative thinking and reported pain during low levels of pain stimulation. However, the authors suggested that further research needs to examine whether prolonged coping skills training (higher frequency of sessions as well as the inclusion of other coping skills such as behavioral components) produces broader effects.

V. N. Thomas et al. (1998), in a pilot study including 30 patients ranging in age from 15 to 35 years, found that regardless of group assignment (CBT group, attention placebo group, wait list control), patients reported high levels of anxiety and depressive symptoms, low levels of pain self-efficacy, and an increase in the use of negative coping strategies. A positive association was found among anxiety, depression, pain, and length of hospital stay such that patients who reported high levels of anxiety and depressive symptoms also experienced greater pain and a longer duration in the hospital. Postintervention examination revealed a trend in the reduction of anxiety and depressive symptoms following CBT that included components of relaxation training, modification of thoughts, feelings, and behaviors, problem solving, and other training in other coping skills. In an extension of the research from the initial pilot study, V. Thomas (2000) found supporting results that revealed significant treatment group differences in favor of the CBT intervention for coping strategies (significant increase in positive coping strategies with significant reduction in negative coping strategies), beliefs in controlling pain, pain self-efficacy, and pain experience.

Powers et al. (2002) investigated the feasibility and outcome of a CBT program for children with SCD. Children aged 9, 10, and 12 years ($N=3$) were included in a pilot study that was comprehensive and multidisciplinary. Both children and their primary caregivers were included. Parents participated in parent educations/skills training and played an active role in helping their children use medications and coping skills optimally and in completing their pain diary data. Children participated in a 6-session intensive cognitive behavioral program that integrated both pharmacological and nonpharmacological strategies (i.e., education about SCD and pain medications, deep breathing, self-monitoring, progressive muscle relaxation, distraction, positive self-talk, and physiological techniques) for pain management. In addition, participants underwent three assessments (pre, post, and 3-month follow-up) and kept daily pain and activity diaries throughout the study. Results of the study indicated that all participants demonstrated a decrease in negative thinking, and one participant showed an increase in active coping attempts. Daily diary data revealed that participants reported having "pain days" from 6% to 20% of the time during the length of the study. During those pain days, children reported that, on average, they used coping strategies 90.3% of the time. Further, they reported that the use of coping strategies was moderately helpful with pain management. On pain days, breathing was most often employed as a means of active coping, followed by relaxation, distraction, and positive self-talk. Individually, each participant exhibited different preferences in coping strategies; one participant clearly favored relaxation, and the other two favored deep breathing and positive self-talk. Daily activity levels remained similar on pain days and no-pain days in some domains (i.e., eating at dinner and playing with friends) but significantly decreased on pain days in other domains (i.e., school attendance). Conclusions were that much remains to be examined in treatment studies of children with SCD. While this study contributed to the literature in numerous ways (i.e., longer follow-up period, parent/caregiver component to the program, multiple assessment periods, combined pharmacological and nonpharmacological approaches), larger sample sizes and clinical trials of comprehensive treatment programs for children with SCD are needed.

## Biofeedback

In a preliminary study, J. E. Thomas, Koshy, Patterson, Dorn, and Thomas (1984) examined the efficacy of using biofeedback therapy for pain management in adults with SCD. Treatment consisted of training in progressive relaxation, thermal biofeedback, cognitive strategies, and self-hypnosis. Participants were asked to attend 15 weekly sessions, with spouses or family members attending twice during the course of therapy. However, most participants did not attend all sessions; in fact, many attended 50% or fewer of the total sessions. Participants were allowed to progress at their own pace, which means that some individuals spent more time with biofeedback, while others spent more time on hypnosis. Data were collected 6 months before and 6 months after the first treatment session. Results indicated a 38.5% reduction in number of emergency room visits, a 31% reduction in number of hospitalizations, a 50% reduction in number of days of inpatient treatment, and a 29% reduction in the quantity of analgesics taken (among those participants who were using medication regularly) between crises during the 6-month period following therapy. The authors reported that it was difficult to motivate participants to come to the therapy appointments between crises. Anecdotal data suggested that many of the participants believed their illness was terminal, and that the therapy offered no hope of a cure but in fact more effort on their part. Even so, all of the participants were able to learn the progressive relaxation skill and received some biofeedback training. Conclusions of the study strongly suggested that, even with these preliminary observations, behavioral self-management techniques may be effectively used for managing mild-to-moderate levels of SCD pain.

Cozzi, Tryon, and Sedlacek (1987) focused strictly on biofeedback-assisted relaxation training utilizing both EMG (Electromyographic) monitoring and thermal biofeedback training in a small sample of children and adolescents. Treatment consisted of 13 structured sessions in which progressive muscle relaxation instructions were delivered by audiotape. Regular practice at home was expected of the participants. Participants were given relaxation tapes, tape recorder, and a liquid crystal Velcro finger thermistor to record temperature readings before and after listening to the tapes. In addition, participants kept daily logs in which they recorded pain and medication usage. Baseline measures (i.e., frequency of emergency room visits and frequency of inpatient hospitalizations) were collected by chart review for the 6 months prior to treatment. At the first visit and posttreatment, self-report measures of anxiety and self-concept were administered. Analyses of self-report data and daily diary data indicated a significant decrease in frontalis muscle tension, an increase in digital temperature, decreases in frequency of headache as a crisis symptom, decreased frequency of analgesic use, reduction in reported pain intensity and frequency of self-treated crises, and reductions in state anxiety. In addition, at 6 months posttreatment, participants reported continued practice of the relaxation exercises taught to them and rated them as "fairly effective" to "very effective."

## Hypnosis

Studies have also examined self-hypnosis training in the management of SCD pain. In clinical case studies, Zeltzer, Dash, and Holland (1979) discussed the impact of self-hypnosis on frequency and intensity of SCD pain crises, analgesia use, frequency of emergency room visits, and frequency and length of hospitalizations in two young adult males with SCD. Hypnosis was induced through eye fixation and progressive relaxation techniques. Instructions to feel increasing sensations of bodily warmth and to visualize blood vessels dilating were repeated several times throughout the relaxed state. A thermal biofeedback device monitored peripheral body temperature throughout the sessions. Results of self-hypnosis training demonstrated both patients evidenced reduced frequency and intensity of pain crises, decreased their need for heavy analgesia, reduced their frequent emergency room visits, and reduced the frequency and length of their hospitalizations for pain. Furthermore, following the intervention, both patients reported participating in daily life events more frequently and were better able to pursue life goals (i.e., increased social activity, participation in work and school).

In another clinical case study (Hall, Chiarucci, & Berman, 1992), a 9-year-old African American female showed decreased need for medication, reduced pain symptoms, and increased school attendance following self-regulation training. This patient initially participated in 9 sessions of self-regulation training, including relaxation and imagery, while peripheral finger temperature was monitored. She practiced frequently and was able to significantly increase her finger temperature. However, after approximately 1 year, she was again having difficulties with pain control. Two follow-up self-regulation sessions were administered, after which the patient was able to return to school and evidenced relatively normal daily function. The authors noted that this patient was very skilled at learning self-regulation strategies and practiced frequently at home. Not all patients are open and willing to engage in learning and implementing self-regulation strategies. A teamwork approach was recommended in both assessment and treatment by professionals, including physicians, psychologists, nurses, and social workers. In addition, the authors speculated that, as in other studies utilizing thermal biofeedback, self-regulation strategies may have potential vasodilation effects that, given the vaso-occlusive episodes hallmark to SCD, may be beneficial in pain management.

Dinges et al. (1997) implemented a cognitive behavioral program that focused on self-hypnosis (i.e., practicing ideomotor exercises like the arm becoming lighter and rising, developing therapeutic metaphors and self-suggestions for pain management). The sample had a broad age range and consisted of children, adolescents, and adults with SCD. There was a baseline component of 4 months during which participants kept daily diaries of pain, sleep, medication use, and missed work/school; once in the treatment phase, which lasted 18 months, the practice of behavioral self-hypnosis exercises was recorded. Group sessions were conducted weekly for the first 6 months, biweekly for the next 6 months, and once every 3 weeks for the remaining 6 months. Caregivers were encouraged to attend as well. Results revealed a significant reduction in pain days, frequency of "bad sleep" nights on pain-free days, and use of pain medications on pain-free days. Participants did report continued disturbed sleep and use of medication on days with SCD pain. Days of school/work missed did not change significantly. Although other nonspecific factors may have contributed to treatment efficacy, the authors stated that the self-hypnosis program demonstrated that adjunctive behavioral treatment can be beneficial in the management of SCD pain.

### Physical Strategies

There are physical strategies that are also recommended to individuals with SCD for prevention and treatment of pain. Unfortunately, very few controlled studies have been conducted of these strategies. Yet, many patients routinely find them helpful (Yaster, Kost-Bylerly, & Maxwell, 2000).

Adequate hydration is one of the most important physical strategies a person with SCD may use to prevent or treat a vaso-occlusive episode. Becoming dehydrated has been associated with the triggering of painful episodes (Yaster et al., 2000). To reduce the sickling of red blood cells that results in vaso-occlusion, increased fluid intake is needed (Benjamin et al., 1999). Therefore, sufficient hydration is necessary to decrease the possibility of a painful episode and further complications of SCD.

Another potential precipitant of a painful episode is extremes or changes of temperature. Cold is associated with increased vasoconstriction and occlusion (Benjamin et al., 1999). Therefore, the application of heat is recommended and often is used to facilitate muscle relaxation and vasodilation.

A third physical strategy that is often reported as helpful is massage (Benjamin et al., 1999). Massage serves to increase relaxation and decrease muscle tension associated with pain. Physical therapy is another strategy that, when applied appropriately, can improve physical fitness, help alleviate forms of musculoskeletal pain, and help prevent deconditioning without precipitating a painful episode. One of the difficulties for patients to follow through with this strategy is that it takes active participation from the individual. In addition, physical therapy can be uncomfortable for some, and patients are fearful that exercise that is uncomfortable or painful will further injure them. This reluctance and mistrust is why accurate assessment of the pain problem is essential, and an individualized treatment plan should be implemented and supervised by a physical therapist or a person knowledgeable about the safety of the exercises and SCD.

The effectiveness of transcutaneous electrical nerve stimulation (TENS) for sickle cell pain has not yet been clearly established through empirical research. However, Wang et al. (1988) reported that, although participants using a TENS unit showed no significant difference in pain ratings or analgesic use compared to a placebo group, there was a significant difference found on the overall value of the TENS unit. The majority (74%) of participants using the TENS unit reported it to be helpful. It has been speculated that the value of TENS in chronic pain reduction might be with greater prolonged use (Chabal, Fishbain, Weaver, & Heine, 1998).

Finally, acupuncture is a physical strategy that has some support as an effective adjunct, alternative therapy, or component of treatment programs for various pain syndromes (National Institutes of Health, 1998). One study by Co, Schmitz, Havdala, Reyes, and Westerman (1979) examined the efficacy of acupuncture for pain relief in 10 adult patients with SCD during 16 pain crises. Overall, acupuncture was beneficial in reducing pain in 15 of the 16 painful episodes. However, there was no significant difference between needling administered to acupuncture points or sham sites. Pain relief was found regardless of which sites were treated. The authors stated that needling, whether at acupuncture sites or sham sites, can be useful for alleviating pain during sickle cell crises.

## Conclusion and Future Directions

Given the complexity of SCD regarding physical, psychological, behavioral, familial, and cultural factors, it is no surprise that SCD research is struggling to address the many significant questions that arise for patients, families, and medical care providers. Although research in SCD has surged, more work needs to be conducted to ensure that treatment options are maximized for patients with SCD. One area of growing focus within SCD research is an examination of the home environment and management of sickle cell-related pain and issues outside the hospital setting. As research is bringing to light, most painful episodes are managed at home. Investigating the home environment, the family's reaction to these painful episodes, how the family facilitates pain control at home, and the stressors on the family and patient necessitate careful and meticulous investigation.

Within the hospital setting, pain management options are increasing and improving in terms of opioid administration, route of administration, and approaches to assessing pain experiences and impact. Clinicians and families continue to struggle in determining the optimal way to manage pain while attending to other physical complications secondary to SCD. Continued efforts to examine attitudes, beliefs, and fears of pain medications, especially opioids, and the impact of these cognitions on the treatment of SCD patients should be a focus in future research and intervention efforts.

Coping styles and variables associated with health, quality of life, and adjustment need continued examination as these variables can have an impact on developing appropriate interventions. Interventions, both individual/group and family, should be a high priority as research has shown that daily life (i.e., school, work, home life), mood, and personal relationships are or can be significantly interrupted or impacted because of SCD pain and symptoms. It is strongly recommended from researchers and clinicians that these interventions be multidisciplinary in integrating both pharmacological and behavioral treatment components.

Finally, one of the most thought-provoking issues in SCD intervention research may be outcome measurement (Powers et al., 2002). The choice of outcome measures raises many questions regarding which variables are most appropriate, most relevant, or most significant in evaluating patient perceptions, progress, and treatments. Dependent measures have included pain variables, health care utilization, quality of life, and psychosocial outcomes. It remains to be determined and debated how the efficacy of interventions can be measured and how treatments can be devised and implemented that will truly make a significant and positive impact on the life of patients with SCD.

In summary, pain is a significant issue for adults and children with SCD. Although research on SCD and related symptoms has increased over the past decade, new paradigms for assessment and treatment have been slow to emerge. Effective management of SCD-related pain in health care settings and in patients' homes should be priorities in the future. In addition, providing culturally sensitive and multidisciplinary care is essential to maximizing health and functioning in patients with SCD. Finally, clinical research and health care delivery/effectiveness research are the keys to advancing the field and to meeting the goals of patients with SCD.

## References


American Pain Society. (1999). *Principles of analgesic use in the treatment of acute pain and cancer pain* (4th ed.). Glenview, IL: Author.

Amrolia, P. J., Almeida, A., Davies, S. C., & Roberts, I. A. (2003). Therapeutic challenges in childhood sickle cell disease. Part 2: A problem-oriented approach. *British Journal of Haematology, 120*, 737–743.

Araujo, J. T., & Comerlatti, L. K. I. (1990). Improvement of sickle cell crisis by dipirone and/ or hydrocortisone [Abstract]. *Blood, 76*, 54a.

Bair, M. J., Robinson, R. L., Eckert, G. J., Stang, P. E., Croghan, T. W., & Kroekne, F. (2004). Impact of pain on depression treatment response in primary care. *Psychosomatic Medicine*, 66, 17–22.

Ballas, S. K. (1998). *Sickle cell pain: progress in pain research and management* (Vol. 2). Seattle, WA: IASP Press.

Ballas, S. K. (2002). Sickle cell anaemia: progress in pathogenesis and treatment. *Drugs, 62*, 1143–1172.

Barbarin, O. A., Whitten, C. F., & Bonds, S. M. (1994). Estimating rates of psychosocial problems in urban and poor children with sickle cell anemia. *Health and Social Work, 19*, 112–119.

Barrett, D. H., Wisotzek, I. E., Abel, G. G., Rouleau, J. L., Platt, A. F., Jr., Pollard, W. E., et al. (1988). Assessment of psychosocial functioning of patients with sickle cell disease. *Southern Medical Journal, 81*, 745–750.

Benjamin, L. J., Dampier, C. D., Jacox, A. K., Odesina, V., Phoenix, D., Shapiro, B., et al. (1999). *Guideline for the management of acute and chronic pain in sickle cell disease* (APS Clinical Practice Guidelines Series, No. 1). Glenview, IL: American Pain Society.

Chabal, C., Fishbain, D. A., Weaver, M., & Heine, L. W. (1998). Long-term transcutaneous electrical nerve stimulation (TENS) use: Impact on medication utilization and physical therapy costs. *Clinical Journal of Pain, 14*, 66–73.

Charache, S., Terrin, M. L., Moore, R. D., Dover, G. J., Barton, F. B., & Eckert, S. V. (1995). Effect of hydroxyurea on the frequency of painful crises in sickle cell anemia. Investigators of the Multicenter Study of Hydroxyurea in Sickle Cell Anemia. *New England Journal of Medicine, 322*, 1317–1322.

Co, L. L., Schmitz, T. H., Havdala, H., Reyes, A., & Westerman, M. P. (1979). Acupuncture: An evaluation in the painful crises of sickle cell anaemia. *Pain, 7*, 181–185.

Compas, B. E., Haaga, D. A. F., Keefe, F. J., Leitenberg, H., & Williams, D. A. (1998). Sampling of empirically supported psychological treatment from health psychology: Smoking, chronic pain, cancer, and bulimia nervosa. *Journal of Consulting and Clinical Psychology, 66*, 89–112.

Conner-Warren, R. L. (1996). Pain intensity and home pain management of children with sickle cell disease. *Issues in Comprehensive Pediatric Nursing, 19*, 183–195.

Cozzi, L., Tryon, W. W., & Sedlacek, K. (1987). The effectiveness of biofeedback-assisted relaxation in modifying sickle cell crises. *Biofeedback and Self-Regulation, 12*, 51–61.

Crain, S. M., & Shen, K. F. (2000). Antagonists of excitatory opioid receptor functions enhance morphine's analgesic potency and attenuate tolerance/dependence liability. *Pain, 84*, 171–181.

Dampier, C. D., Ely, E., Brodecki, D., & O'Neal, P. (2002). Home management of pain in sickle cell disease: A daily diary study in children and adolescents. *Journal of Pediatric Hematology/ Oncology, 24*, 643–647.

Davies, S. (1994). *The foreword. The psychosocial aspects of sickle cell disease*. Oxford: Radcliffe Medical Press.

Davies, S. C., & Roberts, I. A. (1996). Bone marrow transplant for sickle cell disease: An update. *Archives of Disease in Childhood, 75*, 3–6.

Denyes, M. J., & Villarruel, A. M. (1990). *African American Oucher Scale*. Detroit, MI: Wayne State University (Available from the first author).

Dinges, D. F., Whitehouse, W. G., Orne, E. C., Bloom, P. B., Carlin, M. M., Bauer, N. K., et al. (1997). Self-hypnosis training as an adjunctive treatment in the management of pain associated with sickle cell disease. *The International Journal of Clinical and Experimental Hypnosis, 45*, 417–432.

Elander, J., & Midence, K. (1996). A review of evidence about factors affecting quality of pain management in sickle cell disease. *The Clinical Journal of Pain, 12*, 180–193.

Gil, K. M., Anthony, K. K., Carson, J. W., Redding-Lallinger, R., Daeschner, C. W., & Ware, R. E. (2001). Daily coping practice predicts treatment effects in children with sickle cell disease. *Journal of Pediatric Psychology, 26*, 163–173.

Gil, K. M., Carson, J. W., Porter, L. S., Ready, J., Valrie, C., Redding-Lallinger, R., et al. (2003). Daily stress and mood and their association with pain, health-care use, and school activity in adolescents with sickle cell disease. *Journal of Pediatric Psychology, 28*, 363–373.

Gil, K. M., Carson, J. W., Sedway, J., Porter, L. S., Schaeffer, J. J., & Orringer, E. (2000). Follow-up of coping skills training in adults with sickle cell disease: Analysis of daily pain and coping practice diaries. *Health Psychology, 19*, 85–90.

Gil, K. M., Thompson, R. J., Jr., Keith, B. R., Tota-Faucette, M., Noll, S., & Kinney, T. R. (1993). Sickle cell disease pain in children and adolescents: change in pain frequency and coping strategies over time. *Journal of Pediatric Psychology, 18*, 621–637.

Gil, K. M., Williams, D. A., Thompson, R. J., Jr., & Kinney, T. R. (1991). Sickle cell disease in children and adolescents: the relation of child and parent pain coping strategies to adjustment. *Journal of Pediatric Psychology, 16*, 643–663.

Gil, K. M., Wilson, J. J., & Edens, J. L. (1997). The stability of pain coping strategies in young children, adolescents, and adults with sickle cell disease over an 18-month period. *The Clinical Journal of Pain, 13*, 110–115.

Gil, K. M., Wilson, J. J., Edens, J. L., Webster, D. A., Abrams, M. A., Orringer, E., et al. (1996). Effects of cognitive coping skills training on coping strategies and experimental pain sensitivity in African American adults with sickle cell disease. *Health Psychology, 15*, 3–10.

Gil, K. M., Wilson, J. J., Edens, J. L., Workman, E., Ready, J., Sedway, J., et al. (1997). Cognitive coping skills training in children with sickle-cell disease pain. *International Journal of Behavioral Medicine, 4*, 364–377.

Graumlich, S. E., Powers, S. W., Byars, K. C., Schwarber, L. A., Mitchell, M. J., & Kalinyak, K. A. (2001). Multidimensional assessment of pain in pediatric sickle cell disease. *Journal of Pediatric Psychology, 26*, 203–214.

Griffin, T. C., McIntire, D., & Buchanan, G. R. (1994). High-dose intravenous methylprednisolone therapy for pain in children and adolescents with sickle cell disease. *New England Journal of Medicine, 330*, 733–737.

Hall, H., Chiarucci, K., & Berman, B. (1992). Self-regulation and assessment approaches for vaso-occlusive pain management for pediatric sickle cell anemia patients. *International Journal of Psychosomatics, 39*, 28–33.

Hill, H. F., & Mather, L. E. (1993). Patient-controlled analgesia. *Clinical Pharmacokinetics, 24*, 124–140.

Holbrook, C. T. (1990). Patient-controlled analgesia pain management for children with sickle cell disease. *Journal of the Association for Academic Minority Physicians, 1*, 93–96.

Jacob, E., Miaskowski, C., Savedra, M., Beyer, J. E., Treadwell, M., & Styles, L. (2003). Management of vaso-occlusive pain in children with sickle cell disease. *Journal of Pediatric Hematology/Oncology, 25*, 307–311.

Johnson, L. (2003). Sickle cell disease patients and patient-controlled analgesia. *British Journal of Nursing, 12*, 144–153.

Kaslow, N. J., Collins, M. H., Loundy, M. R., Brown, F., Hollins, L. D., & Eckman, J. (1997). Empirically validated family interventions for pediatric psychology: Sickle cell disease as an exemplar. *Journal of Pediatric Psychology, 22*, 213–227.

Kotila, T. R. (2005). Management of acute painful crises in sickle cell disease. Clinical Lab Haematology, 27(4):221–3.

Krueger, R. A. (1998). *Analyzing and reporting focus group results—Focus group kit 6*. Thousand Oaks, CA: Sage.

Masi, C. M., & Woods, K. F. (1993). Variability in inpatient management of sickle cell disease pain crisis [Abstract]. *Clinical Research, 41*, 544a.

McGrath, P. (1990). *Pain in children: Nature, assessment, and treatment*. New York: Guilford Press.

Mitchell, M. J., Lemanek, K., Palermo, T., Powers, S. W., Crosby, L., & Nichols, A. (2003). *Pain in children with sickle cell disease: Integrating parent, family, and cultural perspectives in care.* Unpublished manuscript.

Morrison, R. A., & Vedro, D. A. (1989). Pain management in the child with sickle cell disease. *Pediatric Nursing, 15*, 595–599.

National Association of Health Authorities and Trusts. (1991). *Haemoglobinopathies: Review of services for black and minority ethnic people. Words about Action Bulletin Number 4*. Birmingham, AL: Author.

National Institutes of Health Consensus Panel. *Acupuncture: National Institutes of Health Consensus Development Statement*. National Institutes of Health Web site. Accessed at odp.od.nih.gov/consensus/cons/107/107 statement.htm on December 14, 2004.

Noll, R. B., Vannatta, K., Koontz, K., Kalinyak, K. A., Bukowski, W. M., & Davies, W. H. (1996). Peer relationships and emotional well-being of youngsters with sickle cell disease. *Child Development, 67*, 423–436.

Pallister, C. J. (1992). A crisis that can be overcome: Management of sickle cell disease. *Professional Nurse, 2*, 509–513.

Pegelow, C. (1992). Survey of pain management therapy provided for children with sickle cell disease. *Clinical Pediatrics, 31*, 211–214.

Perlin, E., Finke, H., Castro, O., Rana, S., Pittman, J., Burt, R., et al. (1994). Enhancement of pain control with Ketorolac tromethamine in patients with sickle cell vaso-occlusion crisis. *American Journal of Hematology, 46*, 43–47.

Platt, O. S., Brambilla, D. J., Rosse, W. F., Milner, P. F., Castro, O., Steinberg, M. H., et al. (1994). Mortality in sickle cell disease. Life expectancy and risk factors for early death. *New England Journal of Medicine, 330*, 1639–1644.

Platt, O. S., Thorington, B. D., Brambilla, D. J., Milner, P. F., Rosse, W. F., Vichinsky, E., et al. (1991). Pain in sickle-cell disease: rates and risk factors. *New England Journal of Medicine, 325*, 11–16.

Powers, S. W. (1999). Empirically supported treatments in pediatric psychology: Procedure-related pain. *Journal of Pediatric Psychology, 24*, 131–145.

Powers, S. W., Mitchell, M. J., Graumlich, S. E., Byars, K. C., & Kalinyak, K. A. (2002). Longitudinal assessment of pain, coping, and daily functioning in children with sickle cell disease receiving pain management skills training. *Journal of Clinical Psychology in Medical Settings, 9*, 109–119.

Rees, D. C., Olujohungbe, A. D., Parker, N. E., Stephens, A. D., Telfer, P., & Wright, J. (2003). Guidelines for the management of the acute painful crisis in sickle cell disease. *British Journal of Haematology, 120*, 744–752.

Robinson, B. (1979). Reversal of sickle-cell crisis by dexamethasone [Letter]. *Lancet, 1*, 1088.

Ross, D., & Ross, S. (1984a). Childhood pain: The school-aged child's viewpoint. *Pain, 20*, 179–191.

Ross, D., & Ross, S. (1984b). The importance of type of question, psychological climate and subject set in interviewing children about pain. *Pain, 19*, 71–79.

Schechter, N. L., Berrien, F. B., & Katz, S. M. (1988). PCA for adolescents in sickle cell crisis. *American Journal of Nursing, 88*, 721–722.

Serjeant, G. R. (1992). Sickle Cell Disease: Pathophysiology, Diagnosis, and Management. Oxford: Oxford University Press.

Shapiro, B. S., Benjamin, L. J., Payne, R., & Heidrich, G. (1997). Sickle cell-related pain: Perceptions of medical practitioners. *Journal of Pain Symptom Management, 14*, 168–174.

Shapiro, B. S., & Cohen, D. E. (1993). Patient-controlled analgesia for sickle cell-related pain. *Journal of Pain Symptom Management, 8*, 22–28.

Shapiro, B. S., Dinges, D. F., Orne, E. C., Bauer, N., Reilly, L. B., Whitehouse, W. G., et al. (1995). Home-management of sickle cell-related pain in children and adolescents: natural history and impact on school attendance. *Pain, 61*, 139–144.

Thomas, J. E., Koshy, M., Patterson, L., Dorn, L., & Thomas, K. (1984). Management of pain in sickle cell disease using biofeedback therapy: a preliminary study. *Biofeedback and Self-Regulation, 9*, 413–420.

Thomas, V. (2000). Cognitive behavioural therapy in pain management for sickle cell disease. *International Journal of Palliative Nursing, 6*, 434–442.

Thomas, V. N., Wilson-Barnett, J., & Goodhart, F. (1998). The role of cognitive-behavioural therapy in the management of pain in patients with sickle cell disease. *Journal of Advanced Nursing, 27*, 1002–1009.

Thompson, R. J., Jr., Gil, K. M., Abrams, M. R., & Phillips, G. (1992). Stress, coping, and psychological adjustment of adults with sickle cell disease. *Journal of Consulting and Clinical Psychology, 60*, 433–440.

Thompson, R. J., Jr., Gil, K. M., Keith, B. R., Gustafson, K. E., George, L. K., & Kinney, T. R. (1994). Psychological adjustment of children with sickle cell disease: Stability over a 10 month period. *Journal of Consulting and Clinical Psychology, 62*, 856–866.

Varni, J. W., & Thompson, K. L. (1985). *The Varni/Thompson Pediatric Pain Questionnaire*. Unpublished manuscript.

Vu, T. N. (2004). Current pharmacologic approaches to treating neuropathic pain. *Current Pain Headache Reports*, 8, 15–18.

Walco, G. A., & Dampier, C. D. (1990). Pain in children and adolescents with sickle cell disease: A descriptive study. *Journal of Pediatric Psychology, 15*, 643–658.

Walco, G. A., Sterling, C. M., Conte, P. M., & Engel, R. G. (1999). Empirically supported treatments in pediatric psychology: disease-related pain. *Journal of Pediatric Psychology, 24*, 155–167.

Walco, G. A., Varni, J. W., & Ilowite, N. T. (1992). Cognitive-behavioral pain management in children with juvenile rheumatoid arthritis. *Pediatrics, 89*, 1075–1079.

Wang, W. C., George, S. L., & Wilimas, J. A. (1988). Transcutaneous electrical nerve stimulation treatment of sickle cell pain crises. *Acta Haematology, 80*, 99–102.

Waters, J., & Thomas, V. J. (1995). The nurse's role in the management of sickle cell crisis pain. *The Nursing Times, 91*, 29–31.

Weissman, D. E., & Haddox, J. D. (1989). Opioid pseudoaddiction: an iatrogenic syndrome. *Pain, 36*, 363–366.

Wilson, J. J., & Gil, K. M. (1996). The efficacy of psychological and pharmacological treatment of chronic disease-related and non-disease-related pain. *Clinical Psychology Review, 16*, 573–597.

World Health Organization. (1990). *Cancer pain relief and palliative care* (World Health Organization Technical Report Series 804). Geneva, Switzerland: Author.

Yang, Y. M., Cepeda, M., Price, C., Shah, A., & Mankad, V. (1994). Depression in children and adolescents with sickle cell disease. *Archives of Pediatrics and Adolescent Medicine, 148*, 457–460.

Yaster, M., Kost-Bylerly, S., & Maxwell, L. G. (2000). Acute pain in children: The management of pain in sickle cell disease. *Pediatric Clinics of North America, 47*, 699–711.

Zeltzer, L. K., Dash, J., & Holland, J. P. (1979). Hypnotically-induced pain control in sickle cell anemia. *Pediatrics, 64*, 533–536.

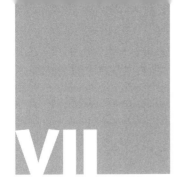

# Training, Funding, and Collaborative Endeavors

Daniel L. Clay and T. David Elkin

# Training in Pediatric Psychosocial Hematology/Oncology

As evidenced by the chapters in this book, psychosocial hematology/oncology (hem/onc) presents a wide array of complex problems and issues for the patients, their families, and the health care team. Because the diseases are unpredictable and often life-threatening, treating the whole child effectively requires a multidisciplinary team of health care professionals working in concert to address the physical, emotional, and spiritual needs of affected families. Working effectively on such a team requires specialized training to manage disease-specific issues such as pain, complexities of multidisciplinary work, and the stress resulting from working with severe and sometimes terminal illnesses. In general, there are many complex roles for psychosocial service providers in the delivery of health care (Brown et al., 2002), and for these reasons, the roles in the hem/onc setting can be even more important and complex.

The purposes of this chapter are to (a) describe the phases of training, (b) discuss issues that have an impact on the training process, and (c) describe key content areas in which training is necessary to reach an acceptable level of competence for working in the area of psychosocial hem/onc. Although the team members consist of various health care professionals and subspecialties such as physicians, nurses, dieticians, psychologists, and social workers, this chapter focuses on graduate and postdoctoral training of psychosocial service providers such as psychologists, social workers, and counselors. However, many of the issues we discuss also apply to training in the other professions at both the preservice and postgraduate levels.

This chapter consists of two main sections: the first section deals with the *process* of training, and the second addresses the *content* of specialized training in hem/onc. The first section begins with a detailed description of training that incorporates a developmental model of knowledge and skill acquisition. We then discuss current trends that have a direct impact on the implementation of training methods and the settings in which clinical training takes place. The second section includes a description of several content areas specific to the needs of patients and health care staff working in hem/onc. These areas address specific knowledge and skill domains and the methods by which these domains can be integrated into the training model.

## The Training Model

Training of psychosocial service providers is usually done in graduate programs designed specifically to prepare practitioners for licensure in their respective field (psychology, social work). These programs typically follow a set of standards for clinical training set forth by accrediting agencies such as the American Psychological Association (APA). Additional guidelines for training have been outlined for working with children (LaGreca & Hughes, 1999) and specifically for domains in pediatric psychology training (Spirito et al., 2003).

For the purposes of this chapter, we assume that trainees will have had a foundation of training in core areas such as assessment and testing, abnormal psychology, health psychology, child development, theories of psychotherapy, and practica in counseling and psychotherapy as outlined by APA accreditation standards. We focus on the acquisition of advanced skills and knowledge in the domains as outlined in Spirito et al. (2003), with specific emphasis on the hem/onc setting. An excellent discussion of pediatric psychology training can be found in the March 2003 special issue of the *Journal of Pediatric Psychology*. A summary of domains of training as outlined in Spirito et al. (2003) is contained in table 28-1. Our goal here is to discuss the specifics of training in hem/onc as they relate to these domains.

Training to effectively work in the hem/onc setting requires an integration of three theoretical or conceptual orientations: psychodynamic/existential, systems, and cognitive behavioral. Clearly, the psychodynamic and existential perspective is critical given the central role of issues such as death, making meaning of the cancer experience, grief, and loss. Use of family systems theory is necessary given the profound impact of hem/onc illnesses and their treatments on immediate and extended family members. Likewise, systems theory is needed to understand and manage the dynamics of the treatment team. Finally, cognitive behavioral theory is used to guide treatment-specific behaviors of the psychosocial service provider. Evidence-based treatments for various problems, such as chronic and procedure-related pain, are typically grounded in cognitive behavioral theory.

Training in psychosocial care is best described from a developmental perspective. As trainees acquire more skills and develop their personal identities, areas of interest and expertise become better defined (Kaslow, McCarthy, Rogers, & Summerville, 1992; Kaslow & Rice, 1985). Consequently, the model described here is a developmental model that consists of four phases of training: entry, skill development, mastery/autonomy, and supervision/teaching. Although the model describes a progression of development, like many areas of development and learning, the process is not always linear. Although trainees may be advanced in some areas (e.g., assessment), they may be at an entry level in other areas (e.g., family therapy). Likewise, trainees may exhibit competency at an advanced level in one area such as consultation but lack the experience and confidence to consistently exhibit competency in that particular area. It is important for supervisors and trainees to understand that the development of skills and competencies will ebb and flow, and with proper supervision and opportunities, trainees will continue to develop the skills and confidence to become effective service providers.

### Phases of Training

#### *Entry Phase*

In the entry phase, trainees typically have little or no experience with service provision to pediatric patients and their families in hem/onc. They should have a solid foundation of basic assessment, counseling, and consultation skills. This foundation of skills is often developed through graduated experiences with clients with less-severe and less-demanding problems than those faced in the hem/onc setting, such as counseling centers and general mental health clinics. Frequently, trainees have completed beginning practicum experiences in other settings. Trainees may be placed in a medical setting for the first time, or they may have limited experiences with health issues. In general, this phase of training involves an introduction to the medical aspects of hem/onc conditions, application of treatment techniques in a new setting, and an introduction to working on a multidisciplinary team. For trainees, the developmental tasks are many and include learning about the hem/onc illnesses and their impact on patients and their families, learning the role of the psychosocial provider on a multidisciplinary team, modifying psychological treatment techniques for highly

**Table 28-1.** Sample Topics Specific to Pediatric Psychology in Each Domain of Training

| *Domains of Training* | *Training Topics* |
|---|---|
| Life span developmental psychology | Effects of disease process and medical regimen on emotional, social, and behavioral development |
| Life span developmental psychopathology | Differentiate emotional distress within normal limits for children with acute and chronic medical conditions |
| Child, adolescent, and family assessment | Experience with the assessment of health-related concerns such as health promotion, health risk, health outcome, and quality of life |
| Intervention strategies | Exposure to and experience with empirically supported interventions specifically applicable in pediatric psychology and delivered in health care settings |
| Research methods and systems evaluations | Exposure to research design issues especially pertinent to pediatric psychology, such as health services research and clinical trials |
| Professional, ethical, and legal issues | Knowledge and experience with issues such as health care delivery, practice of psychology in medical settings, and rights of caregivers versus children when making decisions regarding medical care |
| Diversity | Experience with patients from diverse ethnic and cultural backgrounds, as well as sexual orientations, in health care settings and understanding of nonmainstream health practices influenced by a family's cultural or religious beliefs |
| Role of multiple disciplines in service delivery systems | Experience on multidisciplinary teams delivering health care services |
| Prevention, family support, and health promotion | Understanding the principles of behavior change as they relate to healthy development, health risk behavior, and prevention of disease in adulthood |
| Social issues affecting children, adolescents, and families | Exposure to and experience with advocacy in pediatric health care, including social issues that affect health care delivery |
| Consultation and liaison roles | Exposure to different consultation-liaison models and supervised experience providing consultation in health care settings |
| Disease process and medical management | A basic understanding of various diseases and their medical management |

From "Society of Pediatric Psychology Task Force Report: Recommendations for the Training of Pediatric Psychologists," by A. Spirito et al., 2003, *Journal of Pediatric Psychology, 28,* 85–98. Used with permission.

specialized situations, and understanding vicarious trauma and self-care.

This phase of training can be very stressful and feel overwhelming for the trainee. In many cases, trainees at this stage lack self-confidence and skills, which can lead to high anxiety and dependence on the supervisor (Stoltenberg, McNeill, & Delworth, 1998). Trainees may even articulate that they are not "cut out" for this type of work. Some students, however, may have more experience and skill development prior to entry into hem/onc settings. Even in these cases, the intensity and multiple demands of the hem/onc work environment can be very stressful. Likewise, for many trainees this will be the first experience dealing with death and intense grief in a formal, professional role. Consequently, vicarious trauma and feelings of hopelessness or helplessness are not unusual. In many cases, the other health care team members (nurses, physicians) also are affected, so they may not be a predictable source of support for the trainee.

Good supervision is important at all stages of training, but it is critical in the entry phase. Because of the stress and lack of confidence at this level, trainees often are quite dependent on their supervisors. It is important that supervisor style and behaviors match the developmental needs of the trainee. At this level, supervisors will likely need to be more directive, reassuring, and instrumental in their style (Stoltenberg et al., 1998). Supervision is characterized by trainees asking, What should I do?

The focus is typically on teaching and reinforcing use of specific treatment techniques, such as distraction during painful procedures, coping skills, and methods for dealing with grief. Supervisors also will need to teach the trainee about roles and boundary setting when working on multidisciplinary teams and in many cases will need to model these complex professional behaviors for the trainee. Trainees frequently will want to spend too much time with patients and become overly involved in the treatment of patients, therefore failing to set good boundaries with patients and staff. Consequently, the supervisor will need to pay careful attention to the impact of these experiences on the emotional well-being of the trainee. In supervision, it is often helpful to include a discussion of the emotional impact, coping methods, and steps for appropriate self-care of the trainee. Supervisors disclosing their own struggles with these issues, methods they use for monitoring their own well-being, and strategies for self-care can facilitate a very powerful learning experience for the trainee. It not only normalizes the emotional difficulties associated with this type of work but also gives students examples of specific self-monitoring and self-care strategies.

### Skill Development Phase

With time and experience, trainees become more comfortable in the hem/onc environment. The novelty of the hem/onc environment has diminished, the knowledge about different diseases has increased, and trainees can now "speak the language." They become more proficient at providing many individual interventions (e.g., relaxation training), and they gain more confidence in their abilities. Consequently, the trainees typically begin taking on new and more complex roles within the treatment environment. With less anxiety about competency and mastery of some basic skills, trainees begin to work at a more abstract, systems level. For example, trainees may intervene through more sophisticated family systems approaches. Likewise, a better understanding of systems dynamics may lead to interventions with the health care team, such as reframing of patient or family behaviors to deal with anger of treatment team members.

Although the entry phase typically raises doubts about competencies and the ability to successfully work in the hem/onc environment, the skill development phase often reenergizes trainees. With the successful implementation of some skills, trainees typically are rewarded with experiencing the positive effects of their work with patients and families. It is critical to continue monitoring self-care and boundary setting because early positive experiences in providing care can lead to the trainee becoming enmeshed with the patients. For example, trainees may spend too much time in an inpatient setting, to their own detriment. As the trainee develops more confidence, two additional issues are important to monitor. First, with a newfound confidence trainees may feel overconfident, which can lead to attempting interventions without proper caution. Likewise, overconfidence may lead to the failure of trainees to seek supervision when it is necessary and appropriate.

Supervision during this phase is typically characterized by role transitions within supervision by both the trainee and the supervisor. It is still appropriate for the supervisor to be somewhat directive, but greater emphasis for what occurs during supervision should be placed on the supervisee. For example, supervisors may focus less on informing the trainee what to do and focus more on challenging trainees to think through the choices for interventions, develop a theoretical rationale for the interventions, and support their choices with empirical research. Supervision is characterized by supervisors asking the trainees, What do you think you should do?

The skill development phase can be the most difficult in supervision because the self-confidence and desire for autonomy by the trainee can be temporary, changing from day to day and situation to situation. Likewise, conflict can arise when the trainee desires more autonomy before he or she is developmentally ready. In an attempt to establish this autonomy, trainees may fail to comply with demands of the supervisor, withhold information during supervision, or disregard feedback from the supervisor. The conflict typically plays out in subtle terms. Nonetheless, the back-and-forth struggle for trainees between dependence on the supervisor and desire and demand for autonomy is a very common developmental characteristic of this stage of supervision (Stoltenberg et al., 1998).

### Mastery/Autonomy Phase

Through graduated experiences and good supervision, trainees develop a mastery of a variety of therapeutic interventions at the individual and systems levels. This phase typically occurs at advanced doctoral-level training (e.g., while on predoctoral internship) or even during postdoctoral training. The ability of the trainee to provide timely, efficient, and effective interventions becomes more consistent. Consequently, the trainee may be viewed by others as a more critical member of the health care team. Roles are likely to change again as the trainee takes on more leadership responsibilities on the team. Once the trust of team members is established, other team members may seek out the trainee for very difficult cases or to deal with their own emotional reactions or concerns. Trainees are better able to understand how individual dynamics of team members and overall team functioning have an impact on the quality and consistency of care for the patients and their families.

As a result of the development that occurs through all of these phases, trainee awareness and focus shift from the trainee to the patient. For example, in the entry phase, the trainee often focuses on his or her own abilities, knowledge, and confidence. By the mastery/autonomy phase, the trainee focuses nearly completely on the needs of the patient and the health care team and uses awareness of self as a clinical tool. Trainees are also better able to understand how personal well-being has an impact on their professional competence, and therefore they monitor their own functioning more carefully. These advanced levels of competencies, however, require that trainees understand and accept their own strengths and weaknesses as treatment team members (Stoltenberg et al. 1998).

The trainee typically takes much more responsibility for supervision at this stage. In some cases, regular supervision sessions are not scheduled, and the trainee is expected to seek consultation and supervision as necessary. The process and content covered in supervision is guided by trainees as they develop a greater sense of autonomy. Supervision is characterized by supervisors asking the trainees, "Can you talk about your struggles with determining what to do?" Focus of supervision may also be on personal and professional integration (Stoltenberg et al., 1998). It is critical for the supervisor to gradually allow and encourage greater autonomy in decision making, even if the supervisor may have approached the case issues differently. As long as the trainee has a good rationale and empirical support for decisions, promoting autonomy is the ultimate developmental goal.

#### *Supervision/Mentoring*

The final phase is the supervision or mentoring phase, in which the trainee has obtained a level of competency and mastery that makes him or her competent to supervise others independently. By this time, the "trainee becomes the trainer." That is not to say that everything has been learned, and professional growth has subsided. We view learning and skill acquisition as a lifelong process. Rather, the trainee has gathered enough experiences and developed sufficient skills to effectively teach others who are in earlier phases of development. Mentoring more novice professionals in the provision of services in the hem/onc setting can also be very rewarding and challenging, which seasoned therapists often welcome as a new and different way of having a positive impact. It is critical to effective supervision, however, that the supervisor understand the developmental nature of the learning process outlined above.

## Issues That Have an Impact on Training

Now that we have described the general developmental model of training, it is important to recognize that many factors influence the training process. Health care systems, available resources, and the changing nature of service provision all influence the training process in important ways. Next, we discuss these issues as they relate to the training process. Following the discussion of these issues, the chapter focuses on specific content areas essential to learn for effective psychosocial service provision.

### Managed Care

It is widely accepted that managed care has substantially changed the way that medical services in general, and psychosocial services in particular, are provided in nearly all medical settings. Although changes resulting from managed care have been both negative and positive, most mental health providers report that their practice is more significantly limited and negatively affected (Cashel,

2002). These negative changes include decreased reimbursement amounts for all clinical services, exclusion from provider panels, the need to obtain preapproval for services to be reimbursed, and limits on the amount and types of services, just to name a few.

The most notable impact of managed care on training is the refusal of managed care companies to reimburse for services provided by trainees. Consequently, clinical sites are less likely to invest the staff time and clinic resources in having trainees perform services as part of a practicum experience. Consequently, practicum experiences are limited primarily to academic medical centers. Finding good practicum sites in complex settings such as hem/onc settings is becoming more difficult for academic training programs. Social work training programs may be somewhat less affected than psychology programs, however, because social work departments are often not considered revenue-generating departments within medical centers. Rather, supporting social work as a necessary component of the medical infrastructure (like nursing) results in a decreased need and dependence on reimbursement.

Despite the pervasive impact of managed care, many training programs are not adequately incorporating necessary training in issues related to managed care (Kiesler, 2000). For example, one research study indicated that despite recognizing the need for changes in training, only 40% of accredited psychology programs reported actually making programmatic changes in training (Carlton, 1998). A more recent survey of psychology and social work programs revealed that 60% reported providing some type of training in issues related to managed care (Daniels, Alva, & Olivares, 2002). In general, important managed care issues to address in training include ethical issues in the managed care environment (diagnosis, billing, confidentiality, etc.), understanding the business nature of managed care companies, utilization reviews and provider profiling, use of brief and evidence-based treatments, and demonstration of effect through outcome evaluation. Numerous authors have detailed these needs and recommendations for training more thoroughly elsewhere (e.g., Brokowski, 1995; Charous & Carter, 1996; Cohen, 2003; Cummings, 1995; Patterson, McIntosh-Koontz, Baron, & Bischoff, 1997; Schreter, 1997).

## Evidence-Based Treatments

As a result of managed care and other professional influences, it is clear that students must be trained to provide evidence-based treatments. As psychosocial service providers, particularly in health care settings, it is critical that our practices are based on scientific evidence to support their effectiveness. Increasingly, it is also necessary to provide data to support the cost-effectiveness of our clinical services. As a result, numerous publications have delineated treatments considered "evidence based" as well as treatment guidelines resulting from such research (e.g., Nathan & Gorman, 2002; Parry, Cape, & Pilling, 2004).

Currently, there is significant debate in the psychology profession about whether the profession is overemphasizing the "evidence-based" treatments, but that discussion is clearly beyond the scope of this chapter (for a more thorough discussion of these issues, see Chwalisz, 2003, and the commentaries that follow). What is important to understand is that, as providers of psychosocial services, we are now much more accountable for what we do, and consequently we need to provide data to support our clinical decisions and justify our assessment and treatment choices with insurance companies and managed care companies.

Many of the psychosocial interventions in the hem/onc setting, both at the individual and systems levels, have now amassed a body of empirical support that demonstrate their efficacy. For example, special issues of the *Journal of Pediatric Psychology* have outlined evidence-based approaches for problems like procedural pain. Some of these specific interventions and strategies are outlined in the section describing content areas for training.

By necessity, many interventions are cognitive behavioral and are focused on specific problems. Because it is impossible for trainees to memorize every evidence-based treatment approach for every problem, training needs to focus on assisting trainees to learn how to find and integrate scientific evidence into their clinical practice. Supervisors need to include discussions of the scientific literature, evidence for the usefulness of a range of interventions, and the decision-making process with trainees during supervision. An emphasis on clearly articulating a rationale for treatment decision making, including the data to support the rationale, is critical for trainees to integrate scientific evidence into their clinical decision-making process.

## Cultural Competency

It is critical for psychosocial service providers to be culturally competent practitioners in health psychology in general and specifically when working in hem/onc settings. Many health conditions, including hem/onc conditions such as sickle cell disease, have different prevalence rates and outcomes for people from low-income or minority backgrounds. Issues such as treatment adherence, mortality rates, health care utilization, and functional disability each have been associated with race, ethnicity, socioeconomic status, and other cultural variables (Clay, Mordhorst, & Lehn, 2002; Gotay, 2000). For example, patients may not adhere to treatments for medical conditions if assumptions about the illness or treatments run counter to cultural beliefs or practices. Clay et al. provided a more thorough discussion of cultural variables and their impact on treatment. The APA clearly has delineated the need for training programs to incorporate aspects of multicultural training into their curricula as a necessary component of training (APA, 2003).

A more thorough discussion of cultural issues, training models, and other training issues can be found elsewhere (e.g., Sue & Sue, 2003; Webb, 2001). In general, the development of culturally competent practice involves three critical processes: (a) developing a self-awareness of beliefs, biases, and assumptions; (b) acquiring a body of knowledge about specific racial and cultural groups with which you will be working, including the social and historical contexts of racism and discrimination; and (c) learning specific skills to effectively implement the awareness and knowledge to provide culturally sensitive treatment (Webb, 2001). Liu and Clay (2002) outlined the implementation of these cultural competencies when counseling children. It is important, however, not to overemphasize culture because it may have the same negative affect as ignoring cultural variables.

## Research Training

Many training programs in psychology train doctoral-level practitioners using a scientist-practitioner model. These programs require trainees to develop a set of basic competencies in designing and conducting research studies. Other programs in both psychology and social work adhere to a clinical-scientist model, which requires trainees to develop research skills that allow for an integration of scientific research into clinical practice. As noted, it is critical for trainees to develop the skills necessary to digest the scientific evidence and integrate the resulting knowledge into clinical practice to ensure effective and efficient service provision.

Some research training typically occurs at the predoctoral level and includes courses on statistics, research design, and scientific writing. Programs also typically require trainees to complete a major research project in the form of a thesis or dissertation. More intensive training, however, usually occurs at the postdoctoral level. Many postdoctoral positions are available for specialization in hem/onc that integrate clinical work with systematic, long-term programs of research. Postdoctoral training programs that provide trainees an opportunity to begin their own programs of research are usually necessary for trainees interested in an academic career. Such postdoctoral training programs are housed at academic health sciences centers, federal agencies (e.g., National Institutes of Health, Center for Disease Control), or in private medical facilities.

## Funding for Training

The financial resources necessary to train scientists and practitioners in psychosocial hem/onc are substantial. Because of increasing budget shortfalls at many public institutions, funding for trainees at the doctoral level is decreasing. In addition, insurance companies are less likely to reimburse for services provided by doctoral trainees during their practicum experiences. Consequently, it is becoming increasingly difficult to provide funding for trainees, and they are now often required to obtain student loans to fund training at the predoctoral level. At some academic medical centers, the state government provides some funding for indigent care, so trainees can provide services to this population without the need for additional reimbursement. Faculty in training programs must work closely with hospital managers, hem/onc physicians, clinic psychologists, and social workers to arrange practicum training experiences and supervision. Because supervision is not reimbursed, it is often difficult to obtain adequate supervision time for trainees when supervisors could be seeing patients during that time and billing for it.

Funding is also available from state and federal agencies as well as private foundations in the form of training grants. Most of the available funding comes from federal agencies such as the National Institutes of Health, Centers for Disease Control and Prevention, the Department of Education, and the Health Resource Services Administration. It is these federal agencies that often fund the postdoctoral training programs, although funding programs geared specifically for predoctoral training also exist. In addition, training grants are available through private foundations such as the Robert Wood Johnson Foundation, William T. Grant Foundation, and the American Cancer Society.

Funding priorities are often geared to addressing high-need areas such as the high-incidence conditions, low-income and minority patients, and underserved populations. The competition for training funds from both federal agencies and private foundations is keen, so most of the training grants are awarded to academic institutions that have substantial resources. Training programs, both at the predoctoral and postdoctoral level, will need to continue to search for creative solutions to funding shortages for training in psychosocial hem/onc.

## Core Content Areas

As evidenced by the many different chapters in this book, psychosocial hem/onc by definition covers a wide variety of medical diagnoses and conditions. Each diagnosis has specific risk factors and treatment considerations that will affect the type of assessment and intervention a health care worker may consider. However, an approach to managing psychosocial issues that focuses on individual medical diagnoses by necessity is beyond the scope of this chapter. Consequently, we discuss training issues that generally cover most pediatric hem/onc consultations in an effort to provide a more comprehensive and adaptable set of topics for those involved in psychosocial care.

The setting in which psychosocial care takes place will often determine the areas of proficiency for trainees. Each hem/onc care center has a unique culture. Some of these areas are discussed in the sections below. However, trainees are encouraged to assess the expectations of their own setting so that core areas may be covered and patient care and well-being may be improved.

### *Multidisciplinary Teams*

Initial training in most psychosocial disciplines usually takes the format of one-on-one clinical assessment and intervention. Clinical interaction takes place in a standard therapy room, with few individuals involved in the actual delivery of treatment. The only exposure the trainee has to other professionals involved in the clinical work is that of a supervisor, someone who was not in the therapy room but who has a keen interest in what took place there.

Medical students, in contrast, are taught to think in teams. Their clinical training (i.e., after class work) takes place in rounds, where they are part of a large group of other trainees (typically including fellows, senior residents, first-year residents, and advanced medical students) who follow an attending physician through clinical interactions on a hospital floor. They become accustomed to discussing a particular patient in a group setting, hearing feedback and differing clinical opinions along the way.

Thus, psychosocial care in a medical setting may take place in a setting that is likely very different from initial psychology training models. Multidisciplinary teams are the standard for patient care in the medical model, and the trainee in psychosocial hem/onc should be exposed to this model at an advanced stage of training. Typically, once trainees have gained proficiency in individual clinical care, they can then be exposed to delivering this care in a team setting.

Multidisciplinary teams facilitate clinical care by allowing the members of the team to discuss patient care from a variety of different perspectives. The teams are generally headed by an attending physician and medical residents and may include representatives from psychology, social work, nutrition, nursing, pastoral services, child life, physical/occupational therapy, and hospital-based school teachers. The format of each team may vary from site to site and from clinic to clinic, but in general each member is expected to offer expertise and opinions on the care of the patient being discussed.

This format may be foreign at first to the psychosocial trainee. As discussed, many aspects of professional roles and responsibilities are quite different from the psychology or social work practitioner who works independently. Consequently, particular care should be taken in showing the trainee how clinical information is conveyed in a multidisciplinary team setting. Issues of confidentiality should be considered and should still be paramount. However, general information that will aid the medical team in caring for patients can and should be shared. Good clinical judgment will balance issues of confidentiality and clinical care information.

Another aspect of multidisciplinary teams that may be foreign to psychosocial trainees is the wealth of resources provided by these teams. Trainees may be accustomed to serving as the sole source of external behavioral modifications. However, all members of multidisciplinary teams typically play a significant role in treatment delivery. For example, a child who is disruptive on the hospital floor and not complying with requests from nurses may have privileges such as television and playroom time removed until more adaptive behavior is exhibited. Conversely, a quiet withdrawn child might be targeted by child life for special interventions designed to increase social interactions and improve peer relations. All of these things can be accomplished by other members of the multidisciplinary team, increasing the wealth of clinical resources at the disposal of psychosocial care providers.

One of the greatest difficulties for trainees when they work for the first time as part of a multidisciplinary team is understanding their professional role. The attending physician is typically in charge of treatment, including psychosocial interventions, which is very different from their previous experiences and can be confusing for many trainees. Trainees often have questions such as the following: What am I responsible for? When is my input needed, desired, and appropriate? Why is everyone else doing psychosocial interventions when that is my job? How can I be assertive but respectful of professional boundaries? Who is my real supervisor?

Effectively serving as a member of such complex treatment teams requires advanced levels of professional skills, which often require experience and good supervision to develop. Psychosocial service providers not only treat the individuals with the disease, but also they provide treatments to the patient's family and the treatment team itself. The intensity of many situations encountered on a hem/onc service often leads to problems with the treatment team as well. Team members may experience sadness, grief, anger, and hopelessness, all of which can interfere with effectively serving patients and their families. Understanding when this is happening and determining when and how to intervene with the treatment team requires a great deal of experience and skill. For such interventions to be successful, it also requires trust and respect from other team members. The support that team members offer each other is often instrumental in negotiating these difficult emotional issues and preventing burnout among team members who provide care to these patients.

As mentioned, learning these skills is often facilitated by modeling and direct feedback. Excellent resources are available that outline professional roles in these settings, provide specific suggestions for training activities, and offer different perspectives on the many opportunities for patient care and professional development (Drotar, 1995; Power, Shapiro, & DuPaul, 2003; Roberts, 2003; Spirito et al., 2003).

### *Death, Grief, and Bereavement*

Psychosocial care providers working in pediatric settings inevitably will encounter issues of loss, and this is especially true in hem/onc settings. Although most individual clients seen during early practicum experiences are expected to live and prosper, death and risk of death are pervasive in the hem/onc setting. Although the success rates of treatments have improved substantially for most hem/onc conditions in children, death and the risk of death are a real possibility for a great majority of children in the hem/onc setting. Even when death does not result, loss associated with health impairments, loss of a child's "innocence," and loss of the "normal" family life can be overwhelming for patients and their families. It can be overwhelming for staff as well. Consequently, understanding the impact of loss and death, how it is manifested in different cultures, and how to address it is critical for effective treatment by the psychosocial team member.

There are many good resources that address the theories of grief and bereavement, their psychological and physical manifestations, and specific individual and family interventions. To be effective at addressing these issues, it is important for trainees to have a solid foundation in the general knowledge about these issues. Burnell and Burnell (1989) provided an excellent discussion of the general clinical management of bereavement, including the role of health providers, that provides a good background for trainees. Chochinov and Holland (1989) discussed bereavement issues specific to the oncology setting. Kissane (2000) provided an excellent discussion of a family-based approach to grief with specific intervention techniques that incorporate key aspects of bereavement therapy and family systems therapy.

Trainees need to be comfortable with facing death, grief, and bereavement. It often is necessary for trainees to confront and address their own grief experiences through supervision and their own personal psychotherapy. Trainees should not be afraid or ashamed to mourn with the family, but one wants to make sure that the trainees' needs do not supersede those of the family, or that they do not pose a burden for the family. Trainees should also understand that their job is not to take away grief and bereavement or cure the family of all sorrow, but to begin a process that may take weeks, months, and even years to resolve. Certain techniques, such as distraction, may be the treatment of choice for some families, but emotional expression may work better for others. Cultural practices may dictate widely differing methods for grief, and trainees are encouraged to understand the cultural context of the family's expression of grief. Good clinical insight into tailoring of interventions should be demonstrated so that families may receive the best treatment for their particular situation.

### *Pain*

Trainees should expect that many of their pediatric hem/onc patients will be experiencing pain and discomfort, which are sometimes unfortunate consequences of medical diagnoses and treatments. Although pain may be expected, it can be addressed and reduced through the use of behavioral and cognitive behavioral techniques. Core psychological interventions such as distraction and imagery have been demonstrated to be effective in alleviating pain in this population (Blount, Piira, & Cohen, 2003; Gelfand & Dahlquist, 2003), although some children experience pain that is much more severe and requires pharmacological management. Thus, it is important for trainees to understand the limitations of psychological approaches for pain management.

What is different for the trainee in hem/onc is the context in which these services can be delivered. Psychosocial assessment and intervention may take place in an outpatient clinic, an inpatient hospital room, or in a pain clinic itself. Trainees should demonstrate proficiency in assessing pain location, frequency, intensity, duration, quality, and pain-free periods (McGrath & Hillier, 2002).

In addition, many medical settings now have pain teams designated specifically to address pain management. These teams are usually multidisciplinary and seek to reduce patients' pain experience by using pharmacological and psychological techniques. Although trainees should not be expected to demonstrate knowledge of all analgesic agents used to manage pain, they should be aware how psychosocial techniques can be used together with medical interventions, and that the two treatments are not necessarily mutually exclusive.

### *Relaxation/Distraction*

Although these relaxation and distraction techniques are employed in a wide variety of settings, in a medical setting they are particularly efficacious during medical interventions. They have been demonstrated to be valid in reducing distress during painful procedures such as needle sticks and medication administration.

The trainee should demonstrate competence in using these procedures, both in a traditional setting such as a quiet therapy room and in a medical setting in which interruptions and competing stimuli are the norm. For example, a trainee should be taught that a hospital room is not a private, quiet place; nurses are constantly coming in and out of the room to check on vital signs, other health care professionals are expected to check on the patient, and the like. These interruptions can be seen as problematic for psychosocial treatment delivery, or they can be utilized by the psychologist to the benefit of the patient. Again, the context in which the psychosocial provider works will determine the way in which treatment is delivered. The trainee in psychosocial hem/onc must be able to adapt empirically supported techniques to a novel setting and one that is not necessarily ideal.

### Family Systems

Psychosocial care in a medical setting involves not only the patient, but also the family. Most assessment and treatment interventions will take place in an environment, not a vacuum. Trainees should be made aware that the family system is not merely one modality for conceptualizing psychosocial services but is an overarching theme in the care of the patient. Kazak (2001) has put forth a model for practitioners in this field, demonstrating the "social ecology of pediatric illness."

The way in which the family system is conceptualized and used in the delivery of care in a pediatric hem/onc setting is still underdeveloped. In traditional outpatient therapy, family systems may be understood as complementary and even causal for much of the psychosocial distress observed in the patient. However, in a pediatric hem/onc setting, the family system in all likelihood is not contributory to the development of the disease, but undoubtedly it is affected by the diagnosis and treatment of the disease. In this manner, the family system can serve as both a modifier and a mediator for the psychological distress experienced by the child patient. Careful consideration should be given to how the child's environmental system is affected by the disease and treatment and how this system may be used to assist in overall coping.

### Neuropsychology

Neuropsychology is a specific area of competence and training in psychology that requires specialized training and credentials. However, the trainee should be aware of some of the neurocognitive toxicities associated with the treatment for hem/onc problems. These effects may include decline in overall intellectual abilities, specific aspects of memory, verbal abilities, and executive functioning (Mulhern et al., 1999). The trainee should demonstrate competence in knowing what to assess and the limits of competence in assessment. In other words, the practitioner in this area should know what he or she can assess and when to refer for a full neuropsychological assessment by a credentialed neuropsychologist.

Many of the diseases and treatments encountered by the trainee will involve the central nervous system, frequently leading to debilitating effects, particularly with high doses of chemotherapy and radiation therapy. The research literature has moved from assessment of these late effects to treatment and prophylactic interventions designed to reduce them (Butler & Copeland, 2002; see also chapter 16, this volume). Trainees should have good knowledge of the current literature in neuropsychology, especially as it relates to specific diseases and treatments frequently encountered by the trainee.

### School Integration/Educational Issues

School issues inevitably will arise for children and their families during and after the treatment process. Because school absence is often necessary, prolonged, and unpredictable, parents and educational professionals are often faced with many difficult issues, including if, when, and how to send the child back to school; what to do about all of the missed schoolwork; and how to handle the social implications of returning to school for the child. Teachers must deal with issues such as what to disclose to other children, how to deal with teasing, and managing the emotional reactions of other children. Because research has revealed that teachers feel inadequately prepared to deal with many of these issues (Clay, Mordhorst, & Lehn, 2004), members of the health care team are crucial in serving as a source of support and information for the family and educational professionals.

Educational issues begin in the medical setting during the treatment process. Most hospitals have an education program in place with schoolteachers available to assist in maintaining the patients on their academic trajectory. School planning thus begins in the hospital, and planning to return to school begins not at the end of treatment, but during treatment. Most experts agree that successful school reintegration occurs when the health care team takes an active role in planning for the reintegration. The role of the psychosocial service provider may involve contacting the school, visiting the school, and providing the school with information regarding the diagnosis, effects of treatment, and the general prognosis of the child. Of course, the child and the caregivers must provide consent prior to medical center staff contacting the school setting.

Psychologists, social workers, and child life specialists in hem/onc must have a good working knowledge of educational issues. Clay (2004) provided a thorough integration of psychological and educational issues for children with chronic illness that provides an excellent resource for psychosocial service providers and educators alike. The resource book emphasizes practical strategies to deal with issues such as disclosure of the illness to other children, how to handle teasing, development of special education plans, and strategies for educators to deal with aspects of the illnesses (e.g., pain, medication, adverse side effects).

### *Spirituality, Complementary and Alternative Medicine*

Trainees should be made aware of the burgeoning area of spirituality and complementary medicine. These issues are no longer thought of as fringe aspects of the overall care of the pediatric patient but as important aspects of the patient's overall well-being. An openness to the desires and beliefs of the family and the patient will aid in rapport building and in treatment efficacy. The trainee may not be familiar with all aspects of spirituality and world religion or of all complementary medicine, but these issues should be discussed in a nonjudgmental way in the multidisciplinary setting. Issues of family belief systems and method of interpreting the world and illness can be used to build trust between the patient and the health care team. A basic respect for humans will determine the overall approach in dealing with these issues.

Interventions aimed at alleviating psychological distress have been designed to help mothers of children with cancer develop coping skills to avoid high levels of distress in themselves, which may in turn affect their children's adjustment and disease adaptation. Traditional religious coping may be one such coping skill. Much of the work in this area has been reported by Koenig and colleagues, who found that more religious patients have a significantly faster recovery from depression than those who are less religious (Koenig, 2000; Koenig, Larson, & Larson, 2001). A study reported that the frequency of attendance at religious services is inversely related to distress, according to self-reports. In addition, findings revealed that those who reported regular attendance at religious services also reported experiencing fewer health problems (Ellison, Boardman, Williams, & Jackson, 2001).

This research suggests that mothers' religious involvement may serve as a protective factor against their own psychological distress and may in turn decrease the levels of anxiety and depression in their children with cancer. Maternal religiosity has been found potentially to protect against offspring depression (Miller & Warner, 1997). If mothers are engaging in religious practices, their children may be more likely to maintain lower levels of depressive symptoms, and the religious involvement may also contribute to the child's rate of healing.

In addition to religiosity and spirituality, trainees must have a foundation of knowledge in alternative treatments. The use of alternative treatments such as acupuncture, aromatherapy, massage, and herbal supplements is becoming very common in the general public, specifically in persons with a chronic illness. Despite many of these treatments lacking any empirical evidence, their frequent use makes it important for trainees to understand the available therapies and be able to use the appropriate terminology with patients. Emerging data are providing some support for the beneficial effects of some treatments (e.g., massage, acupuncture). It is critical to keep an open mind and refrain from making judgmental statements to patients when they discuss the use of such alternative treatments.

### *Self-Care and Burnout*

To provide the best possible care for patients and their families, trainees should be taught early on to seek out ways of caring for themselves professionally. Self-care may involve attending national and professional meetings to hone professional skills, develop a social support system to deal with job stress, and seek consultation or even personal counseling to manage personal emotional reactions. Vicarious trauma is not uncommon among health care professionals, especially when working with terminal illness. Longevity is necessary to improve clinical skills, but longevity may be undermined by the very demands of the job itself. Although many trainees may not see burnout as an issue at their career stage, they should be encouraged to begin thinking of this as an important aspect of their professional development, with the ultimate aim better overall care for their patients. In this endeavor, it is important to "take care" of the provider as well as the patient. We discussed these issues more thoroughly in relation to supervision.

## Conclusion

As more and more pediatric hem/onc patients survive diagnosis and treatment, there is an increasing need for more and better trained professionals to provide psychosocial care for them. There should be an increase not only in the quantity of psychosocial trainees, but also the quality of their training and capabilities should increase. As more is known about the acute and chronic effects of hem/onc treatment in pediatrics, psychosocial workers need ever-sharpening levels of skill and training to best assess, intervene, and provide overall care for these patients.

In this chapter, we have provided a suggested outline for both the content and the timing of this training. The unique environment in which pediatric hem/onc services take place demands that trainees receive specialized supervision not only in the basic tenets of psychosocial care, but also in the clinical application of these tenets to patients who need them. Trainees are encouraged to remain consumers of training issues throughout their careers as these issues will influence the quality of care delivered to patients.

## References


American Psychological Association (2003). Guidelines on multicultural education, training, research, practice, and organizational change for psychologists. *American Psychologist, 58(5)*, 377–402.

Blount, R. L., Piira, T., & Cohen, L. L. (2003). Management of pediatric pain and distress due to medical procedures. In M. C. Roberts (Ed.), *Handbook of pediatric psychology* (3rd ed.). New York: Guilford Press (pp. 216–233).

Broskowski, A. T. (1995). The evolution of health care: Implications for the training and careers of psychologists. *Professional Psychology: Research and Practice, 26*, 156–162.

Brown, R. T., Freeman, W. S. Brown, R. A., Belar, C., Hersch, L., Hornyak, L. M., et al. (2002). The role of psychology in health care delivery. *Professional Psychology: Research and Practice, 33*, 536–545.

Burnell, G. M., & Burnell, A. L. (1989). *Clinical management of bereavement: A handbook for healthcare professionals*. New York: Human Sciences Press.

Butler, R. W., & Copeland, D. R. (2002). Attentional processes and their remediation in children treated for cancer: A literature review and the development of a therapeutic approach. *Journal of the International Neuropsychological Society, 8*, 115–124.

Carlton, E. K. (1998). An examination of doctoral-level psychotherapy training in light of the proliferation of managed care. *Professional Psychology: Research and Practice, 29*, 304–306.

Cashel, M. L. (2002). Child and adolescent psychological assessment: Current clinical practices and the impact of managed care. *Professional Psychology: Research and Practice, 33*, 446–453.

Charous, M. A., & Carter, R. E. (1996). Mental health and managed care: Training for the 21st century. *Psychotherapy, 33*, 628–635.

Chochinov, H., & Holland, J. C. (1989). Bereavement: A special issue in oncology. In J. C. Holland & J. H. Rowland (Eds.) *Handbook of Psychooncology: Psychological care of the patient with cancer*. New York: Oxford University Press.

Chwalisz, K. (2003). Evidence-based practice: A framework for 21st-century scientist-practitioner training. *The Counseling Psychologist, 31*, 497–528.

Clay, D. L. (2004). *Helping schoolchildren with chronic health problems in the schools: A practical guide*. New York: Guilford Press.

Clay, D. L., Cortina, S., Harper, D. C., Cocco, K., & Drotar, D. (2004). Teachers' experiences with childhood chronic illness. *Children's Health Care, 33(3)*, 227–239.

Clay, D. L., Mordhorst, M. J., & Lehn, L. (2002). Empirically supported treatments in pediatric psychology: Where is the diversity? *Journal of Pediatric Psychology, 27*, 325–337.

Cohen, J. A. (2003). Managed care and the evolving role of the clinical social worker in mental health. *Social Work, 48*, 34–43.

Cummings, N. A. (1995). Impact of managed care on employment and training: A primer for survival. *Professional Psychology: Research and Practice, 26*, 10–15.

Daniels, J. A., Alva, L. A., & Olivares, S. (2002). Graduate training for managed care: A national survey of psychology and social work programs. *Professional Psychology: Research and Practice, 33*, 587–590.

Drotar, D (1995). *Consulting with pediatricians: Psychological perspectives*. New York: Plenum.

Ellison, C. G., Boardman, J. D., Williams, D. R., & Jackson, J. S. (2001). Religious involvement, stress, and mental health: Findings from the 1995 Detroit area study. *Social Forces, 80*, 215–249.

Gelfand, K. M., & Dahlquist, L. M. (2003). An examination of the relation between child distress and mother and nurse verbal responses during pediatric oncology procedures. *Children's Health Care, 32*, 257–272.

Gotay, C. C. (2000). Culture, cancer, and the family. In L. Baider, C. L. Cooper and A. K. De-Nour (Eds.),

*Cancer and the Family* (2nd Ed.). New York: Wiley, pp. 95–110.

Kaslow, N. J., McCarthy, S. M., Rogers, J. H., & Summerville, M. B. (1992). Psychology postdoctoral training: A developmental perspective. *Professional Psychology—Research and Practice, 23*, 369–375.

Kaslow, N. J., & Rice, D. G. (1985). Developmental stresses of psychology internship training: What training staff can do to help. *Professional Psychology—Research and Practice, 16*, 253–261.

Kazak, A. E. (2001). Comprehensive care for children with cancer and their families: A social ecological framework guiding research, practice, and policy. *Children's Services: Social Policy, Research, & Practice, 44(4), 217–233.*

Kiesler, C. A. (2000). The next wave of change for psychology and mental health services in the health care revolution. *American Psychologist, 55*, 481–487.

Kissane, D. W. (2000). A model of family-centered intervention during palliative care and bereavement: Focused family grief therapy. In L. Baider, C. L. Cooper and A. K. De-Nour (Eds.), *Cancer and the Family* (2nd ed.). New York: Wiley, 175–197.

Koenig, H. G. (2000). Depression in the medically ill: A common and serious disorder. *International Journal of Psychiatry and Medicine, 30,* 2 95–297.

Koenig, H. G., Larson, D. B., & Larson, S. S. (2001). Religion and coping with serious medical illness. *Annals of Pharmacotherapy, 35,* 352–359.

LaGreca, A., & Hughes, J. (1999). United we stand, divided we fall: The education and training needs of clinical child psychologists. *Journal of Clinical Child Psychology, 28*, 435–447.

Liu, W., & Clay, D. L. (2002). Multicultural counseling competencies: Guidelines in working with children and adolescents. *Journal of Mental Health Counseling, 24*, 177–187.

McGrath, P. A., & Hillier, L. M. (2002). A practical cognitive-behavioral approach for treating children's pain. In D. C. Turk & R. J. Gatchel (Eds.), *Psychological approaches to pain management: A practitioner's handbook* (2nd ed.). New York: Guilford Press (534–552).

Miller, L., & Warner, V. (1997). Religiosity and depression: 10-year follow-up of depressed mothers and offspring. *Journal of the American Academy of Child and Adolescent Psychiatry, 36,* 1416–1425.

Mulhern, R. K., Reddick, W. E., Palmer, S. L., Glass, J. O., Elkin, T. D., Kun, L. E., et al. (1999). Neurocognitive deficits in medulloblastoma survivors and white matter loss. *Annals of Neurology, 46*, 834–841.

Nathan, P. E., & Gorman, J. M. (2002). *A guide to treatments that work* (2nd ed.). London: Oxford University Press.

Parry, G., Cape, J., & Pilling, S. (2004). Clinical practice guidelines in clinical psychology and psychotherapy. *Clinical Psychology and Psychotherapy, 10*, 337–351.

Patterson, J. E., McIntosh-Koontz, L., Baron, M., & Bischoff, R. (1997). Curriculum changes to meet challenges: Preparing MFT students for managed care settings. *Journal of Marital and Family Therapy, 23*, 445–459.

Power, T. J., Shapiro, E. S., & DuPaul, G. J. (2003). Preparing psychologists to link systems of care in managing and preventing children's health problems. *Journal of Pediatric Psychology, 28*, 147–155.

Roberts, M. (2003). *Handbook of pediatric psychology* (3rd ed.). New York: Guilford Press.

Schreter, R. K. (1997). Essential skills for managed behavioral health care. *Psychiatric Services, 48*, 653–658.

Spirito, A., Brown, R. T., D'Angelo, E., Delamater, A., Rodrigue, J., & Siegel, L. (2003). Society of Pediatric Psychology task force report: Recommendations for the training of pediatric psychologists. *Journal of Pediatric Psychology, 28*, 85–98.

Stoltenberg, C. D., McNeill, B., & Delworth, U. (1998). *IDM supervision: An integrated developmental model for supervising counselors and therapists*. New York: Jossey-Bass.

Sue, D. W. & Sue, D. (2003). *Counseling the culturally diverse: Theory and Practice*. Hoboken, NJ: John Wiley & Sons, Inc.

Webb, N. B. (2001). Educating students and practitioners for culturally responsive practice. In N. B. Webb (Ed.), *Culturally diverse parent-child and family relationships: A guide for social workers and other practitioners*. New York: Columbia University Press (pp. 351–360).

Stan F. Whitsett, F. Daniel Armstrong, and Brad H. Pollock

# Research Opportunities and Collaborative Multisite Studies in Psychosocial Hematology/Oncology

Over the past several decades, dramatic improvements in outcome have occurred for children treated for cancer. Many of these advances can be attributed to the benefits of multicenter research conducted within the context of a cooperative group clinical trials infrastructure (D'Angio & Vietti, 2001; Pediatric Oncology Group, 1992). Historically, the cooperative groups sponsored by the National Cancer Institute provided pooled expertise, centralized high-quality medical informatics resources, and access to large patient populations. This infrastructure enabled investigators to ask more focused research questions with greater statistical power as well as generalize research findings to the broader population. Although childhood cancer is by no means a rare disease, its incidence in the general population is sufficiently low that few single pediatric oncology treatment centers are likely to treat enough patients, representing an adequately homogeneous sample, to provide a robust evaluation of clinical outcomes. In many respects, multisite research has been *necessary* to acquire adequate sample sizes to allow appropriate statistical evaluations of treatment outcomes and generalization of these outcomes to the larger pediatric oncology population.

Awareness of this fact led first to the development of small consortia of pediatric oncology centers and later to the formation of large multi-institutional cooperative study groups to conduct controlled clinical therapeutic trials for pediatric cancer patients. Ultimately, the four major childhood cancer study groups (the Children's Cancer Group, CCG; the Pediatric Oncology Group, POG; the National Wilms Tumor Study Group; and the Intergroup Rhabdomyosarcoma Study Group) merged in 2000 to form a single collaborative group: the Children's Oncology Group (COG). At present, the 238 institutions that comprise the COG provide the research infrastructure for the majority of pediatric oncology clinical trials conducted in North America, Australia, and parts of Europe. Moreover, because the COG member institutions include all major university and teaching hospitals throughout the United States and Canada, the majority of children diagnosed with cancer in North America will be treated at a COG member institution with the opportunity to be enrolled on a COG protocol.

An early evaluation of referral patterns to the two largest cooperative groups enumerated the observed cancer cases from the CCG and POG cancer incidence registries. The number of observed cases was then compared to the number of expected cases based on age-, sex-, and race-specific incidence rates from the Surveillance and Epidemiologic End Results (SEER) registry applied to the population data from the U.S. Census. It was estimated that 93% of children aged 5–9 years and 84% of those aged 10–14 years were treated at one of the collaborative group centers (Ross, Severson, Pollock, & Robison, 1996). In an updated analysis that directly matched incidence records from CCG and POG with individual records from the SEER registries, it was found that 71% of children under 15 years of age were seen at cooperative group institutions (Liu, Krailo, Reaman, & Bernstein, 2003). Of note is the fact that the proportion of adolescents (those aged 15–19 years) seen at pediatric cooperative institutions was only 24%.

From March 1, 2003, through February 29, 2004, COG enrolled 6,250 childhood cancer patients in its treatment studies, and an estimated 35,000 childhood cancer survivors were actively followed. In many respects, the capacity of the cooperative groups to enroll high percentages of the children diagnosed with cancer in this country and to conduct controlled clinical trials constitutes one of the most influential factors underlying the dramatic improvements in treatment of pediatric oncology patients and in the improved survival rates among these patients ("Progress Against Childhood Cancer," 1992; D'Angio & Vietti, 2001; Pediatric Oncology Group, 1992).

The contributions of cooperative groups to the interdependent goals of clinical research trials and improved treatment of childhood cancers has led to an increasing emphasis on the maintenance of standards of research and clinical excellence within these groups. Rigorous quality control for application of interventions, adherence to research protocols and data acquisition has been implemented to ensure the highest standards of care for children enrolled in cooperative group protocols (Pollock, 1994). Participating centers are required to document all aspects of enrollment and management of protocol patients and must undergo regular on-site auditing of their facilities and data operations. These quality assurance steps have led to significant improvements in research data integrity and are associated with greater accuracy and higher certainty of conclusions drawn from protocol-driven research.

The COG has a quality assurance system in place centered on an Institutional Performance Monitoring Committee. The continuous patient-monitoring criteria are complementary to the group's institutional audit process. On-site institutional auditing is performed on a 3-year cycle even though institutions are at risk for a random audit at any time. If an institution has been found to have a problem on an audit, the frequency of auditing is increased. Data-monitoring reviews are performed every 6 months and include all patient records. Missing data, timeliness of data submission, quality of data, ineligibility, and protocol compliance are evaluated using a numeric scoring system. The group takes action to ensure that individual institutions perform above a certain threshold based on this scoring system. Behavioral research protocols can also be set up to ensure that required tests, data submission, and compliance with other protocol requirements can be evaluated and numerically scored. The completeness of follow-up is monitored for clinical studies. In addition, accrual monitoring is conducted primarily to ensure that institutions comply with a group constitutional requirement that six therapeutic protocol entries and two nontherapeutic protocol entries take place per year based on a 3-year rolling average.

Research on the psychosocial aspects of childhood cancer and its treatment stands to gain equivalent benefit from the establishment of the COG and this conduct of multicenter trials. Historically, much of the early research in psychosocial oncology was based on uncontrolled case reports or very small case series. This approach led to intriguing observations, but the reliability and validity of the findings were always subject to criticism and doubt. These nearly anecdotal reports could not be considered representative of the general pediatric oncology.

To address these limitations, investigators sought to expand their access to larger referred patient populations and to samples more representative of the diverse characteristics inherent in the broader general population of pediatric oncology patients. With more access to larger populations of children with cancer, studies can be conducted with adequate consideration to disease type, cancer treatment approach, age and developmental level of the patients, and cultural influences on psychosocial outcomes. Given these benefits, multicenter research provided a strong research model that could support drawing robust, valid conclusions about various subpopulations of cancer patients while also providing better understanding of the overall psychosocial influence of cancer and its treatment. Today, collaborative multicenter studies provide an efficient means by which these issues can be addressed. The pediatric cooperative group provides a more efficient infrastructure that can be used to better conduct relevant, well-designed psychosocial studies that address questions specific to a particular diagnosis or treatment approach.

With the demonstrated success of improved cure and reduced morbidity associated with multicenter research, it is surprising that more psychosocial research is not presently organized in this manner. At the time this chapter was written, there were only eight open clinical trial protocols that included a psychosocial outcome and only six protocols under review for potential activation. All of these protocols involved assessment of neurocognitive outcome as an outcome of the clinical trial (F. D. Armstrong, personal communication, 2004). There are several plausible explanations for this state of affairs. First, psychologists often are not trained or experienced in the intricacies of multicenter collaborative clinical research. Literature reviews conducted in the development of this chapter revealed very few published discussions on the conduct of multicenter, psychosocial research with pediatric oncology patients (for exceptions, see Armstrong & Drotar, 2002; Armstrong & Reaman, in press). Junior investigators in particular may have had little opportunity to observe or manage the developmental and administrative aspects of multicenter trials. Few of the "strategies" for successful multicenter studies described in the second half of this chapter are included in the academic training of psychologists.

The nature of psychological questions and the data derived to answer these questions represent a second factor that contributes to the paucity of psychosocial research within the collaborative groups. According to the "vision" included in the constitution of the COG, the primary goals are to conduct clinical, laboratory and translational research to optimize treatments for children with cancer and to identify the causes of childhood cancer. In contrast, psychosocial studies have tended to focus more on the long-term emotional, behavioral, and cognitive sequelae of both cancer and its treatment and on the adjustment of children and adolescents to their disease and treatment (Armstrong & Reaman, in press). These two goals are not mutually exclusive, of course, but the mechanics of conducting studies arising from the COG vision are not always compatible with those needed to conduct good psychosocial research. It should be recognized, however, that the dramatic improvements in long-term survival rates for childhood cancer are beginning to make psychosocial outcomes of quality of life, emotional adjustment, and global psychosocial functioning (including cognitive functioning) more important to determination of "optimal treatments" and, for this reason, those that are more consistent with the primary research objectives of the collaborative group.

The success resulting from clinical trials research has led to increased interest in issues of long-term survivorship, including identification of risk factors and development of interventions to prevent or ameliorate psychosocial sequelae. The cooperative group provides investigators interested in survivorship with an infrastructure for tracking long-term survivors while ensuring that health-related privacy is maintained and provides a potentially vast population of children for participation in these types of studies.

The remainder of this chapter provides an overview of the advantages of multicenter psycho-oncology studies, along with strategies that may facilitate the successful conduct of psychosocial multicenter studies within COG. Our collective experience indicates that these studies are not without their challenges, but we are convinced that the opportunities will frequently outweigh the challenges. The potential benefits of high-quality psychosocial research for children with cancer are significant.

## Multicenter Research in Psychosocial Oncology

### Advantages

There are a number of advantages gained by conducting multicenter, psychosocial oncology studies within the cooperative groups. Many of these derive from access to a larger and more varied population of patients, facilitated by having multiple centers involved in the recruitment of patients. Others stem from the cooperative group research infrastructure already put in place to conduct treatment trials.

There are currently 238 member institutions in the COG that provide treatment to more than 70% of children with cancer under age 10 years in the United States (Liu et al., 2003). Involvement of even a limited number of COG centers in a multicenter trial is likely to increase participant accrual dramatically over what most, but not all, single institutions can accomplish. There are several advantages afforded to research conducted in this setting, as well as several disadvantages.

The primary advantage gained by greater participant accrual is primarily statistical; with larger accrual there is a concomitant increase in the statistical power to detect differences between participant groups or within participants arising from an intervention (as in clinical trials). Other advantages include (a) the ability to accrue participants in a relatively short period of time, permitting more rapid acquisition of knowledge and evidence-based and informed modification of treatment; (b) the ability to assess smaller intervention effects with adequate power; (c) access to large numbers of children with similar diseases treated in similar ways as well as large, heterogeneous groups with diverse malignancy diagnoses and treatments; (d) opportunities to examine psychosocial outcomes within a transdisciplinary context; (e) access to an established research participant tracking system; (f) opportunities to engage a broader group of investigators; and (g) access to an efficient system of data collection and analysis (Armstrong & Reaman, in press). Other potential advantages include the enhanced generalizability of large, population-based studies that include diverse or disparate underrepresented groups of children and the improved translation of clinical trial outcomes to practice in community settings.

### Disadvantages

Collaborative, multicenter psychosocial research is not without its disadvantages. Some of these include (a) increased financial cost; (b) difficulties with standardization and quality assurance of data collection procedures across multiple settings; (c) difficulties associated with prioritization of core resource use for research; (d) and issues of authorship and productivity expectations (Armstrong & Reaman, in press)

## Essential Strategies for Successful Multicenter Studies

### Mechanisms for Recruitment and Registration of Participants

Children with new cancer-related symptoms are most often seen initially by their primary care physicians, including pediatricians and family practice physicians. Many of the early symptoms of childhood cancer are nonspecific, and their onset is often insidious. Eventually, these symptoms will warrant a diagnostic workup and generally result in referral to cancer specialists. Although the geographic distribution of primary care services for children is almost ubiquitous, pediatric oncology services tend to be more concentrated in universities, large medical centers, or children's hospitals. Therefore, children with newly detected cancer often have to leave their local residential area for extended periods of time for treatment. Pediatric oncology referral patterns are quite varied across North America; they are influenced not only by physical proximity to referring physicians and patient residential location, but also often by health care financing constraints brought about by restricted access to certain providers in health insurance plans.

On seeing a child for the first time, pediatric oncologists and related childhood cancer subspecialists (neurosurgeons, orthopedic surgeons, etc.) will conduct a diagnostic workup and then determine if there is a cooperative group protocol that is both appropriate for their patient and open to accrual. In some instances, participation in a clinical trial may not be recommended or possible. This may occur because (a) at the time of diagnosis, there is no actively accruing protocol available for the patient's type of cancer; (b) the child does not meet the eligibility criteria for a protocol; or, much less often, (c) the physician prefers another therapy; or (d) the parents or guardians refuse to consider enrolling their child in a research protocol. When a decision is made to enroll a patient on a treatment protocol, written informed consent (and assent if appropriate from the child) is obtained, and then the medical team of the local treating hospital will register the patient in the study.

Historically, all enrollments were completed by local institutional personnel by telephone to the cooperative data centers, where a person at the central office would manually complete the registration, look up the randomization assigned for that patient (for randomized studies), and then convey the treatment assignment to the caller. These transactions were limited to the office hours of the data centers, typically 8:00 a.m. to 5:00 p.m.

Over the years, automated registration procedures have been substituted for the manual telephone calls. One system developed by POG was an automated digitized telephone registration procedure that used the telephone keypad for data entry and a synthetic voice generated by a computer speech card to inform the referring oncologist about the treatment assignment. This successful system was available 24 hours a day, 7 days a week (Krischer et al., 1991).

Several years ago, this system was supplanted with an Internet Web-based registration system. During the registration process, this system allows for all eligibility criteria to be checked, and it allows for a "call-back" Web session by which subsequent randomizations can be performed based on an initial treatment response (e.g., patients with a complete clinical response versus those who are refractory to initial therapy). This automated system allows for nearly instantaneous accrual monitoring and e-mail notification to protocol investigators informing them of new registrations.

## Mechanism for Conveyance and Storage of Data

In a single institution study, the principal investigator has some degree of involvement with virtually every child who is enrolled and with the data acquired for each of those children. Management of the integrity of study data in these cases is typically straightforward. When multiple sites are involved, however, such oversight becomes more complicated, and attention to the acquisition, conveyance, and storage of data becomes more demanding. It is essential that investigators establish the mechanisms for data management prior to enrollment of participants, along with procedures for quality assurance over time.

Multisite clinical trials typically involve the enrollment of small numbers of participants from each of several sites. When data acquisition in these studies is accomplished through administration of pencil-and-paper tests (as is often the case in psychosocial studies), these tests or questionnaires will need to be "scored" for calculation of total and subscale indices. In many cases, the tests/questionnaires used to acquire the data will consist of clinically relevant information that might have broader value for both the participant and the participating center. For example, neuropsychological test batteries are frequently included in study protocols for children with central nervous system tumors, but the results of these tests are also typically needed for development of educational plans useful to the participant's school environment.

In the multicenter studies involving neuropsychological data as part of the study outcome data set, tests will be scored and summary data will be derived at the participating center. Coordinators of such multicenter studies must make certain that the format for data reporting to the central statistical center is clear and describe in detail the data to be accessioned and provided to the coordinating center. Again, using neuropsychological testing as an example, the participating centers will need to know whether to provide individual item, subtest, or total scores; whether the results should be reported as raw scores, standardized scores, or percentiles; and whether detailed qualitative information concerning the specific response pattern of each participant is to be reported.

In some studies, copies of the raw test protocols obtained at each participating site must be provided to the coordinating site. This has historically caused numerous problems, including interpretability of handwritten forms, burdens related to handling a large volume of paper records at the coordinating site, and ethical responsibility for supervision of raw test data. In some cases, this process has been simplified by the use of optically scannable paper forms. If responses to test items can be made directly to the scannable forms, then the accuracy and integrity of the data remain high because the forms (or copies) can be sent directly to the coordinating site. Unfortunately, for many standardized psychological tests, a proprietary response sheet is utilized, and responses on scannable forms must be transcribed from the original test response sheet. The intervening steps involving transcription of test results raise obvious challenges regarding the accuracy of data, not to mention possible copyright violation issues.

Fortunately, with the development of Web-based data collection technologies, the process of capturing data in multisite clinical research has evolved in several fundamental ways that have enhanced the accuracy and timeliness of data acquisition and the maintenance of data integrity (Marks, Conlon, & Ruberg, 2001). The majority of pediatric oncology consortium-based studies now use Web-based technology for direct entry of data and subsequent storage of that data in a single central location. Case record forms identifying all necessary data for each participant are readily accessed by the participating sites and are then subsequently used for entry of data points into specified fields. Data entries can be immediately checked for accuracy to determine that the information entered into that field constitutes a valid value. Completeness can also be checked to ensure that all necessary data are available and entered before the case record form is accepted as complete. Ethical and confidential considerations are addressed directly as part of the internal review board review and consenting process, and computer-based authentication procedures and encryption of data restrict access to data only to authorized personnel.

Through this means of centralized data acquisition, the coordinator and principal investigator of a multicenter study are able to monitor data flow to ensure study progress. Deficiencies in recruitment or attainment of participants, delays in submission of time-sensitive data from participants, and the accuracy and appropriateness of acquired data can all immediately be determined through this centralized process. Such monitoring is far more complicated without the use of some process of remote data capture.

## Establishment of Methodological Standards and Auditing for Quality Control

Each site participating in a multicenter study will bring with it personnel with diverse backgrounds, experiences, and, potentially, alternative methods for accomplishing study tasks. In some cases involving standardized psychological testing, reasonable assumptions can be made that those tests will be administered in a fairly consistent fashion across personnel and sites. However, with the exception of these particularly standardized methods, all other components of the study methodology will need to be operationalized in a manner such that the requirements of each particular task are unambiguous. In addition, it is typically necessary to provide training in those tasks to ensure a uniform approach to measure administration, data collection, data management, and data transfer across participating sites. This training must be offered at the beginning of the study but will need to be available throughout the study duration as new personnel inevitably become involved.

There has been some move to utilize the technology associated with telemedicine to improve the availability of training in multicenter trials (Kennedy et al., 2000). The limitation commonly associated with telemedicine to date is the lack of availability of appropriate videoconferencing equipment in remote locations. When a multicenter trial involves recruitment in remote regions apart from established oncology centers, the utility of this method may be limited. However, because most treatment for childhood cancer is provided through pediatric oncology centers and because most of these centers are associated with larger medical centers or universities, some access to videoconferencing facilities should be available to participating sites for intermittent training purposes. This technology is also appealing because it allows for several sites to be simultaneously involved in training activities, thus allowing investigators to benefit from joint discussion of methods, problems, and solutions.

Once training is complete, it also is essential to monitor continued compliance with study methods. It is well recognized that even highly standardized methods may "drift" with time because of a number of factors. There is no means through which these factors or the speed or extent of drift can be anticipated by study coordinators, making periodic retraining essential for maintaining consistent methodology across sites. Thus, it is more appropriate to provide this retraining on a regular, scheduled basis than to wait until violations with study protocol are identified by accident or audit.

### Development of Incentives for Enrollment of Participants and Continued Participation by Participating Sites

Typically, the principal investigator in a multicenter study will have some explicit incentive for their own involvement in the study. This may come in the form of salary support, academic recognition, or some more intrinsic rewards, such as public identification as a key investigator. Such incentives are more challenging to develop for investigators at the participating sites but are no less essential to ensure their active and continued involvement. There are several strategies that may enhance the participation of these personnel.

For several years, participant enrollment for the pediatric oncology consortium-based studies has provided a per-patient reimbursement. Funds to support research have been provided by grants and contracts from the National Institutes of Health and, on a very limited basis, industry-sponsored support. This reimbursement has typically been directed at clinical trial enrollments and has helped offset the costs of expensive medical procedures, tests, and medications. The Division of Cancer Prevention, National Cancer Institute, through their Community Clinical Oncology Program has provided case reimbursement for intervention-oriented prevention and cancer control trials, but these funds are targeted at defraying institutional data management expenses. It has been rare in the history of consortium-based studies for evaluation of psychological functioning to receive reimbursement, although the desire for this appears to be increasing. Some reimbursement for enrollment of a patient in these studies is justified, particularly for neuropsychological studies that involve extensive batteries of tests (and hence extensive professional time). If this cost can be included in the investigational budget, then it has been found to dramatically increase participant enrollment in the psychological components of multicenter trials and to improve compliance with psychosocial evaluation methodologies.

Regardless of any remuneration for patient enrollment, the motivation of most investigators to become involved and stay involved in multicenter studies will be enhanced if some clear academic benefit may be derived. The most obvious form of academic incentive is authorship on publications or presentations emanating from the research (Armstrong & Drotar, 2000). Depending on the number of centers involved in any particular study, inclusion as a coauthor in publications may or may not appear uniquely rewarding to the investigator. Some publications arising from multicenter trials post such a large number of participating authors that any beyond the first and senior authors are essentially lost in the crowd. If participation of an investigator in the multicenter trial is critical to the success of that trial, then this participation should be recognized in a more meaningful fashion. Rotating authorships of multiple publications with limited coauthors may help to raise the profile of the participating coinvestigators. Similarly, the establishment of investigator specific topics of investigation, couched within the broader research questions, can allow individual investigators to become more fully involved in the development of their own publications. Interested investigators will need access to the study data to allow them to conduct a limited data analysis, although the resultant findings may have great benefit to the larger study group as well as promote scientific advancement of the field.

A final incentive may be found in enhancement of the nonacademic (i.e., clinical) interests of participating investigators. Because many of the investigators at participating sites will be involved in some aspect of the clinical care of the participants, the availability of research findings that have significant clinical relevance should be provide additional rewards for these investigators. This relevance can be focused on immediate care issues, particularly when investigational tools (research protocols) are selected to provide clinically important data about the individual participant. In addition, broader and more long-term clinical relevance can be attained when research methods are tied to clinically important issues—issues that will have meaningful impact on clinical care.

The incentives outlined are intended to promote involvement in multicenter studies through reward and reinforcement of that involvement. However, it should also be noted that the pediatric oncology consortia have strict compliance criteria for centers involved in their studies. As described, to remain members of the cooperative groups, participating centers must undergo regular auditing and data-monitoring assessments, and must ensure high rates of compliance with group protocols.

Those centers found, on the basis of these audits or monitoring evaluation, to be out of compliance may not be allowed to continue their participation in group protocols, a repercussion that most centers work hard to avoid. Psychosocial studies that are included in group protocols may benefit from these compliance criteria and attain better and more continued involvement of investigators at the participating sites.

## Help Inform Site Investigators of Institutional Review Board-Related Matters

Significant changes have occurred in how institutions review and oversee research protocols from the perspective of protection of human subjects and protection of health information privacy under federal Health Insurance Portability and Accountability Act regulations. These changes have resulted in significant regulatory requirements for investigators and represent a real challenge for less-experienced investigators.

The cooperative group provides several levels of support in this area. First, the collaborative process allows senior, experienced investigators to mentor younger investigators, often at different institutions, in the process of writing protocols and appropriately addressing human participants concerns. Second, model protocols and informed consent documents and processes developed for one institution can be provided as templates for multiple institutions, thus reducing the amount of duplicative effort for investigators. Finally, review of protocols at multiple institutions may provide opportunity for development of "best-practice" procedures for human participant protection, resulting in better overall science.

## Select Reliable and Effective Evaluation Tools

It has been suggested that there are as many ideas about the "best" approach to evaluation of a particular psychological outcome as there are psychologists (Armstrong & Drotar, 2000). This becomes highly problematic in multicenter research because all sites must collect identical outcome data. Thus, the development of an outcome protocol in multicenter research often represents a compromise between the ideals of the principal investigator and the recognition of several factors that may mitigate against this ideal. In many cases, the compromise will have to consider the availability and practical utility of evaluation tools at each site. This often leads to what has been referred to as a "lowest common denominator" selection process for the evaluation tools. Psychological tests for multicenter studies (particularly the large cooperative group studies) must be available at all sites for the maximal number of sites to participate. Care must be given in selecting the tests to make certain that each center has access to those tests, and that they are skilled in its administration. Obviously, this may result in some more specialized tests needing to be dropped from the research protocol.

Tests should be selected that will remain valid for the duration of the study. This has posed an ongoing problem within collaborative group studies given the frequency with which major psychological tests are revised and new norms established. Unfortunately, recently published tests may not be available or may not have been incorporated by all centers or sites. This problem has been pronounced in the collaborative group when investigators try to decide on appropriate cognitive measures for a study.

One current example can be seen in the use of global intelligence tests in clinical trials. At the time this chapter was written, the fourth edition of the Wechsler Intelligence Scale for Children (WISC-IV) was just released, ultimately to replace the third edition (WISC-III). Previous prospective outcome trials that include serial evaluations have encountered significant problems when test versions are changed in the middle of the study, often resulting in longitudinal assessments that are not directly comparable and that require the use of complex statistical analysis models (e.g., Wang et al., 2001).

Further compounding this issue are expectations and requirements for the use of specific tests by other agencies and institutions, particularly schools and third-party insurers. These third parties sometimes require use of specific tests for placement or reimbursement, leaving the research psychologist to grapple with compliance with study requirements versus using instruments that facilitate clinical placement or reimbursement for services. This is not a simple issue. Standardized collection of research data may ultimately provide the basis for evidence-based decision making regarding assessment and treatment, and failure to follow the research protocol may interfere with the development of informed clinical decision making in the future. Alternatively, rigid adherence to the research protocol may deny individual children access to services deemed appropriate at the time of the evaluation, and this may constitute a participation risk for those children. This remains an area of concern that has not been resolved in the cooperative group setting.

### Develop a Structure for Communication Between Investigators

Throughout the course of the research—from design and development stages through implementation and data acquisition—mechanisms must be established for rapid and accurate communication between investigators at various sites. Fortunately, with the development of electronic mail (e-mail) and other Internet-based resources, this problem has become considerably easier to surmount. Nevertheless, the infrastructure and specific mechanism for this communication must be developed before the study commences, and all participants in the research should be informed of the structure and its use.

One of the more effective means for accomplishing an opportunity for thorough communication between multiple centers and multiple investigators has been the development of a listserv. This automated e-mail distribution mechanism provides a solution to the dual and often-competing needs of maintaining regular communication regarding study-related issues in a confidential environment. Using a listserv, all participating members of the research team will be immediately informed of any concerns or questions raised by any other member of the research team and of all solutions to those questions. The resource costs for setting up and maintaining a listserv on the group's current informatics system are minimal.

## Conclusion

As is evidenced by material covered in previous chapters in this text, psychosocial research in pediatric oncology has advanced dramatically. Psychosocial research findings have in turn influenced the advancement of medical care for children with cancer as well as enhanced the quality of life of cancer patients, survivors, and their family members. Although some of these advances have occurred because of well-executed research studies conducted at single institutions, the number of patients seen at any single institution and the length of time required to collect data on a small sample of patients have led to the necessity of conducting multicenter studies.

Multicenter research has resulted in many of the more substantive advancements in the field. The large-scale research made possible in the pediatric oncology collective groups provides a platform for even more significant growth in our scientific understanding of the psychological issues arising from cancer and its treatment. The benefits accrued in multicenter and collective group studies are not without their challenges, but many of these issues can be addressed through careful planning and attention to the practical issues inherent in the recruitment of large numbers of participants and the involvement of multiple investigators through a geographically dispersed set of participating institutions. As the implementation of multicenter psychosocial research improves, we can anticipate additional advancement in the knowledge base of psychosocial oncology and direct benefits for the patients and families with whom we all work.

*Acknowledgments.* Preparation of this chapter was supported in part by grant funding from the National Cancer Institute for the Children's Oncology Group (U10-CA30969), the Maternal and Child Health Bureau for the Leadership Education in Neurodevelopmental Disabilities program (MCJ-129147-05-05), the American Cancer Society (RSGPB-03-077-01-PBP), and the Administration on Developmental Disabilities Center for Excellence in Developmental Disabilities Education, Research, and Service (90DD0408).

## References

Armstrong, F. D., & Drotar, D. (2000). Multi-institutional and multidisciplinary research collaboration: Strategies and lessons from cooperative trials. In D. Drotar (Ed.), *Handbook of* research *in pediatric and clinical child psychology: Practical strategies and methods* (pp. 281–303). Dordrecht, Netherlands: Kluwer Academic.

Armstrong, F. D., & Reaman, G. H. (2005). Psychological research in childhood cancer: The Children's Oncology Group perspective. *Journal of Pediatric Psychology, 30*, 89–97.

D'Angio, G. J., & Vietti, T. J. (2001). Old man river. The flow of pediatric oncology. *Hematology-Oncology Clinics of North America, 15*(7), 599–607.

Kennedy, C., Kirwan, J., Cook, C., Roux, P., Stulting, A., & Murdoch, I. (2000). Telemedicine techniques can be used to facilitate the conduct of multicentre trials. *Journal of Telemedicine and Telecare, 6*, 343–347.

Krischer, J. P., Hurley, C., Pillalamarri, M., Pant, S., Bleichfeld, C., Opel, M., et al. (1991). An automated patient registration and treatment randomization system for multicenter clinical trials. *Control Clinical Trials, 12*, 367–377.

Liu, L., Krailo, M., Reaman, G. H., & Bernstein, L. (2003). Childhood cancer patients' access to cooperative group cancer programs: A population-based study. *Cancer, 97*, 1339–1345.

Marks, R. G., Conlon, M., & Ruberg, S. J. (2001). Paradigm shifts in clinical trials enabled by information technology. *Statistics in Medicine, 20*, 2683–2696.

Pediatric Oncology Group. (1992). Progress against childhood cancer: The Pediatric Oncology Group experience. *Pediatrics., 89*(4, Pt. 1), 597–600.

Pollock, B. H. (1994). Quality assurance for interventions in clinical trials. Multicenter data monitoring, data management, and analysis. *Cancer, 74*(9, Suppl.), 2647–2652.

Progress against childhood cancer: The Pediatric Oncology Group experience. (1992). *Pediatrics, 89*(4, Pt. 1), 597–600.

Ross, J. A., Severson, R. K., Pollock, B. H., & Robison, L. L. (1996). Childhood cancer in the United States. A geographical analysis of cases from the Pediatric Cooperative Clinical Trials groups. *Cancer, 77*, 201–207.

Wang, W., Enos, L., Gallagher, D., Thompson, R. J., Jr., Guarini, L., Vichinsky, E., et al. (2001). Neuropsychologic performance in school-aged children with sickle cell disease: A report from the Cooperative Study of Sickle Cell Disease. *Journal of Pediatrics, 139*, 391–397.

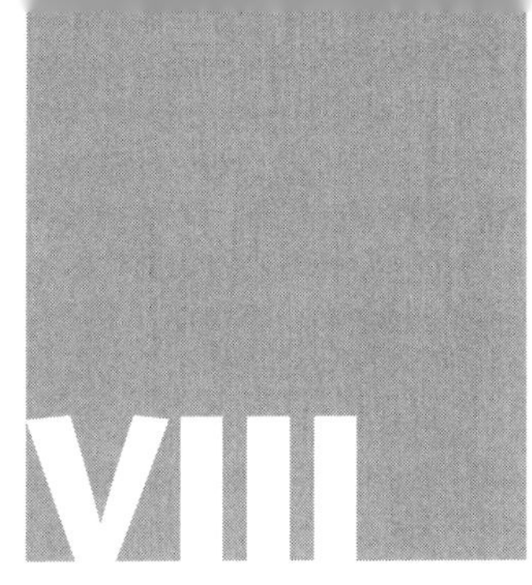


# Prospective and Retrospective View of Pediatric Hematology/Oncology

John J. Spinetta, Giuseppe Masera, and Momcilo Jankovic

# A Prospective and Retrospective View of Pediatric Hematology/Oncology

How does one help a family whose child has been diagnosed with a life-threatening illness? It is a deceptively simple question with complicated answers.

This brief chapter is not meant to be a history of biopsychosocial pediatric oncology, and it does not cover every theme. The explosion of studies on children with cancer over these past decades (Pizzo & Poplack, 2001) renders a retrospective look formidable and subjective. The sole purpose of this retrospective examination into the earliest beginnings is to place into context some of the main themes that have appeared over the past years, so that they can serve as a foundation for our recommendations for future intervention and research in the field. That is our assigned task. Much of the review reflects personal respective experiences beginning in the late 1960s. The chapters that form this volume, written by many of the most experienced psychosocial researchers who have brought the field so far forward over these many years, are the state of the art, tell us where we have been most recently, and tell us in greater detail where we are at the moment.

Where does our psychosocial history begin? What have we done these past many years to help the children and their families cope with the illness and its treatment? With due awareness of the subjectivity and inevitable unfairness of our venture, we undertake the task with due apologies for any omissions that may occur in this retrospective review. As we begin to look in some detail at the main themes formed over the past four decades, we place our review into the context of four preambles: a multidisciplinary and international effort; an alliance between physicians and parents; research and service; and a sharing of the research wealth with economically struggling countries.

## Preamble One: A Multidisciplinary and International Effort

From the earliest years, the effort to care for the child with cancer has been multidisciplinary, multi-institutional, and international, involving a highly cooperative and collaborative effort of physicians, nurses, psychologists, social workers, and allied health care professionals working together across national borders. When, at the beginning, physicians treating the children found themselves struggling with the psychological and social repercussions of the cancer on their young dying patients and their families—issues that ranged far beyond their medical expertise and training—they turned to psychosocial practitioners for help in dealing with these broader human concerns. The pediatric oncologists and hematologists from countries throughout the world began asking for cooperative input from psychiatrists, social workers, nursing care specialists, and psychologists. To the credit of all involved, this cooperative multidisciplinary, multi-institutional, and international effort has been from the very earliest years and continues to be the hallmark of the treatment of childhood cancer (Hewitt, Weiner, & Simone, 2003). The chapters throughout this volume attest to the continuing cooperative multi-institutional and multidisciplinary effort. At the end of each thematic summary, we quote from the series of guidelines written by the International Society of Pediatric Oncology's Psychosocial Committee, for which we have served as chair (Masera) and cochairs (Jankovic and Spinetta) for the past dozen years, and its medical and psychosocial members come from nations worldwide (Masera et al., 1993).

## Preamble Two: An Alliance Between Physicians and Parents

It was clear from the beginning that a hospital health care team could not do it all. As physicians began to modify their protective stance toward the parents regarding patient care and the openness of communication, parents were invited increasingly to participate actively in their child's medical, psychological, and social care. The parents were brought in as part of the decision-making process and support system. Thus began a healthy, cooperative, and open alliance between the parents and the members of the health care team, including the establishment of parent groups for self-help and for raising supplementary and critical funding (Masera, Spinetta, et al., 1998).

## Preamble Three: Research and Service

The primary psychosocial concern in child cancer care has been to help the children and their families cope with the diagnosis of cancer and its aftermath. In the early years, the physicians would typically refer to the division of psychiatry those children and their parents who appeared to have had the most difficult time in coping with the illness. Something had to be done to assist the children and their families. Those professionals, trained in dealing with mental illness, were the first to be called to duty. As psychosocial personnel, we were viewed as firemen and firewomen, at the ready to put out the pathological flames. Even as we became more active members of the health care team, working in the cancer unit, our role continued to center around psychopathology.

Then, we came to realize that the rest of the children and their families, the great majority of whom were struggling with the new diagnosis but who did not show signs of falling apart, also needed our support. As psychosocial team members began facing the unique challenges inherent in the biopsychosocial study of children with cancer and their families, the practice of psychosocial intervention itself took on a new definition. As psychology health care specialists, we began to apply our measurement and research training to the study of issues that practicing pediatric oncologists found pressing: how effectively to help mentally healthy children whose lives had been suddenly turned upside down with the diagnosis of a life-threatening illness. The role of psychology practitioners began to move forward from the view of psychological therapy as helping those suffering from traditional mental illnesses to what would eventually become the field of pediatric psychology and its counterparts in the allied disciplines of nursing and social work (Roberts, 2003).

But physicians did not want the families to wait for intervention until researchers could determine which intervention worked most effectively and validly. What about the immediate needs of the children currently under treatment? Wouldn't it be far better at least to do something to help, even if the intervention had not yet proved to be valid and effective? Thus began the most serious challenge to the psychosocial team, a dilemma that continues to this day: How does one help the child and family who have an immediate here-and-now need for support while pursuing scientifically valid controlled research designed to sort out effective from ineffective interventions? From the beginning then, psychosocial team members working with the children with cancer and their families have worn two hats: of the practitioner and of the researcher.

### Preamble Four: A Sharing of the Research Wealth With Economically Struggling Countries

As we have progressed since the 1960s from the diagnosis of childhood cancer as a death sentence to today's average cure rate approaching 80%, we have come to appreciate the fact that until recently such an enormous success was available to fewer than one fourth of the children with cancer throughout the world. Physicians in the poorer countries—mostly in Asia, Africa, and Latin America—found that their limited resources and inadequate health care infrastructures and training left them ill prepared for the task of treating childhood cancer. Thanks to the generosity and concern of pediatric oncologists from the medically advanced countries, notably from the United States, Europe, and Japan, up-to-date training and financial resources have been made available to physicians from developing countries to help spread further the latest research findings on the treatment of childhood cancer. Many individual childhood cancer centers have taken it on their own to contact other individual centers in Latin America, Asia, and Africa (Global Alliance, 2004; Masera, Baez, et al., 1998; Masera & Biondi, 1999; Naafs-Wilstra et al., 2001). The Pediatric Oncology for Developing Countries program of the International Society of Pediatric Oncology has become an organized clearinghouse for center-to-center twinning efforts to help spread the best childhood cancer research around the world.

Within the context of these four preambles, we begin our retrospective review.

### The Earliest Question, One of Service: Talk to the Child or Not?

During the 1950s and 1960s, the years in which the medical subspecialty of pediatric hematology/oncology came to life, the diagnosis of childhood cancer was typically a diagnosis of impending death. The earliest comments on the psychological reactions of children with cancer that made an appreciable impact were observational, with the physicians who were treating the child and their psychosocial counterparts attempting to bring into focus how best to help the family face the death of the child.

Although many cancer centers began to implement programs for helping the parents cope, very little was done with the patients themselves. There were some programs for teens, but few for the younger children. In fact, no one really knew for sure how much the younger children knew about their illness. The typical approach that was recommended was one of caution when talking to the teenagers and of protective deception when dealing with the younger children. It was thought that, because the fatally ill child under 10 lacked the intellectual ability to formulate a concept of death, the child was not aware of his impending demise, and if the adult did not discuss the issue of the seriousness of the illness with the child, the child would experience little or no anxiety related to the illness.

The earliest written comments reflected this position. Richmond and Waisman (1955) discussed the fatally ill children as reacting to their illness with an air of passive resignation and acceptance, rarely manifesting an overt concern about death. Natterson and Knudson (1960) allowed that anxiety about death might be present in a subtle form in younger children but concluded that only the oldest children actually revealed anxiety or apprehension related to their impending death. In fact, the majority of the authors at the time, following developmental norms of the era, agreed that the older child with a fatal prognosis, especially the adolescent, could be aware of and anxious about impending death, but that the child under 6 years of age was most concerned with separation, and the child from 6 to 10 was most fearful of physical injury and mutilation. An exceptional younger child might be capable of experiencing death anxiety, but in general, fatally ill children were not thought to experience anxiety related to death until well after 10 years of age (Easson, 1970; Evans & Edin, 1968; Friedman, Chodoff, Mason, & Hamburg, 1963; Furman, 1964; Hamovitch, 1964; Morrissey, 1963; Schowalter, 1970; Sigler, 1970; Wiener, 1970).

### The First Major Research Question: Did the Children Know They Were Dying?

The early practitioners initiated research into this arena by focusing on overt expressions concerning impending death as the primary indicators of the child's anxiety. One of the first studies to tackle this issue of what the younger children knew or did not know that dealt directly with the children themselves in a scientifically rigorous manner, rather than merely observing the child, was that of Eugenia Waechter (1971). A nurse-researcher, Waechter in the late 1960s used a set of pictures requesting stories from the children and eliciting indirect and fantasy expression of the child's concern for present and future body integrity and functioning. Waechter (1971) reported a higher number of overtly expressed death themes and a greater degree of concerns with threat to and intrusion into their bodies among the children with cancer than among the comparison controls. She demonstrated that children aged 6 to 10 years with a fatal prognosis not only were aware that they were dying, but also could express that awareness by actual use of words related to death.

Waechter's work provided scientific support to those few of her colleagues who toward the end of the 1960s believed many of the fatally ill children in the group 6–10 years old, if not aware at a conceptual level of their own impending death, were aware at least that something very serious was happening to them (Binger et al., 1969). Among the physicians who believed from their interactions with the children that the younger children did know at some level of understanding that they were dying was Myron Karon (Karon & Vernick, 1968), a pediatric oncologist who in 1969 had just arrived at Children's Hospital of Los Angeles. When the pioneer research of Waechter and her colleagues came to his attention, Karon asked the chief psychologist, David Rigler, if there were additional ways of clearly demonstrating the fact that the younger children could become aware of the fatality of their illness.

Rigler and a young intern took up the challenge, applying rigorous scientific methods, without relying on overt expressions about death, to test the hypothesis that fatally ill children 6 to 10 years old were aware of their impending death (Spinetta, Rigler, & Karon, 1973, 1974). Expanding on Waechter's work, they devised a three-dimensional replica of the children's hospital rooms and asked the children to tell stories about each of four figurines (doctor, nurse, mother, father), which the children placed into the three-dimensional replica. The children related significantly more stories that showed preoccupation with threat to and intrusion into their body functioning than did the chronically ill control children, expressed both more hospital-related anxiety and non-hospital-related anxiety than did the chronically ill children, and placed the four significant figures further away from them in the bed than did the chronically ill children, the distance increasing as the children got closer to their death, reflective of a growing sense of psychological separation of the dying child from the people around them. Thinking that they were protecting their children from further pain by not discussing their impending death, the parents and staff were inadvertently isolating the children and letting them die psychologically alone.

It was clear from these pioneer studies that, despite efforts to keep the children with cancer from becoming aware of the prognosis, the children somehow developed a sense that the illness was very serious and very threatening. Not only were the fatally ill 6- to 10-year-old children concerned about their illness, their fears and anxieties were real, painful, and very much associated with the seriousness of the illness that they were experiencing. Most important, it was shown that a rigorous scientific method could be applied in a nonobtrusive manner in a direct study of what children were experiencing and in determining children's mode of communicating their awareness.

With his intuitive experience so strongly supported, in 1972 Karon applied for and received a major grant from the National Cancer Institute to study exclusively the psychosocial aspects of children with cancer and their families. Despite Karon's untimely death soon after receiving the grant, the door had been opened to the importance of incorporating rigorous research on psychosocial interventions in the treatment of childhood cancer. The National Cancer Institute expanded its funding throughout the 1970s, initiating a fertile multidisciplinary period of research around the United States and Europe on psychosocial intervention for children with cancer and their families.

## The Main Research Themes

As medical treatments for childhood cancer became more effective and the multidisciplinary researchers began applying measurement and research skills to the study of psychosocial interventions, the research questions broadened. As stated clearly throughout this review, the chapters that form this volume detail the most recent underpinnings and precedents of current research and state their histories in today's language. Our task in this chapter is to pull together and integrate the earliest work. The following are the key themes as they have appeared over the years: open communication and family coping; living a normal life by going back to school; pain control using playrooms, doll play, and self-hypnosis; long-term survivors and extended late effects; the once-forgotten siblings; death revisited; consent, compliance, and alternative treatments; burnout; and methodological issues.

## Open Communication and Family Coping

Communicating the diagnosis and how best to do it became the first step in a communicative process and relationship that involved the medical team and the family and that allowed for growth and change over time. As the evidence mounted that the children, siblings, and parents would be best served by being encouraged to bring into the open their anxieties about the illness and its possible consequences, studies devoted greater attention to how parents and medical personnel communicated with the child (Bluebond-Langner, 1977, 1978). The initial diagnosis came to be viewed as a model for all future interchanges of information between the medical professionals and families and between the family members themselves, especially between parent and child (Jankovic, Loiacono, et al., 1994).

As the families of the children diagnosed with cancer struggled to face the new emotional crisis that was challenging the relationships among the family members and the very balance of family life, researchers began to study ways of strengthening the families' coping skills (Kagen-Goodheart, 1977; Kupst et al., 1982; Sourkes, 1977). Aware of the continuing anxieties experienced by the children and their families, G. P. Koocher and O'Malley (1981) researched ways of alleviating that anxiety and offering the type of support the children and families were seeking in specific ways that were most important to the children and families at a given moment.

Basic to effective family coping was the belief that communication of both happy and painful thoughts and feelings, by the parents and by the children, is a healthier state of mental well-being than retaining thought in silence. This belief became a prerequisite to mutual support among family members. It was found that families who allowed open discussion of the illness and its prognosis were able to cope more effectively with the illness within their own family and were able to give and receive the support of other parents in the clinic (Adams, 1980; Kellerman, 1980; Morrow, Hoagland, & Morse, 1982; Mulhern, Crisco, & Camitta, 1981; Slavin, O'Malley, Koocher, & Foster, 1982; Sourkes, 1977; Spinetta & Deasy-Spinetta, 1981; Zeltzer, Kellerman, Ellenberg, Dash, & Rigler, 1980). Today, we take for granted the importance of open communication (Eden, Black, & Emery, 1993; Masera et al., 2003; Masera, Chesler, et al., 1997).

## Living a Normal Life: Back to School

As treatments for childhood cancer became more widely effective, studies began to focus on children treated as outpatients. Although studies demonstrated that the children continued to be aware of the seriousness of their illness (Spinetta & Maloney, 1975), the children dwelled less and less on their illness and were able, while in remission, to live a relatively normal life, somewhat free of their concerns about their illness.

Improvements in the ability of medical care made it possible for children diagnosed with cancer to live longer and, in increasing frequency, to be cured. As children lived and grew older with the disease, parents and professionals realized that they had to help the children face not only the medical concerns that impinged on their child's health and cure, but also the educational and social concerns that accompany typical growth and development. It was not sufficient for young people simply to survive what was once a life-threatening illness. Survival meant that the children had to continue to be educated toward one day becoming fully functioning adult members of society (Lansky, Cairns, & Zwartjes, 1983; Lansky, Lowman, Vats, & Gyulay, 1975).

Thus, parents and professionals faced the increasing responsibility of promoting sound academic and social development as the children went through the treatment process. Attention turned toward the normalizing influence of school.

Programs were developed to help the children return to their typical life as school children, and teachers were trained to treat the children as normally as possible (Chesler & Barbarin, 1987; Deasy-Spinetta, 1980, 1989; Katz, Kellerman, Rigler, Williams, & Siegel, 1977; Masera, Jankovic, Deasy-Spinetta, et al., 1995; Spinetta & Deasy-Spinetta, 1986; van Dongen-Melman et al., 1995).

Today, we take for granted the advice that the family members, children and parents, should continue living as normal a life as the treatments permit (Masera, Jankovic, et al., 1997). We know now that we cannot freeze children for years during treatment while their peers continue to grow and develop, leaving the children with cancer developmentally far behind and in a catch-up mode. We now prepare children for their future. Not only do we give priority to the children continuing to live a normal life during the course of treatment, but also we have in fact come to view childhood cancer as a golden opportunity for the children to learn skills in coping that can give them a running start on their preparation for engaging in a fully functioning adulthood (Parry, 2002; Spinetta, in press).

### Pain Control: Playrooms, Doll Play, and Self-Hypnosis

Researchers began to examine ways of helping the children respond to the treatments less passively and more proactively, with less pain and more equanimity. The earliest child-specific approach was that of helping the child to undergo treatment with the least amount of anxiety and the most support for coping (Hilgard & Le Baron, 1984; Jacobsen et al., 1990; Jay & Elliott, 1990; Jay, Ozolins, Elliott, & Caldwell, 1983; Katz, Kellerman, & Siegel, 1980; Kellerman, Zeltzer, Ellenberg, & Dash, 1983; Walker, 1989; Zeltzer & Le Baron, 1986). As medical procedures advanced, the application of these support strategies—pain control, hypnosis, preparation, doll play, parent training—have become an integral part of childhood cancer treatment programs. The multicenter problem-solving/skills-training studies of Sahler et al. (2005) and Walco (2005) are a testament not only to how far we have come in involving children actively in the control of physical and psychological pain, but also to the cooperative multicentered multidisciplinary effort entailed.

### Long-Term Survivors and Extended Late Effects

How well were the children responding to the increasingly successful treatments? Centers began developing follow-up programs for survivors to measure any potential treatment sequelae (Boman & Bodegard, 2000; Boman, Lindhal, & Bjork, 2003; Kazak & Meadows, 1989; Kupst & Schulman, 1988; Meadows et al., 1993; Meadows, McKee, & Kazak, 1989; Nesbit, Krivit, Robison, & Hammond, 1979; Spinetta, Murphy, Vik, Day, & Mott, 1989; Zeltzer et al., 1980). Programs oriented to the needs of the long-term survivor began when the child went off therapy, with centers focusing on the sequelae specific to each form of illness, treatment, toxicity, and future problems specific to each child's needs. Centers began offering counseling programs for the more serious medical and psychosocial problems, adapted to the need of each individual and local culture. Specialty clinics began to develop, managed by the pediatric oncologist who treated the children and having available a full range of adult and young adult specialists as consulting physicians. Each long-term survivor was monitored for special conditions related to his or her unique history as well as their age-specific developmental concerns. Programs began to include psychological counseling for the survivors experiencing adjustment difficulties and significant adverse side effects from chemotherapy or radiation. Even though the majority of survivors and their families were found to be psychologically healthy, proactive and preventive care programs for all of the families have become routine (Eden, Harrison, Richards, Lilleyman, Bailey, Chessells, et al., 2000; Hewitt et al., 2003; Masera, Jankovic, et al., 1997; Stuber, 1996; Zebrack et al., 2002).

Throughout this time, psychology researchers began to develop instruments for the study of issues specific to children with cancer. As they began to apply these instruments, one of the first problems of which the researchers became increasingly aware was the effect of treatment on the academic functioning of the children. Studies began to assess patterns and difficulties of socially adaptive behavior in the children and, most important, began to document evidence of a strong link between the use of cranial radiation and subsequent learning deficits (Eiser, 1978; Jankovic, Brouwers, et al., 1994; Meadows et al.,

1981; Moss, Nannis, & Poplack, 1981; Pfefferbaum-Levine et al., 1984; Robison et al., 1984).

In addition, researchers found that, as a group, children with cancer functioned at less socially adapted levels in school than peers and had a tendency not to reach out to others, not to initiate activities, not to try new things, and not to express feelings freely. The children retained a self-protective attitude. So, in addition to already being devastated by the emotional stresses associated with a child having cancer and undergoing what to them were extraordinary medical treatments, the parents discovered that the cognitive toxicities of the therapy (i.e., radiation, chemotherapy) placed a large group of the children at a higher risk not only for learning difficulties, but also for subsequent adaptive behavioral problems (Adamoli et al., 1997; Deasy-Spinetta, Spinetta, & Oxman, 1989; Fritz, Williams, & Amylon, 1988).

As medicine continues to achieve an increasingly higher success rate in long-term survival, the cooperative study groups are following survivors for longer periods of time to determine further potential long-term sequelae of treatments used for these children (Eden et al., 2000; Hewitt et al., 2003; Masera et al., 1996; Zebrack et al., 2002).

## The Once-Forgotten Siblings

From the earliest intervention periods, the health care team members had all they could do, first to focus on the needs of the children with cancer, and then on the needs of the parents. The parents were overwhelmed by their concerns for the sick child, giving their immediate and full attention to the medical treatment of their sick child. Without any ill intention on the part of already-overburdened parents, siblings were often inadvertently ignored. They suffered (Binger, 1973; Gogan, Koocher, Foster, & O'Malley, 1977; Sourkes, 1981). Today, siblings are no longer forgotten (Spinetta et al., 1999).

## Death Revisited

Despite the remarkable growth in the percentage of cures and the increasing sense of hope given to newly diagnosed children and their families, many of the children are not able to be cured. Death for some remains a reality (Rando, 1983, 1984; Sahler, 1978). There are three periods of time surrounding this final phase of life that have become the subjects of research. The first is the period when treatment was judged to be no longer effective and the difficult decision made to move from curative intent to the palliative phase of care. The second is the period from the beginning of palliative care to the death of the child. The third is after the child dies, with staff counseling the parents in their grief following the death of their child.

During the palliative phase, the key issues that have become central are the duration and quality of remaining life and the rights of the child to careful, compassionate management with the best palliative care the staff can provide. Along with the extended health care team, the parents of the child have become more actively involved in the decision-making process at the point of transition to the terminal phase. As the child nears death, concern has shifted to ensuring that the child would die without unnecessary physical pain, fear, or anxiety. Whatever the state of the child entering the terminal phase of the illness, it became essential that he or she receive adequate medical, spiritual, and psychological support, and that the child at no point feel abandoned either by the health care team or by the family (Davies, Spinetta, Martinson, McClowry, & Kulenkamp, 1986; Jankovic et al., 1989; Masera et al., 1999; Sourkes, 1996; Spinetta, Swarner, & Sheposh, 1981; Stuber & Mesrkhani, 2001).

During the earliest years, the children died in the hospital. It gradually became evident during the 1980s that many of the children might die more peacefully at home. With the health care team continuing to control emerging symptoms (either directly or through other supportive services, such as home care units and visiting nurses), the parents who wished to have their children die at home or in a hospice setting were given the support to allow them to do so (Martinson, 1979, 1993; Martinson et al., 1977).

After the child dies, hospitals have offered bereavement counseling on the part of physicians and nurses to help clarify past care and guide future grieving. Parents and siblings, when appropriate, have been invited to discuss with the physician both the level of care and the surviving family members' current needs. Health care teams have encouraged bereaved parents and siblings to initiate self-help groups (Jankovic et al., 1989).

## Consent, Compliance, and Alternative Treatments

At the start, compliance with the medical regimens was an unquestioned assumption. How could parents not do all they could to cure their child of the life-threatening cancer? As we began to listen more carefully to the parents, we found that there were many situations that could lead a parent toward noncompliance: the patient's physical discomfort, the parents' fear of losing their parenting role, inadequate information on the child's disease, and uncertainty about the merits of medication, most especially when the child had a recurrence or relapse. As we invited parents more and more to enter into the decision-making process with us, we were able to clarify misunderstandings regarding the illness and treatment (Spinetta et al., 2002). A truly valid informed consent demands no less (Spinetta et al., 2003; Stuber, 1996). A full and adequate explanation from the start can help keep parents from seeking harmful alternative treatments (Jankovic et al., 2004).

## Burnout

In the early years, when so many of the children died, professionals working with the children were very reluctant to admit to one another that treating children with cancer over a long period could have a profound negative effect on staff and could lead to burnout. We lived within a professional culture of never being allowed to complain. We have since become aware of the health benefits in admitting openly to one another that burnout can be caused by the nature of the work itself. Dealing on a daily basis with life-threatening illness, having to assume the emotional burdens of the patients and their families, and seeing many children die can be causes of burnout, especially in susceptible individuals (J. Koocher, 1980; Storlie, 1979). In its more moderate forms, burnout can lead to a loss of energy and dissatisfaction with work. In its more severe forms, burnout can lead to seriously compromised interactions in the work setting with the children and with fellow workers and to disruption of the professional's home life.

Suggestions for prevention and remediation range from modifications in the work environment to maintaining a healthy balance between professional and private life (Spinetta et al., 2000). One serious cause of burnout in the clinic staff are the small-in-number but very-great-in-need families who bring to the diagnosis sufficiently severe premordid problems in adjustment that they typically exhaust the patience and abilities of the clinic team. An effective method for reducing staff burnout is to sort out this small-but-needy percentage of families from the beginning and refer them to out-of-clinic support for their prediagnosis problems (for example, to outside counseling services). Not only can this approach better prepare the families to cope with the treatments, but also it can free up valuable time and energy for the clinic staff to allow them to deal with the remainder of the families. In addition, the health care team members can study the differences in the coping strategies used successfully by the best adapted of the families and develop programs that can help teach some of these skills to the least well adapted of the families once these most-needy families receive the extra outside help they need to deal with prediagnosis problems (Masera, Jankovic, et al., 1997).

## Methodological Issues

As psychosocial researchers began their studies of children with cancer and their families, they struggled with the problem of losing sight of the individual child and family while trying to reach normative conclusions. If the goal of a health care professional's work with the children and their families was to help strengthen the adaptive capabilities specific to each family and to each member of the family, then both research and intervention should be taking into account intraindividual strategies. As they developed new methods of study that combined the best qualities of both intraindividual and normative research strategies, researchers began to find effective ways of understanding individual coping strategies and how to intervene to strengthen them (Kazak, 1993; G. P. Koocher & O'Malley, 1981; Kupst et al., 1982).

Researchers found as well that many of the instruments that had been developed for other purposes, although standardized, often were not able to measure the problems at hand. The use of instruments that had been developed for participants with pathology were inappropriate for studying normally developing children undergoing psychological reactions to the stress event of cancer or for studying their parents. Some of the available instruments specific to children may have been strong yet ill-suited to the study of children with cancer, while those instruments developed specifically to test the problems of children with cancer had first to be standardized to be useful for the research. Further, the most commonly used and most highly standardized instruments typically measured only long-standing qualities of the children. It became essential to develop instruments that would be able to take into account the ongoing changes the child with cancer would undergo depending on disease stage or nondisease factors, such as increasing age with its accompanying changes in the child's level of development (Spinetta, 1984; van Dongen-Melman, DeGroot, Hahlem, & Verhulst, 1996).

The successful progress in updating and fine-tuning research instruments is well demonstrated in the chapters of this book.

## Recommendations for the Future

These are the main themes as we see them, from their earliest beginnings, forming and developing over the years, and continuing actively into the present, as attested to in the chapters throughout this book. Psychosocial interventions have become so fully incorporated into the care of children with cancer that they are now considered not just an appendage, but a critical component and, in some cases, standard of care in the care of the child with cancer.

Where do we go from here? The most detailed and specifically focused recommendations for the future are already clearly drawn at the end of each of the preceding chapters of this book, underscoring the multidisciplinary, multi-institutional, and international cooperative effort that has made the extraordinary biopsychosocial research advances possible. What we recommend in the following suggestions are process rather than content themes.

1. As we health care professionals become more experienced in dealing with the children with cancer and their families, we cannot forget that for each newly diagnosed family, it is truly all brand new. We cannot let our age and experience immunize us from the empathy and understanding the families need and have a right to as they find themselves entering this new and, to them, shocking world of cancer. Each case is individual. We should continue to bring to the newly diagnosed children and their family a fresh sensitivity that acknowledges the newness of their experience.
2. Children, even the youngest, sense the seriousness of their illness. They discern the fears and anxieties of the adults around them. They do their best to communicate with us, at all ages. Even the youngest try to talk to us, often without words, often just by their body language. How well do we listen? Do we truly listen? We need to develop more effective ways of attending to what the children are experiencing and their mode of communicating that awareness.
3. Many of our interventions have proceeded far ahead of our success in measuring their effectiveness. While many new instruments have been developed and older instruments have been creatively applied specific to the study of the children and their families, we need to continue this creative effort and plunge more deeply into the study of the effectiveness of our interventions.
4. Parent groups are critical to the continued success of each clinic's efforts, not only by forming support services for one another on mutual psychosocial needs, but also as importantly in teaming with physicians in raising funds to keep the clinic up to date and growing both in research and in intervention. Health care professionals and parents should strengthen their alliance, making it a priority to continue sharing decision making, not only in individual cases, but also in parental support of the clinic's growth.
5. Among the newly diagnosed families, there will be a small percentage—15% or so—who bring with them prediagnosis problems that can seriously interfere with the child's treatment. We should continue to develop ways to help identify these families at the very beginning so that we can refer them for the extra psychosocial help that they will need to cope with the demands of treatment. With our remaining

resources, we will then be better able to help the families who bring with them a stronger history of coping abilities and who are less encumbered by long-standing behavioral, social, financial, or legal problems.

6. Burnout is a very serious possibility for those working with children with cancer and their families. It is not easy always to be giving one's full attention and empathy to the children and their families, over many months and years. Acknowledging this very real fact and talking about it openly within the health care team can help prevent serious burnout and alleviate the milder and more subtle forms of burnout. Further research and intervention would be most helpful in this much neglected, albeit important, area.
7. Although there is an ongoing need for professionals to publish their findings in refereed journals, it is equally important to translate these findings into readable, clear, and simple booklets or pamphlets for the children, for their parents, and for their teachers. We owe it to the children and their families to continue developing clear and simply written booklets that can help explain some of the complexities of the treatment in ways that they can understand.
8. Much of our psychosocial long-term follow-up study during these past years has focused on potential negative sequelae of the illness and how best to prevent or ameliorate them. The next step in helping the children as they grow into adulthood should be to focus on the potential for growth associated with their illness. The children who are becoming young adults, by overcoming their illness, have a golden opportunity to develop their skills in coping and learning to deal with future life's problems as they enter adulthood (Parry, 2002; Spinetta, 2005; Stuber, 2005).
9. It is essential that pediatric psychosocial researchers continue to maintain a balance between research and intervention efforts. The critical need for the children and parents as a group is that our knowledge grow through our research efforts; the critical need for the individual child and family going through the treatment process is that we be present and attentive to their immediate and pressing individual needs and concerns.
10. Formal therapy should be practiced only by individuals trained to do so. Problems in living that demand a trained therapist should remain in the domain of that trained therapist, just as medical questions should be raised with the treating physician. However, sometimes the child or mother or father may find that they have a greater rapport and ease of communication with someone other than the assigned psychosocial team member. There are times, for example, when the psychosocial person assigned to a family may try to no avail to establish a rapport with a particular child or mother or father, only to find that the child or mother or father talks to the midnight shift nurse by the hour. Or, after failing to communicate with a family member after a long one-to-one counseling session, the assigned psychosocial person may find that the physician has been able to make major psychosocial strides with the same family member with a few brief comments. Rather than become confounded or jealous from such common occurrences, those of us who are the assigned psychiatrist, psychologist, or social worker should feel complimented that our presence on the health care team has had such a profound impact on the ambience of the treatment center that the child, mother, or father feels free to share their common human concerns with the member of the team with whom they feel the most comfortable. Our goal now and in the future should be to continue to support the families in their seeking to discuss the nonmedical aspect of the illness with the team member with whom they are most comfortable.
11. Medicine advances most effectively by narrowing its scope. Psychology advances by broadening its scope and generalizing to theory. Both are necessary in the treatment of the child with cancer. As we continue to develop the research and intervention efforts with the children with oncological and hematological illnesses, we have seen our biopsychosocial efforts become a model for the increasing integration of the psychosocial in the management of children and adolescents with a variety of chronic illnesses (Roberts, 2003). We should continue to disseminate our research

and intervention findings among pediatric practitioners who are negotiating similar issues in different settings and with different chronic childhood illnesses.

12. The area of applied research and intervention that in our opinion remains the most pressing is the sharing of our knowledge and funding with the less economically advantaged countries. Only one of four children with cancer in the world today have access to the 80% cure rates that are common in the medically advanced countries. With relatively little expenditure of funds and effort, the high cure rates can be brought to significantly more of the children with cancer in today's world who do not have access to that level of treatment. Some of the twinning programs described here, with single institutions from the developed countries helping single institutions from some of the poorer countries, can serve both as an example of how to share knowledge and resources and as a stimulus to begin similar programs among institutions not already participating. The need is great; the price is one of personal effort, time, and generosity; the outcome will bring hope to children who today have no hope.

## Summary and Conclusion

We have come a long way since the early beginnings. Over the past several decades, pediatric health care team professionals have approached from a variety of perspectives the question of how to help the children and their families in negotiating the cancer experience. We have approached the issue from the point of view of medicine and biology and from the perspective of family adjustment and coping. We have studied the illness at the point of diagnosis, during the course of treatment, and after treatment is completed. We have dealt with the illness in remission and when the course takes unexpected turns. We have shown that the family's premorbid emotional or physical state affects how the child responds to the treatment process, and we have intervened to help the neediest of the families. We have studied which families engage in nonadherence to treatment demands, and we have tried to reduce that number. We have investigated interventions ranging from very specifically focused behavioral management of pain to the broadly focused role of philosophy and spirituality in helping the family cope. We have studied survivors living with the long-term effects of treatments, and we have determined that one can lead a normal life despite serious physical late effects. We have supported the children through the dying process and tried our best to help the families in their grief. Over the years, we have applied increasingly more rigorous measurements to test the effectiveness of our interventions, and we have tried to do so as nonobtrusively as possible.

As the medical treatment of childhood cancer has moved from an inevitable death sentence to an 80% cure rate, the importance of including the psychosocial in the treatment of the children has now been so integrated that the majority of the pediatric cancer centers now conceptualize treatment as a biopsychosocial process. We have arrived at long last to the fulfillment of what many years ago van Eys (1977) called "the truly cured child"—the child cured medically, psychologically, and socially—what we now refer to as the integrated and interactive biopsychosocial cure of the child with cancer.

## References

Adamoli, L., Deasy-Spinetta, P., Corbetta, A., Jankovic, M., Lia, R., Locati, A., et al. (1997). School functioning for the child with leukemia in continuous first remission: Screening high risk children. *Pediatric Hematology and Oncology, 14*, 121–131.

Adams, D. W. (1980). *Childhood malignancy: The psychosocial care of the child and his family*. Springfield, IL: Thomas.

Binger, C. (1973). Childhood leukemia: Emotional impact on the siblings. In E. J. Anthony & E. Koupernick (Eds.), *The child and his family: Impact of disease and death* (Vol. 2). New York, NY: Wiley.

Binger, C., Ablin, A., Feuerstein, R., Kushner, J., Zoger, S., & Mikkelen, C. (1969). Childhood leukemia: Emotional impact on family. *New England Journal of Medicine, 280*, 414–418.

Bluebond-Langner, M. (1977). Meanings of death to children. In H. Feifel (Ed.), *New meanings of death*. New York: McGraw-Hill.

Bluebond-Langner, M. (1978). *The private worlds of dying children.* Princeton, NJ: Princeton University Press.

Boman, K., & Bodegard, G. (2000). Long-term coping in childhood cancer survivors: Influence of illness, treatment, and demographic background factors. *Acta Paediatrica, 89*, 105–111.

Boman, K., Lindhal, A. & Bjork, O. (2003). Disease-related distress in parents of children with cancer at various stages after the time of diagnosis. *Acta Oncologica, 42*, 137–146.

Chesler, M. A., & Barbarin, O. A. (1987). *Childhood cancer and the family*. New York: Brunner/Mazel.

Davies, B., Spinetta, J. J., Martinson, I., McClowry, S., & Kulenkamp, E. (1986). Manifestations of levels of functioning in grieving families. *Journal of Family Issues, 7*, 297–313.

Deasy-Spinetta, P., & Spinetta, J. J. (1980). The child with cancer in school: Teachers' appraisal. *American Journal of Pediatric Hematology/Oncology*, 2, 89–94.

Deasy-Spinetta, P., & Spinetta, J. J. (1989). Educational issues in the rehabilitation of long-term survivors. In P. A. Pizzo & D. G. Poplack (Eds.), *Principles and practice of pediatric oncology*. Philadelphia: Lippincott.

Deasy-Spinetta, P., Spinetta, J. J., & Oxman, J. B. (1989). The relationship between learning deficits and social adaptation in children with leukemia. *Journal of Psychosocial Oncology*, 6, 109–121.

Easson, W. M. (1970). *The dying child: The management of the child or adolescent who is dying*. Springfield, IL: Thomas.

Eden, O. B., Black, I., & Emery, A. E. (1993). The use of taped parental interviews to improve communication with childhood cancer families. *Pediatric Hematology and Oncology, 10*, 157–162.

Eden, O. B., Harrison, G., Richards, S., Lilleyman, J. S., Bailey, C. C., Chessells, J. M., et al. (2000). Long-term follow-up of the United Kingdom Medical Research Council protocols for childhood acute lymphoblastic leukaemia, 1980–1997. *Leukemia, 14*, 2307–2320.

Eiser, C. (1978). Intellectual abilities among survivors of childhood leukemia as a function of CNS irradiation. *Archives of Diseases of Childhood, 53*, 391–395.

Evans, A. E., & Edin, S. (1968). If a child must die. *New England Journal of Medicine, 278*, 138–142.

Friedman, S. B., Chodoff, P., Mason, J. W., & Hamburg, D. A. (1963). Behavioral observations on parents anticipating the death of a child. *Pediatrics, 32*, 610–625.

Fritz, G. K., Williams, J. R., & Amylon, M. (1988). After treatment ends: Psychosocial sequelae in pediatric cancer survivors. *American Journal of Orthopsychiatry, 58*, 552–561.

Furman, R. A. (1964). Death and the young child, some preliminary considerations. *Psychoanalytic Study of the Child, 19*, 321–333.

Global Alliance for the Cure of Children with Cancer. (2004). Retrieved from http://www.inctr.org/projects/other.shtml

Gogan, J. L., Koocher, G. P., Foster, D. J., & O'Malley, J. E. (1977). Impact of childhood cancer on siblings. *Health and Social Work, 2*, 41–57.

Hamovitch, M. B. (1964). *The parent and the fatally ill child.* Los Angeles: Delmar.

Hewitt, M., Weiner, S. L., & Simone, J. V. (Eds.). (2003). *Childhood cancer survivorship: Improving care and quality of life.* Washington, DC: National Academies Press.

Hilgard, J. R., & LeBaron, S. (1984). *Hypnotherapy of pain in children with cancer.* Los Altos, CA: Kaufman.

Jacobsen, P. B., Manne, S. L., Gorfinke, K., Schorr, O., Rapkin, R., & Redd, W. H. (1990). Analysis of child and parent behavior during painful medical procedures. *Health Psychology, 9*, 559–576.

Jankovic, M., Brouwers, P., Valsecchi, M. G., Van Veldhuizen, A., Huisman, J., Kamphuis, R., et al. (1994). Association of 1800 cGy cranial irradiation with intellectual function in children with acute lymphoblastic leukaemia. *The Lancet, 344*, 224–227.

Jankovic, M., Loiacono, N. B., Spinetta, J. J., Riva, L., Conter, V., & Masera, G. (1994). Telling young children with leukemia their diagnosis: The flower garden as analogy. *Pediatric Hematology and Oncology, 11*, 75–81.

Jankovic, M., Masera, G., Uderzo, C., Conter, V., Adamoli, L., & Spinetta, J. J. (1989). Meetings with parents after the death of their child from leukemia. *Pediatric Hematology and Oncology*, 6, 155–160.

Jankovic, M., Spinetta, J., Martins, A. G., Pession, A., Sullivan, M., D'Angio, G. J., et al. (2004). Nonconventional therapies in childhood cancer: Guidelines for distinguishing non-harmful from harmful therapies. *Pediatric Blood and Cancer, 42*, 106–108.

Jay, S. M., & Elliott, C. H. (1990). A stress inoculation program for parent whose children are undergoing painful medical procedures. *Journal of Consulting and Clinical Psychology, 58*, 799–804.

Jay, S. M., Ozolins, M., Elliott, C. H., & Caldwell, S. (1983). Assessment of children's distress during painful medical procedures. *Health Psychology*, 2, 139–149.

Kagen-Goodheart, L. (1977). Re-entry: Living with childhood cancer. *American Journal of Orthopsychiatry, 47*, 651–658.

Karon, M., & Vernick, J. (1968). An approach to the emotional support of fatally ill children. *Clinical Pediatrics, 7*, 274–280.

Katz, E. R., Kellerman, J., Rigler, D., Williams, K. O., & Siegel, S. E. (1977). School intervention with pediatric cancer patients. *Journal of Pediatric Psychology, 2*, 72–76.

Katz, E. R., Kellerman, J., & Siegel, S. E. (1980). Behavioral distress in children with cancer undergoing medical procedures: Developmental considerations. *Journal of Consulting and Clinical Psychology, 48*, 356–365.

Kazak, A. E. (1993). Psychological research in pediatric oncology. *Journal of Pediatric Psychology, 18*, 313–318.

Kazak, A. E., & Meadows, A. T. (1989). Families of young adolescents who have survived cancer: Social-emotional adjustment, adaptability, and social support. *Journal of Pediatric Psychology, 14*, 175–192.

Kellerman, J. (Ed.). (1980). *Psychological aspects of childhood cancer*. Springfield, IL: Thomas.

Kellerman, J., Zeltzer, L., Ellenberg, L., & Dash, J. (1983). Adolescents with cancer: Hypnosis for the reduction of the acute pain and anxiety associated with medical procedures. *Journal of Adolescent Health Care, 4*, 85–90.

Koocher, J. (1980). Pediatric cancer psychological problems and the high costs of helping. *Journal of Clinical Child Psychology, 10*, 2–5.

Koocher, G. P., & O'Malley, J. E. (Eds.) (1981). *The Damocles syndrome: Psychological consequences of surviving childhood cancer*. New York: McGraw-Hill.

Kupst, M. J., & Schulman, J. L. (1988). Long-term coping with pediatric leukemia: A 6-year follow-up study. *Journal of Pediatric Psychology*, 13, 7–22.

Kupst, M. J., Schulman, J. L., Honig, G., Maurer, H., Morgan, E., & Fochtman, D. (1982). Family coping with childhood leukemia: 1 year after diagnosis. *Journal of Pediatric Psychology, 7*, 157–174.

Lansky, S. B., Cairns, N. U., & Zwartjes, W. (1983). School attendance among children with cancer: A report from two centers. *Journal of Psychosocial Oncology, 1*, 75–82.

Lansky, S. B., Lowman, J. T., Vats, T. S., & Gyulay, J. E. (1975). School phobia in children with malignant neoplasm. *American Journal of the Diseases of Children 129*, 42–46.

Martinson, I. M. (1979). Caring for the dying child. *Nursing Clinics of North America, 14*, 467–474.

Martinson, I. M. (1993). Hospice care for children: Past, present, and future. *Journal of Pediatric Oncology Nursing*, 10, 393–398.

Martinson, I. M., Geis, D., Anglim, M. A., Peterson, E., Nesbit, M., & Kersey, J. (1977). When the patient is dying: Home care for the child. *American Journal of Nursing, 77*, 1815–1817.

Masera, G., Baez, F., Biondi, A., Cavalli, F., Conter, V., Flores, A., et al. (1998). North-south twinning in paediatric haematology-oncology: The La Mascota programme, Nicaragua. *Lancet, 351*, 1923–1926.

Masera, G., Beltrame, F., Corbetta, A., Fraschini, D., Adamoli, L., Jankovic, M., et al. (2003). Audiotaping communication of the diagnosis of childhood leukemia: Parents' evaluation. *Journal of Pediatric Hematology Oncology, 25*(5), 368–371.

Masera, G., & Biondi, A. (1999). Research in low-income countries. *Annals of Oncology, 10*, 137–138.

Masera, G., Chesler, M. A., Jankovic, M., Ablin, A. R., Ben Arush, M. W., Breatnach, F., et al. (1997). SIOP Working Committee on Psychosocial Issues in Pediatric Oncology: Guidelines for communication of the diagnosis. *Medical and Pediatric Oncology, 28*, 382–385.

Masera, G., Chesler, M., Jankovic, M., Eden, T., Nesbit, M. E., Van Dongen-Melman, J., et al. (1996). SIOP Working Committee on Psychosocial Issues in Pediatric Oncology: Guidelines for care of long-term survivors. *Medical and Pediatric Oncology*, 27, 1–2.

Masera, G., Jankovic, M., Adamoli, L., Corbetta, A., Fraschini, D., Lia, R., et al. (1997). The psychosocial program for childhood leukemia in Monza, Italy. *Annals of the New York Academy of Sciences, 824*: 210–220.

Masera, G., Jankovic, M., Deasy-Spinetta, P., Adamoli, L., Ben Arush, M. W., Challinor, J., et al. (1995). SIOP Working Committee on Psychosocial Issues in Pediatric Oncology: Guidelines for school/education. *Medical and Pediatric Oncology*, 25, 321–322.

Masera, G., Spinetta, J. J., D'Angio, G. J., Green, D. M., Marky, I., Jankovic, M., et al. (1993). SIOP Working Committee on Psychosocial Issues in Pediatric Oncology: Critical commentary. *Medical and Pediatric Oncology, 21*, 627–628.

Masera, G., Spinetta, J. J., Jankovic, M., Ablin, A., Buchwall, I., Van Dongen-Melman, J., et al. (1998). SIOP Working Committee on Psychosocial Issues in Pediatric Oncology: Guidelines for a therapeutic alliance between families and staff. *Medical and Pediatric Oncology*, *30*, 183–186.

Masera, G., Spinetta, J. J., Jankovic, M., Ablin, A. R., D'Angio, G. J., Van Dongen-Melman, J., et al. (1999). Guidelines for assistance to terminally ill children with cancer: A report of the SIOP Working Committee on Psychosocial Issues in Pediatric Oncology. *Medical and Pediatric Oncology*, 32, 44–48.

Meadows, A. T., Black, B., Nesbit, M. E., Strong, L. C., Nicholson, H. S., Green, D. M., et al. (1993). Long-term survival: Clinical care, research, and education. *Cancer 71*, (10 Suppl.), 3213–3215.

Meadows, A. T., Massari, D. J., Fergusson, J., Gordon, J., Littman, P., & Moss, K. (1981). Declines in IQ scores and cognitive dysfunctions in children with acute lymphocytic leukemia treated with cranial radiation. *Lancet, 2*, 1015–1018.

Meadows, A. T., McKee, L., & Kazak, A. E. (1989). Psychosocial status of young adult survivors of childhood cancer: A survey. *Medical and Pediatric Oncology, 17*, 466–470.

Morrissey, J. R. (1963). Children's adaptations to fatal illness. *Social Work, 8*, 81–88.

Morrow, G. R., Hoagland, A. C., & Morse, I. P. (1982). Sources of support perceived by parents of children with cancer: Implications for counseling. *Patient Counseling and Health Education, 4*, 36–40.

Moss, H. A., Nannis, E. D., & Poplack, D. G. (1981). The effects of prophylactic treatment of the central nervous system on the intellectual functioning of children with acute lymphocytic leukemia. *American Journal of Medicine, 71*, 47–52.

Mulhern, R. K., Crisco, J. J., & Camitta, B. M. (1981). Patterns of communication among pediatric patients with leukemia, parents, and physicians: Prognostic disagreement and misunderstanding. *Journal of Pediatrics, 99*, 480–483.

Naafs-Wilstra, M., Barr, R., Greenberg, C., Magrath, I., Cardenas, F., Chesler, M., et al. (2001). Pediatric oncology in developing countries: Development of an alliance of stakeholders. *Medical and Pediatric Oncology, 36*, 305–309.

Natterson, J. M., & Knudson, A. G. (1960). Observations concerning fear of death in fatally-ill children and their mothers. *Psychosomatic Medicine*, 22, 456–465.

Nesbit, M. E., Krivit, W., Robison, L., & Hammond, D. (1979). A follow-up report of long-term survivors of childhood acute lymphoblastic or undifferentiated leukemia. A report for Children's Cancer Study Group. *Journal of Pediatrics, 95*, 727–730.

Parry, C. (2002). *The psychosocial experiences of long-term survivors of childhood cancer across the life span.* Unpublished doctoral dissertation, University of Michigan, Ann Arbor.

Pfefferbaum-Levine, B., Copeland, D. R., Fletcher, J. M., Reid, H. L., Jaffe, N., & McKinnon, W. R. (1984). Neuropsychological assessment of long-term survivors of childhood leukemia. *American Journal of Pediatric Hematology/Oncology*, 6, 123–128.

Pizzo, P. A., & Poplack, D. G. (Eds.) (2001). *Principles and practice of pediatric oncology* (4th ed.). Philadelphia: Lippincott, Williams & Wilkins.

Rando, T. (1983). An investigation of grief and adaptation in parents whose children have died from cancer. *Journal of Pediatric Psychology*, 8, 3–20.

Rando, T. A. (Ed.) (1984). *Grief, dying, and death: Clinical interventions for caregivers.* Champaign, IL: Research Press.

Richmond, J. B., & Waisman, H. A. (1955). Psychological aspects of management of children with malignant diseases. *American Journal of the Diseases of Children, 89*, 42–47.

Roberts, M. C. (Ed.). (2003). *Handbook of pediatric psychology* (3rd ed.). New York: Guilford Press.

Robison, L. L., Nesbit, M. E., Sather, N. H., Meadows, A. T., Ortega, J. A., & Hammond, G. D. (1984). Factors associated with IQ scores in long-term survivors of childhood acute lymphoblastic leukemia. *American Journal of Pediatric Hematology/Oncology, 6*, 115–120.

Sahler, O. J. Z. (Ed.). (1978). *The child and death.* St. Louis, MO: Mosby.

Sahler, O. J. Z., Fairclough, D. L., Katz, E. R., Varni, J. W., Phipps, S., Mulhern, R. K., et al. (2005). Problem-solving skills training for mothers of children with newly diagnosed cancer. In R. T. Brown (Ed.), *Pediatric hematology/oncology: A biopsychosocial approach.* Oxford, U.K.: Oxford University Press.

Schowalter, J. E. (1970). The child's reaction to his own terminal illness. In B. Schoenberg, A. Carr, D. Peretz, & A. Kutscher (Eds.), *Loss and grief: Psychological management in medical practice.* New York: Columbia University Press.

Sigler, A. T. (1970). The leukemic child and his family: An emotional challenge. In M. Debuskey (Ed.), *The chronically ill child and his family.* Springfield, IL: Thomas.

Slavin, L., O'Malley, J., Koocher, G., & Foster, D. (1982). Communication of the cancer diagnosis to pediatric patients: Impact on long-term adjustment. *American Journal of Psychiatry, 139*, 179–183.

Sourkes, B. (1977). Facilitating family coping with childhood cancer. *Journal of Pediatric Psychology*, 2, 65–67.

Sourkes, B. (1981). Siblings of the pediatric cancer patient. In J. Kellerman (Ed.), *Psychological aspects of childhood cancer.* Springfield, IL: Thomas.

Sourkes, B. (1996). The broken heart: Anticipatory grief in the child facing death. *Journal of Palliative Care, 12*, 56–59.

Spinetta, J. J. (1984). Development of psychometric assessment methods by life cycle stages. *Cancer, 53*(10, Suppl.), 2222–2226.

Spinetta, J. J. (2005). Resilience in survivors of teenage cancer: A life-adaptive approach. In T.O.B. Eden, R. D. Barr, A. Bleyer, & M. Whiteson (Eds.), Cancer and the Adolescent. Oxford: Blackwell Publishing Co.

Spinetta, J. J., & Deasy-Spinetta, P. (Eds.). (1981). *Living with childhood cancer*. St. Louis, MO: Mosby.

Spinetta, J. J., & Deasy-Spinetta, P. (1986). The patient's socialization in the community and school during therapy. *Cancer, 58*, 512–516.

Spinetta, J. J., Jankovic, M., Ben Arush, M. W., Eden, T., Epelman, C., Greenberg, M. L., et al. (2000). SIOP Working Committee on Psychosocial Issues in Pediatric Oncology: Guidelines for the recognition, prevention, and remediation of burnout in health care professionals participating in the care of children with cancer. *Medical and Pediatric Oncology, 35*, 122–125.

Spinetta, J. J., Jankovic, M., Eden. T., Green, D., Martins, A. G., Wandzura, C., et al. (1999). SIOP Working Committee on Psychosocial Issues in Pediatric Oncology: Guidelines for assistance to siblings of children with cancer. *Medical and Pediatric Oncology, 33*, 395–398.

Spinetta, J. J., & Maloney, L. J. (1975). Death anxiety in the out-patient leukemic child. *Pediatrics, 56*, 1034–1037.

Spinetta, J. J., Masera, G., Eden, T., Oppenheim, D., Martins, A. G., van Dongen-Melman, J., et al. (2002). SIOP Working Committee on Psychosocial Issues in Pediatric Oncology: Refusal, non-compliance, and abandonment of treatment in children and adolescents with cancer. *Medical and Pediatric Oncology, 38*, 114–117.

Spinetta, J. J., Masera, G., Jankovic, M., Oppenheim, D., Martins, A. G., Ben Arush, M. W., et al. (2003). SIOP Working Committee on Psychosocial Issues in Pediatric Oncology: Valid informed consent and participative decision-making in children with cancer and their parents. *Medical and Pediatric Oncology, 40*, 244–246.

Spinetta, J. J., Murphy, J. L., Vik, P. J., Day, J., & Mott, M. A. (1989). Long-term adjustment in families of children with cancer. *Journal of Psychosocial Oncology, 6*, 179–191.

Spinetta, J. J., Rigler, D., & Karon, M. (1973). Anxiety in the dying child. *Pediatrics, 52*, 841–845.

Spinetta, J. J., Rigler, D., & Karon, M. (1974). Personal space as a measure of the dying child's sense of isolation. *Journal of Consulting and Clinical Psychology, 42*, 751–756.

Spinetta, J. J., Swarner, J. A., & Sheposh, J. P. (1981). Effective parental coping following the death of a child from cancer. *Journal of Pediatric Psychology, 6*, 251–263.

Storlie, F. J. (1979). Burnout: The elaboration of a concept. *American Journal of Nursing, 19*, 2108–2111.

Stuber, M. L. (1996). Psychiatric sequelae in seriously ill children and their families. *Psychiatric Clinics of North America, 19*, 481–493.

Stuber, M. L. (2005). Posttraumatic stress and posttraumatic growth in childhood cancer survivors and their parents. In R. T. Brown (Ed.), *Pediatric hematology/oncology: A biopsychosocial approach*. Oxford, U.K.: Oxford University Press.

Stuber, M. L., & Mesrkhani, V. H. (2001). "What do we tell the children?": Understanding childhood grief. *Western Journal of Medicine, 174*, 187–191.

Van Dongen-Melman, J. E., DeGroot, A., Hahlen, K., & Verhulst, F. C. (1996). Commentary: Potential pitfalls of using illness-specific measures. *Journal of Pediatric Psychology, 21*, 103–106.

Van Dongen-Melman, J. E., Pruyn, J. F., De Groot, A., Koot, H. M., Hahlen, K., & Verhulst, F. C. (1995). Late psychosocial consequences for parents of children who survived cancer. *Journal of Pediatric Psychology, 20*, 567–586.

Van Eys, J. (Ed.). (1977). *The truly cured child*. Baltimore, MD: University Park Press.

Waechter, E. H. (1971). Children's awareness of fatal illness. *American Journal of Nursing, 71*, 1168–1171.

Walco, G. (2005). Pain and procedure management. In R. T. Brown (Ed.), *Pediatric hematology/oncology: A biopsychosocial approach*. Oxford, U.K.: Oxford University Press.

Walker, C. (1989). Use of art and play therapy in pediatric oncology. *Journal of Pediatric Oncology Nursing, 6*, 121–126.

Wiener, J. M. (1970). Attitudes of pediatricians toward the care of fatally ill children. *Journal of Pediatrics, 76*, 700–705.

Zebrack, B. J., Zeltzer, L. K., Whitton, J., Mertens, A. C., Odom, L., Berkow, R., et al. (2002). Psychological outcomes in long-term survivors of childhood leukemia, Hodgkin's disease, and non-Hodgkin's lymphoma: A report from the Childhood Cancer Survivor Study. *Pediatrics, 110*, 42–52.

Zeltzer, L., Kellerman, J., Ellenberg, L., Dash, J., & Rigler, D. (1980). Psychologic effects of illness in adolescence. II. Impact of illness in adolescents—crucial issues and coping styles. *Journal of Pediatrics, 97,* 132–138.

Zeltzer, L., & LeBaron, S. (1986). Assessment of acute pain and anxiety and chemotherapy-related nausea and vomiting in children and adolescents. *Hospice Journal,* 2, 75–98.

# Index